GI/LIVER SECRETS

SECRETS

Second Edition

GI/LIVER SECRETS

Second Edition

Peter R. McNally, DO, FACP, FACG

Professor of Medicine
Division of Gastroenterology
University of Colorado Health Sciences Center
Director of Clinical Gastroenterology and Endoscopy
Denver Health Medical Center
Denver, Colorado

HANLEY & BELFUS, INC./Philadelphia

Publisher: **HANLEY & BELFUS, INC.**
                Medical Publishers
                210 South 13th Street
                Philadelphia, PA 19107
                (215) 546-7293; 800-962-1892
                FAX (215) 790-9330
                Web site: http://www.hanleyandbelfus.com

Library of Congress Cataloging-in-Publication Data

GI/Liver secrets / edited by Peter McNally.—2nd ed.
    p. ; cm.—(The Secrets Series®)
  Includes bibliographical references and index.
  ISBN 1-56053-439-7 (alk. paper)
    1. Digestive organs—Diseases—Examinations, questions, etc. I. McNally, Peter R.,
1954- II. Series.
  |DNLM: 1. Digestive System Diseases—Examination Questions. WI 18.2 G428 2001|
RC802.G52 2001
616.3'0076—dc 21

                                                                      00-054272

Disclaimer: The opinions and assertions contained in this book are the private views of the authors and are not to be construed as reflecting the view of the Department of the Army or the Department of Defense.

GI/LIVER SECRETS, 2nd edition   ISBN 1-56053-439-7

Last digit is the print number: 9   8   7   6   5   4   3   2

CONTENTS

CONTRIBUTORS

Amjad Ali, M.D.
Assistant Professor and Director of Laparoscopic Surgery, Department of Surgery, University of Missouri, Kansas City, Missouri

Matthew S. Z. Bachinski, M.D., FACP
Assistant Professor of Medicine, Section of Gastroenterology and Hepatology, Medical College of Georgia, Augusta, Georgia

Bruce R. Bacon, M.D.
James F. King MD Endowed Chair in Gastroenterology, Professor of Internal Medicine, and Director, Division of Gastroenterology and Hepatology, Saint Louis University School of Medicine, St. Louis, Missouri

Francisco J. Baigorri, M.D.
Private Practice, Coral Gables, Florida

Jamie S. Barkin, M.D., FACP, MACG
Professor of Medicine, Division of Gastroenterology, University of Miami; Chief, Division of Gastroenterology, Mount Sinai Medical Center, Miami, Florida

David W. Bean, Jr., M.D.
Diagnostic Radiologist, Medical X-ray Center, P.C., Sioux Falls, South Dakota

Leslie H. Bernstein, M.D., MACG
Professor of Medicine, and Emeritus Chief of Gastroenterology, Albert Einstein College of Medicine, Bronx, New York

Frank Calvin Bigler, M.D., F.A.C.S.
Clinical Staff, Southwest Medical Center, Liberal, Kansas

Bahri M. Bilir, M.D.
Arapahoe Gastroenterology, P.C., Denver, Colorado

Nuray Bilir, M.D.
Arapahoe Gastroenterology, P.C., Denver, Colorado

Aaron Brzezinski, M.D.
Center for Inflammatory Bowel Disease, Department of Gastroenterology, Cleveland Clinic Foundation, Cleveland, Ohio

Bradley G. Bute, M.D.
Private Practice, Advanced Colon and Rectal Surgery, LLC, Bethpage and Commack, New York

Anthony James Canfield, M.D., FACS
Assistant Clinical Professor, Department of Surgery, Uniformed Services University of the Health Sciences F. Edward Herbert School of Medicine, Bethesda, Maryland

Donald O. Castell, M.D.
Kimbal Professor and Chairman, Department of Medicine, Medical College of Pennsylvania–Hahnemann School of Medicine, Philadelphia, Pennsylvania

Frank H. Chae, M.D.
Assistant Professor of Surgery, Department of Surgery, University of Colorado Health Sciences Center, Denver, Colorado

Jeffrey R. Clark, M.D.
Clinical Professor of Surgery, University of Colorado Health Sciences Center, Denver, Colorado

James E. Cremins, M.D., FACP
Washington County Hospital, Hagerstown, Maryland

Albert J. Czaja, M.D.
Professor of Medicine, Division of Gastroenterology and Hepatology, Mayo Medical School and Mayo Foundation, Rochester Minnesota

Dirk R. Davis, M.D.
Northern Utah Gastroenterology and Endoscopy Specialists, Logan, Utah

John C. Deutsch, M.D.
Associate Professor of Medicine, University of Colorado Health Sciences Center, Denver, Colorado

Jack A. DiPalma, M.D.
Professor of Medicine, Chief Division of Gastroenterology, University of South Alabama College of Medicine, Mobile, Alabama

John A. Dumot, D.O.
Associate Staff, Department of Gastroenterology, Cleveland Clinic Foundation, Cleveland, Ohio

Gulchin A. Ergun, M.D.
Associate Professor of Medicine, and Chief, Clinical Section of Gastroenterology, Baylor College of Medicine, Houston, Texas

James E. Fitzpatrick, M.D.
Associate Professor, Department of Dermatology, University of Colorado Health Sciences Center, Aurora, Colorado

Michael G. Fox, M.D.
Staff Radiologist, Department of Radiology, Evans Army Hospital, Colorado Springs, Colorado

Stephen R. Freeman, M.D.
Assistant Clinical Professor of Medicine, Division of Gastroenterology, University of Colorado School of Medicine, Denver, Colorado

William Johnson Georgitis, M.D.
Clinical Professor, Division of Endocrinology, Metabolism and Diabetes, University of Colorado Health Sciences Center, Denver, Colorado

Gregory G. Ginsberg, M.D.
Associate Professor, Director of Endoscopic Services, Department of Medicine, Division of Gastroenterology, University of Pennsylvania School of Medicine, Philadelphia, Pennsylvania

John S. Goff, M.D.
Clinical Professor of Medicine, Division of Gastroenterology, University of Colorado Health Sciences Center, Denver, Colorado

Ian M. Gralnek, M.D., MSHS
Assistant Professor, Department of Medicine, Division of Gastroenterology, UCLA School of Medicine and VA Greater Los Angeles Healthcare System, Los Angeles, California

Carlos Guarner, M.D.
Associate Professor of Medicine, Chief of Liver Section, Gastroenterology Service, Hospital de Sant Pau, Autonomous University of Barcelona, Barcelona, Spain

Jorge L. Herrera, M.D.
Professor of Medicine, Division of Gastroenterology, University of South Alabama College of Medicine, Mobile, Alabama

Colonel Kent C. Holtzmuller, M.D.
Assistant Professor of Medicine, Uniformed Services University of the Health Sciences F. Edward Herbert School of Medicine, Bethesda, Maryland; Division of Gastroenterology, Walter Reed Army Medical Center, Washington, DC

Michael Charles Hotard, M.D., FACS
Assistant Clinical Professor, Department of Surgery, Uniformed Services University of the Health Sciences F. Edward Herbert School of Medicine, Bethesda, Maryland

Prahalad B. Jajodia, M.D.
Department of Gastroenterology, Loma Linda University Medical Center, Loma Linda, California

Dennis M. Jensen, M.D.
Professor of Medicine, Division of Gastroenterology, UCLA Center for the Health Sciences and VA Greater Los Angeles Healthcare System, Los Angeles, California

Brian T. Johnston, M.D.
Royal Victoria Hospital, Belfast, Ireland

Christian Jost, M.D.
Fellow in Gastroenterology, Medical University of South Carolina, Charleston, South Carolina

Peter J. Kahrilas, M.D.
Gilbert H. Marquardt Professor of Medicine, Division of Gastroenterology and Hepatology, Northwestern University Medical School, Chicago, Illinois

Anthony N. Kalloo, M.D.
Associate Professor of Medicine, Division of Gastroenterology, Department of Medicine, Johns Hopkins University School of Medicine, Baltimore, Maryland

Sergey V. Kantsevoy, M.D., Ph.D.
Assistant Professor of Medicine, Division of Gastroenterology, Department of Medicine, Johns Hopkins University School of Medicine, Baltimore, Maryland

James Walter Kikendall, M.D.
GI Program Director, Gastroenterology Service, Walter Reed Army Medical Center, Washington, DC

Bernard Kopchinski, M.D.
Chief Resident in Surgery, William Beaumont Army Medical Center, El Paso, Texas

Burton I. Korelitz, M.D.
Clinical Professor of Medicine, Section of Gastroenterology, New York University School of Medicine, Lenox Hill Hospital, New York, New York

Ronald L. Koretz, M.D.
Chief, Division of Gastroenterology, San Fernando Valley Program, Sylmar, California; Professor of Clinical Medicine, UCLA School of Medicine, Los Angeles, California; and Department of Medicine, Olive View–UCLA Medical Center, Sylmar, California

LTC Jonathan P. Kushner, M.D.
Assistant Professor of Medicine, Uniform Services University of the Health Sciences F. Edward Herbert School of Medicine, Bethesda, Maryland; Staff Gastroenterologist, Madigan Army Medical Center, Tacoma, Washington

Anthony J. LaPorta, M.D.
Associate Professor of Surgery, Uniformed Services University of the Health Sciences F. Edward Herbert School of Medicine, Bethesda, Maryland; Associate Clinical Professor of Surgery, University of Colorado School of Medicine, Denver, Colorado; Chief Surgeon, Evans Army Community Hospital, Fort Carson, Colorado

Nicholas F. LaRusso, M.D.
Chairman and Professor, Department of Medicine, Department of Gastroenterology and Hepatology, Mayo Medical School, Clinic and Foundation, Rochester, Minnesota

Bret A. Lashner, M.D.
Director, Center for Inflammatory Bowel Disease, Department of Gastroenterology, Cleveland Clinic Foundation, Cleveland, Ohio

Steven P. Lawrence, M.D.
Staff Gastroenterologist, Fallon Clinic, Worcester, Massachusetts

Randall E. Lee, M.D., FACP
Assistant Clinical Professor of Medicine, Division of Gastroenterology, Department of Veterans Affairs, Northern California Health Care System, University of California at Davis School of Medicine, Martinez, California

Peter E. Legnani, M.D.
Fellow, Division of Gastroenterology, Mount Sinai School of Medicine, New York, New York

Scot M. Lewey, D.O., FACP, FAAP, FACG
Gastroenterology Associates of Colorado Springs, LLP, Colorado Springs, Colorado

Ramona M. Lim, M.D.
Gastroenterology Fellow, University of Miami School of Medicine, Miami, Florida

Michael F. Lyons, II, M.D.
Clinical Assistant Professor, Department of Medicine, University of Washington School of Medicine, Seattle, Washington

Jeffrey B. Matthews, M.D., FACS
Associate Professor of Surgery, and Chief, Division of General Surgery, Harvard Medical School, Boston, Massachusetts

Colonel Mike McBiles, M.D.
Assistant Professor of Radiology, University of Texas at San Antonio School of Medicine, San Antonio, Texas

Dale L. McCarter, M.D.
Interventional Radiology, Carmel, Indiana

Colonel Peter R. McNally, D.O., FACP, FACG
Professor of Medicine, University of Colorado Health Sciences Center; Director, Clinical Gastroenterology and Endoscopy, Denver Health Medical Center, Denver, Colorado

John H. Meier, M.D.
Private Practitioner, Gastroenterology Associates, P.A., Hickory, North Carolina

John A. Merenich, M.D.
Clinical Associate Professor, Division of Endocrinology, Metabolism and Diabetes, University of Colorado Health Sciences Center, Denver, Colorado

Suzanne Katherine Miller, M.D.
Gastroenterology Fellow, University of Virginia Health Sciences Center, Charlottesville, Virginia

John David Moffat, M.D., FACS
Clinical Staff, Southwest Medical Center, Liberal, Kansas

Klaus E. Mönkemüller, M.D.
Assistant Professor of Medicine, Division of Gastroenterology and Hepatology, University of Alabama School of Medicine, Birmingham, Alabama

Andrew J. Muir, M.D.
Associate Professor, Division of Gastroenterology, Duke University Medical Center, Durham, North Carolina

Satheesh Nair, M.D.
Clinical Assistant Professor of Medicine, Division of Gastroenterology and Hepatology, Tulane University School of Medicine, New Orleans, Louisiana

Jaimie D. Nathan, M.D.
Resident, General Surgery, Department of Surgery, Duke University Medical Center, Durham, North Carolina

Theodore N. Pappas, M.D.
Professor of Surgery, Program Director, General Surgery, Duke University Medical Center, Durham, North Carolina

Pankaj J. Pasricha, M.D.
Associate Professor of Internal Medicine/Gastroenterology, University of Texas Medical Branch, Galveston, Texas

Steve Peck, M.D.
Staff Radiologist, Interventional Radiology, Rose Medical Center, Denver, Colorado

Carlos A. Pellegrini, M.D.
The Henry N. Harkins Professor and Chairman, Department of Surgery, University of Washington School of Medicine, Seattle, Washington

David A. Peura, M.D.
Professor of Medicine, Division of Gastroenterology, University of Virginia Health Sciences Center, Charlottesville, Virginia

Anca I. Pop, M.D.
Department of Medicine, Division of Gastroenterology, James H. Quillen Medical School, East Tennessee State University, Johnson City, Tennessee

Ramona O. Rajapakse, M.D.
Clinical Instructor, Section of Gastroenterology, Department of Medicine, State University of New York at Stony Brook School of Medicine, Stony Brook, New York

Kevin M. Rak, M.D.
Chief, Department of Radiology, Divine Savior Healthcare, Portage, Wisconsin

R. Matthew Reveille, M.D.
Clinical Assistant Professor of Medicine, University of Colorado Health Sciences Center, Denver, Colorado

Caroline A. Riely, M.D.
Professor of Medicine and Pediatrics, Division of Gastroenterology/Hepatology, University of Tennessee Health Science Center, Memphis, Tennessee

Ingram M. Roberts, M.D.
Associate Clinical Professor of Medicine, Yale University School of Medicine, New Haven; Chief, Section of Gastroenterology, Bridgeport Hospital, Bridgeport, Connecticut

Arvey I. Rogers, M.D., FACP, MACG
Professor of Medicine, and Chief, Gastroenterology Division, University of Miami School of Medicine, Miami, Florida

Suzanne Rose, M.D., MS Ed.
Associate Professor of Medical Education and Medicine, Division of Gastroenterology, Department of Medicine; Associate Dean for Student Affairs, Mount Sinai School of Medicine, New York, New York

Bruce A. Runyon, M.D.
Chief, Liver Unit, Rancho Los Amigos/University of Southern California, Downey, California

Paul D. Russ, M.D.
Associate Professor, Department of Diagnostic Radiology, University of Colorado Health Sciences Center, Denver, Colorado

Richard E. Sampliner, M.D.
Professor of Medicine, Division of Gastroenterology, University of Arizona College of Medicine, Tucson, Arizona

Lawrence R. Schiller, M.D.
Clinical Professor of Internal Medicine, Division of Digestive and Liver Diseases, University of Texas Southwestern Medical Center, Dallas, Texas

Steven S. Shay, M.D., FACG, FACP
Staff Gastroenterologist, Department of Gastroenterology, Cleveland Clinic Foundation, Cleveland, Ohio

Kenneth E. Sherman, M.D., Ph.D.
Associate Professor of Medicine, University of Cincinnati College of Medicine, Cincinnati, Ohio

Keith M. Shonnard, M.D.
Interventional Radiology, Carson City, Nevada

Roshan Shrestha, M.D.
Associate Professor of Medicine, Medical Director of Liver Transplantation, Division of Digestive Diseases and Nutrition, University of North Carolina School of Medicine, Chapel Hill, North Carolina

Maria Sjogren, M.D., M.P.H.
Associate Professor, Department of Medicine, Georgetown University School of Medicine; Chief, Department of Clinical Investigation, Walter Reed Army Medical Center, Washington, DC

Julie R. Smith, M.H.S., PA-C
Adjunct Assistant Professor of Physician Assistant Studies, University of South Alabama College of Medicine, Mobile, Alabama

Milton T. Smith, M.D.
Staff Gastroenterologist, Gastroenterology Service, Walter Reed Army Medical Center, Washington, DC

Sandra E. Smith, RD, MS
Nutrition Support Dietitian, Nutrition Care Directorate, Walter Reed Army Medical Center, Washington, DC

Janet K. Stephens, M.D., Ph.D.
Clinical Associate Professor of Pathology, University of Colorado Health Sciences Center, Denver, Colorado

Stephen W. Subber, M.D.
Associate Professor of Radiology, University of Colorado Health Sciences Center, Denver, Colorado

Christina M. Surawicz, M.D.
Professor of Medicine, Department of Medicine, Division of Gastroenterology, University of Washington School of Medicine, Seattle, Washington

Shams Tabrez, M.D.
Fellow in Gastroenterology, Section of Gastroenterology, Bridgeport Hospital, Yale University Affiliated GI Program, Bridgeport, Connecticut

Jayant A. Talwalkar, M.D., M.P.H.
Instructor of Medicine, Department of Gastroenterology and Hepatology, Mayo Medical School, Clinic and Foundation, Rochester, Minnesota

Paul J. Thuluvath, M.D., FRCP
Associate Professor of Medicine, The Johns Hopkins University School of Medicine, Baltimore, Maryland

Neil Toribara, M.D., Ph.D.
Associate Professor of Medicine, University of Colorado Health Sciences Center; Chief, Division of Gastroenterology, Denver Health Medical Center, Denver, Colorado

George Triadafilopoulos, M.D., D.Sc.
Professor of Medicine, Division of Gastroenterology and Hepatology, Stanford University School of Medicine, Stanford, California

James F. Trotter, M.D.
Assistant Professor, Division of Gastroenterology and Hepatology, University of Colorado Health Sciences Center, Denver, Colorado

Thomas E. Trouillot, M.D.
Assistant Professor of Medicine, Gastroenterology and Hepatology, University of Colorado Health Sciences Center, Denver, Colorado

M. Nimish Vakil, M.D., FACP, FACG
Clinical Professor of Medicine, Division of Gastroenterology, University of Wisconsin Medical School, Milwaukee, Wisconsin

Jon A. Vanderhoof, M.D.
Professor of Pediatrics, Section of Pediatric Gastroenterology and Nutrition, University of Nebraska Medical Center/Creighton University, Omaha, Nebraska

Yael Vin, M.D.
Resident in General Surgery, Department of Surgery, Beth Israel Deaconess Medical Center, Boston, Massachusetts

Arnold Wald, M.D.
Professor of Medicine, Division of Gastroenterology, Hepatology, and Nutrition, University of Pittsburgh Medical Center, Pittsburgh, Pennsylvania

Michael B. Wallace, M.D., M.P.H.
Assistant Professor of Medicine, Division of Gastroenterology, Medical University of South Carolina, Charleston, South Carolina

Michael Harry Walter, M.D.
Associate Professor of Medicine, Division of Gastroenterology, Loma Linda University Medical Center, Loma Linda, California

George H. Warren, M.D.
Clinical Associate Professor, Pathology and Medicine, Division of Gastroenterology, University of Colorado Health Sciences Center, Denver, Colorado

Sterling Gaylord West, M.D.
Professor of Medicine, Division of Rheumatology, University of Colorado Health Sciences Center, Denver, Colorado

C. Mel Wilcox, M.D.
Professor of Medicine, Division of Gastroenterology, University of Alabama School of Medicine, Birmingham, Alabama

Rosemary J. Young, R.N., M.S.
Section of Pediatric Gastroenterology and Nutrition, University of Nebraska Medical Center/Creighton University, Omaha, Nebraska

Steven Zacks, M.D., M.P.H.
Clinical Assistant Professor of Medicine, Division of Digestive Diseases and Nutrition, University of North Carolina School of Medicine, Chapel Hill, North Carolina

Arlene J. Zaloznik, M.D.
Associate Professor of Hematology-Oncology, Texas Tech University Health Sciences Center, El Paso, Texas

Bernard E. Zeligman, M.D.
Associate Professor of Radiology, University of Colorado School of Medicine, Denver, Colorado

Gregory Zuccaro, Jr., M.D.
Section Head, Endoscopy and Pancreaticobiliary Diseases, Department of Gastroenterology, Cleveland Clinic Foundation, Cleveland, Ohio

PREFACE

To practice the art of medicine, one must learn the secrets of physiology, disease, and therapy. In this text you will find the answers to many questions about the hepatic and digestive diseases. We hope that medical students, residents, fellows and, yes, even attending physicians will find this book instructive and insightful.

As editor, I am very appreciative of all of my contributors who have parted with their invaluable secrets and made this book an enjoyable and educational experience.

Colonel Peter R. McNally, DO, FACG, FACP

DEDICATION

The editor dedicates this book to his wife, Cynthia; to his children, Alex, Meghan, Amanda, Genevieve, and Bridgette; and to his parents, Jeanette and Rusel.

I. Esophagus

1. SWALLOWING DISORDERS AND DYSPHAGIA

Gulchin A. Ergun, M.D., and Peter J. Kahrilas, M.D.

1. How accurate is patient localization of the site of dysphagia?

Patients with oropharyngeal dysphagia accurately recognize that their swallow dysfunction is in the oropharynx; they may perceive food accumulating uncontrollably in the mouth or an inability to initiate a pharyngeal swallow. Similarly, they generally can recognize aspiration before, during, or after a swallow. Such is not the case, however, with esophageal dysphagia, in which patient identification of the location of obstruction is of limited accuracy. Patients are correct in identifying the location of dysfunction in the esophagus only 60–70% of cases, mistakenly localizing it proximal to the actual site in the remaining cases. Differentiating between proximal and distal lesions may be difficult if only the patient's interpretation is used. Therefore, the identification of associated oropharyngeal symptoms, such as difficulty with chewing, drooling, nasopharyngeal regurgitation, aspiration, or coughing or choking after swallowing can be of great value in placing the problem in the oropharynx vs. the esophagus.

2. What symptoms should you look for in evaluating oropharyngeal dysphagia?
• Nasopharyngeal regurgitation
• Coughing or choking (aspiration) during swallowing
• Inability to initiate a swallow
• Sensation of food getting stuck in the throat
• Changes in speech or voice (nasality)
• Ptosis
• Photophobia or visual changes
• Weakness, especially progressive toward the end of the day

3. Distinguish between globus sensation (globus hystericus) and dysphagia.

Globus sensation is a feeling of a lump in the throat. This sensation should not be confused with dysphagia. Globus sensation is not related to swallowing but is present continually and may even be temporarily alleviated during swallowing. Dysphagia, on the other hand, is difficulty in swallowing and noted by the patient only during swallowing.

4. List the causes of globus sensation in order from most common to least common.
• Gastroesophageal reflux disease
• Anxiety disorder (this diagnosis should not be made without a thorough examination to exclude organic disease)
• Early hypopharyngeal cancer
• Goiter

5. Categorize the causes of oropharyngeal dysphagia.

In the broadest sense, oropharyngeal dysphagia can be viewed as resulting from propulsive failure or structural abnormalities of either the oropharynx or esophagus. Propulsive abnormalities can result from dysfunction of central nervous system control mechanisms, intrinsic musculature, or peripheral nerves. Structural abnormalities may result from neoplasm, surgery, trauma, caustic injury, or congenital anomalies. In some instances, dysphagia occurs in the absence of radiographic findings; motor abnormalities may be demonstrable by more sensitive methods such

1

as electromyography or nerve stimulation studies. However, if all studies are normal, impaired swallowing sensation may be the primary abnormality.

Causes of Oropharyngeal Dysphagia

PROPULSIVE	STRUCTURAL	IATROGENIC
Neurologic	Neoplasm	Oropharyngeal resections
Cerebrovascular accident	Cricopharyngeal bars	Mucositis due to chemothera-
(medulla, large territory cortical)	Hypopharyngeal diverticula	peutic regimens (drugs)
Parkinson's disease	(Zenker's)	Radiation-induced xerostomia
Amyotrophic lateral sclerosis	Cervical vertebral body	Radiation-induced myopathy
Multiple sclerosis	osteophytes	Neck stabilizations (hardware
Degenerative diseases	Bullous skin diseases (epi-	including halo or surgery)
(e.g., Alzheimer's, Huntington's,	dermolysis bullosa, pem-	Steroid myopathy
Friedreich's ataxia)	phigoid, graft vs. host	Tardive dyskinesia
Brain neoplasm (brainstem)	disease	Ill-fitting dental or intraoral
Polio and postpolio syndrome	Lymphadenopathy	prostheses
Cerebral palsy	Caustic injury	
Cranial nerve palsies	Lye	
Recurrent laryngeal nerve palsy	Pill-induced	
Muscular	Infections	
Muscular dystrophy	Abscess	
(Duchenne, oculopharyngeal)	Ulceration	
Myositis and dermatomyositis	Pharyngitis	
Myasthenia gravis	Autoimmune—oral	
Eaton-Lambert syndrome	ulcerations with Crohn's,	
Metabolic	Behçet's disease	
Hypothyroidism with myxedema	Poor dentition/dental	
Hyperthyroidism	anomalies	
Inflammatory/autoimmune		
Systemic lupus erythematosus		
Amyloidosis		
Sarcoidosis		
Infectious		
AIDS with CNS involvement		
Syphilis (tabes dorsalis)		
Botulism		
Rabies		
Diphtheria		
Meningitis		
Viral (coxsackie, herpes simplex)		

6. What sensory cues elicit swallowing?

The sensory cues are not exactly known, but entry of food or fluid into the hypopharynx, specifically the sensory receptive field of the superior laryngeal nerve, is paramount. Swallowing also may be initiated by volitional effort if food is present in the oral cavity. Thus, the required afferent signal for initiation of the swallow response is a mixture of both peripheral sensory input from oropharyngeal afferents and superimposed control from high nervous system centers. Neither is capable of initiating swallowing without some contribution from the other. For this reason swallowing cannot be initiated during sleep when higher centers are turned off or with deep anesthesia of the oral cavity when peripheral afferents are disconnected.

7. What are the most common causes of oropharyngeal dysphagia in elderly patients?

Eighty percent of cases in elderly patients are attributable to neuromuscular disorders rather than structural lesions. Because of the high incidence and prevalence of cerebrovascular disease, cerebrovascular accidents account for most disorders. Parkinson's disease, motor neuron disorders, and skeletal muscle disorders account for the remainder.

8. Can development of dysphagia in later life be related to childhood illness such as polio?

Yes—even if the initial presentation did not include bulbar involvement. The postpolio syndrome is a disorder of the medullary motor neuron resulting from new or continuing instability of previously injured motor neurons. Typically the syndrome consists of new musculoskeletal symptoms, such as weakness and atrophy in previously affected muscles. Patients become symptomatic 25–35 years after the original illness, and even muscular units (limb or bulbar) that appeared untouched in the original infection may develop signs of clinical weakness. Bulbar neuron involvement has been reported in only 15% of patients with the acute infection, but recent studies demonstrate that some bulbar muscle dysfunction can be demonstrated in all patients with postpolio syndrome, although few report dysphagia. Swallowing problems are most severe in patients with bulbar involvement at the onset.

9. What is the appropriate time frame for evaluating stroke-related dysphagia?

About 25–50% of strokes result in oropharyngeal dysphagia. Therefore, most stroke-related swallowing dysfunction improves spontaneously within the first 2 weeks so that unnecessary diagnostic or therapeutic procedures can be avoided. If symptoms persist beyond this period, swallowing function should be evaluated.

10. Brainstem strokes are more likely to cause severe oropharyngeal dysphagia than hemispheric strokes. Why?

The swallowing center is situated bilaterally in the reticular substance below the nucleus of the solitary tract in the brainstem. Efferent fibers from the swallow centers travel either directly or via relay to the motoneurons controlling the swallow musculature located in the nucleus ambiguus. Therefore brainstem strokes are more likely to cause the most severe impairment of swallowing with difficulty in initiating swallow or absence of the swallow response.

11. How should you evaluate a patient who complains of dysphagia that is worse with solids and later in the day, who speaks with a nasal tone, and who has ptosis?

This is a classic presentation of myasthenia gravis, an autoimmune disorder characterized by progressive destruction of acetylcholine receptors at the neuromuscular junction. The most striking feature is fluctuating weakness of certain voluntary muscles, particularly those innervated by brainstem motor nuclei. Consequently, the cranial nerves are almost always involved, particularly the ocular muscles, which accounts for the predilection of ptosis and diplopia as initial symptoms. Muscles of facial expression, mastication, and swallowing are next most frequently involved, and dysphagia is a prominent symptom in more than one-third of cases. The disease is characterized by increasing muscle weakness with repetitive muscle contraction. An anticholinesterase antibody test should be obtained, but it is only about 90% sensitive in diagnosing myasthenia gravis. If myasthenia gravis is strongly suspected, a trial of therapy with an acetylcholinesterase inhibitor, such as tensilon, or a cholinomimetic, such as mestinon, should be considered even in the absence of an anticholinesterase antibody.

12. Is a barium swallow examination adequate to evaluate oropharyngeal dysphagia? Why or why not?

The barium swallow focuses on the esophagus, is done in a supine position, and takes at best a few still images as the barium passes through the oropharynx. Therefore, aspiration may be missed if a conventional barium swallow is ordered. Oropharyngeal dysphagia is best evaluated with a cineradiographic or videofluoroscopic swallowing study. Because the oropharyngeal swallow is quite rapid and transpires in less than 1 second, images must be obtained and recorded at a rate of 15–30/sec to detail adequately the motor events. Moreover, when the swallow is recorded at this rate, the study can be played back in slow motion for careful evaluation. This type of swallowing study is done with the patient upright.

13. Why is simultaneous involvement of the orophyarynx and esophagus extremely unusual for any disease process other than infection?

The oropharynx and the esophagus are fundamentally different in respect to musculature, innervation, and neural regulation.

OROPHARYNX	ESOPHAGUS
Striated muscle	Striated and smooth muscle (proximally) and smooth muscle (middle to distal portion)
Direct nicotinic innervation	Myenteric plexus within longitudinal and circular smooth muscles
Cholinergic	Cholinergic/nitric oxide, vasoactive intestinal peptide

Because most disease processes are specific for a particular type of muscle or nervous system element, it is highly unlikely that they would involve such diverse systems.

14. What are the indications and risks of a cricopharyngeal myotomy?

Indications
- Zenker's diverticulum
- Cricopharyngeal bar with symptoms
- Parkinson's disease?

Risks
- Aspiration in patients with gastroesophageal reflux disease
- Worsening of swallow function

15. What causes of dysphagia should be considered in the patient who has had surgery and other therapy (usually radiation and chemotherapy) for head and neck cancer?
- Radiation myositis and/or fibrosis
- Xerostomia (hyposalivation)
- Anatomic defects due to surgery
- Recurrence of malignancy

16. What is the most difficult substance to swallow (oropharyngeal)?

Water. Swallowing involves several phases. First is a preparatory phase that involves chewing, sizing, shaping, and positioning of the bolus on the tongue. Then, during an oral phase, the bolus is propelled from the oral cavity into the pharynx while the airway is protected. From this location the bolus is transported from the oral cavity into the pharynx and finally the esophagus Water is the most difficult substance to size, shape, and contain in the oral cavity. Similarly, it is the hardest to control as it is passed from the oral cavity into the pharynx. For these reasons, more viscous foods are used to feed patients with oropharyngeal dysphagia.

17. Which patients with which dysfunction are the best candidates for swallow therapy?

Patients: intact mentation, motivated
Dysfunctions: aspiration (during and after swallow), unilateral pharyngeal paresis

18. What are the mechanisms by which gastroesophageal reflux disease is associated with dysphagia? List from most to least common.
1. Inflammation (30% of patients with esophagitis experience dysphagia)
2. Stricture (dysphagia occurs when the lumen diameter is < 11–13 mm)
3. Peristaltic dysfunction (related to severity of disease)
4. Hiatal hernia?

19. Why is "cricopharyngeal achalasia" a misnomer? Contrast with achalasia of the cardia.

The upper esophageal sphincter (UES) is a striated muscle that depends on tonic excitation to maintain contractility. If innervation to the cricopharyngeus is lost, the sphincter becomes flaccid, not contracted. The UES is in direct contrast to the lower esophageal sphincter (LES). In the distal esophagus, achalasia is caused by loss of the inhibitory myenteric plexus neurons, which leaves no mechanism to inhibit myogenic contraction.

	LES	UES
Resting tone	Myogenic	None
Result of denervation	Contraction	Relaxation
Cause of impaired opening	Failure of relaxation	Failure of traction (pulling open)
Source of opening force	Bolus	Supra- and infrahyoid musculature

20. Describe the inheritance pattern and clinical presentation of oculopharyngeal dystrophy.

Inheritance pattern: sex-linked, autosomal dominant; French-Candian ancestry

Clinical presentation: onset in fifth decade, ptosis, less involvement of muscles other than oculopharyngeal, slowly progressive

21. List the common symptoms and causes of xerostomia.

Symptoms	Causes
Dysphagia	Sjögren's syndrome
Dry mouth with viscous saliva	Rheumatoid arthritis
Bad taste in mouth	Drugs (e.g., anticholinergics, antidepressants)
Oral burning	Radiation therapy
Dental decay	
Bad breath	

22. What are the potential extraesophageal manifestations of gastroesophageal reflux disease?

- Asthma
- Laryngitis
- Pharyngitis
- Dental decay with loss of dental enamel
- Globus sensation
- Otitis
- Recurrent sinusitis

23. What is Zenker's diverticulum?

Diverticula can occur throughout the hypopharynx. When they are located posteriorly in an area of potential weakness at the intersection of the transverse fibers of the cricopharyngeus and obliquely oriented fibers of the inferior pharyngeal constrictors (Killian's dehiscence), they are called Zenker's diverticula (see figure at top of following page).

24. Is Zenker's diverticulum a result of an obstructive or propulsive defect?

Previously it was believed that the pathogenesis of the diverticulum was due to abnormally high hypopharyngeal pressures caused by defective coordination of UES relaxation during pharyngeal bolus propulsion. It is now known that Zenker's diverticulum is caused by a constrictive myopathy of the cricopharyngeus (poor sphincter compliance). Increased resistance at the cricopharyngeus and increased intrabolus pressures above this relative obstruction cause muscular stress in the hypopharynx with herniation and diverticulum formation. Thus Zenker's diverticulum is an obstructive rather than propulsive disease.

25. Contrast esophageal and oropharyngeal dysphagia.

ESOPHAGEAL DYSPHAGIA	OROPHARYNGEAL DYSPHAGIA
Associated symptoms: chest pain, water brash, regurgitation	Associated symptoms: weakness, ptosis, nasal voice, pneumonia, cough
Organ-specific diseases (e.g., esophageal cancer, esophageal motor disorder)	Systemic diseases (e.g., myasthenia gravis, Parkinson's disease)
Treatable (e.g., dilation)	Rarely treatable
Expendable organ (only 1 function)	Nonexpendable (functions include speech, respiration, and swallowing)

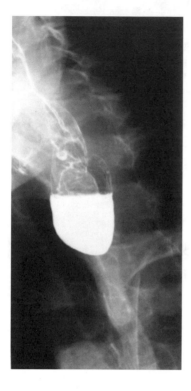

Radiograph of Zenker's diverticulum. (From Ergun GA, Kahrilas PJ: Oropharyngeal dysphagia in the elderly. Pract Gastroenterol 17:9–16, 1993, with permission.)

BIBLIOGRAPHY

1. Alberts MJ, Horner J, Gray L, Brazer S: Aspiration after stroke: Lesion analysis by brain MRI. Dysphagia 7:170–173, 1992.
2. Cook IJ, Blumbergs P, Cash K, et al: Structural abnormalities of the cricopharyngeus muscle in patients with pharyngeal (Zenker's) diverticulum. J Gastroenterol Hepatol 7:556–562, 1992.
3. Cook IJ, Gabb M, Panagopoulos V, et al: Pharyngeal (Zenker's) diverticulum is a disorder of upper esophageal sphincter opening. Gastroenterology 103:1229–1235, 1992.
4. Cook IJ, Kahrilas PJ: AGA technical review of management of oropharyngeal dysphagia. Gastroenterology 116:455–478, 1999.
5. Dodds WJ, Stewart ET, Logemann JA: Physiology and radiology of the normal oral and pharyngeal phases of swallowing. AJR 154:953–963, 1990.
6. Gordon C, Hewer R, Wade D: Dysphagia in acute stroke. BMJ 295:411–414, 1987.
7. Horner J, Massey E, Riski J, et al: Aspiration following stroke: Clinical correlates and outcome. Neurology 38:1359–1362, 1988.
8. Jacob P, Kahrilas PJ, Logemann JA, et al: Upper esophageal sphincter opening and modulation during swallowing. Gastroenterology 97:1469–1478, 1989.
9. Kahrilas PJ, Lin S, Logemann JA, et al: Deglutitive tongue action: Volume accommodation and bolus propulsion. Gastroenterology 104:152–162, 1993.
10. Kahrilas PJ, Logemann JA, Lin S, Ergun G: Pharyngeal clearance during swallowing: A combined manometric and videofluoroscopic study. Gastroenterology 103:128–136, 1992.
11. Logemann J: Evaluation and Treatment of Swallowing Disorders. San Diego, College-Hill Press, 1983.
12. Osserman KE: Myasthenia Gravis. New York, Grune & Stratton, 1958.
13. Robbins J, Hamilton JW, Lof GL, Kempster GB: Oropharyngeal swallowing in normal adults of different ages. Gastroenterology 103:823–829, 1992.
14. Siebens H, Trupe E, Siebens A, et al: Correlates and consequences of eating dependency in the institutionalized elderly. J Am Geriatr Soc 34:192–198, 1986.
15. Sonies BC, Dalakas MC: Dysphagia in patients with the post-polio syndrome. N Engl J Med 324:1162–1167, 1991.
16. Trupe EH, Siebens H, Siebens A: Prevalence of feeding and swallowing disorders in a nursing home. Arch Phys Med Rehabil 65:651–652, 1984.

2. GASTROESOPHAGEAL REFLUX DISEASE

Peter R. McNally, D.O.

1. What is gastroesophageal reflux disease (GERD)? How common is it?

GERD is a pathologic condition of symptoms or histopathologic injury to the esophagus caused by percolation of gastric or gastroduodenal contents into the esophagus. GERD is extremely common. One survey of hospital employees showed that 7% experienced heartburn daily, 14% experienced symptoms weekly and 15% monthly. Other studies have suggested a 3–4% prevalence of GERD among the general population, with a prevalence increase to approximately 5% in people older than 55 years. Pregnant women have the highest incidence of daily heartburn at 48–79%. The distribution of GERD between the sexes is equal, but men are more likely to suffer complications of GERD, esophagitis (2–3:1), and Barrett's esophagus (10:1).

2. What are the typical symptoms of GERD?

Heartburn is usually characterized as a midline retrosternal burning sensation that radiates to the throat and occasionally to the intrascapular region. Patients often place the open hand over the sternal area and flip the wrist in an up-and-down motion to simulate the nature and location of the heartburn symptoms. Mild symptoms of heartburn are often relieved within 3–5 minutes of ingesting milk or antacids. Other symptoms of GERD include the following:
  - **Regurgitation** consists of eructation of gastric juice or stomach contents into the pharynx and often is accompanied by a noxious bitter taste. Regurgitation is most common after a large meal and usually occurs with stooping or assuming a recumbent posture.
  - **Dysphagia** (difficulty in swallowing) usually is caused by a benign stricture of the esophagus in patients with longstanding GERD. Solid foods, such as meat and bread, are often precipitants of dysphagia. Dysphagia implies significant narrowing of the esophageal lumen, usually to a luminal diameter < 13 mm. Prolonged dysphagia, associated with inability to swallow saliva, requires prompt evaluation and often endoscopic removal (see chapter 66).
  - **Waterbrash** is an uncommon symptom but highly suggestive of GERD. Patients literally foam at the mouth as the salivary glands produce up to 10 ml of saliva per minute as an esophagosalivary reflex response to acid reflux.

3. Is gastrointestinal (GI) hemorrhage a common symptom of GERD?

No. Endoscopic evaluation of patients with upper GI hemorrhage has identified erosive GERD as the cause in only 2–6% of cases.

4. What is odynophagia? Is it a common symptom of GERD?

Odynophagia is a painful substernal sensation associated with swallowing that should not be confused with dysphagia. Odynophagia rarely results from GERD. Instead, odynophagia is caused by infections (monilia, herpes simplex virus, and cytomegalovirus), ingestion of corrosive agents or pills (tetracycline, vitamin C, iron, quinidine, estrogen, aspirin, alendronate [Fosamax], or nonsteroidal anti-inflammatory drugs), or cancer.

5. What clues about GERD can be gleaned from the physical exam?

  - **Severe kyphosis** often is associated with hiatal hernia and GERD, especially when a body brace is necessary.
  - **Tight-fitting corsets or clothing** (in men or women) can increase intraabdominal pressure and may cause stress reflux.
  - **Abnormal phonation** may suggest high GERD and vocal cord injury. When hoarseness is due to high GERD, the voice is often coarse or gravelly and may be worse in the morning, whereas in other causes of hoarseness, excessive voice use or abuse leads to worsening later in the day.

- **Wheezing or asthma and pulmonary fibrosis** have been associated with GERD. Patients often give a history of postprandial or nocturnal regurgitation with episodes of coughing or choking caused by near or partial aspiration.
- **Loss of enamel** on the lingual surface of the teeth may be seen in severe GERD, although it is more common in patients with rumination syndrome or bulimia.
- Esophageal dysfunction may be the predominant component of **scleroderma or mixed connective tissue disease**. Inquiry about symptoms of Raynaud's syndrome and examination for sclerodactyly, taut skin, and calcinosis are important.
- **Cerebral palsy, Down syndrome, and mental retardation** are commonly associated with GERD.
- Children with peculiar head movements during swallowing may have **Sandifer's syndrome**.
- Some patients **unknowingly swallow air** (aerophagia) that triggers a burp, belch, and heartburn cycle. The observant clinician may detect this behavior during the interview and physical exam.

6. Do healthy persons have GERD?

Yes. Healthy persons may regurgitate acid or food contents into the esophagus, especially after a large meal late at night. In normal persons, the natural defense mechanisms of the lower esophageal sphincter barrier and esophageal clearance are not overwhelmed, and symptoms and injury do not occur. Ambulatory esophageal pH studies have shown that healthy persons have acid reflux into the esophagus < 2% of the daytime (upright position) and < 0.3% of the nighttime (supine position).

7. How can swallowing and salivary production be associated with GERD?

Reflux of gastric contents into the esophagus often stimulates salivary production and increased swallowing. Saliva has a neutral pH, which helps to neutralize the gastric refluxate. Furthermore, the swallowed saliva initiates a peristaltic wave that strips the esophagus of refluxed material (clearance). During the awake upright period, persons swallow 70 times/hr; this rate increases to 200 times/hr during meals. Swallowing is least common during sleep (< 10 times/hr), and arousal from sleep to swallow during GERD may be reduced by sedatives or alcohol ingestion. Patients with Sjögren's syndrome and smokers have reduced salivary production and prolonged esophageal acid clearance times.

8. What are the two defective anatomic mechanisms in patients with GERD?

Ineffective clearance and defective gastroesophageal (GE) barrier.

9. What clearance defects are associated with GERD?

Esophageal. Normally reflux of gastric contents into the esophagus stimulates a secondary peristaltic or clearance wave to remove the injurious refluxate from the esophagus. The worst case of ineffective esophageal clearance is seen in patients with scleroderma. The lower esophageal sphincter barrier is nonexistent, and there is no primary or secondary peristalsis of the esophagus (hence, no clearance).

Gastric. Gastroparesis may lead to excessive quantities of retained gastroduodenal and food contents. Larger volumes of stagnant gastric contents predispose to esophageal reflux.

10. How may the GE barrier be compromised?

The normal lower esophageal sphincter (LES) is 3–4 cm long and maintains a resting tone of 10–30 mmHg pressure. The LES acts as a barrier against GERD. When the LES pressure is < 6 mmHg, GERD is common; however, the presence of "normal" LES pressure does not predict absence of GERD. In fact, LES pressure < 10 mmHg is found in a minority of people with GERD. Recent studies have shown that transient LES relaxations (tLESRs) are important in the pathogenesis of GERD. During tLESR, the sphincter inappropriately relaxes and free gastric reflux occurs.

11. What factors influence resting LES pressure?

	INCREASED LES PRESSURE	DECREASED LES PRESSURE
Neural agents	Alpha-adrenergic agonists Beta-adrenergic antagonists Cholinergic agonists	Alpha-adrenergic antagonists Beta-adrenergic agonists Cholinergic antagonists
Food	Protein	Fat Chocolate Ethanol Peppermint
Hormones/mediators	Gastrin Motilin Substance P Prostaglandin F_2alpha	Cholecystokinin Secretin Glucagon Gastric inhibitory factor Progesterone Vasoactive intestinal peptide
Medications	Antacids Metoclopramide Cisapride Domperidone	Calcium channel antagonists Theophylline Diazepam Meperidine Morphine Dopamine Diazepam Barbiturates

12. Describe the natural history of GERD.

Most patients with confirmed GERD have experienced symptoms for several years before seeking medical attention. Before the introduction of potent antireflux medications that inhibit the gastric proton pump, it was common for patients to experience recurrent symptoms even on therapy with antacids, H_2 antagonists, and prokinetic drugs. Most patients with GERD can now be successfully managed by the administration of a proton pump inhibitor (PPI), but GERD is recurrent in > 80% of patients within 30 weeks of discontinuation of the drug.

Erosive GERD should be considered a chronic disease. The likelihood of recurrent symptoms after discontinuation of medical therapy is high. The goals of medical therapy should be relief of symptoms and avoidance of the major complications of esophagitis: stricture formation, Barrett's esophagus, and bleeding.

13. What other medical conditions may mimic symptoms of GERD?

The differential diagnosis of GERD includes coronary artery disease, gastritis, gastroparesis, infectious and pill-induced esophagitis, peptic ulcer disease, biliary tract disease, and esophageal motor diseases.

14. How can GERD be distinguished from coronary artery disease?

In the evaluation of patients with retrosternal chest pain, the clinician must always be mindful that patients with GERD do not die, but patients with new-onset angina or an acute myocardial infarction with symptoms mimicking GERD can. Clues that a patient's chest pain is cardiac in origin include radiation of the pain to the neck, jaw, or left shoulder/upper extremity; associated shortness of breath and/or diaphoresis; precipitation of pain by exertion; and relief of pain with sublingual nitroglycerin. Physical findings of new murmurs or gallops or abnormal rhythms are also suggestive of a cardiac origin. Although positive findings on an electrocardiogram (EKG) are helpful in the evaluation of patients with chest pain, the absence of ischemic EKG changes should not discourage the clinician from excluding a cardiac etiology for the patient's symptoms.

15. How should patients with symptoms of GERD be evaluated?

Evaluation of patients with GERD may be guided by the severity of symptoms. Patients without symptoms of high GERD (aspiration or hoarseness) or dysphagia may be given careful instruction about lifestyle modification and a diagnostic trial of H_2 blocker therapy and followed clinically. Diagnostic evaluation is warranted when symptoms of GERD are chronic or incompletely responsive to medical therapy. Esophagogastroduodenoscopy (EGD) is the single best test for evaluation of GERD. Up to 50% of patients with GERD do not have macroscopic evidence of esophagitis at the time of endoscopy. In this group more sensitive GER testing may be necessary or alternative diagnoses considered.

16. Describe the commonly used endoscopic grading system for GERD.

Grade 0	Macroscopically normal esophagus; only histologic evidence of GERD
Grade 1	One or more nonconfluent lesions with erythema or exudate above the GE junction
Grade 2	Confluent, noncircumferential, erosive, and exudative lesions
Grade 3	Circumferential erosive and exudative lesions
Grade 4	Chronic mucosal lesions (ulceration, stricture, or Barrett's esophagus)

17. What are the more sophisticated esophageal function tests? How can they be used appropriately in the evaluation of patients with GERD?

Clinical tests of GERD may be divided into three categories:
1. **Acid sensitivity**
   - Acid perfusion (Bernstein) test
   - 24-hour ambulatory esophageal pH monitoring
2. **Esophageal barrier and motility**
   - Esophageal manometry
   - Gastroesophageal scintiscanning
   - Standard acid reflux (modified Tuttle) test
   - 24-hour ambulatory esophageal pH monitoring
3. **Esophageal acid clearance time**
   - Standard acid reflux clearance test (SART)
   - 24-hour ambulatory esophageal pH monitoring

18. Do all patients with GERD need esophageal function testing?

No. Testing should be reserved for patients who fail medical therapy or in whom the correlation of reflux symptoms is in doubt.

19. How is the Bernstein test performed?

The Bernstein test helps to confirm that symptoms are due to esophageal sensitivity to acid. It is performed by alternatively infusing sterile water and dilute 0.1 N HCL in the distal esophagus.

20. When is ambulatory 24-hour esophageal pH monitoring helpful?

Ambulatory 24-hour esophageal pH monitoring is helpful in evaluating patients refractory to standard medical therapy. Acid hypersecretion is often seen in patients with GERD, and esophageal pH monitoring may be helpful in titrating the dose of H_2 blocker or PPI. Persistence of acid reflux on "adequate" doses of a PPI should raise the possibility of patient noncompliance or Zollinger-Ellison syndrome. Some authoritites have reported that ambulatory 24-hr pH monitoring with distal and proximal esophageal pH electrodes is helpful in the evaluation of patients with atypical reflux symptoms, such as hoarseness, throat tightness, asthma, and interstitial lung disease.

21. When are esophageal manometry and scintiscanning helpful?

Esophageal manometry is helpful in evaluating the competency of the LES barrier and the body of the esophagus for motor dysfunction. Severe esophagitis may be the sole manifestation of early scleroderma. When ambulatory pH testing is not available, scintiscanning has been shown to be helpful.

22. Define the various types of medical therapy for GERD and give a logical approach to prescription therapy for patients with longstanding GERD.

For patients with mild, uncomplicated symptoms of heartburn, empiric H_2 blocker therapy without costly and sophisticated diagnostic testing is reasonable. For patients recalcitrant to conventional therapy or with complications of high GERD (aspiration, asthma, hoarseness), Barrett's esophagus, or stricture, diagnostic and management decisions become more complicated. Medical or surgical therapy depends on patient preference, health care cost, risk of medical or surgical complications, and other related factors.

Medical Therapy for GERD

TOPICAL	DOSAGE	SIDE EFFECTS
Antacids	1–2 tablets after meals and at bedtime, as needed	Diarrhea (magnesium-containing) and constipation (aluminum- and calcium-containing)
Sucralfate	1 gm 4 times/day	Incomplete passage of pill, especially in patients with esophageal strictures; constipation; dysgeusia
H_2 blockers		
Cimetidine	400–800 mg 2–4 times/day	Gynecomastia, impotence, psychosis, hepatitis, drug interactions with warfarin, theophylline
Ranitidine	150–300 mg 2–4 times/day	Same, less common
Famotidine	20–40 mg 1–2 times/day	Same, less common
PPIs		
Omeprazole	20–60 mg/day	Drug interaction due to cytochrome p-450 (warfarin, phenytoin, diazepam)
Lansoprazole	30 mg/day	CYP-1A2 inducer; decreases theophylline levels
Rabeprazole	20 mg/day	Probably none
Pantoprazole	40 mg/day	Probably none
Esomeprazole	20–40 mg/day	Probably none
Prokinetic agents		
Bethanechol	10–25 mg 4 times/day or at bedtime	Urinary retention in patients with detrusor-external sphincter dyssynergia or prostatic hypertrophy, worsening asthma
Metoclopramide	10 mg 3 times/day or at bedtime	Extrapyramidal dysfunction, Parkinsonian-like reaction; cases of irreversible tardive dyskinesia have been reported
Cisapride	10–20 mg 3 times/day and at bedtime	FDA recall, because of potential fatal arrhythmia Available only on compassionate basis.

PPIs = proton pump inhibitors, FDA = Food and Drug Administration.

23. Describe the commonly recommended approach to graded treatment of GERD.

Stage I	Lifestyle modifications
	Antacids, prokinetics, over-the-counter H_2 blockers, or sucralfate
Stage II	H_2 blocker therapy
	Reinforce need for lifestyle modifications
Stage III	PPIs
	Reinforce need for lifestyle modifications
Stage IV	Surgical antireflux procedure

The author favors initiation of aggressive lifestyle modification (especially weight reduction and dietary changes) and pharmacologic therapy to achieve endoscopic healing of esophagitis (usually a PPI). When esophagitis is healed, an effective dose of an intermediate-potency H_2 blocker is substituted for the PPI. Then the patient is counseled about the risks, benefits, and alternatives to long-term medical therapy. Surgery is encouraged for the fit patient who requires chronic high doses of pharmacologic therapy to control GERD or dislikes taking medicines.

24. Do patients scheduled for surgical antireflux procedures need to undergo sophisticated esophageal function testing before surgery?

There is no absolute correct answer. However, it is prudent to do esophageal motility studies to ensure that esophageal motor disease is not present. Patients with scleroderma may have a paucity of systemic complaints, and the diagnosis may go undetected without esophageal manometry. Generally, surgical antireflux procedures are avoided or modified in such patients. In addition, esophageal motility studies and ambulatory 24-hour pH monitoring may confirm or refute that the patient's symptoms are attributable to GERD before performance of a surgical procedure.

25. What are the most serious long-term complications of GERD?

Esophageal stricture and Barrett's esophagus.

26. How should esophageal strictures be managed?

- Prevention of peptic stricture with early institution of effective medical or surgical therapy appears to be particularly important for patients with scleroderma.
- For patients suffering symptoms of dysphagia due to peptic stricture, esophageal dilation is effective. Dilation can be accomplished using mercury-filled, polyvinyl, Maloney bougies, wire-guided hollow Savary-Gulliard or American dilators, or through-the-scope (TTS) pneumatic balloons. Usually the esophagus is dilated to a diameter of 14 mm or 44 French. After successful dilation of a peptic stricture the patient should be placed on chronic PPI therapy to avoid recurrent stricture formation.
- Surgery, is an effective method of managing esophageal strictures. Usually pre-and intra-operative dilation is combined with a definitive antireflux procedure.

27. What is Barrett's esophagus? How is it managed?

Barrett's esophagus is a metaplastic degeneration of the normal esophageal lining, which is replaced with a premalignant, specialized columnar epithelium. It is seen in roughly 5–7% of patients with uncomplicated reflux but in up to 30–40% of patients with scleroderma or dysphagia.

Currently, there is no proven method to eliminate Barrett's esophagus. Preliminary studies of laser or bicap ablation of the metaplastic segment followed by alkalization of the gastroesophageal refluxate are encouraging. The need for cancer surveillance is discussed elsewhere in this book.

28. List some of the atypical symptoms and signs of GERD.

- Asthma
- Chest pain
- Cough
- Hiccups
- Hoarseness
- Lingual dental erosions
- Recurrent otitis in children
- Throat-clearing
- Throat tightness

29. Does the presence of heartburn symptoms predict a GERD-related cough etiology?

No. There is poor correlation between symptoms of heartburn and cough. Between 43–75% of patients with GERD-related cough do not have heartburn symptoms. Both medical treatment with PPIs and surgical antireflux procedures have been reported to be effective for GERD-related cough. Caveats include:

- 35% response rate to omeprazole 40 mg 2 times/day after 2 weeks
- Results of surgical antireflux procedures are best when preoperative esophageal manometry is normal and response to PPI is positive.

30. What is the best method to evaluate for possible GERD-related cough?

The first step is to exclude non–GERD-related etiologies: angiotensin-converting inhibitors, environmental irritants, smoking, parenchymal lung disease, allergic rhinitis and pneumonitis, and asthma and sinusitis, which are often "silent." Symptom relief after a 2-week trial of omeprazole, 40 mg 2 times/day, is a cost-effective approach. Patients who do not respond should be considered for further evaluation, including esophageal manometry/pH testing and/or EGD.

31. What laryngeal conditions are associated with GERD?

The most common laryngeal manifestation of high reflux or esophagopharyngeal reflux (EPR) is hoarseness. Other laryngeal conditions associated with EPR are listed below.

- Arytenoid fixation
- Carcinoma of the larynx
- Contact ulcers and granuloma
- Globus pharyngeus
- Hoarseness

- Laryngomalacia
- Pachydermia laryngitis
- Paroxysmal laryngospasm
- Recurrent leukoplakia
- Vocal cord nodules

32. How often do people with EPR and hoarseness relate symptoms of heartburn?

The prevalence of GERD symptoms among patients with reflux laryngitis is low (6–43%).

33. What is the most efficient, cost-effective method to evaluate hoarse patients for EPR?

The first step in the evaluation of hoarseness should be exclusion of structural ear, nose, and throat (ENT) disorders, including neoplasm. The next step is an empiric trial of double-dose PPI for 2–3 months. Most EPR-related hoarseness improves with acid suppression (60–96%). Patients responding to PPIs may stop the medication and be monitored for recurrence of symptoms. Hoarse patients with a negative ENT evaluation who fail PPI therapy should undergo formal esophageal pH analysis.

34. Can gastroesophageal reflux worsen asthma?

Yes. Numerous studies have shown that reflux symptoms are common among asthmatics (65–72%) and that medical and surgical antireflux treatment may improve pulmonary function.

35. How does gastroesophageal reflux worsen asthma?

Several mechanisms are theorized to explain GERD-induced bronchospasm:

1. Asthmatics with GERD have been shown to have autonomic dysregulation with heightened vagal response, which is presumed to be responsible for the decrease in LES pressure and more frequent transient relaxations of the LES, which promote reflux

2. Esophageal reflux may incite a vagal-mediated esophagobronchial reflex of airway hyperreactivity.

3. Microaspiration of gastric juice has been shown to activate a local axonal reflex involving release of substance P, which leads to airway edema. The finding of lipid-laden alveolar macrophages among asthmatics demonstrates aspiration of gastric material into the pulmonary tree.

36. Which patients with GERD should be considered for a surgical antireflux procedure?

Any young, healthy patient with chronic GERD requiring lifelong PPI medical therapy may be considered for an antireflux procedure. Other indications include failed medical therapy, complicated GERD (e.g., bleeding, recurrent strictures), medical success at excessive cost in young, otherwise healthy patients, and problematic symptoms due to regurgitation (asthma, hoarseness, cough).

37. Which patients are poor candidates for a surgical antireflux procedure?

- Elderly patients with substantial comorbid disease
- Patients with poor or absent esophageal peristalsis
- Patients with highly functional symptoms

Lack of available surgical expertise is also a contraindication for antireflux procedures.

38. What is the best surgical antireflux procedure?

Rapid advances in endoscopic and laparoscopic surgery make this question unanswerable. The Bard endoscopic sewing system (BESS) procedure is a novel endoscopic surgical technique used to "tighten" the LES. New laparoscopic devices, such as oblique telescopes and curvilinear articulating devices, are making laparoscopic fundoplication technically easier (see chapters 79 and 85). Comparison studies are needed to determine the role of these new antireflux procedures.

39. What cytochrome p-450 (CYP-450) systems are involved in the metabolism of PPIs?

All of the PPIs undergo some hepatic metabolism through the CYP-450 system. The CYP-2C19 and CYP-3A4 microsomal enzymes are responsible for the majority of PPI hepatic metabolism. Genetic polymorphism with CYP-2C19 is common; about 5% of Americans and 20% of Asians are deficient in this enzyme. Omeprazole decreases the metabolism of phenytoin and warfarin R-isomer (CYP-2C9), diazepam (CYP-2C19), and cyclosporine (CYP-3A4).

40. How do esomeprazole (Nexium) and omeprazole (Prilosec) differ?

Omeprazole is a racemic mixture of both the S- and R-isomers, whereas esomeprazole is a pure form of the S-isomer. Less esomeprazole (S-isomer) is metabolized by the CYP-2C19 pathway, leading to greater area under the curve and better intragastric acid suppression for 24 hours. Esomeprazole is the only PPI shown to be stastically superior to omeprazole in healing erosive esophagitis at 8 weeks (90–94% efficacy rate).

BIBLIOGRAPHY

1. Bainbridge ET, Temple JG, Nicholas SP, et al: Symptomatic gastroesophageal reflux in pregnancy: A comparative study of white Europeans and Asians in Birmingham. Br J Clin Pract 37:53, 1983.
2. Brunnen PL, Karmody AM, Needham CD: Severe peptic esophagitis. Gut 10:831, 1969.
3. Collen MJ, Lewis JH, Benjaman SB: Gastric acid hypersecretion in refractory gastroesophageal reflux disease. Gastroenterology 98:654, 1990.
4. Deemester TR, Wang CI, Wernly JA, et al: Technique, indications, and clinical use of 24 hour esophageal pH monitoring. J Thorac Cardiovasc Surg 79:656, 1980.
5. DeVault KR: Overview of therapy for the extraesophageal manifestations of gastroesophageal reflux disease. Am J Gastroenterol 95:S39–S44, 2000.
6. Dodds WJ, Kahrilas PJ, Dent J, et al: Analysis of spontaneous gastroesophageal reflux and esophageal acid clearance in patients with reflux esophagitis. J Gastrointest Motil 2:79, 1989.
7. Graham DY, Smith JL, Patterson DJ: Why do apparently healthy people use antacid tablets? Am J Gastroenterol 78:257–260, 1983.
8. Harding SM, Sontag SJ. Asthma and gastroesophageal reflux. Am J Gastroenterol 95:S23–32, 2000.
9. Irwin RS, Richter JE. Gastroesophageal reflux and chronic cough. Am J Gastroenterol 95:S9–S14. 2000.
10. Johnson LF: Gastroesophageal reflux. In Spittell JA Jr (ed): Clinical Medicine. New York, Harper & Row, 1982, pp 1–39.
11. Kahrilas PJ, Gupta RR: The effect of cigarette smoking on salivation and esophageal acid clearance. J Lab Clin Med 114:431, 1989.
12. Kahrilas PJ, Hogan WJ: Gastroesophageal reflux. In Sleisenger MH, Fordtran JS (eds): Gastrointestinal Disease, 5th ed. Philadelphia, W. B. Saunders, 1993, pp 379–401.
13. Korsten MA, Rosman AS, Fishbein S, et al: Chronic xerostomia increases esophageal acid exposure and is associated with esophageal injury. Am J Med 90:701, 1991.
14. Lazarchick DA, Filler SJ: Dental erosion: Predominant oral lesion in gastroesophageal reflux disease. Am J Gastroenterol 95:S33–S38, 2000.
15. Martinez-Serna T, Davis RE, Mason R, et al: Endoscopic valvuloplasty for GERD. Gastrointest Endosc 52:663–670, 2000.
16. McNally PR, Maydonovitch CL, Prosek RA, et al: Evaluation of gastroesophageal reflux as a cause of idiopathic hoarseness. Dig Dis Sci 34:1900–1904, 1989.
17. Meier JH, McNally PR, Freeman SR, et al: Does omeprazole (Prilosec) improve asthma in patients with gastroesophageal reflux: A double blind crossover study. Dig Dis Sci 39:1900–1904, 1994.
18. Nebel OT, Fornes MF, Castell DO: Symptomatic gastroesophageal reflux: Incidence and precipitating factors. Am J Dig Dis 21:953, 1976.
19. Ogrek CP: Gastroesophageal reflux. In Haubrich WS, Schaffner F (eds): Bockus Gastroenterology, 5th ed. Philadelphia, W. B. Saunders, 1995, pp 445–463.
20. Ott DJ: Barium esophagram. In Castell DO, Wu WC, Ott DJ (eds): Gastroesophageal Reflux Disease. Mt Kisco, NY, Futura, 1985, pp 109–128.
21. Richter JE. Extraesophageal presentations of gastroesophageal reflux disease: An overview. Am J Gastroenterol 95:S1–S3, 2000.
22. Richter JE, Castell DO: Gastroesophageal reflux. Pathogenesis, diagnosis, and therapy. Ann Intern Med 97:93, 1982.
23. Sontag SJ, O'Commell S, Khandelwal S, et al: Most asthmatics have gastroesophageal reflux with or without bronchodilator therapy. Gastroenterology 99:613, 1990.
24. Spencer CM, Faulds D: Esomeprazole. Drugs 60:321–327, 2000.
25. Winnan GR, Meyer CT, McCallum RW: Interpretation of Bernstein test: A reappraisal. Ann Intern Med 96:320–322, 1982.
26. Wong RKH, Hanson DG, Waring PJ, Shaw G: ENT manifestations of gastroesophageal reflux. Am J Gastroenterol 95:S15–S22, 2000.

3. ESOPHAGEAL INFECTIONS

Dirk R. Davis, M.D.

1. What are the typical symptoms from patients with infectious esophagitis?

Odynophagia and, to a lesser degree, dysphagia are by far the most common symptoms. Nausea, dysgeusia, heartburn, chest pain, fever, bleeding, and even hiccups also can be present.

2. What is the most common cause of infectious esophagitis in the general population?

Candida albicans. This virtually ubiquitous yeast is found in normal oral flora. Infection is a two-step process. The first step is colonization, which involves mucosal adherence and proliferation. It is estimated that 20% of asymptomatic people have fungal colonization of the esophagus. The second step, infection, usually is associated with impaired host defenses. Infection is characterized by invasion of the mucosa with budding yeast and the presence of hyphae on microscopic examination. Creamy white adherent plaques or exudates are seen endoscopically.

3. How helpful is the finding of oral thrush in diagnosing fungal esophagitis in patients with esophageal symptoms?

Although 75% of patients with candidal esophagitis have coincident oral infection, the absence of thrush does not exclude the diagnosis and a high degree of suspicion should be maintained, especially in an immunocompromised patient.

4. Is empiric therapy for fungal esophagitis reasonable in patients with typical symptoms?

In an immunocompromised population, an empiric trial of fluconazole, 100–200 mg/day for 10–14 days, is warranted. If symptoms do not improve within 5–7 days, upper endoscopy should be performed for diagnostic evaluation.

5. Is there any benefit to prophylaxis for fungal esophagitis in HIV-infected patients?

Recurrences of candidal esophagitis are common in HIV patients. Prophylaxis with fluconazole, 150 mg/week orally, can be recommended. This treatment reduces the number of yeast in host flora, making colonization and infection less likely.

6. Describe the appropriate therapy for candidal esophagitis.

Although nonabsorbable (topical) agents such as nystatin and clotrimazole are essentially free of side effects and drug interactions, the orally administered imidazole antifungals are preferred. Fluconazole has advantages over the other agents and is the treatment of choice at a dose of 100 mg orally for 10–14 days. Nystatin is effective at a "swish-and-swallow" dose of 500,000 units 5 times/day for 7–14 days. Clotrimazole can be given as a 10-mg buccal troche 5 times/day, or a 100-mg vaginal suppository can be dissolved in the mouth and swallowed (3 times/day for 10–14 days). Because ketoconazole has unpredictable absorption and lower efficacy, it is no longer recommended.

7. What is the first-line therapy in granulocytopenic patients with fungal esophagitis?

Granulocytopenic patients should receive intravenous amphotericin B because of the high risk of fungal dissemination. Dose and duration of treatment are based on severity of infection; febrile patients with extensive esophagitis or disseminated infection should receive 0.5 mg/kg/day. Patients with milder infections may be treated with doses of 0.3mg/kg/day.

8. What other fungal organisms should be considered in esophageal infections?

Although less likely, *Candida* species other than *C. albicans* can cause esophagitis. Non-candidal fungi cause primary esophageal infections only in severely immunocompromised patients. Examples include *Histoplasma, Cryptococcus, Blastomyces,* and *Aspergillus* species.

9. What commonly used drugs may predispose to fungal esophagitis?

Systemic and topical-inhaled corticosteroids are associated with an increased risk of candidal infection because of effects on mucosal immunity. Antibiotics that affect normal oral flora change the competitive milieu, predisposing to candidal proliferation and infection. Acid suppressive therapies, both H_2 receptor blockers and proton pump inhibitors, increase the incidence of esophageal colonization with *C. albicans*, probably as a result of loss of the cleansing effect of spontaneous gastroesophageal reflux events.

10. What medical illnesses are known to be associated with an increased risk of candidal esophagitis?

Diseases associated with impaired immunity, primarily HIV infection and hematologic malignancies, increase the prevalence of fungal esophagitis. Nonhematologic malignancy is also associated with an increased risk for candidal infection. Diabetes mellitus, adrenocortical (Cushing's) disease, alcoholism, and diseases affecting peristalsis (achalasia/scleroderma) increase the likelihood of monilial esophagitis. Achlorhydria secondary to gastric surgery or atrophy also is associated with a higher risk for fungal esophagitis.

11. What is the most common viral cause of esophagitis?

In the general population, herpes simplex virus (HSV) is the most common cause and typically is seen in conjunction with orolabial infection. The clinical course usually mirrors that of the orolabial lesions and, in an immunocompetent patient, may not require treatment.

12. What is the first-line therapy for HSV esophagitis?

In severely symptomatic patients or patients with known immunocompromise, intravenous acyclovir should be initiated at a dose of 250 mg/m² every 8–12 hours for 7–10 days.

13. What is the most common viral esophagitis in immunocompromised patients?

Cytomegalovirus (CMV). Endoscopic biopsies of esophageal lesions demonstrate CMV in up to 40% of cases. CMV infection can be newly acquired through transfusions or organ transplantation, or it can result from reactivation of latent infection. It is usually a widespread visceral infection, not limited to the esophagus.

14. How common are coinfections with *Candida* spp. and CMV in HIV-infected patients?

Both organisms can be identified in 20% of esophageal infections. It may be difficult to diagnose CMV disease until the fungal infection has been adequately treated. Epstein-Barr (EBV) virus and HSV infections also occur coincidentally with monilial infection but much less commonly.

15. Describe the initial therapy for CMV esophagitis.

Two drugs are effective in treating CMV disease in immunocompromised patients: ganciclovir and foscarnet. Ganciclovir, 5 mg/kg intravenously every 12 hours for 2 weeks, is effective in 80% of cases. The most common side effect is granulocytopenia, especially if used in conjunction with anti-HIV drugs such as zidovudine. Because it is much less expensive than foscarnet, it is considered first-line therapy. In granulocytopenic patients or patients who have failed ganciclovir, foscarnet should be administered at a dose of 90 mg/kg intravenously every 12 hours for 3–4 weeks. The most significant adverse effect of foscarnet is renal toxicity. Recurrences of CMV esophagitis in the setting of immunocompromise are common, and maintenance therapy may be required.

16. Can HSV and CMV infections be differentiated endoscopically?

Although the diagnosis of viral esophagitis must be made histologically or by culture, endoscopic appearance may suggest an etiology. Early in HSV infection, typical small vesicles are seen. They may progress, forming circumscribed ulcers up to 2 cm in diameter with raised yellowish edges—the classic "volcano ulcers." Typical CMV lesions are usually linear, serpiginous ulcers in the middle and/or distal esophagus and may coalesce to form giant ulcers. Concomitant infections with both organisms have been reported.

17. Differentiate HSV and CMV microscopically.

HSV infects squamous epithelium. Biopsies from the ulcer margins demonstrate multinucleated giant cells with ballooning degeneration of squamous cells, margination of chromatin, and characteristic ground-glass nuclei. Cowdry type A intranuclear inclusions are pathognomonic for HSV infection. CMV is found in submucosal fibroblasts and vascular epithelium, which require deep biopsies from the ulcer crater for diagnosis. The classic histologic features of CMV infection are large cells with both intracytoplasmic inclusions and amphophilic intranuclear inclusions. Biopsies should be placed in viral transport media; culture remains the standard for diagnosis.

18. Does HIV infect the esophagus primarily?

Uncertain and controversial. Large ulcers in the esophagus have been reported in patients with HIV infection when biopsies, brushings, and cultures fail to identify known pathogens. Viral particles from biopsies of the ulcer margin, consistent with HIV, have been demonstrated by electron microscopy. Symptoms may resolve rapidly with ulcer healing in response to corticosteroid therapy. Prednisone, 40 mg/day orally, can be given until symptoms resolve; then the dose is tapered by 10 mg/week. Treatment with corticosteroids increases the risk of other opportunistic infections, primarily *Candida* spp. and CMV. Failure to respond to corticosteroids should raise suspicions.

19. List three other possible viral causes for ulcerative esophagitis.

Epstein-Barr virus has been reported to cause esophageal ulcers in patients with AIDS as well as in immunocompetent patients with infectious mononucleosis. The esophageal ulcers respond to treatment with acyclovir but in patients with AIDS often recur after therapy is discontinued. **Varicella zoster virus** (VZV) can also cause severe esophagitis in severely immunocompromised patients. The diagnosis is made easier when the typical dermatologic varicelliform lesions are present. Disseminated visceral VZV can be present without the typical skin manifestations of disease. Acyclovir is the first-line therapy. **Human papilloma virus** can also infect the esophagus in both normal and immunocompromised people but is seldom symptomatic. It does not cause significant inflammation but small macules. Florid, even fatal esophageal papillomatosis has been reported.

20. Are patients with HIV/AIDS at significant risk for bacterial esophagitis?

In general, bacterial esophagitis is rare. The most significant risk factor is granulocytopenia. Patients with HIV disease have relatively preserved granulocyte populations but are still at increased risk because of overall immunocompromise. Patients receiving chemotherapy for malignant disease are at the greatest risk for bacterial infection.

21. How is the diagnosis of bacterial esophagitis established?

Tissue Gram stain of mucosal biopsies documents invasion of the esophageal mucosa with sheets of bacterial organisms. Infection is usually polymicrobial, most typically with gram-positive organisms found in normal oral flora, but gram-negative species are also seen. Hemotoxylin stains are not helpful. Cultures of tissue biopsies are usually not of benefit because of contamination of the endoscope. Concomitant fungal and viral infections must be excluded.

22. Describe the recommended treatment for bacterial esophagitis.

Because bacterial esophagitis is most common in granulocytopenic patients, the risk of overwhelming sepsis warrants aggressive treatment. A beta-lactam antibiotic, given intravenously in combination with an aminoglycoside, is appropriate; adjustments are based on clinical course.

23. Does it make sense to stain for acid-fast organisms in evaluating esophageal ulcers?

A shallow linear ulcer with smooth edges and a necrotic base, usually in the middle third of the esophagus, is suggestive of *Mycobacterium tuberculosis* (TB). TB is seldom a primary infection in the esophagus, but cases have been reported. It more often results from direct extension from adjacent mediastinal lymph nodes in patients with pulmonary tuberculosis. *Mycobacterium-avium* complex is commonly reported in patients with AIDS and tends to be widely disseminated at the time of diagnosis. Esophageal involvement is rare but should be considered in the differential diagnosis; appropriate tissue stains and culture should be obtained. As is the case with TB, treatment is difficult, requiring multidrug regimens over months.

BIBLIOGRAPHY

1. Baehr PH, McDonald GB: Esophageal infections: Risk factors, presentation, diagnosis and treatment. Gastroenterology 106:509, 1994.
2. Dieterich DT, Wilcox CM: The Practice Parameters Committee of the American College of Gastroenterology: Diagnosis and treatment of esophageal diseases associated with HIV infection. Am J Gastroenterol 91:2265, 1996.
3. Laine L: The natural history of esophageal candidiasis after successful treatment in patients with AIDS. Gastroenterology 107:744, 1994.
4. Rabeneck L, Laine L: Esophageal candidiasis in patients infected with the human immunodeficiency virus. Arch Intern Med 154:2705, 1994.
5. Raufman JP: Esophageal infections. In: Yamada T (ed): Textbook of Gastroenterology, 2nd ed. Philadelphia, J.B. Lippincott, 1995, p 1243.
6. Sutton FM, Graham DY, Goodlame RW: Infectious esophagitis. Gastrointest Endosc Clin North Am 4:713, 1994.
7. Wilcox CM, Straub RF, Clark WS: Prospective evaluation of oropharyngeal findings in human immunodeficiency virus-infected patients with esophageal ulceration. Am J Gastroenterol 90:1938, 1995.

4. ESOPHAGEAL CAUSES OF CHEST PAIN

Brian T. Johnston, M.D., and Donald O. Castell, M.D.

1. When should the clinician consider an esophageal cause of chest pain?

Esophageal disease is a common problem, but esophageal causes of chest pain are rarely life-threatening and do not necessitate emergency diagnosis. Therefore, the initial approach must be to exclude coronary artery disease (CAD). In the United States 1.5 million patients/year suffer an acute myocardial infarction, and one-fourth of all deaths are attributed to myocardial infarction.

A normal electrocardiogram (EKG) during the episode of pain is reassuring. However, a pain episode sufficiently severe to warrant admission to hospital merits serial EKGs and assessment of cardiac enzyme levels. Further investigations after the acute episode include an exercise stress test (EST), thallium EST, or coronary angiography. Because a routine EST has a false-negative rate of 34%, only the last two investigations reliably exclude coronary artery disease. At this stage, esophageal chest pain may be considered.

The concept of the esophagus as the origin of chest pain is not new. A century ago, Sir William Osler hypothesized that esophageal spasm represented one cause of chest pain in soldiers during wartime. A recent multicenter study reported that 55% of patients seen in emergency departments across the United States were shown not to be having cardiac pain.

2. Does exclusion of CAD exclude all cardiac diagnoses?

No. Cardiac abnormalities other than CAD can be found in patients with chest pain, including mitral valve prolapse and microvascular angina. Exclusion of mitral valve prolapse requires echocardiography, whereas microvascular angina can be excluded only by the complicated procedure of measuring coronary artery resistance during stimulation with ergonovine and rapid atrial pacing.

However, studies suggesting that pain is no more common in patients with mitral valve prolapse or microvascular angina than in the general population question whether in fact these abnormalities produce pain. If so, the mechanism is unclear. Furthermore, the prognosis is excellent; the mortality rate is no different from that of the general population. Finally, a positive association between these abnormalities and esophageal motility disorders suggests a common or associated cause—either a generalized smooth muscle defect or heightened visceral nociception. It is therefore appropriate to search first for an esophageal cause, which may be more common and more responsive to treatment.

3. Does history help to discriminate cardiac from esophageal chest pain?

Yes and no. A sharp pain localized by one finger at the fifth intercostal space in the midclavicular line with onset at rest in a 20-year-old woman is unlikely to be caused by coronary artery disease. Certain features in a patient's presenting history clearly help to differentiate between causes. However, many studies have shown sufficient overlap of all features to preclude certain diagnosis on the basis of symptoms alone. The description of pain by some patients with a known esophageal source and no cardiac disease mimics exactly the classical description of angina pectoris, including pain on exertion. One study from Belgium documented normal coronary angiograms in 25% of patients regarded by cardiologists as having myocardial ischemia on the basis of symptoms. In one-half of these patients, a probable esophageal cause could be identified.

4. What are the noncardiac causes of chest pain? How common are they?

Gastroesophageal reflux disease (GERD) is the most frequent esophageal cause of chest pain. In most studies it accounts for up to 50% of all cases of unexplained chest pain. Esophageal dysmotility can be diagnosed in another 25–30% of cases. Of the remaining 20–30%, one-third to one-half can be explained by a musculoskeletal source, such as costochondritis (Tietze's syndrome) and chest-wall pain syndromes. Psychologic disorders, acting either independently or as cofactors, are responsible for many of these pain syndromes. Panic disorder, in particular, must be considered.

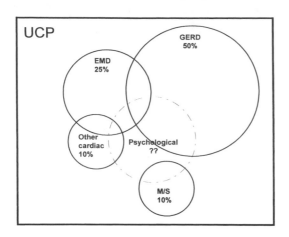

FIGURE 1. Venn diagram of the various causes of unexplained chest pain (UCP) and their frequency of diagnosis. EMD = esophageal motility disorders, M/S = musculoskeletal.

5. Because GERD is the most likely diagnosis, is a trial of acid suppression acceptable?

A therapeutic trial of acid suppression is relatively inexpensive, noninvasive, and easy to perform and may avoid further investigation. However, adequate doses of appropriate medication must be used. Currently, we recommend a proton pump inhibitor (omeprazole, 20 mg; lansoprazole, 30 mg; rabeprazole, 20 mg; or pantoprazole, 40 mg) given twice daily before meals for a period of 4–8 weeks. This test produces both false-negative and false-positive results. In patients who do not have relief of symptoms, the tendency is to conclude that GERD is not the cause of the pain. This conclusion cannot be made without ambulatory monitoring of intragastric and intraesophageal pH while the patient continues proton pump inhibitor (PPI) therapy. False positives may occur because of a placebo response, especially in patients with unexplained chest pain (UCP). One study of patients with presumed esophageal chest pain noted a placebo response in 36%.

6. What is the most useful esophageal investigation?

Because GERD is the most common cause of UCP, it should be the first diagnosis considered. Ambulatory pH monitoring of the esophagus is the gold standard for diagnosing GERD and is the test most likely to yield a positive result in patients with UCP. It remains the appropriate initial investigation even when a trial of acid suppression has appeared ineffective.

If ambulatory pH monitoring is abnormal (see below), esophagogastroduodenoscopy (EGD) may be indicated to exclude the more serious consequences of GERD, such as esophagitis and Barrett's esophagus. An EGD should be considered when the total esophageal acid exposure for a 24-hour period exceeds 10% or when supine acid exposure is above normal limits. If ambulatory pH monitoring is negative, investigation for esophageal motility abnormalities is indicated.

Unexplained chest pain
↓
Exclude cardiac disease (of epicardial vessels)
↓
Trial of acid suppression
↓
Esophageal pH monitoring*
↓
Baseline manometry and provocation testing
(Bernstein, edrophonium, balloon distention)
↓
Consider other causes

*EGD is indicated for severe reflux on pH monitoring (see text).

Other more unusual causes of UCP, such as biliary tract disease and gastric or duodenal ulceration, have been reported. Therefore, further gastrointestinal investigation, including abdominal ultrasound, occasionally is warranted, especially if the history points to such diagnoses.

7. How is esophageal pH monitoring performed?

Esophageal pH monitoring is performed after an overnight fast. The level of acidity is measured by an intraesophageal electrode of either glass or antimony. The electrode is traditionally placed 5 cm above the upper border of the lower esophageal sphincter (LES), as previously determined by manometry.

An antimony electrode is thinner (2-mm diameter) but requires the use of a silver/silver chloride reference electrode attached to the patient's chest. The electrode is passed transnasally, and pH is recorded for a minimum of 16 hours. Patients are encouraged to follow their usual routine. Data are recorded on a portable recording device with marker buttons that allow the patient to indicate timing of meals, bedrest, and symptoms. A diary card is also completed to corroborate the timings. All information is transferred to a computer on completion of the study and analyzed both visually and by specialized software.

8. What abnormalities may be found with pH monitoring?

Analysis of the tracing includes both duration of esophageal acid exposure (i.e., time when esophageal pH is < 4) and its association with symptoms. Objective GERD is diagnosed when the duration of acid exposure for the total time or for either the upright or recumbent periods exceeds the 95th percentile of normal values. In our laboratory, these limits are defined as exposures to a pH < 4 for 4.2% of the total time, 6.3% of the upright period, and 1.2% of the recumbent period.

Although an abnormal degree of acid reflux suggests the cause of the patient's symptoms, the case is not proved. Thus, the occurrence of symptoms during the monitoring period is extremely valuable. If symptoms strongly coincide with episodes of acid reflux, the diagnosis can be made even when absolute levels of acid exposure do not exceed the 95th percentile of normal. Similarly, failure of all symptoms to correlate with acid reflux is strong evidence against reflux-related chest pain.

The situation is more difficult when some but not all symptoms are associated with episodes of acid reflux. Various "symptom indices" have been introduced in an attempt to quantify the symptom-reflux association. The simplest index uses the total number of symptoms as its denominator and symptoms that coincide with acid reflux as its numerator:

$$\text{Symptom index} = \frac{\text{No. of symptoms occurring during acid reflux}}{\text{Total no. of symptoms during pH monitoring}}$$

A value of 50% or greater (e.g., two of four symptoms occur during episodes of acid reflux) is regarded as positive (Fig. 2). The approach to reflux-induced chest pain is no different from the normal management of GERD (see chapter 2).

9. If reflux has been excluded, which esophageal motility abnormalities may be found in patients with chest pain?

Abnormal esophageal motility may be found in 25–30% of patients with UCP. They may be categorized into the following types:

1. **Nutcracker esophagus** is the most common manometric abnormality. It has been so named because of the extremely high pressures generated during esophageal peristalsis. The diagnosis requires an average peristaltic amplitude > 180 mmHg during 10 wet swallows over both distal channels (Fig. 3).

2. **Nonspecific esophageal dysmotility** is a diagnostic category that includes patients with weak or poorly conducted waves; it is the second most common manometric finding. This terminology is being replaced with the more specific category, ineffective esophageal motility.

3. **Diffuse esophageal spasm** is diagnosed when at least 2 of 10 water swallows produce simultaneous contractions instead of normal peristalsis. It also may be associated with other abnormalities, such as multipeaked or prolonged duration contractions. Although frequently suggested as a diagnosis clinically, this manometric pattern is found in only approximately 3% of patients with UCP (Fig. 4).

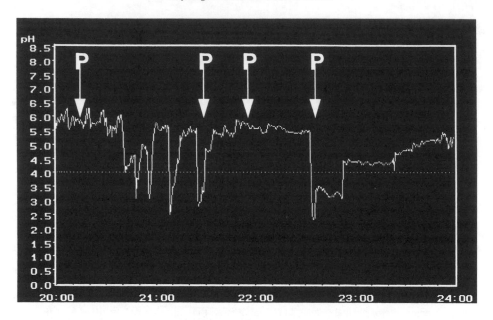

FIGURE 2. A 4-hour sample of esophageal pH monitoring. During this period 2 of 4 symptoms (P) were associated with episodes of acid reflux, yielding a symptom index of 2/4 (50%).

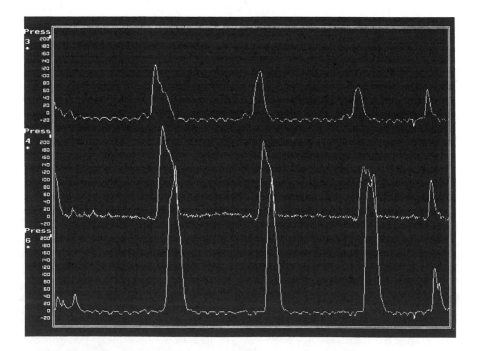

FIGURE 3. Nutcracker esophagus. The patient's average peristaltic amplitude was 250 mmHg. She experienced pain synchronous with most of her swallows.

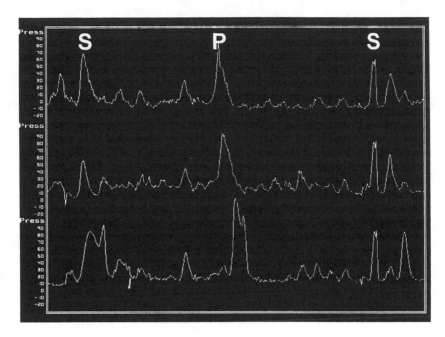

FIGURE 4.   Diffuse esophageal spasm. Both simultaneous (S) and peristaltic (P) contractions occur in response to water swallows.

4. **An abnormally high basal LES pressure** is also on occasions associated with UCP; the "hypertensive LES."

5. **Achalasia** occasionally presents with chest pain and is further discussed in chapter 5.

The relative frequencies of different diagnoses in patients with an esophageal dysmotility cause for chest pain are as follows: nutcracker esophagus 48%, nonspecific esophageal dysmotility 36%, diffuse esophageal spasm 10%, hypertensive lower esophageal sphincter 4%, achalasia 2%.

10. What is the relationship of esophageal motility abnormalities to chest pain?

The mechanism or mechanisms by which motility abnormalities may cause chest pain are poorly understood. Specific mechanoreceptors have been identified in the esophageal mucosal and muscle layers. Abnormal contractions per se may be sufficient to stimulate these receptors and cause pain. Alternatively, the mechanoreceptors may be stimulated by esophageal distention, secondary to failed LES relaxation or retention of the bolus within the esophageal body. Yet another possibility is alteration of the threshold for esophageal sensation, which "tunes in" the patient to changes in esophageal pressure. A final theory is that high tension in the esophageal wall inhibits esophageal blood flow, causing myoischemia. However, the esophagus has an extensive blood supply, and contractions are unlikely to be sufficiently prolonged to induce ischemia. It is possible that dysmotility per se is not the cause of pain. Rather, it may represent an epiphenomenon that, like pain, is induced by another, unrecognized process.

11. What is esophageal provocation testing?

As with GERD, the demonstration of an esophageal motility abnormality is not conclusive proof that dysmotility is the source of the pain. Occasionally, during routine manometry, a patient develops pain coincident with abnormal waveforms. More typically, the patient remains asymptomatic.

In an attempt to provoke symptoms, additional measures analogous to the exercise stress test used by cardiologists may be used to stimulate the esophagus. Options include acid infusion, pharmacologic stimulation, and intraesophageal balloon distention. For many years, it was believed that GERD caused chest pain by inducing dysmotility. Although this theory does not appear to be correct, acid perfusion (Bernstein test) is still used as a diagnostic test in UCP. Typically, 60–80 ml of 0.1 N hydrochloric acid are infused into the esophagus at a rate of 6–8 ml/min without the patient's knowledge, followed by a similar infusion of saline. The test is positive only if (1) it reproduces the patient's typical symptoms during acid infusion and (2) the symptoms disappear or do not recur during saline infusion. Chemoreceptors are present in the esophageal mucosa. Patients with a positive Bernstein test demonstrate acid sensitivity and should be treated for GERD-induced chest pain. Ambulatory pH monitoring with specific evaluation of symptom associations with pH decreases has largely made the Bernstein test obsolete!

Various pharmacologic agents have been used to stimulate the esophageal smooth muscle. The current choice is the cholinesterase inhibitor, edrophonium (80 mg/kg intravenously). After injection, even in normal subjects, esophageal smooth muscle responds with increased peristaltic amplitude and duration during swallows. The test is regarded as positive only if it reproduces the patient's typical pain.

Intraesophageal balloon distention (IEBD) involves the graduated inflation of a latex balloon within the esophagus until pain or a predetermined maximal volume is reached. This test has the advantage of being specific to the esophagus and may reproduce the pain by a mechanism not dissimilar to that of dysmotility. It is positive only if it induces a patient's typical pain at an inflation volume that does not induce pain in normal subjects. Balloon distention has been shown to be reproducible and has the highest yield of all available provocation tests. Of the three forms of provocation, acid and edrophonium typically induce symptoms in 20% of cases; balloon distention has double this yield (Fig. 5).

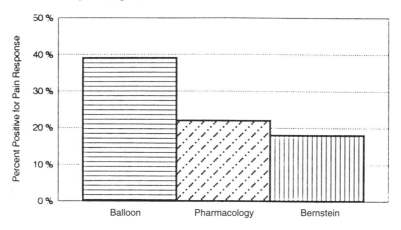

FIGURE 5.   Mean values of seven reported studies of the percentage of positive pain response achieved by provocation with balloon distention, edrophonium, and acid in patients with unexplained chest pain.

12. How does provocation testing compare with combined ambulatory monitoring of both motility and pH?

All esophageal provocation tests have one major drawback—they are not physiologic. In an attempt to record the motility tracing during spontaneous chest pain, longer periods of manometry have been performed. Technology has now made it possible to record esophageal motility over a 24-hour period in an ambulatory fashion.

Such a recording provides a large quantity of data. Currently, however, the best method of analysis is unclear. Whatever method is adopted, it must somehow compare the tracing during symptomatic and asymptomatic periods. Although ambulatory monitoring demonstrates the physiologic association between pain and dysmotility, it has not superseded the bank of esophageal provocation testing in most laboratories. Practitioners who have the most experience with ambulatory monitoring suggest that it should be reserved until after provocation testing has been performed and used only in patients with a positive result to delineate further the exact nature of the disorder.

13. What is visceral hypersensitivity? Define the "irritable esophagus."

Many patients with UCP have lower thresholds to pain in response to IEBD than normal individuals. This finding is believed to be due to visceral hypersensitivity or altered nociception. For some patients, the problem may not be due to abnormal contractions but rather to abnormal perception of normal events, including peristaltic muscle contractions, physiologic quantities of acid reflux, and luminal distention by air or food. Combined pH and manometric monitoring has identified patients who are sensitive to both acid and motility events. This condition is described as the irritable esophagus. Research analyzing cerebral evoked potential responses to esophageal stimulation suggests that the abnormality is due to central interpretation rather than abnormal firing of the peripheral nociceptors.

14. Does UCP have a psychological component?

All disease has a psychological element; illness is interpreted according to personality and previous experiences. This maxim appears to be particularly true for UCP. Psychological abnormalities have been documented in 34–59% of patients with UCP and are present in all of the causes described above. Psychiatric diagnoses are probably most prevalent in patients with esophageal motility abnormalities (84% in one study). Psychological factors, therefore, must be considered in the management of patients with UCP, including the likely possibility of panic attacks. Patients with high psychological scores are particularly susceptible to an initial placebo response to most medication, but in the long term treatment is ineffective; if such patients are identified, specific therapies can address the problem. Patients with high psychological scores have a worse prognosis and experience increased disability attributed to the illness.

15. What are the treatment options for nonreflux esophageal chest pain?

Medical treatment of diagnoses other than achalasia may target the motility abnormalities or the visceral hypersensitivity. Treatment for psychological factors also needs consideration. Finally, if medical therapy fails, more aggressive options may be considered for some patients.

Calcium antagonists, nitrates, and anticholinergic agents are the primary treatments aimed at motility dysfunction, i.e., the spastic component. If the pain is only occasional, short-acting nitrates or calcium antagonists may be taken sublingually as needed. More frequent episodes of chest pain are better managed by regular therapy with a long-acting preparation. Although such medications may have a dramatic effect on esophageal pressures, their symptomatic efficacy is often disappointing. Benzodiazepines both reduce skeletal muscular contractions and modify sensory pathways. They have had limited success in esophageal motility abnormalities. Of the other drugs used to modify sensory pathways, including anxiolytics and antidepressants, imipramine and other tricyclic antidepressants recently have been shown to be effective in low doses, suggesting that the effect is not due primarily to antidepressant activity.

Various psychological and behavioral therapies have been tried in small-scale studies. Relaxation therapy has met with some success and can easily be taught to patients who are willing to acknowledge the psychological element in their disease. Reassurance is available to all physicians. The ability to demonstrate a definite esophageal abnormality as an explanation for chest pain is of significant therapeutic benefit. The frequency of both pain and office visits for treatment of pain decreases after such reassurances.

Both empiric dilatation with a bougie and more specific targeting of a hypertensive LES with pneumatic dilatation have had limited success in some patients. Surgical myotomy may be of benefit to some patients with diffuse esophageal spasm or nutcracker esophagus. However, such interventions have documented complications and should be reserved for the rare severely disabled patient. The treatment of achalasia is discussed in chapter 5.

16. Can abnormal belching or aerophagia cause chest pain?

Esophageal distention, whether by reflux of gastric contents, impaction of a food bolus, or entrapment of air, can cause chest pain. In several well-documented cases gaseous esophageal distention was secondary to an abnormal belch reflex. Normally, the UES relaxes in response to distention with air. When this response fails, pain may occur.

17. What is the prognosis for patients with UCP?

Patients with UCP have a poor functional outcome. They consult a physician or visit the emergency department an average of twice per year, with an average of one hospitalization per year. If the patient does not have coronary artery disease, a positive esophageal diagnosis significantly reduces such behavior. Despite ongoing morbidity, the mortality rate of these patients (<1% per annum) is the same as for the general population.

BIBLIOGRAPHY

1. Cannon RO, Cattau EL, Yakshe PN, et al: Coronary flow reserve, esophageal motility, and chest pain in patients with angiographically normal coronary arteries. Am J Med 88:217–222, 1990.
2. Cannon RO III, Quyyumi AA, Mincemoyer R, et al: Imipramine in patients with chest pain despite normal coronary angiograms. N Engl J Med 330:1411–1417, 1994.
3. Castell DO: Chest pain of undetermined etiology. Proceedings of a symposium. Am J Med 92(Suppl 5A), 1992.
4. Castell DO, Castell JA (eds): Esophageal Motility Testing, 2nd ed. Norwalk, CT, Appleton & Lange, 1994.
5. Chambers J, Bass C: Chest pain and normal coronary anatomy: A review of natural history and possible etiologic factors. Progr Cardiovasc Dis 33:161–184, 1990.
6. Gignoux C, Bost R, Hostein J, et al: Role of upper esophageal reflux and belch reflex dysfunctions in noncardiac chest pain. Dig Dis Sci 38:1909–1914, 1993.
7. Katz PO, Dalton CB, Richter JE, et al: Esophageal testing of patients with noncardiac chest pain or dysphagia. Results of three years' experience with 1161 patients. Ann Intern Med 106:593–597, 1987.
8. Kemp HG, Kronmal RA, Vlietstra RE, Frye RL: Seven year survival of patients with normal or near normal coronary arteriograms: A CASS registry study. J Am Coll Cardiol 7:479–483, 1986.
9. Lam HG, Dekker W, Kan G, et al: Acute noncardiac chest pain in a coronary care unit. Evaluation by 24-hour pressure and pH recording of the esophagus. Gastroenterology 102:453–460, 1992.
10. Lantinga LJ, Sprafkin RP, McCroskery JH, et al: One-year psychosocial follow-up of patients with chest pain and angiographically normal coronary arteries. Am J Cardiol 62:209–213, 1985.
11. MacKenzie J, Belch J, Land D, et al: Oesophageal ischaemia in motility disorders associated with chest pain. Lancet ii:592–595, 1988.
12. Mayou R: Invited review: Atypical chest pain. J Psychosom Res 33:393–406, 1989.
13. Pope JH, Aufderheide TP, Ruthazer R, et al: Missed diagnoses of acute cardiac ischemia in the emergency department. N Engl J Med 342:1163–1170, 2000.
14. Prakash C, Clouse RE: Long-term outcome from tricyclic antidepressant treatment of functional chest pain. Dig Dis Sci 44:2372–2379, 1999.
15. Richter JE: The esophagus and noncardiac chest pain. In Castell DO (ed): The Esophagus. Boston, Little, Brown, 1992; pp. 715–746.
16. Richter JE, Barish CF, Castell DO: Abnormal sensory perception in patients with esophageal chest pain. Gastroenterology 91:845–852, 1986.
17. Semble E, Wise CM: Chest pain: A rheumatologist's perspective. South Med J 81:64–68, 1988.
18. Shapiro LM, Crake T, Poole-Wilson PA: Is altered cardiac sensation responsible for chest pain in patients with normal coronary arteries? Clinical observation during cardiac catheterization. BMJ 296:170–171, 1988.
19. Smout AJPM, DeVore MS, Dalton CB, Castell DO: Cerebral potentials evoked by oesophageal distension in patients with non-cardiac chest pain. Gut 33:298–302, 1992.
20. Spears DF, Koch KL: Esophageal disorders in patients with chest pain and mitral valve prolapse. Am J Gastroenterol 81:951–954, 1986.
21. Vantrappen G, Janssens J, Ghillebert G: The irritable oesophagus—a frequent cause of angina-like pain. Lancet I:1232–1234, 1987.
22. Ward BW, Wu WC, Richter JE, et al: Long-term follow-up of symptomatic status of patients with noncardiac chest pain: Is diagnosis of esophageal etiology helpful? Am J Gastroenterol 82:215–218, 1987.

5. ACHALASIA

Pankaj Jay Pasricha, M.D.

1. Define achalasia.

The term *achalasia* (Greek = lack of relaxation) describes the pathophysiologic hallmark of the disease: failure of the lower esophageal sphincter (LES) to relax. This term has replaced the previous designation *cardiospasm*, which implies an exaggerated state of contraction. The second cardinal feature is aperistalsis of the body of the esophagus. However, LES dysfunction is more important, because all available treatment is directed at removing the functional obstruction at this level so that gravity can compensate for the lack of pumping ability in the body of the esophagus.

2. How common is achalasia?

Achalasia is a relatively uncommon disorder with a prevalence estimated at about 10 in 10,000 and an incidence rate in the range of 0.5 new cases/year/100,000 population.

3. Define vigorous achalasia.

The term *vigorous* is applied to cases of achalasia in which prominent contractions can be noticed in the body of the esophagus, either on radiography or by manometry. These contractions are simultaneous and therefore fulfill the manometric definition of aperistalsis required for the diagnosis of achalasia. They should be distinguished from isobaric waves, which can be seen in patients with achalasia and represent bolus-induced passive fluctuations in pressure within the common cavity of the dilated esophagus.

4. What is the relationship between diffuse esophageal spasm (DES) and achalasia?

DES may be regarded as a "cousin" of achalasia. The primary manometric distinction between DES and vigorous achalasia is the presence of at least some normal peristalsis in the former. LES dysfunction is seen often, but to a lesser degree than in achalasia. Some evidence suggests that in a small subset (about 5% or less) of patients, DES may evolve into classic achalasia.

5. What is the major pathologic lesion in achalasia? How does it produce the disease?

Although other lesions have been described, including degeneration of the vagus nerve and changes in its dorsal motor nucleus, the myenteric plexus appears to be the major site of disease. The characteristic finding is loss of ganglion cells, which appears to be selective for inhibitory neurons (those producing nitric oxide and/or vasoactive intestinal peptide [VIP]) with relative sparing of the cholinergic (stimulatory) limb. Thus the normal balance of excitatory and inhibitory neural input to smooth muscle is upset. The loss of inhibition, coupled with a relative preservation of the excitatory stimulus, may be responsible for the LES abnormalities. An inflammatory infiltrate, characteristically mononuclear, is also commonly seen in the myenteric plexus. It is speculated that unchecked inflammation at this site leads to neuronal destruction and eventually to the clinical manifestations of achalasia.

6. What is the suspected cause of achalasia?

Earlier studies raised the possibility of a virus, particularly one belonging to the herpes family (because of the predilection of herpes viruses for squamous mucosa). However, subsequent investigations, using the polymerase chain reaction to detect different markers, found no evidence for any known viral cause. More recently, attention has focused on a possible autoimmune basis, with reports of circulating antineuronal antibodies. These suspicions are given further credence by the finding that achalasia may be particularly associated with certain class II HLA antigens such as Dqw1. Nevertheless, the cause of achalasia remains a mystery.

7. Is achalasia an acquired or congenital disease?

Most cases of achalasia are acquired. Achalasia is uncommon before the age of 25, with a clear-cut age-related increase thereafter. Most commonly the disease occurs in middle adult life (30–60 years of age) and affects both sexes and all races nearly equally. Rare cases of familial achalasia have been described. Occasionally, achalasia may be found as part of a congenital syndrome such as triple-A syndrome (achalasia, alacrimia, and resistance to adrenocorticotropic hormone), Alport's syndrome, or other rare conditions.

8. Describe the dysphagia associated with achalasia.

In general, the dysphagia due to motor disorders of the esophagus occurs with solids as well as liquids. However, many patients with achalasia complain predominantly, if not exclusively, of solid food dysphagia. The converse, dysphagia for liquids only, is almost never seen. Patients often localize the dysphagia to the region of the LES. Regurgitation of food, either active or induced by the recumbent position or bending, should raise the suspicion of achalasia, particularly if it occurs early in the course of symptoms. Patients often complain of waking up in the mornings with remnants of the previous night's supper in their mouth.

9. What other symptoms may be associated with achalasia?

Weight loss is common but not invariable. Pulmonary symptoms (e.g., pneumonia, lung abscesses from aspiration) are much less common than in the past because of earlier diagnosis and treatment. Two surprisingly common symptoms may lead to the wrong diagnosis: chest pain and heartburn (seen in up to 50% and 25% of patients, respectively). At least two different types of chest pain are experienced by patients with achalasia. The obstructive type is associated with swallowing a food bolus and resolves with passage of food into the stomach. The second type is unrelated to eating and is more often seen in patients with vigorous achalasia. However, it is not necessarily related to esophageal contractions and may reflect abnormalities in the sensory pathway, similar to those in patients with spastic motility disorders. Heartburn is indistinguishable from that in patients with gastroesophageal reflux disease (GERD), including response to antacids. In fact, some patients with achalasia have been mistakenly diagnosed with GERD for several years. Whether heartburn results from lactic acid production due to bacterial breakdown of retained food or true acid reflux is not clear.

10. Does achalasia involve any other parts of the gastrointestinal tract?

The stomach and pyloric sphincter.

11. What is the best way to diagnose achalasia?

Achalasia should be considered in all patients with a history of dysphagia for both solids and liquids. A definitive diagnosis requires two steps: (1) confirmation of the underlying pathophysiology (best done by manometry) and (2) exclusion of cancer at the GE junction, which can produce a similar picture (pseudoachalasia); this requires endoscopy with particular emphasis on the retroflexed view.

12. What are the characteristic radiologic features of achalasia?

An atonic and dilated body of the esophagus is often seen; however, occasional early cases present with a normal-sized esophagus and prominent (nonperistaltic) contractions. The "sigmoid esophagus" is an elongated, dilated organ seen in patients with longstanding disease. Epiphrenic diverticula may accompany this picture. In most cases of achalasia, the GE junction is smoothly narrowed, giving rise to the classic "bird's beak" and allowing only very small amounts of contrast to pass through to the stomach. Previous dilatation or surgery may alter this typical appearance.

13. What is required for the manometric diagnosis of achalasia?

(1) Lack of peristalsis in the body (the smooth muscle portion) of the esophagus, and (2) abnormal or absent LES relaxation in response to swallowing (with normal relaxation being more than 90%).

14. What is the most important potential pitfall in the manometric diagnosis of achalasia?

An occasional patient with otherwise typical features of achalasia may demonstrate complete or near-complete relaxation of the LES, but this appearance may be artifactual due to relative movement between the side-hole/point sensor in the manometry catheter and the LES. This problem can be avoided by the use of a Dent sleeve catheter, which incorporates a 6-cm long sensor device for measurement of LES pressures.

15. Describe the typical endoscopic features of achalasia.

Endoscopy may be reported as normal in a surprising number of patients in whom achalasia is not suspected before the procedure. In more obvious cases, esophageal dilation, varying amounts of food material or secretions, and either a lack of contractions or multiple simultaneous contractions are seen. The esophageal mucosa may demonstrate various changes, from mild erythema to frank erosions or even ulceration. Candidiasis and retained medications may cause some of these lesions; in other cases, stasis of retained material may give rise to an edematous and nodular mucosa.

A tight but relatively elastic feel as the endoscope passes (or "pops") through the GE junction is characteristic of achalasia but may be easily overlooked if the diagnosis is not specifically entertained. The inability to pass the scope despite moderate amounts of pressure is highly suggestive of an inflammatory or neoplastic stricture. Of interest, resistance also may be encountered at the pyloric outlet in patients with achalasia, giving rise to the "difficult pylorus" sign.

16. What is the difference between secondary achalasia and pseudoachalasia?

Although achalasia is most often idiopathic, it has been described in association with various diseases, such as cancer, Chagas' disease, amyloidosis and other infiltrative disorders, mixed connective tissue disorders, endocrine disorders, and intestinal pseudoobstruction. Such cases are called secondary achalasia. Pseudoachalasia refers to an achalasia-like syndrome that is produced by infiltrating cancer of the GE junction.

17. How can pseudoachalasia be diagnosed?

A high index of suspicion should be maintained in patients presenting with what looks like achalasia but with marked weight loss and short duration of symptoms. However, these and other features, such as the age of the patient, are not highly specific. Endoscopy remains the crucial diagnostic test because the clinical history, radiographic appearance of barium study, and even manometric analysis may not distinguish pseuodoachalasia from the idiopathic form. A careful examination of the GE region, including a retroflexed view from the stomach, is absolutely mandatory. Biopsies should be taken of any suspicious area or lesion. Even so, the sensitivity of this method in excluding underlying cancer is reported to be around 80% or less. Endoscopic ultrasound (EUS) may provide additional value, but this has yet to be convincingly demonstrated.

18. Is achalasia a premalignant condition?

Cancer in the setting of achalasia may result from longstanding stasis and secondary changes in the epithelium. When cancer develops, it is usually of the squamous variety and arises in the dilated middle part of the esophagus, rendering it relatively silent until a late stage. Although earlier studies suggested an incidence as high as 20%, a recent large, population-based study demonstrated only a 16-fold increase in cancer risk during years 2–24 after the diagnosis of achalasia.

19. Should patients with achalasia undergo periodic endoscopic surveillance?

A surveillance strategy would require 406 endoscopies to detect one cancer in males and 2220 endoscopies to detect one cancer in females. The American Society of Gastrointestinal Endoscopy recommends the following guidelines for surveillance: (1) For the rare untreated patient, periodic endoscopic surveillance after 15 years is justified; (2) if effective dilation or myotomy was performed early in the course of the disease, there may be no need for endoscopic surveillance; and (3) patients who are treated later in the course of the disease appear to be at increased risk for malignancy, and the role of endoscopic surveillance has not been determined.

20. What treatment options are available for achalasia? Describe their rationale.

All of the therapeutic options available for achalasia are palliative. Their goal is to decrease the resistance to bolus transit created by the dysfunctional LES. Traditional pharmacologic therapy does so by inducing smooth muscle relaxation. Botulinum toxin injections block the excitatory neural input to the LES by inhibiting the release of acetylcholine from nerve endings. The theoretical rationale for balloon dilation is to achieve a partial tear of the LES muscle, but this option is somewhat speculative because the few animal studies that evaluate this method have shown no histologic evidence of damage despite marked reductions in LES pressure. Surgical myotomy has the most straightforward rationale of all treatment options but comes at a price (see below).

21. Discuss the various pharmacologic options for palliation of achalasia.

Nitrates are probably more effective than calcium channel blockers but have significant adverse side effects that lead to discontinuation of the drug in up to one-third of patients. Isosorbide dinitrate (5–10 mg sublingually before meals) begins to act within 15 minutes, and effects may persist for as long as 90 minutes. Symptoms are improved in 75% to 85% of patients. Nifedipine, which may be more effective than diltiazem or verapamil, lowers LES pressure by 30–40%. The effects peak within 30–45 minutes and last more than 1 hour. Contrary to popular belief, nifedipine is poorly absorbed sublingually. Oral doses of 10–20 mg have been reported to improve symptoms in 50–70% of patients. In most cases, however, the use of pharmacotherapy is at best temporizing. Most patients require additional forms of treatment after 6 months or so because of side effects, progression of disease, or development of tolerance.

22. What does Viagra have to do with achalasia?

Sildenafil (Viagra) blocks phosphodiesterase type 5 (the enzyme responsible for degradation of cyclic guanosine monophosphate [cGMP]), which results in increased cGMP levels within smooth muscle and consequent relaxation. It is effective in short-term reduction of LES pressures in patients with achalasia, but its clinical role has yet to be reported.

23. What is the single most permanent treatment of achalasia?

The answer is clearly surgery, with short-term (5 years or less) efficacy around 90%. Long-term results are less positive, with only about two-thirds of patients reporting good-to-excellent outcomes. This is probably due in large part to the sequelae of the reflux disease that invariably accompanies successful myotomy (see below).

24. What is the major problem with surgery?

In the past, surgery was associated with considerable morbidity, whether done via a thoracic or abdominal approach. Recent advances in laparoscopic techniques have enabled a minimally invasive approach to myotomy, with significant reductions in perioperative pain, morbidity, and length of hospitalization. However, the major problem remains unchanged: long-term GERD, which can be particularly damaging in an atonic esophagus. Although most surgeons using an abdominal approach incorporate a "loose" antireflux procedure along with the myotomy, its effectiveness in preventing GERD remains controversial. Two long-term studies, one with and one without an antireflux procedure, were comparable in that only two-thirds of patients in either study were still doing well 10 years or beyond. Although such results are not yet available after laparoscopic surgery, there is no good basis to think that they will be different.

25. How can postoperative GERD be avoided?

The best advice to give patients after myotomy is that they need to be followed carefully for GERD. A very low threshold should be used for initiation of antireflux medications, preferably proton-pump inhibitors.

26. How is balloon dilation of the LES accomplished?

Using a whalebone as a dilator, Sir Thomas Willis first described dilation of the LES in a patient with achalasia. Forceful dilation of the LES is achieved by stretching it to at least 30 mm or more (for adults): this obviously requires more than simple bougies and is best accomplished using a specially designed balloon catheter. The most commonly available device (Rigiflex by Microvasive) is passed over a guidewire and requires fluoroscopic monitoring. A less common device is the Witzl dilator, which consists of a polyethylene balloon mounted on a forward viewing endoscope that is inflated under direct visualization (with the endoscope in the retroflexed position in the stomach). It has the advantage of not requiring fluoroscopy. Otherwise there is little science to dilation. A good stretch requires obliteration of the balloon waist: however, considerations of duration, pressure, number of inflations, presence of blood on the dilator, or induction of chest pain are of little, if any, importance in determining efficacy.

27. What can be done if symptoms do not respond to the first dilation?

A larger balloon (available in 5 mm increments up to 40 mm) may be used to attempt further stretching of the LES—the so-called progressive method. An alternative method, championed by vanTrappen and colleagues but seldom practiced in the U.S, is repeated dilation (regardless of the initial symptomatic response) until certain objective parameters of esophageal emptying (usually determined radiographically) are met. Regardless of the method used, if the patient fails 3 dilations, most authorities recommend surgery.

28. What are the results of pneumatic dilation?

The overall immediate response rate to pneumatic dilation is 75–80%; long-term results show that up to one-half of patients require one or more dilations over a 5-year period. Beyond this time, about 50–70% of patients continue to do well. Up to 20% or more, however, may eventually need surgery.

29. How does pneumatic dilation compare with surgery?

A classic randomized, controlled trial of surgery and dilation clearly favored surgery in terms of long-term results. However, it is not clear whether this is the most cost-effective approach, considering the long-term and cumulative costs of surgery (estimated at nearly $2\frac{1}{2}$ times more than the cost of pneumatic dilation), even in view of the perforation rate and need for retreatment associated with pneumatic dilation.

30. What is the major disadvantage of forceful dilation? How can it be prevented?

The major risk of dilation is perforation (estimated rate = 1–10% or even higher). Because of the empirical way in which dilation is performed, this risk appears to be inherent; there are few ways to prevent this complication. It is important to exclude stricture (malignant or benign), to ensure a near-empty esophagus, and to perform all manipulations of the balloon under fluoroscopic control. Relative contraindications cited in the literature include a tortuous sigmoid shape, previous myotomy, epiphrenic diverticula, and large hiatal hernias, but most experts do not view these as absolute. Larger balloons are expected to increase the risk for perforation, but comparative data are not available. GERD is believed to be uncommon after forceful dilation, with an incidence of around 2%.

31. How is perforation treated in patients with achalasia?

Treatment is controversial. Perforations after achalasia dilatation tend to be small and well contained. Thus many authorities advocate conservative treatment (i.e., antibiotics and parenteral alimentation); good results are reported in the literature. However, it is difficult to predict the outcome with this form of treatment in individual cases. Surgery is definitely indicated in patients with large perforations and free flow of contrast into the mediastinum or with evidence of sepsis. When surgery is performed early, the clinical outcome and long-term course appear similar to elective myotomy.

32. Which patients are particularly likely to respond to dilation?

In general, older patients (> 40–50 years) do significantly better after dilation than younger patients.

33. What objective parameters should be followed after dilation?

The most consistent and important parameter determining long-term response after pneumatic dilation is post-treatment LES pressure. The best results are obtained when LES pressure is < 10 mmHg. It is theoretically possible that a treatment regimen based on "optimization" of esophageal emptying rather than symptomatic response alone may lead to better long-term results. Nevertheless, this theory has yet to be convincingly demonstrated by an appropriately designed clinical trial.

34. How is botulinum toxin (BoTox) injection administered?

BoTox is available through most hospital pharmacies in vials containing 100 units of the lyophilized powder. For use in achalasia, it can be diluted in 5 ml of normal saline to yield a solution containing 20 U/ml. Flexible upper endoscopy is performed using routine sedation, and the toxin is injected via a 5-mm sclerotherapy needle into the LES region, piercing the mucosa about 1 cm above the Z-line and slanting the needle approximately 45°. The injections are administered in 4 aliquots distributed circumferentially in 4 different quadrants. The original dose of 80 U was chosen empirically; there is no good reason why the contents of an entire vial (100 U) cannot be administered. Precise location of the injection site may not be necessary because diffusion may take care of any minor variations. Others advocate the use of EUS to help guide injections; it is not clear whether EUS results in better outcomes than the traditional method.

35. What are the results with BoTox treatment?

Only about two-thirds of patients show sustained improvement (beyond the first month or so). Older patients do better, and patients with vigorous achalasia may have a more favorable response than those with the classic form. Patients who respond to an initial injection remain in remission for several months (range = 4 months to > 1 year). When symptoms return, patients usually respond to repeat injections of botulinum toxin. Larger doses of BoTox at the time of initial injection have not been proved to improve the response rate.

36. Discuss the major drawbacks of botulinum toxin treatment.

Overall BoTox is a relatively safe and simple treatment with few if any major complications. The major drawback is cost, coupled with the need for multiple injections. Some surgical reports suggest that repeat injections of BoTox may cause fibrosis and obliteration of the submucosal plane at the GE junction, making myotomy somewhat more difficult technically. However, outcomes after surgery appear not to be affected, whether or not BoTox had been used.

37. What is the overall best treatment for achalasia?

Because no treatment is curative, there is no real answer. It is best for the physician to become familiar with the advantages and disadvantages of each option and present them to the patient. The final choice depends on several factors, including patient preference and risk tolerance as well as local availability of technical expertise. Regardless of the treatment, patients need to be followed carefully and therapeutic strategies revisited on a periodic basis.

BIBLIOGRAPHY

1. Annesse V, Basciani M, Perri F, et al: Controlled trial of botulinum toxin injection versus placebo and pneumatic dilation in achalasia. Gastroenterology 111:1418–1424, 1996.
2. Csendes A, Baghetto I, Henriquez A, Cortes C: Late results of a prospective randomized study comparing forceful dilation and esophagomyotomy in patients with achalasia of the esophagus. Gut 30:299, 1989.
3. Eckardt VF, Aignherr C, Bernhard G: Predictors of outcome in patients with achalasia treated with pneumostatic dilatation. Gastroenterology 103:1732–1738, 1992.
4. Ellis FH Jr, Watkins E Jr, Gibb SP, Heatley GJ: Ten to 20-year clinical results after short esophagomyotomy without an antireflux procedure (modified Heller operation) for esophageal achalasia. Eur J Cardiothorac Surg 6:86–90, 1992.
5. Goldblum JR, Whyte RI, Orringer MB, Appelman HD: Achalasia: A morphologic study of 42 resected specimens. Am J Surg Pathol 18:327–337, 1994.
6. Malthaner RA, Todd TR, Miller L, Pearson FG: Long-term results in surgically managed esophageal achalasia. Ann Thorac Surg 58:1343–1347, 1994.
7. Mearin F, Mourelle M, Guarner F, et al: Patients with achalasia lack nitric oxide synthase in the gastro-oesophageal junction. Eur J Clin Invest 23:724–728, 1993.

8. Orr WC, Allen ML, Mellow M, et al: Differential effects of calcium channel blocking and anticholinergic agents on esophageal function. Gastroenterology 86:A1202, 1984.
9. Parkman HP, Reynolds JC, Ouyang A, et al: Pneumatic dilation or esophagomyotomy treatment for idiopathic achalasia: Clinical outcomes and cost analysis. Dig Dis Sci 38:75–85, 1993.
10. Pasricha PJ, Rai R, Ravich WJ, et al: Botulinum toxin for achalasia: Long-term follow-up and predictors of outcome. Gastroenterology 110:1410–1415, 1996.
11. Pasricha PJ, Ravich WJ, Hendrix TR, et al: Treatment of achalasia with intrasphincteric injection of botulinum toxin. A pilot trial. Ann Intern Med 121:590–591, 1994.
12. Pasricha PJ, Ravich WJ, Hendrix TR, et al: Intrasphincteric botulinum toxin for the treatment of achalasia. N Engl J Med 332:774–778, 1995.
13. Patti MG, Pellegrini CA: Minimally invasive approaches to achalasia. Semin Gastrointest Dis 5:108–112, 1994.
14. Reynolds JC, Parkman HP: Achalasia. Gastroenterol Clin North Am 18:223–255, 1989.
15. Rosati R, Fumagalli U, Bonavina L, et al: Laparoscopic approach to esophageal achalasia. Am J Surg 169:424–427, 1995.
16. Spiess AE, Kahrilas PJ: Treating acahalasia. From whalebone to laparoscope. JAMA 280:638–642, 1998.
17. Traube M, Dubovik S, Lange RC, McCallum RW: The role of nifedipine in achalasia: Results of a randomized double-blind placebo-controlled study. Am J Gastroenterol 84:1259, 1989.
18. Triadafilopoulos G, Aaronson M, Sackel S, Burakoff R: Medical treatment of esophageal achalasia. Double-blind crossover study with oral nifedipine, verapamil, and placebo. Dig Dis Sci 36:260, 1991.
19. van Harten J, Burggraaf K, Danhof M, et al: Negligible sublingual absorption of nifedipine. Lancet 2:1363–1365, 1987.
21. Vantrappen G, Jannsens J: To dilate or operate? That is the question. Gut 24:1013–1019, 1983.
20. Vantrappen G, Hellemans J: Treatment of achalasia and related motor disorders. Gastroenterology 79:144–154, 1980.

6. ESOPHAGEAL CANCER

Nimish Vakil, M.D.

1. What is the incidence of esophageal cancer in the United States and is it changing?

Esophageal cancer is relatively infrequent in the United States. The annual incidence is < 10/100,000 patients, whereas in some areas of China the annual incidence is > 100/100,000. Over the past 3 decades, the incidence of distal esophageal adenocarcinoma has increased sharply in North America, whereas the incidence of squamous cell carcinoma of the esophagus has fallen. The rise in esophageal adenocarcinoma has been most marked in white men. Recent studies suggest that the incidence of esophageal adenocarcinoma is rising in African American and Hispanic males. For unknown reasons, the disease remains rare in women. Although the absolute numbers of cases of esophageal cancer remains low, there has been a remarkable rise in the incidence of distal esophageal cancer over the past 3 decades in most developed countries, making it one of the most rapidly growing cancers in the United States. The decline in distal gastric cancers over the same period has been correlated with a decline in the prevalence of *Helicobacter pylori* infection in the U.S.

2. What are the risk factors for the development of esophageal cancer?

Smoking and alcohol use have been associated with the development of squamous cell carcinoma of the esophagus, but they do not appear to be major risk factors for the development of esophageal adenocarcinoma. Squamous cell carcinoma is much more frequent in African Americans than in whites, whereas adenocarcinoma is much more frequent in whites. Frequent, longstanding heartburn is an important risk factor for the development of esophageal adenocarcinoma. In some studies, obesity has been shown to be an independent risk factor, and obese patients with reflux disease are at particularly high risk for the development of esophageal cancer. Recent studies have drawn an epidemiologic link between the widespread use of drugs that affect the lower esophageal sphincter and the increasing risk of esophageal cancer. A true cause and effect relationship has not been established.

3. What are the current recommendations for screening and surveillance of esophageal cancer in patients at risk?

Screening. Currently there is no acceptable screening method for esophageal cancer in the U.S. Some economic models have suggested that a one-time screening endoscopy to identify Barrett's esophagus may be cost-effective in patients with longstanding reflux esophagitis, but the assumptions for the risk of developing cancer in Barrett's esophagus may be too high. There is no direct clinical evidence to support this practice at present.

Surveillance. Surveillance is recommended in patients with Barrett's esophagus. The American College of Gastroenterology guidelines recommend that patients undergo surveillance endoscopy and biopsy every 2–3 years. The frequency with which endosocopy should be performed has not been determined in clinical trials but is based on cost models and expert opinion.

4. How is esophageal cancer diagnosed?

Endoscopy and biopsy are necessary for the diagnosis of esophageal cancer. Staging has become important in the management of patients with esophageal cancer. Staging helps to determine the choice of treatment and is an important determinant of prognosis. Computed tomography (CT) of the chest and abdomen is the recommended initial test for staging.

5. Discuss the role of endoscopic ultrasound in the diagnosis and staging of esophageal cancer.

In patients who appear to have limited local disease on computed tomography and no evidence of distant metastases, endoscopic ultrasound may be helpful in regional staging. Esophageal cancer is seen as a hypoechoic interruption of the layers of the esophagus. Endoscopic ultrasound is better than CT at staging the depth of insertion. This factor becomes important in deciding between different methods of curative therapy. For example patients with cancer localized to the mucosa can be considered for mucosal resection, but deeper levels of invasion make this therapy inappropriate. Endoscopic ultrasound has better results in regional staging than the newest spiral CT scanners. Magnetic resonance imaging (MRI) has not been particularly helpful in imaging the depth of local invasion. Endoscopic ultrasound also may be helpful in the evaluation of mediastinal lymph nodes. Large nodes (>10 mm) that are uniformly hypoechoic are suspicious. Fine-needle aspiration under ultrasound guidance may help to establish lymph node involvement.

6. How is esophageal cancer staged? Why is staging important?

Esophageal cancer staging is performed according to the tumor-node-metastasis (TNM) classification. Accurate staging is important to establish prognosis and treatment approach. Treatment, as in all malignant disorders, is based on the risk of the therapy balanced against the likelihood of a good outcome. Patient preference and local expertise also may determine the choice of treatment. Rational choices can be based on the stage of esophageal cancer, as discussed below.

Staging of Esophageal Cancer

Primary tumor

Tx	Primary tumor cannot be assessed
T0	No evidence of primary tumor
Tis	Carcinoma in situ
T1	Tumor invades lamina propria or submucosa
T2	Tumor invades muscularis propria
T3	Tumor invades adventitia
T4	Tumor invades adjacent structures

Regional lymph nodes

For the cervical esophagus, cervical and supraclavicular lymph nodes are considered regional; for the thoracic esophagus, mediastinal and perigastric lymph nodes (excluding celiac nodes) are considered regional.

Nx	Regional nodes cannot be assessed
N0	No regional lymph node metastases
N1	Regional lymph node metastases

Distant metastases

MX	Cannot be assessed
M0	No distant metastases
M1	Distant metastases

Stages

Stage 0	Tis, N0, M0
Stage 1	T1, N0, M0
Stage IIA	T2, N0, M0; T3, N0, M0
Stage IIB	T1, N1, M0; T2, N1, M0
Stage III	T3, N1, M0; T4, any N, M0
Stage IV	Any T, any N, M1

7. What curative therapies are available for esophageal cancer?

Treatment guidelines from the American College of Gastroenterology recommend stage directed therapy. Treatment options are summarized by stage below:

Stage 0, I, IIA (early-stage disease). Patients with early-stage disease generally are treated with curative surgery alone. Endoscopic mucosectomy using a suction cap fitted with a snare may be curative in stages 0 and I. Experience with this modality is increasing in the U.S., but controlled data are lacking. Other ablative therapies also have been used, including electrocautery, argon plasma coagulation, and photodynamic therapy. Chemotherapy and radiation are not used as adjuvants for early-stage disease. Surgical therapy consists of resection of the tumor with anastomosis of the stomach with the cervical esophagus (gastric pull-up) or interposition of the colon to reestablish gastrointestinal continuity. Results are better in hospitals that perform this surgery frequently and poorer in small hospitals that perform the surgery infrequently.

Stage IIB and III (regionally advanced disease). The results of single-modality (surgery, chemotherapy, or radiation) therapy are limited. Less than 10% of patients are cured by surgery alone. The results of radiation and chemotherapy also are limited. Recent studies have shown that a multimodality approach consisting of chemotherapy and radiation with surgery (triple therapy) offers the best likelihood of cure. Triple therapy is aggressive and expensive and has a high side-effect rate. Patients who are in poor general condition may elect to have palliative therapy after balancing the low probability of cure against the morbidity of treatment.

Stage IV (distant metastases). Distant metastases make esophageal cancer incurable; therapy is palliative. Radiation and chemotherapy are frequently used and may offer small increases in survival rates with the trade-off of systemic side effects. In patients with dysphagia, a number of palliative measures are possible but do not prolong survival.

8. What are the endoscopic methods for the palliation of esophageal cancer?

A number of endoscopic methods are available for the palliation of esophageal cancer. Endoscopic dilation causes temporary relief of dysphagia and is not effective as long-term therapy. Expandable metal stents provide rapid palliation of dysphagia, but late complications can be a problem. Membrane-covered metal stents were developed to prevent the problems associated with tumor ingrowth. A number of tumor ablative therapies are also available. Injection of absolute alcohol into the tumor has been reported but is inexpensive. There is little control of the degree of necrosis, and tracking of the sclerosant beyond the esophagus can cause perforation and chemical mediastinitis. Argon plasma therapy and Nd YAG laser can restore luminal patency by tumor ablation. Argon plasma coagulation is considerably less expensive than laser therapy and as effective. The principal disadvantage of these modalities is that they may require multiple treatments (and therefore multiple visits to the hospital), which is undesirable in patients who have a short time to live. Photodynamic therapy is a recent development in the palliation of esophageal cancer. A light-sensitive drug (Photofrin) is injected intravenously and selectively accumulates in the tumor tissue. Specially developed catheters are used to deliver light to the tumor and cause necrosis of the tumor. The procedure is safe and well tolerated. Its principal disadvantages are cost and development of cutaneous photosensitivity.

9. What does the future hold for patients at risk for development of esophageal cancer?

The future of esophageal cancer lies in prevention. Symptoms develop late in the disease, and most patients are incurable at presentation. Because of the low absolute numbers of patients developing the disease, widespread screening programs in the general population are unlikely to be cost-effective. One-time endoscopic screening for Barrett's esophagus has been proposed as a method for identifying patients at risk, but timing, cost-effectiveness, and efficacy remain unproven.

BIBLIOGRAPHY

1. Bosset JF, Gignoux M, Triboulet J et al: Chemoradiotherapy followed by surgery compared with surgery alone in squamous cell cancer of the esophagus. N Engl J Med 337:161–167, 1997.
2. Herskovic A, Martz K, Al-Saraf M et al: Combined chemotherapy and radiotherapy compared with radiotherapy alone in patients with cancer of the esophagus. N Engl J Med 326:1593–1598, 1992.
3. Knyrim K, Bethge N, Wagner J, Keymling M, Vakil N: A prospective controlled randomized trial of expandable metal stents in malignant esophageal obstruction. N Engl J Med 329:1302–1307, 1993.
4. Lightdale C: Practice guidelines: Esophageal cancer. Am J Gastroenterol 94:20–29, 1999.
5. Pera M, Cameron A, Trastek V et al: Increasing incidence of adenocarcinoma of the esophagus and esophago-gastric junction. Gastroenterology 104:510–513, 1993
6. Provenzale D, Kemp JA, Arora S, et al: A guide for surveillance of patients with Barrett's esophagus. Am J Gastroenterol 89:670–680, 1994.
7. Sibille A, Lambert R, Souquet JC, et al: Long-term survival after photodynamic therapy for esophageal cancer. Gastroenterology 108:337–344, 1995.

7. PILL-INDUCED AND CORROSIVE INJURY OF THE ESOPHAGUS

Matthew Bachinski, M.D., F.A.C.P., and James Walter Kikendall, M.D., F.A.C.P

1. Who is affected by pill-induced esophageal injury?

Anyone of any age who ingests caustic pills is susceptible to pill-induced injury. Reported cases range from 5–89 years old. Women outnumber men by a ratio of 1.5:1. It is not uncommon for pills to stick in a normal esophagus during transit. One study showed that 36 of 49 normal subjects who assumed a supine position after swallowing a round, nonsticky barium tablet with 15 ml of water retained the tablet in the esophagus for 5–45 minutes. A more sticky gelatin tablet remained in the esophagus for more than 10 minutes in over one-half of normal subjects who ingested the pill in a supine position. Esophageal dysmotility or structural abnormalities, such as rings or strictures, are clearly not required for pill-induced injury.

2. What factors contribute to esophageal retention of pills?

Esophageal clearance is determined by several factors, some of which can be modified to decrease the risk of pill-induced injury. Upright posture improves esophageal clearance of pills. The volume of water ingested with pills also affects clearance, although no study has identified the volume required to ensure passage through the esophagus. One study showed that 11 of 18 patients retained a barium pill swallowed with 15 ml of water compared with 3 of 18 who swallowed the pill with 120 ml of water. Other partially modifiable factors include structural abnormalities such as rings or strictures, which can be dilated as needed. Abnormal esophageal · motility sometimes is improved with pharmacologic agents, but motility usually is normal in patients with pill-induced injury. Taking the pill with inadequate fluid and lying down immediately afterward are often the only identifiable risk factors.

3. What are the risk factors for pill-induced injury?

Anyone who takes a caustic pill is at risk, but some patients are at particular risk for severe pill-induced esophageal injury, including those with structural abnormalities of the esophagus, both pathologic (stricture, tumor, ring) and physiologic (hiatal hernia, narrowing of the esophagus secondary to compression from the left atrium, aortic arch, left mainstem bronchus). Cardiac disease is a risk factor because of esophageal compression by a dilated left atrium and frequent use of inherently caustic medications (e.g., aspirin, potassium chloride, quinidine). Patients who have undergone thoracotomy are at increased risk because they are bedridden and may develop adhesions and fibrosis that trap the esophagus between the aorta and vertebral column, making it more susceptible to compression by an enlarged left atrium and thus decreasing esophageal clearance. Supine positioning during pill ingestion impairs esophageal clearance and places patients at risk. The stickiness of the pill surface, the inherent caustic nature of certain drugs, and the volume of liquid consumed with pills affect risk. Elderly patients and patients with underlying gastroesophageal reflux disease (GERD) are at increased risk. GERD may cause a more acid environment; because many drugs, including nonsteroidal anti-inflammatory drugs (NSAIDs), are weak acids, their absorption into tissues is increased in an acidic environment.

4. Describe the typical presentation of patients with pill-induced injury.

The typical patient has no prior history of esophageal disease and presents with the sudden onset of retrosternal pain, which may have awakened the patient from sleep (particularly if pills were ingested with little liquid just before or while lying down) and may be exacerbated by swallowing. The pain may be mild or so severe that swallowing is impossible. The pain typically increases over the first 3–4 days before gradually subsiding. Painless dysphagia is uncommon

(20%) and may suggest an alternative diagnosis. Less common symptoms and signs include dehydration, weight loss, fever, and hematemesis. Patients with preexisting esophageal problems such as GERD frequently present with worsening symptoms of heartburn, regurgitation, and dysphagia.

5. How is the diagnosis of pill-induced esophageal injury made?

The diagnosis of pill-induced esophageal injury may be suspected on the basis of history alone when typical symptoms suddenly appear soon after the ingestion of a pill known to cause esophageal injury. In a typical and uncomplicated case, an invasive diagnostic test may not be required, and the diagnosis can be made on the basis of history and physical exam. A diagnostic study is indicated when symptoms are severe, persist longer than 3–4 days, have atypical features, or suggest a complication (stricture, hemorrhage) or when the history suggests an alternative diagnosis (e.g., foreign body obstruction, infectious esophagitis in an immunocompromised host). Upper endoscopy is the most sensitive test; results are abnormal in almost all cases of pill-induced esophageal injury. In addition, it allows the most accurate assessment of alternate diagnoses such as severe GERD, infectious esophagitis, or malignancy.

6. What does the typical pill-induced lesion look like at time of endoscopy?

The typical lesion of pill-induced esophageal injury is one or more discrete ulcers with normal surrounding mucosa. Ulcers range in size from pinpoint to circumferential lesions that may be several centimeters long. Ulcers may have local surrounding inflammation. Pill fragments have been seen in ulcer craters.

7. What are the potential complications of pill-induced esophageal ulcers?

Typical ulcers involve only the mucosa, but deeper lesions may occur. Torrential hemorrhage has resulted from erosions into vascular structures, including the left atrium. Cases with penetration to the mediastinum have been reported. Deep circumferential ulceration may result in formation of a circumferential fibrotic stricture, but this occurs in less than 10% of reported cases. Probably the true incidence of stricture formation is much less, because severe or atypical cases are more likely to be reported.

8. What pills are frequently implicated or particularly injurious?

Antibiotic pills are frequent offenders, accounting for more than one-half of all reported cases of pill-induced esophageal injury because of the large number of prescriptions written and the caustic nature of the pills themselves. Doxycycline and tetracycline accounted for 293 of 454 reported cases of pill-induced esophageal injury in one recent review. Although frequent offenders, antibiotics rarely cause complicated injury to the esophagus. Patients with antibiotic-associated injury almost always present with acute, severe pain and local, circumscribed tissue injury due to mucosal ulceration. The ulceration is believed to be secondary to a single trapped pill.

Cardiac and vascular medications, including antihypertensives and antiarrhythmics, compose a large group of caustic drugs. Quinidine alone has been reported in 13 cases of pill-induced injury; 7 of the 13 patients later developed strictures, making quinidine a particularly injurious substance. An unusual feature of quinidine-induced injury is its tendency to form profuse, irregular exudate that is sufficiently thick and adherent, appearing as a filling defect suggestive of carcinoma on barium swallow. On endoscopy the exudate can be washed away and has not been shown to be predictive of late fibrotic stricture formation.

Anti-inflammatory medications are relatively uncommon agents in pill-induced esophageal injury. A recent review reported only 71 cases of injury attributable to this class of drugs. In part because they are so widely prescribed, 22 different antiinflammatory agents have been reported to cause injury, but approximately 45% of these reports are secondary to aspirin, doleron, and indomethacin. No hallmark lesion is associated with NSAIDs.

9. Do any new drugs on the market deserve special notice?

Alendronate sodium (Fosamax, Merck & Co., West Point, PA) is an oral aminobiphosphonate that inhibits osteoclast activity in the bones. It is used to treat and prevent osteoporosis in postmenopausal women. It can cause significant esophageal injury. The package insert for Fosamax advises how to administer the medication to maximize esophageal clearance. These factors include consuming 6–8 oz of water with the pill and staying upright for 30 minutes after taking the pill. The manufacturer advises that abnormalities of the esophagus which delay esophageal emptying and the inability to stand or sit upright for 30 minutes after ingestion are contraindications for prescription. Endoscopy reveals a classic esophageal lesion with Fosamax. Like quinidine, it causes a circumscribed ulceration covered by a thick, white, loosely adherent exudate. Histology confirms a leukofibrinous exudate similar to pseudomembranous colitis.

10. What other mechanisms have been proposed to explain pill-induced injury?
Animal studies have demonstrated that certain pills placed in direct contact with esophageal tissue can cause ulceration. This finding has been verified in humans by esophagogastroduodenoscopy (EGD), which revealed an esophageal ulcer containing a retained pill and circumscribed to the location of the pill. It is believed that pills must be inherently caustic to cause injury. Local acid burn is proposed for pills (e.g., doxycycline, tetracycline, ascorbic acid, ferrous sulfate) that produce an acidic solution with a pH < 3 when dissolved in 10 ml of water. Phenytoin dissolved in 10 ml of saliva raises the pH to 10.4, suggesting that it may cause an alkaline burn. Other proposed mechanisms of injury include induction of gastroesophageal reflux (theophylline and anticholinergics) and production of localized hyperosmolarity capable of tissue desiccation and vascular injury (potassium chloride). Finally, some medications appear to be absorbed locally into the esophageal mucosa, causing toxic intramucosal concentrations (doxycycline, nonsteroidal anti-inflammatory drugs [NSAIDs], alprenolol).

11. What are the postulated mechanisms of NSAID-induced injury?
Thirty million people use NSAIDs each day, and approximately 16% of patients report gastrointestinal side effects. Gastric injury is most common, although cases of esophageal injury are well-documented. In one study, all patients with NSAID-induced esophageal injury who were tested with 24-hour pH monitoring had gastroesophageal reflux disease (GERD). In the presence of GERD associated with a pH < 4, NSAIDs may enter the mucosa and cause direct toxicity. NSAIDs may cause injury by inhibiting synthesis of mucosal prostaglandins. Prostaglandins are known to have a cytoprotective role in gastric mucosa, but it is unclear whether the same effect applies to esophageal mucosa. The role of the mucus and bicarbonate layer in protecting the esophagus is also unclear, but the deleterious effect of NSAIDs on the mucosal barrier of the stomach secondary to prostaglandin inhibition may occur also in the esophagus. Finally, NSAIDs may negatively affect lower esophageal sphincter pressure and function, thereby increasing GERD and potentiating their own absorption.

12. Where are the areas of physiologic narrowing of the esophagus?
The normal esophagus has areas, generally minor, of external compression and narrowing at the sphincters. Pills may be more likely to hang up and cause injury in these areas. Degenerative arthritis of the cervical spine may cause external compression of the esophagus, which often worsens with age. The aortic arch and the left mainstem bronchus may cause compression of the esophagus. The left atrium varies in size, depending on underlying heart disease, and may cause significant compression of the esophagus. Such compression is particularly troublesome because the medications often used to treat diseases associated with left atrial enlargement, such as potassium chloride in conjunction with diuretics and quinidine for atrial fibrillation, are particularly caustic agents.

13. Does alcohol consumption play a role in pill-induced esophageal injury?
Alcohol appears to act synergistically with caustic agents to induce esophageal injury. In one study, healthy volunteers took 8 aspirins/day for 2 weeks. EGD showed no esophageal mucosal damage. After the same volunteers consumed a single dose of aspirin combined with alcohol, 33% had erythema and/or esophageal hemorrhage. Alcohol may affect the esophagus by interfering with esophageal clearance and thus prolonging aspirin contact with the mucosa. Alcohol is believed to decrease primary and secondary contractions of the esophagus.

14. What are the options for treating pill-induced esophageal injury?

Most cases of pill-induced injury heal without active intervention in 3 days to several weeks. Therapy starts with avoidance of the initial drug responsible for the injury and all other caustic drugs, when possible. When avoidance is not possible, every effort must be made to decrease the potential for reinjury by using elixir or other liquid preparations, administering medications in the upright position with at least 4 ounces of liquid, and maintaining an upright posture for at least 10 minutes after ingestion.

Medications that buffer acid, decrease production of acid, or create a barrier coat for the esophagus are frequently prescribed (antacids, H_2 blockers, sucralfate) but are of questionable value unless GERD contributes to symptoms. The use of topical anesthetics in various combinations (Bemylid-Benadryl, Mylanta, and lidocaine in equal parts) may decrease symptoms, but their use is limited by potential systemic toxicity.

Patients with such severe symptoms that they cannot eat or drink require hydration. If symptoms persist, they may require parenteral nutrition and analgesia. Other supportive measures may also be required for treatment of complications (e.g., blood products for hemorrhage and antibiotics for bacterial superinfection).

Acute inflammatory stenosis may resolve spontaneously, but chronic stricture formation may require repeated esophageal dilation. Strictures that prove to be recalcitrant to repeated dilation may require surgical correction, but this complication is rare.

15. Discuss the epidemiology of caustic ingestion in the United States.

Chemical ingestion remains an important problem despite improvements in packaging (e.g., child-proof containers), product labeling, and warnings. Approximately 26,000 caustic ingestions occur per year. Adolescents and adults who willfully ingest caustic agents as a suicidal gesture in general consume a larger volume and therefore have more serious injury than children, who ingest the agent accidentally and often expectorate most of it before swallowing. Children often have minimal esophageal damage, but their oral, pharyngeal, and laryngeal injury may be more severe. Approximately 80% of caustic ingestions occur accidentally in children less than 5 years of age, who most often consume household cleaners.

16. What are the common caustic agents? Where are they found?

Caustic agents are present in many common household products. The severity of the damage depends largely on the corrosive properties and concentration of the ingested agents. The caustic agents most often responsible for serious injury are strong alkaline cleaning products, such as drain cleaners and lye soaps. Severe alkaline burns also result from the ingestion of disc batteries that contain concentrated sodium or potassium hydroxide. Concentrated acid compounds also cause severe injury but are not common household items; thus they are encountered less often. The severity of esophageal and gastric injury secondary to caustic ingestion depends not only on the concentration and corrosive properties of the agent but also on the quantity consumed.

Caustic Agents Found in Common Household Products

CLASS	CAUSTIC AGENT	PRODUCT CONTAINING AGENT
Strong alkalis	Ammonia Lye (sodium hydroxide, potassium hydroxide)	Cleaning products Clinitest tablets Disc batteries Drain cleaners Nonphosphate detergents Paint removers Washing powders
Strong acids	Hydrochloric acid	Muriatic acid Soldering fluxes Swimming pool cleaners Toilet bowl cleaners

Table continued on following page

Caustic Agents Found in Common Household Products (Continued)

CLASS	CAUSTIC AGENT	PRODUCT CONTAINING AGENT
Strong acids *(cont.)*	Nitric acid	Gun barrel cleaners
	Oxalic acid	Antirust compounds
	Phosphoric acid	Toilet bowl cleaners
	Sulfuric acid	Battery acid
		Toilet bowl cleaners
Miscellaneous	Sodium hypochlorite	Liquid bleach

17. Lye (sodium hydroxide) is a common caustic ingestion. How has its formulation changed over the past 30 years? How has this change affected the pattern of injury?

Before the 1960s caustic ingestion frequently involved solid or crystalline lye products with concentrations > 50%. Such products were extremely corrosive and caused extensive damage on contact with the mucosa, but the immediate burning pain on contact with the oral mucosa often caused the victim to spit out the solid material. Injury was usually limited to the mouth, pharynx, and esophagus and rarely affected the stomach. Reports vary, but free esophageal perforation and mediastinitis were common complications. Such experiences led to the belief that lye injured the esophagus with relative sparing of the stomach compared with acids. This dictum did not hold true with concentrated liquid lye preparations, which can be swallowed more easily and quickly than solid lye. In the late 1960s such products were introduced as drain cleaners in concentrations of 25–36%. They caused devastating injury. Complications included respiratory compromise, esophageal and gastric perforations, septicemia, and death. Patients who survived often developed esophageal stricture as a later complication of ingestion. By the mid 1970s highly concentrated liquid products had been replaced in the U.S. by moderately concentrated (< 10%) liquid drain cleaners. If ingested in sufficient quantity, such products are strong enough to cause severe esophageal and gastric injury, including visceral perforation. More often a smaller volume is ingested, and the patient recovers from the acute injury; later, however, strictures may develop. Caustic materials currently available for industrial usage often are much more concentrated than household products. Children occasionally encounter cleaning products containing highly concentrated lyes or acids, particularly around farms, construction sites, and swimming pools.

18. Describe the pathophysiology of acute alkali esophagitis.

When tissue is exposed to strong alkali, the immediate result is liquefactive necrosis, the complete destruction of entire cells and their membranes. Cell membranes are destroyed as their lipids are saponified and cellular proteins are denatured. Thrombosis of the local blood vessels also contributes to tissue damage. Tissue destruction and organ penetration progress rapidly until the alkali is diluted and neutralized by dilution with tissue fluids. Transmural necrosis of organs exposed to strong alkali occurs rapidly. Experimental exposure of cat esophagus to 5 ml of a 30.2% sodium hydroxide solution for only 3 seconds causes perforation and impending death.

The severity of caustic injury to the esophagus can be graded as first-, second-, or third-degree, using a system similar to that for classifying burns of the skin. The table below correlates the degree of burn with the endoscopic and pathologic findings. Endoscopy within the first 24 hours may underestimate the severity of esophageal injury.

Degree of Esophageal Injury and Associated Findings

DEGREE	ENDOSCOPIC FINDINGS	PATHOLOGY
First	Erythema and edema of mucosa only	Sloughing of superficial layers of mucosa
Second	Ulceration with membranous exudate	Ulcer extends through mucosa and submucosa to muscularis tissue
Third	Deep ulceration with penetration, black discoloration	Transmural injury, erosions into mediastinum or peritoneal structures

19. What are the three phases of injury and healing associated with lye?

Experimental lye injury may be divided into three phases: the acute or liquefaction phase (approximately days 1–4), the subacute or reparative phase (days 5–14), and the scar retraction or cicatrization phase. The acute phase is characterized by liquefactive necrosis, vascular thrombosis, and progressive inflammation. Mucosal erythema and edema are intense, but even severely injured tissue may not exhibit sloughing or ulceration during the first 24 hours. The hallmark of the subacute or reparative phase is sloughing of the necrotic areas with obvious ulceration and development of granulation tissue. Fibroblasts appear, and collagen deposition peaks during the second week but may continue for months. Mucosal reepithelialization begins, and the wall of the esophagus is thinnest and most vulnerable during this period. The cicatrization phase, which begins about the end of the second week, is marked by continued proliferation of fibroblasts and further deposition of collagen. The recently formed collagen contracts both circumferentially and longitudinally, resulting in esophageal shortening and stricture formation. Reepithelialization is generally complete by 1–3 months after lye ingestion. The table below summarizes the phases of lye injury. The evolution and outcome of a given lye ingestion involve a spectrum of events that may not follow the exact time course outlined above.

Phases of Lye Injury

PHASE	PATHOLOGY	COMMENTS
Acute (days 1–4)	Liquefactive necrosis	Sloughing or ulcer not apparent < 24 hr Vascular thrombosis Increased inflammation
Subacute (days 5–14)	Sloughing of casts	Esophageal wall is thinnest Granulation tissue Fibroblast begin Collagen deposition
Cicatrization (day 15–3 months)	Fibroblasts proliferate Further collagen deposition Stricture formation	Reepithelialization in 1–3 months

20. Contrast the effects of acid ingestion with the effects of lye ingestion.

Concentrated acid solutions cause more severe pain on contact with the oropharyngeal mucosa than liquid alkalis, which often are swallowed before protective mechanisms can take effect. This property tends to limit the amount of acid that is ingested by accident. In past decades it often was noted that acid caused the greatest damage in the stomach, whereas alkali preferentially injured the esophagus. This observation was largely due to the fact that granular or solid lye usually was swallowed in small quantities and failed to reach the stomach in sufficient volume to cause serious gastric injury. The highly concentrated liquid alkalis introduced in the 1970s were likely to cause penetrating injury to both esophagus and stomach. The moderately concentrated liquid acids and alkalis available today are less likely to cause acute perforation of either organ but often lead to late stricture formation.

Histologic examination of tissue exposed to acid reveals coagulation necrosis with clumping and opacification of the cellular cytoplasm. The cell boundaries are usually recognizable in contrast to the complete cellular destruction of the liquefactive necrosis induced by strong alkali. The coagulum formed during coagulative necrosis consists in part of consolidated connective tissue, thrombosis of vessels, and clumping of blood proteins. This coagulum may limit the depth of penetration of the acid. However, esophageal perforations due to acid ingestion have been reported.

21. Do acute signs and symptoms predict the severity and extent of caustic injury?

Clinicians should be aware when evaluating patients with caustic ingestion that early signs and symptoms are not reliable indicators of the severity of caustic injury. Caustic agents (acids and crystalline lye) frequently cause immediate pain on contact with the mucosa of the oropharynx and may be expectorated before they are swallowed. Therefore, patients who ingest such agents may exhibit signs and symptoms of damage to the oropharynx with no injury to the esophagus. In contrast, lethal esophageal burns may occur with minimal evidence of oropharyngeal damage. Therefore, signs and symptoms of injury to the oropharynx do not reliably indicate the severity of damage to the esophagus or stomach. The distribution and severity of injury with acid or alkali depend as much on the physical characteristics of the product (solid versus liquid, volatility, titratable acid or base) as the volume ingested and the duration of exposure.

22. Describe the presentation of a typical case of caustic ingestion.

The typical clinical course of uncomplicated caustic ingestion has three phases that closely parallel the phases of experimental caustic injury: acute, latent, and retractive. In the acute phase, immediate oral burning pain often limits the volume of ingestion. Caustic burns to the epiglottis and larynx may lead to immediate or delayed wheezing, cough, stridor, hoarseness, dyspnea, or aphonia. Dyspnea also may result from aspiration with damage to the bronchial tree and lung parenchyma. If a significant volume of the agent is swallowed, chest pain, dysphagia, or odynophagia may develop within minutes. Secretions may not be handled because of injury to and swelling of the posterior pharynx; drooling may occur. Retching and emesis may follow, and vomitus may contain blood or tissue. Pain and dysphagia in the uncomplicated course are largely due to dysmotility and edema and may subside over 3–4 days.

The patient with more complex injury may have additional symptoms and a worsening course. Persistent substernal pain or back pain may indicate a third-degree burn of the esophagus with mediastinitis. Perforation of the esophagus or stomach may cause peritonitis with abdominal rigidity and rebound tenderness. Perforation may evolve over the first few days and manifest as increasing pain, fever, and shock.

23. Describe the common features of the patient's course after acute ingestion.

Initial pain and dysphagia may remit after a few days, ushering in the latent phase. Both physician and patient may be lulled into a false sense of security. The third phase, scar retraction, may begin as early as the end of the second week and last for several months. Clinically apparent esophageal strictures develop in 10–30% of patients with documented esophageal injury. Eighty percent of strictures become apparent during weeks 2–8, but occasionally patients may become symptomatic from stricture many months after the initial ingestion. Early strictures often progress rapidly, advancing from mild dysphagia to the inability to handle secretions in only a few days. The rapid progression of early strictures necessitates rapid evaluation and therapy to avoid the formation of dense, tight, constricting lesions. Therapy for such strictures is careful bougienage, as needed to maintain esophageal patency.

24. What is the mortality rate associated with caustic ingestion?

The mortality rate has decreased markedly over the past three decades from approximately 20% to 1–3%. The decreased mortality is probably due to improvements in supportive care (antibiotics and nutritional support), advances in surgery, anesthesia, and intensive care management as well as substitution of less concentrated alkali and acids for the highly concentrated products available in the 1950s and before.

25. What is the cancer risk to a patient with stricture after lye ingestion?

The association between esophageal cancer and caustic ingestion is strong. The expected incidence of esophageal carcinoma is higher in patients with caustic ingestion than in the general population. Approximately 1–7% of patients with carcinoma of the esophagus have a history of caustic ingestion. The latent period is long and in one study was on average 41 years. Currently no screening is recommended after lye ingestion.

26. Describe the emergency department management of a patient with caustic ingestion.

The initial steps in the management of a suspected caustic injury are similar to those used on an emergency basis to manage any toxic ingestion. First, airway, breathing, and circulation

(ABCs) must be controlled. Patients with caustic ingestion may present with respiratory compromise and require endothracheal intubation to protect the airway and to provide adequate oxygenation. Intubation should be performed only under direct visualization and should not be attempted in a blind manner. Next, hypotension must be addressed with adequate fluid support and resuscitation, as needed. If obvious signs of mediastinitis or peritonitis suggest perforation of a viscus, the patient should be prepared for surgery.

When respiratory and hemodynamic status have been addressed and the patient is stable, an attempt should be made to determine the quantity and type of caustic agent and time of ingestion as well as any coingestions (more often with suicidal attempts than accidental ingestion). It is helpful to obtain the container of the caustic agent, which lists all active substances as well as concentrations of caustics. If the clinician is not familiar with management of poison ingestion or if the content of the caustic is in question, a poison control center should be contacted. Emesis should not be induced, because it will reexpose the esophagus and perhaps larynx to caustic materials. If a solid caustic has been ingested, a few sips of water may help to dislodge the solid particles from the esophageal mucosa and dissolve them in a larger volume of water in the thicker-walled stomach. This, of course, should not be done in patients at risk of aspiration or with clinical evidence of perforation.

By the time victims of ingestion present to the physician, it is usually too late to intervene effectively to reduce internal burns. Because of the rapid action of alkali agents, efforts to neutralize caustic substances are not likely to be effective in limiting injury. In addition, an attempt to neutralize the alkali agent may be dangerous. Neutralization may release significant amounts of heat and add thermal injury to chemical injury. Oral administration of any substance also may increase the risk of vomiting and aspiration. With acid injury, large volumes of water or milk within minutes of ingestion may dilute and neutralize the acid.

27. Should gastric lavage be performed on patients with caustic ingestion?

The answer is controversial. Patients most likely to benefit from gastric lavage present shortly after ingestion when a significant amount of caustic material may still be present in the stomach. In addition, patients with suspected coingestion of pills may benefit from lavage to decrease absorption. Such benefits must be weighed against the risks. Nasogastric intubation may induce retching and vomiting with recurrent exposure of the esophagus and oropharynx to caustics. Because the nasogastric tube may perforate the esophagus or stomach, strong consideration should be given to placement under fluoroscopic guidance. If the tube is placed, gastric contents should be aspirated before lavage. The stomach should be lavaged with cold water to dissipate any heat that is produced.

28. What is the role of endoscopic evaluation in patients with caustic ingestion?

Flexible upper endoscopy has a role in the early, emergent and later, subacute management of caustic ingestion. Patients in whom perforation (diagnosed either radiographically or clinically) requires surgical exploration should undergo complete upper endoscopy to identify the extent of disease. For example, in patients with a normal esophagus but injured stomach, surgery may be limited to the abdomen. The risk of upper endoscopy is acceptable once the decision to operate has been made.

If surgery is not indicated, endoscopy still should be performed to identify uninjured patients who do not require prolonged hospital observation and to define the severity of burns in injured patients. Timing of endoscopy is based on clinical suspicion of severe injury. If significant esophageal injury is unlikely, EGD should be performed promptly to provide rapid reassurance and to avoid hospital observation. More than 50% of patients with a history of caustic injury are found on endoscopy to have no injury. If internal injury is likely but signs of perforation are absent, a delay of 48–72 hours permits development of the inflammatory reaction (little inflammation may be present in the first 24 hours) and easier assessment of the true extent of injury. Although endoscopic evaluation identifies the location of the mucosal injury, it may not accurately predict the depth of invasion.

Endoscopy classifies injuries into four categories, as outlined in the table below. The findings influence hospital stay and likelihood of stricture formation.

Classification of Injury by Endoscopic Findings

ENDOSCOPIC FINDINGS	HOSPITAL STAY	RISK OF STRICTURE
No injury	No observation in hospital	None
Gastric only	Observe 24–48 hours	None
Linear esophageal injury, oriented longitudinally	Observe 24–48 hours	Low
Circumferential esophageal injury	Observe at least 48 hours	High

29. What is the role of corticosteroids in the treatment of caustic ingestion?

Patients in whom endoscopy demonstrates near-circumferential or circumferential esophageal burns are at risk for strictures. Since the 1950s, corticosteroids have been the mainstay of prophylaxis against stricture formation. The rationale for their use was based on animal studies showing that steroid therapy begun within 24 hours after lye injury and continued for 6–8 weeks reduced the incidence of strictures by inhibiting formation of granulation tissue. This effect may be observed when corticosteroids are used as late as 4–7 days after caustic ingestion. Follow-up was short, however, and early death from septicemia was much more common in steroid-treated animals.

A prospective, randomized, controlled trial in children with caustic ingestion, performed by Anderson in 1990, showed that corticosteroids did not decrease stricture formation. The study, however, had a small number of patients, and although formation of esophageal stricture did not seem to be affected by corticosteroids, the need for total esophagectomy was decreased in the steroid-treated group (4 vs. 7 untreated patients).

Clearly there is no consensus. If steroids are to be used, they should be reserved for patients with circumferential esophageal burns, who are at greatest risk of stricture formation. The dosage and length of therapy for corticosteroids have not been defined. Prednisone, 1.5–2.0 mg/kg/day with a tapering period of 2 months, has been recommended.

In patients with significant caustic ingestion and clinical evidence of impending airway compromise, corticosteroids may help to decrease inflammation of the bronchopulmonary tree. Dexamethasone (pediatric dosage = 0.5–1.0 mg/kg; adult dosage = 2.0–3.0 mg/kg) is given intravenously to patients who have a high probability of impending airway compromise and may need intubation, cricothyrotomy, or tracheostomy for treatment of airway obstruction.

The negative aspects of corticosteroids, including increased risk of infection and systemic side effects, also must be considered.

30. What is the role of antibiotics in the treatment of caustic ingestion?

Empirical antibiotic therapy is even less established. It was originally advocated because antibiotics reduced the early mortality rate in animals treated with steroids for esophageal burns. In addition, antibiotics originally were thought to decrease long-term stricture formation, but this effect has not been reproducible in animal or human studies. The patients most likely to benefit are those who are treated with corticosteroids and appear to be at increased risk of systemic infection. Gram-positive organisms are most commonly implicated, but broad-spectrum coverage is generally prescribed.

Empirical therapy has not been shown to be more efficacious than monitoring for clinical signs of infection and using broad-spectrum antibiotics at their first appearance. If empirical therapy is chosen, antibiotics may be stopped after 5–7 days of infection-free observation.

31. Discuss the prophylactic role of bougienage.

Once the acute injury has resolved, the next complication is likely to be stricture of the esophagus in patients who had circumferential burns. If such patients are left untreated, a long narrow stricture may develop. Such strictures may not be amenable to dilation and may require surgery. To avoid stricture formation, patients may undergo prophylactic dilation with a Maloney dilator or esophageal stenting. Dilation should be avoided during the acute phase of injury because of the increased risk of perforation. Dilation should be initiated in patients with circumferential burns at about the third week, before the stricture becomes symptomatic. Dilation is accomplished with a single pass of a moderately large (42-French) dilator several times a week. If resistance is encountered, the dilator is not forced through. Instead, progressive dilations are initiated, starting with the largest dilator that passes without resistance. This method generally maintains patency of the esophageal lumen. Although some risk is associated with dilation, the procedure may prevent formation of the long narrow stricture commonly associated with caustic ingestion. An alternative to prophylactic dilation is close personal observation and questioning so that therapeutic dilation can be instituted at the onset of symptomatic dysphagia. Unfortunately, many injured patients are too young or too unreliable to be managed with this wait-and-see approach.

32. What is the role of computed tomography (CT) scanning?

Available data support CT scan with contrast as a predictor of the number of sessions of dilation that will be required to maintain a patent esophagus. Maximal esophageal wall thickness (> 9 mm) in the area of the stricture was shown on multivariate analysis to be independently associated with the number of sessions of dilation required by the patient.

33. Discuss the role of esophageal stents.

The use of prophylactic esophageal stents to maintain lumen patency during the healing process is controversial and should be limited to centers with experience in placing stents and ongoing research interests. Stents are placed endoscopically or surgically and left in place for approximately 3 weeks. The theory is that stenting allows esophageal healing without cicatrization and stenosis. After 3 weeks the stent is removed. The stents are uncomfortable, and appreciable risk is associated with placement and removal. No randomized data evaluate the efficacy of stents, but anecdotal data have shown that most patients require subsequent esophageal dilation.

34. What factors contribute to the controversies associated with treatment of caustic ingestions?

Currently many sources promote different invasive and noninvasive therapies for caustic ingestions. Fortunately, the number of severe caustic ingestions seems to be decreasing. Because of decreasing experience and ethical concerns about testing experimental therapies on humans, few well-controlled data are available to guide the clinician. Withholding therapy, however, is also an ethical concern.

35. What are the advantages and disadvantages of nasogastric intubation?

Advantages: Nasogastric tubes (NGTs) provide a mechanism to deliver adequate nutritional support and needed medications. They also allow the esophagus to rest and prevent wound trauma that may be associated with bolus food ingestion. Finally, NGTs maintain a lumen that can be used to assist dilation.

Disadvantages: NGTs may cause continuous irritation and inflammation of the healing esophagus and lead to increased fibrosis and stricturing.

Overall recommendation: A fluoroscopically placed, flexible NGT seems to be beneficial for the first 2 weeks in patients who are seriously ill and unlikely to maintain adequate nutrition.

36. What is the role of total parenteral nutrition (TPN)?

Total parenteral nutrition (TPN) has been advocated to allow complete esophageal rest and maintain maximal nutrition for healing. No prospective data support TPN in all patients. Clear candidates are patients at high risk of aspiration and patients in whom passage of an NGT is contraindicated because of the severity of esophageal injuries.

37. Why is prophylactic dilation controversial?

The final area of controversy is the use and timing of prophylactic dilation. Most agree that oral esophageal dilation is the cornerstone of stricture prophylaxis. Others argue that repeated trauma to esophageal mucosa from dilation causes increased fibrosis and encourages stricture formation. Prophylactic dilation of all patients with caustic ingestion clearly subjects some patients to unneeded, potentially hazardous procedures. No data are available to resolve this issue. Because strictures rarely manifest before the second week after ingestion, it seems wise to wait 10–14 days before beginning bougienage.

BIBLIOGRAPHY

1. Anderson KD, Rouse TM, Randolph JG: A controlled trial of corticosteroids in children with corrosive injury of the esophagus. N Engl J Med 323:10, 1990.
2. Bozymski EM, London JF: Miscellaneous diseases of the esophagus. In Sleisinger MH, Fordtran JS (eds): Gastrointestinal Diseases, 5th ed. Philadelphia, W.B. Saunders, 1993.
3. Browne JD, Thompson JN: Caustic injuries of the esophagus. In Castell DO(ed): The Esophagus. Boston, Little, Brown, 1992.
4. Byrne WJ: Foreign bodies, bezoars, and caustic ingestions. Gastrointest Endosc Clin North Am 4:99–119, 1994.
5. Gumaste VV, Pradyuman BD: Ingestion of corrosive substances by adults. Am J Gastroenterol 87:1–5, 1991.
6. Kikendall JW: Caustic injury of the esophagus and stomach. In Current Therapy in Gastroenterology and Liver Disease, 3rd ed. Philadelphia, B.C. Decker, 1990.
7. Kikendall JW: Caustic ingestion injuries. Gastroenterol Clin North Am 20:847–857, 1991.
8. Kikendall JW, Johnson LF: Pill-induced esophageal injury. In Castell DO (ed): The Esophagus. Boston, Little, Brown, 1995.
9 Kochhar R, Ray JD, Sriram PVJ, et al: Intralesional steroids augment the effect of endoscopic dilation in corrosive esophageal strictures. Gastrointest Endosc 49:135–141, 1999.
10. Lahoti D, Broor SL, Basu PP, et al: Corrosive esophageal strictures: Predictors of response to endoscopic dilation. Gastrointest Endosc l41:86–91, 1995.
11. Loeb PM, Eisenstein AM: Caustic injury to the upper gastrointestinal tract. In Scharschmidt BF (ed): Gastrointestinal Diseases, 5th ed. Philadelphia, W.B. Saunders, 1993, pp 293–301.
12. Minocha A, Greenbaum DS: Pill-esophagitis caused by nonsteroidal antiinflammatory drugs. Am J Gastroenterol 86:1086–1089, 1991.
13. Ribeiro A, DeVault KR, Wolfe J, Stark ME: Alendronate-associated esophagitis: Endoscopic and pathologic features. Gastrointest Endosc 47:216–221, 1998.
14. Semble EL, Wu WC, Castell DO: Nonsteroidal antiinflammatory drugs and esophageal injury. Semin Arthritis Rheum 19:99–109, 1989.
15. Spechler SJ: Caustic ingestions. In Taylor MB (ed): Gastrointestinal Emergencies. Baltimore, Williams & Wilkins, 1990, pp 13–21.

8. BARRETT'S ESOPHAGUS

Richard E. Sampliner, M.D.

1. What is Barrett's esophagus?

Barrett's esophagus is a metaplastic change in the lining of the normally squamous-lined esophagus. As a result of gastroesophageal reflux disease, the esophagus is lined with intestinal metaplasia, a premalignant epithelium.

2. How is Barrett's esophagus diagnosed?

The ultimate criterion for histologic diagnosis is the presence of goblet cells. Currently, two techniques are necessary: endoscopy to recognize abnormal-appearing esophageal epithelium and biopsy to detect intestinal metaplasia.

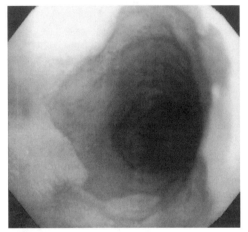

Endoscopic appearance of Barrett's esophagus. The lighter-colored proximal mucosa is normal squamous epithelium. The darker distal mucosa is Barrett's-appearing epithelium.

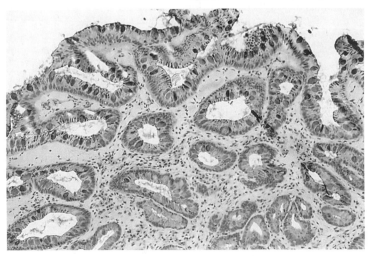

Histology of intestinal metaplasia. The dark-stained, barrel-shaped structures are the goblet cells, the hallmark of intestinal metaplasia.

3. Why is Barrett's esophagus important?

It is the premalignant lesion for adenocarcinoma of the esophagus and presumably for a proportion of adenocarcinomas of the gastric cardia. The cancer with the most rapidly rising incidence in the United States and Western Europe over the past 3 decades has been adenocarcinoma of the esophagus in white males.

4. Does short-segment Barrett's esophagus need to be identified?

Yes. Barrett's esophagus ranges from short tongues of intestinal metaplasia in the distal esophagus to circumferential intestinal metaplasia of nearly the entire length of the esophagus. In the mid 1970s, before the recognition of the importance of intestinal metaplasia, Barrett's esophagus was defined as a "columnar-lined esophagus" of at least 3 cm in length. However, it is now recognized that short-segment Barrett's esophagus can develop dysplasia and adenocarcinoma.

5. What is the risk of cancer associated with Barrett's esophagus?

Recent prospective series have documented a lower risk for the development of cancer than former series. Rather than a 1–2% risk per year, the risk appears to be 0.4–0.5% per year. This difference may be due to the larger, prospective series with longer follow-up. This lower incidence has been documented in higher-risk patients—predominantly Caucasian males. However, the most important question for the individual patient is his or her specific risk. An evidence-based answer has not yet been developed.

6. Who should be screened for Barrett's esophagus?

People at highest risk for the development of adenocarcinoma should be screened. Clues are available from the epidemiology of adenocarcinoma: older white males, patients with long-standing reflux symptoms, smokers, and the obese. Specific criteria to select individual patients have not been defined by prospective studies. In clinical practice, however, the movement has been toward the concept of once-in-a-lifetime endoscopy for patients with chronic gastroesophageal reflux to detect Barrett's esophagus. Focusing on patients at highest risk of developing cancer would be more effective.

7. What is the therapy for Barrett's esophagus?

Standard clinical therapy is pharmacologic (proton pump inhibitor) and surgical (laparoscopic fundoplication). Both techniques are highly effective in controlling reflux symptoms and healing erosive esophagitis. For younger patients who are noncompliant or do not wish to take daily medication, surgery may be preferable. For patients with prominent regurgitation, inadequately controlled with proton pump inhibitors, surgery should be considered. A higher failure rate for laparoscopic fundoplication has been recognized in patients with Barrett's esophagus compared with patients with non-Barrett's reflux.

Goals of Therapy for Barrett's Esophagus

1. Control reflux symptoms.
2. Heal erosive esophagus.
3. Prevent adenocarcinoma.

8. Does Barrett's esophagus reverse with medical therapy?

Rarely. In published series, which typically use high doses of proton pump inhibitor, Barrett's esophagus was eliminated in only 2% of 151 patients. Even if esophageal acid exposure is nearly eliminated, the estimated decrease in the area of Barrett's esophagus over an interval of 2 years is only 8%.

9. Does Barrett's esophagus reverse with surgical therapy?

Rarely. Barrett's esophagus has been eliminated in < 4% of 449 patients having antireflux surgery in large series in the 1990s. If the elimination of all refluxate by successful fundoplication does not reverse Barrett's esophagus and eliminate the risk of cancer, it is unlikely that medical therapy other than chemoprevention will do so.

10. Discuss the appropriate surveillance of patients with Barrett's esophagus.

The database for developing guidelines for surveillance of this premalignant mucosa is limited, but gastroenterologists must deal with this issue in everyday practice. Surveillance intervals are based on the detection of dysplasia with the goal of early intervention to improve the survival rates associated with adenocarcinoma. The surveillance intervals have been increasing and probably will continue to do so with improved understanding of the natural history of dysplasia. Currently a patient with two endoscopies with systematic biopsies showing no dysplasia can be surveyed every 3 years. If low-grade dysplasia is associated with no greater abnormality on follow-up endoscopy with biopsy, surveillance can be performed every year for 3 years, then every 2 years, until no dysplasia is found.

11. Summarize the evolution of Barrett's esophagus to adenocarcinoma.

Intestinal metaplasia
↓
Low-grade dysplasia
↓
High-grade dysplasia
↓
Adenocarcinoma

12. Describe the management of high-grade dysplasia.

Management of high-grade dysplasia is one of the most controversial issues in the treatment of Barrett's esophagus. Current alternatives include more frequent surveillance (every 3 months) until cancer is detected, experimental endoscopic reversal therapy, and esophagectomy. The problems with conventional esophagectomy include the operative mortality rate, especially in low-volume centers; the high frequency of morbidity; and the permanent impact on eating and nutrition. Many patients are elderly and are not good surgical candidates because of comorbidity. It is also not uncommon for patients to refuse surgery even after consultation with a surgeon.

13. Can the development of adenocarcinoma of the esophagus be prevented in patients with Barrett's esophagus?

Prevention is the major challenge to clinicians. Given the lack of reversal of Barrett's esophagus with standard medical and surgical therapy, it is not clear that we can prevent the development of adenocarcinoma. It has been argued that control of reflux into the esophagus will prevent the progression from metaplasia to dysplasia and subsequent adenocarcinoma. However, this argument is far from proven, and only retrospective data can be brought to bear upon the issue. There are exciting developments in experimental endoscopic therapy to eliminate the presence of intestinal metaplasia. Even with validation of these techniques and more widespread clinical application, it will remain a major challenge to document the prevention of adenocarcinoma or at least the reduction of the risk of developing adenocarcinoma in patients with Barrett's esophagus.

14. What advances can we anticipate in the management of Barrett's esophagus?

Progress in our understanding of the genetic changes involved in the progression of Barrett's esophagus to adenocarcinoma has been dramatic. The technical advances that continue to be made in endoscopy offer the opportunity for major advances in clinical management of Barrett's esophagus. We can look forward to unsedated endoscopy with smaller-caliber endoscopes for cheaper and easier detection of Barrett's esophagus. There is even the potential to develop non-endoscopic techniques to recognize Barrett's esophagus. Optical methods for identifying dysplasia without biopsy add the possibility of real-time recognition. Newer endoscopic techniques to remove dysplastic and metaplastic epithelium will make our current attempts look primitive.

Preventing adenocarcinoma may well require the validation of biomarkers that define the sub-group of patients at highest risk for developing cancer. This approach will focus surveillance on patients at highest risk, leading to cost savings and greater clinical effectiveness. Chemoprevention may well offer opportunities for cancer prevention that transcend the possibilities of technical advances.

BIBLIOGRAPHY

 1. Begg C, Cramer L, Hoskins W, Brennan M: Impact of hospital volume on operative mortality for major cancer surgery. JAMA 280:1747–1751, 1998.
 2. Csendes A, Braghetto I, Brudiles P, et al: Long-term results of classic antireflux surgery in 152 patients with Barrett's esophagus: Clinical, radiologic, endoscopic, manometric and acid reflux test analysis before and late after operation. Surgery 123:645–657, 1998.
 3. Devesa S, Blot W, Fraumeni J: Changing patterns in the incidence of esophageal and gastric carcinoma in the United States. Cancer 83:2049–2053, 1998.
 4. Drewitz D, Sampliner R, Garewal H: The incidence of adenocarcinoma in Barrett's esophagus: A prospective study of 170 patients followed 4.8 years. Am J Gastroenterol 92:212–215, 1997.
 5. Farrell T, Smith C, Metreveli R, et al: Fundoplication provides effective and durable symptom relief in patients with Barrett's esophagus. Am J Surg 178:18–21, 1999.
 6. Fass R, Sampliner R, Malagon I, et al: Failure of oesophageal acid control in candidates for Barrett's oesophagus on a very high dose of proton pump inhibitor. Aliment Pharmacol 14:597–602, 2000.
 7. Haag S, Nandurkar S, Talley N: Regression of Barrett's esophagus: The role of acid suppression, surgery, and ablative methods. Gastrointest Endosc 50:229–240, 1999.
 8. O'Connor J, Falk G, Richter J: The incidence of adenocarcinoma and dysplasia in Barrett's esophagus. Am J Gastroenterol 94:2037–2042, 1999.
 9. Ouatu-Lascar R, Triadafilopoulos G: Complete elimination of reflux symptoms does not guarantee normalization of intraesophageal acid reflux in patients with Barrett's esophagus. Am J Gastroenterol 93:711–716, 1998.
10. Overholt B, Panjehpour M, Haydek J: Photodynamic therapy for Barrett's esophagus: Follow-up in 100 patients. Gastrointest Endosc 49:1–7, 1999.
11. Peters F, Ganesh S, Kuipers E, et al: Endoscopic regression of Barrett's oesophagus during omeprazole treatment: A randomised double blind study. Gut 45:489–494, 1999.
12. Sampliner R: The Practice Parameters Committee of the American College of Gastroenterology. Practice guidelines on the diagnosis, surveillance, and therapy of Barrett's esophagus. Am J Gastroenterol 93:1028–1032, 1998.
13. Sharma P, Morales T, Bhattacharyya A, et al: Dysplasia in short segment Barrett's esophagus: A prospective 3-year follow-up. Am J Gastroenterol 92:2012–2016, 1997.
14. Sharma P, Morales T, Sampliner R: Short segment Barrett's esophagus: The need for standardization of the definition and of endoscopic criteria. Am J Gastroenterol 93:1033–1036, 1998.
15. Sharma P, Sampliner R, Camargo E: Normalization of esophageal pH with high dose proton pump inhibitor therapy does not result in regression of Barrett's esophagus. Am J Gastroenterol 92:582–585, 1997.
16. Weston A, Krmpotich P, Makdisi W, et al: Short segment Barrett's esophagus: Clinical and histological features, associated endoscopic findings, and association with intestinal metaplasia. Am J Gastroenterol 91:981–986, 1996.

9. ESOPHAGEAL ANOMALIES

John H. Meier, M.D.

1. A patient with dysphagia is found to have a web by barium studies. What blood disorder must be investigated?

Esophageal webs are often, but not universally, associated with iron deficiency anemia.

2. What is the best therapy for the dysphagia?

Esophageal bougienage is the preferred therapy, although many webs probably are ruptured unwittingly at endoscopy. Webs are thin, typically less than 2 mm in diameter.

3. Define Plummer-Vinson syndrome. Is it common?

The full syndrome, also known as Paterson-Brown-Kelly syndrome, consists of iron deficiency, angular cheilitis, glossitis, and post-cricoid web. The full syndrome is rare and may be decreasing in frequency.

4. Describe the usual mucosal layers of a web.

Resected specimens consist of mucosa, submucosa, and connective tissue.

5. What is the best way to confirm a suspected web?

Videofluoroscopy with lateral views. Standard barium swallow allows only brief visualization, and the lesion can be missed.

6 What other findings may be associated with webs?

Webs have been associated with inlet patches with gastric mucosa and with graft-vs.-host disease.

7. For which cancer are patients with esophageal webs reportedly at increased risk?

Esophageal webs are associated with squamous cell carcinoma of the hypopharynx and upper esophagus, although the degree of risk is not well-defined.

8. When should you suspect an esophageal duplication cyst? How can it be diagnosed?

Esophageal duplication cysts are exceedingly rare but may present as a submucosal mass or extrinsic compression. Communication with the esophagus is unusual but may occur at either or both ends of the esophagus. Endoscopic ultrasound may be suggestive, but surgery is currently required to rule out cystic neoplasm.

9. Describe the three types of esophageal rings.

The three types of esophageal rings are cleverly named A, B, and C. The A ring occurs about 2 cm proximal to the gastroesophageal junction, is muscular in origin, and is usually asymptomatic. The B ring, also known as a Schatzki ring, is mucosal and occurs at the squamocolumnar junction. The C ring is a nonpathologic radiographic anomaly caused by diaphragmatic indentation on the esophagus. C rings are never symptomatic.

10. What causes A and B rings?

The precise cause is not known. A rings may be associated with esophageal dysmotility. B rings may be reflux-related, but the literature is contradictory. Recent radiology literature suggests that B rings may be more common in children than previously thought, which raises the possibility that they are congenital. Not many children are symptomatic, however—a finding that is unexplained.

11. Are all Schatzki's rings symptomatic? What is the typical history of the symptomatic patient?

Schatzki's rings are usually symptomatic only when the luminal diameter is < 13 mm. Symptomatic patients usually describe only intermittent solid-food dysphagia induced by hurrying a meal or anxiety. Patients may present initially with foreign-body impaction.

12. How are Schatzki's rings treated?

Usually with large-diameter bougie. Repeat treatment may be needed over time.

13. Describe the three types of esophageal diverticula.

1. Upper esophageal, also called Zenker's diverticulum (which is arguably a hypopharyngeal lesion—this could be a trick question).
2. Midesophageal, also called a traction diverticulum.
3. Distal esophageal, also called an epiphrenic diverticulum.

14. What is the typical history of Zenker's diverticulum?

Patients may complain of regurgitation of undigested food, bad breath, a visible lump on the side of the neck, and dyphagia in the lower neck area.

15. What causes Zenker's diverticulum?

The cause has been long debated, with initially contradictory studies. The lesion is more common in elderly patients. Impaired cricopharyngeal compliance, usually due to fibrotic changes, causes increased intrabolus pressure with swallowing. Relaxation of the upper esophageal sphincter (UES) is usually normal. The result is increased hypopharyngeal pressure, with herniation at a weak point just above the cricopharyngeus.

16. What is Killian's dehiscence?

The weak point just above the cricopharyngeus is called Killian's dehiscence. It is a triangular area where the oblique fibers of the inferior pharyngeal constrictors and the transverse fibers of the cricopharyngeus overlap.

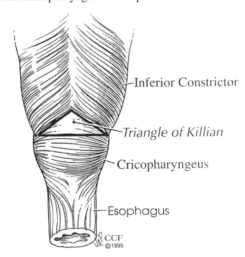

Killian's triangle and dehiscence. (From Castell DO (ed): The Esophagus. Philadelphia, Lippincott Williams & Wilkins, 1999, p 302, with permission.)

17. How is Zenker's diverticulum treated?

Symptomatic Zenker's diverticula require surgery. Most surgeons perform diverticulectomy because of the small risk of squamous cell carcinoma and persistent symptoms. Cricopharyngeal myotomy also should be done; otherwise, the recurrence rate is significant.

18. Why are midesophageal diverticula called traction diverticula?

It was previously thought that midesophageal diverticula were formed by adhesion of the esophagus to tuberculous mediastinal lymph nodes. Most are now thought to result from esophageal motility disorders or to represent a forme fruste of tracheoesophageal fistula. Few cause symptoms or need treatment.

19. Should all epiphrenic diverticula be surgically treated?

No. Unusually large diverticula or those producing symptoms such as regurgitation or aspiration should be resected. Because of the high association with motility disorders, manometry should be performed. Results of manometry often change the surgical approach to include long myotomy or myotomy of the lower esophageal sphincter (LES), as appropriate. Recurrence is common with diverticulectomy alone.

20. Is surgery required for the cricopharyngeal "bar" or "achalasia" that radiologists sometimes describe?

No! This finding may or may not be the cause of symptoms. Because the bar can result from poor hypopharygeal bolus propulsion, hypertrophy, or decreased opening capacity, caution must be exercised before recommending myotomy. Surgery occasionally causes severe reflux. Bougienage can be effective in relieving symptoms in some cases.

21. What is esophageal felinization? Does it cause symptoms?

This radiographic finding—with transient, delicate, transverse folds—is reminiscent of the cat esophagus. Although possibly related to reflux, it usually is asymptomatic. It may represent contractions of the muscularis mucosa.

22. Define dysphagia lusoria. What is the most common type?

Lusoria means "a trick of nature," and dysphagia lusoria refers to impingement of aberrant vasculature on the proximal esophagus. Most patients with aberrant vasculature are asymptomatic, but some have dysphagia. The most common type involves an aberrant right subclavian artery, which arises from the left side of the aortic arch and compresses the esophagus. Double aortic arch, right aortic arch, and several other anomalies are reported.

23. What sort of preoperative evaluation should be done in patients with dysphagia lusoria?

Magnetic resonance imaging (MRI) is believed to be the most accurate modality for defining the lesion. Patients also should undergo manometry and barium swallow with marshmallow or barium pill to be certain that symptoms are caused by the vascular anomaly.

24. What causes esophageal atresia with tracheoesophageal fistula?

Atresia occurs when embryonic foregut fails to recanalize to form an esophagus. The tracheoesophageal (TE) fistula is due to lack of separation of lung bud from the foregut. The exact insult causing these anomalies is not known.

25. What is the most common type of esophageal atresia with TE fistula? Describe its presentation.

The most common type of TE fistula with atresia is the lower-pouch fistula. Because the esophagus has not fully formed (atresia), the upper and lower pouches are not in continuity. This anomaly may cause intrauterine polyhydramnios. After birth, regurgitation after feeding and weight loss are seen. The fistula between the distal part of the esophagus and the trachea can cause pneumonia due to reflux of stomach contents.

26. What is the least common type of esophageal atresia with TE fistula? Describe its presentation.

The least common form is congenital esophageal stenosis, a forme fruste of atresia, which can present as late as adulthood. The differential diagnosis includes bullous skin disorders, radiation injury to the esophagus, caustic ingestion, and prolonged nasogastric suction. Congenital stenosis typically presents with lifelong dysphagia to solid foods and prolonged meals and low body weight. Barium radiographs may show a fixed segment of narrowing, usually midesophageal, and endoscopy may demonstrate multiple cartilaginous rings.

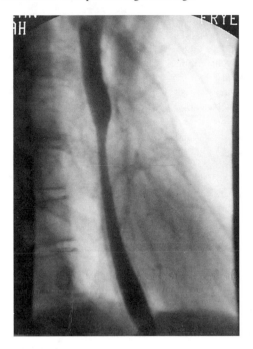

Barium esophagram showing segmental narrowing consistent with congenital esophageal stenosis.

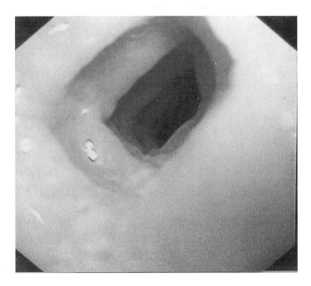

Endoscopic view of the same patient demonstrating cartilaginous rings at endoscopy.

27. How is esophageal atresia with TE fistula treated?

For patients presenting in childhood, surgical repair is usually possible. With modern techniques, mortality is due to associated cardiac anomalies rather than the surgery itself. Congenital esophageal stenosis is generally treatable with cautious bougienage.

28. What is intramural pseudodiverticulosis?

Formed by dilation of submucosal esophageal glands, small pseudodiverticula are commonly associated with candidal esophagitis (50%). Many patients have esophageal motor disorders, and many have esophageal strictures. The inciting event is unknown, but the lesion has been seen after corrosive ingestion. Treatment with stricture dilation and medications can be effective. Some have identified an increased risk of esophageal cancer and recommend periodic surveillance, although the cost-effectiveness of this approach is not established.

BIBLIOGRAPHY

1. Achkar E: Esophageal diverticula. In Castell DO (ed): The Esophagus. Philadelphia, Lippincott Williams & Wilkins, 1999, pp 301–314.
2. Beekman RP, Hazekamp MG: A new diagnostic approach to vascular rings and pulmonary slings: The role of MRI. Magn Res Imag 16:137–45, 1998.
3. Boyce GA, Boyce HW: Esophagus: Anatomy and structural anomalies. In Yamada T (ed): Textbook of Gastroenterology, 2nd ed. Philadelphia, J.B. Lippincott, 1995, pp 1156–1173.
4. Buckley K, Buonomo C, Husain K, Nurko S: Schatzki ring in children and young adults: Clinical and radiologic findings. Pediatr Radiol 28:884–886, 1998.
5. Harford W: Diverticula of the hypopharynx and esophagus, the stomach, and the small bowel. In Feldman M, Scharschmidt B, Sleisenger M (eds): Sleisenger and Fordtran's Gastrointestinal and Liver Disease, 6th ed. Philadelphia, W. B. Saunders, 1998, pp 309–316.
6. Long J, Orlando R: Anatomy and developmental and acquired anomalies of the esophagus. In Feldman M, Scharschmidt B, Sleisenger M (eds): Sleisenger and Fordtran's Gastrointestinal and Liver Disease, 6th ed. Philadelphia, W. B. Saunders, 1998, pp 457–466.
7. Pokieser P, Schima W, Schober E, Levine M: Congenital esophageal stenosis in a 21-year-old man: Clinical and radiographic findings. AJR 170:147–148, 1998.
8. Shand A, Papachrysostomou M, Ghosh S: Dysphagia in oesophageal intramural pseudo-diverticulosis: Fibrosis, dysmotility, or web? Eur J Gastroenterol Hepatol 11:1331–1333, 1999.
9. Tobin R: Esophageal rings and webs. In Castell DO (ed): The Esophagus. Philadelphia, Lippincott Williams & Wilkins, 1999, pp 295–300.
10. Tobin R: Esophageal rings, webs, and diverticula. J Clin Gastroenterol 27:285–295, 1998.
11. Tsai JY, Berkery L, Wesson DE, et al: Esophageal atresia and tracheoesophageal fistula: Surgical experience over two decades. Ann Thorac Surg 64:778–783, 1997.
12. Uygur-Bayramicli O, Tuncer K, Dolapcioglu C: Plummer-Vinson syndrome presenting with an esophageal stricture. J Clin Gastroenterol 29:291–292, 1999.
13. Waring JP, Wo JM: Cervical esophageal web caused by an inlet patch of gastric mucosa. South Med J 90:554–555, 1997.
14. Wilkinson JM, Euinton HA, Smith LF, et al: Diagnostic dilemmas in dysphagia aortica. Eur J Cardio-Thorac Surg 11:222–227, 1997.

II. Stomach

10. GASTRITIS
R. Matthew Reveille, M.D.

1. What are the cardinal symptoms of gastritis?

Symptoms associated with gastritis include dyspepsia (epigastric discomfort or burning), nausea, vomiting, postprandial fullness or bloating, and occasionally GI bleeding. Many people with histologic evidence for gastritis are asymptomatic. Chronic gastritis increases in frequency with age, and about 60% of adults have histologic evidence of a nonspecific chronic gastritis.

2. Describe the endoscopic and histologic appearance of acute gastritis.

Acute gastritis is usually seen endoscopically as scattered mucosal erosions and foci of intramucosal hemorrhage, termed "erosive" and "hemorrhagic" gastritis, respectively. Histologically, the minimal inflammatory component is confined to the mucosa.

3. What causes acute gastritis?

Most cases of acute gastritis involve chemical or ischemic injury. Viruses that produce a gastroenteritis syndrome (e.g., enteroviruses, rotavirus, Norwalk agent) typically do not cause true gastritis. Rarely, invasive bacterial infections cause an acute phlegmonous or emphysematous gastritis, which can be lethal. Common causes are listed below:

Alcohol	Viruses
Aspirin	Cytomegalovirus
Nonsteroidal anti-inflammatory drugs	Herpes viruses
(cyclo-oxygenase 2 and nonselective	Bacteria
cyclo-oxygenase inhibitors)	Alpha-hemolytic streptococci
"Stress" gastritis	Clostridium septicum
Corrosive (alkali) ingestion	Uremia
Bisphosphonates	Radiation exposure

4. In what clinical circumstances should you be concerned about stress gastritis?

The risk factors for stress gastritis include respiratory failure requiring mechanical ventilation, underlying liver or renal disease with coagulopathy, sepsis, extensive surgery or trauma, burns, and central nervous system injury. The erosions of stress gastritis often develop within 24 hours of a physiologic insult and can produce overt GI bleeding in up to 30% of patients, with potentially life-threatening hemorrhage in about 3% of cases. Unique lesions called Curling's ulcers are seen with burns; they appear to have a higher risk of bleeding and perforation, especially in the duodenum. In major head trauma, Cushing's ulcers often develop. They are particularly aggressive, because of acid hypersecretion due to hypergastrinemia, and often deep. Cushing's ulcers bleed and perforate more often than any other form of stress gastropathy. The importance of identifying true high-risk patients and initiating prophylaxis against stress gastritis to prevent bleeding and perforation cannot be overstated.

5. What are the options for prophylaxis of stress gastritis in the intensive care setting?

A principal goal of stress prophylaxis has been to raise gastric luminal pH above 4.0. At pH > 4, the proteolytic enzyme pepsin is inactivated and blood coagulation is enhanced. Various prophylactic methods are now acceptable. Antacids instilled into the stomach via a nasogastric (NG) tube every 2–4 hours, with periodic monitoring of the gastric pH, is still effective. Administration of intravenous H_2 blockers via bolus or continuous infusion is used most commonly. Whether the use of H_2 blockers increases the risk of nosocomial pneumonia in patients on ventilators remains controversial. An alternative to H_2 blockers is gastric instillation of sucralfate suspension, 1 gm every 4 hours via an NG tube. Misoprostol, a prostaglandin analog, has been used at 200 μg via NG every 4 hours. This dose results in mucosal protection and acid suppression. Periodic monitoring of gastric pH is probably prudent, with the addition of antacids to titrate the pH level back above 4.0.

6. What new approach may soon become the method of choice?

Intravenous proton pump inhibitors (PPIs), which are expected to provide long-duration acid suppression. It is likely that they will replace all other options for the prevention of stress gastritis. Monitoring of gastric pH will not be necessary.

7. Describe a classification scheme for the causes of chronic gastritis.

Classification continues to be controversial. The Sydney classification scheme of 1990 attempted to bring together endoscopic, anatomic, and histologic findings, but it is not widely accepted. From a pathophysiologic perspective, chronic gastritis is classified as follows:

Classification of Chronic Gastritides

Chemical gastritis	Hypertrophic gastropathies
Alkaline/bile reflux	Ménétrier's disease
NSAIDs (?)	Gastric pseudolymphoma
"Specific" gastritis	Zollinger-Ellison syndrome
Eosinophilic gastritis	Normal variant
Eosinophilic granuloma	Portal hypertensive/congestive gastropathy
Eosinophilic gastroenteritis	(not a true gastritis)
Collagenous gastritis	"Nonspecific" gastritis
Granulomatous gastritis	Nonerosive types
Crohn's disease	Type A autoimmune gastritis
Tuberculosis	Type B environmental gastritis
Histoplasmosis	*Helicobacter pylori*-related chronic gastritis
Syphilis	Erosive types
Sarcoidosis	Lymphocytic gastritis (*H. pylori*, sprue)
Foreign body	Varioliform gastritis
Parasitic	
Idiopathic	

8. What is the significance of chronic gastritis?

Chronic gastritis of the nonspecific, nonerosive type is associated with a risk of developing ulcer disease during the patient's lifetime. Some forms of specific chronic gastritis result in hypo/achlorhydria and vitamin B12 deficiency. Still other forms of gastritis are signs of more widespread GI disorders, such as Crohn's disease and eosinophilic gastroenteritis. The major clinical significance of chronic gastritis is that it is considered by many to be a very early premalignant lesion that progresses in time through atrophy and intestinal metaplasia to carcinoma. Fortunately, most patients in the U.S. with chronic gastritis do not develop gastric carcinoma. Chronic gastritis also appears to be a risk factor for primary gastric lymphoma.

9. How are types A and B of chronic nonspecific gastritis distinguished on anatomic and etiologic grounds?

Early in their course, the two disorders have an anatomic predilection for specific sites of inflammation. In **type A gastritis**, inflammation is associated with antiparietal cell antibodies and thus is autoimmune. It involves the fundus and corpus of the stomach. With time, atrophy and loss of intrinsic factor production occur, with B12 deficiency as a consequence. Patients develop achlorhydria and typically have hypergastrinemia.

In **type B gastritis**, or antral gastritis, the inflammatory process and subsequent atrophy and metaplasia are largely confined to the antrum. Infection of the antrum with the ulcer-causing bacterium *Helicobacter pylori* accounts for approximately 80% of all cases of type B gastritis. In other parts of the world, environmental exposures, such as diets high in nitrates and deficient in green vegetables, have been implicated in chronic type B gastritis. Type B gastritis is associated with gastric carcinoma and lymphoma.

Of interest, the anatomic distinctions between types A and B tend to blur with time. Advanced cases of either type can involve virtually the entire stomach and lead to diffuse atrophy and metaplasia. Both forms are associated with the formation of gastric hyperplastic polyps and adenomas.

10. In what clinical setting is portal hypertensive (congestive) gastropathy encountered?

Portal hypertensive gastropathy, as the name implies, refers to mucosal and submucosal changes in the stomach as a result of cirrhosis and portal hypertension. Development of this gastropathy is common after successful eradication of esophagogastric varices by endoscopic means. Endoscopically, gastric folds appear prominent and erythematous, with punctate intramucosal hemorrhages and a reticulated or "mosaic" mucosal pattern. Histologically, superficial capillary congestion, vascular ectasia, and perivascular fibrosis are seen, with no significant inflammatory component.

11. How is GI bleeding from congestive gastropathy managed?

GI blood loss can be either acute or chronic. Acute bleeding often is managed like variceal bleeding—with an intravenous infusion of either vasopressin or octreotide (somatostatin analog). H_2 blockers or PPIs are often given as well, although the benefits of antisecretory therapy have not been proved. For chronic blood loss, if no other cause is identified and there are no contraindications, a frequently effective approach is administration of a beta-blocker (e.g., propranolol, nadolol) in divided doses, titrated to produce a resting pulse of 60 bpm. Rarely do patients with blood loss from portal hypertensive gastropathy require portosystemic shunt surgery, unless they have refractory or rebleeding varices that need surgical decompression.

12. Define alkaline reflux gastritis.

Alkaline or bile reflux gastritis refers to mucosal injury caused by reflux of duodenal or jejunal contents into the stomach. This condition is seen most commonly after vagotomy and antrectomy for ulcer disease with either a Billroth I or II anastomosis. The gastritis is nonerosive. Histologic exam reveals hyperplasia of gastric foveolar glands, islands of lipid-containing histiocytes, and, occasionally, cystic dilatations of the glands, along with edema in the lamina propria and minimal to mild chronic inflammation. The term *bile reflux gastritis* is probably more accurate, because chronic exposure of gastric mucosa to bile can produce such changes.

13. What are the treatment options for patients with symptomatic alkaline reflux gastritis?

Most patients are asymptomatic from the gastritis per se, but some complain of burning epigastric pain unrelieved by random use of antacids, worsened by meals, and associated with bilious vomiting. Various medical treatments have been tried, none with universal success. Rational treatments are based on attempts to neutralize the effects of refluxed bile, alter bile components, promote prompt gastric emptying, or divert bile from entering the stomach. Aluminum-containing antacids and sucralfate taken after meals and at bedtime bind bile acids and may offer protection for the mucosa, although they are seldom effective. Ursodiol, a component of bear bile, has been used to alter bile composition to more water-soluble forms, which are less injurious to the mucosa. Bile acid binders, such as cholestyramine and colestipol, are useful, but caution must be used in patients with prior vagotomy with gastric stasis so that bezoars do not form. Prokinetic drugs (e.g., metoclopramide, bethanechol, domperidone, erythromycin) enhance gastric emptying and may be worth trying. If medical therapy fails to relieve symptoms, surgical diversion by Roux-en-Y gastrojejunostomy may be necessary.

14. Outline the approach to the patient with chronic dyspepsia and gastritis.

See algorithm on next page.

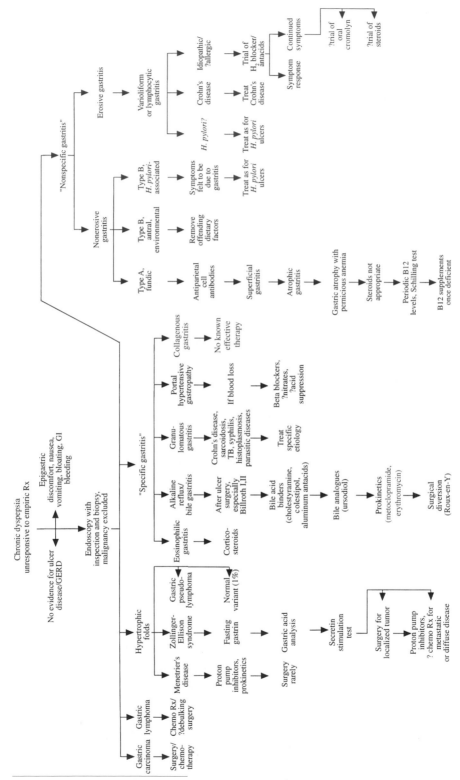

Evaluation and management of chronic gastritis.

BIBLIOGRAPHY

1. Antonioli DA: Chronic gastritis: Classification. In Bayless TM (ed): Current Therapy in Gastroenterology and Liver Disease, 4th ed. St. Louis, Mosby, 1994.
2. Correa P: Chronic gastritis: A clinico-pathological classification. Am J Gastroenterol 83:504, 1988.
3. Cote JF, et al: Collagenous gastritis revealed by severe anemia in a child. Hum Pathol 29:883, 1998.
4. DeCross AJ, McCallum RW: Chronic gastritis: Management. In Bayless TM (ed): Current Therapy in Gastroenterology and Liver Disease, 4th ed. St. Louis, Mosby, 1994.
5. Deprez P: Who? When to treat? Gastritis, particular histological lesions, NSAID therapy and extradigestive diseases. Acta Gastroenterol Belg 61:307, 1998.
6. Dixon MF, et al: Reflux gastritis: Distinct histopathological entity. J Clin Pathol 39:524, 1986.
7. Dixon MF, et al: Lymphocytic gastritis-relationship to *Campylobacter pylori* infection. J Pathol 153:125, 1989.
8. Dooley CP, et al: Prevalence of *Helicobacter pylori* infection and histologic gastritis in asymptomatic persons. N Engl J Med 321:1562, 1989.
9. Ectors NL, Dixon MF, Geboes KJ, et al: Granulomatous gastritis: A morphological and diagnostic approach. Histopathology 23:55, 1993.
10. Elta FG, Appelman HD, Behler EM, et al: A study of the correlation between endoscopic and histologic diagnoses in gastroduodenitis. Am J Gastroenterol 82:749, 1987.
11. Gostout CJ, Viggiano TR, Balm RK: Acute gastrointestinal bleeding from portal hypertensive gastropathy: Prevalence and clinical features. Am J Gastroenterol 88:2030, 1993.
12. Graham DY, Go MF: *Helicobacter pylori*: Current status. Gastroenterology 105:279, 1993.
13. Haot J, et al: Lymphocytic gastritis: Prospective study of its relationship with varioliform gastritis. Gut 31: 282, 1990.
14. Laine L, Weinstein WM: Histology of alcoholic hemorrhagic "gastritis": A prospective evaluation. Gastroenterology 94:1254, 1988.
15. McCormack TT, et al: Gastric lesions in portal hypertension: Inflammatory gastritis or congestive gastropathy? Gut 26:1226, 1985.
16. Reveille RM: Chronic gastritis. In Levine JS (ed): Decision Making in Gastroenterology, 2nd ed. St. Louis, Mosby, 1992.
17. Rubin CE: Histological classification of chronic gastritis: An iconoclastic view. Gastroenterology 102:360, 1992.
18. The Sydney System: A new classification of gastritis: The Working Party Report of the World Congresses of Gastroenterology. J Gastroenterol Hepatol 6:207, 1991.
19. Wu TT, Hamilton SR. Lymphocytic gastritis: association with etiology and topology. Am J Surg Pathol 23:153, 1999.

11. GASTRIC CANCER

John C. Deutsch, M.D.

1. What are the histologic types of gastric cancer?

Over 80% of gastric cancers are adenocarcinomas. Less common are gastric lymphomas, gastric stromal tumors (e.g., leiomyosarcomas), carcinoid tumors, and metastatic tumors (e.g., melanoma, breast cancer).

2. What is the ethnic and geographic distribution of distal gastric adenocarcinoma?

Distal gastric adenocarcinoma is one of the most common malignancies worldwide. Approximately 600,000 deaths per year are due to gastric cancer worldwide. There is a high incidence in Asia and South America. Scandinavian countries have a higher incidence than the U.S.

3. What is the role of *Helicobacter pylori* in gastric adenocarcinoma?

Despite some conflicting reports, people with *H. pylori* infection appear to have a twofold increase in the risk of acquiring gastric adenocarcinoma.

4. What is the role of achlorhydria in gastric cancer?

Achlorhydria is generally caused by immune destruction of the parietal cells. Antiparietal cell antibodies and elevated gastrin levels can be found in the serum, and patients have associated B12 deficiency. Other causes include destruction after long bouts of infection with *H. pylori*. People with achlorhydria have a 4–6-fold increase in the incidence of gastric cancers.

5. Who should be screened for gastric cancer?

Screening is performed in Japan in middle-aged people and is recommended on an annual basis over the age of 50 years. There are no screening recommendations for distal gastric adenocarcinoma in the United States, and no recommendations are widely accepted for the screening of immigrants from high risk areas. Screening for proximal gastric cancer is probably warranted in people with a longstanding history of reflux symptoms.

6. What is gastric stump cancer?

After partial gastric resection, the incidence of gastric cancers at the sight of the intestinal-gastric anastomosis appears to be increased by about twofold greater. However, this increase is not apparent until at least 15 years after surgery. In the initial 5 years after partial gastrectomy, there may be an actual decrease in cancer risk. These data suggest a certain background rate of gastric cancer formation. If part of the stomach is removed, less mucosa is at risk for malignant transformation. However, the surgery then imparts a procancer effect, and over time more and more cancers start to form in the remaining mucosa.

7. How is the incidence of gastric adenocarcinoma changing?

Gastric adenocarcinoma has two major sights of presentation—either proximally in the stomach near the esophagogastric junction or distally in the stomach in the antrum. Worldwide, adenocarcinoma of the distal stomach is one of the most common malignancies; in the United States, however, this presentation has markedly decreased over the past several decades. Conversely, proximal gastric adenocarcinoma has been increasing rapidly increasing in the United States, probably in relation to reflux of gastric contents.

8. Describe the staging scheme for gastric adenocarcinoma.

Tumor-node-metastasis (TNM) staging is generally used. T-stage is primarily determined by the relation of the tumor to the muscularis propria (above, into, or through). N-stage is determined by the number and location of affected nodes. M-stage is determined by whether distant metastases are present.

9. What is the role of surgery in treating localized gastric adenocarcinoma?

Surgery is a potential curative therapy for localized gastric adenocarcinoma. The prognosis is based on TNM staging. The extent of resection is somewhat controversial. Japanese literature suggests that an extended lymphadenectomy plus omentectomy (D2 operation) is superior to a limited lymphadenectomy with omentectomy (D1 procedure) or limited lymphadenectomy (D0 procedure). In a randomized European study, patients undergoing D2 resection had twice the operative mortality as those undergoing D1 resection. There was no survival benefit.

10. What is the role of neoadjuvant therapy in gastric adenocarcinoma?

Neoadjuvant therapy is treatment given prior to an attempt at curative surgical resection to make the primary tumor smaller and possibly to treat small foci of disease outside the operative field. Although the concept is attractive, definitive studies demonstrating the utility of neoadjuvant therapy for gastric cancer have not been performed.

11. What is the role of adjuvant therapy in gastric adenocarcinoma?

Adjuvant therapy is additional treatment given to patients after attempted curative surgery. Adjuvant treatment is given if there is no evidence of remaining disease, but the risk of relapse is high. Several Japanese studies have shown a benefit for postoperative adjuvant therapy in gastric cancer, usually with mitomycin-containing regimens. In western studies, however, adjuvant therapy has not yet been shown to provide a definite advantage. Studies are ongoing.

12. What is the usual therapy for metastatic gastric adenocarcinoma?

Chemotherapy can be used with modest benefits. Several regimens have activity in gastric adenocarcinoma, using drugs such as 5-fluorouracil, etoposide, platinum-containing drugs, and taxanes.

13. What is a MALToma?

MALTomas are **m**ucosal-**a**ssociated **l**ymphoid **t**umors. They can occur in any mucosal location, both within and outside the gastrointestinal tract. MALTomas are often low-grade B-cell lymphomas but also may be high-grade aggressive tumors.

14. What is special about gastric MALTomas?

Gastric MALTomas, unlike MALTomas in other locations, often are associated with infection by H. pylori. Lymphoid tissue is not a normal part of gastric epithelium, and infection with *H. pylori* seems to drive lymphoid proliferation and tumor development.

15. What is the role of antibiotic therapy in gastric MALTomas?

Treatment of *H. pylori* infection usually leads to regression of low-grade B-cell gastric MALToma. It is believed that the low-grade tumors retain responsiveness to *H. pylori* antigen stimulation. Complete responses can take up to 18 months after antibiotic therapy. High-grade gastric MALTomas and those with more acquired chromosomal abnormalities do not respond well to antibacterial therapy.

16. Describe the staging scheme for gastric lymphoma.

Several staging systems are used for gastric lymphoma, including TNM staging (as for gastric adenocarcinoma). A clinical staging system used for non-Hodgkin's lymphoma (the Ann Arbor Classification) is also available. The Ann Arbor system identifies the primary site of lymphoma as nodal or extranodal and assesses extent of disease based on number of sites involved, relation of the tumor to the diaphragm, and whether disease has metastasized to nonlymphoid organs. In the Ann Arbor system, a lymphoma involving both the stomach and a lymph node may be stage 2E (two sites with extranodal primary) or stage 4 (nodal primary with metastasis to the stomach). A new staging system that combines TNM staging with Ann Arbor criteria has recently been recommended for gastrointesintal lymphomas.

17. What is the best therapy for aggressive (non-MALT) gastric lymphoma?

Therapy is determined somewhat by stage. For most cases of Ann Arbor stages I and II, surgery can be curative. However, recent data suggest that chemotherapy with or without radiation therapy can be equally effective. T-stage is also important because of the possibility of perforation when chemotherapy is used for T3 or T4 tumors. The trend is away from surgery for all stages.

18. What are gastric carcinoid tumors?

Gastric carcinoid tumors are growths of neuroendocrine cells that may be benign or malignant. They stain for chromogranin. As a rule, even the malignant tumors are slow growing. Tumors > 1 cm in diameter are generally more aggressive, whereas smaller tumors are not and may represent endochromagraffin cell hyperplasia. Tumors > 2 cm often have metastasized. Management depends on whether an elevated gastrin level is present and the size of the primary tumor. High gastrin levels confer a more benign prognosis than tumors in patients with low gastrin levels. As a rule, large tumors often require gastrectomy, whereas smaller tumors can be managed endoscopically.

19. What causes gastric carcinoid tumors?

Two processes appear to lead to gastric carcinoid: de novo malignant transformation and loss of normal growth regulation in response to chronic elevation of serum gastrin levels. Tumors arising from de novo malignant transformation are usually single, larger, and more aggressive, whereas those arising from elevated gastrin levels are often multiple and smaller. It is important to distinguish between the two types.

20. What is the role of diet in the development of gastric cancer?

Dietary factors appear to be important in the development of gastric cancer. In general, the incidence of gastric cancer is higher when a higher proportion of the diet is obtained from salted or smoked meats or fish. Fruits and vegetables appear to be protective. Tobacco smoking appears to increase the risk of gastric cancer. Dietary factors are thought to explain a large part of the variation in incidence of gastric cancers from country to country. Immigration from high-incidence countries to lower-incidence countries decreases the risk of gastric cancer risk.

BIBLIOGRAPHY

1. American Joint Committee on Cancer. Handbook for Staging of Cancer. In Beahrs OH, Henson DE, Hutter RVP, Kennedy BJ (ed): The Manual for Staging of Cancer. Philadelphia, J.B. Lippincott, 1998, pp 72–80.
2. Blot WJ, Devesa SS, Kneller RW, Fraumeni JF Jr: Rising incidence of adenocarcinoma of the esophagus and gastric cardia [see comments]. JAMA 265:1287–1289, 1991.
3. Crump M, Gospodarowicz M, Shepherd FA: Lymphoma of the gastrointestinal tract. Semin Oncol 26:324–337, 1999.
4. Cuschieri A, Fayers P, Fielding J, et al: Postoperative morbidity and mortality after D1 and D2 resections for gastric cancer: Preliminary results of the MRC randomised controlled surgical trial. The Surgical Cooperative Group [see comments]. Lancet 347:995–999, 1996.
5. Devesa SS, Blot WJ, Fraumeni JF Jr: Changing patterns in the incidence of esophageal and gastric carcinoma in the United States. Cancer 83:2049–2053, 1998.
6. El-Serag HB, Sonnenberg A: Ethnic variations in the occurrence of gastroesophageal cancers [see comments]. J Clin Gastroenterol 28:135–139, 1999.
7. Eslick GD, Lim LL, Byles JE, et al: Association of *Helicobacter pylori* infection with gastric carcinoma: A meta-analysis. Am J Gastroenterol 94:2373–2379, 1999.
8. Fuchs CS, Mayer RJ. Gastric carcinoma [see comments]. N Engl J Med 333:32–41, 1995.
9. Granberg D, Wilander E, Stridsberg M, et al: Clinical symptoms, hormone profiles, treatment, and prognosis in patients with gastric carcinoids. Gut 43:223–228, 1998.
10. Hanazaki K, Sodeyama H, Mochizuki Y, et al: Efficacy of extended lymphadenectomy in the noncurative gastrectomy for advanced gastric cancer. Hepatogastroenterology 46:2677–2682, 1999.
11. Isaacson PG: Gastric MALT lymphoma: From concept to cure. Ann Oncol 10:637–645, 1999.
12. Kelsen DP: Adjuvant and neoadjuvant therapy for gastric cancer. Semin Oncol 23:379–389, 1996.
13. Kulke MH, Mayer RJ: Carcinoid tumors [see comments]. N Engl J Med 340:858–868, 1999.

14. Lauffer JM, Zhang T, Modlin IM: Review article: Current status of gastrointestinal carcinoids. Aliment Pharmacol Ther 13:271–287, 1999.
15. Lowy AM, Leach SD: Adjuvant/neoadjuvant chemoradiation for gastric and pancreatic cancer. Oncology (Huntington) 13:121–130, 1999.
16. Moradi T, Delfino RJ, Bergstrom SR, et al: Cancer risk among Scandinavian immigrants in the US and Scandinavian residents compared with US whites, 1973–89. Eur J Cancer Prev 7:117–125, 1998.
17. Pisani P, Parkin DM, Bray F, Ferlay J: Estimates of the worldwide mortality from 25 cancers in 1990. Int J Cancer 83:18–29, 1999.
18. Reed PI: Diet and gastric cancer. Adv Exp Med Biol 348:123–132, 1993.
19. Rohatiner A, d'Amore F, Coiffier B, et al. Report on a workshop convened to discuss the pathological and staging classifications of gastrointestinal tract lymphoma. Ann Oncol 5:397–400, 1994.
20. Rotterdam H: Carcinoma of the stomach. In Rotterdam H, Enterline HT (eds): Pathology of the Stomach and Duodenum. New York, Springer-Verlag, 1989, pp 142–204.
21. Safatle-Ribeiro AV, Ribeiro U Jr, Reynolds JC: Gastric stump cancer: What is the risk? Dig Dis 16:159–168, 1998.
22. Svendsen JH, Dahl C, Svendsen LB, Christiansen PM: Gastric cancer risk in achlorhydric patients: A long-term follow-up study. Scand J Gastroenterol 21:16–20, 1986.
23. Vanagunas A: Eradication of *Helicobacter pylori* and regression of B-cell lymphoma. Biomed Pharmacother 51:156–160, 1997.
24. Vaquerano J, Esemuede N, Odocha O, Leffall LD: Gastric carcinoma in African Americans: A 10-year single center analysis. In Vivo 10:233–235, 1996.
25. Wils J: The treatment of advanced gastric cancer. Semin Oncol 23:397–406, 1996.
26. Zinzani PL, Magagnoli M, Galieni P, et al: Nongastrointestinal low-grade mucosa-associated lymphoid tissue lymphoma: Analysis of 75 patients. J Clin Oncol 17:1254–1260, 1999.

12. PEPTIC ULCER DISEASE AND HELICOBACTER PYLORI

Suzanne Miller, M.D., and David A. Peura, M.D.

1. What is *Helicobacter pylori*?

H. pylori (previously classified as *Campylobacter pylori*) is a spiral-shaped, gram-negative bacterium, 0.5 microns in width and 2–6.5 microns in length. Its main distinguishing features are multiple sheathed, unipolar flagella and potent urease activity. The organism's shape and flagella allow penetration of and movement through the gastric mucus layer. Its urease activity appears essential for colonization and survival. Urease also forms the basis for diagnostic testing for infection. Although gastric bacteria were first described in the human stomach at the turn of the century, their importance in peptic ulcer disease and chronic gastritis was not appreciated until the early 1980s. *H. pylori* was first successfully cultured in 1982 by Marshall and Warren.

2. Do any other *Helicobacter*-like organisms cause disease?

A number of other *Helicobacter* species have been identified, mostly in animals. *H. hepaticus* and *H. bilis* induce inflammatory bowel disease in mice. Studies to determine the possible association with this disease in humans are under way. *H. pullorum* and *H. hepaticus* are associated with hepatitis in chickens and mice, respectively. In ferrets, *H. mustelae* causes gastritis. Other *Helicobacter* species isolated in humans include *H. fennelliae, H. westmeadii,* and *H. cinaedi*, grown from blood cultures of bacteremic patients. In Chile a *Helicobacter* species has been isolated from gallbladder mucosa of patients with chronic cholecystitis. *H. heilmanni* has been shown to cause gastritis, gastric ulcers, and rarely mucosa-associated lymphoid tissue (MALT) lymphoma. The relevance of *Helicobacter* species in human disease is an increasing area of research.

3. What is the worldwide prevalence of *H. pylori*?

H. pylori infection is estimated to be present in 50% of the world's adult population. The geographic distribution of *H. pylori* is closely correlated with socioeconomic development (see figure on following page). In developing countries, the prevalence of infection may reach levels of 80–90% by 20 years of age. This prevalence remains constant for the rest of adult life. In contrast, in developed countries the prevalence of *H. pylori* infection is less than 20% in people below the age of 25 years and increases about 1% per year to about 50–60% by age 70. Incidence data from developing countries appear to be subject to generational bias; primary infection is acquired during childhood, but each successive birth cohort is less likely to develop infection. Within a given geographic area, incidence appears to be affected by racial and ethnic factors. For example, in the United States, African-Americans and Hispanics acquire infection earlier in life and more frequently than Caucasians.

4. Are children ever infected by *H. pylori*?

Most infection is probably acquired during childhood, usually by the age of 5 years. Anti-*Helicobacter* antibodies have been demonstrated in neonates, but they probably represent placental transfer of maternal antibodies rather than primary infection. Familial clustering of *H. pylori* infection is common, and siblings and parents of infected children are more likely to be infected. Members of the same family have been demonstrated to be infected with the same strain of *H. pylori*.

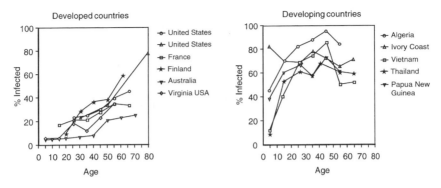

Seroprevalence of *H. pylori* infection in developed and developing countries. (From Marshall BJ, et al: *H. pylori* in Peptic Ulceration and Gastritis. Boston, Blackwell, 1991, pp 46–58. Reprinted with permission of the American Digestive Health Foundation.)

5. What are the risk factors for *H. pylori* infection?

Low socioeconomic status, crowded living conditions, and suboptimal sanitary conditions appear to be major risk factors. Gastroenterologists have a higher than expected prevalence of infection, possibly from contact with infected gastric secretions and endoscopic equipment. Such transmission is less likely now that most physicians adhere to universal precautions during endoscopic procedures. No evidence links *H. pylori* infection to gender, smoking, alcohol, or particular diet. Studies in monozygotic and dizygotic twins raised in the same and different environments have supported genetic susceptibility to infection.

6. How is infection transmitted?

The exact mode of transmission is not known, but most data support fecal-oral or oral-oral routes. The higher than anticipated prevalence in institutionalized people, familial clustering of infection, association with crowded living conditions, and documented transmission from contaminated devices such as endoscopes suggest person-to-person spread. Humans appear to be the major reservoir of *H. pylori,* although the organism has been isolated from domestic cats and primates. The organism remains viable in water for several days and thus municipal water supplies may serve as a source of infection.

7. Where in the gastrointestinal (GI) tract does *H. pylori* live?

H. pylori primarily colonizes the stomach and is well adapted to survive in this otherwise hostile environment. The organism lives within or beneath the gastric mucus layer, somewhat protected from stomach acid, and generally does not invade the epithelial cells. *H. pylori* has potent urease activity, which hydrolyzes urea to ammonia and bicarbonate and increases its resistance to the stomach's low pH environment. *H. pylori* recognizes and binds to specific receptors expressed by gastric epithelial cells and, therefore, is able to adhere tightly to the epithelial cell surface. The organism has been found adherent to ectopic gastric epithelium throughout the GI tract, i.e., esophagus (Barrett's esophagus), duodenum (gastric metaplasia), small intestine (Meckel's diverticulum), and rectum (ectopic patches of gastric mucosa).

8. What invasive tests can be used to diagnose *H. pylori* infection?

Histopathologic examination is widely available, and specimens are easy to store. Organisms can be detected with standard hematoxylin and eosin stains or special stains, such as Giemsa or Warthin-Starry, which make the organisms easier to identify. The sensitivity and specificity of histopathology for *H. pylori* are greater than 95% but may be influenced by sampling error, number of organisms present, use of certain medications, and experience of the pathologist.

Rapid urease testing relies on the potent urease activity of *H. pylori* when a gastric biopsy specimen is placed in medium containing urea and a colored pH indicator. If the organism is present, the urease hydrolyzes urea to bicarbonate and ammonia, increasing the pH and changing the color of the pH indicator. The number of organisms present, use of certain medications, and sampling error may influence urease testing. The sensitivity of the rapid urease test is ~90%; its specificity is 100%.

9. What is the role of culure of *H. pylori* from gastric biopsy?

Culture of *H. pylori* from gastric biopsy is difficult, requiring incubation for 3–5 days in special medium in a controlled microaerophilic environment. With easier diagnostic methods available, culture is not clinically useful for diagnosis and is reserved for determining antibiotic sensitivities in resistant organisms.

10. How is *H. pylori* diagnosed noninvasively?

Serology involves obtaining a serum sample from the patient. IgG or IgA antibodies directed at various bacterial antigens can be detected by enzyme-linked immunosorbent assay (ELISA). In addition, several office-based serologic methods are commercially available. Serologic methods detect evidence of primary *H. pylori* infection in untreated people with sensitivity and specificity > 90%. Although antibody levels may fall after successful bacterial eradication, they remain elevated for up to 3 years. This "serologic scar" limits the usefulness of serology in assessing treatment and determining reinfection.

Urea blood or breath tests are ideally suited to make a primary diagnosis of infection, to monitor treatment response, and to assess reinfection, because they are positive only in a setting of active infection. The patient ingests a small amount of carbon-labeled (13C or 14C) urea. The urease of *H. pylori* hydrolyzes the urea and liberates labeled carbon dioxide, which is absorbed and exhaled in the breath. Labeled carbon dioxide can be collected and quantified in blood or breath samples. Sensitivity and specificity of urea blood or breath testing are > 95%.

Stool antigen testing is becoming increasingly popular. It is accurate (sensitivity and specificity = 90% and 98%, respectively) and inexpensive. The test is based on polymerase chain reaction amplification of specific *H. pylori antigens* in stool samples. Stool antigen testing is useful in primary diagnosis and confirmation of eradication of the organism after antibiotic treatment.

Diagnostic Test for H. pylori

TEST	SENSITIVITY (%)	SPECIFICITY (%)	RELATIVE COST
Noninvasive			
Serology	88–99	86–95	$
Urea breath test	90–97	90–100	$$
Stool antigen test	90	98	$
Invasive			
Rapid urease assay	89–98	93–98	$$$$*
Histology	93–99	95–99	$$$$$*
Culture	77–92	100	$$$$$*

* Includes cost of endoscopy.
Reprinted with permission of the American Digestive Health Foundation. (Adapted from Brown K, Peura D: Diagnosis of *Helicobacter pylori* infection. Gastroenterol Clin North Am 22:105– 116, 1993.)

11. Do any medications affect diagnostic *H. pylori* testing?

Use of antibiotics, bismuth-containing compounds, or proton pump inhibitors (PPIs) can suppress *H. pylori*, leading to false-negative results with rapid urease testing, histopathology, urea blood or breath testing, and stool antigen testing. Ideally diagnostic testing should be performed at least 4 weeks after the discontinuance of any antibiotics and 2 weeks after the discontinuation of proton pump inhibitors. Multiple biopsies from two regions or more of the stomach can improve the sensitivity of histologic examination or rapid urease testing when patients are taking any of these agents at the time of testing.

12. What is the association of *H. pylori* with histologic gastritis?

Infection with *H. pylori* produces an active chronic gastritis with intraepithelial and interstitial neutrophils in addition to lymphocytes and plasma cells. In most people, gastritis remains confined to the antrum. In others, however, it may progress to involve the entire stomach. Patients with antral gastritis alone are more likely to develop subsequent duodenal ulcers, whereas patients with pangastritis, especially in association with atrophy and intestinal metaplasia, are at risk for gastric ulcers and adenocarcinoma.

13. Does *H. pylori* play a role in gastric ulcers?

Most gastric ulcers (60–90%) occur in the setting of *H. pylori* gastritis. *H. pylori* makes the gastric mucosal layer more susceptible to acid injury through various mechanisms. Direct adherence of the organism to epithelial cells, ammonia produced by the urease enzyme, and bacterial cytotoxins may damage epithelial cell membranes. Other bacterial enzymes disrupt the protective mucus barrier, rendering the underlying mucosal surface more susceptible to acid injury. Further damage may result from the local and systemic inflammatory response to infection.

14. Describe the association of *H. pylori* with duodenal ulcer disease.

The association is quite strong. Infection increases serum gastrin levels, which results in increased gastric acid production by parietal cells. Excessive acid production leads to damage of duodenal mucosa over time with subsequent development of duodenal gastric metaplasia. *H. pylori* may infect these duodenal "patches" of gastric mucosa, leading to duodenitis and eventual duodenal ulceration. Elimination of either gastric acid or infection can prevent duodenal ulcers due to *H. pylori*.

15. Does *H. pylori* play a role in gastric cancer?

Gastric cancer is the second most common cancer in the world. Unfortunately it still carries a poor prognosis, and treatment options are limited. Patients with *H. pylori* infection have been repeatedly reported to have a 3–6-fold higher incidence of gastric cancer. The World Health Organization has classified *H. pylori* as a group I carcinogen. The chronic gastritis produced by *H. pylori* results in increased DNA turnover and free radical generation. Infection with *H. pylori* also results in decreased secretion of vitamin C, a known antioxidant, in gastric juice. Over time these factors lead to mutation of gastric epithelial cells and development of adenocarcinoma.

16. Describe the association of *H. pylori* with MALT lymphoma.

The association is strong. It is believed that the chronic inflammation produced by the organism leads to a monoclonal neoplasm of inflammatory cells. Eradication of *H. pylori* infection results in regression of or cure of this type of tumor in 90% of patients when it is superficial and of low histologic grade.

17. What may cause ulcers besides *H. pylori*?

Most *H. pylori*-negative gastric ulcers are associated with NSAIDs. However, both adenocarcinoma and lymphoma can cause gastric ulceration and should be excluded. As the prevalence of *H. pylori* decreases, *H. pylori*-negative duodenal ulcers are more commonly encountered and now account for 20–40% of duodenal ulcers. They are often due to NSAIDs, hypersecretory conditions such as Zollinger-Ellison syndrome, or unusual manifestations of conditions such as Crohn's disease. True idiopathic duodenal ulcers may be genetically determined and are characterized by hypersecretion of acid, rapid gastric emptying, poor response to traditional treatment, frequent recurrence, and clinical complications.

18. Can infected people develop symptoms even without a detectable ulcer?

Nonulcer dyspepsia (NUD) is a poorly defined clinical entity, probably with multiple causes. Evidence that *H. pylori* gastritis causes dyspepsia in the absence of an ulcer has been difficult to obtain, because no specific symptoms separate *H. pylori*-related dyspepsia from other forms of nonulcer dyspepsia. In addition, the effect of treatment for *H. pylori* infection on NUD symptoms has been unreliable. Nevertheless, a subset of patients with NUD certainly has symptoms related to infection and responds to treatment. Unfortunately, at present we cannot reliably identify such patients.

19. Why do only a few infected people develop clinical disease?

All infected people develop histologic evidence of active chronic gastritis. However, only a minority develop clinically obvious symptoms. At present, it is unknown whether host factors, such as immune response or genetic susceptibility, or infection with more virulent bacterial strains is the major determinant of clinical illness. Recent data suggest that specific pleomorphism of IL1-B can be a genetic risk for *H. pylori*, resulting in low acid output and subsequent development of gastric cancer.

20. In what situation is it appropriate to eradicate *H. pylori* infection?

Patients with active or past ulcer disease should be tested for *H. pylori* and treated if positive. Patients who experience any ulcer-related complication also should be tested and treated if positive. Patients with low-grade MALT lymphoma should be tested and treated becuause eradication of *H. pylori* may result in a cure of the lymphoma. Controversial areas are patients younger than age 50 with dyspepsia and patients at increased risk of gastric cancer (i.e., positive family history or gastric metaplasia on prior biopsies). Current data are insufficient to recommend treatment of all infected patients with nonulcer dyspepsia or asymptomatic people to prevent subsequent ulcer disease or gastric neoplasia. Treatment decisions should be made on a case-by-case basis.

21. What role does treatment of *H. pylori* infection play in complicated ulcer disease?

Complications such as bleeding from peptic ulcers are associated with significant morbidity and mortality. Data suggest that once complicated ulcers have healed, maintenance antisecretory therapy reduces the likelihood of recurrent complication; preliminary studies show that eradicating *H. pylori* also may be effective in preventing ulcer complications. However, many complicated ulcers are due to NSAIDs and not *H. pylori* alone; therefore, patients who require chronic NSAID therapy may be at risk for recurrent complications despite the eradication of *H.pylori*. Such patients may be best treated with *H. pylori* eradication and chronic antisecretory therapy or with the new COX-2 inhibitors.

22. What treatment regimens have been used to eradicate *H. pylori*?

The FDA has approved both dual and triple drug therapies. The dual therapies consist of one antibiotic with a PPI. Triple therapies consist of two antibiotics and a PPI. Antibiotics studied include amoxicillin, clarithromycin, tetracycline, and metronidazole. Even though approved by the FDA, dual therapies have lower efficacy than triple therapies and have no role in first-line treatment of *H. pylori*. First-line therapy should consist of a PPI, clarithromycin, and amoxicillin (PCA). In patients allergic to penicillin, a PPI, clarithromycin, and metronidazole (PCM) can be used. Bismuth, metronidazole, tetracycline, and a PPI (BMT+PPI) are considered second-line therapy. The dose of metronidazole in BMT+ PPI therapy should be increased to 500 mg 4 times/day to overcome *H. pylori* resistance to metronidazole. The choice of eradication therapy should be based on efficacy, ease of compliance, side-effect profile and cost.

Therapeutic Options

REGIMEN	DRUGS	DOSAGE	DURATION
First-line therapy			
Standard triple therapy	PPI (Omeprazole)	20 mg 2 times/day	2 weeks
	Clarithromycin	500 mg 2 times/day	2 weeks
	Amoxicillin or	1 gm 2 times/day	2 weeks
	Metronidazole	500 mg 2 times/day	
	(if penicillin allergic)		
	or		
Prevpac (prepackaged triple therapy)	Lansoprazole	30 mg 2 times/day	2 weeks
	Amoxicillin	1 gm 2 times/day	
	Clarithromycin	500 mg 2 times/day	

Table continued on following page

Therapeutic Options (Continued)

REGIMEN	DRUGS	DOSAGE	DURATION
Second-line therapy			
Standard triple therapy plus PPI	Pepto-Bismol	2 tablets 4 times/day	2 weeks
	Metronidazole	250 mg 4 times/day	
	Tetracycline or	500 mg 4 times/day or	
	Amoxicillin	500 mg 4 times/day	
	Plus Lansoprazole or	30 mg 2 times/day	
	Omeprazole	20 mg 2 times/day	
Standard triple therapy plus ranitidine *(acute ulcer)*	To standard triple therapy, add H_2RA	Full dose at bedtime	2 weeks, then 4–6 weeks treatment with H_2RA alone
Dual therapy with acid pump inhibitor	Omeprazole	20 mg 2 times/day	
	Amoxicillin (dosed concurrently) *or*	500–750 mg 4 times/day	2 weeks
	Omeprazole	20 mg 2 times/day	
	Clarithromycin (dosed concurrently	500 mg 3 times/day	
Dual therapy with acid pump inhibitor *(acute ulcer)*	Omeprazole	20 mg twice daily	2 weeks
	Amoxicillin (dosed concurrently) *or*	500–750 mg 4 times/day	
	Omeprazole	20 mg twice daily	2 weeks, then 2 weeks treatment with omeprazole alone (20 mg/day) *or* 4–6 weeks treatment with full-dose H_2RA
	Clarithromycin (dosed concurrently)	500 mg 3 times/day	

From *Helicobacter pylori*: The New Factor in Management of Ulcer Disease, 1994, Digestive Health Initiative.

23. How should eradication of *H. pylori* be confirmed?

Once therapy for *H. pylori* eradication is complete, cure of the infection should be confirmed noninvasively unless confirmation of ulcer healing is clinically necessary as well. Urea blood or breath testing and stool antigen testing are appropriate for this purpose.

24. What happens to peptic ulcer disease when *H. pylori* infection is eradicated?

The annual recurrence rate of healed gastric ulcers in *H. pylori*-infected patients is 59%. The rate of recurrence of duodenal ulcers after healing is approximately 67%. The rate can be reduced to 25% with chronic acid suppression therapy. If *H. pylori* is eradicated, recurrence of gastric and duodenal ulcers has been reported to be approximately 4% and 6% per year, respectively. However, data from United States trials suggest that the true recurrence rate after cure of infection may be closer to 20% for duodenal ulcer.

25. Is reinfection a common problem?

Rates of reinfection after eradication vary geographically, but even in developing countries the annual recurrence rate is typically less than 5%. In developed countries, such as the U.S., once infection has been eliminated, the annual rate of reinfection is very low (0.5–3%).

26. What is the role of vaccination in the prevention of *H. pylori*?

Vaccines against *H. pylori* have proved effective in preventing infection in animals, but no safe vaccine is available for large-scale human use. This is an important area of research.

27. What role does *H. pylori* play in gastroesophageal reflux disease (GERD)?

H. pylori may be protective against GERD or reduce its severity, because the ammonia it produces may buffer gastric acid. The bacteria also appear to augment the effect of antisecretory drugs, H2 blockers, and proton pump inhibitors. Some patients who have no reflux symptoms and peptic ulcer disease may develop GERD once treated with an eradication regimen for *H. pylori*.

28. Is *H. pylori* associated with any diseases outside the GI tract in humans?

Many studies report an association between *H. pylori* and ischemic heart disease. Although the studies vary in methods and results, there appears to be a consistent 10–20% excessive risk of ischemic heart disease in patients infected with *H. pylori*. It is theorized that higher serum cytokine levels induced by *H. pylori* infection lead to increased systemic inflammatory responses and atherosclerosis. Idiopathic chronic urticaria, as well as acne rosacea and alopecia areata, have been linked to *H. pylori* infection. In some patients, urticaria has improved with the eradication of *H. pylori*, but the results with alopecia and rosacea are less striking. Raynaud's phenomenon and migraine headaches have been observed to improve with treatment of *H. pylori*, although no controlled studies have been performed in these or any other extraintestinal conditions.

BIBLIOGRAPHY

 1. Blecker U, Lanciers S, Mahta D, et al: Familial clusters of *Helicobacter pylori* infections. Clin Pediatr 33:307–308, 1994.
 2. Brown K, Peura D: Diagnosis of *Helicobacter pylori* infection. Gastroenterol Clin North Am 22:105– 116, 1993.
 3. Chang MC, Wu MS, Wang Hp, Lin JT: *Helicobacter pylori* stool antigen (HpSA) test: A simple, accurate, and non-invasive test for detection of *Helicobacter pylori* infection. Hepatogastroenterology 46:299–302, 1999.
 4. Ciocola AA, McSorley DJ, Turner K, et al: *Helicobacter pylori* infection rates in duodenal ulcer patients in the U.S. may be lower than previously estimated. Am J Gastroenterol 94:1834–1840, 1999.
 5. Dixon MF: Pathophysiology of *Helicobacter pylori* infection. Scand J Gastroenterol 29(Suppl 201):7– 10, 1994.
 6. El-Omar EM, Carrington M, Chow W, et al: Interleukin-1 polymorphisms associated with increased risk of gastric cancer. Nature 404:398–402, 2000.
 7. Fallone CA, Barkun AN, Friedman G, et al: Is *Helicobacter pylori* eradication associated with gastroesophageal reflux disease? Am J Gastroenterol 95:914–920, 2000.
 8. Forbes GM, Gluner ME, Cullen DJ, et al: Duodenal ulcer treated with *H. pylori* eradication: Seven-year follow-up. Lancet 343:258–260, 1994.
 9. Gasbarrini A, Franceschi F, Armuzzi A, et al: Extra digestive manifestations of *Helicobacter pylori* gastric infection. Gut 45(Suppl I):I9–12, 1999.
10. Laine L, Estrada R, Trujillo M, et al: Effect of proton-pump inhibitor therapy on diagnostic testing for *Helicobacter pylori*. Ann Intern Med 129:547–550, 1998.
11. Marshall BJ, Warren JR: Unidentified curved bacilli in the stomach of patients with gastritis and peptic ulceration. Lancet 1:1311–1315, 1984.
12. Marshall BJ, et al (eds): *Helicobacter pylori* in Peptic Ulceration and Gastritis. Boston, Blackwell Scientific, 1991.
13. McColl K: *Helicobacter pylori*: Clinical aspects. J Infect 34:7–13, 1997.
14. Moss SF, Calam J: Acid secretion and sensitivity to gastrin in patients with duodenal ulcer: Effect of eradication of *H. pylori*. Gut 34:888–892, 1993.
15. NIH Consensus Development Panel on *Helicobacter pylori* in Peptic Ulcer Disease: *Helicobacter pylori* in peptic ulcer disease. JAMA 272:65–69, 1994.
16. Northfield TC, Mendall M, Goggin PM (eds): *Helicobacter* Infection: Pathophysiology, Epidemiology and Management. Boston, Kluwer Academic, 1993.
17. McColl K, Murray L, El-Omar E, et al: Symptomatic benefit from eradicating *Helicobacter pylori* infection in patients with non-ulcer dyspepsia. N Engl J Med 339:1869–1874, 1998.
18. Peura D: *Helicobacter pylori*: Rational Management Options. Am J Med 105:424–430, 1998.
19. Rathbone BJ, Heathley RV (eds): *Helicobacter pylori* and Gastrointestinal Disease. Boston, Blackwell Scientific, 1992.
20. Walsh JH, Peterson WI: The treatment of *Helicobacter pylori* infection in the management of peptic ulcer disease. N Engl J Med 333:984–991, 1995.

13. GASTRIC POLYPS AND THICKENED GASTRIC FOLDS

Gregory G. Ginsberg, M.D.

1. What are gastric polyps?

Gastric polyps are any abnormal growth of epithelial tissue arising from the otherwise smooth surface of the stomach. Gastric polyps may be sessile or pedunculated. **Hyperplastic** polyps (Fig. 1) account for 70–90% of gastric polyps. **Adenomatous, fundic gland** (Fig. 2), and **hamartomatous** polyps make up the remainder. Early **gastric cancers** may present as polypoid lesions. Gastric polyps may be singular or multiple. Although endoscopic features may predict histology, accurate discrimination of polyp type can be achieved only with tissue sampling and, in some cases, only after complete resection of the polyp.

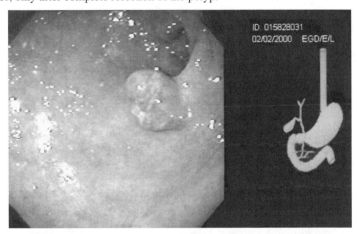

FIGURE 1.   Sessile hyperplastic polyp with superficial inflammatory changes is seen in the antrum.

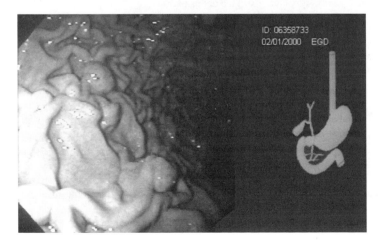

FIGURE 2.   Two fundic gland polyps are seen among normal-appearing gastric rugae in the fundus.

73

2. Describe the histologic features of each type of gastric polyp.

Hyperplastic polyps consist of hyperplastic, elongated gastric glands with abundant edematous stroma. There is often cystic dilation of glandular portions but no alteration of the original cellular configuration. **Adenomatous** polyps are true neoplastic growths composed of dysplastic epithelium not normally present in the stomach. They are composed of cells with hyperchromatic, elongated nuclei arranged in picket-fence patterns with increased mitotic figures. **Fundic gland** polyps are composed of hypertrophied fundic gland mucosa and are considered a normal variant. **Hamartomatous** polyps have branching bands of smooth muscle surrounded by glandular epithelium; the lamina propria is normal.

3. What is the risk of malignancy associated with gastric polyps?

The risk of malignant transformation in **hyperplastic** polyps is low (0.6–4.5%). **Adenomas** are true neoplasms. The risk of malignant transformation is as high as 75% and size-dependent; size > 2.0 cm is critically significant, although carcinoma arising in adenomatous polyps < 2.0 cm is well reported. Fundic gland polyps are generally benign; however, rare cases of malignant transformation have been reported in large fundic gland polyps and in association with familial adenomatous polyposis (FAP) syndromes. Gastric **hamartomas** are thought to have no malignant potential.

4. How should gastric polyps be managed?

Because polyp histology cannot be reliably distinguished by endoscopic appearance or forceps biopsy sampling, most gastric epithelial polyps should be entirely excised endoscopically if feasible. Gastric epithelial polyps with a diameter of 3–5 mm may be removed entirely by multiple forceps biopsies. Sessile and pedunculated polyps > 5.0 mm in diameter should be excised by **snare resection** and tissue retrieved for histologic evaluation. Endoscopic ultrasound (EUS) may be used adjunctively to confirm the epithelial origin of the lesion before resection. Larger, broad-based polyps that cannot be safely removed endoscopically should undergo surgical excision. When numerous gastric polyps are present, resection or biopsy should be performed on the largest lesions, and a sufficient number sampled to confirm benignity and uniformity of histology. Hyperplastic and adenomatous gastric polyps occur against a background of chronic gastritis and, in some instances, intestinal metaplasia. Thus the risk of cancer in the gastric mucosa apart from the polyp is increased. This association is greater with adenomatous than hyperplastic gastric polyps and increases with age. Therefore, in addition to removing all polyps, a careful exam should be performed to evaluate the remaining gastric mucosa, and biopsies should be obtained from any areas displaying surface abnormalities.

5. Is surveillance indicated for patients with gastric polyps?

Although data are insufficient to demonstrate a long-term benefit from endoscopic surveillance, in selected patients it is appropriate. The detection of intestinal metaplasia in the surrounding gastric mucosa—and even more so atypia or dysplasia—must be considered. Endoscopic surveillance, if undertaken, should be performed no less than every 2–3 years in the absence of dysplasia.

6. Describe the relationships between gastric polyps and other conditions.

Gastric adenomatous and hyperplastic polyps commonly appear against a background of chronic gastritis and are late manifestations of *Helicobacter pylori* infection or type A chronic gastritis (pernicious anemia). Multiple mucosal biopsies should be obtained to determine the presence and severity of underlying gastritis with the emphasis on identifying the presence and type of intestinal metaplasia. *H. pylori* eradication should be attempted for patients with *H. pylori* gastritis and gastric polyps, although it is uncertain whether eradication positively affects polyp recurrence or metaplasia.

Gastric hyperplastic, adenomatous, and fundic gland polyps have an increased prevalence in patients with FAP and attenuated FAP syndromes. The relationship between FAP and fundic gland polyps appears more prominent in Japanese than Western populations.

Several reports have proposed a possible causal relationship between the long-term use of proton pump inhibitors and the development of gastric fundic gland and hyperplastic polyps.

7. What is meant by thickened gastric folds?

Thickened gastric folds appear larger than normal and do not flatten with insufflation of air at endoscopy. Radiographically, large gastric folds are > 10 mm in width after distention of the stomach with contrast material during upper GI series.

8. List the differential diagnosis for intrinsic causes of thickened gastric folds.

Lymphoma	Lymphocytic gastritis
Mucosa-associated lymphoid	Eosinophilic gastritis
tissue (MALT)	Gastric antral vascular ectasia (GAVE) syndrome
Linitis plastica	Gastritis cystica profunda
Gastric adenocarcinoma	Gastric anisikiasis
Ménétrier's disease	Kaposi's sarcoma
H. pylori gastritis (acute)	Gastric varices
Zollinger-Ellison syndrome	Sentinel fold

9. What systemic diseases may be associated with thickened gastric folds or granulomatous gastritis?

Gastric Crohn's disease and sarcoidosis are the most commonly encountered granulomatous gastropathies. Other potential causes of granulomatous gastritis include histoplasmosis, candidial infection, actinomycoses, and blastomycoses. Secondary syphilis may present with *Treponema pallidum* infiltration, producing a perivascular plasmacytic response in the gastric mucosa. Disseminated mycobacteria in tuberculosis may result in gastric infiltration. Systemic mastocytosis, in addition to facial flushing, may be associated with hyperemic thickened gastric folds. Rarely, amyloidosis may cause gastric wall infiltration with thickened gastric folds.

10. EUS displays the gastric wall in five alternating hyperechoic and hypoechoic bands. Histologically, to what wall layers do they correlate?

Correlation of EUS Bands and Wall Layers

WALL LAYER	EUS BANDS	HISTOLOGIC CORRELATION
1st	Hyperechoic	Superficial mucosa
2nd	Hypoechoic	Deep mucosa, including the muscularis mucosa
3rd	Hyperechoic	Submucosa
4th	Hypoechoic	Muscularis propria
5th	Hyperechoic	Serosa

11. Describe the role of EUS in the evaluation of thickened gastric folds.

EUS is the most accurate diagnostic imaging study for the evaluation of thickened gastric folds. Although EUS cannot differentiate between histologically benign and malignant processes, it is discriminatory in the differential diagnosis of large gastric folds. EUS allows selection of patients in whom further investigation is warranted with large-particle endoscopic biopsy, snare biopsy, EUS-guided fine-needle aspiration, or full-thickness biopsy at laparotomy. EUS is the most sensitive means for identifying gastric varices, thereby avoiding the potential risk of endoscopic biopsy. When EUS demonstrates enlargement limited to the superficial layers, multiple large-capacity forceps biopsies should confirm the histologic diagnosis. Conversely, when EUS documents thickening and wall layer disruption primarily of the deeper layers (i.e., the submucosa or muscularis propria), endoscopic biopsies are apt to be nondiagnostic. This appearance on EUS, however, is highly suggestive for malignant invasion; therefore, surgery is recommended to obtain a full-thickness biopsy when endoscopic tissue sampling is negative (Fig. 3).

12. What are the clinical features of high-grade non-Hodgkin's gastric lymphoma?

High-grade non-Hodgkin's gastric lymphomas account for 3% of all gastric malignancies but make up the largest group second to adenocarcinoma. The stomach is the most common site

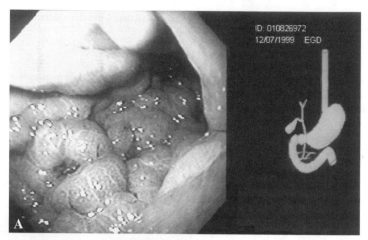

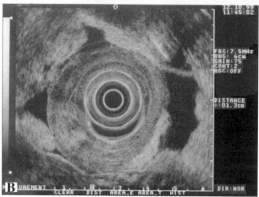

FIGURE 3. Thickened gastric folds in a patient with linitis plastica. The gastric lumen fails to distend on insufflation, and the folds do not flatten out *(A)*. EUS may show wall thickening (13 mm), elimination of the normal wall layer pattern, and ascites, as seen here *(B)*.

of extranodal lymphoma, accounting for 10%. B-cell lymphomas make up the largest pathologic group of gastric lymphomas, followed by T-cell phenotype and other varieties. Endoscopically they may present as a discrete polypoid lesion, an ulcerated mass, or a diffuse submucosal infiltration with enlarged rugal folds. The most common presenting symptoms are abdominal pain, weight loss, nausea, anorexia, and hemorrhage. Standard biopsy techniques frequently do not yield a diagnosis. When gastric lymphoma is suspected, large-particle biopsies, snare biopsies, and needle aspirates should be attempted. EUS is useful in identifying abnormalities of the submucosal wall layers and in establishing nodal involvement. When endoscopic biopsy techniques are unrevealing, surgical full-thickness biopsy should be obtained (Fig. 4).

13. Define MALToma.

Low-grade gastric mucosa-associated lymphoid tissue (MALT) lymphoma is classified as an extranodal marginal zone lymphoma. MALT is characterized histologically by numerous enlarged lymphoid follicles, a dense B-cell lymphocytic infiltrate, infiltrates of plasma cells, and the presence of lymphoepithelial lesions. Gastric MALTomas may present with bleeding due to ulceration or simply as thickened folds seen on endoscopy or CT scan. Mucosal biopsies, preferably from large-particle forceps, are usually satisfactory for diagnosis. The majority (> 80%) of gastric MALT lymphomas are associated with *H. pylori* infection. The median age of detection is in the fifth decade, but it can occur at any age. The majority of MALTomas are low-grade and run an indolent course, however, they may bleed and/or progress to invasive lymphoma. (Fig. 5).

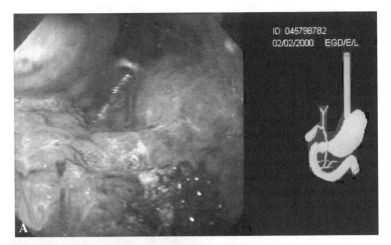

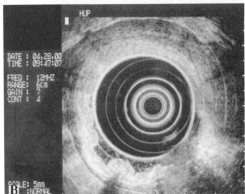

FIGURE 4. In a patient with gastric lymphoma, endoscopy demonstrates expansive focal thickening of folds, erosions and hyperemia *(A)*. EUS demonstrates focal mural thickening (12 mm) and disruption of the normal wall layer pattern superiorly *(B)*. The normal wall layer pattern and thickness (5.4 mm) are preserved inferiorly.

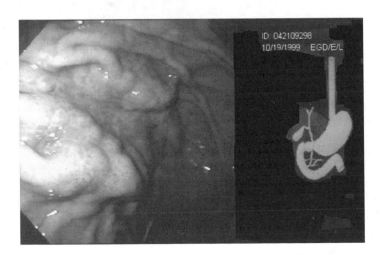

FIGURE 5. MALToma detected on endoscopy in a patient with dyspeptic symptoms. There is focal thickening of the folds in contrast to normal surrounding gastric mucosa.

14. How are MALTomas managed?

After forceps biopsy has raised consideration of the diagnosis, gastric mapping by biopsies and EUS should be performed to assess the extent and nature of involvement. Gastric mapping should be done to assess for *H. pylori* and to establish the presence and distribution of the MALT, chronic active gastritis, atrophic gastritis, and intestinal metaplasia. EUS should be performed to assess the depth of wall-layer involvement and presence of wall-layer disruption. Low-grade MALTomas demonstrate only focal thickening of the mucosal and submucosal layers without wall-layer disruption or surrounding adenopathy. Transmural thickening and wall-layer disruption indicates high-grade MALToma.

Treatment options include surgery, radiation, chemotherapy, and *H. pylori* eradication. Numerous studies indicate that if *H. pylori* infection is eradicated in low-grade disease limited to the submucosa, regression of tumor occurs in 60–75% of patients. EUS is useful to measure regression of disease objectively.

15. Define Ménétrier's disease.

Ménétrier's disease is a rare condition characterized by giant gastric rugal folds that often spare the antrum. The histologic features are marked foveolar hyperplasia with cystic dilations that may penetrate into the submucosa. Symptoms may include abdominal pain, weight loss, gastrointestinal blood loss, and hyperalbuminemia. The cause is unclear. The diagnosis can be confirmed by EUS findings of thickening of the deep mucosal layer and large-particle biopsy specimens demonstrating the characteristic histology. Treatment with H_2 receptor antagonists is successful in some patients (Fig. 6).

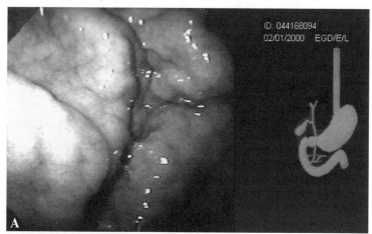

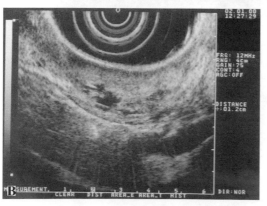

FIGURE 6. In Ménétrier's disease, giant gastric folds are commonly seen. They are soft and pliable on palpation with a probe *(A)*. EUS demonstrates marked thickening of the submucosa (12 mm) with cystic dilations *(B)*.

16. How is Ménétrier's disease different in children and adults?

Unlike Ménétrier's disease in adults, which is characterized by chronicity of symptoms, Ménétrier's disease in children is generally self-limited. Recurrence and sequelae are rare. Clinically, pediatric patients present with abrupt onset of vomiting associated with abdominal pain, anorexia, and hypoproteinemia. Gradual onset of edema and ascites results from this protein-losing enteropathy. Hypoalbuminemia, peripheral eosinophilia, and mild normochromic, normocytic anemia are often seen. Radiographic findings include thickened gastric folds in the fundus and body of the stomach, often with antral sparing. Such findings are confirmed by an upper GI barium meal, ultrasonography, and endoscopy. Histologically the gastric mucosa is hypertrophic with elongation of gastric pits and glandular atrophy. In children, however, intranuclear inclusion bodies consistent with cytomegalovirus (CMV) infection are common; culture of gastric tissue is often positive for CMV. Pediatric patients generally respond to supportive, symptomatic treatment with complete resolution.

17. What is the differential diagnosis for a submucosal mass seen on endoscopy?

Common	*Less Common*	*Rare*
Leiomyoma	Carcinoid	Leiomyoblastoma
Lipoma	Leiomyosarcoma	Liposarcoma
Aberrant pancreas	Granular cell tumor	Schwannoma
Gastric varices	Lymphoma	
External compression	Splenic remnant	
by liver or spleen	Submucosal cyst	
	Splenic artery aneurysm	

18. Discuss the role of EUS in evaluating submucosal lesions.

Although EUS does not provide a histopathologic diagnosis, it allows reliable characterization of certain lesions based on their location relative to the sonographic pattern of the gut wall and their EUS appearance. EUS is accurate in differentiating true submucosal tumors from extraluminal compression by adjacent organs. EUS may determine whether a lesion is vascular and is highly accurate in confirming isolated gastric varices, thereby avoiding the risk of biopsy. Leiomyomas are seen as hypoechoic structures arising from the fourth (hypoechoic) sonographic layer, which corresponds to the muscularis propria. Although no unique sonographic differences in size, shape, or appearance distinguish leiomyoma from leiomyosarcoma, the risk of malignancy is considered low if the lesion is < 3 cm in diameter. Gastric lipomas appear as hyperechoic lesions within the submucosal layer. Gastric wall cysts are seen as echo-free structures within the submucosa. Other less common submucosal lesions, such as pancreatic rests, carcinoids, fibromas, and granular cell tumors, can be identified but have not been described in sufficient numbers to allow description of distinctive EUS findings. EUS findings in submucosal gastric lesions serve as a guide to therapeutic decisions based on lesion size. One management scheme is to follow asymptomatic lesions < 3 cm in diameter that have no evidence of invasion or enlargement by serial endosonography. A significant change in size of the lesion by EUS should be considered an indication for surgery. Larger lesions should be considered for de novo resection (Fig. 7).

19. A submucosal mass was identified during upper endoscopy. EUS demonstrates a hypoechoic lesion arising from the fourth wall layer or muscularis propria. What is the most likely diagnosis?

The most common lesion with such EUS findings is leiomyoma. However, leiomyosarcoma, although less common, may have similar characteristics. In addition, other rare lesions, such as schwannoma, liposarcoma and myxosarcoma, may arise from the muscularis propria and have a similar EUS appearance. EUS is not a substitute for histologic confirmation. When the lesion is well circumscribed, small (< 3 cm), and without evidence of surrounding tissue invasion or adenopathy, its size may be followed for interval stability, which confirms benignity. Lesions that are > 3–4 cm, increase in size, or invade surrounding tissue should be considered for resection.

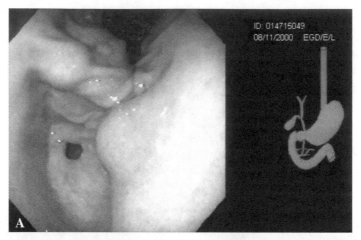

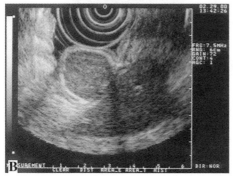
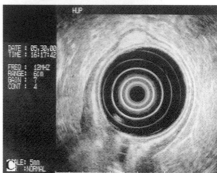

FIGURE 7. Multiple large and small submucosal lesions are seen on endoscopy *(A)*. EUS demonstrates typical characteristics of leiomyoma *(B)* and lipoma *(C)*.

20. A 65-year-old woman presents with self-limited, coffee-ground emesis. Endoscopy reveals a single, pedunculated, 1-cm polyp in the gastric body. What is the best option for management?

Most gastric polyps are epithelial in origin; of these, 70–90% are hyperplastic and 10–20% are adenomatous. Although gastric polyps may cause abdominal pain or bleeding, up to 50% are asymptomatic. Complete removal of the lesion by snare polypectomy for histologic evaluation is both diagnostic and curative. Although the risk of complications is greater than for colonoscopic polypectomy, snare polypectomy is generally safe and well tolerated. An epinephrine solution diluted to 1:10,000 can be injected into the stalk of large polyps to lessen the risk of postpolypectomy bleeding. Glucagon may be used to prevent peristalsis from inhibiting retrieval. An overtube should be considered to avoid accidental dislodgement of the polyp into the airway during retrieval. An alternative retrieval technique uses the Roth net, which satisfactorily secures the resected polyp. A 6–8-week course of a proton pump inhibitor is generally recommended to promote healing.

21. A patient with FAP has multiple gastric polyps on surveillance endoscopy. What is the most likely histology of such polyps? What is their malignant potential? What other significant upper GI lesions may be detected at the time of upper endoscopy?

Nearly all patients with FAP have polyps in the upper GI tract. Most polyps are found in the proximal stomach or fundus; they are small, multiple, and hyperplastic. Although they carry no risk for carcinomatous conversion, they may cause bleeding. Forty to ninety percent of patients, however, have adenomatous polyps in the distal stomach, antrum, or duodenum, particularly in the periampullary region. Risk of adenocarcinoma of the gastric antrum is not increased in U.S. families with adenomatous polyposis but appears to be increased in Japanese families. The relative risk of duodenal, particularly periampullary, cancer is markedly increased in patients with FAP and duodenal or ampulary adenomas.

22. Describe the manifestations of gastric polyps in the other hereditary GI polyposis syndromes.

Patients with Gardner's syndrome have a preponderance of hyperplastic polyps in the proximal stomach. Patients with Peutz-Jeghers syndrome and juvenile polyposis syndromes may have hamartomatous polyps in the stomach. Although hamartomas may cause bleeding, an increased cancer risk is not apparent.

23. What is the relationship between carcinoid tumors of the stomach and atrophic gastritis?

Carcinoid tumors of the stomach occur primarily in the fundus and body. They are generally submucosal and often appear polypoid. Although they can be observed in otherwise normal stomachs, they are found with much higher frequency in patients with achlorhydria secondary to atrophic gastritis. Carcinoids are thought to develop as a result of high concentrations of circulating gastrin, which is trophic for the enterochromaffin cells of the proximal stomach. Although carcinoids have been detected in rats given high doses of omeprazole for long periods, no such lesions have been observed in humans treated with long-term acid suppressive therapy. Gastric carcinoids in the setting of achlorhydria and hypergastrinemia may be treated with antrectomy to remove the source of gastrin. Carcinoids that are not the result of hypergastrinemia should undergo appropriate gastric resection for removal of large tumors. The stomach is the location of approximately 2–3% of all carcinoids, but carcinoids represent only 0.3% of all gastric tumors. Gastric carcinoids do not produce symptoms related to vasoactive peptides, and their discovery is frequently incidental. Complete excision is the treatment of choice, and many, if not most, can be removed endoscopically either with multiple forceps biopsies or snare resection. EUS is useful to assess the gastric wall layer of origin and depth of invasion when endoscopic excision is considered. When EUS confirms that the lesion is within the submucosal layer, submucosal injection of saline may be performed to enable endoscopic snare resection.

24. Endoscopy performed on a man with AIDS to evaluate abdominal pain reveals a serpiginous, reddish-purple, thickened fold in the body of the stomach. The patient has similar-appearing lesions on the roof of the mouth and lower extremities. What does this lesion represent? What is the risk of bleeding at biopsy? What histologic characteristics are the biopsies likely to reveal?

The lesion is most likely Kaposi's sarcoma (KS). Upper endoscopy or flexible sigmoidoscopy reveals GI lesions in 40% of patients with AIDS who have KS of the skin and lymph nodes. Endoscopic appearance is characteristic. There is no increased risk of bleeding from biopsies. Histologic confirmation is possible in only 23% of visibly inspected luminal KS because of the submucosal location. Because the vascular lesion is deep to the submucosa and not reached by biopsy forceps, the technique is safe, but the results are nonspecific. Symptoms include pain, dysphasia, and occasionally bleeding and obstruction.

25. A 60-year-old woman is referred with nocturnal epigastric pain and secretory diarrhea. Fasting serum gastrin level is > 1,000 pg/ml. Endoscopy demonstrates diffusely thickened hyperemic antral folds with antral erosions. Forceps biopsies are nondiagnostic. Thiazin stain for *H. pylori* is negative. What is the differential diagnosis? What series of tests should be ordered next?

Hypergastrinemia has several possible causes. The absence of a history of gastric surgery excludes the consideration of retained antrum syndrome. Spurious use of H_2 blockers or proton pump inhibitors may cause elevation of the serum gastrin level. Type A atrophic gastritis associated with pernicious anemia results in hypergastrinemia due to disinhibition of gastrin production.

Finally, the patient may have antral gastrin cell hyperplasia or gastrinoma as part of Zollinger-Ellison syndrome. The endoscopic appearance is consistent only with the last two diagnoses. Gastric acid analysis identifies the presence of gastric acid hypersecretion, distinguishing hypergastrinemia from Zollinger-Ellison syndrome and appropriate hypergastrinemia in response to achlorhydria. Patients with Zollinger-Ellison syndrome fail to respond to exogenous secretin and show no decrease in serum gastrin level. However, a secretin stimulation test need not be done when gastric acid hypersecretion > 1000 pg/ml accompanies hypergastrinemia.

26. A 40-year-old man has a history of chronic pancreatitis complicated by pseudocysts requiring drainage. He presents with a self-limited upper GI bleed. Endoscopy demonstrates a normal esophagus and duodenum. What is the most likely diagnosis? What therapeutic options should be considered?

The patient has isolated gastric varices secondary to splenic vein thrombosis. Splenic vein thrombosis is a potential complication of acute and chronic pancreatitis, pancreatic carcinoma, lymphoma, trauma, and hypercoagulable states. The left gastric veins empty via the splenic vein. Esophageal venous flow is unaffected. Because endoscopic therapy is generally not effective for the prevention of gastric variceal bleeding, surgery with splenectomy is required. Gastric varices are submucosal or deep to the submucosa, whereas the esophageal varices lie superficial in the lamina propria. Gastric variceal bleeding accounts for 10–20% of acute variceal hemorrhage. The incidence of gastric variceal bleeding is 10–20% among patients with bleeding from esophagogastric varices. Acute bleeding may be treated endoscopically. However, rebleeding is the rule, and the mortality rate is as high as 55%. When bleeding is due to portal hypertension, transjugular intrahepatic or surgical shunting is effective. European and Canadian experience with intravascular injection of cyanoacrylate has been encouraging, but the drug is not currently available in the U.S. When not actively bleeding, gastric varices may be difficult to distinguish from benign prominent folds. EUS identifies hypoechoic, tortuous dilated blood vessels in the submucosa that are characteristic for gastric varices.

27. A 65-year-old woman is referred for evaluation of chronic iron deficiency anemia and Hemoccult-positive stool. Colonoscopy and upper GI series are negative. Findings of an upper endoscopy are noted in the figure below. Identify the immediately apparent diagnosis and appropriate treatment.

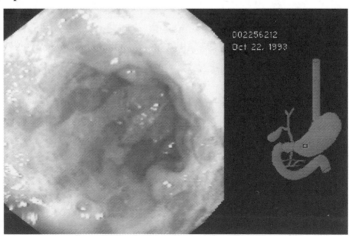

The striking endoscopic appearance of raised, convoluted thickened folds that radiate spoke-like from a pylorus covered by friable vascular malformations is characteristic of "watermelon stomach," also known as gastric antral vascular ectasia (GAVE). The endoscopic appearance is diagnostic. GAVE is a rare source of chronic occult GI bleeding; its incidence in the general population is unknown. It occurs more frequently in women and often is associated with autoimmune or connective tissue disorders. Underlying atrophic gastritis with hypergastrinemia and pernicious anemia may be present. The pathogenesis is unclear. Histologic features include dilated mucosal capillaries with focal thrombosis; dilated, tortuous submucosal venous channels; and fibrous fibromuscular hyperplasia. Chronic GI blood loss responds to endoscopic coagulation therapy. The best experience has been with Nd:YAG laser. Lesions may recur but usually respond to repeat endoscopic therapy.

28. What is the most likely diagnosis for the lesion in the figure below?

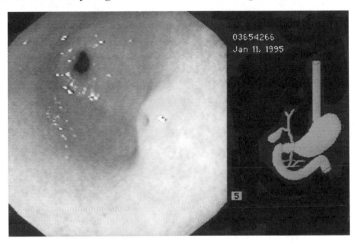

The lesion is a pancreatic rest, also called aberrant or heterotopic pancreas. Such lesions occur typically in the prepyloric antrum and often have central umbilication. Endoscopic appearance is usually diagnostic. EUS findings are variable but may demonstrate a relatively hyperechoic lesion arising from the mucosa or submucosa, with a central ductal structure in some cases. Pancreatic rests rarely produce symptoms.

BIBLIOGRAPHY

1. Amer MH, el-Akkad S: Gastrointestinal lymphoma in adults: Clinical features and management of three hundred cases. Gastroenterology 106:846, 1994.
2. Caletti GC, Brocchie E, Baraldini M, et al: Assessment of portal hypertension by endosonography. Gastrointest Endosc 34:154–155, 1988.
3. Choudhry U, Boyce HW Jr, Coppola D: Proton pump inhibitor-induced gastric polyps: A retrospective analysis of their frequency, and endoscopic, histologic, and ultrastructural characterisitics. Am J Clin Pathol 110:615–621, 1998.
4. Cristallini E, Ascani S, Bolis G: Association between histologic type of polyp and carcinoma of the stomach. Gastrointest Endosc 38:481–484, 1992.
5. D'Amore F, Brincker H, Gronback K: Non-Hodgkin's lymphoma of the gastrointestinal tract: A population-based analysis of incidence, geographic distribution, clinical pathologic presentation features, and prognosis. J Clin Oncol 12:1673, 1994.
6. Deppish LM, Rona VT: Gastric epithelial polyps: A ten year study. J Clin Gastroenterol 11:110–115, 1989.
7. el-Zimaity HM, Jackson FW, Grahm DY: Fundic gland polyps developing during omeprazole therapy. Am J Gastroenterol 92:1858–1860, 1997.
8. Friedman SL, Wright, TL, Altman DF: Gastrointestinal Kaposi's sarcoma in patients with AIDS: Endoscopic and autopsy findings. Gastroenterology 89:102, 1985.
9. Frucht H, Howard JM, Slaff JL, et al: Secretin and calcium provocative tests in Zollinger-Ellison syndrome. Ann Intern Med 111:697–699, 1989.
10. Gilliam JH, Geisinger KR, Wu WC, et al: Endoscopic biopsies diagnostic of gastric antral vascular ectasia: The watermelon stomach. Dig Dis Sci 34:885–888, 1989.
11. Ginsberg GG, Al-Kawas FH, Fleischer DE, et al: Gastric polyps: Relationship of size and histology to cancer risk. Am J Gastroenterol 91(4):714–17, 1996.

12. Gostout CJ, Ahlquist DA, Radford CM, et al: Endoscopy laser therapy for watermelon stomach. Gastroenterology 96:1462–1465, 1989.
13. Hughes R: Diagnosis and treatment of gastric polyps. Gastrointest Endosc Clin North Am 2:457–467, 1993.
14. Kimmey ND, Martin RW, Haggit RC, et al: Histologic correlates of gastrointestinal ultrasound imaging. Gastroenterology 94:433, 1989.
15. Mendis RE, Gerdes H, Lightdale CJ, Botete JF: Large gastric folds: A diagnostic approach using endoscopic ultrasonography. Gastrointest Endosc 40:437–441, 1994.
16. Nobre-Leitao C, Lage P, Cravo S, et al: Treatment of gastric MALT lymphoma by *Helicobacter pylori* eradication: A study controlled by endoscopic ultrasonography. Am J Gastroenterol 93:732–736, 1998.
17. Ohkusa T, Takashimizu I, Fujiki K, et al: Dissappearance of hyperplastic polyps in the stomach after eradication of Helicobacter pylori. A randomized clinical trial. Ann Intern Med 129:712–715, 1998.
18. Okada M, Lizuka Y, Oh K, et al: Gastritis cystica profunda presenting as giant gastric mucosal folds: The role of endoscopic ultrasonography and mucosectomy in the diagnostic work-up. Gastrointest Endosc 40:640–644,1994.
19. Rustgi AK: Hereditary gastrointestinal polyposis in non-polyposis syndromes. N Engl J Med 331:1694–1702, 1994.
20. Scharschmidt B. The natural history of hypertrophic gastropathy (Ménétrier's disease). Am J Med 63:644–652,1997.
21. Steinbach G, Ford R, Glober G, et al: Antibiotic treatment of gastric lymphoma-associated lymphoid tissue: An uncontrolled trial. Ann Int Med 131:88–95,1999.
22. Tio TL, Tytgat GNJ, der Hartog Jager FZA: Endoscopic ultrasonography for the evaluation of smooth muscle tumors in the upper gastrointestinal tract: An experience with 42 cases. Gastrointest Endosc 36:343–350, 1990.

14. GASTROPARESIS

Prahalad Jajodia, M.D., and Michael H. Walter, M.D.

1. Define gastroparesis.

Gastroparesis is a motility disorder of the stomach that often is associated with other intestinal motility disorders. It results from impairment of the normal gastric emptying mechanism.

2. What factors determine gastric motility and emptying?

(1) Composition of the meal, (2) neuroregulators, and (3) hormonal regulators. Liquids and solid meals empty from the stomach at different rates, and content further influences emptying (e.g., fat slows emptying). Neural innervation is complex but largely involves the vagus nerve. Hormones also affect gastric smooth muscle. Motilin and neurotensin accelerate, whereas secretin and cholecystokinin delay, gastric emptying.

3. Describe the electric pacesetter in the stomach.

The rate of contraction of the stomach is controlled by a pacemaker located on the greater curve of the stomach, which oscillates at 3 cycles/minute. The cells with the highest frequency determine the 3-per-minute. Stomach potentials differ from those in the heart: because of neurohormonal influences, not every potential results in a contraction.

4. What is the interdigestive myoelectric cycle (IDMEC)?

In the fasting state, the GI tract undergoes cycles of contractions with cycle lengths of 90–120 minutes. Most of this time is spent in the quiet phase (phase I). Muscle contractions begin to appear in phase II and build to a crescendo of maximal contractility in phase III, which lasts about 5 minutes. Phase III is a forceful burst of contractions that sweeps the antrum and continues along the entire GI tract. This is the migrating motor complex (MMC). Phase III is sometimes followed by a brief period of decreasing activity (phase IV).

5. Describe gastric motility and emptying.

The stomach serves as a reservoir for food and allows it to pass into the duodenum at a controlled rate. The proximal half of the stomach serves as the reservoir, with the volume governed by the muscular tone of the stomach. Distention of the esophagus or stomach relaxes the muscular tone. This reflex, called receptive relaxation, means that the volume of the stomach can be increased without a rise in pressure.

The contractions in the distal half of the stomach from the circumferential bands of muscle are forceful and culminate in terminal antral contracts (TACs). TACs result in a to-and-fro movement that grinds food into smaller pieces. These hydrodynamic forces cause a sieving process whereby 1-mm particles are selectively propelled more rapidly and pass the pylorus before it and the antrum close at the end of the TAC.

Liquid emptying is volume-dependent and follows first-order kinetics. During the first 30 minutes emptying is rapid. From 30–120 minutes emptying is constant but slower than the first 30 minutes. Solid emptying is volume-independent. Initially, while solids are reduced in size, there is no emptying. This is followed by a prolonged linear phase. Overall, gastric emptying is controlled by the activity in the proximal and distal halves of the stomach as well as the pyloric outlet, all of which act in sequence with one another.

6. What causes gastroparesis?

As gastric motility becomes better understood, associated disorders increase. Some of these disorders are well established, whereas others are of uncertain significance. Idiopathic gastroparesis remains the most common cause of delayed gastric emptying.

7. Define idiopathic gastroparesis.

Many patients with nausea, bloating, and early satiety have delayed gastric emptying with no clear predisposing factor. Idiopathic gastroparesis may be sudden in onset or present with insidious development of symptoms. Nausea, fever, myalgias, and diarrhea may be present in some cases, suggesting viral etiologies. Transient slowing of gastric emptying has been reported after acute viral gastroenteritis and after infection with parvovirus-like agents (Norwalk agents).

8. Describe the natural history of idiopathic gastroparesis.

Although some patients with idiopathic gastroparesis exhibit persistent symptoms, many improve spontaneously to the point that medical therapy is no longer required. Patients with symptoms believed to be of viral etiology report gradual improvement, weight gain, and little or no disability, whereas those without a viral prodrome experience a more progressive course with worsening pain, early satiety, anorexia, and overall lower quality of life. In patients with delayed gastric emptying of uncertain etiology and abdominal pain, it is important to exclude structural disorders that mimic idiopathic gastroparesis.

9. What is diabetic gastroparesis?

The most recognizable disorder of delayed gastric emptying is diabetic gastroparesis. Nausea, vomiting, and early satiety are quite common in patients who have had diabetes for several years. Although advanced diabetes also may affect small intestinal motility, impaired gastric motor function is more common. It is traditionally believed that abnormal gastric emptying develops in diabetes (usually type I) of more than 10 years' duration complicated by peripheral and autonomic neuropathy. In diabetics on hemodialysis, development of gastroparesis correlates with duration of diabetes, orthostatic hypotension, prior myocardial infarction, cerebrovascular accident, and extremity gangrene. Abnormal gastric emptying is more commonly recognized by scintigraphy. Prevalence among long-standing type I diabetics ranges from 27–58%. Gastroparesis does not necessarily correlate with presence of symptoms. Some asymptomatic diabetics exhibit markedly delayed gastric emptying, whereas others with severe nausea have normal gastric scintigraphy. Periods of poor glycemic control have been correlated with delays in emptying, suggesting that the motor defect is not fixed and can be modulated by other factors.

10. Describe the pathogenesis of diabetic gastroparesis.

The pathogenesis of diabetic gastroparesis is poorly understood. Vagal neuropathy has been proposed to impair gastric motility in diabetes. Diabetics produce only one-third of the normal gastric acid output in response to sham feeding, a vagal-mediated reflex. Many diabetics with gastroparesis exhibit evidence of autonomic dysfunction, including postural hypotension or loss of vagotonic reflexes that slow the heart. Abnormal jejunal contractions in human diabetics are similar to those in dogs after sympathectomy, suggesting that aberrant sympathetic nervous function may play a role in diabetic gut complications. Hyperglycemia alone, in the absence of underlying neuropathy or myopathy, can alter gastric motor function by disrupting both normal fasting and postprandial antral contractions. There is a strong correlation with delayed gastric emptying of liquids when the blood glucose exceeds 270 mg/dl. Likewise, delays in solid emptying during periods of hyperglycemia in type I diabetics improve during euglycemia. In addition to its effects on gastric motor function, hyperglycemia can alter gastric sensory function.

11. Which surgical procedures are associated with postoperative gastroparesis?

Vagotomy. Approximately 5% of patients who undergo vagotomy and drainage for peptic ulcer disease or malignancy experience nausea, vomiting, and early satiety caused by postoperative gastric stasis in the absence of anatomic obstruction. Some patients who undergo highly selective vagotomy, including procedures performed by a laparoscopic approach, may develop gastroparesis.

Roux-en-Y gastrojejunostomy. Some patients may experience intractable nausea, vomiting, and abdominal pain after construction of a Roux-en-Y gastrojejunostomy. Symptoms of retention may result from either gastric, spastic, or retroperistaltic Roux limb motor abnormalities.

Fundoplication. Nausea and bloating may develop after surgery for gastroesophageal reflux disease, including the newer laparoscopic fundoplication.

Gastric bypass surgery. Gastroplasty and gastric bypass are performed in some morbidly obese patients who fail dietary methods of weight control. Gastroplasty (gastric partitioning) creates a 50-ml fundic pouch that is continuous with the distal stomach through a 10-mm stoma. Gastric bypass divides the stomach into two compartments, with the proximal compartment draining through a 12-mm gastroenterostomy. These procedures produce delayed gastric emptying of solids and fundic distention, leading to early satiety, loss of appetite, and weight reduction.

Other surgeries. Esophagectomy with gastric pull-through into the thoracic cavity may be curative for esophageal malignancy, but delays in gastric emptying are reported with colonic interposition after esophagectomy. Delayed gastric emptying in up to 50% of cases complicates pylorus-preserving Whipple procedures performed for pancreatic cancer and chronic pancreatitis. Gastroparesis is a common sequela of lung and heart-lung transplantation and may predispose to microaspiration into the transplanted lung.

12. Which conditions cause selective gastric motor dysfunction that leads to gastroparesis?

Gastroesophageal reflux disease. Delays in solid- or liquid-phase gastric emptying can be seen in some patients with gastroesophageal reflux. Delays correlate poorly with symptoms, lower esophageal sphincter pressure, and 24-hour pH monitoring.

Intra-abdominal malignancy. Nausea, vomiting, and early satiety are common with upper GI malignancies and lead to poor food intake. Delayed gastric emptying is seen in up to 60% of patients with nonobstructing pancreatic carcinoma and bilateral breast cancer. Indirect immunofluorescence study of serum shows positive staining of Purkinje cell nuclei, suggestive of an immune cause for the gastric motor defect. Immune mechanisms also have been proposed in intestinal pseudoobstruction in patients with small cell lung carcinoma. Because of the frequent poor response to medications, patients with gastroparesis from malignancy often require a surgical drainage procedure, such as gastrojejunostomy.

Radiation-induced gastric stasis. Severe nausea, vomiting, and intolerance of both liquid and solid meals are common after abdominal irradiation.

Atrophic gastritis. Delayed gastric emptying of solids but not liquid meals may be seen in patients with atrophic gastritis with or without pernicious anemia. This condition may be caused in part by poor intragastric processing of food. Decreased gastric secretions increase the time needed to fragment solid foods to tiny particles because of deficient peptic digestion.

13. Which disorders with diffuse abnormalities of GI motor activity cause gastroparesis?

Rheumatologic disorders. GI symptoms such as dysphagia, heartburn, nausea, and vomiting are common in patients with scleroderma and presumed to result from motility abnormalities of the upper gut. Characteristic manometric findings are observed in both the stomach and small intestine. Delayed gastric emptying or gastric atony is also observed in other rheumatologic diseases, such as polymyositis, dermatomyositis, and systemic lupus erythematosus.

Chronic intestinal pseudoobstruction. Nausea, vomiting, bloating, and early satiety result from gastric and small intestinal motor impairment. Chronic pseudoobstruction is familial in many cases, resulting from an inherited visceral myopathy or neuropathy. The diagnosis is suggested by delayed transit and luminal dilation on barium radiography and characteristic neuropathic or myopathic patterns on manometry. It is confirmed by full-thickness biopsy of the small intestinal wall.

Infectious disorders. GI motor activity is disrupted in Chagas disease, because the myenteric plexus is damaged by *Trypanosoma cruzi* infection. Gastroparesis, megaduodenum, and chronic intestinal pseudoobstruction as well as several extraintestinal manifestations may be seen. Other infections that disrupt gut motor activity include varicella zoster, Epstein-Barr virus, and *Clostridium botulinum*. Gastric emptying is often markedly delayed in patients with human immunodeficiency virus who have pathogenic GI infections.

Miscellaneous conditions. Delayed gastric emptying also is seen in smooth muscle disorders such as myotonic dystrophy and progressive muscular dystrophy. Primary or secondary amyloidosis can cause neuropathic or myopathic intestinal pseudoobstruction. Solid-phase gastric emptying may be delayed in patients with idiopathic slow-transit constipation, idiopathic megarectum, and achalasia. Furthermore, voluntary suppression of defecation can delay gastric emptying in healthy volunteers.

14. Which drugs affect gastric emptying?
Prescription and over-the-counter medications can modify gastric emptying rates.

Effects of Medications on Gastric Emptying

Delay gastric emptying		
Alcohol (high concentration)	Glucagon	Phenothiazine
Aluminum hydroxide antacids	Interleukin-1	Progesterone
Atropine	L-dopa	Propantheline bromide
Beta agonists	Lithium	Sulcralfate
Calcitonin	Omeprazole	Tetrahydrocannabinol
Calcium channel blockers	Ondansetron	Tobacco
Dexfenfluramine	Opiates	Tricyclic antidepressants
Diphenhydramine		
Accelerate gastric emptying		
Beta blockers	Domperidone	Metoclopramide
Cisapride	Erythromycin	Naloxone
Diazepam	Histamine H$_2$	Prostaglandin E$_2$

From Yamada T, Alpers DH, et al (eds): Textbook of Gastroenterology, 3rd ed. Philadelphia, Lippincott Williams & Wilkins, 1999, with permission.

15. List the conditions that have an established association with delayed gastric emptying.
1. **Diabetes mellitus.** GI symptoms are common but not always associated with gastroparesis. Although most authorities believe that gastroparesis is a neuropathy, it is difficult to be certain about its relationship to duration of disease, associated nausea, vomiting, neuropathy, retinopathy, and type of diabetes.
2. **Anorexia nervosa.** Delayed gastric emptying is common. Nausea, vomiting, gastric dilation, and even perforation on feeding have been reported.
3. **Gastric surgery.** Gastric atony may occur after gastric surgery. This uncommon complication affects about 5% of patients, ranging from 1.25% of patients who undergo vagotomy and pyloroplasty to 9% of patients who undergo vagotomy and subtotal gastrectomy. Surgery should not be done acutely on a dilated, obstructed stomach, because atony is more likely to occur.
4. **Gastric dysrhythmias**, usually of an idiopathic nature, may delay gastric emptying. Various dysrhythmias have been described and may be measured with electrogastrography (see figure on following page). Tachygastria is associated with delayed gastric emptying. Secondary gastric dysrhythmias are associated with anorexia nervosa and motion sickness. They also have been reported in gastric ulcers and gastric cancers.
5. **Obesity** slows gastric emptying because of the inverse relationship between body size and gastric emptying.
6. **Various kinds of stress** through the CNS modulate gastric emptying, including stress from pain or anxiety.
7. **Neurologic disorders**, including strokes, brain tumors, headaches, and high intracranial pressures, alter gastric emptying.
8. **Diseases that involve the gastric wall** may slow gastric emptying, including scleroderma, amyloidosis, systemic lupus erythematosus, and dermatomyositis.
9. **Abdominal cancer** may delay gastric emptying by direct involvement of the stomach wall or by invading the surrounding nerves. Gastroparesis also may be a paraneoplastic effect.

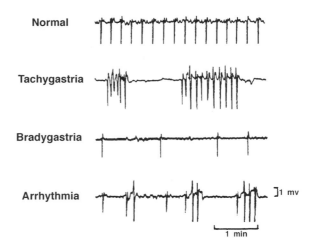

Normal

Tachygastria

Gastric arrhythmias that may delay gastric emptying are measured with electrogastrography.

Bradygastria

Arrhythmia

]1 mv

1 min

16. What is the differential diagnosis of chronic nausea and vomiting?

Differential Diagnosis of Chronic Nausea and Vomiting

Gastric disorders
1. Causes of mechanical gastric outlet obstruction
   • Chronic peptic ulcer disease
   • Acute pyloric channel ulcer
   • Gastric carcinoma
   • Gastric lymphoma
   • Duodenal carcinoma
   • Pancreatic disease
   • Crohn's disease
2. Functional gastric outlet obstruction
   • Gastroparesis: diabetes, scleroderma, metabolic, idiopathic
   • Drug-induced
   • Viral infection
   • Gastric surgery
   • Anorexia nervosa

Small intestine disorders
1. Mechanical obstruction: usually presents acutely or with intermittent acute symptoms
2. Motility disorder/intestinal pseudoobstruction
   • Scleroderma
   • Diabetes
   • Jejunal diverticulosis
   • Amyloidosis
   • Peritoneal studding with metastases
   • Oat cell tumor of the lung with paraneoplastic neuropathy involving intestine
   • Familial visceral myopathy
   • Familial visceral neuropathy
   • Hypothyroidism

Psychogenic disorders
1. Bulimia
2. Psychogenic, without bulimia

Central nervous system disorders
1. Increased intercranial pressure secondary to tumor
2. Pseudotumor

Drugs
1. Narcotics
2. Cardiac glycosides
3. Theophylline derivatives

Pregnancy
1. Nausea and vomiting of pregnancy
2. Hyperemesis gravidarum

Metabolic/endocrine disorders
1. Hyperthyroidism
2. Addison's disease

Other: idiopathic cyclic vomiting (motility disorder)

From Yamada T, Alpers DH, Owyang C, et al (eds): Textbook of Gastroenterology, 2nd ed. Philadelphia, J.B. Lippincott, 1995.

17. What are the symptoms of gastroparesis?

Gastroparesis is part of the differential diagnosis of chronic nausea and vomiting. Symptoms, therefore, are nonspecific and include nausea, vomiting, early satiety, abdominal bloating, and weight loss.

18. What parts of the history and physical exam are important in establishing a diagnosis of gastroparesis?

The nonspecific symptoms listed in question 17 suggest gastroparesis. Nausea may be insidious and without vomiting. The timing of vomiting also may be important. Patient with gastroparesis may vomit undigested food several hours after eating. Patients with regurgitation do not have true nausea; therefore, other diagnoses should be considered. Associated symptoms, such as pain, fever, and diarrhea, are indicative of other causes. Gastric outlet obstruction and its causes should be considered before making a diagnosis of gastroparesis. A drug history is important because many drugs slow gastric emptying, including pain medications and any drug with anticholinergic properties. A psychological history is important because patients with bulimia and anorexia nervosa may be quite difficult to differentiate from patients with primary gastroparesis.

19. What tests should be done in patients suspected of having gastroparesis?

Tests for Gastric Emptying

TEST	DESCRIPTION	COMMENTS
Radiographs		
Upper GI series	Barium sulfate suspension	Insensitive; not quantitative
Barium burger	Barium-impregnated food	More sensitive; not quantitative
Radiopaque tubes	Barium-filled plastic	Sensitive; quantitative
Intubation		
Saline load	Saline	Semiquantitative; insensitive
Serial test meal	Liquid nutrients	Quantitative; somewhat sensitive; impractical
Double sampling dye dilution	Liquid nutrients	Quantitative; somewhat sensitive
Intestinal dye dilution	Liquid or mixed meals	Quantitative; sensitive; cumbersome
Scintigraphy		
Scanner or single crystal	Liquid or mixed meals	Semiquantitative; sensitive
Gamma camera	Liquid or mixed meals; nondigestible	Quantitative; sensitive; most versatile; now standard technique
Real-time ultrasound		
To measure gastric volume	Liquid meals	Quantitative; erect posture only; nonobese only
To measure gastric emptying time (antral cross-section)	Liquid or mixed meals	Semiquantitative; erect posture only; nonobese only
Gastric impedance		
Nontomographic; limited Electrodes	Nonionic liquid or homogenized mixed meals	Quantitative; needs H_2 blockers
Tomographic	Nonionic liquid or homogenized mixed meals	Quantitative; needs H_2 blockers
Ferromagnetic study	Iron suspension	Little experience

From Yamada T, Alpers DH, Owyang C, et al (eds): Textbook of Gastroenterology, 2nd ed. Philadelphia, J.B. Lippincott, 1995.

20. Outline an approach to the diagnosis of gastroparesis.

Gastroparesis is often a diagnosis of exclusion. A pregnancy test, along with tests to rule out Addison's disease and hyperthyroidism, should be done. An upper endoscopy is necessary to exclude gastric outlet obstruction. The presence of > 100 ml of fluid in a fasting stomach is abnormal and indicates gastroparesis. Partial small bowel obstruction also needs to be considered.

A quantitative gastric emptying study should be done next. Several tests are available. Gamma scintigraphy is the standard because of its precision, simplicity, and reproducibility. Because gastric emptying of solids is a better indicator of disease, a solid-meal study should be done. A convenient measure is T50%, or the time it takes for one-half of the test meal to leave the stomach. The nature of the early emptying phase also may be important.

Antroduodenal manometry also may be used to measure gastric contractions as they progress along the antrum and into the duodenum. This test is more difficult to perform, is not as widely available, and gives different information from the nuclear medicine study of gastric emptying. Electrogastrography (EGG) is becoming more readily available and measures the pacesetter potential at a frequency of 3 contractions per minute. Tachygastria correlates with gastroparesis, but more needs to be learned about this test before it can be used as a clinical tool.

Regardless of the method or measurement, many variables influence gastric emptying, including the type of marker, size and kind of meal composition, meal temperature, time of day at which the test is done, position of patient, age, sex, drug intake, and history of smoking.

21. Once gastroparesis is diagnosed, how should it be treated?

Electrolytes should be corrected, and any drug that potentially slows gastric emptying should be stopped. Several prokinetic drugs that facilitate gastric motility are available:

Bethanechol is a cholinergic drug that stimulates muscarinic receptors. Antral contractions increase, but phase III activity does not. Its usefulness in gastroparesis is limited.

Metoclopramide is a dopamine antagonist with potent cholinergic effects. It acts mainly on the proximal GI tract. In the stomach it increases antral contractions and relaxes the pylorus. It also has antiemetic properties. The usual dosage is 10 mg 4 times/day, and it may be given orally or intravenously. Side effects are common, including drowsiness, dystonic reactions, and nervousness.

Cisapride is a benzamide derivative that facilitates acetylcholine release at the myenteric plexus. It affects the entire GI tract and does not have the CNS side effects of metoclopramide. Cisapride was recently taken off the market because of life-threatening arrhythmias in some patients but may be obtained directly from Janssen Pharmaceutica if certain criteria are met

Domperidone is a benzimidazole derivative with clinical effects similar to metoclopramide. It acts primarily on the proximal GI tract and has fewer side effects than metoclopramide. It is not yet available in the U.S.

Erythromycin in doses of 50 mg IV induces phase III contractions in the antrum and upper small bowel. It acts as a motilin agonist, and the effect on the stomach has been described as pharmacologic antrectomy. Its effect becomes less dramatic after 4 weeks. More information is needed before its therapeutic role is established.

22. What are the prokinetic medication options for refractory gastroparesis?

A few patients may be unresponsive to or intolerant of oral prokinetic pills. In such cases, a liquid form of prokinetic agents can be prescribed because liquid emptying may be near normal in gastroparesis. Metoclopramide is efficacious in gastroparesis when given subcutaneously. A metoclopramide nasal spray is being tested for chemotherapy-induced nausea.

23. Summarize the complications of gastroparesis.

Nausea and vomiting may be sufficiently severe to lead to significant weight loss and malnutrition, GI hemorrhage from Mallory-Weiss tears, and aspiration pneumonia. Nutritional deficiencies are commonly seen in patients with postvagotomy gastric stasis. A common complication is development of phytobezoar in the stomach. Phytobezoars can cause ulceration, small intestinal obstruction, and gastric perforation.

24. How do you eliminate bezoars in patients with gastroparesis?

Bezoars can be eliminated by mechanical means, such as endoscopic destruction, and lavage and dietary measures, such as exclusion of foods high in indigestible residue. Enzymatic digestion may be accomplished with papain or cellulase or agents such as N-acetylcysteine, which dissolves the mucus components of the bezoar.

25. Describe the surgical managementof medically refractory gastroparesis.

Surgery is the therapeutic option of last resort in patients with gastroparesis. Surgical jejunostomy with enteric feeding can improve overall health in some patients with diabetic gastroparesis, resulting in improvement in GI symptoms and nutrition and reduction in hospitalization rates. Additional gastrostomy placement can drain gastric secretions during severe symptom flares. Finally, diabetic patients with gastroparesis and renal failure show greater improvement in gastric function after combined pancreas-kidney transplantation than after kidney transplantation alone, suggesting that the enhancement of glycemic control provided by the pancreatic graft provides significant benefit. Surgical placement of electrical leads on the gastric wall for electrical pacing has been proposed. In preliminary studies of humans with gastroparesis, gastric pacing reduces the frequency of nausea and vomiting, with acceleration of liquid emptying and variable effects on gastric emptying of solids.

BIBLIOGRAPHY

1. Bardhan PK, Salam MA, Molla AM: Gastric emptying of liquid in children suffering from acute rotaviral gastroenteritis. Gut 33:26, 1992.
2. Benini L, Sembenini C, Castellani G, et al: Gastric emptying and dyspeptic symptoms in patients with gastroesophageal reflux. Am J Gastroenterol 91:1351, 1996.
3. Bensen ES, Jaffe KM, Tarr PI: Acute gastric dilatation in Duchenne muscular dystrophy: A case report and review of the literature. Arch Phys Med Rehabil 77:512, 1996.
4. Bitytskiy LP, Soykan I, McCallum RW: Viral gastroparesis: A subgroup of idiopathic gastroparesis clinical characteristics and long-term outcomes. Am J Gastroenterol 92:1501, 1997.
5. Caras S, Laurie S, Cronk W, et al: Case report: Pancreatic cancer presenting with paraneoplastic gastroparesis. Am J Med Sci 312:34, 1996.
6. Cucchiara S, Salvia G, Borrelli O, et al: Gastric electrical dysrhythmias and delayed gastric emptying in gastroesophageal reflux disease. Am J Gastroenterol 92:1103, 1997.
7. Eisenberg B, Murata GH, Tzamaloukas AH, et al: Gastroparesis in diabetics on chronic dialysis: Clinical and laboratory associations and predictive features. Nephron 70:296, 1995.
8. Foltynova V, Brousil J, Velatova A, et al: Swallowing function and gastric emptying in patients undergoing replacement of the esophagus. Hepatogastroenterology 40:48, 1993.
9. Fontana RJ, Barnett JL: Jejunostomy tube placement in refractory diabetic gastroparesis: A retrospective review. Am J Gastroenterol 91:2174, 1996.
10. Fujuwara Y, Nakagawa K, Tanaka T, Utsunomiya J: Relationship between gastroesophageal reflux and gastric emptying after distal gastrectomy. Am J Gastroenterol 91:75, 1996.
11. Gattuso JM, Kamm MA, Morris G, Britton KE: Gastrointestinal transit in patients with idiopathic megarectum. Dis Colon Rectum 39:1044, 1996.
12. GEMS Study Group: Report of a multicenter study on electrical stimulation for the treatment of gastroparesis [abstract]. Gastroenterology 112:A735, 1997.
13. Hathaway DE, Abell T, Cardoso S, et al: Improvement in autonomic and gastric function following pancreas-kidney versus kidney-alone transplantation and the correlation with quality of life. Transplantation 57:816, 1994.
14. Haubrich WS, Schaffner F, Berk JE (eds): Bockus Gastroenterology, 5th ed. Philadelphia, W.B. Saunders, 1995.
15. Hunter RJ, Metz DC, Morris JB, Rothstein RD: Gastroparesis: A potential pitfall of laparoscopic Nissen fundoplication. Am J Gastroenterol 91:2617, 1996.
16. Konturek JW, Fischer H, van der Voort IR, Domschke W: Disturbed gastric motor activity in patients with human immunodeficiency virus infection. Scand J Gastroenterol 32:221, 1997.
17. Lyrenas EB, Olsson EH, Arvidsson UC, et al: Prevalence and determinants of solid and liquid gastric emptying in unstable type I diabetes. Relationship to postprandial blood glucose concentrations. Diabetes Care 20:413, 1997.
18. MacDonald A, Baxter JN, Bessent RG, et al: Gastric emptying in patients with constipation following childbirth and due to idiopathic slow transit. Br J Surg 84:1411, 1997.
19. McCallum RW, Chen JDZ, Lin Z, et al: Gastric pacing improves emptying and symptoms in patients with gastroparesis. Gastroenterology 114:456, 1998
20. Merio R, Festa A, Bergmann H, et al: Slow gastric emptying in type I diabetes: Relation to autonomic and peripheral neuropathy, blood glucose, and glycemic control. Diabetes Care 20:419, 1997.
21. Nakamura T, Takebe K, Ishii M, et al: Study of gastric emptying in patients with pancreatic diabetes (chronic pancreatitis) using acetaminophen and isotope. Acta Gastroenterol Belg 59:173, 1996.
22. Neild PJ, Nijram K, Sharpstone D, et al: Gastric emptying in HIV-infected patients; correlation with weight loss, autonomic function and gastrointestinal infection [abstract]. Int Conf AIDS 11:107, 1996.
23. Sleisenger MH, Fordtran JS, (eds): Gastrointestinal and Liver Disease: Pathophysiology, Diagnosis, Management, 6th ed. Philadelphia, W.B. Saunders, 1998.
24. Tobi M, Holtz T, Carethers J, Owyang C: Delayed gastric emptying after laparoscopic anterior highly selective and posterior truncal vagotomy. Am J Gastroenterol 90:810, 1995.
25. Troncon LE, Oliveira RB, Romanello LM, et al: Abnormal progression of a liquid meal through the stomach and small intestine in patients with Chagas disease. Dig Dis Sci 38:1551, 1993.
26. Yamada T, Alpers DH, Laine L, et al (eds): Textbook of Gastroenterology 3rd ed. Philadelphia, Lippincott Williams & Wilkins, 1999.

III. Liver and Biliary Tract Disorders

15. EVALUATION OF ABNORMAL LIVER TESTS

Kenneth E. Sherman, M.D., Ph.D.

1. What are liver tests?

Usually the term refers to the routine chemistry panel that includes alanine aminotransferase (ALT), aspartate aminotransferase (AST), gamma glutamyl transpeptidase (GGT), alkaline phosphatase (AP), bilirubin, albumin, and protein. Other terms for the same tests are liver function tests (LFTs) and liver-associated enzymes (LAEs), but neither is totally accurate. Only the first four are properly called enzymes, and only the last two provide a measure of liver function. These tests help to characterize injury patterns and provide a crude measure of the synthetic function of the liver. Various combinations can be helpful in diagnosing specific disease processes, but generally these tests are not diagnostic. Other LFTs are described below. Finally, certain tests help to define specific causes of liver disease. They may be serologic (e.g., hepatitis C antibody) or biochemical (e.g., alpha-1 antitrypsin level) but generally are not used as screening assays or as part of general health profiles.

2. What are the true liver function tests?

True LFTs evaluate the liver's synthetic capacity or measure the ability of the liver either to uptake and clear substances from the circulation or to metabolize and alter test reagents. **Albumin** is the most commonly used indicator of synthetic function, although it is not highly sensitive and may be affected by poor nutrition, renal disease, and other factors. In general, low albumin levels indicate poor synthetic function. The **prothrombin time** (PT) is another simple measure of the liver's capacity to synthesize clotting factors. The PT may be related to decreased synthetic ability or vitamin K deficiency. A high PT that does not correct with oral administration of vitamin K (5–10 mg for 3 days) may indicate liver disease, unless ductal obstruction or intrahepatic cholestasis prevents bile excretion into the duodenum and thus limit absorption of vitamin K. Administration of a subcutaneous or intravenous injection of vitamin K (10 mg) may correct the defect and suggests that vitamin K absorption rather than synthetic dysfunction is responsible for the PT abnormality.

Various uptake and excretion tests profess to define liver function, including bromosulphothalein (BSP), indocyanine green, aminopyrine, caffeine, and monoethylglycinexylidide (MEGX). Research laboratories frequently use such tests to determine severity of liver disease and to predict survival outcomes, but currently they are not part of routine clinical practice.

3. What is the difference between cholestatic and hepatocellular injury?

The two main mechanisms of liver injury are damage or destruction of liver cells, which is classified as hepatocellular, and impaired transport of bile, which is classified as cholestatic. Hepatocellular injury is most often due to viral hepatitis, autoimmune hepatitis, and various toxins and drugs. Transport of bile may be impaired by extrahepatic duct obstruction (e.g., gallstone, postsurgical stricture), intrahepatic duct narrowing (e.g., primary sclerosing cholangitis), bile duct damage (e.g., primary biliary cirrhosis), or failed transport at the canalicular level (e.g., chlorpromazine effect). In some cases, elements of both types of damage are involved; this scenario is often called a "mixed injury" pattern.

4. What is the most specific test for hepatocellular damage?

The most specific test for hepatocellular damage is the ALT level. The AST level also may be elevated but is not as specific.

5. How is cholestatic injury best diagnosed?

Cholestatic injury is best diagnosed by an elevated AP level. Bile acids stimulate AP production, but duct obstruction or damage prevents bile acid excretion into the duodenum. Therefore, the AP level in serum rises dramatically. Serum AP levels may be slightly increased in early hepatocellular disease, but this increase is due to release of cellular enzyme without excessive stimulation of new enzyme. Because AP can be derived from other body tissue (e.g., bone, intestine), a concurrent elevation of GGT or 5'-nucleosidase helps to support a cholestatic mechanism.

6. What are serum transaminases?

The two serum transaminases commonly assayed in clinical practice are ALT and AST. Many laboratories still use older terminology that refers to ALT as serum glutamic pyruvate transaminase (SGPT) and to AST as SGOT (serum glutamic oxaloacetic transaminase). The newer terms reflect more accurately their enzymatic action, which involves the transfer of amino groups from one structure to another. As noted above, elevation of ALT and/or AST reflects the presence of hepatocellular injury. It is important to understand how the assays are performed and what confounding factors may alter interpretation of test results.

7. How is ALT assessed?

The most commonly used test reaction for ALT is as follows:

$$\text{Alanine} + \text{alpha-ketoglutarate} \leftrightarrow \text{pyruvate} + \text{L-glutamate}$$

This reaction requires ALT and pyridoxal phosphate (vitamin B6). A crucial point is that enzyme assays do not measure how much enzyme is present; instead, they indirectly measure the catalytic activity of the enzyme in performing a particular function. Therefore, the assay does not indicate how much ALT is present but how quickly it causes the above reaction to take place. The assumption is that the faster the reaction, the greater the amount of ALT. To complicate matters further, the assay does not measure the amount of reaction product that is created. Instead, a linked enzyme reaction is used:

$$\text{Pyruvate} \leftrightarrow \text{lactic acid}$$

This reaction occurs in the presence of another enzyme, lactate dehydrogenase. The reaction requires the oxidation of reduced nicotinamide adenine dinucleotide (NADH) and creates the unreduced form (NAD+) as an additional reaction product. NAD+ absorbs light at a 340-nm wavelength. This absorption, as measured by a spectrophotometer, is used to determine ALT activity. Therefore, the end-point measurement is several steps removed from the quantitative measurement of interest. The speed of a reaction, however, may be affected by several components of the process, including temperature, substrate concentration, amount of enzymes or cofactors, interfering substances in the reaction mix, and sensitivity of the spectrophotometer. For example, if a patient is deficient in pyridoxal phosphate and this cofactor is not added in excess of the amount needed for the test reaction, the reaction rate is slowed, and the final result is a falsely low ALT activity. This confounding effect is probably common in malnourished alcoholics, in whom deficiency of vitamin B6 rather than ALT level is the limiting step in the reaction.

8. How are normal and abnornmal levels of ALT determined?

This determination is generally made by the local laboratory in an arbitrary manner. A small set of so-called healthy patients is selected, often from a blood bank. The ALT is determined in all members, and a mean and standard deviation are calculated. Arbitrary cut-offs are assigned, usually at values representing the top and bottom 2.5% of the sample population. This technique is unfortunate, because many demographic factors play a role in ALT level. Men have higher ALT levels than women, obese women have higher ALT levels than people close to ideal body weight, and certain racial groups have higher ALT activity than others. In addition, patients who donate blood may not in fact be free of liver disease. Therefore, if the random test population consists mainly of thin Caucasian women who donate blood at an office drive, the cut-off values may be very low. Thus many overweight men may have ALT levels in the "high" range, even in the absence of disease. This problem applies to all of the enzyme tests described in this chapter. Therefore, the further a test result is from normal, the more likely that disease in fact exists. Conversely, patients with significant silent liver disease may have normal ALT levels.

The ALT level, therefore, is an imperfect marker of the liver process. In diseases that involve massive liver damage, such as acute viral hepatitis, acetaminophen or solvent toxicity, or amanita mushroom poisoning, ALT may be increased to very high levels. For example, an ALT ≥ 2000 IU/L (50 times the upper limit of normal) is frequently seen in significant acetaminophen overdoses. This value reflects significant loss of ALT from damaged hepatocytes. In patients with chronic viral hepatitis, levels tend to be lower and frequently are 2–10 times normal.

9. What makes the AP level rise?

AP is a group of enzymes that catalyze the transfer of phosphate groups. Different isoenzymes can be identified from multiple sites in the body, including liver, bone, and intestine. Most hospital labs do not have the facilities to identify the source. This inability may pose a problem for clinicians. In one large study of hospitalized patients, only about 65% of elevated AP was from the liver. When the source is the liver, the mechanism appears to be related to stimulation of enzyme synthesis associated with local increases in bile acids. This finding results from drug-associated cholestasis and intrahepatic and extrahepatic obstruction. The problems associated with determining enzyme activity and establishing a normal range are analogous to those described for serum transaminases. The association of elevated AP with either GGT or 5'-nucleosidase helps to establish a liver source and suggests the presence of a cholestatic process.

10. What does an elevated bilirubin mean?

Bilirubin, a breakdown product of red blood cells, exists in two forms: conjugated and unconjugated. Unconjugated bilirubin appears in the serum when blood is broken down at a rate that overwhelms the processing ability of the liver. This finding is most common in patients with hemolysis. Several genetically acquired enzyme deficiencies result in improper or incomplete bilirubin conjugation in the liver. The most common is Gilbert's syndrome, which is characterized by a relative deficiency of glucuronyl transferase. Recently, the specific gene defect that accounts for a significant proportion of the observed phenotypic abnormality has been described. Patients often have high-normal to borderline-elevated bilirubin levels. When they fast or decrease caloric intake (e.g., patients with viral gastroenteritis), the bilirubin rises, primarily because of increases in the unconjugated form. If a bilirubin fractionation is not done, a patient with abdominal pain, nausea and vomiting, and an elevated bilirubin may be misdiagnosed as having cholecystitis. The resulting cholecystectomy could easily have been avoided by obtaining the fractionation.

11. How is bilirubin level determined?

The most common test for bilirubin involves a biochemical reaction over time. Most labs report only total bilirubin. By stopping the reaction at a particular time and subtracting the result from the total bilirubin, the lab arrives at the indirect bilirubin, which is an approximation of unconjugated bilirubin. Exact measurement requires the use of chromatography, which is not routinely performed in clinical labs. Conjugated bilirubin is elevated in many diseases, including viral, chemical, and drug- and alcohol-induced hepatitis; cirrhosis; metabolic disorders; and intrahepatic and extrahepatic biliary obstruction.

12. What tests are used to evaluate hemochromatosis?

Hemochromatosis is a disease of iron overload in the liver and other organs. The defect is probably in a regulatory mechanism for iron absorption in the small intestine. Over many years, patients build up stored iron in the liver, heart, pancreas, and other organs. The most common screening test for hemochromatosis is **serum ferritin**; an elevated level suggests the possibility of iron overload. Unfortunately, ferritin is also an acute-phase reactant and may be falsely elevated in various inflammatory processes. If ferritin is elevated (usually > 400 mg/L), serum iron and total iron binding capacity (TIBC) should be assessed. If the serum iron divided by TIBC is

> 50–55%, hemochromatosis should be strongly suspected instead of secondary iron overload (hemosiderosis).

Until recently, the definitive test was a quantitative assessment of iron. A **liver biopsy** specimen is used to determine the amount of iron in liver tissue. From a calculation based on the patient's age and iron content in liver, an index, called the iron-age index, was used to determine the presence or absence of hemochromatosis. This test may not be as reliable as previously thought, based on the recent availability of genetic testing. Three major **gene defects** have been described. They involve single amino acid mutations, which result in altered iron absorption. The most important gene is designated C282Y; H63D also may have a role in some populations. These genes are bi-allelic; that is, each parent contributes one-half of the patient's complement. Therefore, patients may be homozygote wildtype, heterozygote, or homozygote with mutation. Only patients with both mutated alleles are thought to have genetic hemochromatosis.

Studies suggest that **magnetic resonance imaging** of the liver also may be helpful in evaluating hepatic iron content and in the future may reduce the need for liver biopsy. However, most radiologists are not trained to interpret the results.

13. Describe the role of alpha-1 antitrypsin.

Alpha-1 antitrypsin is an enzyme, made by the liver, that helps to break down trypsin and other tissue proteases. Multiple variants are described in the literature. The variant is expressed as an allele from both parents. Therefore, a person may have one or two forms of alpha-1 antitrypsin in the blood. One particular variant, called Z because of its unique electrophoretic mobility on gel, is the product of a single amino acid gene mutation from the wild-type protein (M). The Z protein is difficult to excrete from the liver cell and causes local damage that may result in hepatitis and cirrhosis.

14. What three tests are used to diagnose alpha-1 antitrypsin deficiency?

1. Serum protein electrophoresis (SPEP). When blood proteins are separated on the basis on electrical migration in gel, several bands are formed. One of these, the alpha-1 band, consists mostly of alpha-1 antitrypsin. Therefore, an alpha-1 antitrypsin deficiency results in a flattening of the alpha-1 band on SPEP.

2. Direct assay that uses a monoclonal antibody against alpha-1 antitrypsin. The degree of binding can be measured in a spectrophotometer by rate nephelometry.

3. Alpha-1 antitrypsin phenotype. Only a few labs in the U.S. run this test, which designates the allelic protein types in the serum (e.g., MM, ZZ, MZ, FZ). Patients with protein of the ZZ type are said to be homozygotic for Z-type alpha-1 antitrypsin deficiency. This is the form most frequently associated with significant liver disease. If Z protein is trapped in hepatocytes, it can be seen in liver tissue as small globules that stain with the periodic acid-Schiff (PAS) reaction and resist subsequent digestion with an enzyme called diastase. An immunostain is also available in some institutions.

15. What is Wilson's disease?

Wilson's disease, a disorder of copper storage, is associated with deficiency of an enzyme derived from liver cells. Like iron, copper may accumulate in many tissues in the body. Its storage sites are somewhat different, however. Deposition may be seen in the eye (Kayser-Fleischer rings) and parts of the brain. Many cholestatic diseases of the liver (e.g., primary biliary cirrhosis) also result in aberrant copper storage but not to the degree seen in true Wilson's disease.

16. How is Wilson's disease diagnosed?

The main screening test is the serum ceruloplasmin level, which is low in over 95% of patients with Wilson's disease. Ceruloplasmin is also an acute-phase reactant and may be falsely elevated into a low-normal range in patients with an inflammatory process. Follow-up tests include assessments of urine and serum copper levels. A quantitative assessment of copper in liver tissue from liver biopsy provides definitive diagnosis. Copper is stained in the tissue with special stain processes (e.g., rhodanine stain).

17. Summarize the tests for common metabolic disorders of the liver.

DISEASE	PRIMARY TEST	SUPPORTIVE TEST	DEFINITIVE TEST
Hemochromatosis	Serum ferritin > 400 mg/L	Iron saturation > 55% Iron age index > 2	C282Y, H63D homo-zygosity
Alpha-1 antitrypsin deficiency	SPEP or Al-AT level	Phenotype (Pi type)	Liver biopsy with PAS-positive diastase-resistant granules
Wilson's disease	Ceruloplasmin < 10 mg/dl	Urine/serum copper >80 mg/24 hr	Liver biopsy with quantitative copper >50 mg/g wet weight

SPEP = serum protein electrophoresis, PAS = periodic acid-Schiff test.

There are numerous other hereditary diseases of the liver, including Gaucher's disease, Niemann-Pick disease, and hereditary tyrosinemia. These rare diseases are usually diagnosed in children. Specific tests are beyond the scope of this chapter.

18. What are autoimmune markers?

Autoimmune markers are tests used to determine the presence of antibodies to specific cellular components that have been epidemiologically associated with the development of specific liver diseases. Autoimmune markers include antinuclear antibody (ANA), antismooth muscle antibody (ASMA; also called anti-actin antibody), liver-kidney microsomal antibody type 1 (LKM-1), antimitochrondrial antibody (AMA), soluble liver antigen (SLA), and antiasialoglycoprotein receptor antibody. ANA, ASMA, and AMA are the most readily available tests and help to define the probability of the more common classes of autoimmune liver disease. Currently SLA is not easily obtained in the U.S.

19. How are the common antibody tests performed and interpreted?

The common antibody tests are performed by exposure of the patient's serum to cultured cells and labeling with a fluorescein-tagged antibody against human antibodies. The cells are examined by fluorescent microscopy and graded according to intensity of the signal and which part of the cell binds the antibody. Therefore, reading of antibody levels and determination of positive or negative results are highly subjective, and most hepatologists require positive results in dilution titers > 1:80 or 1:160 before considering the tests as part of a diagnostic algorithm. ANA and ASMA are particularly common in older people, women, and patients with a wide spectrum of liver diseases. Therefore, the diagnosis of autoimmune liver disease depends on a broad clinical picture that takes into account age, sex, presence of other autoimmune processes, gammaglobulin levels, and liver biopsy findings. In addition, the overlap in antibodies in different autoimmune liver diseases is considerable. The table below provides a crude representation of one classification scheme. A newer scoring system that tries to take into account the variables noted above also has been proposed.

Classification of Autoimmune Liver Disease

DISEASE	ANTIBODY
Type I classic lupoid hepatitis	Antinuclear antibody and/or antismooth muscle antibody
Type II autoimmune hepatitis	Liver-kidney microsomal antibody type I
Type III autoimmune hepatitis	Soluble liver antigen
Primary biliary cirrhosis	Antimitochondrial antibody

20. When should screening or diagnostic tests be ordered for patients with suspected liver disease?

The transaminases, bilirubin, and alkaline phosphatase serve as screening tests when liver disease is suspected. The history, physical exam, and estimation of risk factors help to determine which specific diagnostic tests should be ordered. Some patients have occult liver disease with normal or near-normal enzymes, and occasionally patients with isolated enzyme elevations have no identifiable disease. In general, patients should have at least two sets of liver enzyme tests to eliminate lab error before a full work-up for liver disease is begun. Many diseases (hepatitis B and hepatitis C) generally require proof of chronicity (abnormality > 6 months) before therapy is initiated or confirmatory and staging liver biopsies are obtained. The severity of enzyme abnormality and the likelihood of finding a treatable process may modify the typical waiting period. For example, a female patient with transaminase levels 10 times normal, a history of autoimmune thyroid disease, and an elevated globulin fraction probably has a flare of previously unrecognized chronic autoimmune hepatitis. An autoimmune profile and early liver biopsy may help to support this hypothesis and lead to prompt treatment with steroids and other immunosuppressants.

BIBLIOGRAPHY

1. Bacon BR, Olynyk JK, Brunt EM, et al: HFE genotype in patients with hemochromatosis and other liver disease. Ann Intern Med 130:953–962, 1999.
2. Bassett ML, Halliday JW, Powell LW: Value of hepatic iron measurements in early hemochromatosis and determination of the critical iron level associated with fibrosis. Hepatology 6:24–29, 1986.
3. Brensilver HL, Kaplan MM: Significance of elevated liver alkaline phosphatase in serum. Gastroenterology 68:1556–1562, 1975.
4. Buffone GS, Beck JR: Cost-effectiveness analysis for evaluation of screening programs: Hereditary hemochromatosis. Clin Chem 40:1631–1636, 1994.
5. Eriksson S, Carlson J, Velez R: Risk of cirrhosis and primary liver cancer in alpha-1 antitrypsin deficiency. N Engl J Med 314:736–739, 1983.
6. Kaplan MM: Laboratory Tests in Diseases of the Liver, 6th ed. Philadelphia, J.B. Lippincott, 1987, pp 219–260.
7. Scharschmidt BF, Goldberg HI, Schmid R: Approach to the patient with cholestatic jaundice. N Engl J Med 308:1515–1519, 1983.
8. Sherman KE: Alanine aminotransferase in clinical practice: A review. Arch Intern Med 151:260–265, 1991.
9. Wroblewski F: The clinical significance of transaminase activities of serum. Am J Med 27:911–923, 1959.

16. VIRAL HEPATITIS

Kenneth E. Sherman, M.D., Ph.D.

1. What are the types of hepatitis viruses?

There are currently five identifiable forms of viral hepatitis: A, B, C, D, and E. All of these viruses are hepatotrophic; that is, the liver is the primary site of infection. Other viruses also infect the liver, but it is not their primary site of replication and cellular damage. Examples include cytomegalovirus (CMV), herpes simplex virus (HSV), Epstein-Barr virus (EBV), and many of the arthropod-borne flaviviruses (e.g., dengue virus, yellow fever virus). Other viruses may be hepatotrophic, but their pathogenic potential is unclear. Examples include the TT virus and hepatitis G.

Key Characteristics of the Hepatitis Viruses

TYPE	NUCLEIC ACID	GENE SHAPE	ENVELOPE	SIZE (NM)
A	RNA	Linear	No	28
B	DNA	Circular	Yes	42
C	RNA	Linear	Yes	(?) 40–50
D	RNA	Circular	Yes	43
E	RNA	Linear	No	32

2. What is the difference between acute and chronic hepatitis?

All hepatitis viruses can cause acute infection, which is defined as the presence of clinical, biochemical, and serologic abnormalities for up to 6 months. Hepatitis A and E are cleared from the body within 6 months and do not cause persistent infection for a longer period. In contrast, hepatitis B, C, and D can lead to chronic infection, which is more likely to be associated with development of cirrhosis. An increased risk of primary hepatocellular carcinoma occurs in patients chronically infected with hepatitis B, C, and D.

3. How common is chronic hepatitis B?

The risk of chronicity for hepatitis B is highly dependent on the person's age at infection and immunologic status. Neonates infected with hepatitis B have a chronicity rate approaching 100%. The rate decreases to about 70% for young children. Healthy young adults probably have chronicity rates less than 1%, but patients taking steroids or with chronic illness (e.g., renal disease) are less likely to clear the viral infection.

4. When does chronic hepatitis D develop?

Hepatitis D chronicity occurs only in the presence of simultaneous hepatitis B infection. In patients with chronic hepatitis B who become superinfected with hepatitis D, the risk of chronicity approaches 100%.

5. How common is chronic hepatitis C?

Hepatitis C chronicity may occur in up to 85% of patients. It is frequently associated with the development of histologically identifiable hepatitis. A small number of patients may have a chronic, nonfibrotic carrier state. A liver biopsy is essential to determine whether fibrogenic potential is present.

6. How are hepatitis viruses transmitted?

Hepatitis A and E are transmitted via a fecal-oral route. Both agents are prevalent in areas where sanitation standards are low. Large epidemics of both diseases frequently occur after floods and other natural disasters that disrupt already marginal sanitation systems. Hepatitis A is endemic in the United States and much of the world, whereas hepatitis E is not endemic in the United States. Large outbreaks of hepatitis E have been seen in Central and South America, Bangladesh, and India. The fecal-oral transmission route includes not only direct contamination of drinking water and food, but viral concentration and enteric acquisition by eating raw shellfish from sewage-contaminated waters.

7. Describe the symptoms of hepatitis.

The classic symptoms of acute hepatitis include anorexia, nausea, vomiting, severe fatigue, abdominal pain, mild fever, jaundice, dark urine, and light stools. Some patients may have a serum sickness-like presentation that includes arthralgias, arthritis, and skin lesions; this presentation is more common in **hepatitis B** than in other forms of acute viral hepatitis and may be seen in up to 20% of infected patients. It is associated with formation of immune complexes between antigen and antibody. Many patients with acute viral hepatitis do not have disease-specific symptoms. All forms of viral hepatitis may present as a mild-to-moderate flulike illness. In a recent national survey of the U.S. population, approximately 30% of participants had serologic evidence of past **hepatitis A** infection, but few were diagnosed with hepatitis A or reported an illness with classic hepatitis features.

Patients with chronic **hepatitis B or C** report fatigue as the leading symptom. Other common manifestations include arthralgias, anorexia, and vague, persistent right upper quadrant pain. Jaundice, easy bruisability, or prolonged bleeding after shaving or other small skin breaks usually mark the development of end-stage liver disease and often signify the presence of scarring and irreversible liver dysfunction.

8. What biochemical abnormalities are associated with viral hepatitis?

Elevation of serum transaminases (alanine aminotransferase [ALT], aspartate aminotransferase [AST]) is the hallmark of acute liver damage and identifies the presence of various processes caused by viral hepatitis. ALT is more specific than AST. AST may be elevated in association with muscle injury. In patients with acute hepatitis A, B, D, or E, elevations of transaminases to several thousand are not uncommon; they usually are accompanied by more modest increases in alkaline phosphatase and gamma-glutamyl-transferase (GGT). As the disease progresses, the transaminases decrease. As the levels decrease slowly over a period of weeks, bilirubin often rises and may peak weeks after the transaminases peak. Bilirubin levels usually subside by 6 months after infection. Hepatitis C is not as frequently associated with a notable acute hepatitis, and transaminases rarely exceed 1000 IU/L.

9. What biochemical findings indicate chronic infection?

Abnormalities that persist for longer than 6 months define the process as chronic. In this stage of disease, transaminases range from mildly elevated to 10–15 times the upper limit of normal. Bilirubin is often normal or mildly elevated, as are alkaline phosphatase and GGT. Sudden elevations of transaminases in the chronic period often signify a viral flare rather than development of a new process superimposed on the preexisting chronic viral state. However, superinfection with hepatitis D in a patient with chronic hepatitis B is frequently observed.

10. How is hepatitis A diagnosed?

The diagnosis of hepatitis A depends on identifying a specific IgM antibody directed against the viral capsid protein. This is often identified as a HAVAB-M test (hepatitis A viral antibody-IgM class) on lab order sheets. The IgM antibody appears early in infection and persists for 3–6 months. The other available lab test detects the IgG form of the antibody, which diagnoses past infection and does not have a role in routine clinical practice. Some laboratories offer a combined (total) IgM + IgG, which complicates interpretation of positive results.

11. How is hepatitis B diagnosed?

The incorrect interpretation of hepatitis B serologic markers is common and leads to many inappropriate laboratory tests and specialty consultations. It is important to understand the sequence of marker appearance and disappearance and the information that each marker provides. Tests of hepatitis B include both serologic and molecular markers: hepatitis B surface antigen (HBsAg) and hepatitis B surface antibody (HBsAb), hepatitis B anticore antibody (HBcAb), hepatitis B e antigen (HBeAg) and hepatitis B e antibody (HBeAb), DNA polymerase assay, hybridization assays, bDNA assays, and polymerase chain reaction (PCR).

12. Describe the HBsAg and HBsAb tests.

HBsAg, a protein that forms the outer coat of the hepatitis B virus, is produced in great excess during viral replication and aggregates to form noninfectious spherical and filamentous particles in the serum. It is detected by a radioimmunoassay (RIA) or enzyme-linked immunosorbent assay (ELISA) and indicates the presence of either acute or chronic infection. Its disappearance from the serum indicates viral clearance.

The **HBsAb** test detects an antibody directed against the surface antigen. This neutralizing antibody binds with and helps to clear the virus from the circulation. Its presence, therefore, indicates past infection with hepatitis B, which has been successfully cleared. The surface antibody also may appear in patients who are successfully vaccinated with the currently available recombinant hepatitis B vaccines. Its presence at a titer > 10 mIU/ml of serum confers protection against active infection.

13. How is the HBcAb test interpreted?

This test detects antibody formation against the core protein of the hepatitis B virus. The core protein surrounds the viral DNA and is surrounded by HBsAg in the complete virion, which is called the Dane particle. No commercial assay for HB core antigen is available. An ELISA assay is used to detect the antibody (HBcAb). The specific test comes in three forms, which must be differentiated to understand the meaning of the results: an IgG form, an IgM form, and a total form that measures both IgG and IgM. Most laboratories include the total test in hepatitis screening profiles, but it is important to find out which test is routinely run. A positive total HBcAb indicates either current or past hepatitis B infection. A positive HB anti-HBc IgM usually indicates an acute hepatitis B infection, although it also may indicate viral reactivation associated with immunosuppression or chronic illness. In contrast, a positive HB anticore IgG is consistent with either resolved past infection or, if present in conjunction with HBsAg, a chronic carrier state. Rarely, the presence of anti-HBc without anti-HBs suggests an occult infectious process.

14. What do the HBeAg and HBeAb tests indicate?

The e antigen is a soluble protein encoded by a portion of the core coding domain. Its presence suggests active replication. Therefore, HBeAg is seen in both acute infection and actively replicating chronic hepatitis B. In patients with acute infection, ordering of this test is not necessary. In patients with chronic infection, a positive result indicates a replicative form of the disease. Only when HBsAg is present, and chronic liver disease is suspected does this test help in decision making related to treatment and treatment outcomes. In a patient with resolved acute infection or relatively inactive (nonreplicative) chronic hepatitis B infection, HBeAg disappears and anti-HBe appears. Some patients with a point mutation in the precore coding region of the hepatitis B genome cannot make HBe and therefore do not develop an antibody response after resolution. The clinical significance of this mutation remains unclear, but it is quite prevalent in certain parts of the world.

15. Describe the DNA polymerase assay.

The polymerase assay was one of the earliest molecular assays used to detect hepatitis B DNA in serum. It was based on the finding that the hepatitis B virus carries its own DNA polymerase enzyme within the core. The assay measures the enzyme activity as it directs the incorporation of radioactive-tagged nucleotides into new viral DNA. The test is not highly sensitive and is not in routine clinical use. However, it is frequently referenced in research about hepatitis B from the 1970s and 1980s as a marker of viral activity.

16. What are hybridization assays?

Hybridization assays include various specific techniques that use a probe complementary to specific portions of the hepatitis B DNA genome. The actual hybridization may be performed on a filter paper matrix (dot blot) or in a column filled with beads that are impregnated with the probe material. The assay detects a marker substance on the probe, which sticks to the viral DNA. The marker is often a radioactive tracer (e.g., radioactive phosphorus [32P]) but also may be a chemical reactant (e.g., horseradish peroxidase). The sensitivity of these assays is not as great as amplification techniques, but most detect HBV DNA in a range of 1.5–20 pg/ml of serum. This range seems to provide a good marker for distinguishing replicative from non-replicative disease.

17. Describe the bDNA assay.

In this hybridization assay the viral nucleic acid hybridizes with complementary bDNA (branched- chain DNA) attached to a microtiter well. The hybridized viral DNA is then further hybridized to specific complementary DNAs in a reaction mixture, which are arrayed in a manner analogous to a multibranched tree. On the tree are pods of a marker molecule that emit light in a chemiluminescent reaction that can be detected by a luminometer. Because the light emission is proportionate to the amount of bound DNA, the test provides a highly reliable quantitative assay that is more sensitive than standard hybridization assays.

18. What are PCR assays?

Whereas the bDNA assay amplifies the signal generated by hybridization, PCR amplifies a portion of the DNA itself and makes it more detectable. PCR is the most sensitive technique available for detection of hepatitis DNA. Unfortunately, this sensitivity has little clinical relevance. Regardless of whether the carrier state is replicative or nonreplicative, DNA is always detected by PCR amplification. There is a high correlation between PCR positivity and the presence of HBsAg in serum. The HBsAg assay is cheaper and more reliable and should be the key test to determine whether active hepatitis B infection is present. Therefore, the health care provider must specify which DNA test is required, because many clinical labs default to PCR-based tests if not instructed otherwise.

19. How is hepatitis C diagnosed?

The screening assay for hepatitis C is an ELISA (also called EIA) assay that detects the presence of antibody to two regions of the hepatitis C genome. The currently available assay is in its second generation or third generation, depending on the manufacturer, and future modifications are likely. The test is highly sensitive but not specific; therefore, it gives many false-positive reactions. In populations with a low pretest probability of carrying hepatitis C, more than 40% of repeatedly reactive specimens are false positives. The antibody that is detected is nonneutralizing; that is, its presence does not confer immunity. If antibody is detected and the reaction is not a false positive, the patient almost always has active viral infection. Clearly, it is important to separate false positives from true positives. The cause of most false-positive reactions is binding of nonspecific immunoglobulin on the ELISA well surface. To avoid the use of serum, which requires obtaining drawn blood, oral fluid collection has been demonstrated to be an alternative screening modality to screen populations for HCV.

20. How is a positive result on the ELISA confirmed?

To support a true-positive reaction, the most commonly used test is a recombinant immunoblot assay (RIBA), which involves exposing the patient's serum to a nitrocellulose strip impregnated with bands of antigen. The currently available version (HCV RIBA 3.0, Chiron Corp, Emeryville, CA) has multiple antigens on the test strip as well as controls for nonspecific immunoglobulin binding and superoxide dismutase antibodies, which may confound the test results. The RIBA is not as sensitive as the ELISA, however, and therefore should not be used as a screening test for hepatitis C infection.

21. What other assays are available for hepatitis C?

Other assays in specialized laboratories include a bDNA quantitative assay for hepatitis C RNA and a PCR assay (see hepatitis B tests). The PCR is more sensitive but less amenable to clinical laboratory testing. In the past, both bDNA assays and PCR-based assays were reported in terms of copies of HCV RNA/ml. Efforts are under way to encourage universal use of an international unit assay standard, which will facilitate interpretation of different assays. The presence of hepatitis C RNA in serum or liver tissue is the gold standard for diagnosis of hepatitis C infection. Recent data suggest that quantitative evaluation of hepatitis C RNA levels in serum may have prognostic value in determining who is likely to respond to therapeutic intervention and in following the course of a treatment cycle. Preliminary data suggest that the most sensitive qualitative assay for HCV may be performance of transcription mediated amplification (TMA), but further field evaluation is indicated before routine implementation in clinical laboratories.

22. How is hepatitis D diagnosed?

Hepatitis D is diagnosed by an ELISA assay that detects the presence of antibody to hepatitis D in serum or plasma. The presence of the antibody in serum correlates with ongoing hepatitis D replication in the liver. Detection of hepatitis D antigen in liver tissue generally adds little to the diagnostic process. Early in the course of infection, acute hepatitis D may be detectable only by performing a test for the IgM form of the antibody. A PCR-based assay also may be performed to detect the presence of RNA from hepatitis D in serum or tissue. This assay is not commercially available, and its use seems to add little to the antibody testing. Because hepatitis D occurs only with concurrent acute hepatitis B infection or as a superinfection of chronic hepatitis B, there is little utility in testing for its presence at the initial work-up for viral causes of liver enzyme abnormalities.

23. How is hepatitis E diagnosed?

The original assays relied on a technique called an antibody-blocking assay, in which freshly infected primate tissue was exposed first to serum from the patient and then to serum from a known positive patient. If antibody is present in the unknown serum, it binds to the tissue and blocks the attachment of the second known antibody. This technique was difficult and is supplanted by a commercial ELISA. Hepatitis E does not seem to occur naturally in the United States. However, there should be a high index of suspicion in patients who have an acute hepatitis A-like illness, test negative for hepatitis A antibody IgM, and have traveled to an endemic area.

24. Are there other hepatitis viruses not yet discovered?

Probably. Several lines of evidence suggest that there are more hepatotrophic viruses than are currently recognized. Epidemiologic studies suggest that a small percentage of posttransfusion cases and a higher percentage of community-acquired cases of hepatitis have no identifiable viral infection, even when molecular detection techniques are used. Forms of liver disease (e.g., giant cell hepatitis) have been associated with paramyxovirus infection, although its role remains speculative at best. The cause of fulminant hepatic failure, hepatitis-associated aplastic anemia, and cryptogenic cirrhosis cannot be defined in a significant proportion of cases. Such findings point to the presence of one or more as yet unidentified agents. In recent years, three new agents have been extensively studied: the TT virus, hepatitis G virus and SEN-V. All may be associated with serum transaminase abnormalities in certain circumstances, but their exact role in acute and chronic disease has not been delineated.

25. What is the treatment of acute viral hepatitis?

The primary treatment of acute hepatitis of any type is mainly supportive. Patients generally do not require hospitalization unless the disease is complicated by significant hepatic failure, as evidenced by encephalopathy, coagulopathy with bleeding, renal failure, or inability to maintain adequate nutrition and fluid intake. Efforts must be made to identify the form of hepatitis and, if necessary, to ensure that the patient is removed from situations in which he or she is a high risk to others. For example, a food-handler should be removed from the workplace when hepatitis A is diagnosed, and health authorities must be notified.

26. Are specific antiviral agents available?

Specific antiviral treatment has been attempted in acute hepatitis cases. Recent literature about use of alpha and beta interferon in acute hepatitis C infection is conflicting. By general agreement, early drug intervention leads to a response in terms of both ALT level and viral load. Whether the rate of viral persistence associated with chronic HCV infection is lowered remains unclear. Because most patients with acute HCV infection are not identified, large-scale trials may be impossible, except in special populations such as health care workers with contaminated needlestick exposure. Alpha interferon also has been studied in patients with acute hepatitis D infection and fulminant hepatitis due to either coinfection or superinfection with hepatitis B. It appears to have little value in this setting.

27. Is chronic viral hepatitis treatable?

Yes. The chronic forms of hepatitis B, C, and D have been studied with regard to a number of treatment modalities. Alpha interferon has been tested in multiple randomized, controlled trials and has been found to be effective for all three agents. Interferon plus ribavirin is the most effective approved therapy for chronic hepatitis C. Lamivudine (3TC) is a nucleotide analog that is highly effective in suppression of hepatitis B and is FDA approved as well.

28. Which patients with chronic hepatitis B are candidates for therapy?

Patients with chronic hepatitis B, well-compensated liver disease, and evidence of viral replication (HBV DNA or HBeAg) are candidates for therapy. The goal of therapy is to reduce the level of replication and to change the infection to a relatively inactive disease. The clearance of HBsAg is not the immediate goal of therapy, although some evidence suggests that this may occur more frequently in successfully treated patients than in those that do not respond over subsequent years.

29. Describe the standard treatment and its side effects.

The standard treatment is alpha interferon 2b at a dose of 30–35 MU/week for 16 weeks. Longer treatment regimens are under evaluation. Patients seem to tolerate a dosing of 5 MU 6 days/week better than other dosing schemes. Side effects include a flu-like syndrome, which is occasionally quite severe. Often platelet count and absolute neutrophil count decrease significantly; thus the patient must be monitored closely and dose adjustments made.

30. What is the response rate to treatment of chronic hepatitis B?

Response rates range up to 60%, although in some groups it may be as low as 5%. Poor response is seen in patients with chronic, longstanding infection since childhood and in patients with HIV infection or other immunosuppression. The ideal patients, in terms of response outcomes are women with recent chronic infection, ALT > 200 IU/L, and viral load < 100 pg/ml by hybridization assay. Treatment with lamivudine at a dose of 100 mg/day results in complete viral suppression in nearly 100% of treated patients within a few months. Unfortunately, mutant virus emerges at a rate of 10–20% per year, and future therapies may require multidrug regimens. Several class-related agents are under evaluation. At least one of these, adefovir, may not be associated with cross-resistant mutants with lamivudine.

31. Describe the treatment of chronic hepatitis C. How effective is it?

Treatment of chronic hepatitis C is also interferon-based, although a lower dose is generally used. To date, three interferon products have been approved by the Food and Drug Administration for chronic hepatitis C. The standard treatment in patients with well-compensated liver disease consist of interferon alpha 2b, 3 MU 3 times/week, and ribavirin, 1000–1200 mg/day orally for 24–48 weeks. Although the side-effect profile is the same as for hepatitis B treatment, this regimen is usually better tolerated because of the lower interferon dosing. Use of this regimen in genotype 1 patients for 1 year leads to sustained viral clearance (no virus 6 months after completion of therapy) in 25–30% of treated patients. If the viral genotype is classified as non-1, there is little benefit to continued therapy beyond 6 months and response rates approach 60%. The role of long-term suppressive therapy in interferon-ribavirin nonresponders remains to be determined.

32. Describe the side effects of ribavirin.

Certain patients may be at risk of complications with ribavirin use. Ribavirin causes a dose-dependent hemolysis in approximately 80% of treated patients. Patients with underlying cardiac disease who cannot tolerate anemia may not be suitable candidates. Furthermore, ribavirin is teratogenic. Adequate birth control should be used during and for 6 months after treatment.

33. What is PEG-interferon?

Addition of a polyethylene glycol (PEG) moiety to interferon results in a PEG-interferon product that has a prolonged half-life with higher potency against the hepatitis C virus. PEG-interferons will replace nonpegylated interferons when regulatory approvals are provided.

34. What alternative therapies for hepatitis C are under investigation?

Alternative therapies for hepatitis C under investigation in many clinical research centers include combinations with interferon such as thymosin alpha-1, ursodeoxycholic acid, histamine dihydrochloride, and phlebotomy in patients with borderline iron overload. Although results in early trials are encouraging, none of these alternatives can be recommended as standard therapy at present. Newer-generation therapies, including protease and helicase inhibitors and ribozymes active at internal ribosomal entry site of the virus, are also under development.

35. How is hepatitis D treated?

Hepatitis D also may be treated with interferon. Doses of 9 MU 3 times/week for 48 weeks were associated with a 50% response rate in one randomized, controlled trial. Relapse at the end of therapy was common, however.

36. How can be hepatitis A be prevented?

Hepatitis A infection can be prevented by the use of pooled gammaglobulin after acute exposure or a vaccine for long-term protection. A vaccine previously used in Europe, Canada, and elsewhere became available in the United States in 1995. The vaccine is prepared from an attenuated strain of the virus grown on tissue culture cells. It is chemically inactivated and seems to confer immunity in 80-90% of treated subjects. The vaccine has not been tested in young (< 2 year old) children but is recommended for people who travel to hyperendemic areas with poor sanitation, child-care workers, deployable military personnel, and other high-risk individuals. Universal vaccination has not been studied adequately to determine its cost-benefit ratio. For individuals exposed in local outbreaks (shellfish, food-handler), gamma globulin should be adequate for short-term protection.

37. Describe the vaccine for hepatitis B.

A vaccine for hepatitis B has been available since the early 1980s. It was originally prepared by isolation of the surface antigen protein. The current forms most widely used in the United States are surface antigen proteins made by recombinant techniques. The vaccine is more than 90% effective in providing long-term immunity after 3 doses. In 20–30% of vaccinated people, antibody titers drop to < 10 mIU/ml within 5 years. This titer is believed to be the critical protective level. Current Public Health Service recommendations do not mandate either follow-up testing or boosters, except in dialysis patients. These recommendations may change as future data become available. Acute hepatitis B exposure in nonvaccinated individuals requires treatment with hepatitis B immunoglobulin (HBIG). This hyperimmune gamma globulin has high-titer antibodies against hepatitis B surface antigen. It may be administered simultaneously with the first dose of vaccine; this regimen is often followed in infants of HBsAg-positive mothers.

38. Can hepatitis C be prevented?

No vaccine is available for hepatitis C. Because of rapid mutation in the envelope region of the genome, a multivalent vaccine probably will be required and may take several years to develop and test before it is available for routine use. There is some interest in development of virus-free pooled globulin products, which may mediate the infectious process, particularily in patients infected with hepatitic C virus after liver transplant.

CONTROVERSY

39. Should all patients with hepatitis C undergo liver biopsy?

For: Liver biopsy is the gold standard for evaluation of activity and fibrosis in the liver. Surrogate markers, including imaging with liver-spleen scan, SPECT, CT, MR, and ultrasound as well as lab tests for procollagen, have not been reliable markers. Standard liver tests are also frequently not helpful. A liver biopsy helps (1) to determine whether treatment should be started, (2) to decide aggressiveness of therapy, and (3) to provide factual evidence of an otherwise often asymptomatic condition, which encourages patients to continue treatment. The risk of biopsy in experienced hands is low, and until treatments are highly effective in all treated patients, it should be a mandatory part of the work work-up.

Against: Almost all patients with HCV infection deserve at least one course of therapy, regardless of the level of activity or fibrosis. Biopsies are a barrier to treatment, relegating patient care to a limited pool of practitioners who perform liver biopsies. Therefore, liver biopsy is not indicated in routine management.

BIBLIOGRAPHY

1. Alter MJ, Margolis HS, Krawczynski K, et al: The natural history of community-acquired hepatitis C in the United States. N Engl J Med 327:1899–1905, 1992.
2. Centers for Disease Control: Hepatitis B virus: A comprehensive strategy for eliminating transmission in the United States through universal childhood vaccination: Recommendations of the Immunization Practices Advisory Committee (ACIP). MMWR 40(no. RR-13), 1991.
3. Choo QL, Richman KH, Han JH, et al: Genetic organization and diversity of the hepatitis C virus. Proc Natl Acad Sci USA, 88:2451–2455, 1991.
4. Davis GL, Balart LA, Schiff E, et al: Treatment of chronic hepatitis C with recombinant interferon alfa. N Engl J Med 321:1501–1506, 1989.
5. Dawson GJ, Chau KH, Cabal CM, et al: Solid phase enzyme linked immunosorbent assay for hepatitis E virus IgG and IgM antibodies utilizing recombinant antigens and synthetic peptides. J Virol Meth 38:175–186, 1992.
6. Di Bisceglie AM, Martin P, Kassianides C, et al: Recombinant interferon alfa therapy for chronic hepatitis C: A randomized, double-blind, placebo-controlled trial. N Engl J Med 321:1506–1510, 1989.
7. Di Bisceglie AM, Shindo M, Fong T-L, et al: A study of ribavirin therapy for chronic hepatitis C. Hepatology 16:649–654, 1992.
8. Dienstag JL, Schiff ER, Wright TL, et al: Lamivudine as initial treatment for chronic hepatitis B in the United States. N Engl J Med 341:1256–1263, 1999.
9. Farci P, Mandas A, Coina A, et al: Treatment of chronic hepatitis D with interferon alfa-2a. N Engl J Med 330:88–94, 1994.
10. Houghton M, Weiner A, Han J, et al: Molecular biology of the hepatitis C viruses: Implications for diagnosis, development and control of viral disease. Hepatology 14:381–388, 1991.
11. Kaneko S, Miller RH, Di Bisceglie AM, et al: Detection of hepatitis B virus DNA in serum by polymerase chain reaction: Application for clinical diagnosis. Gastroenterology 99:799–804, 1990.
12. Koretz RL, Abbey H, Coleman E, Gitnick G: Non-A, non-B post-transfusion hepatitis: Looking back in the second decade. Ann Intern Med 119:110–115, 1993.
13. Krawczynski K, Bradley DW: Enterically transmitted non-A, non-B hepatitis. Identification of virus-associated antigen in experimentally infected cynomologus macaques. J Infect Dis 159:1042–1049, 1989.
14. Laras A, Koskinas J, Avigidis K, Hadziyannis SJ: Incidence and clinical significance of hepatitis B precore gene transaltion initiation mutants in e antigen-negative patients. J Viral Hepatitis 5:241–248, 1988.
15. McHutchison JG, Gordon SC, Cort S, Albrecht JK: Interferon alfa-2b alone or in combination with ribavirin as initail treatment for chronic hepatitis C. N Engl J Med 339:1485–1492, 1998.
16. Perrillo RP, Regenstein FG, Peters MG, et al: Prednisone withdrawal followed by recombinant alpha interferon in the treatment of chronic type B hepatitis: A randomized, controlled trial. Ann Int Med 109:95–100, 1988.
17. Seeff LB, Ruskell-Bales Z, Wright EC, et al: Long-term mortality after transfusion-associated non-A, non-B hepatitis. N Engl J Med 327:1906–1911, 1992.
18. Sherman KE, Creager RL, O'Brien J, et al: The use of oral fluid for hepatitis C antibody screening. Am J Gastroenterol 89:2025–2027, 1994.
19. Zaaijer HL, Borg F, Cuypers HTM, et al: Comparison of methods for detection of hepatitis B virus DNA. J Clin Microbiol 32:2088-2091, 1994.

17. ANTIVIRAL THERAPY FOR HEPATITIS C INFECTION

Julie R. Smith, M.H.S., PA-C, and Jorge L. Herrera, M.D.

1. What are the indications for antiviral therapy in patients with chronic hepatitis C?

Hepatitis C progresses in all chronically infected patients but at different rates. The average time for development of cirrhosis is 30 years, but there is a wide range of variability. Only about 20% of patients progress to cirrhosis. Because it is difficult to predict who will progress, everyone who is chronically infected should be evaluated for possible treatment. Many factors can speed progression of fibrosis, including alcohol consumption, coinfection with hepatitis B or human immunodeficiency virus (HIV), iron overload, and concomitant liver disease such as alpha-1-antitrypsin deficiency, Wilson's disease, or autoimmune hepatitis.

Patients with extrahepatic manifestations of hepatitis C infection should be considered for antiviral treatment. Mixed cryoglobulinemia, leading to leukocytoclastic vasculitis, may be a systemic manifestation of hepatitis C infection and may respond to antiviral therapy. Renal disease, joint inflammation, or central nervous system complications may result from microvascular injury.

2. What is the recommended evaluation of patients with chronic hepatitis C before therapy is begun?

The initial history and physical should include identification of possible risk factors in an effort to assess the duration of infection. Laboratory evaluation is geared toward confirming the infection, excluding other possible causes of liver disease, and detecting coinfection. Recommended laboratory tests are listed in the table below.

Some experts recommend testing for immunity against hepatitis B (hepatitis B surface antibody [HBsAb]) and hepatitis A (anti-HAV); in patients who are not immune, vaccination to prevent hepatitis A and B should be considered. In the absence of obvious advanced disease, a liver biopsy is advised to assess severity of disease, estimate prognosis, and determine urgency of antiviral therapy.

Recommended Pretreatment Evaluation of Patients with Chronic Hepatitis C Infection

TEST	PURPOSE
HCV-RNA by PCR	Confirm viremia
Serum albumin, bilirubin, PT	Assess liver function
Iron, transferrin, ferritin	Assess for iron overload
Antinuclear antibody	Detect autoimmune hepatitis
Alpha-1-antitrypsin phenotype	Detect alpha-1-antitrypsin deficiency
Ceruloplasmin (age <45 years)	Detect Wilson's disease
HBsAg, HIV antibody test	Detect viral coinfection
Hepatitis C genotype	Assess likelihood of response to therapy
Liver biopsy	Determine severity of disease and urgency for therapy

HCV = hepatitis C virus, PCR = polymerase chain reaction, PT = prothrombin time, HBsAg = hepatitis B surface antigen, HIV = human immunodeficiency virus.

3. Should hepatitis C genotype testing be performed before initiation of therapy?

Based on genomic sequencing of the hepatitis C virus, several genotypes (or strains) have been identified. They are classified as genotypes 1 through 6, with several subtypes denoted as 1a, 1b, 2a, and so forth. The various genotypes exhibit geographic variability. In the United States, genotype 1 accounts for approximately 70% of infections. Genotypes 2 and 3 account for the remaining 30%. In Europe, the proportion of genotype 2 and 3 infections is greater than in the United States. In the Middle East, genotype 4 predominates, and genotype 6 is seen most commonly in Asia.

Determining the genotype before therapy is important because it helps to predict likelihood of response and length of antiviral therapy. For example, patients infected with genotype 2 without cirrhosis have a greater than 60% chance of achieving a sustained response and need to be treated only for 6 months. In contrast, the probability of response to therapy is much less likely in genotype 1 infections, which require treatment for 1 year to maximize the chance of sustained remission. The genotype, however, has no value in predicting severity of disease or likelihood of progression to cirrhosis.

4. Is a liver biopsy mandatory before initiation of antiviral therapy?

A liver biopsy is not required to diagnose chronic hepatitis C but evaluates the level of hepatic inflammation and fibrosis. No other test makes this determination accurately. Liver function tests, such as prothrombin time and albumin or bilirubin level, become abnormal only when extensive damage has occurred. Likewise, liver enzymes, viral load, and genotype do not correlate with severity of liver disease. An adequate biopsy sample is the best way to assess the severity of liver disease.

5. What are the treatment options for hepatitis C infection?

The immune modulator interferon (IFN) was the first medication approved by the Food and Drug Administration (FDA) for treatment of hepatitis C. There are three types: IFN alpha-2a, IFN alpha-2b, and consensus IFN. They differ in amino acid configuration but are similar in efficacy. In most cases, they are administered subcutaneously for 6–12 months.

Ribavirin, an oral nucleoside analog, recently has been approved for the treatment of hepatitis C. Used alone, it is not effective as an antiviral agent against hepatitis C, but in combination with IFN alpha, efficacy improves by 10–20%.

At present, combination therapy with interferon and ribavirin is the treatment of choice for patients who have not been previously treated and patients who have relapsed after initial treatment with interferon monotherapy. Patients who fail to respond to interferon monotherapy also may benefit from a trial of combination therapy.

6. How is response to antiviral therapy assessed?

A decrease or normalization of liver enzymes usually indicates a positive response and is classified as a biochemical response to treatment. Such changes correlate with decreased hepatic inflammation as assessed by repeat liver biopsy. A biochemical response to treatment is not always associated with a virologic response. Liver enzymes should be monitored monthly, and viral load should be assessed at 3 and 6 months of treatment. If during therapy HCV-RNA becomes undetectable by a sensitive polymerase chain reaction (PCR) assay, a virologic response has been achieved. If the virus is still undetectable at the end of therapy, it is considered an end-of-treatment response. Patients who remain negative for the virus at 6 months after treatment are considered sustained responders. Sustained responses are durable; over 95% of patients continue to be HCV-RNA–negative in blood and liver 5–10 years after completing therapy. Patients who become negative during treatment but then are found to be viremic after discontinuation of treatment are termed relapsers.

7. How often should viral load be measured during treatment?

Baseline quantitation of HCV-RNA should be performed before treatment. A PCR-based assay with low sensitivity (100–600 copies/ml) is recommended. Because of marked variability among laboratories measuring viral load, it is recommended that the same laboratory and assay be used to monitor response to therapy over time. As an alternative, a nonquantitative HCV-RNA PCR assay may be used. This assay is usually more sensitive than the quantitative assay and less subject to interlaboratory variability, but it does not quantify the amount of virus in blood.

The timing and frequency of HCV-RNA level monitoring depends on the therapeutic regimen. Patients receiving interferon monotherapy should have a repeat HCV-RNA determination after 3 months of therapy. If the virus is detectable, further therapy at the same dose is unlikely to achieve a response; the patient should discontinue therapy or change to a different treatment regimen. Patients who have achieved viral eradication after 3 months should complete 12 months of interferon therapy and be reevaluated at the end of therapy and 6 months after discontinuation with HCV-RNA testing to confirm a sustained response or to detect relapse.

In contrast, patients undergoing combination therapy with interferon/ribavirin should receive 6 months of therapy before virologic response is assessed. If after 6 months of therapy HCV-RNA is still detectable in serum, continued therapy at the same dose is unlikely to achieve a sustained remission. Discontinuation of therapy should be considered. Patients who are found to be HCV-RNA–negative at 6 months can either discontinue therapy or complete a 1-year regimen, depending on pretreatment characteristics. Once therapy is completed, a repeat HCV-RNA 6 months later is recommended to confirm sustained virologic response or to detect relapse.

8. What pretreatment characteristics predict a favorable response to antiviral therapy?
1. Viral load < 2 million copies/ml
2. Infection with HCV genotype 2 or 3
3. Liver biopsy with little or no fibrosis
4. Age < 40 years at time of treatment
5. Female gender

Genotype is the most important predictive factor of response to therapy. Patients infected with genotype 2 or 3 without fibrosis on liver biopsy need to receive combination therapy for only 6 months.

9. What is the efficacy of interferon monotherapy for chronic hepatitis C?
Considering all patients treated for hepatitis C, approximately 10–20% achieve sustained response after 12 months of IFN monotherapy. This percentage is reduced in patients infected with genotype 1 or with substantial fibrosis on liver biopsy. A patient with advanced fibrosis and genotype 1 has less than a 5% chance of obtaining sustained response to IFN monotherapy. Approximately 35–45% of patients achieve normal liver enzyme levels during therapy but relapse after treatment discontinuation.

10. What is the efficacy of combination interferon and ribavirin?
Combining ribavirin with interferon for 12 months increases the rate of virologic sustained response up to 40% for all patients. A subset of patients, particularly those infected with genotype 2 or 3 without fibrosis, have a > 60% chance of achieving a sustained response with only 6 months of combination therapy. Patients infected with genotype 1 have a lower response rate of 10–30%, depending on pretreatment viral load and presence or absence of fibrosis on biopsy.

11. What are the side effects of interferon therapy? How should the patient be monitored?
Interferon suppresses bone marrow, potentially resulting in life-threatening leukopenia or thrombocytopenia. Complete blood counts are monitored periodically, and the dose is adjusted as needed. Other side effects that can diminish quality of life include flulike symptoms, headaches, fever, depression, anxiety, sexual dysfunction, hair loss, insomnia, and fatigue. Evening administration or pre-injection acetaminophen or ibuprofen can reduce the flulike symptoms.

Depression requires close monitoring. Patients with a history of severe depression or suicidal ideation or attempts should not be treated with interferon. Patients who have required pharmacologic therapy for mild depression in the past may benefit from initiation of antidepressants before treatment with interferon. Selective serotonin reuptake inhibitors usually are successful in reversing interferon-associated depression.

Hypothyroidism is an irreversible side effect of interferon. Levels of thyroid-stimulating hormone (TSH) should be determined before initiation of therapy and at regular intervals during treatment.

12. What are the side effects of ribavirin therapy? How should the patient be monitored?

Ribavirin can cause hemolysis and rapidly lead to symptomatic anemia. A reduction in hemoglobin to 10 gm/dl or less should trigger a decrease in the daily dose. If the hemoglobin decreases to 8.5 gm/dl or less, discontinuation of therapy is advised. For patients with known ischemic cardiac disease, closer monitoring is recommended, with reduction or discontinuation of therapy if the hemoglobin decreases by more than 2 gm/dl compared with baseline.

Other side effects from ribavirin include rash, shortness of breath, nausea, sore throat, and glossitis. The rash may be severe and require discontinuation of the medication. The other side effects are generally not life-threatening and can be treated symptomatically.

Because ribavirin is teratogenic, male and female patients should be advised to practice effective contraception during therapy and for 6 months after completion.

13. What are the contraindications to interferon therapy?

1. Interferon should not be used in patients who already have leukopenia or thrombocytopenia because of the potential for bone marrow suppression. It is not recommended for patients with decompensated cirrhosis because it is rarely effective and may cause further decompensation of liver disease.

2. Patients with severe depression, history of suicide attempt or ideation, psychosis, or personality disorders should not be treated, or should receive treatment only under the close monitoring of a psychiatrist. Patients with manic depression do poorly with interferon therapy and should not be treated.

3. Patients who continue to drink alcohol on a daily basis do not respond to antiviral therapy. Complete abstinence from alcohol during therapy is recommended. For patients who drink excessive amounts of alcohol, abstinence for a minimum of 6 months before initiation of therapy is required to maximize benefits of therapy.

4. Autoimmune diseases pose a relative contraindication to therapy. Psoriasis can worsen during therapy.

5. Interferon therapy should not be administered during pregnancy. If hepatitis C infection is diagnosed during pregnancy, treatment should be initiated only after delivery and breast-feeding have been completed.

6. Patients with advanced comorbid conditions should not be offered antiviral therapy for hepatitis C. Hepatitis C infection progresses slowly over time. If the patient has a serious comorbidity that is likely to be fatal within 5–10 years, treating the hepatitis C infection is not likely to be of benefit.

14. What are the contraindications to ribavirin therapy?

Because ribavirin must be used with interferon, all contraindications to interferon apply to treatment with ribavirin. In addition, there are specific contraindications to ribavirin:

1. Pregnancy is an absolute contraindication because of the teratogenic potential.

2. Anemia and hemoglobinopathies should be considered relative contraindications. Extreme care should be exercised in treating such patients. As a rule, females with a hemoglobin < 12 gm/dl, or males with < 13gm/dl before therapy are at high risk of developing severe anemia during therapy.

3. Patients with known ischemic heart disease should be treated with caution and monitored closely.

4. Patients with renal insufficiency should not be treated with ribavirin because the development of severe, long-lasting, and life-threatening hemolysis is common.

15. Should patients with cirrhosis secondary to hepatitis C infection be treated with antiviral therapy?

Patients with compensated cirrhosis (normal albumin and bilirubin levels, normal prothrombin time, and no ascites, encephalopathy, or history of variceal bleeding) are excellent candidates for antiviral therapy. They are most likely to benefit from viral eradication. Once liver insufficiency develops or complications of portal hypertension become clinically evident, antiviral therapy is relatively contraindicated. Evaluation for liver transplantation is a better option for such patients.

For patients with compensated disease, the main concern about antiviral therapy is worsening of preexisting thrombocytopenia or leukopenia due to hypersplenism. Although sustained viral response in patients with cirrhosis is less common than in noncirrhotic patients, normalization of liver enzymes and reduction in viral load during treatment result in overall improvement of liver disease and possibly delayed need for liver transplantation or development of hepatocellular carcinoma. Long-term treatment with interferon to minimize inflammation and improve fibrosis is being explored in this group of patients.

16. Should patients with hepatitis C and normal liver enzyme levels be treated with antiviral therapy?

As a group, patients who test positive for HCV-RNA in blood and have persistently normal levels of alanine aminostransferase over time tend to have mild disease on liver biopsy. Such is not the case in all patients, however, and up to 20% may have evidence of significant necroinflammatory disease on biopsy or even fibrosis. For this reason, the approach should be individualized. In general, the natural history of the disease should be discussed with the patient. A liver biopsy should be offered to stage severity of disease. If the liver biopsy shows mild or minimal disease, continued observation without therapy is a reasonable option. For patients with more advanced disease on liver biopsy, antiviral therapy has been shown to be as effective as in patients with elevated liver enzymes.

17. Should patients with HCV/HIV coinfection receive antiviral therapy for hepatitis C infection?

Coinfection with HIV and HCV results in marked acceleration of progression of liver disease. With the advent of newer, more effective antiretroviral agents, patients infected with HIV are living longer, and more are developing end-stage liver disease from HCV infection. For this reason, patients coinfected with HIV and HCV should be considered candidates for antiviral therapy against HCV.

Anti-HCV therapy is most likely to be effective if the patient is first placed on antiretroviral therapy, the HIV viral load is controlled, and the CD4 count is reconstituted. In general, patients with a CD4 count < 400/mm^3 do not respond to antiviral therapy for HCV.

Anti-HCV therapy in patients receiving anti-HIV medications is complicated by the additive bone marrow suppression as well as other gastrointestinal side effects. Close monitoring of the blood count is needed. Monitoring of HIV blood levels also is recommended because of concern about a possible negative interaction between ribavirin and some antiretroviral medications.

18. How should patients with HCV/HBV coinfection be treated?

Because most patients with HCV/HBV coinfection have quiescent hepatitis B infection, the antiviral therapy need be directed only at the hepatitis C virus. If active hepatitis B and C infection are present, as evidenced by a positive HCV-RNA and HBV-DNA (non-PCR assay), the patient should be treated with the recommended dose of interferon for hepatitis B in conjunction with ribavirin for hepatitis C. A flare of hepatitis is not unusual when treating patients with hepatitis B infection.

19. What are the options for patients who do not respond to combination therapy with interferon and ribavirin?

Currently, there are no established guidelines for the treatment of such patients. Those who were treated for only 6 months, achieved a response, and then relapsed may benefit from retreatment with the same regimen for 1 year. In contrast, those who did not respond to 1 year of combination therapy are unlikely to respond to additional therapy. Long-acting forms of interferon, also known as pegylated (PEG) interferon, are under development. These formulations are injected subcutaneously once a week and achieve stable blood levels of interferon. Preliminary trials have shown that PEG interferon is more effective than regular interferon in achieving a sustained response. It is hoped that PEG interferon in combination with ribavirin will be more active than currently available therapies. Antiviral products aimed directly at the hepatitis C virus genome, such as proteases, helicases, and ribozymes, are currently under development and may increase the percentage of patients who achieve a sustained response to therapy.

20. What is the role of antiviral therapy in acute hepatitis C?

The role for antiviral therapy in acute hepatitis C is unclear. Acute infections are usually asymptomatic and found incidentally, such as needlestick injuries in health care workers. More than 70% of acute hepatitis cases become chronic, indicating the need for some form of treatment in the early stages. Some studies have shown that early treatment with IFN or combination therapy decreases the chronicity rate in patients with acute hepatitis C. Although the current antiviral regimens for hepatitis C are not FDA-approved for the treatment of acute hepatitis C, strong consideration should be given to early initiation of antiviral therapy when acute hepatitis C is diagnosed.

BIBLIOGRAPHY

1. Gish RG: Standards of treatment in chronic hepatitis C. Sem Liv Dis 19(Suppl 1):35–47, 1999.
2. McHutchison JG, Gordon SC, Schiff ER, et al: Interferon alfa-2b alone or in combination with ribavirin as initial treatment for chronic hepatitis C. N Engl J Med 339:1485–1492, 1998.
3. Poynard T, Marcellin P, Lee S, et al: Randomized trial of interferon alfa 2-b and ribavirin for 48 weeks or for 24 weeks versus interferon alfa 2b plus placebo for 48 weeks for treatment of chronic infection with hepatitis C virus. Lancet 352:1426–1432, 1998.
4. Davis GL, Esteban-Mur R, m Rustgi V, et al: Interferon alfa-2b alone or in combination with ribavirin for the treatment of relapse of chronic hepatitis C. N Engl J Med 339:1493–1499, 1998.
5. Heathcote EJ, Keeffe EB, Lee SS, et al. Retreatment of chronic hepatitis C with consensus interferon. Hepatology 27:1136–1143, 1998.
6. Keeffe EB, Hollinger FB: Therapy of hepatitis C: Consensus interferon trials. Hepatology 26(Suppl 1):101S–107S, 1997.
7. Poynard T, McHutchison J, Goodman Z, et al: Is an "a la carte" combination interferon alfa-2b plus ribavirin regimen possible for the first line treatment in patients with chronic hepatitis C? Hepatology 31:211–218, 2000.
8. Morishima C, Gretch DR: Clinical use of hepatitis C virus tests for diagnosis and monitoring during therapy. Clinics in Liv Dis 3:717–740, 1999.
9. Dieterich DT, Purow JM, Rajapaksa R: Activity of combination therapy with interferon alfa-2b plus ribavirin in chronic hepatitis C patients co-infected with HIV. Sem Liv Dis 19:(Suppl 1):87–94, 1999.
10. Maddrey WC: Safety of combination interferon alfa-2b/ribavirin therapy in chronic hepatitis C-relapsed and treatment-naïve patients. Sem Liv Dis 19(Suppl 1):67–75, 1999.
11. Rossine A, Ravaggi A, Biasi L, et al: Virological response to interferon treatment in hepatitis C virus carriers with normal aminotransferase levels and chronic hepatitis. Hepatology 26:1012–1017, 1997.
12. Vogel W: Treatment of acute hepatitis C virus infection. J Hepatol 31(Suppl 1):189–192, 1993.
13. Zarski JP, Bohn B, Bastie A: Characteristics of patients with dual infection by hepatitis B and C viruses. J Hepatol 28:27–33, 1998.

18. ANTIVIRAL THERAPY FOR HEPATITIS B

Jorge L. Herrera, M.D., and Julie R. Smith, M.H.S., PA-C

1. Is antiviral therapy recommended for acute hepatitis B?

No. Acute hepatitis B, defined as a positive test for hepatitis B surface antigen (HBsAg) and the presence of hepatitis B core antibody-immunoglobulin M (HBcAb-IgM), is a self-limited disease in 90–95% of adults and resolves without specific antiviral therapy within 3–6 months after the onset of clinical symptoms. For this reason, only supportive care is offered to patients with acute hepatitis B infection. Antiviral therapy is considered only for patients with chronic hepatitis B (positive HBsAg test for more than 6 months).

2. Do all patients with chronic hepatitis B benefit from therapy?

No. Only patients with high viral load and evidence of ongoing hepatic necrosis, such as elevated liver enzyme levels or liver biopsy demonstrating active inflammation, should be considered for therapy. Typical candidates for antiviral therapy test positive for hepatitis B e antigen (HBeAg) and negative for HBe antibodies (HBeAb); they also have detectable levels of hepatitis B virus DNA (HBV-DNA) by liquid hybridization assays. In contrast, chronic hepatitis B carriers (HBsAg-positive), who are characterized by normal levels of liver enzymes, negative HBeAg, positive HBeAb, and nondetectable HBV-DNA by liquid hybridization assay, do not require antiviral therapy.

Antiviral Therapy for Patients with Chronic Hepatitis B Infection

SEROLOGIC PATTERN	INTERPRETATION	COURSE OF ACTION
HBsAg-positive, HbcAb-IgM-positive	Acute hepatitis B	Observe; resolution likely in 90–95% of adults
HBsAg-positive > 6 mo, HBeAg-positive, HBeAb-negative, HBV-DNA–positive, elevated ALT level	Chronic infection with high-grade viremia	Initiate antiviral therapy
HBsAg-positive >6 mo, HBeAg-negative, HBeAb-positive, HBV-DNA-negative, normal ALT level	Chronic carrier	Observe
HBsAg-positive >6 mo, HBeAg-negative, HBeAb-positive, HBV-DNA-positive, elevated ALT level	Chronic infection with HBeAg mutant	Consider antiviral therapy

HBsAg = hepatitis B surface antigen, HBcAb-IgM = hepatitis B core antibody-immunoglobulin M, HBeAg = hepatitis B e antigen, HBeAb = hepatitis e antibody, HBV-DNA = hepatitis B virus DNA, ALT = alanine aminotransferase.

3. What assay should be used to measure HBV-DNA in assessing patients with chronic hepatitis B for possible therapy?

In contrast to other chronic viral illnesses, HBV-DNA should be measured by the nonpolymerase chain reaction (non-PCR) assay to assess the need for antiviral therapy. The PCR assay is too sensitive and detects small quantities of circulating hepatitis B virus, which usually are not clinically significant. In contrast, HBV-DNA hybridization assays have a lower sensitivity of about 10^6 (1 million) viral copies and detect only clinically significant levels of hepatitis B virus. Patients with less than 10^6 copies of HBV usually have normal liver enzyme levels, minimal or no inflammation on liver biopsy, and an excellent prognosis. The need to treat chronic hepatitis B infection should be based on the presence of HBV-DNA by hybridization—not by PCR.

4. Should patients with chronic hepatitis B who test negative for HBeAg be treated with antiviral therapy?

Traditionally, a positive HBeAg has been used as the hallmark of high viral load and an indication for antiviral therapy; thus, the absence of HBeAg implies a low viral load and no need for therapy. To complicate matters, an increasing number of patients who are HBeAg-negative and HBeAb-positive are found to have high levels of viremia due to mutation of the virus. The mutant strains are incapable of producing the e-antigen. When the evaluation of patients with chronic unexplained elevation of liver enzyme tests reveals only HBsAg positivity, consider infection with HBV-mutant strain. The only way to identify such patients is to measure HBV-DNA by hybridization, which is positive. Patients infected with the HBeAg mutants should be treated, but they are more resistant to therapy. Long-term remission is less common compared with patients infected with the HBeAg-producing or "wild" strain. In contrast, patients who test negative for HBeAg, positive for HBeAb, and negative for HBV-DNA by hybridization do not require therapy.

5. Is liver biopsy required before therapy is started?

A liver biopsy is not needed to establish the diagnosis of hepatitis B infection; however it is the only tool available to determine severity of disease. Because the treatment of hepatitis B can exacerbate hepatic inflammation, it is important to know the severity of liver disease before initiating therapy. Patients who already have extensive fibrosis or cirrhosis on biopsy are less likely to tolerate a flare of hepatitis during treatment than patients with milder histologic disease. In addition, the detection of cirrhosis on liver biopsy selects a group of patients who require closer observation as well as screening for hepatocellular carcinoma and esophageal varices.

6. What are the options for treating chronic hepatitis B infection?

Currently, two medications have been approved for the treatment of chronic hepatitis B infection: interferon alpha-2b and lamivudine. Interferon alpha-2b is an injectable immunomodulatory medication that enhances clearance of the hepatitis B virus by improving the immune response. Lamivudine is an oral nucleoside analog that directly inhibits viral replication without stimulating an immune response. Lamivudine inhibits the reverse transcriptase activity of HBV-DNA polymerase and halts viral replication. Interferon is dosed at either 10 million units subcutaneously 3 times/week or 5 million units subcutaneously daily for 16 weeks. Lamivudine is given as one 100-mg tablet by mouth once a day for 1–2 years.

7. What are the endpoints of antiviral therapy?

The goals of antiviral therapy are to eradicate the virus (or at least to lower HBV-DNA to undetectable levels by hybridization assay), to normalize liver enzyme levels, and to induce e-antigen seroconversion (defined as achieving HBeAg-negative, HBeAb-positive status). Once e-antigen seroconversion is achieved, antiviral therapy may be discontinued. Remission is usually long-lasting, but as long as the patient continues to test positive for HBsAg, he or she is at risk of reactivation and should be monitored closely.

HBsAg rarely, if ever, clears during antiviral therapy. With continued follow-up after successful antiviral therapy, however, a percentage of patients lose HBsAg and develop HBsAb. HBsAg clearance occurs in 10–15% of patients within the first year after treatment. After 4 years of observation, as many as 65% lose HBsAg and acquire HBsAb. Once HBsAg is cleared and the surface antibody appears, long-lasting remission and immunity to hepatitis B are likely.

8. What is the expected response to interferon therapy?

Because interferon stimulates the immune response, increased clearance of the hepatitis B virus is expected during therapy. Clearance of the virus is achieved by necrosis of infected hepatocytes. Thus, a flare of hepatitis is common during treatment with interferon. Usually it occurs soon after initiation of interferon therapy and is manifested by elevated levels of alanine aminostransferase (ALT) and aspartate aminotransferase (AST). The flare may be accompanied by jaundice and signs and symptoms typical of acute viral hepatitis but usually is associated with reduction or disappearance of HBV-DNA in blood. As the liver enzyme levels return to normal, the HBeAg assay becomes negative, followed by seroconversion to positive HBeAb. Once seroconversion is achieved, therapy can be discontinued. The virologic response is usually long-lasting. If after 16 weeks of interferon therapy e-antigen seroconversion has not been achieved, response to further interferon therapy is unlikely and it should be discontinued.

9. What is the expected response to lamivudine therapy?

In contrast to interferon, lamivudine inhibits viral replication but does not stimulate immune clearance of the virus. For this reason, immune-mediated hepatocyte necrosis is unusual, and biochemical flare of hepatitis is rarely seen with lamivudine therapy. In most patients, the HBV-DNA serum levels decrease dramatically or become undetectable soon after initiating therapy. This decrease is associated with normalization of liver enzyme levels. Seroconversion from HBeAg-positive to HBeAg-negative and from HBeAb-negative to HBeAb-positive is less common and often requires prolonged therapy for 1–3 years. During lamivudine therapy, HBeAg becomes negative in 32% of patients treated for 1 year and induces a positive HBeAb in about 17% after 1 year.

Prolonged therapy with lamivudine has been associated with the emergence of escape mutants, also known as YMDD or M552 mutants. The incidence of lamivudine escape mutants increases with duration of therapy and is estimated to occur in 16–32% of patients during the first year, 38–50% after 2 years of therapy, and 49% or higher after the third year. The emergence of these mutants usually is signified by a resurgence of detectable HBV-DNA levels as measured by hybridization detection of HBV-DNA. Because these mutants are less pathogenic than the "wild" strain, continuation of lamivudine therapy is recommended to prevent resurgence of the "wild" strain.

10. What are the advantages of interferon therapy for chronic hepatitis B infection?

Therapy with interferon is of short duration (16 weeks in most cases) and is successful in 30–40% of selected patients. Successful response is durable, and relapses are rare once interferon is discontinued. Once the HBV infects the liver cell, the HBV genome localizes to the nucleus of the hepatocyte and is converted to covalently closed circular DNA (cccDNA). Clearance of this HBV-DNA is needed to achieve HBsAg seroconversion and can be achieved only by immune-mediated lysis of infected hepatocytes. Cases of HBsAg seroconversion (HBsAg becomes negative and HBsAb becomes positive) have been documented years after inducing e-antigen seroconversion by interferon. Finally, "interferon escape mutants" have not been described.

11. What are the disadvantages of interferon therapy?

Interferon therapy is associated with significant side effects, including flulike syndrome, fever, depression, insomnia, irritability, and bone marrow suppression (see Chapter 17). The interferon-induced flare of hepatitis may be severe and is particularly dangerous in patients with advanced liver disease and cirrhosis, who may not be able to tolerate a flare of hepatitis. For this reason, interferon therapy is relatively contraindicated in patients with cirrhosis caused by chronic hepatitis B infection.

Another disadvantage is that patients with persistently normal liver enzyme levels and patients who acquired the disease at birth are unlikely to respond to interferon therapy. Finally, patients infected with the hepatitis B e-antigen mutant are less likely to achieve a lasting response to interferon.

12. Which parameters predict a good response to interferon therapy?

Patients likely to respond to interferon therapy are characterized by elevated liver enzymes (ALT > 150 U/dl), low viral load (HBV-DNA< 200 pg/ml), positive HBeAg status, female sex, and acquisition of infection during adulthood. Such patients have a 30–40% chance of achieving e-antigen seroconversion after a 16-week course of interferon. In contrast, patients with normal or minimal elevations of liver enzymes have a < 5% chance of achieving sustained remission.

13. What is the role of "prednisone priming" before initiation of interferon therapy?

To enhance response to interferon among patients with normal ALT levels, prior treatment with prednisone has been proposed. The rationale for this approach is based on the observation that withdrawal of corticosteroid therapy frequently results in an acute hepatitis-like elevation of serum aminotransferases that is thought to represent an immunologic rebound against the virus. This flare is associated with a transient decrease in HBV-DNA and elevations of ALT, two features that predict a good response to interferon therapy. Increased likelihood of response to interferon has been noted among patients with normal ALT levels who receive corticosteroids before receiving interferon therapy.

14. What are the advantages of lamivudine therapy?

Lamivudine is taken orally once daily and is associated with minimal to no side effects. Lamivudine therapy rarely induces a flare of hepatitis and can be used in patients with cirrhosis. In most patients, it significantly reduces HBV-DNA levels and normalizes liver enzymes. Patients with normal ALT levels appear to respond to lamivudine therapy as well as those with elevated ALT. Finally, patients infected with hepatitis e-antigen mutants also appear to respond well to lamivudine. Although the treatment course is 1 year or longer, 1 year of lamivudine therapy is less costly than 16 weeks of high-dose interferon.

15. What are the disadvantages of lamivudine therapy?

The treatment course is long, lasting 1–3 years. To approach the efficacy rates of interferon in inducing e-antigen seroconversion, treatment for 1 year or longer is needed. The development of resistant lamivudine escape mutants increases with longer duration of therapy. Finally, because lamivudine acts at the reverse transcriptase level in the cytoplasm and does not affect the cccDNA in the nucleus, HBsAg seroconversion is less likely and has not been documented with lamivudine therapy, raising concerns about the durability of response.

16. Should patients with advanced, decompensated cirrhosis secondary to hepatitis B receive antiviral therapy or be referred for liver transplantation without a trial of therapy?

Although patients with decompensated disease cannot be treated with interferon, treatment with lamivudine is beneficial and often life-saving. In many such patients, evidence of severe decompensation reverses, and patients no longer need to be listed for liver transplantation after a response to lamivudine therapy. In addition, lamivudine therapy, when continued after transplantation, is associated with a decreased chance of recurrence of infection in the graft. In general, patients with severe liver disease due to hepatitis B infection, even if listed for transplantation, should be considered potential candidates for treatment with lamivudine.

17. How are lamivudine escape mutants detected? What should be the course of action if they develop?

Mutations that cause HBV resistance to lamivudine develop frequently and usually begin to appear after 8–9 months of treatment, with a progressive increase in rate of detection over time. Mutations develop in approximately 16–50% of patients treated for 1–3 years. The development of the mutant strain can be detected clinically by the reappearance of HBV-DNA in serum in a patient who had become HBV-DNA–negative upon initiation of lamivudine therapy. Occasionally, mild elevation of ALT is noted with the emergence of the mutant strain. Fortunately, the mutant strain replicates less efficiently and is less virulent than the "wild" strain. For that reason, continuation of lamivudine therapy, despite the emergence of a mutant strain, is recommended. If the lamivudine is discontinued, re-emergence of the more pathogenic strain is likely.

New antiviral agents, including adefovir dipivoxil, are under study for the treatment of lamivudine-resistant mutants. Early investigations suggest that these mutants are sensitive to adefovir. In the future, combination therapy with lamivudine and adefovir may enhance response and prevent the emergence of resistant mutant strains.

18. Is combination therapy with interferon and lamivudine better than either agent alone?

No advantage to combination therapy has been shown in randomized controlled trials. At present, combination therapy is not recommended. Studies of combination therapy initially used lamivudine as a single agent, then added interferon to the regimen. It is not known whether using both agents simultaneously at the beginning of therapy or starting with interferon and adding lamivudine is more effective than either agent alone.

19. What is the role of famciclovir in the treatment of hepatitis B?

Famciclovir is effective in reducing HBV-DNA levels; however, less than 10% of patients achieve e-antigen seroconversion after 1 year of therapy with famciclovir. Fortunately, famciclovir-resistant strains appear to be sensitive to lamivudine, but famciclovir is not effective against lamivudine-resistant strains. Famciclovir is likely to be more effective if used as part of a multidrug cocktail to treat HBV infection. The combination of famciclovir with lamivudine appears to be additive in its ability to suppress viral load, but preliminary studies have not shown an increased e-antigen seroconversion rate.

20. What is the role of lamivudine therapy after liver transplantation?

Lamivudine is the agent of choice for the treatment of hepatitis B after transplant. Interferon is not effective in this setting, because the immune suppression needed to prevent rejection makes interferon ineffective in clearing the virus. In contrast, lamivudine induces a sustained inhibition of viral replication and normalizes serum transaminases in the majority (> 70%) of posttransplant patients with hepatitis B. Loss of HBsAg can be achieved in a substantial number of patients treated soon after transplantation.

BIBLIOGRAPHY

1. Perillo R, Schiff ER, Davis GL, et al: A randomized, controlled trial of interferon alfa-2b alone and after prednisone withdrawal in the treatment of chronic hepatitis B. N Engl J Med 232:295–301, 1990.
2. Perillo RB, Mason AL: Therapy for hepatitis B virus infection. Gastroenterol Clin North Am 23:581– 601, 1994.
3. Locarnini Stephen, Birch C: Antiviral chemotherapy for chronic hepatitis B infection: Lessons learned from treating HIV-infected patients. J Hepatol 30:536–550, 1999.
4. Perillo RP, Regenstein FG, Peters M, et al: Prednisone withdrawal followed by recombinant alfa interferon in the treatment of chronic type B hepatitis. A randomized, controlled trial. Ann Intern Med 109:98–100, 1988.
5. Wong DK, Cheung AM, O'Rourke K, et al: Effect of alfa-interferon treatment in patients with hepatitis B e antigen-positive chronic hepatitis B: A meta-analysis. Ann Intern Med 119:312–323, 1993.
6. Lai CL, Chien RN, Leung NW, et al: A one-year trial of lamivudine for chronic hepatitis B. N Engl J Med 339:61–68, 1998.
7. Tassopoulos NC, Volpes R, Patore Giuseppe, et al: Efficacy of lamivudine in patients with hepatitis B e-antigen negative/hepatitis B virus DNA-positive (precore mutant) chronic hepatitis B. Hepatology 29:889–896, 1999.
8. Dienstag JL, Schiff ER, Mitchell M, et al: Extended lamivudine retreatment for chronic hepatitis B: Maintenance of viral suppression after discontinuation of therapy. Hepatology 30:1082–1087, 1999.
9. Hussain M, Lok ASF: Mutations in the hepatitis B virus polymerase gene associated with antiviral treatment for hepatitis B. J Viral Hep 6:183–194, 1999.
10. Villeneuve JP, Condreay LD, Willems B, et al: Lamivudine treatment for decompensated cirrhosis resulting from chronic hepatitis B. Hepatology 31:207–210, 2000.
11. Kapoor D, Guptan RC, Wakil SM, et al: Beneficial effects of lamivudine in hepatitis B virus related decompensated cirrhosis. J Hepatol 33:308–312, 2000.
12. Perillo R, Rakela J, Dienstag J, et al: Multicenter study of lamivudine therapy for hepatitis B after liver transplantation. Hepatology 29:1581–1586, 1999.
13. Perillo R, Schiff E, Yoshida E, et al: Adefovir dipivoxil for the treatment of lamivudine-resistant hepatitis B mutants. Hepatology 32:129–134, 2000.
14. Xion X, Flores C, Ynag H, Toole J, Gibbs C: Mutations in hepatitis B DNA polymerase associated with resistance to lamivudine do not confer resistance to adefovir in vitro. Hepatology 28:1669–1673, 1998.

19. AUTOIMMUNE HEPATITIS

Albert J. Czaja, M.D.

1. What is autoimmune hepatitis?

Autoimmune hepatitis is an unresolving inflammation of the liver of unknown cause that is characterized by interface hepatitis on histologic examination, autoantibodies in serum, and hypergammaglobulinemia. Cirrhosis, portal hypertension, liver failure, and death are possible consequences. Diagnosis requires the exclusion of the disorders listed below. A careful clinical history, selected laboratory tests, and expert histologic examination establish the diagnosis in most instances.

Differential Diagnosis and Discriminative Tests

POSSIBLE DIAGNOSES	DIAGNOSTIC TESTS	DIAGNOSTIC FINDINGS
Wilson disease	Copper studies	Low ceruloplasmin
		Low serum copper level
		High urinary copper
		Increased hepatic copper
	Slit lamp eye exam	Kayser-Fleischer rings
Primary sclerosing cholangitis	Cholangiography	Focal biliary strictures
	Liver biopsy	Fibrous obliterative cholangitis
Primary biliary cirrhosis	Antimitochondrial antibodies	AMA > 1:40
		Antipyruvate dehydrogenase-E2
	Liver biopsy	Florid duct lesion
		Increased hepatic copper
Autoimmune cholangitis	Liver biopsy	Cholangitis
		Ductopenia
Chronic hepatitis C	Viral markers	Anti-HCV/RIBA positive
		HCV RNA present
	Liver biopsy	Portal lymphoid aggregates
		Steatosis
Drug-induced hepatitis	Clinical history	Exposure to minocycline, isoniazid, nitrofurantoin, propylthiouracil, α-methyldopa
Hemochromatosis	Genetic testing	C282Y, H63D mutations
	Iron/ferritin	Increased
	Liver biopsy	Iron overload
		Hepatic iron index>1.9
Alpha-1 antitrypsin deficiency	Phenotype	ZZ or MZ
	Liver biopsy	Hepatic inclusions
Nonalcoholic steatohepatitis	Clinical findings	Obesity, diabetes, drugs, hyperlipidemia
	Ultrasonography	Hepatic hyperechogenicity
	Liver biopsy	Macrosteatosis

2. What are its predominant features?

Autoimmune hepatitis affects mainly women (71%). It may occur at any age (9 months to 77 years), but typically it is diagnosed before the fourth decade. An acute, even fulminant, presentation is possible, and the disease may be mistaken for acute viral or toxic hepatitis. Concurrent immunologic diseases are present in 38% of patients. Examples include autoimmune thyroiditis, ulcerative colitis, Graves' disease, and synovitis. Cirrhosis is present in 25% of patients at presentation, and the disease may have an indolent, subclinical stage. Smooth muscle antibodies (SMAs) and antinuclear antibodies (ANAs) are the most common serologic markers. In 64% of patients, SMAs and ANAs are present together. Autoantibody titers fluctuate and may disappear. Patterns of seropositivity also change during the disease, and one autoantibody may disappear as another appears. There is no minimal titer of significance, but autoantibody titers in adults should be >1:40. Serum titers >1:80 increase diagnostic confidence. Hypergammaglobulinemia, especially elevation of the serum immunoglobulin G level, is a hallmark of the disease, and the diagnosis is suspect without it. Marked cholestatic features are incompatible with the diagnosis, and a predominant serum alkaline phosphatase abnormality, pruritus, hyperpigmentation, and/or bile duct lesions on histologic examination suggest other diseases, such as primary biliary cirrhosis, primary sclerosing cholangitis, or autoimmune cholangitis. Similarly, serologic evidence of active infection with hepatitis A, B, or C viruses, Epstein-Barr virus, or cytomegalovirus argues against the diagnosis.

Immunologic Diseases Associated with Autoimmune Hepatitis

Autoimmune thyroiditis*	Lichen planus
Celiac sprue	Myasthenia gravis
Coombs'-positive hemolytic anemia	Neutropenia
Cryoglobulinemia	Pericarditis
Dermatitis herpetiformis	Peripheral neuropathy
Erythema nodosum	Pernicious anemia
Fibrosing alveolitis	Pleuritis
Focal myositis	Pyoderma gangrenosum
Gingivitis	Rheumatoid arthritis*
Glomerulonephritis	Sjögren's syndrome
Graves' disease*	Synovitis*
Idiopathic thrombocytopenic purpura	Systemic lupus erythematosus
Insulin-dependent diabetes	Ulcerative colitis*
Intestinal villous atrophy	Urticaria
Iritis	Vitiligo

*Most common association.

3. What are the characteristic histologic findings in autoimmune hepatitis?

Interface hepatitis (piecemeal necrosis or periportal hepatitis) implies disruption of the limiting plate of the portal tract by inflammatory infiltrate and it is a requisite finding (Fig. 1). Interface hepatitis, however, is not pathognomonic; the same pattern may be seen in acute and chronic hepatitis associated with viruses, drugs, alcohol, and toxins. Lobular hepatitis, which is characterized by prominent cellular infiltrates that line sinusoidal spaces in association with degenerative or regenerative changes, is another common but nondiagnostic histologic manifestation (Fig. 2). Marked plasma cell infiltration of the portal tracts also characterizes the disease (Fig. 3). In contrast, prominent portal lymphoid aggregates and steatosis suggest the diagnosis of chronic hepatitis C (Fig. 4); ground-glass hepatocytes are characteristic of chronic hepatitis B; and marked bile duct damage or loss connotes a cholangiopathy. Unusual histologic features associated with autoimmune hepatitis include centrilobular (zone 3) necrosis and hepatocytic giant cells.

4. What are the different types of autoimmune hepatitis?

Patients with autoimmune hepatitis are classified according to the type of autoantibodies associated with their disease. **Type 1 autoimmune hepatitis** is characterized by SMA and/or ANA. It is the most common form in the United States and western Europe. Antibodies to actin (anti-actin), a subgroup of SMA, also may be present and support the diagnosis.

Type 2 autoimmune hepatitis is characterized by antibodies to liver/kidney microsome type 1 (anti-LKM1). These antibodies rarely coexist with SMA or ANA. Patients with type 2 autoimmune hepatitis are typically young (2–14 years). They frequently have concurrent immunologic diseases,

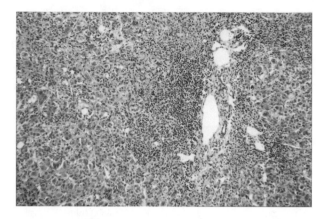

FIGURE 1. Interface necrosis. The limiting plate of the portal tract is disrupted by inflammatory infiltrate (H & E; original magnification ×100).

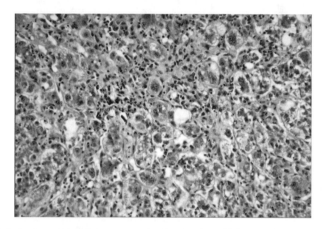

FIGURE 2. Lobular hepatitis. Inflammatory cells line the sinusoidal spaces in association with liver cell regenerative or degenerative changes (H & E; original magnification × 200).

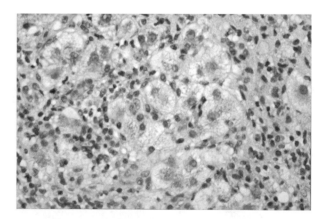

FIGURE 3. Plasma cell infiltration. Plasma cells infiltrate the periportal region (H & E; original magnification × 400).

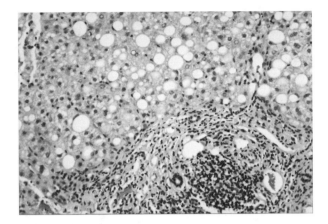

FIGURE 4.   Chronic hepatitis C. Small lymphocytes aggregate in the portal tract, and vacuoles of lipid are present within the cytoplasm of hepatocytes (H & E; original magnification × 200).

such as autoimmune thyroiditis, vitiligo, insulin-dependent diabetes, and ulcerative colitis, and commonly express organ-specific antibodies, such as antibodies to thyroid, islets of Langerhans, and parietal cells. Serum immunoglobulin A levels may be low, and a fulminant presentation is possible. Preliminary studies that suggested a more aggressive liver disease than type 1 autoimmune hepatitis have not been substantiated. Type 2 autoimmune hepatitis is found in only 4% of adults with autoimmune hepatitis in the United States, and surveys of pediatric patients also indicate a low occurrence.

Type 3 autoimmune hepatitis is the least established form. It is characterized by the presence of antibodies to soluble liver antigen/liver-pancreas (anti-SLA/LP). Eleven percent of patients with type 1 autoimmune hepatitis have anti-SLA/LP and cannot be distinguished from seronegative counterparts. Type 3 autoimmune hepatitis, as defined by anti-SLA/LP, may be a variant of type 1 autoimmune hepatitis rather than a separate entity.

Types of Autoimmune Hepatitis

FEATURES	TYPE 1	TYPE 2
Autoantibodies	Smooth muscle Nucleus Actin Asialoglycoprotein receptor Perinuclear antineutrophil cytoplasm	Liver/kidney microsome 1 Liver cytosol type 1 Recombinant P450 IID6 254-271 core motif Asialoglycoprotein receptor
Organ-specific antibodies	Possible (especially antibodies to thyroid)	Common (antibodies to thyroid, parietal cells, islets of Langerhans)
Autoantigen	Unknown	P450 IID6 (CYP2D6)
HLA phenotype	B8, DR3, DR4	DR7
Predominant age	Adult	Child
Fulminant onset	Possible	Possible
Concurrent immune disease	38%	34%
Low IgA level	No	Possible
Progression to cirrhosis	36%	82%
Corticosteroid-responsive	Yes	Yes

5. What are the diagnostic criteria?

Definite diagnosis requires histologic evidence of interface hepatitis with or without lobular hepatitis or bridging necrosis and absence of biliary lesions, granulomas, copper deposits, or other changes suggestive of a different etiology. The serum aminotransferase level must be abnormally increased and dominate the biochemical profile. Total levels of serum globulin, gamma globulin, or immunoglobulin G must be greater than 1.5 times the upper limit of normal, and serum titers of SMA, ANA, or anti-LKM1 must be greater than 1:80. There must be no history of parenteral exposure to blood or blood products, recent use of hepatotoxic drugs, or excessive alcohol consumption (<35 gm/day in men and <25 gm/day in women). Active viral infection must be excluded, and serum levels of alpha-1 antitrypsin, copper, and ceruloplasmin must be normal. **Probable diagnosis** is made when similar findings are less pronounced.

The scoring system has been revised recently by the International Autoimmune Hepatitis Group. It balances clinical, laboratory, and histologic manifestations and provides an objective measure of the net strength of the diagnosis. The scoring system is useful for evaluating conditions with mixed or inconsistent features. Response to corticosteroid therapy is scored, and the treatment outcome can upgrade or downgrade the diagnosis. Chronicity no longer requires 6 months of disease activity; the designation of autoimmune hepatitis can be made at its first manifestation.

Scoring System for the Diagnosis of Autoimmune Hepatitis*

CLINICAL FEATURE	SCORE	CLINICAL FEATURE	SCORE
Female	+2	Average alcohol intake	
Alkaline phosphatase:aspartate		< 25 g/day	+2
aminotransferase ratio		> 60 g/day	–2
< 1.5	+2	Histologic findings	
1.5–3.0	0	Interface hepatitis	+3
> 3.0	–2	Lymphoplasmacytic infiltrate	+1
Serum gamma globulin or IgG level		Rosette formation	+1
above normal limit		None of above	–5
> 2.0	+3	Biliary changes	–3
1.5–2.0	+2	Other changes	–3
1.0–1.5	+1	Concurrent immune disease	+2
< 1.0	0	Novel autoantibodies	+2
ANA, SMA or anti-LKM1		HLA DR3 or DR4	+1
> 1:80	+3	Response to corticosteroids	
1:80	+2	Complete	+2
1:40	+1	Relapse after drug withdrawal	+3
< 1:40	0		
AMA positive	–4	**Aggregate score before treatment**	
Hepatitis markers		Definite autoimmune hepatitis	> 15
Positive	–3	Probable autoimmune hepatitis	10–15
Negative	+3		
Drug history		**Aggregate score after treatment**	
Positive	–4	Definite autoimmune hepatitis	> 17
Negative	+1	Probable autoimmune hepatitis	12–17

*Revised proposal of the International Autoimmune Hepatitis Group, J Hepatol 31:929-938, 1999.

6. Are ANA, SMA, and anti-LKM1 pathogenic autoantibodies?

SMA, ANA and anti-LKM1 are the bases for subclassifying patients with autoimmune hepatitis, but they have no pathogenic properties. Autoantibody behavior does not correlate with disease activity or treatment response. Autoantibody determinations should be used only for diagnostic purposes.

Antinuclear antibodies typically produce homogeneous or speckled patterns by indirect immunofluorescence on HEp-2 cell lines, but they also may produce diffuse granular, centromeric, nucleolar, and mixed patterns in type 1 autoimmune hepatitis. The individual patterns of indirect immunofluorescence do not have diagnostic or prognostic implications.

Smooth muscle antibodies reflect the presence of antibodies to actin and/or nonactin components (tubulin, vimentin, desmin, and skeletin). Reactivity by indirect immunofluorescence against actin cables in cultured fibroblasts has high specificity for the diagnosis. Polymerized F-actin, the target of this reactivity, is closely associated with the hepatocyte membrane. There is no direct evidence, however, that SMAs induce liver cell injury.

Antibodies to liver/kidney microsome type 1 are reactive against a 50-kDa microsomal antigen in the liver and kidney that has been identified as the cytochrome monooxygenase, P450 IID6 (CYP2D6). Antibodies to LKM1 inhibit P450 IID6 activity in vitro but not in vivo, and their pathogenicity has not been established. An 8-amino acid core motif within P450 IID6, either in isolation or as part of sequences extending up to 33 amino acids, has been identified as the epitope of anti-LKM1. Reactivity at the site between amino acids 254 and 271 of the recombinant P450 IID6 molecule distinguishes patients with autoimmune hepatitis and anti-LKM1 from those with chronic hepatitis C and anti-LKM1.

Autoantibodies Associated with Autoimmune Hepatitis

AUTOANTIBODY SPECIES	IMPLICATION(S)
Nuclear	Type 1 autoimmune hepatitis
	Not disease-specific
	Reactive to multiple nuclear antigens
Smooth muscle	Type 1 autoimmune hepatitis
	Reactive to actin and nonactin components
	Frequently concurrent with antinuclear antibodies
Actin	Type 1 autoimmune hepatitis
	Diagnostic specificity
	Commonly young patients
	Possibly more aggressive disease
	Unsettled assay
Liver/kidney microsome 1	Type 2 autoimmune hepatitis
	Inhibits P450 IID6 in vitro
	May occur in chronic hepatitis C
Asialoglycoprotein receptor	Generic marker of autoimmune hepatitis
	Correlates with inflammatory activity
	Possible barometer of treatment response
	Persistence identifies propensity to relapse
	Possible marker of important autoantigen
Liver cytosol type 1	Type 2 autoimmune hepatitis
	Young patients
	Possibly worse prognosis
	Commonly discounts hepatitis C virus infection
	Directed against formiminotransferase cyclodeaminase and/or argininosuccinate lyase
Soluble liver antigen	Type 3 autoimmune hepatitis
	Glutathione S-transferases disputed as autoantigens
	Useful in evaluating seronegative autoimmune hepatitis
	Commonly present with markers of type 1 disease
	Reactivities same as antibodies to liver-pancreas
Liver-pancreas	Type 3 autoimmune hepatitis
	Reactivities same as antibodies to soluble liver antigen
	Useful in evaluating seronegative autoimmune hepatitis
Perinuclear antineutrophil cytoplasm	Common in type 1 autoimmune hepatitis
	Absent in type 2 autoimmune hepatitis
	Mainly IgG1 isotype
	Actin disputed as autoantigen
	Useful in evaluating seronegative autoimmune hepatitis

7. What other autoantibodies are important?

Multiple autoantibodies have been described in autoimmune hepatitis, but none has been shown to be pathogenic or clinically versatile. Their characterization may help to identify the autoantigens responsible for the disease, and some may prove to be valuable diagnostic and prognostic instruments. Currently, tests are not generally available.

Antibodies to soluble liver antigen (anti-SLA) react with liver cytokeratins 8 and 18. Glutathione S-transferases have been proposed as the autoantigenic targets, but this association is disputed. Anti-SLAs are found only in autoimmune hepatitis but do not define a clinically distinct subgroup. Their greatest clinical value may be to rediagnose some cases of cryptogenic chronic hepatitis as autoimmune hepatitis.

Antibodies to liver-pancreas (anti-LP) are present in 17% of patients with type 1 autoimmune hepatitis. In contrast, they are detected in 33% of patients who are seronegative for conventional autoantibodies. Antibodies to liver-pancreas may define another subtype of autoimmune hepatitis or be useful in reclassifying patients with cryptogenic chronic hepatitis. Recently, anti-LP and anti-SLA have been found to have similar reactivities, and the antibodies are now referred to as anti-SLA/LP.

Antibodies to liver cytosol type 1 (anti-LC1) have specificity for autoimmune hepatitis and were used initially to differentiate anti-LKM1-positive patients with and without hepatitis C viral infection. They occur mainly in young patients, typically < 20 years old, and their presence has been associated with more severe disease. Antibodies to liver cytosol type 1 are detected in only 32% of anti-LKM1–positive patients. They are best regarded as supplemental markers of type 2 autoimmune hepatitis. In 14% of patients with autoimmune hepatitis, they are the sole markers of disease and may be useful in evaluating young patients who lack conventional autoantibodies. Formiminotransferase cyclodeaminase and argininosuccinate lyase have been proposed as the target autoantigens.

Antibodies to asialoglycoprotein receptor (anti-ASGPR) are specific for autoimmune hepatitis. They are present in all types of autoimmune hepatitis, including 82% of patients with SMA and/or ANA, 67% of patients with anti-LKM1, and 67% of patients with anti-SLA. The autoantibodies are directed against a transmembrane hepatocytic glycoprotein that can capture, display, and internalize potential antigens, induce T-cell proliferation, and activate cytotoxic T-cells. The occurrence of antibodies to human ASGPR in 88% of patients with autoimmune hepatitis compared with 7% of patients with chronic hepatitis B, 8% with alcoholic liver disease, and 14% with primary biliary cirrhosis indicates diagnostic specificity. Autoantibody reactivity also correlates with inflammatory activity, and these autoantibodies disappear during successful therapy. Loss of anti-ASGPR during treatment may identify patients who are less likely to relapse after drug withdrawal.

Perinuclear antineutrophil cytoplasmic antibodies (pANCA) are present in 50–93% of patients with type 1 autoimmune hepatitis. Preliminary studies suggest that the pANCAs of autoimmune hepatitis differ from those of primary sclerosing cholangitis by being higher in titer and of the IgG1 isotype. Actin has been proposed as the target autoantigen, but this association is disputed. Perinuclear antibodies do not occur in type 2 autoimmune hepatitis. Their most valuable clinical application may be in the assessment of seronegative patients with presumed type 1 autoimmune hepatitis.

8. What is the significance of antimitochondrial antibodies in autoimmune hepatitis?

Antimitochondrial antibodies (AMAs) can be demonstrated by indirect immunofluorescence in 20% of patients with autoimmune hepatitis, but serum titers are typically low (<1:160 in 88% of cases). The histologic findings in such patients are indistinguishable from those in patients without AMA, and tissue copper stains by rhodanine are negative or only mildly positive. Responsiveness to corticosteroids can be anticipated.

Patients with high titers of AMA may have primary biliary cirrhosis, an overlap syndrome between autoimmune hepatitis and primary biliary cirrhosis, or anti-LKM1, which has been mistaken for AMA. Recognition of AMA by indirect immunofluorescence requires reactivity to the distal tubules of the murine kidney and parietal cells of the murine stomach. Recognition of anti-LKM1 requires reactivity to the proximal tubules of the murine kidney and murine hepatocytes. An exuberant reaction against the renal tubule may obscure these distinctions, and anti-LKM1 reactivity may be reported as AMA positivity.

The antibodies that are specific against the mitochondrial autoantigens of primary biliary cirrhosis are the E2 subunits of pyruvate dehydrogenase and/or branched-chain ketoacid dehydrogenase. They occur in only 8% of patients with autoimmune hepatitis and may indicate an incorrect original diagnosis, a disorder with mixed features (overlap syndrome), or a rare instance of false seropositivity.

9. Can autoimmune hepatitis exist in the absence of conventional autoantibodies?

Thirteen percent of patients with severe chronic hepatitis lack a confident etiologic diagnosis. Such patients are diagnosed with cryptogenic chronic hepatitis, but they may have an autoimmune hepatitis that has escaped diagnosis by conventional serologic testing. Patients with cryptogenic chronic hepatitis are frequently similar in age, gender, HLA phenotype, laboratory findings, and histologic features to patients with type 1 autoimmune hepatitis. They also respond well to corticosteroid therapy, entering remission as commonly (83% vs. 78%) and failing treatment as rarely (9% vs. 11%) as patients with conventional markers. They may have "autoantibody-negative autoimmune hepatitis." Some patients may express SMA and/or ANA later in their course or have less conventional autoantibodies, such as anti-SLA/LP, anti-LC1, or pANCA. The scoring system is the best method of securing the diagnosis. If indicated, patients should be treated with corticosteroids.

10. What are the pathogenic mechanisms?

The pathogenic mechanisms of autoimmune hepatitis are unknown, but two theories prevail. One theory proposes an **antibody-dependent cell-mediated form of cytotoxicity**. A defect is postulated in the modulation of B-cell production of immunoglobulin G. The immunoglobulin adheres to normal hepatocytic membrane proteins and creates an antigen-antibody complex on the hepatocyte surface. This complex is then targeted by natural killer cells that have Fc receptors for the immunoglobulin. The natural killer cells do not require previous exposure to the target antigen for activation; they accomplish liver cell injury by cytolysis.

The other theory proposes a **cellular form of cytotoxicity**. A disease-specific autoantigen is displayed on the surface of antigen-presenting cells in association with HLA class II antigens. Immunocytes that are HLA-restricted are sensitized to the self-antigen, and clonal expansion of the antigen-primed lymphocytes follows. Activated cytotoxic T-lymphocytes infiltrate the liver tissue and destroy the hepatocytes displaying the target autoantigen. Lymphokines facilitate cell-to-cell communication, promote neoexpression of HLA class II antigens, enhance autoantigen presentation, activate the immunocytes, and intensify tissue damage by direct action (Fig. 5).

Common to both theories are host predisposition to heightened immunoreactivity that is genetically determined and uncertainty about the nature or need of a triggering agent. Viral infections, drug exposures, and environmental factors have been proposed as triggering mechanisms that can activate a final common pathway of pathogenesis.

11. What are the autoantigens?

Cytochrome monooxygenase, P450 IID6 (CYP2D6), is the target autoantigen of type 2 autoimmune hepatitis. The target autoantigen of type 1 autoimmune hepatitis is unknown, but asialoglycoprotein receptor is an excellent candidate. Each antigen is expressed on the hepatocyte surface, and each is associated with tissue-infiltrating, antigen-sensitized lymphocytes. CD4 T-helper cells predominate in the portal tracts and scar tissue; antigen-sensitized suppressor/cytotoxic lymphocytes congregate near areas of interface hepatitis; and B-cells and natural killer cells are scant in all regions. These findings suggest that a cell-mediated form of cytotoxicity is the most important mechanism of liver cell injury in autoimmune hepatitis and implicate CD8 cytotoxic T lymphocytes as the most likely effectors.

P450 IID6 (CYP2D6) is a 50-kDa microsomal enzyme that metabolizes at least 25 different drugs, including antihypertensive agents, beta blockers, antiarrhythmic drugs, and antidepressants. Asialoglycoprotein receptor is a transmembrane hepatocytic glycoprotein that can process and display multiple intrinsic and extrinsic antigens. Each is capable of transforming a variety of peptides into immunoreactive molecules. Other candidate autoantigens may exist and should be sought in the periportal regions of the liver tissue where the inflammatory infiltrate predominates.

Cell-mediated cytotoxicity

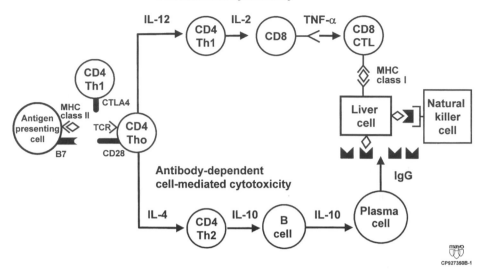

FIGURE 5. Putative pathogenic mechanisms. Activation of CD4 T-helper cells requires ligation of its T-cell antigen receptor (TCR) with the antigenic peptide displayed by the class II molecule of the major histocompatibility complex (MHC) (first signal) and coupling of B7 and CD28 (second signal). The activated CD4 T-helper cell (Th0) then differentiates in accordance with the predominant cytokine milieu. Cell-mediated cytotoxicity is favored by a type 1 (Th1) cytokine response mediated by interleukin (IL)-12, IL-2, and tumor necrosis factor-alpha (TNFα). Cytotoxic T lymphocytes (CD8 CTL) undergo activation by interaction with processed antigenic peptides presented by class-I MHC molecules. Sensitized cytotoxic T lymphocytes injure liver cells by the release of lymphokines. Antibody-dependent cell-mediated cytotoxicity is favored by a type-2 (Th2) cytokine response mediated by IL-4 and IL-10. Plasma cells are activated to produce immunoglobulin G (IgG), which forms complexes with normal membrane constituents of the hepatocyte. The Fc receptors of natural killer cells bind to the antigen–antibody complexes and cause cytolysis.

12. Do viruses cause autoimmune hepatitis?

Multiple viruses can trigger autoimmune hepatitis, including hepatitis A, hepatitis B, and hepatitis C. The lack of a confident animal model for the disease, the long lag time between exposure and clinical manifestation, and the likely persistence of autoimmune hepatitis after disappearance of its trigger have hampered efforts to define etiologic factors. Currently, the definite diagnosis of autoimmune hepatitis requires the exclusion of viral infection, and patients with true viral infection and low-titer autoantibodies are considered to have viral disease with nonspecific features of autoimmunity. The multiplicity of viruses that have been implicated as triggers suggests that a final common pathway of pathogenesis can be initiated by various agents.

13. Do drugs cause autoimmune hepatitis?

Drugs can produce the clinical syndrome of autoimmune hepatitis and must be excluded at the time of presentation. A recently implicated drug is minocycline. Other medications that can mimic the syndrome are nitrofurantoin, isoniazid, propylthiouracil, and α-methyldopa. Identification of a drug-induced syndrome is important because discontinuation of the drug ameliorates the disease.

14. Why does autoimmune hepatitis affect mainly women?

The basis for the female propensity for autoimmune hepatitis is unknown. Hormonal factors are inadequate explanations in children and postmenopausal women. Sex-linked immunoregulatory genes have been proposed but not identified.

15. What are the genetic predispositions to autoimmune hepatitis?

Susceptibility in Caucasoid northern Europeans and Americans relates to the human leukocyte antigens (HLA) DR3 and DR4. HLA DR3 is the principal risk factor; HLA DR4 is a secondary but independent risk factor. Eight-five percent of American patients with type 1 autoimmune hepatitis are positive for HLA DR3, HLA DR4, or both. HLA DR7 characterizes patients with type 2 autoimmune hepatitis. The HLA phenotype identifies patients with a predisposition for autoimmune hepatitis, but it does not predict emergence of the disease. Autoimmune hepatitis does not have a strong penetrance in families, and familial occurrence is rare.

Effects of Class II MHC Alleles on Disease Expression and Behavior

	ASSOCIATED CLASS II MHC ALLELES	
DISEASE EXPRESSION AND BEHAVIOR	*DRB1*0301*	*DRB1*0401*
Earlier age onset	+	−
More frequent confluent necrosis and/or cirrhosis	+	−
Lower frequency of remission during therapy	+	−
Higher frequency of treatment failure	+	−
Higher frequency of relapse after drug withdrawal	+	−
More frequent liver transplantation	+	−
Associated with tumor necrosis factor-α polymorphism *(TFNA*A)*	+	−
Associated with cytotoxic T lymphocyte antigen-4 polymorphism involving guanine for alanine substitution	+	−
Older age onset	−	+
More common in women	−	+
More commonly associated with concurrent immune disorders	−	+
Higher frequency of remission during therapy	−	+
Higher serum levels of gamma globulin and immunoglobulin G	−	+
More frequently associated with smooth muscle antibodies	−	+
More frequently associated with high titer antinuclear antibodies	−	+

16. Has a susceptibility gene been identified?

A single susceptibility gene has not been described, and autoimmune hepatitis is probably a polygenic disorder. High-resolution DNA-based techniques have indicated that the class II allele, *DRB1*0301*, of the major histocompatibility complex (MHC) is the principal risk factor, and the allele, *DRB1*0401*, is the secondary risk factor in Caucasoid northern Europeans and Americans. In contrast, *DRB1*1501* protects against the disease in this population. Susceptibility alleles for type 1 autoimmune hepatitis in various ethnic groups are different. They include *DRB1*0405* in Japan, *DRB1*0405* in Argentine adults, *DRB1*1301* in Argentine children and Brazilian patients, and *DRB1*0404* in Mestizo Mexicans.

17. How do different susceptibility alleles produce the same disease?

Each susceptibility allele for autoimmune hepatitis encodes an amino acid sequence in the antigen binding groove of the HLA DR molecule and this sequence influences recognition of the autoantigen by the T cell receptor (TCR) of CD4 T helper cells. The sequence is 6 amino acids long and in a critical position on the lip of the antigen binding groove. The sequence encoded by *DRB1*0301* and *DRB1*0401* in Caucasoid northern Europeans and Americans is denoted as LLEQKR at positions 67–72 of the DRβ polypeptide chain. Lysine (K) at position DRβ71 is the critical residue. Different susceptibility alleles that encode the same or similar short amino acid sequence in this critical location carry the same risk for autoimmune hepatitis ("shared motif hypothesis").

DRB1*0404 in the Mestizo Mexicans and *DRB1*0405* in the Japanese encode an arginine for a lysine at position DRβ71. Arginine is positively charged like lysine, and its substitution has little effect on the presentation of antigenic peptide. Both alleles, therefore, are expected to confer similar susceptibilities to autoimmune hepatitis. In contrast, *DRB1*1501* encodes an alanine for a lysine at DRβ71, and the substitution of this neutral, nonpolar amino acid for either lysine or arginine at DRβ71 has a major effect on antigen binding and TCR recognition. As a result, *DRB1*1501* is protective against autoimmune hepatitis.

The "shared motif hypothesis" does not account for all ethnic differences in susceptibility. The association between *DRB1*1301* and type 1 autoimmune hepatitis in South America remains unexplained.

18. What other factors promote autoimmune hepatitis?

Multiple autoimmune promoters contribute to disease expression and severity. They may be genetically acquired and not disease-specific. A polymorphism of the gene governing production of tumor necrosis factor-α, *TFNA*2*, has been described in type 1 autoimmune hepatitis. This polymorphism may result in high inducible and constitutive levels of tumor necrosis factor-α and thereby favor a type 1 cytokine response and expansion of cytotoxic T cells.

Similarly, a polymorphism involving substitution of a guanine for an alanine at position 49 in the gene encoding cytotoxic T-lymphocyte antigen-4 (CTLA-4) has been described in type 1 autoimmune hepatitis. This polymorphism may impair downregulation of the immunocyte response and foster cellular hyperreactivity. Other autoimmune promoters, including those governing cytokine levels, autoantibody production, adhesion molecule display, and Fas/Fas ligand interactions, are unstudied.

19. Do the HLA phenotypes influence disease expression and outcome?

In Caucasoid patients with type 1 autoimmune hepatitis, both HLA DR3 and HLA DR4 have been associated with different clinical manifestations and outcomes. Patients with HLA DR3 are younger and have more active disease, as assessed by serum aminotransferase levels and histologic findings of confluent necrosis and cirrhosis, than other patients. Similarly, they relapse more frequently after drug withdrawal, enter remission less commonly, deteriorate more often, and require liver transplantation more frequently than patients with other phenotypes. In contrast, patients with HLA DR4 are older and more commonly female than patients with HLA DR3. They have higher serum levels of gamma globulin, a greater frequency of concurrent immunologic diseases, and a greater likelihood of entering remission during therapy. The expression of SMA and high-titer ANA also may be associated with HLA DR4. High-resolution DNA-based techniques have indicated that the same alleles *(DRB1*0301* and *DRB1*0401)* that affect susceptibility also affect outcome.

20. What are the determinants of prognosis?

The severity of inflammatory activity, as reflected in conventional biochemical indices and histologic assessment, is the principal determinant of immediate prognosis. Sustained serum aspartate aminotransferase (AST) activity of at least 10-fold normal or more than 5-fold normal in conjunction with a hypergammaglobulinemia of at least twice normal is associated with a 3-year survival rate of 50% and 10-year survival rate of 10%. Lesser degrees of biochemical activity are associated with better prognoses. In such patients, the 15-year survival exceeds 80%, and the probability of progression to cirrhosis is less than 50%.

Histologic findings at presentation also reflect disease severity and immediate prognosis. Extension of the inflammatory process between portal tracts or between portal tracts and central veins (bridging necrosis) is associated with a 5-year mortality rate of 45% and an 82% frequency of cirrhosis. Similar consequences occur in patients who have destruction of entire lobules of liver tissue at presentation (multilobular necrosis). The 5-year mortality rate of cirrhosis is 58%; 20% die of variceal hemorrhage within 2 years.

In contrast, patients with interface hepatitis (piecemeal necrosis or periportal hepatitis) on histologic examination have a normal 5-year life expectancy and a low frequency of cirrhosis (17%). Spontaneous resolution of inflammatory activity may occur unpredictably in 13–20% of patients, regardless of disease activity at accession. No findings at presentation, including hepatic encephalopathy and ascites, preclude a satisfactory response to corticosteroid therapy.

21. What therapies are effective?

Prednisone in combination with azathioprine and a higher dose of prednisone alone are the established therapies. Both regimens are equally effective in inducing clinical, biochemical, and histologic remission and prolonging immediate life expectancy. The combination regimen is preferred because it is associated with a lower frequency of drug-related side effects (10% vs. 44%).

Postmenopausal women and patients with labile hypertension, brittle diabetes, emotional instability, exogenous obesity, acne, or osteoporosis are ideal candidates for the combination regimen. Women who are pregnant or contemplating pregnancy and patients with active neoplasia or severe cytopenia are candidates for the single-drug regimen. The single-drug regimen also may be used in patients in whom a short treatment trial (6 months or less) is anticipated.

The treatment schedules have been established only in patients with type 1 autoimmune hepatitis, but the same regimens are applied to all types.

Recommended Treatment Regimens

		COMBINATION	
INTERVAL ADJUSTMENTS	PREDNISONE (mg/day)	PREDNISONE (mg/day)	AZATHIOPRINE (mg/day)
Week 1	60	30	50
Week 2	40	20	50
Week 3	30	15	50
Week 4	30	15	50
Daily maintenance until end point	20	10	50

Indications for Corticosteroid Therapy and Criteria for Treatment Selection

INDICATIONS FOR TREATMENT	CRITERIA FOR TREATMENT SELECTION
Absolute	**Prednisone regimen**
AST ≥ 10-fold normal	Severe cytopenia
AST ≥ 5-fold normal and gamma globulin	Thiopurine methyltransferase deficiency
≥ 2-fold normal	Pregnancy or contemplation of pregnancy
Histologic findings of bridging necrosis	Active neoplasia
or confluent necrosis	Short-term trial (≤ 6 months)
Incapacitating symptoms	
	Combination regimen
Relative	Preferred therapy
Persistent symptoms	Postmenopausal women
Disease progression	Obesity
Mild-to-moderate laboratory changes	Osteopenia
	Brittle diabetes
None	Labile hypertension
Interface hepatitis and no symptoms	Acne
AST < 5-fold normal	Long-term treatment (> 6 months)
Inactive or minimally active cirrhosis	
Liver failure with minimal inflammatory activity	

22. What are the indications for treatment?

The benefits of corticosteroid therapy have been demonstrated only in patients with severe inflammatory activity. Therapy in patients with less active disease has an uncertain benefit-risk ratio. The absolute indications for treatment are incapacitating symptoms, bridging necrosis or multilobular necrosis on histologic examination, and sustained severe biochemical abnormalities. Other findings do not compel therapy. In such instances, the treatment decision must be individualized. Treatment is not indicated in patients with inactive or minimally active cirrhosis, patients with decompensated liver disease and mild or no inflammatory activity, and patients who are asymptomatic with histologic features of mild interface hepatitis.

23. Are there any predictors of response to treatment?

No findings at presentation predict response to treatment, and no patient with absolute indications for therapy should be denied treatment, even in the presence of cirrhosis, ascites, or hepatic encephalopathy. The principal indices of response are the levels of serum aspartate aminotransferase, bilirubin, and gamma globulin. At least 90% of patients demonstrate improvement in at least one parameter within 2 weeks of therapy, and this improvement predicts immediate survival with 98% accuracy. Failure to improve pretreatment hyperbilirubinemia within 2 weeks of therapy in a patient with multilobular necrosis invariably predicts death within 6 months; such patients should be assessed for liver transplantation. Patients who fail to enter remission within 2 years of treatment have a 43% frequency of subsequent hepatic decompensation, and the frequency of decompensation increases to 69% after 4 years of continuous therapy without remission. Typically, the first feature of decompensation is the formation of ascites. This finding compels evaluation for liver transplantation. Long-term prognosis relates to the ability to induce remission and prevent features of liver failure.

24. What are the results of corticosteroid therapy?

Sixty-five percent of patients achieve clinical, biochemical, and histologic remission within 3 years of treatment. The average duration of therapy until remission is 22 months. The probability of entering remission increases at a constant annual rate during the first 3 years of therapy, and most patients who enter remission (87%) do so within this period. Patients with and without histologic cirrhosis at presentation have 10-year life expectancies that exceed 90%, and their survival rate is similar to that of age- and sex-matched normal individuals from the same geographic region.

Thirteen percent of patients develop drug-related side effects that prematurely limit treatment (drug toxicity). The most common serious complication is intolerable obesity or cosmetic change (47%). Osteoporosis with vertebral compression (27%), brittle diabetes (20%), and peptic ulceration (6%) restrict therapy less frequently. Patients with cirrhosis develop serious side effects more commonly than others, possibly because they have higher serum levels of unbound prednisolone as a consequence of prolonged hyperbilirubinemia and/or hypoalbuminemia. No findings at presentation predict a serious side effect, and all previously untreated patients with absolute indications for therapy, including postmenopausal women, should be managed aggressively. Serum thiopurine methyltransferase levels may be valuable in assessing candidates for azathioprine therapy, especially those who have preexistent or evolving cytopenia.

Deterioration despite compliance with therapy (treatment failure) develops in 9% of patients, and an incomplete response occurs in 13%. Cirrhosis develops in 36% of patients within 6 years. Relapse after drug withdrawal occurs in as many as 86% of patients who enter remission, and only 14% of patients have sustained inactivity after cessation of therapy. The risk of extrahepatic malignancy in patients receiving long-term immunosuppressive therapy is 1.4-fold greater than that in an age- and sex-matched controls (95% confidence limits, 0.6- to 2.9-fold normal). This realization underscores the importance of adhering to rigid criteria for treatment.

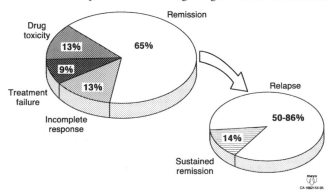

FIGURE 6.   Responses to initial course of corticosteroid therapy.

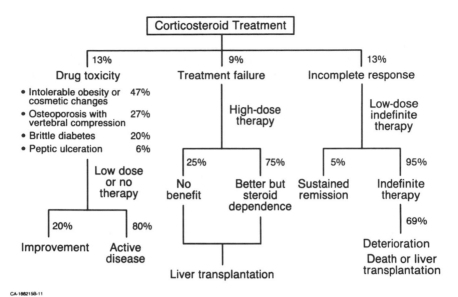

FIGURE 7.   Frequency and consequences of suboptimal responses to corticosteroid therapy.

25. What are the endpoints of treatment?

Conventional treatment should be continued until remission, drug toxicity, clinical deterioration (treatment failure), or confirmation of an incomplete response. Remission connotes absence of symptoms, resolution of laboratory indices of active inflammation, and histologic improvement to normal, inactive cirrhosis, or portal hepatitis. Improvement of the serum aspartate aminotransferase level to twice normal or less is compatible with remission if the other criteria are met. Liver biopsy assessment before drug withdrawal is essential to establish remission because histologic activity may be present in 55% of patients who satisfy other requirements. Typically, histologic improvement lags behind clinical and biochemical resolution by 3–6 months. Treatment should be extended for at least this period.

Treatment failure connotes progressive worsening of laboratory tests, persistent or recurrent symptoms, ascites formation, or features of hepatic encephalopathy despite compliance with therapy. These changes justify an alternative treatment strategy. The emergence of serious drug-related side effects and failure to induce remission after protracted treatment also compel modifications in therapy. The risk of serious drug toxicity exceeds the likelihood of inducing remission after 3 years of continuous administration. In such patients, an incomplete response is established, and a decreasing benefit-risk ratio justifies termination of conventional treatment.

26. When should liver biopsy be performed?

Liver biopsy should be performed at presentation to establish the diagnosis and stage the disease. Liver biopsy also is indicated after clinical and biochemical resolution during therapy. It is typically done 3–6 months after disappearance of the clinical and laboratory features and before drug withdrawal. The presence of interface hepatitis justifies continuation of treatment for at least 6 months. Reversion of liver architecture to normal is the ideal treatment endpoint; it is associated with the lowest frequency of relapse after drug withdrawal. Progression to cirrhosis during therapy identifies patients who relapse after drug withdrawal, and a long-term maintenance strategy with low dose prednisone or azathioprine alone can be implemented. Liver biopsy is justified at any time when signs and symptoms worsen despite compliance with treatment. Tissue examination may disclose a superimposed insult or the emergence of a variant syndrome.

27. Does corticosteroid treatment prevent cirrhosis?

Cirrhosis develops in 36% of patients within 6 years despite corticosteroid treatment. Typically, it eventuates during the early, most active stages of disease and is less likely after induction of remission. The mean annual incidence of cirrhosis is 11% during the first 3 years of illness and 1% thereafter, despite relapse and retreatment. The presence of histologic cirrhosis during or after treatment does not diminish survival or increase morbidity. The 10-year life expectancy of such patients is 93%; the probability of esophageal varices is 13%; and the likelihood of upper gastrointestinal bleeding is 6%. Progression to cirrhosis undoubtedly reflects the difficulty in obtaining complete, rapid, and sustained suppression of inflammatory activity.

28. Does hepatocellular carcinoma develop?

Hepatocellular cancer may develop in patients with autoimmune hepatitis who have cirrhosis, but it is rare. Only 1 of 212 patients (0.5%) developed hepatocellular cancer during 1732 patient-years of follow-up. Among patients with cirrhosis at presentation or subsequently, the incidence of hepatocellular cancer has been only 1 per 1002 patient-years of observation. Among patients with histologic cirrhosis for at least 5 years, the incidence of primary hepatic malignancy has been only 1 per 965 patient years. The efficacy of a surveillance program in detecting early treatable tumors is uncertain, and implementation of such a program is empiric. Serum alpha fetoprotein levels are abnormally increased in 35% of patients with severe autoimmune hepatitis, but these abnormalities are typically mild (range = 19.6–262 ng/ml) and commonly resolve during corticosteroid therapy. Late elevation of the serum alpha fetoprotein level suggests neoplasm, but normal levels do not exclude the diagnosis.

29. What is the most common treatment problem?

Relapse after drug withdrawal is the most common management problem. Fifty percent of patients who enter remission relapse within 6 months after termination of treatment, and 70% relapse within 3 years. The frequency of relapse can be as high as 86% and increases after each subsequent retreatment and drug withdrawal. The risk of relapse diminishes with duration of sustained remission but never disappears. A sustained remission of a least 6 months is associated with only an 8% frequency of relapse.

The principal causes of relapse are premature withdrawal of medication due to anxiety about drug-related side effects or reliance on clinical and laboratory indices to define the endpoint of treatment. Patients who have interface hepatitis at termination of therapy and patients who have developed cirrhosis during treatment invariably relapse after drug withdrawal. Relapse occurs in 50% of patients with portal hepatitis at remission and 20% of patients with normal liver tissue.

The inability to prevent relapse probably reflects failure of corticosteroid therapy to eliminate the pathogenic mechanisms. Patients with the HLA A1-B8-DR3 phenotype and those with persistence of antibodies to asialoglycoprotein receptor may relapse more commonly than counterparts without these findings.

30. How should relapse be managed?

The major consequence of relapse and retreatment is the development of drug-related side effects. The frequency of complications after the first relapse and retreatment is similar to that after the original treatment (33% vs. 29%). The frequency increases to 70% after a second relapse and retreatment.

Two regimens have been used successfully in the management of multiple relapse. The objective of **indefinite low-dose prednisone therapy** is to control symptoms and maintain serum aspartate aminotransferase levels below 5-fold normal on the lowest dose possible. The daily dose of prednisone is reduced by 2.5 mg each month until these goals are achieved. Eighty-seven percent of patients can be managed on 10 mg of prednisone daily or less (median dose = 7.5 mg daily). Side effects that occurred during conventional therapy improve in 85%; new side effects do not develop; and mortality is similar to that of patients treated with full-dose conventional regimens (9% vs. 10%).

The objective of **indefinite azathioprine therapy** is to sustain the remission achieved during conventional corticosteroid treatment by using nonsteroidal medication. Azathioprine (2 mg/kg/day) is sufficient to control clinical and biochemical manifestations of the disease as prednisone is withdrawn. Cytopenia compels dose reduction in only 9% of patients; corticosteroid-induced side effects improve; and arthralgias associated with steroid withdrawal eventually resolve. The two regimens have not been compared head-to-head, and no objective evidence suggests that one is better than the other.

31. How should treatment failure be managed?

High-dose prednisone (60 mg/day) or prednisone (30 mg/day) in conjunction with azathioprine (150 mg/day) induces clinical and biochemical remission in 75% of patients within 2 years. The doses of medication are reduced with each month of clinical and biochemical improvement until conventional maintenance doses are achieved. Histologic remission occurs in less than 20% of patients, and the majority who fail treatment become corticosteroid-dependent and are at risk for disease progression and drug-related complications. Limited studies suggest the advantage of 6-mercaptopurine (6-MP) over azathioprine in treatment failure. Different absorption characteristics or metabolic pathways may favor its use. The initial dose of 12.5–25 mg/day can be increased as tolerated to 1.5 mg/kg/day. Pharmacokinetic studies in patients with cirrhosis have not demonstrated a sufficient disturbance in the conversion of prednisone to prednisolone to justify use of the latter drug.

Liver transplantation is an excellent treatment for patients with decompensated disease. The 5-year life expectancy after transplantation is 92%, and the autoantibodies disappear within 2 years. Disease recurs in as many as 30% of patients. Typically, recurrence is associated with inadequate immunosuppression and controlled by adjustments in this regimen. Progression to cirrhosis and graft failure have been reported, and patients with autoimmune hepatitis may be at increased risk to develop acute rejection, steroid resistant rejection, and chronic rejection.

32. What strategy is best for patients with drug toxicity or incomplete response?

There are no confident treatment guidelines for patients with drug toxicity or incomplete response. Management is empiric, and outcomes must be monitored closely. In patients with **drug toxicity**, the dose of the offending medication is reduced to the lowest possible level or withdrawn completely. Disease activity is controlled by the alternative, presumably tolerated, medication (prednisone or azathioprine), and its dose is adjusted in accordance with response.

In patients with **incomplete response**, the medication is reduced to the lowest level possible to prevent symptoms and maintain serum aspartate aminotransferase levels below 5-fold normal. Patients eventually may decompensate and require liver transplantation. Novel therapies for steroid intolerance, such as cyclosporine (5–6 mg/kg/day), have been used anecdotally, and results after 1 year have been encouraging. Indefinite therapy with cyclosporine may be necessary, and patients have an uncertain risk for serious long-term complications.

33. What about variant syndromes?

Codification of the diagnostic criteria for autoimmune hepatitis has highlighted the presence of many conditions with autoimmune features that lack classical findings or have mixed manifestations. Disorders with features of two different diseases are designated "overlap syndromes." Examples include patients with autoimmune hepatitis and primary biliary cirrhosis and patients with autoimmune hepatitis and primary sclerosing cholangitis. Disorders with features that are inconsistent with the diagnosis of autoimmune hepatitis or insufficient for classification in another diagnostic category are "outlier syndromes." Examples include patients with autoimmune cholangitis and cryptogenic chronic hepatitis ("autoantibody-negative autoimmune hepatitis"). The variant syndromes are detectable in 18% of patients with autoimmune liver disease and should be sought in all patients with autoimmune features who respond poorly to corticosteroid therapy.

The principal manifestation of a variant syndrome is cholestasis in conjunction with hepatitis. Antimitochondrial antibodies, inflammatory bowel disease, pruritus, disproportionate elevation of the serum alkaline phosphatase level, hyperlipidemia, and histologic changes that suggest bile duct destruction and/or loss are clues to its presence. The cholestatic findings justify cholangiography and a management strategy suited for the predominant manifestations. Marked hepatocellular disease justifies corticosteroid therapy; marked cholestatic disease warrants treatment with ursodeoxycholic acid (13-15 mg/kg/day); and comparably mixed hepatocellular and cholestatic disease justifies combination therapy with corticosteroids and ursodeoxycholic acid. Treatments are empiric and continued as a 3–6-month trial. None has been shown effective, especially in reversing the histologic findings, and serum alkaline phosphatase levels greater than two-fold normal identify patients who are unlikely to benefit from corticosteroid treatment.

34. What about patients with mixed autoimmune and viral features?

Most patients with mixed autoimmune and viral features have true viral infection and low-titer autoantibodies that have no diagnostic, clinical or therapeutic relevance. Such patients have chronic viral hepatitis with autoimmune features, and antiviral therapy should be instituted as indicated. Rarely, patients with autoimmune hepatitis have either false-positive markers for viral infection or true coincidental viral infection. Patients with false-positive viral markers respond well to corticosteroids, and the false-positive virologic reactions usually disappear. Patients with true viral infection and high titers of SMA and/or ANA (titers > 1:320) and histologic changes of moderate-to-severe interface hepatitis with portal lymphoplasmacytic infiltration have two diseases. Treatment must be directed against the predominant disorder; corticosteroids are justified if the diagnosis is autoimmune hepatitis. Antiviral therapy may be instituted later if viral-predominant manifestations emerge and corticosteroids are withdrawn.

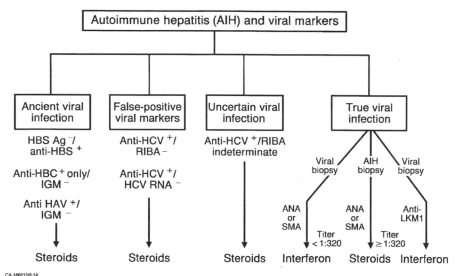

FIGURE 8.   Treatment strategies for patients with autoimmune hepatitis (AIH) and viral markers. Patients with true viral infection require liver biopsy assessment to establish the presence of histologic patterns consistent with viral infection (viral biopsy) or autoimmune hepatitis (AIH). Clinical, laboratory and histologic changes of AIH, including high-titer autoantibodies, suggest AIH with coincidental viral infection. Empiric treatment of the predominant syndrome with corticosteroids can be instituted and monitored closely.

35. What new immunosuppressant therapies are promising?

Cyclosporine (5–6 mg/day) has been used empirically for corticosteroid-recalcitrant and corticosteroid-intolerant disease. The net benefit-risk ratio and indications for its use remain unclear.

Tacrolimus (0.075 mg/kg/day) has reduced serum aspartate aminotransferase and bilirubin levels by 50% of baseline in open-labeled treatment trials. Additional clinical studies are necessary to establish its ability to induce clinical, biochemical, and histologic remission and to allay concerns about renal insufficiency, oncogenicity, and increased hepatic fibrogenesis.

Ursodeoxycholic acid (13–15 mg/kg/day) is a rational choice if it can alter aberrant HLA class I expression, impair cytokine production, and reduce apoptosis. Preliminary studies have shown biochemical improvement in treatment-naïve patients with mild disease, but it has not been found superior to placebo in the treatment of problematic patients.

Budesonide (3 mg thrice daily) is a second-generation glucocorticoid with a high first-pass clearance by the liver and metabolites devoid of glucocorticoid activity. Its potential for rapid delivery to the target tissue and low risk of side effects has not been realized in a small pilot study of problematic patients. Future studies must assess its value in treatment-naïve patients with mild disease.

Deflazacort, a derivative of prednisolone, is less diabetogenic than prednisone. Preliminary studies in 16 patients have indicated an efficacy comparable to prednisone. Its major theoretical advantage is a lower risk of side effects, but analyses of safety are not complete.

Mycophenolate mofetil is metabolized by hepatic esterases to the active metabolite, mycophenolic acid. Mycophenolic acid, in turn, inhibits inosine monophosphate dehydrogenase and thereby prevents de novo synthesis of purines during lymphocyte activation. Its lymphocyte-specific actions may have greater impact on the immune response than azathioprine, and anecdotal studies have indicated its potential value and favorable side-effect profile.

Rapamycin is structurally similar to tacrolimus but inhibits activation and proliferation of T cells by interleukin (IL)-2, IL-4, and IL-6. It has more theoretical appeal than practical use in autoimmune hepatitis.

Summary of New Therapies Offering Blanket Immunosuppression

AGENT	PUTATIVE ACTIONS	EXPERIENCE
Cyclosporine	Inhibits lymphokine release Prevents cytotoxic T cell expansion	Anecdotal in steroid-intolerant or recalcitrant disease
Tacrolimus	Prevents effector cell expansion Inhibits IL-2 receptor Impairs antibody production	Limited open trial benefit Never used to remission Stimulates experimental fibrogenesis
Ursodeoxycholic acid	Suppresses class I HLA display Impairs cytokine production Inhibits apoptosis	Anecdotal benefit in treatment-naive mild disease No advantage in problematic patients
Budesonide	Second-generation steroid High hepatic first-pass clearance Metabolites devoid of steroid activity	Anecdotal benefit in treatment-naive mild disease No advantage in problematic patients Steroid side effects
Deflazacort	Prednisolone derivative Less diabetogenic	Efficacy comparable to prednisone in open-label trial Uncertain side-effect profile
Mycophenolate mofetil	Pro-drug metabolized to mycophenolic acid Prevents purine synthesis during lymphocyte activation Lymphocyte-specific actions	Anecdotal success in steroid recal- citrance
Rapamycin	Similar to tacrolimus Blocks IL-2, IL-4 and IL-6 signals Prevents effector cell expansion	Theoretical value Untested
6-Mercaptopurine	Metabolite of azathioprine Possibly better absorption Different metabolic pathways	Anecdotal success in treatment failure and steroid intolerance

36. What new site-specific treatment interventions are promising?

Greater knowledge about the pathogenesis of autoimmune hepatitis has suggested certain site-specific interventions that require further testing:

Promising New Therapies Based on Site-specific Interventions

AGENT	PUTATIVE ACTIONS	EXPERIENCE
Blocking peptides	Displace autoantigenic peptide from antigen-binding groove of class II HLA DR molecule and should blunt immunocyte activation and immune reaction.	Theoretical Untested
Soluble CTLA-4	Blocks second signal important in immunocyte activation by binding with B7 ligand expressed by antigen-presenting cell and preventing its union with the CD28 ligand of immunocyte.	Successful in preventing rejection after mismatched bone marrow transplantation
T-cell vaccination	Eliminates cytotoxic T-cell clones; requires identification of T-cell clone responsible for autoimmune hepatitis in humans.	Effective in prevention and treatment of experimental hepatitis in animals
Oral tolerance	Induces nonresponsiveness to fed antigen. Causes suppression or clonal anergy, depending on antigen dose. Low doses of antigen selectively recruit CD4 T-helper cells that produce IL-4, IL-10, and transforming growth factor-beta, which inhibit T1 cytokine responses. High doses inundate the mesenteric lymph nodes and inactivate CD4 T-helper cells by induction of T-cell anergy and/or apoptosis. Should be ideal for autoimmune hepatitis because it depends on hepatic portal circulation and uptake by immunocytes within liver.	Limited success in experimental and human autoimmune encephalitis, diabetes, rheumatoid arthritis
Recombinant interleukin-10	Bolsters type-2 cytokine response. May downregulate cytotoxic type-1 cytokine response.	Theoretical Untested
Antibodies to tumor necrosis factor-alpha (TNFα)	Suppress proinflammatory cytokine. May impair cytotoxic type 1 cytokine response. High inducible and constitutive levels of TNFα are predicted by the presence of polymorphism, *TFNA*2*, in autoimmune hepatitis. Modulation of these levels may influence disease behavior.	Theoretical Untested Funtional consequences of *TFNA*2* are unknown; it is premature to unbalance immunoregulatory network with monoclonal antibodies.
Gene therapy	Replaces or counteracts critical single amino acid substitution in susceptibility gene, autoimmune promoter gene, or immunocyte activator gene Identification of critical single amino acid substitutions in antigen- binding groove of HLA DR molecule, T-cell receptor, and/or cytokine genes affords opportunities for correction by gene therapy.	Theoretical Untested

BIBLIOGRAPHY

1. Czaja AJ: Diagnosis, prognosis, and treatment of classical autoimmune chronic active hepatitis. In Krawitt EL, Wiesner RH (eds): Autoimmune Liver Disease. New York, Raven Press, 1991, pp 143–166.
2. Czaja AJ: Chronic active hepatitis: The challenge for a new nomenclature. Ann Intern Med 119:510–517, 1993.
3. Czaja AJ: Autoimmune hepatitis and viral infection. Gastroenterol Clin North Am 23:547–566, 1994.
4. Czaja AJ: Autoimmune hepatitis: current therapeutic concepts. Clin Immunother 1:413– 429, 1994.
5. Czaja AJ: Autoimmune hepatitis: evolving concepts and treatment strategies. Dig Dis Sci 40:435–456, 1995.
6. Czaja AJ: The variant forms of autoimmune hepatitis. Ann Intern Med 125:588–598, 1996.
7. Czaja AJ, Strettel MDJ, Thomson LJ, et al: Associations between alleles of the major histocompatibility complex and type 1 autoimmune hepatitis. Hepatology 25:317–323, 1997.
8. Czaja AJ: Frequency and nature of the variant syndromes of autoimmune liver disease. Hepatology 28:360–365, 1998.
9. Czaja AJ: Drug therapy in the management of type 1 autoimmune hepatitis. Drugs 57:49–68, 1999.
10. Czaja AJ: Behavior and significance of autoantibodies in type 1 autoimmune hepatitis. J Hepatol 30:394–401, 1999.
11. Czaja AJ, Cookson S, Constantini PK, et al: Cytokine polymorphisms associated with clinical features and treatment outcome in type 1 autoimmune hepatitis. Gastroenterology 117:645–652, 1999.
12. Czaja AJ, Donaldson PT: Genetic susceptibilities of immune expression and liver cell injury in autoimmune hepatitis. Immunological Rev 174:250–259, 2000.

20. PRIMARY BILIARY CIRRHOSIS AND PRIMARY SCLEROSING CHOLANGITIS

Jayant A. Talwalkar, M.D., M.P.H., and Nicholas F. LaRusso, M.D.

1. Define primary biliary cirrhosis and primary sclerosing cholangitis.

Primary biliary cirrhosis (PBC) and primary sclerosing cholangitis (PSC) are chronic cholestatic liver diseases of unknown etiology in adults. PBC mainly affects women in the fifth decade of life and is characterized by destruction of interlobular and septal bile ducts. PSC mainly affects men in the fourth decade of life and is characterized by diffuse inflammation and fibrosis of the entire biliary tree. Both PBC and PSC eventually progress to end-stage liver disease, requiring consideration for liver transplantation.

2. Is PBC an autoimmune disorder?

The underlying cause of PBC is unknown. Evidence for an autoimmune etiology includes the following:
- Frequent association with other autoimmune diseases such as Sjögren's syndrome, rheumatoid arthritis, scleroderma/CREST (the syndrome consisting of **c**alcinosis, **R**aynaud phenomenon, **e**sophageal disease, **s**clerodactyly, and **t**elangiectasia), thyroiditis, lichen planus, discoid lupus, and pemphigoid
- Presence of circulating serum autoantibodies, such as antimitochondrial antibodies (AMA), antinuclear antibody (ANA), anti-smooth muscle antibody (ASMA), extractable nuclear antigen (ENA), rheumatoid factor, and thyroid specific antibodies
- Histologic features, including lymphoplasmacytic cholangitis with portal tract expansion indicative of immunologic bile duct destruction
- Familial clustering among patients with PBC
- Increased prevalence of circulating serum autoantibodies in relatives of patients with PBC
- Increased frequency of class II major histocompatibility complex (MHC) antigens in PBC

3. Is PSC an autoimmune disorder?

The evidence supporting an immunogenic origin for PSC includes the following:
- 70–80% prevalence of inflammatory bowel disease among patients with PSC worldwide
- Increased incidence of PSC and chronic ulcerative colitis in families of patients with PSC
- Evidence for immune system dysregulation, including increased serum levels of immunoglobulin M, serum autoantibodies such as ANA, ASMA, and peripheral antineutrophil cytoplasmic antigen (p-ANCA), circulating immune complexes, and abnormalities in peripheral blood lymphocyte subsets
- Increased frequency of human leukocyte antigens (HLA) B8, DR3a, and DR4
- Aberrant expression of HLA class II antigen on bile duct epithelial cells.

4. Do viral infections have a role in the development of PSC?

Viral agents such as respiratory enteric orphan (REO) virus type III and cytomegalovirus capable of infecting the biliary tree have been implicated in the development of PSC. A hypothesis of viral-mediated immune system activation with subsequent immunologically mediated bile duct destruction has been proposed. However, no direct evidence has linked these or other viruses to the development of PSC.

5. What are the clinical features of PBC and PSC?

The clinical presentations of both PBC and PSC may be similar, although the demographics differ. Eighty-five to 90% of patients with PBC are women presenting in the fourth to sixth decade of life, whereas 70% of patients with PSC are men with an approximate age of 40 years at diagnosis. Despite an increasing frequency of asymptomatic or subclinical disease probably due to greater awareness, each generally presents with the gradual onset of fatigue and pruritus. Right upper quadrant pain and anorexia also may be present at diagnosis. Although uncommon, steatorrhea in PBC and PSC is usually due to bile salt malabsorption, pancreatic exocrine insufficiency, or concomitant celiac disease. Jaundice as a primary manifestation of PBC remains uncommon yet often heralds the presence of advanced histologic disease. In PBC, jaundice before pruritus is unusual but may be the most common presenting complaint in men. In PSC, the development of cholangitis characterized by recurrent fever, right upper quadrant pain, and jaundice may occur. A history of previous reconstructive biliary surgery, the presence of dominant extrahepatic biliary strictures, or the development of a superimposed cholangiocarcinoma may be responsible. The symptoms of end-stage liver disease, such as gastrointestinal bleeding, ascites, and encephalopathy, occur late in the course of both diseases.

6. What are the common findings on physical examination?

Physical examination may reveal jaundice and excoriations from pruritus in both disorders. Xanthelasmas (raised lesions over the eyelids from cholesterol deposition) and xanthomas (lesions over the extensor surfaces) are occasionally seen in the late stages of both diseases, particularly PBC. Hyperpigmentation, especially in sun-exposed areas, and vitiligo may be present. The liver usually is enlarged and firm to palpation. The spleen also may be palpable if portal hypertension from advanced disease has developed. Characteristics of end-stage liver disease, including muscle wasting, spider angiomata, ascites, and hepatic encephalopathy, appear in the advanced stages of both diseases and are rare as presenting features.

7. What diseases are associated with PBC ?

Up to 80% of patients with PBC also have coexistent extrahepatic autoimmune diseases, such as sicca (Sjögren's) syndrome, scleroderma/CREST, rheumatoid arthritis, dermatomyositis, mixed connective tissue disease, keratoconjunctivitis sicca, and systemic lupus erythematosus. Autoimmune thyroiditis and renal tubular acidosis also have been described with PBC.

8. What diseases are associated with PSC?

Chronic ulcerative colitis (CUC) and less frequently Crohn's colitis are present in at least 70–80% of patients with PSC. CUC usually appears before the onset of PSC but may be diagnosed simultaneously or after recognition of PSC. The disease activity of CUC associated with PSC is usually quiescent; in 80% of patients, CUC is either asymptomatic or mildly symptomatic when PSC is diagnosed. Although an increased prevalence of extrahepatic autoimmune disorders has been observed for PSC, they are much less common than in PBC.

9. What important biochemical abnormalities are associated with PBC and PSC?

In both disorders, alkaline phosphatase usually is elevated 3–4 times above normal with mild-to-moderate elevations in alanine aminotransferase (ALT) and aspartate aminotransferase (AST). In PBC, serum bilirubin values are usually normal initially. In PSC, serum bilirubin values are modestly increased in up to 50% of patients at the time of diagnosis. Tests reflective of synthetic liver function, including serum albumin and prothrombin time, remain normal unless the disease is advanced. Serum immunoglobulin M (IgM) is elevated in 90% of patients with PBC. Tests related to copper metabolism are virtually always abnormal in both diseases, reflecting chronic cholestasis. The widespread use of automated blood chemistries has resulted in the diagnosis of an increasing number of presymptomatic patients with PBC and PSC.

10. What is the lipid profile in patients with PBC? Are they at increased risk for developing coronary artery disease?

Serum cholesterol levels are usually elevated in PBC. In the early stages of disease, increases in high-density lipoprotein (HDL) cholesterol exceed those of low-density lipoprotein (LDL) and very-low-density lipoprotein (VLDL). With disease progression, the concentration of HDL decreases, whereas LDL concentrations become markedly elevated. The hyperlipidemia associated with PBC, however, does not appear to place patients at increased risk for atherosclerotic disease.

11. What serum autoantibodies are associated with PBC?
Circulating AMA is found in up to 95% of patients with PBC. Although considered non–organ-specific as well as non–species-specific, AMA usually is detected by an enzyme-linked immunsorbent assay (ELISA). However, antibodies directed against a specific group of antigens on the inner mitochondrial membrane (M2 antigens) are present in 98% of patients with PBC. This subtyping of serum AMA increases the sensitivity and specificity for disease detection.
Other AMA subtypes related to PBC react with antigens on the outer mitochondrial membrane. Anti-M4 occurs in association with anti-M2 in patients with features of both chronic autoimmune hepatitis and PBC. Anti-M8, when present with anti-M2, may be associated with a more rapid course of PBC in select patients. Anti-M9 has been observed with and without anti-M2 and may be helpful in the diagnosis of early-stage PBC.

12. What serum autoantibodies are associated with PSC?
In PSC, serum AMA is rare and, if present, usually is seen in very low titers. However, low but detectable titers of ANA and/or ASMA have been found in PSC. Peri-antineutrophil cytoplasmic antibody (p-ANCA) has been observed in up to 65% of patients with PSC. However, the finding of p-ANCA among patients with ulcerative colitis and no evidence of PSC limits its diagnostic utility.

13. What are the cholangiographic features of the biliary tree in PSC?
The biliary evaluation of PSC by endoscopic or transhepatic cholangiography demonstrates diffuse stricturing of both intrahepatic and extrahepatic ducts with subsequent saccular dilatation of intervening areas. These abnormalities result in the characteristic "beads-on-a-string" appearance. Twenty percent of patients have only intrahepatic and hilar involvement with sparing of the remaining extrahepatic ducts. The presence of a dominant stricture should raise the question of cholangiocarcinoma as a complication of PSC.

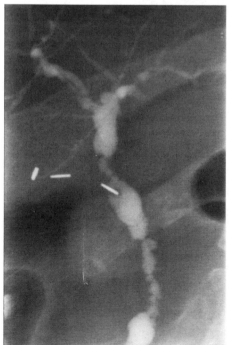

Retrograde cholangiogram exhibiting classic features of PSC, including diffuse stricturing and beading of intra- and extrahepatic bile ducts. (From LaRusso NF, et al: Primary sclerosing cholangitis. N Engl J Med 310:899–903, 1984, with permission.)

14. Is it important to evaluate the biliary tree in PBC?

In PBC, ultrasound examination of the biliary tree is usually adequate to exclude the presence of extrahepatic biliary obstruction. However, in patients with atypical features such as male gender, AMA-negative status, or associated inflammatory bowel disease, an endoscopic cholangiogram should be considered to distinguish PBC from PSC and other disorders causing biliary obstruction. Increasing experience with magnetic resonance cholangiography suggests this noninvasive diagnostic approach as an alternative.

15. What are the hepatic histologic features of PBC and PSC?

Histologic abnormalities on liver biopsy are highly characteristic of both PBC and PSC in the early stages of disease. In PBC, the diagnostic finding is described as a "florid duct lesion," which reveals bile duct destruction and granuloma formation. An often marked lymphoplasmacytic inflammatory cell infiltrate in the portal tracts is accompanied by the segmental degeneration of interlobular bile ducts (chronic nonsuppurative destructive cholangitis).

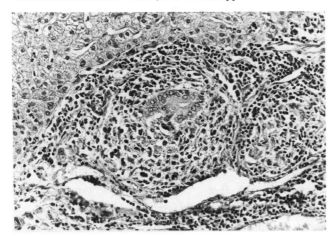

Florid duct lesion (granulomatous bile duct destruction) in PBC. A poorly formed granuloma surrounds and destroys the bile duct in an eccentric fashion.

Early histologic changes in PSC include enlargement of portal tracts by edema, increased connective tissue, and proliferation of interlobular bile ducts. The diagnostic morphologic abnormality in PSC is termed *fibrous obliterative cholangitis*, which leads to the complete loss of interlobular and adjacent septal bile ducts from fibrous chord and connective tissue deposition. The histologic findings at end stages of both diseases are characterized by a paucity of bile ducts and biliary cirrhosis.

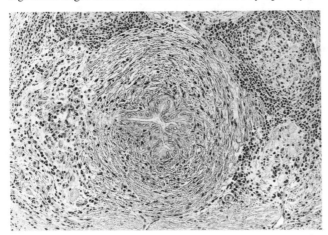

Fibrous obliterative cholangitis in PSC. The interlobular bile duct shows a typical fibrous collar, and epithelium seems undamaged.

16. Do asymptomatic patients with PBC have a normal life expectancy?

Most patients with PBC experience a progressive clinical course resulting in eventual cirrhosis. Asymptomatic patients appear to have a longer median survival than symptomatic patients. However, a reduction in median survival compared with age- and sex-matched healthy populations also is observed. Estimates of overall median survival without liver transplantation range between 10 and 12 years from the time of diagnosis; advanced histologic disease imparts a median survival approaching 8 years. Elevations of total bilirubin above 8–10 mg/dl have been associated with a median life expectancy of 2 years without liver transplantation.

17. Do asymptomatic patients with PSC have a normal life expectancy?

Although some symptomatic or minimally symptomatic patients with PSC may do well for many years, most published investigations to date support the contention that PSC is a progressive disease, which can ultimately lead to liver failure and death without liver transplantation. A median survival of 9–12 years from the time of diagnosis among all patients with PSC appears to be independent of geographic and environmental influences. Rates of survival for asymptomatic and symptomatic patients with PBC or PSC compared with healthy controls are similar.

18. What is the role of mathematical models in estimating survival for PBC and PSC?

The development of mathematical models for both PBC and PSC has improved estimation of rates of disease progression and survival without liver transplantation on an individual basis. They are useful for stratifying patients by survival risk, developing endpoints of treatment failure, and designing therapeutic trials. The use of these models in defining the optimal selection of patients and timing for liver transplantation is the subject of current investigations.

Prognostic models for PBC developed at the Mayo Clinic rely on parameters such as serum bilirubin, albumin, prothrombin time, presence or absence of peripheral edema, and patient age. In PSC, the important variables that predict survival include patient age, serum bilirubin, presence of splenomegaly, and hepatic histologic stage. A revision of the Mayo Clinic PSC model (substituting a history of variceal bleeding for histologic stage) provides prognostic information in the absence of invasive procedures such as a liver biopsy.

19. What vitamin deficiencies are associated with PBC and PSC?

Patients with PBC and PSC are susceptible to fat-soluble vitamin deficiencies, especially in advanced stages of disease. The development of diminished visual acuity at night can be attributed to vitamin A deficiency. Vitamin D deficiency occurs commonly in association with marked steatorrhea, which is related to a decrease in duodenal bile acid concentration. Vitamin D deficiency may contribute to metabolic bone disease. Prolongation of serum prothrombin time is associated with vitamin K deficiency. Finally, vitamin E deficiency may uncommonly cause neurologic abnormalities affecting the posterior columns, characterized by areflexia or loss of proprioception and ataxia.

20. What bone disease is associated with PBC and PSC?

Metabolic bone disease (i.e., hepatic osteodystrophy), which may lead to disabling pathologic fractures, is a serious complication of both PBC and PSC. It is related to osteoporosis and rarely to vitamin D deficiency. Severe bone pain in an acute or chronic setting related to avascular necrosis (AVN) also may occur in PBC and PSC.

21. What liver-related complications are specific to PSC?

Complications specific to PSC include recurrent bacterial cholangitis, dominant stricturing of the extrahepatic bile ducts, and cholangiocarcinoma. Cholangitis is frequent in patients with a history of previous biliary surgery or dominant stricture formation of the extrahepatic bile duct. Dominant strictures of the biliary tree occur in approximately 15–20% of patients with PSC during the natural history of disease. They often involve the hilus but can equally affect both hepatic ducts as well as the common bile duct. Dominant strictures frequently are associated with the acute onset of jaundice, pruritus, and bacterial cholangitis.

Ten to 15% of patients with PSC develop cholangiocarcinoma during the course of disease. The highest incidence apparently occurs in patients with long-standing CUC and cirrhotic-stage PSC. Early detection of cholangiocarcinoma remains difficult because of the insensitivity of current techniques such as mucosal biopsy or brush cytology. The measurement and detection of an elevated serum CA-19-9 level in select patients with PSC may be a signal to pursue the exclusion of cholangiocarcinoma.

22. What is the differential diagnosis of PBC and PSC?
The differential diagnosis of PBC and PSC includes other causes of chronic cholestasis, including extrahepatic biliary obstruction due to biliary stones, iatrogenic strictures, and tumors. Although ultrasound or computed tomography may suggest the presence of biliary dilation, the performance of cholangiography is required to render a definitive diagnosis of PSC. Drug-induced cholestasis secondary to phenothiazines, estrogens, androgens, and a number of other drugs also should be considered as alternative diagnoses.

23. Define autoimmune cholangitis. How is it related to PBC?
Recent observations have documented a group of patients with PBC and no detectable serum AMA. The presence of significant titers (> 1:40) of serum ANA and/or ASMA are often observed as well. The terms *autoimmune cholangitis* and *AMA-negative PBC* have been applied to such patients. The clinical course and response to therapy with ursodeoxycholic acid (UDCA), however, are the same as in patients with AMA-positive PBC.

24. What is meant by an overlap or variant syndrome in PBC and PSC?
The presence of features consistent with both autoimmune hepatitis (AIH) and PBC is defined as an overlap or variant syndrome. Both ANA and AMA are often positive by serologic testing. Piecemeal necrosis and coexistent periductal/portal inflammation with bile duct destruction are commonly seen. This group appears to benefit from immunosuppresive treatment as well as UDCA.
Similar overlap occurs in PSC and AIH in both adult and pediatric populations. The biliary stricturing and dilation typical of PSC often are accompanied by histologic lesions seen in AIH. High-titer ANA serologic status, which is also seen in this condition, may warrant the use of immunosuppressive therapy for potential benefit. In patients with AIH and inflammatory bowel disease, cholangiography is recommended to exclude PSC, especially in the presence of abnormal serum liver biochemistries reflective of cholestasis.

25. Describe the treatment of pruritus in patients with PBC and PSC.
Pruritus is a frequent complication of both diseases and creates difficult management options in cholestatic liver disease. Cholestyramine relieves the itching associated with PBC and PSC by reducing serum bile acid levels in patients with cholestasis. In addition, it increases intestinal excretion of bile acids by preventing their absorption. It is administered in 4-gm doses (mixed with liquids) with meals or after breakfast for a total daily dose of 12–16 gm. Cholestyramine should be given 1½ hours before or after other medications to avoid nonspecific binding and diminished intestinal absorption. Once the itching remits, the dosage should be reduced to the minimal amount that maintains relief.
Rifampin at a dose of 300-600 mg/day also has been effective in relieving pruritus due either to p450 enzyme induction or inhibition of bile acid uptake. For refractory cases, phenobarbital may be added in a dose of 120–160 mg/day. Experimental approaches for severe or refractory pruritus include phototherapy and charcoal hemoperfusion for the removal of bile acids.

26. How is osteopenia treated in patients with PBC and PSC?
There is no effective therapy for the osteopenia associated with PBC and PSC. As mentioned earlier, this metabolic bone disease is due most often to osteoporosis and infrequently to osteomalacia. However, low serum vitamin D levels can be corrected by administering 50,000 units of vitamin D up to 3 times/week.
Estrogen replacement therapy, especially when instituted soon after menopause, has been associated with the slowing of bone loss in women. In cholestatic patients, estrogen therapy was

previously thought to be contraindicated because of the risk for drug-induced cholestasis. However, this problem does not appear to be associated with standard estrogen replacement therapy, which was shown to improve osteoporosis in a recent retrospective study. It is prudent, however, to institute clinical and biochemical monitoring of treated patients within 2–3 months after starting estrogen therapy.

27. Describe the treatment of fat-soluble vitamin deficiency in PBC and PSC.

Problems with night vision due to vitamin A deficiency may be alleviated by replacement therapy. Decreased serum levels can be corrected with the oral administration of vitamin A (25,000–50,000 units) 2 or 3 times/week. Because excessive vitamin A intake has been associated with hepatotoxicity, serum levels should be monitored. In patients with low vitamin E levels, replacement therapy with 400 units/day can be instituted, although replacement is not always effective. Prolongation of prothrombin time (PT) also can be associated with hepatic failure. If PT levels improve after a trial of water-soluble vitamin K (5–10 mg/day for 1 week), patients should be maintained on this regimen indefinitely.

28. Do lipid-lowering agents have a role in treatment of PBC and PSC?

Because patients with PBC and PSC do not appear to have an increased risk of atherosclerotic disease despite high serum cholesterol levels, lipid-lowering agents usually are not recommended. In some patients with xanthelasma, cholestyramine may stabilize or even decrease the size of subcutaneous lipid deposits.

29. Describe the treatment of bacterial cholangitis in PSC.

Bacterial cholangitis in PSC should be treated with broad-spectrum antibiotics. Ciprofloxacin reaches high biliary concentrations and has broad gram-negative and gram-positive coverage. Similar results can be observed with other fluoroquinolones, such as norfloxacin and levofloxacin. Prophylactic therapy with oral fluoroquinolone therapy may reduce the frequency of bacterial cholangitis in patients with PSC and a history of recurrent bacterial cholangitis.

30. What are the therapeutic options for biliary strictures in PSC?

Balloon dilation of dominant strictures by either transhepatic or endoscopic retrograde approaches can relieve biliary obstruction in PSC. Balloon dilation is most effective in patients with acute elevations in serum bilirubin level or recent onset of bacterial cholangitis. It appears less effective in patients with longstanding jaundice or history of recurrent bacterial cholangitis. The role for long-term endoscopic stent placement and exchange for recurrent PSC-related strictures, however, has not been assessed in a prospective clinical trial setting.

31. Describe the role of transjugular intrahepatic portosystemic shunt (TIPS) in PBC and PSC.

TIPS rapidly decompresses the portal system with subsequent reduction in local venous pressure within both esophageal and gastric varices. TIPS placement is indicated for refractory variceal bleeding or recalcitrant ascites from end-stage liver disease in general. In patients with PSC who have undergone proctocolectomy because of ulcerative colitis, the development of peristomal varices with subsequent transfusion-dependent bleeding has been shown to resolve after TIPS placement. Serial Doppler ultrasound examinations every 3–6 months are required to exclude the possibility of shunt stenosis or occlusion.

32. What medical agents have been tried for the treatment of PBC?

A number of potential treatments for PBC have been evaluated to date with the primary goal of stabilizing or halting disease progression. Pharmacologic agents such as colchicine, corticosteroids, cyclosporine, azathioprine, and methotrexate have demonstrated marginal clinical benefit and significant adverse effects. Randomized, placebo-controlled clinical trials in patients with PBC at the Mayo Clinic and elsewhere provide substantial experience with the use of ursodeoxycholic acid (UDCA). At doses of 13–15 mg/kg/day, UDCA prolongs the time to treatment failure, improves overall survival, reduces the risk of developing esophageal varices and cirrhosis, and remains a cost-effective therapy.

33. What medical agents have been tried for the treatment of PSC?

Because of the variable nature of disease progression in PSC, the development of randomized clinical trials for the assessment of medical therapies has been difficult. As a potential consequence, no acceptable medical therapy is available for the treatment of PSC. As with PBC, the use of pharmacologic agents such as d-penicillamine, colchicine, corticosteroids, and immunosuppressive agents have not conferred significant clinical benefit. UDCA in standard doses (13–15 mg/kg/day) appears to improve biochemical parameters, but no significant effect on histology or survival has been observed. Higher doses of UDCA (25–30 mg/kg/day) are currently under investigation.

34. Describe the mechanism of action for UDCA in PBC.

UDCA is a hydrophilic, nonhepatotoxic compound that acts by attenuating the effect of endogenous hydrophobic bile acids, some of which are believed to be hepatotoxic. Alterations in the bile acid pool may occur by competition for ileal uptake sites or by direct action at the hepatocyte level. In addition, UDCA may reduce class I and class II HLA antigen expression on hepatocytes and biliary epithelial cells.

35. What is the role of reconstructive biliary tract surgery in PSC?

Choledochoduodenostomy and choledochojejunostomy are palliative measures to alleviate symptoms related to biliary obstruction. Reconstructive surgery does not have a beneficial effect on the natural history of PSC, particularly in patients with advanced liver disease. The development of postoperative bacterial cholangitis appears to occur in > 60% of patients. In addition, an increased risk for technical difficulty and inability to perform liver transplantation have been associated with previous biliary reconstruction. At most centers, however, reconstructive surgery is rarely performed for PSC because of improvements in endoscopic or transhepatic modalities.

36. Does proctocolectomy in patients with PSC and CUC favorably affect hepatobiliary disease?

Proctocolectomy has not been shown to have a beneficial effect on clinical outcome or survival in PSC. Currently, there is no indication to remove the colon in a patient with PSC in anticipation of a beneficial effect on liver disease. If carcinoma or precancerous lesions in the colon develop, a proctocolectomy is indicated. The development of peristomal varices after ileostomy creation is associated with considerable morbidity after proctocolectomy. Creation of an ileal pouch-anal anastomosis is recommended to avoid this significant complication.

37. Do patients with PBC and PSC have an increased risk for hepatocellular carcinoma?

Recent information suggests a higher-than-expected rate of cancer among patients with PBC, including hepatocellular carcinoma (HCC), which previously was thought to occur infrequently. Surveillance procedures, including abdominal ultrasound with serum alpha fetoprotein (AFP) levels every 12 –24 months, may be useful for exclusion or early detection of HCC in such patients. No systematic investigation of the risk for HCC in patients with PSC has been reported, but it appears to occur infrequently.

38. What is the role of liver transplantation in PBC and PSC?

The treatment of choice for patients with end-stage PBC and PSC is liver transplantation. Five- and 10-year survival rates of 85% and 70%, respectively, are among the highest for all individuals after liver transplantation. Factors that influence the consideration for liver transplantation are deteriorating hepatic synthetic function (defined as a Child-Turcotte-Pugh score ≥ 7), intractable symptoms, and diminished quality of life. Refractory ascites, progressive hepatic encephalopathy, uncontrolled or recurrent variceal bleeding, spontaneous bacterial peritonitis, and hepatorenal syndrome are also indications for consideration of liver transplantation. In addition to increased survival, a number of published reports have documented improvements in quality of life after liver transplantation.

39. Do PBC and PSC recur after liver transplantation?

A positive AMA persists in most patients with PBC after liver transplantation. Seven percent of posttransplant patients have evidence of histologic recurrence of PBC (florid duct lesion) in the hepatic allograft. No significant impact on survival, however, has been associated with recurrent histologic disease. The role of UDCA in preventing disease progression among liver transplant recipients with early-stage, recurrent PBC remains unknown.

Recurrent allograft disease with PSC has been reported, yet its true prevalence depends on establishing well-defined diagnostic criteria and the rigor of excluding patients with chronic ischemic biliary tract strictures after liver transplantation. For example, subclinical bacterial cholangitis from the Roux-en-Y biliary anastomosis in patients with PSC may be associated with the development of bile duct strictures. In addition, the presence of rejection, ABO mismatch, and possibly cytomegalovirus have been hypothesized to contribute to biliary stricturing. Nevertheless, recent data suggest that approximately 20% of patients transplanted for PSC develop recurrent disease and generally not of serious clinical significance.

40. What are the complications in PSC patients after liver transplantation?

Patients with PSC appear to have an increased incidence of chronic ductopenic rejection, graft loss from rejection, and biliary stricturing.

BIBLIOGRAPHY

1. Balan V, Batts KP, Porayko MK, et al: Histologic evidence for recurrence of primary biliary cirrhosis after liver transplantation. Hepatology 18:1392–1398, 1993.
2. Batts KP, Ludwig J: Histopathology of autoimmune chronic active hepatitis, primary biliary cirrhosis, and primary sclerosing cholangitis. In Krawitt EL, Wiesner RH (eds): Autoimmune Liver Diseases. New York, Raven Press, 1991, pp 75–92.
3. Cangemi JR, Wiesner RH, Beaver SJ, et al: Effect of proctocolectomy for chronic ulcerative colitis on the natural history of primary sclerosing cholangitis. Gastroenterology 96:790–794, 1989.
4. Crippin JS, Lindor KD, Jorgensen R, et al: Hypercholesterolemia and atherosclerosis in primary biliary cirrhosis: What is the risk? Hepatology 15:858–862, 1992.
5. Dickson ER, Grambsch PM, Fleming TR, et al: Prognosis in primary biliary cirrhosis: Model for decision making. Hepatology 10:1–7, 1989.
6. Dickson ER, Murtaugh PA, Wiesner RH, et al: Primary sclerosing cholangitis: Refinement and validation of survival models. Gastroenterology 103:1893–1901, 1993.
7. Graziadei IW, Wiesner RH, Batts KP, et al: Recurrence of primary sclerosing cholangitis following liver transplantation. Hepatology 29:1050–1056, 1999.
8. Graziadei IW, Wiesner RH, Marotta PJ, et al: Long-term results of patients undergoing liver transplantation for primary sclerosing cholangitis. Hepatology 30:1121–1127, 1999.
9. Hay JE, Lindor KD, Wiesner RH, et al: The metabolic bone disease of primary sclerosing cholangitis. Hepatology 14:257–261, 1991.
10. Kim WR, Ludwig J, Lindor KD: Variant forms of cholestatic diseases involving small bile ducts in adults. Am J Gastroenterol 95:1130–1138, 2000.
11. LaRusso NF, Wiesner RH, Ludwig J, MacCarty RL: Primary sclerosing cholangitis. N Engl J Med 310:899–903, 1984.
12. Lindor KD: Ursodiol for primary sclerosing cholangitis. Mayo Primary Sclerosing Cholangitis-Ursodeoxycholic Acid Study Group. N Engl J Med 336: 691–695, 1997.
13. Lindor KD, Dickson ER, Baldus WP, et al: Ursodeoxycholic acid in the treatment of primary biliary cirrhosis. Gastroenterology 106:1284–1290, 1994.
14. MacCarty RL, LaRusso NF, Wiesner RH, Ludwig J: Primary sclerosing cholangitis: Findings on cholangiography and pancreatography. Radiology 149:39–44, 1983.
15. Maddrey WC: Bone disease in patients with primary biliary cirrhosis. Prog Liver Dis 9:537–554, 1990.
16. Markus BH, Dickson ER, Grambsch PM, et al: Efficacy of liver transplantation in patients with primary biliary cirrhosis. N Engl J Med 320:1709–1713, 1989.
17. Nichols JC, Gores GJ, LaRusso NF, et al: Diagnostic role of CA 19-9 for cholangiocarcinoma in patients with primary sclerosing cholangitis. Mayo Clin Proc 68:874–879, 1993.
18. Nijhawan PK, Therneau TM, Dickson ER, et al: Incidence of cancer in primary biliary cirrhosis: The Mayo experience. Hepatology 29:1396–1398, 1999.
19. Rosen CB, Nagorney DM, Wiesner RH, et al: Cholangiocarcinoma complicating primary sclerosing cholangitis. Ann Surg 213:21–25, 1991.
20. Wiesner RH: Liver transplantation for primary biliary cirrhosis and primary sclerosing cholangitis: Predicting outcomes with natural history models. Mayo Clin Proc 73:575–588, 1998.

21. HEPATITIS VACCINES AND IMMUNOPROPHYLAXIS

Maria J. Sjogren, M.D., COL, MC

1. Discuss the concept of immunization (vaccination).

During the past century major progress in the control of infectious diseases has become possible because of the remarkable developments in microbiology. The success of immunization in humans rests on one major concept: humans have specific immunologic mechanisms that can be programmed to provide a defense against infectious agents. The body's immune mechanism is stimulated by direct introduction of infectious agents or smaller components in the form of vaccines.

2. Outline briefly the history of vaccination.

In 1798 Edward Jenner described his work with cowpox vaccination. He demonstrated that a person inoculated and infected with cowpox was protected against smallpox. The procedure, which he termed "vaccination," represented the first use of a vaccine for prevention of disease. The word "vaccine" is derived from the Latin word for cow; cows were host to the first true vaccine virus, cowpox. The evolution into the golden era of vaccine development began in 1949 with the discovery of virus propagation in cell culture. The first product developed by using the new cell culture technique was the Salk trivalent formalin-inactivated polio vaccine. After its success, vaccines to prevent human hepatitis A and B were developed rapidly, considering that the viral agents were discovered in 1973 and 1965, respectively.

3. Distinguish between active and passive immunization.

Active immunization involves the introduction of a specific antigen to provoke an antibody response that will prevent disease. **Passive immunization** or **immunoprophylaxis** is the introduction of antibodies produced by immunization or prior natural infection (of a suitable animal or human host) to prevent or modify the natural infection in a susceptible person.

4. What are the major categories of vaccines?

Two categories of vaccines are widely available: (1) **inactivated or killed vaccines**, in which the infectious agent is incapable of multiplying in the host but retains antigenic properties and evokes an antibody response, and (2) **live, attenuated vaccines**, which are prepared with live, viable agents. Because of attenuation, however, the agents are incapable of inducing clinical disease. The end result is development of antibody and prevention of infection. The live vaccines generally contain relatively low concentrations of the infectious agent. Ideally, only one administration is required with live vaccines, and the immunity is long-lasting. With killed vaccines, the immunologic response correlates with the concentration of the antigenic component. Inactivated vaccines commonly require a series of doses to stimulate a long-lasting immunologic response.

5. Describe the basic characteristics of immunoprophylaxis.

Immunoprophylaxis affords a relatively brief period of protection (weeks to a few months). Before the development of hepatitis A and B vaccines, immunoprophylaxis was the mainstay of preventing infection. Passive immunization occurs naturally in humans when maternal antibodies of the immunoglobulin G (IgG) class are passed to neonates. Such antibodies provide protection against many communicable bacterial and viral diseases for a period of months, during the period when the immune system has not yet fully developed. They disappear within the first year of life.

At the beginning of passive immunization therapy, the antibody-containing serum (e.g., horse serum) was administered directly. Currently, the antibody of interest is isolated and concentrated by means of fractionation of serum.

6. Which immunoglobulins are available for human use?

PRODUCT	SOURCE	USE
Immune serum globulin	Pooled human plasma	Prevents measles Prevents hepatitis A
Measles immunoglobulin	Pooled human plasma	Prevents measles
Hepatitis B immunoglobulin	Pooled plasma donors with high antibody titer	Used in accidental needlestick or sexual exposure
Rabies immunoglobulin	Pooled plasma from hyper-immunized donors	Immunotherapy for rabies
Botulism	Specific equine antibody	Treatment and prophylaxis for botulinum toxin

7. Which viral agents are mainly responsible for acute and chronic viral hepatitis?

ACUTE HEPATITIS	CHRONIC HEPATITIS	MAIN ROUTE OF TRANSMISSION	VACCINE STATUS
Hepatitis A virus (HAV)	No	Fecal-oral	Commercially available
Hepatitis B virus (HBV)	Yes	Bloodborne	Commercially available
Hepatitis C virus (HCV)	Yes	Bloodborne	Not available
Hepatitis D virus (HDV)	Yes	Bloodborne	Not available
Hepatitis E virus (HEV)	No	Fecal-oral	IND status

IND = investigational new drug.

8. What kind of immunoprophylaxis is available for hepatitis A?

Although hepatitis A vaccine is the first line of preventive therapy, administration of serum IgG is still of value to prevent hepatitis A infection in certain circumstances. Immunoglobulin may be used to provide short-term protection in persons who require immediate immunity and in children too young to receive the vaccine. The recommended dose of IgG for adults is 0.02 ml/kg for preexposure when the period of exposure will not exceed 3 months. If the period of exposure is prolonged, 0.06 ml/kg every 5 months is recommended. IgG affords excellent prophylaxis but is impractical because protection lasts only a few months. Although considered safe, it may cause fever, myalgias, and considerable pain at injection sites.

9. What vaccines are available for hepatitis A?

Two vaccines are commercially available in the United States: VAQTA, manufactured by Merck, Sharp, & Dohme, and HAVRIX, manufactured by SmithKline Biologicals. A single dose of VAQTA has 100% protective efficacy. The initial trial included 1037 children aged 2–16 years and took place in an upstate New York community with a 3% annual incidence of acute hepatitis A. Children were randomized to receive one intramuscular injection of a highly purified, formalin-inactivate HAV vaccine or placebo. From day 50 until day 103 after injection, 25 cases of clinically apparent hepatitis developed in the placebo group and 0 in the vaccine group (p < 0.001). The vaccine gave a calculated 100% efficacy rate. HAVRIX, when tested against placebo in more than 40,000 Thai children, gave a calculated 97% rate of protective efficacy after three doses. Two doses of either vaccine provide long-term immunity. Both are approved in the U.S. for subjects older than 2 years.

10. Compare the major characteristics of VAQTA and HAVRIX.

	VAQTA	HAVRIX
Type	Inactivated vaccine	Inactivated vaccine
HAV strain	Attenuated CR326F′	Attenuated HM175
Cell culture	Cultured in MRC-5 cells	Cultured in MRC-5 cells

Table continued on following page

	VAQTA	HAVRIX
Adjuvant	Aluminum hydroxide	Aluminum hydroxide
Standards met	FDA, WHO	FDA, WHO
Immunity	Promotes anti-HAV in serum	Promotes anti-HAV in serum
Route of administration	Intramuscular	Intramuscular
Adult doses	1 ml (50 U) at 0 and 6 months	1 ml (1440 U) at 0 and 6–12 months
Pediatric doses (2–17 yr)	0.5 ml (25 U) at 0 and 6–18 months	0.5 ml (720 U) at 0 and 6–12 months

FDA = Food and Drug Administration, WHO = World Health Organization.

11. Who should be immunized against hepatitis A?
- Travelers
- Military personnel
- People living in or relocating to areas of high endemicity
- Native people from Alaska (cyclical epidemics)
- Homosexually active men
- Users of illicit drugs
- Residents of communities experiencing a hepatitis A outbreak
- Persons with clotting factor disorders
- Certain institutional workers
- Employees of child day-care centers
- Laboratory workers who handle live HAV
- Handlers of primates that may harbor HAV

12. What side effects have been observed with the hepatitis A vaccine?
1–10%: local reactions at injection site, such as induration, redness, and swelling; systemic reactions, such as fatigue, fever, or malaise; anorexia; nausea.

< 1%: hematoma at injection site, pruritus, skin rash, pharyngitis, upper respiratory tract infections, abdominal pain, diarrhea, vomiting, arthralgia, myalgia, lymphadenopathy, insomnia, photophobia, vertigo.

13. Do nonresponders to hepatitis A vaccine exist?
HAV vaccines are highly immunogenic in most healthy people. Some nonhealthy populations have a shown a lower anti-HAV titer after immunization, such as HIV-infected people and people with chronic liver disease.

14. What is the lowest protective anti-HAV serum level after immunization?
The lowest anti-HAV protective titer has not been established, but the Advisory Committee on Immune Practices defines the minimum as 20 mIU/ml.

15. Does the concurrent administration of hepatitis A vaccine influence the immune response to other traveler's vaccines?
Recent studies of 396 travelers who received vaccines against hepatitis A, poliomyelitis, hepatitis B, diphtheria, tetanus, yellow fever, Japanese encephalitis, typhoid fever, or rabies (according to individual needs) showed that concurrent administration of hepatitis A vaccine did not compromise the immune response to the hepatitis A or other vaccines.

16. What kind of immunoprophylaxis is available for hepatitis B?
1. **Active immunization:** hepatitis B vaccine, first licensed in the U.S. in 1981, is recommended for both pre- and postexposure prophylaxis.

2. **Passive immunization:** hyperimmune globulin (HBIG) provides temporary passive protection and is indicated in certain postexposure situations.

17. What is the recommended dose of HBIG for adults and children?

HBIG contains high concentrations of anti-HBs, whereas regular immunoglobulin is prepared from plasma with varying concentrations of anti-HBs. In the U.S., HBIG has an anti-HBs titer > 1:100,000 by radioimmunoassay.

Recommended Treatment after Exposure to Hepatitis B Virus

	HBIG		VACCINE	
Exposure	Dose	Timing	Dose	Timing
Perinatal	0.5 ml IM	Within 12 hours of birth	0.5 ml at birth	Within 12 hours of birth; repeat at 1 and 6 months
Sexual	0.6 ml/kg IM	Single dose within 14 days of sexual contact	Same time as HBIG	Start immunization at once

IM = intramuscularly.

18. How many hepatitis B vaccines are available in the U.S.? Are they comparable?

Three vaccines have been licensed in the U.S. For practical purposes, they are comparable in immunogenicity and efficacy rates, although the preparations are different:

1. **Heptavax-B** (Merck, Sharp & Dohme) became available in 1986 and is no longer manufactured in the U.S. It consists of hepatitis B surface antigen (HBsAg) purified from the plasma of chronically infected humans and evokes antibodies to the group a determinant of HBsAg, effectively neutralizing the various subtypes of HBV. Abundant evidence supports it efficacy, but it is expensive to prepare, and a number of physical and chemical inactivation steps are needed for purification and safety. Because of these problems, alternate approaches based on recombinant DNA technology were developed. Each milliliter of plasma-derived vaccine has 20 mg of HBsAg.

2. **Recombivax-HB**, also manufactured by Merck Sharp & Dohme (West Point, PA) became available in 1989. It is a noninfectious, nonglycosylated HBsAg vaccine, subtype adw, made by recombinant DNA technology. Yeast cells (*Saccharomyces cerevisiae*) expressing the HBsAg gene are cultured, collected by centrifugation, and broken by homogenization with glass beads. HBsAg particles are purified and absorbed in aluminum hydroxide. Each milliliter has 10 mg of HBsAg.

3. **Engerix-B**, manufactured by SmithKline Biologicals (Rixensart, Belgium), is a noninfectious recombinant DNA vaccine. It contains purified HBsAg obtained by culturing genetically engineered *Saccharomyces cerevisiae* cells, which carry the surface antigen gene of HBV. This surface antigen is purified from the cells and adsorbed on aluminum hydroxide. Each milliliter has 20 mg of HBsAg.

19. What is the immunization schedule for HBV vaccine in adults and children?

Recombivax -HB Vaccine

GROUP	FORMULATION	INITIAL	1 MONTH	6 MONTHS
Birth to 10 years	Pediatric dose: 0.5 ml	0.5 ml	0.5 ml	0.5 ml
Adults and older children	Adult dose: 10 mg/1.0 ml	1.0 ml	1.0 ml	1.0 ml
Dialysis patients	Special dose: 40 mg/1.0 ml	1.0 ml	1.0 ml	1.0 ml

Engerix-B Vaccine

GROUP	FORMULATION	INITIAL	1 MONTH	6 MONTHS
Birth to 10 years	Pediatric dose: 10 mg/0.5 ml	0.5 ml	0.5 ml	0.5 ml
Adults and older children	Adult dose: 20 mg/1.0 ml	1.0 ml	1.0 ml	1.0 ml
After needlestick injury	20 mg/1.0 ml	1.0 ml at 0, 1, and 2 months		
Hemodialysis patients	40 mg/2.0 ml	2.0 ml at 0, 1, 2, and 6 months		

20. What is the recommended regimen for infants born to HBsAg-positive mothers?

TREATMENT	BIRTH	WITHIN 7 DAYS	1 MONTH	6 MONTHS
Recombivax-HB (pediatric dose)	0.5 ml	0.5 ml	0.5 ml	0.5 ml
HBIG	0.5 ml	None	None	None

21. Is a booster needed after immunization? If so, how often?

Booster shots are not recommended for healthy adults or children. For immunocompromised patients (e.g., hemodialysis patients), a booster dose should be administered when anti-HBs levels drop to 10 mIU/ml or less.

22. Summarize the evidence for long-term immunization after vaccination.

The persistence of antibody directly correlates with the peak level achieved after the third dose. Follow-up of adults who were immunized with plasma-derived hepatitis B vaccine demonstrated that the antibody levels had fallen to undetectable or very low levels in 30–50% of recipients. Long-term studies of adults and children indicate that protection lasts at least 9 years, despite loss of anti-HBs in serum. After 9 years of follow-up, anti-HBs loss ranged from 13–60% in a group of homosexual men and Alaskan Eskimos, two groups at high risk of infection. However, vaccine recipients were virtually 100% protected from clinical illness, despite the absence of booster immunization. Among people without detectable anti-HBs, breakthrough infections have been noted in later years, based on the detection of hepatitis B core antibody. However, clinical illness did not occur, and HBsAg was not detected. The infection is assumed to be without consequence and to confer permanent immunity.

23. Is it possible that the vaccine will not protect against HBV infection?

Hepatitis B vaccines effectively evoke neutralizing antibodies to the group a determinant of HBsAg, which is believed to be formed by the highly conformational structure between amino acids 124 and 127. Some diversity has been demonstrated but probably does not affect neutralization of HBsAg. Hepatitis B mutants have been reported. Probably they arose randomly and were not corrected because of an intrinsic failure of the polymerase enzyme. Significant variants have been described in HBV vaccines, initially in Italy but also in Japan and Gambia. Italian investigators reported that 40 of 1600 immunized children showed evidence of HBV infection despite adequate antibody response to the HBV vaccine. The mutant virus had substitutions in amino acids 145 (Italy), 126 (Japan), and 141 (Gambia). Whether HBV mutants have substantial clinical significance is not known. Large-scale epidemiologic studies of the incidence, prevalence, and clinical correlation have not been performed.

24. Is it harmful to give hepatitis B vaccine to known hepatitis B carriers?

No deleterious effects were observed in 16 chronic carriers of HBsAg who received at least 6 monthly injections of hepatitis B vaccine. The vaccine was administered in an attempt to eliminate the chronic carrier status. However, no such result was observed. None of the volunteers lost HBsAg or developed anti-HBs. This finding simplified the design of hepatitis B vaccination programs.

25. Is it possible to immunize people simultaneously against hepatitis A and B?

To date, over 1000 subjects have received a combined product of both vaccines. Twinrix (SmithKline Biologicals), which is commercially available in Europe, elicits antibodies to HAV and HBV in more than 80% of recipients by month 2. Limited long-term follow-up reports a 100% anti-HAV and a 95% anti-HBV response by 2 years after immunization. The combined vaccine appears to be safe, well tolerated, and highly immunogenic. The side-effect profile is reportedly similar to that of the individual vaccines.

26. Is immunoprophylaxis advisable for hepatitis C?

No firm recommendation can be made for postexposure prophylaxis for hepatitis C. Study results are equivocal. Some experts recommend administration of immunoglobulin (0.06 mg/kg) after a bona-fide percutaneous exposure. The immunoglobulin should be administered as soon as possible. However, work in chimpanzees has shown a lack of protectiveness when animals that received prophylaxis with immunoglobulin were challenged with HCV. Moreover, recent data show that in humans the neutralizing antibody evoked after infection with HCV is short-lived and does not protect against reinfection. Immunoprophylaxis for hepatitis C seems to be quite difficult. It is problematic to design a vaccine because of the multiple viral genotypes. Moreover, the hepatitis C genotypes do not afford cross-protection.

27. Is a vaccine available for hepatitis E?

Experimental hepatitis E vaccines consisting of recombinant HEV open reading frame 2 have been shown to be efficacious in preclinical trials in animal models and are undergoing phase II evaluation in humans.

28. Shjould patients with chronic liver disease be immunized against hepatitis A and hepatitis B?

Acute hepatitis A has resulted in higher moribidty and mortality rates in healthy people over the age of 40 years and in people with chronic hepatitis C. HAV vaccine is safe and effective in people with chronic liver disease and may prevent additional injury to an already compromised liver. Acute hepatitis B has not been shown to induce high mortality rates in people with chronic liver disease; however, preventing further hepatic injury seems logical and wise. Cost-effectiveness of these measures is still uncertain.

BIBLIOGRAPHY

 1. Bock HL, Kruppenbacher JP, Bienzle U, et al: Dose the concurrent administration of an inactivated hepatitis A vaccine influence the immune response to other travelers' vaccines? J Travel Med 7:74–78, 2000.
 2. Carman WF, Zanetti AR, Karayaiannis P, et al: Vaccine-induced escape mutants of hepatitis B virus. Lancet 336:325–329, 1990.
 3. Centers for Disease Control and Prevention: Hepatitis B virus: A comprehensive strategy for eliminating transmission in the United States through universal childhood vaccination. MMWR 40/RR-13:10, 1991.
 4. Centers for Disease Control and Prevention: Prevention of hepatitis A through active or passive immunization. MMWR 48/RR-12, 1999.
 5. Centers for Disease Control and Prevention:Update: Recommendations to prevent hepatitis B virus transmission—United States. MMWR 48:33–34, 1999.
 6. Chen HL, Chang MH, Ni YH, et al: Seroepidemiology of hepatitis B virus infection in children: Ten years of mass vaccination in Taiwan. JAMA 276:906–908, 1996.
 7. Fan PC, Chang MH, Lee PI, et al: Follow-up immunogenicity of an inactivated hepatitis A vaccine in healthy children: Results after 5 years. Vaccine 16:232–235, 1998.
 8. Hadler SC, Francis DP, Maynard J, et al: Long-term immunogenicity and efficacy of hepatitis B vaccine in homosexual men. N Engl J Med 315:209–214, 1986.
 9. Keefe EB, Iwarson S, McMahon BJ, et al: Safety and immunogenicity of hepatitis A vaccine in patients with chronic liver disease. Hepatology 27:881–886, 1998.
10. Lee PI, Chang LY, Lee CY, et al: Detection of hepatitis B surface gene mutation in carrier children with or without immunoprophylaxis at birth. J Infect Dis 176:427–430, 1997.
11. Parkman PD, Hopps HE, Meyer HM: Immunoprevention of infectious diseases. In Nohmias AJ, O'Reilly RJ (eds): Immunology. New York, Plenum, 1982, pp 561–583.
12. Plotkin S, Plotkin S: A short history of vaccine. In Plotkin S, Mortimer E (eds): Vaccines, 2nd ed. Philadelphia, W.B. Saunders, 1988, pp 1–7.
13. Ryan ET, Kain K: Health advice and immunization for travelers. N Engl J Med 342:1716–1725, 2000.
14. Thoelen S, Van Damme P, Leentvaar-Kuypers A, et al: The first combined vaccine against hepatitis A and B: An overview. Vaccine 17:1657–1662, 1999.
15. Wainwright RB, McMahon B, Bulkow L, et al: Duration of immunogenicity and efficacy of hepatitis B vaccine in a Yupik Eskimo population. JAMA 261:2362–2366, 1989.
16. Whittle HC, Inskip H, Hall AJ, et al: Vaccination against hepatitis B and protection against viral carriage in the Gambia. Lancet 337:747–750, 1991.

22. LIVER PROBLEMS IN PREGNANCY

Anca I. Pop, M.D., and Caroline A. Riely, M.D.

1. What are the structural and functional hepatic adaptations during pregnancy?

Liver size and histology do not change. Maternal blood volume and cardiac output increase significantly, without a corresponding increase in hepatic blood flow, with a net decrease in fractional blood flow to the liver. An enlarging uterus makes venous return via the inferior vena cava progressively more difficult toward term. Blood is shunted via the azygous system with possible development of esophageal varices.

2. Does liver function change during pregnancy?

Hepatic function remains normal during pregnancy, but the normal range of laboratory values changes because of hormonal changes and an increase in blood volume with subsequent hemodilution. Aspartate aminotransferase (AST), alanine aminotransferase (ALT), gamma-glutamyl transpeptidase (GGTP), bilirubin, and prothrombin remain within normal limits. Total alkaline phosphatase (AP) is elevated. The placenta is the major source of AP; levels return to normal within 20 days after delivery. Increased fibrinogen synthesis leads to a significant rise in serum levels, which is attributed to the action of estrogens, along with increases in other coagulation proteins (factors VII, VIII, IX, and X), a gradual increase in ceruloplasmin levels, and increased serum-binding proteins for thyroxine, vitamin D, folate, corticosteroids, and testosterone. Also attributed to estrogen effects are the significant increases in serum concentration of major lipid classes (triglycerides, low-density and very-low-density lipoproteins, and cholesterol), which may be twice the normal limit for nonpregnant women of the same age. Serum albumin decreases slightly, contributing to the ~ 20% decline in total serum protein concentration.

3. Is the serum ceruloplasmin level a good diagnostic marker in pregnant women at term who are suspected of having Wilson's disease?

No. Ceruloplasmin levels increase gradually during pregnancy, reaching the maximum at term. The patient's usual low level may be misleadingly normal (> 20 mg/dl during pregnancy).

4. Can we assume the presence of chronic liver disease in a pregnant patient with angiomas and palmar erythema on physical examination and small esophageal varices detected endoscopically?

No. Spider angiomas and palmar erythema are common and appear in about two-thirds of pregnant women without liver disease. Small esophageal varices are present in approximately 50% of healthy pregnant women without liver disease because of the increased flow in the azygous system.

5. What is the most common liver disorder unique to pregnancy?

Intrahepatic cholestasis of pregnancy.

6. What is the most common cause of jaundice in pregnancy?

Viral hepatitis.

7. What is the expected clinical and biochemical course after delivery for patients with intrahepatic cholestasis of pregnancy?

Pruritus should improve promptly after delivery (within 24 hours). Jaundice is rare and, if present, may persist for days. Biochemical abnormalities may persist for months.

8. What biochemical changes are noted in cholestasis of pregnancy?

Serum bile acids, often measured as cholyglycine, increase by 10–100-fold. Serum levels of AP rise by 7–10-fold, along with a modest rise in serum levels of 5'-nucleotidase (confirming the hepatic source of AP). AST, ALT, and direct bilirubin also rise. No evidence of hemolysis is found. GGTP is normal, as is prothrombin time (PT), unless cholestyramine treatment leads to malabsorption.

9. What is the major clinical manifestation of intrahepatic cholestasis of pregnancy?

Severe pruritus with onset in the second or, more commonly, third trimester (> 70% of cases).

10. What is a possible cause for abnormal bleeding in a postpartum woman previously diagnosed with intrahepatic cholestasis of pregnancy? What is the treatment?

Malabsorption of liposoluble vitamins, including vitamin K, especially in patients treated with cholestyramine for pruritus. The international normalized ratio (INR) corrects with parenteral administration of vitamin K.

11. What is the effect of intrahepatic cholestasis of pregnancy on the fetus?

Fetal distress requiring cesarean section develops in about 30–60% of cases. Prematurity occurs in about 50% of cases and fetal death in up to 9% of affected pregnancies. All of these effects are more likely if the disorder begins early in pregnancy.

12. What is the therapy for intrahepatic cholestasis of pregnancy?

Alleviating pruritus is the main goal. Therapeutic agents include:
• Ursodeoxycholic acid, 8–10 mg/kg/day
• Cholestyramine, 4 gm 4 or 5 times/day (bile acid-binding resin)
• Hydroxyzine hydrochloride (Atarax) or pamoate (Vistaril) (antihistamines)
• Phenobarbital ,100 mg/day (choleretic and centrally acting sedative)
• Phototherapy with ultraviolet B light

Vitamin K before delivery is highly recommended to minimize the risk of postpartum hemorrhage. Mother and fetus should be observed closely. Elective induction is recommended at 36–38 weeks if the fetal lungs have matured.

13. Can intrahepatic cholestasis of pregnancy recur?

Yes. About 40–70% of subsequent pregnancies show evidence of mild intrahepatic cholestasis. The same pattern can be seen with use of estrogen-containing contraceptives.

14. What atypical signs and symptoms make the diagnosis of intrahepatic cholestasis of pregnancy doubtful?

Fever, hepatosplenomegaly, pain, jaundice preceding or without pruritus, and pruritus after delivery or before 21 weeks of pregnancy, especially with a singleton pregnancy, should prompt the search for an alternate diagnosis.

15. What biochemical changes suggest an alternate diagnosis?

• Normal AST and ALT levels
• Elevated AP and GGTP
• Predominantly unconjugated hyperbilirubinemia.

16. What are the clinical and laboratory features of acute fatty liver of pregnancy?

Acute fatty liver of pregnancy (AFLP) is a rare disorder with an incidence of 1:13,000–1:16,000 pregnancies. Onset occurs in the second half of pregnancy, usually during the third trimester, although occasionally postpartum onset is reported. Clinical manifestations include nausea and vomiting, jaundice, malaise, thirst, and altered mental status. Severe cases progress rapidly to hypoglycemia, disseminated intravascular coagulation (DIC), renal insufficiency, coma, and death. Signs of coexistent preeclampsia may be present, such as moderately increased arterial blood pressure, proteinuria, and hyperuricemia. Laboratory abnormalities consist of moderate AST/ALT elevations (usually < 1000), conjugated hyperbilirubinemia, elevated PT, fibrin split products, and D-dimers, along with low platelet count, elevated levels of ammonia and serum uric acid, and leukocytosis. Hypoglycemia is a sign of extreme severity; blood glucose levels must be monitored closely.

17. Is biopsy pathognomonic for AFLP?

Biopsy is confirmatory, but not pathognomonic or indispensable in making the diagnosis. Histology is characterized by microvesicular fatty infiltration, mostly in centrilobular zones. In general, lobular and trabecular architecture is preserved, and inflammatory infiltrates and cell necrosis are mild, if present at all. AFLP is a systemic disorder. Similar fatty changes have been noted in pancreatic acinar cells and tubular epithelial cells of the kidneys. The same prominent microvesicular steatosis is seen in other conditions such as Reye's syndrome, sodium valproate toxicity, Jamaican vomiting sickness, and congenital defects of urea cycle enzymes or beta-oxidation of fatty acids.

18. How do we diagnose and treat AFLP?

High clinical suspicion is crucial for early recognition and appropriate management. AFLP is suggested by hepatic failure at or near term or shortly after delivery in the absence of risk factors or serology suggesting viral hepatitis. Thirst, a symptom of underlying vasopressin-resistant diabetes insipidus, is specific to AFLP or HELLP syndrome (see question 24). Biopsy, if feasible, is diagnostic in the appropriate clinical context. Treatment consists of admission to hospital, close monitoring by a multidisciplinary team (hepatologist, maternal-fetal medicine specialist, intensive care specialist) and immediate delivery. Recovery is usually complete, although it may be delayed in patients with significant clinical complications before delivery (e.g., DIC, renal failure, infections).

19. Describe the pathogenesis of AFLP.

AFLP is a fetal–maternal interaction. The fetus has an isolated deficiency of long chain 3-hydroxyacyl-CoA dehydrogenase (LCHAD), which leads to a disorder of mitochondrial fatty-acid oxidation. The inheritance pattern is recessive and involves a mutation from glutamic acid to glutamine at amino-acid residue 474 (Glu474Gln) on at least one allele. It is hypothesized that in the presence of this mutation in homozygous or compound heterozygote fetuses, long-chain fatty acid metabolites produced by the fetus or placenta accumulate in the mother and are highly toxic to the maternal liver. The mother is phenotypically normal; her genotype does not correlate with development of AFLP.

20. Does AFLP recur in subsequent pregnancies?

The disorder is recessive, affecting 1:4 fetuses. The rate of recurrence of maternal liver disease is 15–25%.

21. What is the outcome of a child whose mother has AFLP?

Previously reported fetal mortality rates of 75–90% have been significantly reduced by better awareness, earlier diagnosis, availability of neonatal intensive care units, and institution of close monitoring and dietary treatment through childhood. Children present at a mean age of 7.6 months (range = 0–60 months) with acute hepatic dysfunction (incidence of 79%). They may experience hypoketotic hypoglycemia, hypotonia, hepatomegaly, hepatic encephalopathy, high transaminases, and fatty liver. The condition may progress rapidly to coma and death. Frequent feedings of a low-fat diet in which the fats are medium-chain triglycerides prevent hypoketotic hypoglycemic liver dysfunction. According to recent studies, 67% of children treated with dietary modification are alive, and most attend school.

22. Is genetic testing indicated in women diagnosed with AFLP?

All women with AFLP, as well as their partners and children, should undergo molecular diagnostic testing. Testing for Glu474Gln only in the mother is not sufficient to rule out LCHAD deficiency in the fetus or other family members.

23. What is the spectrum of liver involvement in preeclampsia?

Liver involvement in preeclampsia ranges from subclinical, with biopsy evidence of fibrino-gen deposition along hepatic sinusoids, to several possibly severe disorders. In patients with HELLP syndrome (see question 24), the chief complaint is abdominal pain, which usually pre-sents in the second half of gestation but may occur up to 7 days after delivery (almost 30% of af-fected women). Hepatic infarction is another rare manifestation of liver involvement in preeclampsia. Patients present in the third trimester or early after delivery with unexplained fever, leukocytosis, abdominal or chest pain, and extremely elevated aminotransferases (> 3,000). The diagnosis depends on visualization of hepatic infarcts on computer tomographic (CT) contrast images or magnetic resonance imaging (MRI). Subcapsular hematomas and hepatic rupture are life-threatening complications with high morbidity and mortality rates. A high index of suspicion and early CT imaging allow diagnosis and prompt intervention.

24. How common is HELLP syndrome?

The incidence of HELLP syndrome (hemolysis, elevated liver enzymes, low platelets) is 0.2–0.6% in all pregnancies and 4–12% in preeclamptic patients. The incidence is higher in mul-tiparous, white, and older women (mean age = 25 years).

25. Describe the incidence and prognosis of spontaneous intrahepatic hemorrhage.

Spontaneous intrahepatic hermorrhage occurs in about 1–2% of patients with preeclampsia, with an estimated incidence of 1 in 45,000 live births. Prognosis improves with awareness, early diagnosis by imaging studies, and aggressive surgical management. Recent reported maternal mortality rates range from 33% to 49%. Fetal mortality remains high (~60%).

26. What findings typically lead to the diagnosis of HELLP syndrome?

Diagnosis relies on typical laboratory evidence of liver involvement with associated throm-bocytopenia. Not all patients have clinical hypertension or proteinuria at presentation. Liver test abnormalities are hepatocellular. Liver function is normal. Thrombocytopenia is present, usually < 100,000/mm^3. Hemolysis is mild, with microangiopathic findings on peripheral smear. Biopsy is characteristic but may be extremely risky and is not needed for diagnosis. It shows periportal hemorrhage, fibrin deposition, and necrosis, possibly with steatosis and/or deposition of fibrino-gen along sinusoids with focal parenchymal necrosis. A normal biopsy does not exclude the diag-nosis, because involvement may be patchy.

27. What is the treatment for severe preeclamptic liver disease?

The initial priority is to stabilize the mother, by administering intravenous fluids, correcting any concurrent coagulopathy, administering magnesium for seizure prophylaxis, and treating severe hypertension. Early hepatic imaging is indicated to rule out infarcts or hematomas. Fetal functional status should be determined. Fetal outcome is related mostly to gestational age. Beyond 34 weeks of gestation with evidence of fetal lung maturity, delivery is the recommended therapy. If fetal lungs are immature, the fetus can be delivered 48 hours after administration of two doses of steroids. Termination of pregnancy should be attempted immediately with evidence of fetal or maternal distress. In cases of ruptured subcapsular hematoma, massive transfusions and immediate surgical intervention are required.

28. Does HELLP recur in subsequent pregnancies?

Possibly. Studies report recurrence risks as low as 3.4 % and as high as 25%.

29. What information helps to differentiate AFLP from HELLP?

At presentation, AFLP and HELLP may be difficult to differentiate. Hypertension is usually but not invariably associated with HELLP syndrome. Patients with HELLP have mild, predomi-nantly unconjugated hyperbilirubinemia due to hemolysis, along with severe thrombocytopenia, but no laboratory values suggestive of hepatic failure. Laboratory abnormalities are significantly more severe in AFLP; evidence of hepatic synthetic failure manifests as prolonged PT and significant hypoglycemia in advanced stages. Fibrinogen is low, and ammonia is elevated. Biopsy shows microvesicular steatosis, predominantly in the central zone, in patients with AFLP, whereas patients with HELLP show predominantly periportal fibrin deposition, necrosis, and hemorrhage.

30. Can gestational age differentiate between different liver diseases in pregnancy?

Most definitely. Hyperemesis gravidarum presents in the first trimester of pregnancy. Patients have severe nausea and vomiting, and about one-half have associated elevations of bilirubin, AST, or ALT. Cholestasis of pregnancy, viral hepatitis, and abnormal liver chemistries due to cholelithiasis may present at any point in gestation, from the first to the third trimester. Acute fatty liver of pregnancy and preeclamptic liver disease (HELLP, hepatic infarct, and hepatic rupture) are specifically encountered in the third trimester of pregnancy. Herpes simplex virus or hepatitis E virus is exacerbated in pregnancy and presents usually with or without hepatic failure in the third trimester, close to term. Budd-Chiari syndrome presents from the second half of pregnancy to 3 months after delivery.

31. What signs and symptoms suggest the diagnosis of Budd-Chiari syndrome?

The clinical triad of sudden onset of abdominal pain, hepatomegaly, and ascites, near term or shortly after delivery. Ascitic fluid shows a high protein content in about one-half of cases. Biopsy typically shows centrilobular hemorrhage and necrosis, along with sinusoidal dilation and erythrocyte extravasation into the space of Disse. Hepatic scintigraphy and CT typically show compensatory hypertrophy of the caudate lobe due to its separate drainage into the inferior vena cava. Doppler analysis of portal and hepatic vessels and MRI establish hepatic vein occlusion.

32. How severe is the course of viral hepatitis acquired during pregnancy?

Hepatitis A, B, and C run a similar course in pregnant and nonpregnant patients. On the other hand, hepatitis E runs a different course in pregnancy. It is fulminant in up to 20% of patients, compared with less than 1% of nonpregnant women. The fatality rate is 1.5% during the first trimester, 8.5% during the second trimester, and up to 21% during the third trimester compared with 0.5–4% in nonpregnant women. Fetal complications and neonatal deaths are increased if infection is acquired in the third trimester of pregnancy. Herpes simplex hepatitis also can be fulminant in pregnancy and associated with high mortality rates. Patients present in the third trimester with fever, systemic symptoms, and possibly vesicular cutaneous rash. Associated pneumonitis or encephalitis may be present. Liver biopsy is characteristic, showing necrosis and inclusion bodies in viable hepatocytes, along with few or no inflammatory infiltrates. Response to acyclovir therapy is prompt; there is no need for immediate delivery of the baby.

33. Can we maintain a woman with Wilson's disease on therapy during pregnancy?

Absolutely. Therapy must continue during pregnancy; otherwise, the mother is at risk for hemolytic episodes associated with fulminant hepatic failure. Agents approved by the Food and Drug Administration are D-penicillamine, trientine, and zinc. Evidence indicates that penicillamine and trientine (tissue copper-chelating agents) are teratogenic in animal studies, and there are reports of penicillamine effects in humans, including cutis laxis syndrome or micrognathia, low-set ears, and other abnormalities. According to the current consensus, penicillamine and trientine are safe in doses of 0.75–1 gm/day during the first two trimesters; the dose should be reduced to 0.5 gm/day during the last trimester and in nursing mothers. Zinc therapy is an attractive alternative with a different mechanism of action; it induces synthesis of metallothionein, which sequesters copper in enterocytes, blocking its absorption. No teratogenic effects have been reported in animals or humans. The recommended doses are 50 mg 3 times/day for patients with 24-hour urinary copper values over 0.1 mg and 25 mg 3 times/day for patients with lower urinary copper values. Close monitoring of urinary copper and zinc levels is suggested; the zinc dose should be adjusted accordingly.

34. What methods of contraception are available for patients with liver disease?

Patients with advanced or untreated liver disease commonly experience amenorrhea and infertility. If clinical improvement leads to restoration of fertility, multiple methods of contraception are available, including barrier methods and intrauterine devices. Tubal ligation may be used in women who have completed their families. Estrogen-based contraceptive agents are generally contraindicated, especially for patients with acute liver disease, but progestin contraceptives are safe alternatives. Numerous formulations and delivery systems are available.

35. How should patients with preexistent liver disease be managed if pregnancy occurs?

Patients are best managed by a multidisciplinary team that includes a maternal-fetal medicine specialist, perinatologist, and hepatologist. They have an increased risk for maternal complications along with a higher incidence of fetal wastage and prematurity. In general, patients should be maintained on the previous therapy that was successful in controlling liver disease and restoring fertility. Women with autoimmune hepatitis should be continued on corticosteroids alone or in combination with azathioprine, which is not teratogenic at the usual dose. Patients with Wilson's disease should be continued on the anticopper agent. Patients with portal hypertension should have a baseline endoscopy. If they have never bled and medium or large varices are present, they are at increased risk for variceal hemorrhage during pregnancy. Primary prophylaxis with a nonselective beta blocker or isosorbide mononitrate should be instituted. The fetus should be monitored for bradycardia or growth retardation if the mother is maintained on beta blockers. Variceal bleeding is safely managed with variceal band ligation or sclerotherapy. Octreotide in customary doses is safe in pregnancy. Performing surgical portacaval shunts for patients with well-preserved liver function is possible. Placement of a transjugular intrahepatic portosystemic shunt and splenectomy (in patients with massive splenomegaly, varices, and thrombocytopenia) also have been reported.

36. What are the effects of pregnancy on the mother with portal hypertension?

The morbidity rate is 30–50% because of possible onset of hepatic encephalopathy, spontaneous bacterial peritonitis, and progressive liver failure. The indicence of variceal hemorrhage is 19–45%, especially in the second trimester and during labor. Postpartum hemorrhage is seen in 7–10% of women, most frequently in those with cirrhotic portal hypertension; thrombocytopenia plays a major role. The mortality rate of the above complications is 4–7% in noncirrhotic and 10–18% in cirrhotic patients with portal hypertension.

37. What is the effect of the maternal portal hypertension on pregnancy?

Spontaneous abortion rates for patients with cirrhosis range from 15–20%. Most cases occur in the first trimester. Of interest, patients with extrahepatic portal hypertension and patients with well-compensated cirrhosis who underwent surgical shunting before conception have abortion rates similar to the general population. The incidence of premature termination of pregnancy in the second and third trimesters is similar in all of the above groups. Fetal mortality rates are around 50% if the mother requires emergent surgical intervention for variceal hemorrhage. Perinatal mortality rates in cirrhotic mothers are as high as 11–18% becaues of premature delivery, stillbirth, and neonatal death, but they are similar to those for the general population in noncirrhotic patients with portal hypertension and patients who underwent previous portal surgical decompressive procedures.

38. When can a liver transplant recipient actively seek conception?

A 1-year waiting period is advisable. Case reports suggest that conception close to the transplant date may result in increased maternal and fetal morbidity and mortality.

39. Are immunosuppressive agents safe during pregnancy?

Corticosteroids, azathioprine, cyclosporine, tacrolimus, and OKT3 have no apparent teratogenic potential. All may contribute to low birth weights and fetal prematurity. Tacrolimus crosses the placenta and may contribute to transient perinatal hyperkalemia and mild, reversible renal impairment.

There are no reports of allograft loss as a result of pregnancy in the tacrolimus-treated group of 35 patients at the University of Pittsburgh. The Philadelphia-based cyclosporine registry reports an allograft rejection rate of 17% and a graft loss rate of 5.7% in 35 patients taking cyclosporine.

40. How may vertical transmission of viral hepatitis A be prevented?

Maternal infection with the hepatitis A virus (HAV) is not associated with fetal wastage or teratogenic effects. Vertical transmission of HAV is rare. Passive immunization with immuno-globulin and HAV vaccine is safe and recommended in pregnant women.

41. How may vertical transmission of viral hepatitis B be prevented?

The hepatitis B virus (HBV) may be transmitted vertically. If the mother acquires HBV in the first trimester of pregnancy, there is a 10% risk that the infant will test positive for hepatitis B surface antigen (HBsAg) at birth. The percentage dramatically increases to 80–90% if the acute maternal infection develops during the third trimester. In mothers who have chronic hepatitis B and test positive for the hepatitis B early antigen (HBeAg), 90% of neonates develop chronic hepatitis B without prophylaxis. If the mother has HBeAg- and HBeAb-negative chronic hepatitis B, 40% of neonates develop chronic hepatitis B infection without prophylaxis. The rate decreases to < 5% if the mother is HBeAg-negative and HBeAb-positive. Antepartum serum HBsAg testing is mandatory. Neonates of HBs Ag-positive mothers or HBsAg-unknown mothers are treated with HBV human hyperimmune globulin (HBIG), 0.5 ml intramuscularly, at delivery. At the same time they are given the first dose of HBV vaccine. The second dose is administered at 1 month of age and the third dose at 6 months of age. If the mother is HBsAg-negative, the child should be vaccinated only with the three-dose regimen, with the first inoculation at birth. The regimen is about 85% effective in preventing chronic hepatitis B in neonates and is ineffective in cases of hematogenous transplacental transmission, which are seen in about 15% of pregnancies as a result of small placental tears. Hepatitis B vaccination is safe in pregnant women.

42. What about vertical transmission of viral hepatitis C?

Vertical transmission of the hepatitis C virus (HCV) is possible when maternal serum levels of HCV RNA are high. Levels of RNA ≥ 1,000,000 copies/ml are reportedly associated with vertical transmission rates as high as 50%. High levels frequently are seen in patients coinfected with HIV. No prophylaxis is recommended. Immunoglobulin therapy is ineffective.

43. Is it possible to prevent vertical transmission of viral hepatitis D and G?

Perinatal transmission of the hepatitis D virus (HDV) is rare. There are no documented cases of vertical transmission of HDV in the United States. No clinical data about hepatitis G infection during pregnancy are available, and no studies of vertical transmission have been done.

44. Are HCV-infected women allowed to breastfeed?

HCV-infected women should be told that hepatitis C transmission via breast-feeding has not been documented. Current available studies show that the average rate of infection is 4%, similarly for breastfed and bottle-fed infants. According to the Centers for Disease Control and Prevention (CDC) and to a 1997 consensus statement from the National Institutes of Health, "breastfeeding is not contraindicated for HCV-positive mothers," and "the maternal to baby transmission of HCV infection through breast milk has not been documented."

45. Does the mode of delivery influence hepatitis C transmission?

Current data are limited but indicate that infection rates are similar in infants delivered vaginally and cesarean-delivered infants.

46. How can perinatal HCV infection be diagnosed?

Infants passively acquire maternal antibodies that can persist for months. Anti-HCV antibodies after 12 months of age or positive HCV-RNA, which can be detected as early as 1 or 2 months, is diagnostic of perinatal transmission of HCV. Recent CDC data probably will change the current guidelines and recommend testing only at 24 months of age.

BIBLIOGRAPHY

1. Barton JR, Sibai BM: HELLP and the liver diseases of preeclampsia. Clin Liver Dis 3:31–49, 1999.
2. Barton JR, Sibai BM: Care of the pregnancy complicated by HELLP syndrome. Gastroenterol Clin North Am 21:937–950, 1992.
3. Brewer GJ, Johnson VD, Dick RD, et al: Treatment of Wilson's disease with zinc. XVII: Treatment during pregnancy. Hepatology 31:364–370, 2000.
4. Centers for Disease Control and Prevention: Recommendations for prevention and control of hepatitis C virus (HCV) infection and HCV-related chronic disease. MMWR 47(RR-19), 1998.
5. Connoly TJ, Zuckerman AL: Contraception in the patient with liver disease. Semin Perinatol 22:178–182, 1998.
6. Everson GT: Liver problems in pregnancy: Distinguishing normal from abnormal hepatic changes. Medscape Women's Health 3(2):3, 1998.
7. Ibdah JA, Bennett MJ, Rinaldo P, et al: A fetal fatty-acid oxidation disorder as a cause of liver disease in pregnant women. N Engl J Med 340:1723–1731, 1999.
8. Jain A, Venkataramanan R, Fung JJ, et al: Pregnancy after liver transplantation under tacrolimus. Transplantation 64:559–565, 1997.
9. Knox TA: Evaluation of abnormal liver function in pregnancy. Semin Perinatol 22:98–103, 1998.
10. Kochhar R, Kumar S, Goel R, et al: Pregnancy and its outcome in patients with noncirrhotic portal hypertension. Digest Dis Sci 44:1356-1361, 1999.
11. Misra S, Sanyal AJ: Pregnancy in a patient with portal hypertension. Clin Liver Dis 3:147–163, 1999.
12. Molmenti EP, Jain AB, Marino N, et al: Liver transplantation and pregnancy. Clin Liver Dis 3:163–173, 1999.
13. Polywka S, Schroter M, et al: Low risk of vertical transmission of hepatitis C virus by breast milk. Clin Infect Dis 29:1327–1329, 1999.
14. Radomski JS, Ahlswede BA, Jarrell BE, et al: Outcomes of 500 pregnancies in 335 female kidney, liver and heart transplant recipients. Transplant Proc 27:1089, 1995.
15. Radomski JS, Moritz MJ, Munoz SJ, et al: National Transplantation Pregnancy Registry: Analysis of pregnancy outcomes in female liver transplant recipients. Liver Transplant Surg 1:281, 1995.
16. Reinus JF, Leikin EL: Viral hepatitis in pregnancy. Clin Liver Dis 3:115–131, 1999.
17. Reyes H: Acute fatty liver of pregnancy: A cryptic disease threatening mother and child. Clin Liver Dis 3:69–83, 1999.
18. Riely CA, Fallon HJ: Liver diseases. In Burrow GN, Duffy TP (eds): Medical Complications during Pregnancy, 5th ed. Philadelphia, W.B.Saunders, 1999, pp 269–294.
19. Riely CA: Liver diseases in pregnancy. In Reece EA, Hobbins JC (eds): Medicine of the Fetus and Mother, 2nd ed. Philadelphia, Lippincott-Raven, 1999, pp 1153–1163.
20. Rinaldo P, Raymond K, Al-Odaib A, Bennett MJ: Clinical and biochemical features of fatty acid oxidation disorders. Curr Opin Pediatr 10:615–621, 1998.
21. Rosa FW: Teratogen update: Penicillamine. Teratology 33:127–131, 1986.
22. Sheikh RA, Yasmeen S, Pauly MP, Riegler JL: Spontaneous intrahepatic hemorrhage and hepatic rupture in the HELLP syndrome. J Clin Gastroenterol 28:323–328, 1999.
23. Solomon L, Abrams G, Dinner M, Berman L: Neonatal abnormalities associated with D-penicillamine treatment during pregnancy. N Engl J Med 296:54–55, 1977.
24. Sternlieb I: Wilson's disease and pregnancy [editorial]. Hepatology 31:531–532, 2000.

23. RHEUMATOLOGIC MANIFESTATIONS OF HEPATOBILIARY DISEASES

Sterling G. West, M.D.

1. List the diseases of the liver that may present with rheumatic manifestations.
- Viral hepatitis
- Autoimmune chronic active hepatitis
- Primary biliary cirrhosis
- Hemochromatosis

2. Which viral hepatitis is most commonly associated with rheumatic manifestations?
Approximately 25% of patients with hepatitis B antigenemia develop a rheumatic syndrome. Up to 50% of patients with hepatitis C develop an autoimmune syndrome.

3. What are the most common extrahepatic rheumatologic manifestations of hepatitis B infection?
- Acute polyarthritis-dermatitis syndrome
- Polyarteritis nodosa (PAN)
- Membranous glomerulonephritis
- Cryoglobulinemia: usually associated with hepatitis C; only 5% of all essential mixed cryoglobulinemia is due to hepatitis B alone.

4. Describe the clinical characteristics of the polyarthritis-dermatitis syndrome associated with hepatitis B infection.
The polyarthritis is acute, severe, and symmetric, involving both small and large joints. A classically urticarial rash usually accompanies the arthritis. Both arthritis and rash precede the onset of jaundice and/or elevated liver-associated enzymes by several days. The arthritis improves with nonsteroidal anti-inflammatory drugs (NSAIDs) and resolves with onset of jaundice. This syndrome is due to deposition of circulating immune complexes.

5. What is the typical presentation of hepatitis B-associated PAN?
Approximately 25% of all patients with PAN have the hepatitis B antigen. They may present with a combination of fever, arthritis, mononeuritis multiplex, abdominal pain, renal disease, and/or cardiac disease. Although liver enzymes may be abnormal, symptomatic hepatitis is not a prominent feature.

6. How is PAN associated with hepatitis B antigenemia diagnosed?
The diagnosis is made on the basis of a consistent clinical presentation coupled with an abdominal or renal angiogram showing vascular aneurysms and corkscrewing of blood vessels. The gold standard is a tissue biopsy showing medium-vessel vasculitis. (See figure at top of next page.)

7. How is hepatitis B-associated PAN treated?
Patients typically are quite ill and will die without aggressive corticosteroid and cytotoxic drug therapy. Adjunctive antiviral and plasmapheresis therapy may be beneficial. The overall 5-year survival rate is 50–75%.

8. What are the most common hepatitis C virus (HCV)-related autoimmune disorders?
- Mixed cryoglobulinemia (10–60% of HCV-infected patients)
- Membranoproliferative glomerulonephritis

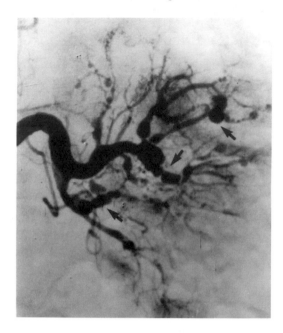

Renal angiogram showing vascular aneurysms in a patient with hepatitis B-associated
polyarteritis nodosa *(arrows)*.

- Nonerosive polyarthritis (5–10%): intermittent, mono- or oligoarthritis affecting large and medium-sized joints.
- Autoantibody production: rheumatoid factor, antinuclear antibodies (ANA), anticardiolipin antibodies, anti-smooth muscle antibodies, and antithyroid antibodies. Anti-LKM-1 may be seen in children with type II autoimmune hepatitis.
- Porphyria cutanea tarda: metabolic disorder due to reduced hepatic activity of uroporphyrinogen decarboxylase.

9. Describe the relationship between viral hepatitis and cryoglobulinemia.

Approximately 80–90% of patients with essential mixed cryoglobulinemia (type III more often than type II) are positive for HCV. HCV is concentrated up to 1000-fold in the cryoprecipitate. Infected patients are prone to develop autoimmune and lymphoproliferative diseases due to the predilection of HCV to infect B cells, resulting in recombination of the proto-oncogene *bcl-2*, which inhibits apoptosis and leads to extended lymphocyte survival. The result is increased autoantibody formation and/or neoplastic transformation (non-Hodgkin's B-cell lymphomas).

10. Describe the typical clinical features of cryoglobulinemia associated with HCV infection.

Patients present with a combination of fever, arthritis, renal disease, paresthesias, petechial rash predominantly on the lower extremities, positive rheumatoid factor, and low complement levels. Hepatitis is not a prominent feature. Patients have been treated successfully with combined corticosteroids, interferon alpha, and plasmapheresis.

11. What is lupoid hepatitis?

Patients with lupoid hepatitis, now called type I autoimmune hepatitis (AIH), are young (< 40 years) and predominantly female (70%). They have clinical (arthralgias) and laboratory manifestations that resemble systemic lupus erythematosus (SLE). Patients commonly have positive ANA, antibodies against smooth muscle antigen (F1 actin), and occasionally LE cells.

12. To what degree is lupoid hepatitis similar to SLE?

Comparison of Systemic Lupus Erythematosus and Lupoid Hepatitis

	SLE	LUPOID HEPATITIS
Young women	+	+
Polyarthritis	+	+
Fever	+	+
Rash	+	+
Nephritis	+	–
Central nervous system disease	+	–
Photosensitivity	+	–
Oral ulcers	+	–
Antinuclear antibody	99%	70–90%
Lupus erythematosus cells	70%	40–50%
Polyclonal gammopathy	+	+
Anti-Smith antibodies	25%	0
Positive anti-ds DNA	70%	Rare–40%
Positive anti-F1 actin	Rare	60–95%

SLE = systemic lupus erythematosus.

13. What is the difference between anti-Sm and anti-SM antibodies?
Anti-Sm antibodies are antibodies against the Smith antigen, which is an epitope on small nuclear ribonuclear proteins. It is highly diagnostic of SLE. Anti-SM antibody is an antibody against the smooth muscle antigen (F1 actin). It is highly diagnostic of autoimmune hepatitis.

Anti-Smith vs. Anti-Smooth Muscle Antibodies

	SLE	AUTOIMMUNE HEPATITIS
Anti-Smith (Sm) antibodies	Yes	No
Anti-smooth muscle (SM) antibodies	No	Yes

14. List the common autoimmune diseases associated with primary biliary cirrhosis (PBC).
Up to 80% of patients with PBC have one or more of the following disorders:
• Keratoconjunctivitis sicca (Sjögren's syndrome)   66%
• Autoimmune thyroiditis (Hashimoto's disease)   20%
• Scleroderma/Raynaud's disease   20%
• Rheumatoid arthritis   10%

15. Compare and contrast the arthritis that may occur with PBC and rheumatoid arthritis.

	PBC ARTHRITIS	RHEUMATOID ARTHRITIS
Frequency in patients with PBC	10%	10%
Number of joints	Polyarticular	Polyarticular
Symmetry	Symmetric	Symmetric
Inflammatory	Yes	Yes
Rheumatoid factor	Sometimes	Yes (85%)
Erosions on radiograph	Rare	Common

16. What other musculoskeletal manifestations may occur in patients with PBC?
- Osteomalacia due to fat-soluble vitamin D malabsorption
- Osteoporosis due to renal tubular acidosis
- Hypertrophic osteoarthropathy

17. What autoantibodies commonly occur in patients with PBC?
- Antimitochondrial antibodies   80%
- Anticentromere antibodies   20%*

* Most patients also have manifestations of the CREST variant of scleroderma. (CREST = **c**alcinosis, **R**aynaud's phenomenon, **e**sophageal disease, **s**clerodactyly, and **t**elangiectasia).

18. How commonly does arthritis occur in patients with hemochromatosis?
Approximately 40–75% of patients have a noninflammatory degenerative arthritis, most commonly involving the second and third metacarpophalangeal joints (MCPs), proximal interphalangeal joint, wrists, knees, and hips. Of importance, this arthropathy may be the presenting complaint of hemochromatosis and is frequently misdiagnosed as seronegative rheumatoid arthritis.

19. Describe the radiographic features suggestive of hemochromatotic arthropathy.
Suggestive radiographic features include subchondral sclerosis, cyst formation, irregular joint space narrowing, and osteophyte formation consistent with degenerative arthritis of involved joints. The key is finding degenerative changes in the MCP joints (typically second and thirrd) with hooklike osteophytes. This finding is important, because the MCPs and wrists rarely develop degenerative joint disease without an underlying cause such as hemochromatosis.

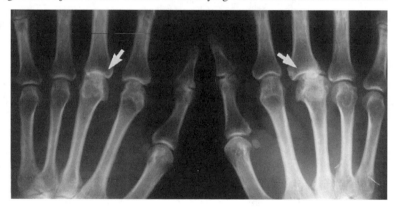

Radiograph of hands showing degenerative arthritis with hooklike osteophytes of the second and third metacarpophalangeal joints in a patient with hemochromatosis *(arrows)*.

20. Describe the relationship between calcium pyrophosphate disease and hemochromatosis.
Chondrocalcinosis of the triangular fibrocartilage at the ulnar side of the wrist and the hyaline cartilage of the knees is seen in 20–50% of patients with hemochromatosis. Crystals of calcium pyrophosphate may shed into the joints, causing superimposed flares of inflammatory arthritis (i.e., pseudogout).

21. Discuss the genetics of hemochromatosis.
Hemochromatosis is among the most common genetic disorders in Caucasians of European descent. Nearly 90% of patients with hereditary hemochromatosis are homozygous for the same mutation (C282Y) in the HFE gene. The homozygote frequency in the Caucasian population is 0.3–0.5%, and carrier frequency is 7–10%. The HFE gene is located on chromosome 6 near the locus of the major histocompatibility complex (MHC). It encodes for a MHC class-I like protein that complexes with the transferrin receptor, decreasing its affinity for transferrin, a key protein

involved in iron transplant. The mutation of HFE gene results in a protein that does not bind well to the transferrin receptor and thus results in increased iron uptake.

22. Compare and contrast the features of hemochromatotic arthropathy (HA) and rheumatoid arthritis (RA).

	HEMOCHROMATOTIC ARTHROPATHY	RHEUMATOID ARTHRITIS
Sex	M > F (10:1)	F > M (3:1)
Age of onset	> 35 yr	All ages
Joints	Polyarticular	Polyarticular
Symmetry	Symmetric	Symmetric
Inflammatory signs/symptoms	Only with pseudogout attack	Yes
Rheumatoid factor	Negative	Positive (85%)
Gene	HFE (90%)	HLA DR4 (70%)
Synovial fluid	Noninflammatory	Inflammatory
Radiographs	Degenerative changes	Inflammatory, erosive disease

23. Is phlebotomy effetive in halting the progression of HA?
Phlebotomy does not halt the progression of the arthropathy.

24. What is the correlation between the severity of arthropathy and severity of liver disease in hemochromatosis?
There is no correlation.

25. Why does hemochromatosis cause a degenerative arthritis?
The arthropathy is characterized by hemosiderin deposition in synovium and chondrocytes. The presence of iron in these cells may lead to increased production of destructive enzymes (e.g., collagenase) that cause cartilage damage. Other mechanisms also may be possible; the precise pathway by which chronic iron overload leads to tissue injury has not been fully established.

26. What other musculoskeletal problems may occur in patients with hemochromatosis?
- Osteoporosis due to gonadal dysfunction from pituitary insufficiency caused by the iron overload state.
- Osteomalacia due to vitamin D deficiency due to liver disease.
- Hypertrophic osteoarthropathy: cirrhosis of any cause including hemochromatosis can be associated with periosteal reaction involving shafts of long bones.

BIBLIOGRAPHY

1. Beutler E: Targeted disruption of the HFE gene. Proc Natl Acad Sci USA 95:2033–2034, 1998.
2. Bothwell TH, MacPhail AP: Hereditary hemochromatosis: Etiologic, pathologic, and clinical aspects. Semin Hematol 35:55–71, 1998.
3. Duffy J: Arthritis and liver disease. In Koopman W (ed): Arthritis and Allied Conditions, 13th ed. Philadelphia, Lea & Febiger, 1997, pp 1265–1278.
4. Ferri C, La Civita L, Longombardo G, et al: Mixed cryoglobulinemia: A cross-road between autoimmune and lymphoproliferative disorders. Lupus 7:275–279, 1998.
5. Fomberstein B, Yerra N, Pitchumoni CS: Rheumatological complications of GI disorders. Am J Gastroenterol 91:1090–1103, 1996.
6. Gumber SC, Chopra S: Hepatitis C: A mulifaceted disease: Review of extrahepatic manifestations. Ann Intern Med 123:615–620, 1995.
7. Hall S, Czaja AJ, Kaufman DK, et al: How lupoid is lupoid hepatitis? J Rheumatol 13:95–98, 1986.
8. Inman RD: Rheumatoid manifestations of hepatitis B infections. Semin Arthritis Rheum 11:406–420, 1982.
9. Lamprecht P, Gause A, Gross WL: Cryoglobulinemic vasculitis. Arthritis Rheum 42:2507–2516, 1999.
10. Marx WJ, O'Connell DJ: Arthritis of primary biliary cirrhosis. Arch Intern Med 139:213–216, 1979.
11. Rivera J, Garcia-Monforte A, Pineda A, Millan Nunez-Cortes J: Arthritis in patients with chronic hepatitis C virus infection. J Rheumatol 26:420–424, 1999.

24. EVALUATION OF FOCAL LIVER MASSES

Steven P. Lawrence, M.D.

1. Describe the initial work-up for a patient with a liver mass.

The first step is an accurate history and physical examination. Age, sex, and birthplace are important clues to etiology. Risk factors for viral hepatitis or a history of cirrhosis increases the possibility of a primary malignant process. A previously diagnosed neoplasm heightens suspicion for metastatic disease. Use of oral contraceptives or anabolic steroids, alcohol intake, and potential occupational exposure to carcinogens should be noted. Hepatomegaly and/or splenomegaly, abdominal pain, or stigmata of chronic liver disease, such as palmar erythema, spider angiomata, or gynecomastia, may be present.

Liver-associated enzymes, with the exception of gamma-glutamyl transpeptidase (GGT), are usually normal with benign liver tumors. Serum alkaline phosphatase levels are often elevated with hepatic metastases, but not in all cases. An increase in serum transaminases may signify chronic hepatitis or cirrhosis. Positive hepatitis B or C serologies or iron studies may identify an underlying cause of liver dysfunction or cirrhosis.

Differential Diagnosis of Focal Liver Masses in Adults

BENIGN	MALIGNANT
Epithelial tumors	
Hepatic adenoma	Hepatocellular carcinoma
Bile duct adenoma	Cholangiocarcinoma
Biliary cystadenoma	Biliary cystadenocarcinoma
	Squamous carcinoma
Mesenchymal tumors	
Cavernous hemangioma	Angiosarcoma
Fibroma	Epithelioid hemangioendothelioma
Leiomyoma	Fibrosarcoma
Lipoma	Leiomyosarcoma
	Liposarcoma
	Rhabdomyosarcoma
	Primary hepatic lymphoma
Other lesions	
Focal nodular hyperplasia	Metastatic tumors
Liver abscess	
Macroregenerative nodules in cirrhosis	
Focal fatty infiltration	
Focal sparing with diffuse fatty liver	
Simple hepatic cyst	
Microhamartoma (von Meyenbrug complex)	

Modified from Kew MC: Tumors of the liver. In Zakim D, Boyer TD (eds): Hepatology: A Textbook of Liver Disease, 2nd ed. Philadelphia, W.B. Saunders, 1990, pp 1206–1239.

2. What tumor markers are useful in the evaluation of focal liver lesions?

Serum alpha-fetoprotein (AFP) and tumor-associated antigen CA 19-9 are markers of primary hepatic malignancy and are used when radiographic studies indicate a focal neoplasm originating in the liver.

AFP is the best diagnostic marker for hepatocellular carcinoma (HCC) and also plays a role in screening programs of at-risk populations. AFP levels above 200 ng/ml are highly suggestive of HCC, whereas lesser elevations may be due to benign chronic hepatitis. A universally accepted cutoff value for AFP in the diagnosis of HCC has not been established, and some authorities use a level > 400 ng/ml. Not all hepatomas secrete AFP, and approximately one-third of patients have a normal AFP value, especially when the tumor is smaller than 2 cm. AFP levels should decrease or normalize with successful treatment.

CA 19-9 is used in the diagnosis of cholangiocarcinoma, a malignancy originating in the bile ducts. CA 19-9 levels > 100 U/ml are found in over 50% of patients and values > 1,000 suggest unresectability. This marker is more sensitive in patients with primary sclerosing cholangitis, a risk factor for cholangiocarcinoma. Significant false-positive elevations in CA 19-9 can occur with bacterial cholangitis. CA 19-9 also serves as a tumor marker for pancreatic carcinoma.

3. What imaging modalities are used in the detection and characterization of focal liver masses?

Recent advances in computed tomography (CT) and magnetic resonance imaging (MRI) allow detailed assessment of focal liver lesions. These imaging studies have largely supplanted previously used nuclear medicine-based protocols for the characterization of liver masses.

Helical (spiral) CT, which is now widely available, offers substantial improvement in hepatic imaging because of its rapid scan time within a single breath-hold. This feature eliminates respiratory motion and allows contrast injection to be viewed in both arterial (early) and portal or venous phases of perfusion. Lesions that derive their vascular supply from the hepatic artery, such as HCC and hypervascular metastases, are prominent during the arterial phase. The venous or portal phase of helical CT provides maximal enhancement of normal liver parenchyma and optimizes detection of hypovascular lesions.

MRI scanning has undergone similar refinements, with breath-hold T1-weighted images and fast (turbo) spin-echo T2-weighted sequences that eliminate motion artifacts and make use of contrast agents in a manner analogous to helical CT. Gadolinium-enhanced MRI should be considered in patients with contraindications to iodine-based CT, such as contrast allergies or renal insufficiency.

Many focal liver masses are found incidentally on **ultrasound** examination of the abdomen. Although liver ultrasound often cannot fully characterize the lesion, it has a role in verifying simple hepatic cysts, which may have nonspecific radiographic patterns on CT or MRI.

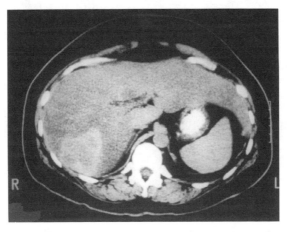

Unenhanced CT appearance of a cavernous hemangioma in the right lobe of the liver.

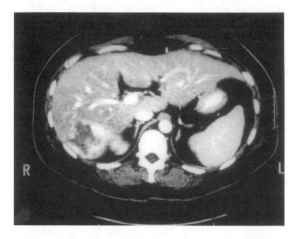

Enhanced CT appearance of a cavernous hemangioma in the right lobe of the liver.

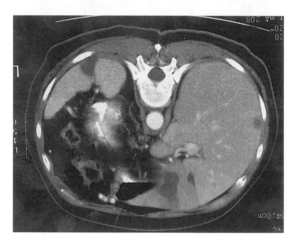

Contrast-enhanced helical CT scan showing multiple nodules in both liver lobes, consistent with hepatic metastasis.

4. What is the most common benign cause of a focal liver lesion?

Cavernous hemangiomas are the most common benign hepatic tumor, occurring in up to 20% of the population. They occur in all age groups, more commonly in women, as solitary (60%) or multiple asymptomatic masses. Most are < 3 cm and usually occur in the posterior segment of the right hepatic lobe. The term *giant hemangioma* is sometimes used when the size exceeds 6 cm. Microscopically, hemangiomas consist of blood-filled vascular sinusoids separated by connective-tissue septae. Occasionally, hemangiomas are large enough to cause abdominal pain, but the risk of tumor growth or bleeding is minimal and does not justify surgical removal unless the patient is significantly symptomatic.

5. Why is oral contraceptive use important in the differential diagnosis of focal liver masses?

Most cases of hepatic adenomas directly relate to the use of oral contraceptive pills (OCPs). This benign tumor was rarely seen before oral contraceptive agents came into common usage in the 1960s. Risk correlates with duration of use and age > 30 years. Hepatic adenomas most commonly occur in young and middle-aged women, with an incidence of 3–4 per 100,000. Men infrequently develop adenomas, although cases have been reported with anabolic steroid use.

Hepatic adenomas are well-demarcated, fleshy tumors with prominent surface vasculature. Microscopically, they consist of monotonous sheets of normal or small hepatocytes with no bile ducts, portal tracts, or central veins.

6. Why is surgical resection of hepatic adenomas recommended?

Spontaneous rupture and intraabdominal hemorrhage can occur in up to 30% of patients with hepatic adenoma, especially during menstruation or pregnancy. HCC also can develop within adenomas. Approximately 25% of patients with these tumors have abdominal pain, usually a result of bleeding within the adenoma. Adenomas have been known to regress with discontinuation of birth control pills, which should be recommended, but surgical resection remains the management of choice.

7. What is focal nodular hyperplasia?

Focal nodular hyperplasia (FNH) is a round, nonencapsulated mass, usually exhibiting a vascular central scar. Fibrous septae radiate from the scar in a spokelike fashion. Hepatocytes are arranged in nodules or cords between the septae, and the mass includes bile ductules, Kupffer cells, and chronic inflammatory cells. FNH is theorized to result from a hyperplastic tissue response to a congenital arterial malformation.

FNH is the second most common benign liver tumor. Over 90% occur in women and usually are diagnosed between 20 and 60 years of age. Oral contraceptives are not considered a causative agent of FNH but occasionally may enhance their growth.

8. List the differences between hepatic adenomas and FNH.

	HEPATIC ADENOMA	FOCAL NODULAR HYPERPLASIA
Size (mean)	10 cm	8 cm
Kupffer cells	No	Yes
Central scar	Rare	Common
Symptoms	Common	Rare (only with large lesions)
Complications	Bleeding, malignancy	Rare lesions may grow in size
Treatment	Surgical resection	Resection not necessary
Sulfur-colloid liver scan	Cold defect	Positive uptake in 60–70%

9. What is the most frequent malignancy in the liver?

Metastatic disease to the liver is much more common than primary hepatic tumors in the United States and Europe. Cancers arising in the colon, stomach, pancreas, breast, and lung are the most likely to metastasize to the liver. Esophageal, renal, and genitourinary neoplasms also should be considered when searching for the primary site. Multiple defects in the liver suggest a metastatic process: only 2% present as solitary lesions. Involvement of both lobes is most common; 20% are confined to the right lobe alone and 3% to the left lobe.

10. What is the most common primary liver cancer?

Hepatocellular carcinoma (HCC) is by far the most common malignancy originating in the liver, accounting for approximately 80% of primary liver cancers. The incidence in the United States ranges from 2–3 cases per 100,000. Geographic location influences both the age of peak occurrence (> 55 years in the U.S.) and male-to-female incidence ratios. High-incidence areas in Asia and Africa, related to hepatitis B, have a much younger average age of onset and a higher male predominance. Worldwide, men are more likely than women to develop HCC by a factor of 4:1. HCC usually occurs within a cirrhotic liver; approximately 80% of patients diagnosed with HCC have cirrhosis.

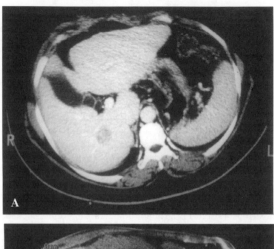

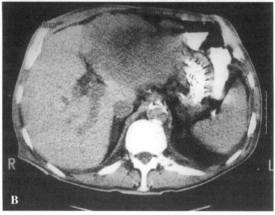

Variable CT presentations of hepatocellular carcinoma. *A* (with contrast) shows a single nodular hypodense area with some peripheral enhancement in the right lobe. *B* (noncontrast) demonstrates the massive type with replacement of the left lobe.

11. Describe the various presenting forms of HCC.

Nodular: most common; multiple nodules of varying size scattered throughout the liver.

Solitary (or massive): occurs in younger patients; large, solitary mass, often in the right lobe.

Diffuse: rare; difficult to detect on imaging; widespread infiltration of minute tumor foci.

12. What types of cirrhosis most commonly are associated with HCC?

Autopsy studies indicate that 20–40% of patients dying with cirrhosis harbor HCC. The etiologies of cirrhosis most commonly related to HCC, in order of decreasing risk, are as follows:

1. Chronic hepatitis C
2. Chronic hepatitis B
3. Hemochromatosis
4. Alpha-1-antitrypsin deficiency
5. Alcoholic cirrhosis (alcohol potentiates the carcinogenic risk in viral cirrhosis)

13. What clinical and laboratory findings should raise suspicion for HCC?

1. New abdominal pain or weight loss
2. Hepatomegaly
3. Hepatic bruit

4. Acute hemoperitoneum
5. Blood-tinged ascitic fluid
6. Persistent fever
7. Sudden increase in serum alkaline phosphatase
8. Increasing ratio of aspartate aminotransferase to alanine aminotransferase
9. Polycythemia or persistent leukocytosis
10. Hypoglycemia
11. Hypercalcemia
12. Hypercholesterolemia

Findings 9–12 are paraneoplastic syndromes associated with HCC.

14. What primary liver tumor occurs in young adults without underlying cirrhosis?

The fibrolamellar variant of HCC is a distinctive, slow-growing subtype of hepatic neoplasm, occurring at a mean age of 26. Patients seldom have a history of prior liver disease. Unlike typical HCC, men and women are equally affected. Fibrolamellar tumors usually present with abdominal pain, due to a large, solitary mass, most often in the left lobe (75%). The AFP level is normal.

The term *fibrolamellar* characterizes the microscopic appearance of this lesion; thin layers of fibrosis separate the neoplastic hepatocytes. A **fibrous central scar** may be seen on imaging studies. Recognition of this variant is important because nearly one-half are resectable at the time of diagnosis.

15. What factors predispose to the development of cholangiocarcinoma?

Cholangiocarcinomas, which account for about 10% of primary liver cancers, arise as adenocarcinomas from bile duct epithelium. Jaundice is the most frequent clinical presentation of this tumor. Risk factors for cholangiocarcinoma include:

• Primary sclerosing cholangitis   • Liver fluke infestation
• Chronic ulcerative colitis   • Congenital cystic liver diseases, choledochal cysts

16. What is a Klatskin tumor?

Cholangiocarcinomas at the hilar bifurcation of the hepatic ducts are referred to as Klatskin tumors. Peripheral (or intrahepatic) and extrahepatic bile duct cholangiocarcinomas are other subtypes. The characteristic desmoplastic reaction accompanying these tumors often makes them poorly visible on imaging studies and difficult to diagnose on biopsy. Delayed tumor enhancement on CT after IV contrast is noted in approximately 75% of intrahepatic cholangiocarcinomas. Only about 25% of cholangiocarcinomas occur in the setting of cirrhosis. Most are unresectable when diagnosed and thus require palliative drainage of obstructive jaundice by endoscopic, percutaneous, or surgical methods.

17. How do primary and metastatic hepatic lymphomas differ?

Primary hepatic lymphomas are much less common than secondary liver involvement from Hodgkin's and non-Hodgkin's lymphomas. Primary lymphoma typically presents as a large, solitary mass, whereas secondary spread is characterized by multiple nodules or hepatomegaly. In one-third of secondary hepatic lymphomas the disease is so diffusely infiltrative that imaging studies appear normal. Organ transplantation and AIDS increase the risk of primary lymphoma formation.

18. When should liver transplantation be considered in patients with HCC?

(1) Solitary lesion < 5 cm *or* (2) < 3 nodules, each < 3 cm *and* (3) no metastatic or regional lymph node involvement

19. When should resection be considered in patients with HCC?

HCC is resectable in only ~10% of patients in the United States. Five-year survival rates with surgical treatment range between 17% and 40%. Most patients succumb to intrahepatic recurrence of tumor. The multifocal nature of HCC carcinogenesis explains this poor prognosis. Selection criteria for resectability of HCC include:

• Child-Pugh class A cirrhosis
• Solitary lesion < 5 cm

• Hepatic wedge pressure gradient < 10 mm Hg
• Lack of vascular invasion or extrahepatic spread

20. What palliative therapies are available for the management of HCC?

Percutaneous ethanol (or acetic acid) injection and transcatheter arterial chemoembolization are commonly used for the local control of HCC. Radiofrequency thermal ablation is a newer therapy under study for inoperable HCC. Percutaneous injection and chemoembolization also are used to delay tumor progression in patients awaiting liver transplantation.

Chemoembolization involves the selective administration of chemotherapy, followed by embolization, into the hepatic artery branch feeding the tumor. Although this treatment slows tumor growth, it may not improve survival. Combining injection or ablation therapy with chemoembolization in patients with unresectable HCC may prove to be the most beneficial approach.

21. Who should be screened for HCC? Describe a typical screening strategy.

Patients with cirrhosis, especially those at high risk of HCC, should be screened. Screening is done routinely in people with viral-induced cirrhosis (hepatitis B and C) and cirrhosis-related to metabolic liver disease.

Serial AFP measurements and hepatic ultrasound studies are the most commonly used screening tools. Optimal screening intervals are not established, but AFP levels every 3–4 months and ultrasound every 6 months are common practice. Although surveillance may not have a definite impact on mortality rate, it allows more tumors to be amenable to curative resection.

22. What benign tissue abnormality may simulate a focal liver mass?

Focal fatty infiltration may appear similar to the focal hepatic lesions described above. Focal fatty liver is often seen in alcoholism, obesity, diabetes mellitus, malnutrition, corticosteroid excess or therapy, and AIDS. MRI imaging may be necessary to fully characterize this entity. An interesting aspect of focal fat is its rapid disappearance once the inciting disease process is corrected.

23. What new imaging techniques are under development to evaluate focal liver masses?

MRI imaging with recently developed contrast agents termed ferumoxides are used with increasing frequency in place of angiographically assisted CT scanning. Ferumoxides are dextran-coated iron oxide particles given by intravenous infusion and taken up by Kupffer cells in normal liver as well as lesions such as FNH and focal fat. They provide a dark background (negative contrast) on T2-weighted MRI imaging and improve lesion detection by enhancing contrast differences between normal liver and hepatic masses. Clinical trials suggest that ferumoxide-enhanced MRI can identify 20–40% more lesions than conventional MRI and CT. Ferumoxides are particularly useful in the detection of metastatic disease and HCC, although cirrhosis may sometimes reduce their efficacy.

Lipiodol CT is sometimes used in the detection of HCC. Lipiodol CT involves the injection of an iodized oil contrast medium into the hepatic artery; CT scanning is carried out several days later. Because hepatomas cannot clear the contrast, the resolution of very small lesions is greater.

24. Why is fine-needle biopsy of hepatic masses controversial?

Establishing a diagnosis for a focal liver mass by fine-needle aspiration (FNA) cytology is more problematic than one would think, owing to subtle histopathologic differences between normal hepatocytes and benign lesions or even well-differentiated hepatomas. The literature reveals a wide range of sensitivity for FNA-based diagnosis of primary hepatic lesions. The most optimistic studies report sensitivities and specificities > 95%. Hemangiomas, FNH, and HCC appear to be more difficult to diagnose accurately by FNA; sensitivity ranges between 60% and 70% in many series. Rigorous protocols making use of two or more imaging studies to characterize a benign lesion can have an accuracy and sensitivity as high as 80–90%. When HCC is suspected, the use of MRI, lipiodol CT, and angiography (in selected cases) can confirm the diagnosis in > 95% of patients without the use of FNA.

Another controversy about the use of FNA in HCC is the risk of needle-tract seeding and tumor spread into the circulation, a risk that may be as high as 5%. With the increasing use of liver transplantation in the treatment of HCC, this complication can have grave consequences.

FNA plays a dominant role in the setting of suspected metastatic disease to the liver and inoperable primary cancers. When surgical resection of a lesion, based on clinical and imaging findings, is deemed necessary, preoperative biopsy is generally not advocated.

25. Outline a logical approach to the evaluation of a focal hepatic mass.

The work-up of a focal liver mass must occur in the context of a carefully considered differential diagnosis. Associated symptoms, presence of underlying liver disease or extrahepatic malignancy, drug and occupational exposures, and laboratory abnormalities must be assessed before proceeding with further radiographic studies. Symptomatic lesions and lesions noted incidentally are likely to have different etiologies. The patient's age and sex are important clues. Cirrhosis requires a modified approach because of the increased likelihood of HCC.

Incidental lesions
Simple cysts → verify with ultrasound

Hemangiomas → helical CT with contrast → gadolinium-enhanced MRI

FNH → helical CT with contrast → ferumoxide-enhanced MRI

Hepatic adenoma → history of OCPs → rule out hemangioma and FNH → ? biopsy → resection (outlined above)

Symptomatic lesions
Hepatic adenoma → history of OCPs → rule out hemangioma/FNH → resection

Liver abscess → sepsis → ultrasound → helical CT with contrast (rim enhancement)

Cirrhosis or risk factors for cholangiocarcinoma
HCC → AFP → helical CT or MRI with contrast → lipiodol CT

Cholangiocarcinoma → CA 19-9 → delayed-phase helical CT with contrast

History of malignancy
Metastases → helical CT with contrast → if resection is considered → ferumoxide-enhanced MRI (to rule out multiple metastasis)

BIBLIOGRAPHY

1. Bennett WF, Bova JG: Review of hepatic imaging and a problem-oriented approach to liver masses. Hepatology 12:761–775, 1990.
2. Craig JR, Peters RL, Edmondson HA, Omata M: Fibrolamellar carcinoma of the liver: A tumor of adolescents and young adults with distinctive clinico-pathologic features. Cancer 46:372–379, 1980.
3. de Groen PC, Gores GJ, LaRusso NF, et al: Biliary tract cancers. N Engl J Med 341:1368–1378, 1999.
4. Fernandez MP, Redvanly RD: Primary hepatic malignant neoplasms. Radiol Clin North Am 36:333–348, 1998.
5. Kerlin P, Davis GL, McGill DB, et al: Hepatic adenoma and focal nodular hyperplasia: Clinical, pathologic, and radiologic features. Gastroenterology 84:994–1002, 1983.
6. Kew MC: Tumors of the liver. In Zakim D, Boyer TD (eds): Hepatology: A Textbook of Liver Disease, 2nd ed. Philadelphia, W.B. Saunders, 1990, pp 1206–1239.
7. Mergo PJ, Ros PR: Benign lesions of the liver. Radiol Clin North Am 36:319–331, 1998.
8. Mor E, Kaspa RT, Sheiner P, Schwartz M: Treatment of hepatocellular carcinoma associated with cirrhosis in the era of liver transplantation. Ann Intern Med 129:643–653, 1998.
9. Patel AH, Harnois DM, Klee GG, et al: The utility of CA 19-9 in the diagnosis of cholangiocarcinoma in patients without primary sclerosing cholangitis. Am J Gastroenterol 95:204–207, 2000.
10. Peng YC, Chan CS, Chen GH: The effectiveness of serum a-fetoprotein level in anti-HCV positive patients for screening hepatocellular carcinoma. Hepato-Gastroenterol 46:3208–3211, 1999.
11. Reddy KR, Schiff ER: Approach to a liver mass. Semin Liver Dis 13:423–435, 1993.
12. Ros PR, Davis GL: The incidental focal liver lesion: Photon, proton, or needle? Hepatology 27:1183–1190, 1998.
13. Souto E, Gores GJ: When should a liver mass suspected of being a hepatocellular carcinoma be biopsied? Liver Transpl 6:73–75, 2000.
14. Takamori R, Wong LL, Dang C, Wong L: Needle-tract implantation from hepatocellular cancer: Is needle biopsy of the liver always necessary? Liver Transpl 6:67–72, 2000.
15. Torzilli G, Minagawa M, Takayama T, et al: Accurate preoperative evaluation of liver mass lesions without fine-needle biopsy. Hepatology 30:889–893, 1999.
16. Weimann A, Ringe B, Klempnauer J, et al: Benign liver tumors: Differential diagnosis and indications for surgery. World J Surg 21:983–991, 1997.

25. DRUG-INDUCED LIVER DISEASE

Peter R. McNally, D.O.

1. How common is drug-induced liver disease?

More than 600 medicines have been reported to cause liver injury. Drug-induced liver disease accounts for 2–5% of hospital admissions for jaundice in the United States and 10–20% of cases of fulminant liver failure.

2. How are the three patterns of drug-induced liver injury distinguished?

Hepatocellular, cholestatic, and mixed injury patterns typically are distinguished by alanine aminotransferase (ALT) and alkaline phosphatase (AP) values and ratios.

Patterns of Drug-Induced Liver Disease

	ALT	AP	ALT:AP RATIO
Hepatocellular injury	≥ 2-fold increase	Normal	High (≥ 5)
Cholestatic injury	Normal	≥ 2-fold increase	Low (≤ 2)
Mixed injury	≥ 2-fold increase	≥ 2-fold increase	2–5

3. Describe the typical chronologic association between drug exposure and onset of hepatitis or cholestasis.

Cholestatic or hepatocellular liver injury typically occurs 5–90 days after initial exposure. On withdrawal of the drug, biochemical improvement in hepatocellular injury usually is seen within 2 weeks, whereas cholestatic or mixed injury may not improve for 4 weeks. Persistence of abnormal liver biochemistries beyond these intervals suggests a coexistent or independent cause of liver disease (e.g., viral or autoimmune liver disease, primary biliary cirrhosis, primary sclerosing cholangitis).

4. What is the differential diagnosis of drug-induced liver disease?

Diagnosis of a drug-induced cause of liver injury requires exclusion of viral, toxic, cardiovascular, inheritable, and malignant causes. Careful history, review of past laboratory testing, and physical examination are often helpful. When drug-induced liver injury is suspected, withdrawal of the offending agent and close observation often provide adequate circumstantial evidence for the diagnosis. Liver biopsy should be reserved for situations in which discontinuation of the medication is not followed by prompt improvement, the cause of liver disease remains in question, or the severity necessitates intervention (organ transplantation, corticosteroids).

5. Explain the two most common mechanisms of drug-induced liver injury.

1. **Intrinsic** (hepatotoxin with direct or indirect toxicity to hepatocytes). Examples include phosphorus, carbon tetrachloride, acetaminophen, and chloroform. Intrinsic hepatotoxins cause direct damage to the liver by covalently binding to cellular macromolecules, such as hydrogen peroxide, hydroxyl radicals, or lipid peroxides. These, in turn, interrupt cell membranes or inactivate critical cellular enzyme systems.

2. **Idiosyncratic** hyperimmune reaction. Examples include phenytoin, isoniazid, ticrynafen, halothane, and valproic acid. Idiosyncratic hepatotoxins are dose-independent, and hepatic injury cannot be reproduced in animal models. Clinical features of hypersensitivity (rash, fever, and eosinophilia) are common.

6. What variables appear to influence susceptibility to drug-induced hepatic injury?

Age. Young people are more susceptible to aspirin and valproic acid. Old people are more susceptible to isoniazid, halothane, and acetaminophen.

Sex. Women are more susceptible to all drug-induced liver disease, probably because of lower body mass and susceptibility to autoimmune hepatitis (e.g., alcohol, methyldopa, nitrofurantoin).

Route of administration. Tetracycline toxicity occurs primarily with the parenteral route.

Drug–drug interactions. Valproic acid increases chlorpromazine-induced cholestasis. Rifampin potentiates isoniazid hepatotoxicity. Chronic alcohol ingestion potentiates acetaminophen and isoniazid hepatotoxicity.

Malnutrition. Low glutathione level potentiates acetaminophen hepatotoxicity.

7. Name the two most common causes of drug-induced liver disease.
Alcohol and acetaminophen.

8. How is acetaminophen toxic to the liver?
Acetaminophen is toxic to the liver only in excessive doses or when the protective-detoxifying pathway in the liver is overwhelmed. Accumulation of the toxic metabolite, N-acetyl-p-benzoquinone, is responsible for the death of hepatocytes. Acetaminophen is the second most common cause of death from poisoning in the United States.

9. At what dose is acetaminophen toxic?
Acetaminophen is hepatotoxic in nonalcoholic patients at doses > 7.5 gm. A potentially lethal effect is seen with ingestion of > 140 mg/kg (10 gm in a 70-kg man). Chronic alcoholics are at greater risk of acetaminophen injury because of alcohol induction of the cytochrome P450 system and attendant malnutrition with low levels of glutathione, an intracellular protectant naturally found in hepatocytes.

10. How is acetaminophen toxicity treated?
The Rumack-Matthew nomogram helps to predict the likelihood of liver injury from acetaminophen and to direct therapy. The antidote for acetaminophen overdose is N-acetylcysteine (NAC). The oral dose of NAC is 140 mg/kg, followed by 17 maintenance doses of 70 mg/kg every 4 hours. NAC can be administered intravenously for 48 hours with equal or better efficacy than the oral route. Ipecac is given if the time of ingestion can be verified to be < 4 hours. Use of activated charcoal is controversial, because it can interfere with the adsorption of oral NAC.

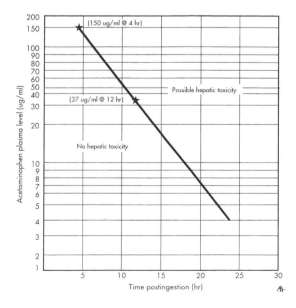

Rumack-Matthew nomogram.

11. What are the clinical findings of chlorzoxazone hepatotoxicity?

Chlorzoxazone (Parafon Forte) is a centrally acting muscle relaxant. Hepatotoxic effects are rare, but severe hepatitis, including fulminant hepatic failure, has been reported. Onset of injury may occur within 1 week of initiation or up to several years later. The transaminase elevation may exceed 1,000 IU/L. Most patients also exhibit hyperbilirubinemia. Discontinuation of the medication is usually the only intervention necessary.

12. What commonly used "recreational" drugs are associated with hepatotoxicity?

Cocaine. An estimated 30 million Americans have experimented with cocaine, and 5 million abuse it habitually. Patients with cocaine hepatotoxicity may present with jaundice or fatigue and generalized malaise. The aminotransferase elevations can be in the 5,000-IU/L range. Cocaine toxicity also may cause coagulopathy, rhabdomyolysis, and disseminated intravascular coagulation (DIC). The mechanism of hepatotoxicity is unknown. Liver biopsy typically shows zone III injury, suggesting related ischemia. In this setting, liver injury may be multifactorial and include coexistent viral liver disease (hepatitis B, C, and delta) and acetaminophen or alcohol use.

Ecstasy. This synthetic amphetamine (3,4-methylene dioxymethamphetamine) is commonly used as a "weekend" drug. It makes users euphoric and more sociable and eliminates fatigue. Initially thought to have little toxicity, Ecstasy has been reported to cause various systemic effects, including cardiac arrythmias, DIC, acute renal failure, hyperthermia and fulminant hepatitis. Physicians should suspect Ecstasy use in a young adult with acute hepatitis but no identifiable cause.

13. What anesthetic agents are associated with hepatocellular injury?

Halothane, enflurane, methoxyflurane, and isoflurane. Whenever hepatitis occurs postoperatively, nonanesthetic causes must be considered (e.g., viral hepatitis, drug-induced hepatitis, bile duct injury, cholestasis of total parenteral nutrition or sepsis, transfusion hepatitis, ischemic hepatopathy).

14. How common is halothane hepatitis? Describe the clinical signs and prognosis.

The risk for halothane hepatitis is 1/10,000 patients but increases to 7/10,000 after two or more exposures. Over 75% of patients with halothane liver injury present within 2 weeks of exposure with fever, nausea, rash, arthralgias, and diffuse abdominal discomfort. Laboratory abnormalities include eosinophilia, AST and ALT elevations in the range of 500–1,000-IU/L, and AP elevation (usually < 2 times normal). The mechanism appears to be related to development of sensitization to both the oxidative metabolite of halothane, trifluoroacetyl halide, and autoantigens (including CYP2D6). Prognostic factors for poor outcome include short latent period from exposure to jaundice, obesity, age > 40 years, hepatic encephalopathy, and prolongation of the prothrombin time. Corticosteroids and exchange transfusions are not helpful, and the mortality rate of fulminant halothane hepatitis is nearly 80% without liver transplantation.

15. Who is at risk for liver toxicity from isoniazid (INH) therapy?

INH hepatitis may present insidiously from 4–6 months after initiation of therapy. Some patients experience influenza-like symptoms. Abnormal AST and ALT elevations develop in up to 20% of patients taking INH, but aminotransferase activity usually subsides to normal spontaneously. The risk for frank hepatitis is 0.3% at ages 20–34 years, 1.2% at ages 35–49, and 2.3% at ages > 50. Coadministration of rifampin increases the likelihood of INH toxicity. Acetaminophen toxicity is increased by INH because it induces the cytochrome P450 enzyme system.

16. How is INH toxicity prevented?

Current recommendations include screening patients for ethanol abuse and preexisting liver or renal disease. The presence of chronic liver disease is not an absolute contraindication to the use of INH, but the indications should be scrutinized and therapy monitored more closely. The American Thoracic Society recommends dispensing only one month's supply of INH to ensure close monitoring. Patients should be advised to report prodromal symptoms immediately. All patients older than 35 years should have serial monitoring of ALT, and the use of INH should be reconsidered when ALT elevations persist or remain > 100 IU/L.

17. **Describe the clinical features of phenytoin hepatotoxicity.**
Phenytoin causes allergic hepatitis, cholestasis, granulomatous liver disease, and even frank fulminant hepatic failure. Symptoms of hepatotoxicity usually occur within the first 8 weeks of administration. The incriminated metabolite is arene oxide. Systemic symptoms include pharyngitis, lymphadenopathy, and atypical lymphocytosis (so-called pseudolymphoma syndrome). There are some favorable reports of treating acute phenytoin hepatitis with corticosteroids.

18. **What drugs have been reported to cause chronic hepatitis and cirrhosis?**
Isoniazid, methotrexate, methyldopa, nitrofurantoin, oxyphenisatin, perhexiline maleate, and trazodone.

19. **What are the clinical features of methyldopa (Aldomet) hepatocellular injury?**
Liver injury usually occurs within 6–12 weeks of initiation of methyldopa therapy. Aminotransferase values should be obtained periodically during the first 4 months of drug administration. Women appear to be more susceptible to methyldopa hepatotoxicity, and the clinical presentation may mimic autoimmune "lupoid" hepatitis.

20. **Describe the clinical features of nitrofurantoin hepatocellular injury.**
A cholestatic pattern of liver injury is usually seen with nitrofurantoin. Clinical symptoms of fever, rash, and eosinophilia are common. Over 100 cases of chronic active hepatitis secondary to nitrofurantoin have been reported, most in women taking the drug for > 6 months. Laboratory findings consist of high aminotransferase values, increased gamma globulin, HLA-B8 histocompatibility markers, and, often, positive autoimmune markers (antinuclear antibody).

21. **What laxative is associated with chronic hepatitis?**
Oxyphenisatin. Laxatives containing oxyphenisatin are no longer available in the U.S.

22. **What antiarthritic drugs have been reported to cause liver injury?**
Sulindac (Clinoril). Over 400 cases of sulindac-induced hepatitis have been reported. A cholestatic hepatitis is seen in most patients. Common clinical manifestations include fever, rash, and Stevens-Johnson syndrome. A "trapped" common bile duct causing cholestasis has been reported after sulindac-induced pancreatitis.
Diclofenac (Voltaren). The pattern of injury, uniquely more common in women than men, is primarily hepatitis. Fulminant hepatitis and death have been reported.
Phenylbutazone (Butazolidin). An immunologic type of injury is usually seen, with fever, rash, and eosinophilia. Illness usually starts within 6 weeks of initiating the drug. The hepatic injury seen is variable; acute hepatitis, cholestasis, and granulomatous hepatitis have been reported.
Ibuprofen (Motrin, Advil). Hepatic injury due to ibuprofen is relatively uncommon. Over-the-counter doses of ibuprofen have not been reported to cause clinically apparent liver injury.
Piroxicam (Feldene). Lethal hepatitis and cholestasis have been reported, but overall liver injury appears to be uncommon.
Celecoxib (Celebrex). Acute pancreatitis and hepatitis have been reported.

23. **Name the two types of cholestatic drug-induced hepatic injury.**
Inflammatory and bland cholestasis.

24. **List the common causes of drug-induced cholestasis.**

Inflammatory cholestasis	Bland cholestasis
Allopurinol	Anabolic steroids
Amitriptyline	Androgens
Azathioprine	Estrogens
Captopril	Oral contraceptives
Carbamazepine	Phenytoin

25. What chemotherapeutic agent is associated with a sclerosing cholangitis pattern of injury?

Floxuridine. Selective hepatic artery infusion has been associated with a large bile duct injury and cholestasis in up to 30% of patients.

26. List the drugs associated with mixed cholestatic-hepatitis type of liver injury.

Amitriptyline	Flutamide	Ranitidine
Amoxicillin	Ibuprofen	Sulfonamides
Ampicillin	Imipramine	Sulindac
Captopril	Nitrofurantoin	Toxic oil syndrome
Carbamazepine	Phenylbutazone	Trimethoprim-sulfamethoxazole
Cimetidine	Quinidine	Naproxen

27. Which drugs cause the three types of drug-induced steatosis ("fatty liver")?

MICROVESICULAR STEATOSIS	MACROVESICULAR STEATOSIS	PHOSPHOLIPIDOSIS
Aspirin (Reye's syndrome)	Acetaminophen	4,4'-Diethylamino ethyl hexestrol
Ketoprofen	Cisplatin	Perhexiline maleate
Tetracycline	Corticosteroids	Amiodarone
Valproic acid	Methotrexate	Trimethroprim-sulfamethoxazide
Zidovudine (AZT)	Tamoxifen	Parenteral nutrition

28. How is the hepatic injury caused by amiodarone unique?

Amiodarone is an iodine-containing benzofuran used in Europe as an antianginal and antiarrhythmic agent. Amiodarone accumulates within the lysosome, where it complexes with phospholipids and inhibits lysosomal phospholipases.

29. How should patients receiving chronic methotrexate (MTX) be monitored for chronic hepatitis and cirrhosis?

MTX has been used in patients with refractory psoriasis and rheumatoid arthritis. In patients with psoriasis, many advocate an index liver biopsy after 2–4 months of MTX therapy, followed by serial repeat biopsies after every 1.0–1.5 gm of cumulative dose. In patients with rheumatoid arthritis, MTX appears to be somewhat less hepatotoxic. The American College of Rheumatology does not recommend a pretreatment liver biopsy in the absence of preexisting liver disease, but liver-associated enzymes should be monitored. Reevaluation of MTX safety is advised when AST or ALT levels exceed 3 times the baseline values. Liver biopsies are advised every 2 or 3 years (or every 1.5 gm of cumulative dose).

30. What are the histologic grades of MTX liver injury?

Histologic Grades of Methotrexate Liver Injury

GRADE	FIBROSIS	FATTY INFILTRATION	NUCLEAR VARIABILITY	PORTAL INFLAMMATION
I	None	Mild	Mild	Mild
II	None	Moderate to severe	Moderate to severe	Portal expansion, lobular necrosis
IIIA	Mild (septa extending into lobules)	Moderate to severe	Moderate to severe	Portal expansion, lobular necrosis
IIIB	Moderate to severe	Moderate to severe	Moderate to severe	Portal expansion, lobular necrosis
IV	Cirrhosis			

31. Outline the recommendations for change in MTX therapy based on liver biopsy findings.

I   Continue therapy; repeat biopsy after 1–1.5 gm of cumulative dose.

II   Continue therapy; repeat biopsy after 1–1.5 gm of cumulative dose.

IIIA   Continue therapy, but repeat biopsy in 6 months.

IIIB   No further MTX; exceptional cases need close histologic follow-up.

IV   No further MTX; exceptional cases need close histologic follow-up.

32. What is veno-occlusive disease (VOD)? What drugs have been implicated as causes?

VOD is an occlusive disease that affects terminal hepatic venules and veins. Patients typically present with hepatomegaly, ascites, weight gain, peripheral edema, jaundice, and pain from capsular distention of the liver. Aminotransferase values may be normal or modestly elevated. Liver biopsy is often required for the diagnosis and shows histologic features of perivenular sclerosis, blood-filled congested sinuses, and hemorrhagic necrosis. Drugs causing VOD include vincristine, 6-thioguanine, carmustine (BCNU), azathioprine, radiotherapy, 6-mercaptopurine, doxorubicin, aflatoxin, and pyrrolizidine alkaloids (bush tea).

33. What drugs are associated with the development of hepatic adenomas?

Before the availability of oral contraceptives, hepatic adenomas were rare. After 5 years of oral contraceptive use, the relative risk of developing a hepatic adenoma has been estimated to increase 116-fold. Hepatic adenomas often regress when exogenous estrogen is removed and can recur during pregnancy. Anabolic steroids also have been reported to cause hepatic adenomas. Hepatic adenomas are usually asymptomatic but can be associated with abdominal fullness, pain, hepatomegaly, and hemorrhage.

34. Define peliosis hepatis. With what drugs is it associated?

Peliosis hepatis describes small venular cavities or lakes within the liver that arise from injury to sinusoids. The condition is generally asymptomatic but may result in hemorrhage or liver failure. Anabolic steroids and oral contraceptives have been shown to cause peliosis hepatitis.

35. Which three vascular injuries to the liver can be caused by drugs?

Hepatic VOD	Pyrrolizidine alkaloids, antineoplastic drugs
Peliosis hepatis	Anabolic steroids, oral contraceptives
Hepatic vein thrombosis	Oral contraceptives

36. What are the three most common drug-induced hepatic neoplasms?

• Hepatic adenoma: oral contraceptives, anabolic steroids

• Hepatocellular carcinoma: anabolic steroids, oral contraceptives, thorium oxide (Thorotrast), vinyl chloride

• Angiosarcoma: thorium oxide (Thorotrast), vinyl chloride, arsenic, anabolic steroids

37. Over 50 drugs have been cited as causing hepatic granulomas. Name the most common.

Allopurinol	Phenylbutazone	Isoniazid	Chlorpromazine
Quinidine	Nitrofurantoin	Diazepam	Sulfonamides
Penicillin	Gold	Aspirin	Phenytoin
Mineral oil	Oral contraceptives	Quinine	Oxicillin
Diltiazem	Tolbutamide		

38. Which drugs commonly used to treat endocrine disease have been reported to cause liver injury?

Troglitazone is a new type of oral antihyperglycemic drug that reduces hepatic glucose output and promotes insulin-dependent glucose metabolism in skeletal muscle without altering insulin secretion. Several cases of fulminant hepatic failure have been reported with use of troglitazone. Aminotransferase levels should be monitored monthly for the first 6 months and every 2 months for the balance of the first year of treatment.

Sulfonylureas include chlorpropamide, glipizide, tolazamide, tolbutamide acetohexamide, and glyburide. The pattern of injury is cholestatic for chlorpropamide, glipizide, tolazamide, and tolbutamide and hepatocellular or mixed with the remainder. A hypersensitivity reaction is thought to be responsible. Hypersensitivity to chlorpropamide does not predict the same response to tolbutamide.

Thiourea derivatives (propylthiouracil, methimazole) may cause hepatocellular or cholestatic injury.

Steroid derivatives (anabolic steroids, oral contraceptives, tamoxifen, danazol, glucocorticoids) are reported to cause cholestasis or canalicular type of liver injury.

Lipid-lowering agents include niacin and HMG-CoA reductase inhibitors. Niacin (nicotinic acid) may cause mixed cholestatic-hepatic injury. Injury is more common with the sustained-release form or at doses >3 gm/day for the regular-release form. Serial monitoring of liver enzymes is recommended, and the drug should be discontinued if elevations are detected. Lovastatin is the most commonly prescribed of the HMG-CoA reductase inhibitors used to treat hypercholesterolemia. Mild elevations in aminotransferases are common, but levels usually return to normal on drug withdrawal.

39. What commonly used cardiovascular drugs have been reported to cause liver injury?

Quinidine. Liver injury has been reported after a single dose. The predominant injury is hepatocellular with focal necrosis, but diffuse granulomas also have been seen.

Procainamide. Injury to the liver is rare, but hepatocellular, cholestatic, and granulomatous injuries have been reported.

Verapamil and nifedipine. Hepatitis has been reported to develop within 2–3 weeks of drug administration. Cholestatic, hepatocellular, and mixed injuries have been reported. A pseudoalcohol pattern of steatosis and Mallory's hyaline has been reported with use of nifedipine.

Methyldopa. Asymptomatic elevations in aminotransferases are seen in up to 5% of patients taking methyldopa. Women are especially susceptible. Both acute and chronic forms of hepatitis have been reported.

Hydralazine. Hepatocellular and granulomatous injury have been reported.

Captopril. Hypersensitivity symptoms usually herald jaundice. Cholestasis usually ameliorates rapidly after drug removal.

Enalapril. Scattered cases of hepatitis and cholestasis have been reported.

Ticrynafen. This uricosuric diuretic was removed from the U.S. market shortly after its introduction because of the significant incidence of liver injury. The hepatitis can be fatal.

Amiodarone. This antianginal and antiarrhythmic drug is widely used in Europe. A characteristic injury of phospholipidosis is seen.

40. What commonly used antimicrobial agents have been shown to cause liver injury?

Tetracycline. Liver injury is seen almost exclusively with parenteral administration and is more common in women, especially during pregnancy. Microvesicular steatosis is the characteristic histologic finding.

Erythromycin estolate. Initially liver injury was thought to occur only with the estolate form, but the ethylsuccinate form has recently been implicated as a cause of cholestatic hepatitis. A hypersensitivity picture is usually seen within days to 2 weeks after exposure.

Chloramphenicol. Rare cases of cholestasis and jaundice have been reported.

Penicillin. Both cholestatic and hepatitis-like patterns have been reported. Hypersensitivity is the mechanism of injury.

Amoxicillin, clavulanic acid. Cholestatic hepatitis has been seen during or within weeks of administration.

Sulfonamides cause mixed hepatocellular injury that usually is heralded by rash, fever, and eosinophilia.

Pyrimethamine-sulfadoxine. Hepatocellular injury is most common, but fulminant hepatitis and death have been reported.

Sulfasalazine, which is used to treat inflammatory bowel disease, may cause the same injury as sulfonamides.

Nitrofurantoin. Hallmarks of hypersensitivity are common, with both cholestatic and hepatocellular injury reported. Chronic active hepatitis has been reported, usually in women older than 40 years with HLA-B8 histocompatibility.

Isoniazid is associated with an age-related risk for toxicity. Fulminant hepatitis with death has been reported (see question 15.)

Rifampin potentiates the hepatotoxity of isoniazid, presumably by induction of cytochrome P450. Women older than 50 years are especially susceptible.

Griseofulvin. Hepatitis is rare, but the drug can precipitate attacks of acute intermittent porphyria.

Ketoconazole. Toxic hepatitis more common in women older than 40 years. Fulminant hepatitis has been reported. Periodic monitoring of liver enzymes is recommended to detect early injury.

Flucytosine. Transaminase elevations are common; significant hepatitis is rare.

41. Can herbal remedies injure the liver?

Yes and no. Comfrey and chaparral leaf are known to be hepatotoxic. Because the composition of herbal remedies is variable and unregulated, persons with preexisting liver disease should be cautious and consult their doctor. Milk thistle (*Silybum marianum*) is a safe substance that has been used for centuries to remedy liver disease. Many patients with liver disease self-medicate with milk thistle. Although aminotranferase levels commonly improve, no good evidence suggess that it improves the liver disorder. Silymarin plus thioctic acid and penicillin has been successfully used in the treatment of *Amanita* mushroom poisoning.

BIBLIOGRAPHY

1. Andreu V, Mas A, Bruguera M, et al: Ecstasy, a "recreational" amphetamine, was a significant cause of hepatotoxicity in young adults. J Hepatol 29:394–397, 1998.
2. Burgquest SR, Felson DT, Prashker MJ, Freedberg KA: The cost of liver biopsy in rheumatoid arthritis patients treated with methotrexate. Arthritis Rheum 38:326–333, 1995.
3. Gitlin N, Julie NL, Spurr CL, et al: Two cases of severe clinical and histologic hepatotoxicity associated with troglitazone. Ann Intern Med 129:36–38, 1998.
4. Kremer JM, Alaarcon GS, Lightfoot RW, et al: Methotrexate for rheumatoid arthritis: Suggested guidelines for monitoring liver toxicity. Arthritis Rheum 37:316–328, 1994.
5. Lindberg MC: Hepatobiliary complications of oral contraceptives. J Gen Intern Med 7:199–209, 1992.
6. Neuberger J. Halothane hepatitis. Eur J Gastroenterol Hepatol 10:631–633, 1998.
7. Nolan CM, Goldberg SV, Buskin SE: Hepatotoxicity associated with isoniazid preventive therapy: A 7-year survey from a public health tuberculosis clinic. JAMA 281:1014–1018, 1999.
8. Ranek L, Dalhoff K, Poulsen HE, et al: Drug metabolism and genetic polymorphism in subjects with previous halothane hepatitis. Scand J Gastroenterol 28:677–680, 1993.
9. Roy AK, Mahoney HC, Levine RA: Phenytoin-induced chronic hepatitis. Dig Dis Sci 38:740–743, 1993.
10. Scully LJ, Clarke D, Barr RJ: Diclofenac-induced hepatitis: Three cases with features of autoimmune chronic active hepatitis. Dig Dis Sci 38:774–751, 1993.
11. Sherlock S, Dooley J: Drugs and the liver. In Sherlock S (ed): Disease of the Liver and Biliary System, 9th ed. Oxford, Blackwell, 1993, pp 322–356.
12. Stickel F, Egerer G, Seitz HK: Hepatotoxicity of botanicals. Public Health Nutr 3:113–124, 2000.
13. Tarzi EM, Harter JG, Zimmerman HJ, et al: Sulindac-associated hepatic injury: Analysis of 91 cases reported to the Food and Drug Administration. Gastroenterology 104:569–574, 1993.
14. West SG: Methotrexate hepatotoxicity. Rheum Dis Clin North Am 23:883–915, 1997.
15. Zimmerman HJ, Maddrey WC: Toxic and drug-induced hepatitis. In Schiff L, Schiff ER (eds): Diseases of the Liver, 7th ed. Philadelphia, J.B. Lippincott, 1993, pp 707–783.

26. ALCOHOLIC LIVER DISEASE

Thomas E. Trouillot, M.D.

1. How does one identify a patient with a pathologic pattern of alcohol consumption?

Alcohol is ubiquitous in western society. Over 95% of people have tried an alcoholic beverage in their lifetime. The overall prevalence of alcohol abuse in the general population is 9.4%. The clinician is challenged with identifying the pathologic patterns of alcohol consumption in his or her patients before long-term consequences develop. Ultimately, the total amount of alcohol consumed per weight determines who is at risk for alcohol-related disease. Identifying patients who have developed tolerance to alcohol is often facilitated by the **CAGE** question mnemonic. A positive answer to any of the four questions helps identify a patient who is at risk for alcohol abuse and may require further counseling or intervention:

C   Have you ever felt you should **C**ut down on your drinking?
A   Did you ever get **A**ngry when someone asked you about your alcohol consumption?
G   Did you ever feel **G**uilty about your drinking habits?
E   Did you ever have an **E**ye-opener in the morning to steady your nerves or get rid of a hangover?

2. Describe the pathologic patterns of alcohol consumption.

The pathologic patterns of alcohol consumption include episodic or binge drinking associated with periods of inebriation followed by extended periods of sobriety. Daily consumption of alcohol amounting to > 45 grams/day is associated with progressive liver injury. It is postulated that women require less daily alcohol to develop liver injury due, in part, to a lower body mass compared with men.

3. What terms for alcohol-related disease are included in the Diagnostic and Statistical Manual of the American Psychiatric Association (DSM-IV)?

Alcohol dependency is a maladaptive pattern of substance abuse leading to clinically significant impairment or distress, as manifested by three or more of the following within the same 12-month period: (1) tolerance, (2) withdrawal, (3) alcohol taken in larger amounts or for longer periods than intended, (4) persistent desire to cut down use, (5) great deal of time spent in activities surrounding alcohol, (6) giving up important social, occupational, or recreational activities, and (7) continued use despite knowledge of adverse physical or psychological problems related to alcohol.

Alcohol abuse is a maladaptive pattern of substance abuse leading to clinically significant impairment or distress, as manifested by one or more of the following within the same 12-month period: (1) recurrent use resulting in a failure to fulfill major role obligations at work, school, or home; (2) recurrent use in situations in which alcohol is physically hazardous; (3) recurrent substance-related legal problems; and (4) continued use despite having persistent or recurrent social or interpersonal problems caused or exacerbated by the effects of alcohol.

4. How does the body metabolize alcohol?

Alcohol is metabolized primarily through the liver. Once alcohol is ingested and absorbed through the gut, it is metabolized by both gastric and hepatic alcohol dehydrogenase to acetaldehyde. This, in turn, is oxidized by the liver, using aldehyde dehydrogenase and the microsomal ethanol-oxidizing system, cytochrome P450 2E1 (CYP2E1).

5. What liver enzyme is a potential target for drug intervention to discourage alcohol consumption?

Aldehyde dehydrogenase (ALDH) is the enzyme responsible for variable rates of alcohol clearance based on the genetic inheritance of an aberrant allele. It enables oxidation of acetaldehyde to acetate. Certain Asian populations carry an aberrant allele that results in impaired enzyme activity, accumulations of acetaldehyde, and secondary symptoms of flushing, tachycardia, and severe nausea and vomiting. To take advantage of this reaction, disulfiram (Antabuse), a competitive inhibitor of ALDH, is used as a deterrent to consume alcohol. Accumulation of acetaldehyde results in the typical reaction of skin flushing, anxiety, nausea, and vomiting.

6. What is considered heavy alcohol consumption?

Beer (12 oz), wine (5 oz), and hard liquor (1.5 oz of 80-proof) contain approximately 14 grams of ethanol. Moderate alcohol consumption is considered < 20 gm/day in women and < 40 gm/day in men. Heavy alcohol consumption is considered > 20 gm/day in women and > 80 gm/day in men. The incidence of cirrhosis is significantly increased in men who consume > 40–60 gm/day. Approximately 20% of men drinking > 12 beers/day develop cirrhosis in 10 years.

7. How does acute alcohol toxicity manifest?

Large quantities of alcohol consumed over a short period can result in acute liver toxicity as well as a more general syndrome called acute alcohol poisoning. Patients usually have evidence of recent alcohol ingestion with clinically relevant behavioral and psychological changes. The average alcoholic beverage raises blood alcohol concentration by 15–20 mg/dl, the amount metabolized by the liver in 1 hour.

BLOOD ALCOHOL LEVEL (MG/DL)	EXPECTED EFFECT
20–99	Impaired coordination, euphoria
100–199	Ataxia, decreased mentation, poor judgment, labile mood
200–299	Marked ataxia and slurred speech, poor judgment, labile mood, nausea and vomiting
300–399	Stage I anesthesia, memory lapse, labile mood
> 400	Respiratory failure, coma, death

8. Describe the most common form of alcoholic liver disease and its clinical manifestations.

Fatty liver or hepatic steatosis is the most common form of alcoholic liver disease and is reversible with abstinence from alcohol intake. Its first clinical manifestation is typically asymptomatic hepatomegaly. As a consequence of preferential alcohol oxidation, the liver develops fatty deposition. In turn, there is a slight-to-moderate elevation in liver transaminases with a typical ratio of aspartate aminotransferase to alanine aminotransferase (AST:ALT) of 2:1. This transaminitis usually resolves after several days of abstinence.

9. Describe the features of alcoholic hepatitis.

The clinical manifestations of alcoholic hepatitis range from anicteric hepatomegaly to fulminant liver failure. Alcoholic hepatitis usually is associated with heavy alcohol consumption for more than 10 years. The clinical features include jaundice, fever, elevated white blood cell count, hepatomegaly, frequently infection, and moderate elevation of AST to 2–5 times the upper limits of normal. The pathophysiology of alcoholic hepatitis is related to the toxic effects of acetaldehyde production from the hepatic metabolism of alcohol. Liver histology is characterized by hepatocellular disarray; polymorphonuclear cell infiltration in the parenchyma; Mallory's hyaline bodies (approximately 30% of cases), which are clumps of intermediary cytokeratin filaments due to tubulin-acetaldehyde adducts; and some degree of steatosis cholestasis, fibrosis, and necrosis. Approximately 25% of patients with alcoholic hepatitis present with infection and manifestations of portal hypertension (ascites or varices) without cirrhosis. In addition, an estimated 30% of patients with alcoholic hepatitis are infected with hepatitis C virus.

10. When is it appropriate to use corticosteroids for alcoholic hepatitis?

The use of corticosteroids to treat patients with acute alcoholic hepatitis has been studied in a number of clinical trials. Although the pathophysiology to explain their efficacy is not well understood, their use may attenuate immune processes that activate or perpetuate alcohol hepatitis, possibly by decreasing cytokine production. Most studies support the use of corticosteroids when a patient develops severe alcoholic hepatitis characterized by hepatic encephalopathy and/or a high discriminant function (DF) value.

11. How is DF value calculated?

$$[4.6 \times (\text{prothrombin time seconds} - \text{control time})] + \text{serum bilirubin mg/dl}$$
or
$$[4.6 \times (\text{prothrombin time seconds} - \text{control time})] + \text{serum bilirubin mmol/L/17}.$$

A DF value > 32 is associated with severe alcoholic hepatitis and a high short-term mortality rate (within approximately 1 month). The usual treatment is prednisolone or prednisone, 40 mg once daily for 30 days. Patients with mild alcoholic hepatitis or more severe clinical manifestations complicated by significant GI bleeding or sepsis are not likely to benefit from corticosteroids.

12. What other treatments may be used for alcoholic hepatitis?

Pentoxifylline, a nonselective phosphodiesterase inhibitor of tumor necrosis factor production, recently was shown in a randomized, placebo-controlled trial to decrease mortality by 40% in patients with severe alcoholic hepatitis (DF > 32), particularly by decreasing the incidence of hepatorenal syndrome.

Other medications, such as polyenylphosphatidylcholine, colchicine, and propylthiouracil, may decrease the inflammatory response to alcoholic liver injury and inhibit or reverse hepatic fibrosis.

Nutritional support is important because many alcoholic patients are malnourished with depleted vitamin stores and low hepatic glutathione levels (an important liver compound used to metabolize drugs and toxins).

Note: All treatment for alcoholic hepatitis is predicated on complete abstinence from alcohol. No therapy shows any benefit in patients who continue to drink heavily.

13. Why can moderate doses of acetaminophen be toxic to patients with alcoholic liver disease?

Because alcohol induces the cytochrome P-450 system, hepatic metabolism of acetaminophen can result in the development of toxic intermediates. Normally, these toxic intermediates are conjugated with glutathione, which protects against oxidative injury. Typically alcoholics have poor nutrition and depleted glutathione stores. Alcohol-induced cytochrome P-450 and depleted glutathione stores porbably explain why alcoholics are more susceptible to acetaminophen hepatoxicity.

14. What is the most advanced form of chronic alcoholic liver disease?

Cirrhosis, which accounts for approximately 75% of deaths due to alcoholism. It is characterized by the formation of severe hepatic fibrosis (scarring), typically in a micronodular pattern. This, in turn, leads to (1) loss of liver cell mass, which impairs liver synthetic function (development of hepatic encephalopathy, hypoalbuminemia, and coagulopathy), and (2) development of portal hypertension and its clinical complications (esophageal and gastric varices, ascites, and spontaneous bacterial peritonitis). Patients who develop these clinical complications are considered to have decompensated liver function. The 5-year survival rate is upward of 90% in patients with alcoholic liver disease and cirrhosis when they have compensated liver disease and maintain abstinence. When patients develop hepatic decompensation and continue to drink heavily, the 5-year survival rate drops to approximately 30%. Life-threatening complications of cirrhosis include infection, variceal bleeding, and hepatorenal syndrome.

15. List the important extrahepatic manifestations of alcoholic liver disease.

Ascites	Spider angiomata	Dupuytren's contractures	Peripheral neuropathy
Splenomegaly	Asterixis	Korsakoff's syndrome	Hypogonadism
Caput medusae	Palmar erythema	Wernicke's encephalopathy	Gynecomastia

16. When is a patient with advanced alcoholic liver disease a suitable candidate for liver transplantation?

When a patient with alcoholic liver disease and cirrhosis develops hepatic decompensation, liver transplantation should be considered. Manifestations of chronic liver failure that are considered indications for liver transplant evaluation include hepatic encephalopathy, ascites, spontaneous bacterial peritonitis, bleeding esophageal or gastric varices, and/or liver biochemical deterioration with a prolonged protime or international normalized ratio, elevated total bilirubin, or low serum albumin. Patients with alcoholic liver disease who actively consume alcohol are not immediate liver transplant candidates. However, a somewhat arbitrary rule of 6-month sobriety has been used as a guideline by most liver transplant centers. Definitive data are lacking to determine the ideal candidates, intervention, and period of abstinence to ensure sobriety after liver transplantation.

BIBLIOGRAPHY

1. Abittan CS, Lieber CS: Alcoholic liver disease. Clinical Perspectives in Gastroenterology. 1999, pp 257–263.
2. Akriviadis E, Botla R, Briggs W, et al: Pentoxifylline improves short-term survival in severe acute alcoholic hepatitis: A double-blind, placebo-controlled trial. Gastroenterology 199:1637–1648, 2000.
3. Gish RG, Olden K: Alcohol and liver disease: Should liver transplantation be offered? Practical Gastroenterology. 1997, pp 9–23.
4. Imperiale TF, McCullough AJ: Do corticosteroids reduce mortality from alcoholic hepatitis? A meta-analysis of the randomized trials. Ann Intern Med 113:299–307, 1990.
5. Keeffe EB: Assessment of the alcoholic patient for liver transplantation: Comorbidity, outcome, and recidivism. Liver Transplant Surg 2:12–20, 1996.
6. Lieber CS: Alcoholism: A disease encompassing all of medicine. Resident Staff Physician 41:15–28, 1995.
7. Mathurin P, Duchatelle V, Ramond MJ, et al: Survival and prognostic factors in patients with severe alcoholic hepatitis treated with prednisolone. Gastroenterology 110:1847–1853, 1996.
8. Mayfield D, McLeod G, Hall P: The CAGE questionnaire: Validation of a new alcoholism screening instrument. Am J Psychiatry 131:1121–1123, 1974.
9. Raymond MJ, Poynard T, Reuff B, et al: A randomized trial of prednisolone in patients with severe alcoholic hepatitis. N Engl J Med 326:507–512, 1992.
10. Schuckit MA: Drug and Alcohol Abuse. A Clinical Guide to Diagnosis and Treatment, 4th ed. New York, Plenum, 1995.
11. Weinrieb RM, Van Horn DH, McLellan AT, Lucey MR: Interpreting the significance of drinking by alcohol-dependent liver transplant patients: Fostering candor is the key to recovery. Liver Transplant 6.769–776, 2000.

27. VASCULAR LIVER DISEASE

Bahri M. Bilir, M.D., Nuray Bilir, M.D., M.S., and Peter R. McNally, D.O.

1. Describe the important vascular anatomy of the liver.

The liver constitutes 5% of body weight in adults but receives 20% of cardiac output via the hepatic artery and portal vein. The **hepatic artery** is a branch of the hepaticoduodenal artery from the celiac axis. It carries approximately 30% of the afferent flow but delivers more than 50% of the oxygen used in the resting state.

The **portal vein** is a valveless vein that carries 70–80% of total liver blood flow and delivers a little less than 50% of needed oxygen. It is formed at the level of the pancreas where the splenic veins join the superior mesenteric vein. At the liver hilum, both the portal vein and hepatic artery divide into right and left branches and subdivide further up to the level of the porta hepatis. Both hepatic arterioles and portal venules drain into the sinusoids from this point onward. At this level, hepatic arteries have sphincters that dynamically regulate the blood flow. Sphincters within the sinusoid also help to regulate blood flow and distribution. These sphincters are important in the physiologic regulation of blood flow to the liver through the hepatic artery. A reduction in portal vein flow leads to an immediate increase in hepatic arterial flow. Nonetheless, portal vein flow is relatively constant and is not influenced by hepatic arterial flow.

At the end of the sinusoid, blood enters into the central venule, which forms the hepatic venule. There are three major **hepatic veins**: right, middle, and left. The branches of the three main hepatic veins have a distribution that is quite different from the distribution of the hepatic artery and portal vein. Therefore, surgical and vascular anatomy of the liver differs from the four macroscopic lobes (right, left, caudate, and quadrate lobes). Vascular anatomy, as described by Coinaud, divides the liver into eight segments. Each of these eight segments has its own afferent and efferent blood supply. This anatomy is particularly important in the resection of liver masses. The caudate lobe is drained through a variable number of small veins (dorsal hepatic veins) that directly enter into the superior vena cava. This information is important in understanding the compensatory hypertrophy of the caudate lobe in Budd-Chiari syndrome.

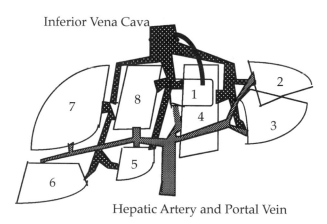

Vascular and surgical anatomy of the liver. According to Coinaud, there are eight functional segments in the liver, which receive blood supply via the portal vein and hepatic artery. Efferent drainage is through the right, middle, and left hepatic veins. The caudate lobe (segment 1) has a separate and direct outflow to the inferior vena cava via the dorsal hepatic veins. This vascular anatomy is particularly useful in the resection of liver masses.

2. Describe the microarchitecture of the liver, including the microcirculation.

The basic element in the liver's structure is the liver cell plate, which consists of 15–20 hepatocytes lined up between the portal area and hepatic veins. The hepatocytes near the hepatic veins are called perivenular or pericentral hepatocytes. Perivenular hepatocytes are subject to more hypoxia than other hepatocytes because they are at the end of the unidirectional sinusoidal blood flow.

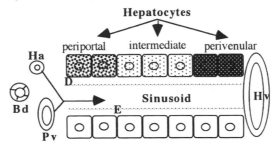

Hepatic microarchitecture. Blood from the portal vein (Pv) and hepatic artery (Ha) join and traverse the sinusoids, eventually leaving the liver from the hepatic venules (Hv). The low-pressure circulation in the sinusoids allows plasma to pass through the fenestrated epithelium (E) and reach the space of Disse (D), where, through direct contact with hepatocytes, exchange of nutrients and metabolites takes place. The hepatocytes near the portal triad are called periportal, and those near the hepatic veins are called perivenular hepatocytes.

In diseases such as vaso-occlusive disease or Budd-Chiari syndrome, when the outflow tract is occluded, perivenular hepatocytes are the first to be damaged. This area is also known as zone III in Rappaport's concept of the liver lobule. Zone I hepatocytes are close to the portal tract and also are called periportal hepatocytes. Zone II or intermediate hepatocytes are between the periportal and perivenular hepatocytes. There are no absolute boundaries between these zones and hepatocytes. The metabolic function of these cells, as well as their susceptibility to injury, changes gradually, depending on their position within the liver cell plate. Zone II and III hepatocytes are involved in drug metabolism and rich in cytochrome P450 enzymes. The toxic effects of most drugs metabolized by these microsomal enzymes are seen in zone II and III hepatocytes, with relative sparing of zone I.

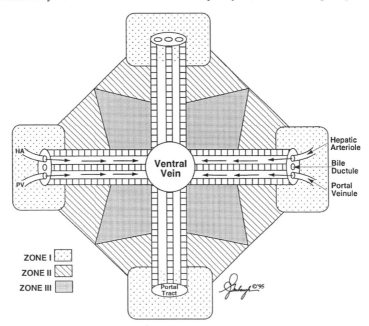

3. Define Budd-Chiari syndrome (BCS). What are the predisposing conditions?

BCS is thrombosis of the hepatic veins. The associated conditions are abdominal trauma; myeloproliferative syndromes; paroxysmal nocturnal hemoglobinuria; conditions associated with lupus, anticoagulants, antithrombin III deficiency, and protein C and S deficiency; tumors of the pancreas, adrenal glands, and kidneys; hepatocellular carcinoma; pregnancy; and drugs that cause hypercoagulability, such as oral contraceptives and dacarbazine. Presence of the factor V Leiden mutation portends a high relative risk for BCS. The factor V Leiden mutation may be responsible for about 25–30% of cases of BCS considered to be "idiopathic."

4. What are the symptoms and presenting complaints in BCS?
- Ascites (>90% of patients) is the cardinal feature.
- Abdominal pain (up to 80% of patients) is localized to the right upper quadrant.
- Hepatosplenomegaly is a common physical finding.
- Jaundice, when present, is slight and not a dramatic feature.
- Hepatic encephalopathy and variceal bleeding are less common (10–20% incidence) and usually are observed late in the disease.

5. How is BCS diagnosed?

The diagnosis can be made in about 75% of patients with Doppler ultrasound of the hepatic veins. The ultrasound may show the clot in the lumen as echogenic material, decreased or absent flow, or a hyperechogenic cord replacing one or more of the main hepatic veins. Caudate lobe hypertrophy may be inaccurately interpreted as a liver mass. Hepatic vein catheterization and angiography are highly sensitive and specific procedures in diagnosing BCS and are accepted as gold standards. They also allow therapeutic measures, such as the use of streptokinase, in acute disease. Magnetic resonance angiography is a research tool that may become a useful noninvasive test in the future.

6. Why do some patients with BCS have an enlarged caudate lobe?

Approximately one-half of patients with BCS develop compensatory hypertrophy in the caudate lobe of the liver, which has separate hepatic veins (dorsal hepatic veins) that drain directly into the inferior vena cava. If the obstruction is below the level of these veins, they remain patent, whereas the hepatic veins draining the right and left lobes are thrombosed. The caudate lobe hypertrophies to compensate for the function of the failing liver. This hypertrophy may be quite marked and can cause a characteristic indentation in the inferior venogram.

7. Describe the pathologic features of BCS in liver biopsies.

In the acute event, centrilobular congestion and dilatation of the perivenular sinusoid are seen in the liver biopsy. In severe cases, zone III necrosis may be quite evident. Centrilobular fibrosis develops with 4 weeks, and within 4 months regenerative nodules and cirrhosis develop. Examination of the hepatic veins and inferior vena cava may show concentric thickening in the vein wall with no inflammation. Both subintimal fibrosis and an organizing thrombus in the lumen may contribute to the occlusion of the outflow track.

8. How is BCS treated?

Treatment of BCS depends to a great degree on the acuity of onset and associated conditions. In acute presentations with clearly documented recent thrombosis (i.e., after abdominal trauma or recurrence of BCS after liver transplantation), heparinization and thrombolytic therapy probably have a role. Both tissue plasminogen activator and streptokinase have been used with inconclusive results. Percutaneous transluminal and surgical angioplasty also have been tried, but initial success was handicapped by a high rate of reclosure. In patients with myeloproliferative disorders, rapid and aggressive treatments with hydroxyurea and other agents in conjunction with heparinization have provided favorable outcomes. Symptomatic treatments, such as paracentesis and diuretics, are also quite useful.

9. What is the prognosis of BCS?

Despite all of these available treatments, the long-term prognosis remains poor, and most patients (> 90% in one study) die within 3.5 years. The only treatment that has changed this poor outcome is liver transplantation. Although it is still controversial, liver transplantation with post-transplant anticoagulation has been used successfully in many institutions, with a 5-year survival rate of over 60%. Some centers, however, report a 20% recurrence rate. If transplantation is not an option, surgical portacaval shunts are among the options and have similar recurrence rates.

10. Does BCS caused by factor V Leiden mutation preclude liver transplantation?
No. The resistance to activated protein C caused by factor V Leiden mutation is corrected once the liver allograft is functioning. Some transplant centers recommend screening for protein C resistance among cadaveric donors with a history of venous thrombosis to avoid transmitting a thrombophilic condition to the recipient.

11. What is hepatic veno-occlusive disease (VOD)?
Hepatic VOD is the nonthrombotic occlusion of small hepatic veins by connective tissue and collagen. Large-sized hepatic veins are disease-free. VOD is associated with centrilobular congestion with or without hepatocellular necrosis. The disease frequently progresses into extensive perivenular fibrosis, central-to-central bridging, and eventually cirrhosis.

12. Name the conditions associated with hepatic veno-occlusive diseases.
Ingestion of plants containing pyrrolizidine alkaloids, cancer chemotherapy, bone marrow transplantation, hepatic irradiation, and arsphenamine and urethane therapy have been reported to cause hepatic VOD. The incidence of VOD after bone marrow transplantation varies from 2% to 64%, depending on the autologous or allogeneic nature of the transplant and the aggressiveness of induction chemotherapy.

13. When should you suspect hepatic VOD after bone marrow transplantation?
The first signs and symptoms of VOD may appear as early as the first week after exposure to the toxic insult. VOD after bone marrow transplantation presents with weight gain and ascites within the first week or two. Most cases are diagnosed within 1–2 months. The most common features at presentation are jaundice, hepatomegaly, abdominal pain, and ascites. Transjugular biopsies at this stage are essential for early diagnosis. The biopsy shows perivenular sinusoidal dilatation, fibrosis, zone III necrosis, central venular occlusion, and phlebosclerosis.

14. Which cardiac conditions can cause liver dysfunction?
Hepatic congestion has been found in all forms of heart disease, both acquired and congenital, that cause congestive heart failure. Coronary artery disease, hypertension, rheumatic valve disease, cor pulmonale, congenital disease, constrictive pericarditis, scleroderma, and late syphilis have been reported to cause hepatic congestion and dysfunction. The common pathway in the pathogenesis is pump failure, which results in stasis of flow above the level of the hepatic veins.

15. Describe the clinical manifestations of hepatic congestion due to right ventricular failure.
Patients with right ventricular failure may have mild-to-severe discomfort in the right upper quadrant and occasionally mild jaundice. Physical examination reveals hepatomegaly with hepatojugular reflux, ascites, and peripheral edema.

16. What kind of liver chemistry abnormalities are found in hepatic congestion?
In acute cardiac failure, such as shock states, the liver can be severely affected. Findings include very high levels (> 1,000 IU) of aspartate aminotransferase (AST) and alanine aminotransferase (ALT), with ALT usually higher than AST; increased prothrombin time; and gradually rising bilirubin levels. In some patients with shock, the liver may never recover; they may have full clinical and biochemical signs of acute liver failure. In chronic cardiac congestion, AST and ALT levels are slightly elevated, and bilirubin and alkaline phosphatase levels are high.

17. Describe the pathologic changes associated with liver congestion.
Centrilobular congestion manifests as a dilated central vein, dilated sinusoids, and drop-out of perivenular hepatocytes in liver biopsies. If untreated, the stasis slowly progresses to perivenular

fibrosis, bridging fibrosis between the central veins, and eventually cirrhosis. Of note, most patients die of cardiac complications before they develop complications of liver cirrhosis.

18. What is the most common vascular tumor of the liver?
Hemangiomas are the most common vascular tumors of the liver. Autopsy studies suggest that they are present in about 2–5% of the population. The incidence is similar in males and females, but tumors are larger in females, suggesting a proliferative effect of female hormones. Most patients are asymptomatic and do not require treatment. In large hemangiomas, disseminated intravascular coagulation (DIC), thrombocytopenia, and hypofibrinogenemia may occur (Kasabach-Merritt syndrome). The most specific diagnostic technique is [99m]technetium-labeled red blood scan, which works best if the hemangioma is > 2 cm. In small hemangiomas, MRI or angiography may be helpful. Liver biopsy, unless indicated for another reason, should not be performed. Hemangiomas usually grow little, if any, in adults. Treatment, which is usually resection, is reserved for patients with DIC or bleeding complications.

19. How common is angiosarcoma of the liver?
It is extremely rare: 1 in 50,000 in autopsy studies. Angiosarcoma of the liver usually occurs in the sixth or seventh decade of life and is more common in men than women. Angiosarcomas originate from the endothelial lining of the sinusoid. Histologic examination reveals characteristic spindle-shaped tumor cells with hyperchromatic nuclei. Exposures to thorium oxide (Thorotrast), vinyl chloride, and arsenic are among the predisposing factors. Prognosis is dismal, and most patients die within 6 months of diagnosis.

20. Which vascular tumors of the liver synthesize factor VIII-related antigen?
Histologically, there are two cells types: epithelioid and dendritic. These cells are located in a mixed stroma that is fibrotic and, at times, calcified. Many dendritic cells may have characteristic vacuoles that help in the diagnosis. Most patients present with constitutional symptoms (45%), anorexia, fatigue, and right upper quadrant pain. Alpha fetoprotein is usually normal. The diagnosis is made with CT and biopsy. Angiography, if performed, usually reveals a vascular mass, and [99m]technetium-tagged red blood cell scan is negative. Although in some patients the clinical course is long, such tumors should be resected, if possible. In nonresectable tumors, liver transplantation has been performed. Recurrence after liver transplantation also has been reported.

21. What are the common causes of portal vein thrombosis?
The most common cause of portal vein thrombosis in children is infectious thrombosis due to omphalitis. In adults, portal vein thrombosis is seen in low-flow states such as portal hypertension in cirrhosis; hypercoagulable states associated with BCS; surrounding inflammation, such as retroperitoneal infections or pancreatitis; or procedure-related traumatic complications, such as postoperative or postangiography events.

22. Describe the presentation of portal vein thrombosis. How is it diagnosed and treated?
In the acute phase, patients present with abdominal pain, fever, ileus, and liver failure. In the more chronic form, patients present with ascites, splenomegaly, and variceal bleeding. Portal venography is the diagnostic test of choice. Heparin and thrombolytic agents have been tried in the acute phase, but the success rate is not very good. If the portal vein thrombosis extends to the splenic or superior mesenteric veins, the transplantation becomes technically impossible. Prognosis is poor.

BIBLIOGRAPHY

1. Blendis LM: Circulation in liver disease. Transplant Proc. 25:1741–1743, 1993.
2. Chu G, Farrell GC: Portal vein thrombosis associated with prolonged ingestion of oral contraceptive steroids. J Gastroenterol Hepatol 8:390–393, 1993.
3. Deltenre P, Denninger MH, Hillarie S, et al: Factor V Leiden related Budd-Chiari syndrome. Gut 48:264–268, 2001.
4. Dilawari JB, Bambery P, Chawla Y, et al: Hepatic outflow obstruction (Budd-Chiari syndrome): Experience with 177 patients and review of the literature. Medicine 73:21–36, 1994.

5. Gertsch P, Matthews J, Lerut J, et al: Acute thrombosis of the splanchnic veins. Arch Surg 128:341–345, 1993.
6. Glassman AB, Jones E: Thrombosis and coagulation abnormalities associated with cancer. Ann Clin Lab Sci 24:1–5, 1994.
7. Janssen HL, Meinardi JR, Vleggaar FP, et al: Factor V leiden mutation, prothrombin gene mutation, and deficiencies in coagulation inhibitors associated with Budd-Chiari syndrome and portal vein thrombosis: Results of case-control study. Blood 96:2364–2368, 2000.
8. MuCuskey RS, Reilly FD: Hepatic microvasculature: Dynamic structure and its regulation. Semin Liver Dis 13:1–12, 1993.
9. Naschitz JE, Solbodin G, Lewis RJ, et al: Heart diseases affecting the liver and liver diseases affecting the heart. Am Heart J 140:111–120, 2000.
10. Panis Y, Belghiti J, Valla D, et al: Portosystemic shunt in Budd-Chiari syndrome: Long-term survival and factors affecting shunt patency in 25 patients in Western countries. Surgery 115:276–281, 1994.
11. Seeto RK, Fenn B, Rockey DC. Ischemic hepatitis: Clinical presentation and pathogenesis. Am J Med 109:109–113, 2000.
12. Shulman HM, et al: Veno-occlusive disease of the liver after marrow transplantation. Histological correlates of clinical signs and symptoms. Hepatology 19:1171–1180, 1994.
13. Tan HP, Markowitz JS, Maley WR, et al: Successful liver transplantation in a patient with Budd-Chiari syndrome caused by homozygous factor V leiden. Liver Transplant 6:654–656, 2000.
14. Toledo-Pereyra LH, Suzuki S: Cellular and biomolecular mechanisms of liver ischemia. Transplant Proc 26:325–327, 1994.

28. NONALCOHOLIC STEATOHEPATITIS

Steven Zacks, M.D., M.P.H., and Roshan Shrestha, M.D.

1. Define nonalcoholic steatohepatitis (NASH).

It is the presence of macrovesicular fatty changes (steatosis) and lobular inflammation in the absence of alcoholism. Although inflammation is necessary for the diagnosis of NASH, NASH is part of a spectrum of nonalcoholic fatty liver disease ranging from steatosis (fatty infiltration without inflammation) to steatosis with inflammation (NASH) to NASH with fibrosis and cirrhosis.

2. How is NASH diagnosed?

The diagnosis of primary NASH depends on convincing evidence of negligible (< 20 gm/day) alcohol consumption and must include a negative evaluation for chronic hepatitis C virus infection (antibody to hepatitis C virus) and hepatitis B virus infection (hepatitis B surface antigen). Ceruloplasmin and α_1-antitrypsin levels are usually normal. Idiopathic genetic hemochromatosis must be excluded because in one series elevated levels of serum ferritin and transferrin saturation were found in up to 58% of patients with NASH. Autoimmune serology (antimitochondrial antibody, antinuclear antibody, antismooth muscle antibody, and antiliver/kidney microsomal antibody) should remain negative, although some patients may have low titers of antinuclear antibodies (ranging from 1:40 to 1:320). A substantial portion of cases of cryptogenic cirrhosis may be "burnt-out" NASH, because a high proportion are associated with obesity, type 2 diabetes, or hyperlipidemia.

3. Discuss the prevalence of NASH.

There are few data about the prevalence of NASH in the United States. In the recent National Health and Nutrition Examination Survey (NHANES-3), 2.6% of the U.S. population had raised values of serum alanine aminotransferase (ALT) for which no cause of chronic liver disease could be found, suggesting a diagnosis of NASH. Raised ALT concentration was significantly associated with increased waist-to-hip ratio and indices of insulin resistance.

Using the presence of a hyperechoic liver on ultrasound as a diagnostic criterion, 14% of 2574 randomly selected Japanese subjects had fatty liver. Because ultrasound can detect only fat, not all of these patients had the inflammation necessary for a diagnosis of NASH. Autopsy studies demonstrate NASH in 18.5% of obese subjects and 2.7% of normal-weight people. In the U.S., 20% of apparently normal people evaluated as donors for living-related liver transplants had fatty liver and 7.5% had NASH. In Japan, fatty liver was detected in 9.2% subjects assessed for living donation.

4. How can you distinguish between NASH and alcoholic steatohepatitis?

An alcohol history is the key to distinguishing the two entities. Because patients may not be honest about alcohol consumption, a number of tests have been devised to detect excessive alcohol consumption. Among several indicators of excessive alcohol consumption, the ratio of desialyted transferrin to total transferrin is the best single marker.

5. Describe the natural history of NASH.

It was thought that NASH had a benign course, with few patients progressing to decompensated cirrhosis, but more recent studies suggest that up to 40% of patients with fibrosis may develop cirrhosis. Prognosis correlates with the amount of inflammatory change seen on biopsy. Patients with a significant inflammatory activity on biopsy are more likely to progress to cirrhosis. In patients who developed cirrhosis and/or had a liver related death, ninety percent had ballooning degeneration or ballooning degeneration with polymorphonuclear cell infiltration, Mallory's hyaline, or fibrosis.

NASH may be less serious than alcoholic hepatitis. During a follow-up period of 1–7 years, the progression to cirrhosis occurred in approximately 8–17% of patients with NASH compared with 38–50% of patients with alcoholic hepatitis.

6. What factors predict the presence of steatosis and fibrosis in NASH?

In one retrospective study of 144 patients with NASH, older age, obesity, presence of diabetes mellitus, and an aspartate aminotransferase (AST)/ALT ratio > 1 were significant predictors of severe liver fibrosis (bridging/cirrhosis). Body mass index was the only independent predictor of the degree of fat infiltration. Increased transferrin iron saturation correlated positively with the severity of fibrosis in univariate analysis. Female patients tended to have more advanced fibrosis. Neither iron transferrin saturation nor gender was significant after controlling for age, obesity, diabetes, and AST/ALT ratio in the multivariate analysis.

7. Describe the pathogenesis of NASH.

It is unknown. Accumulation of fat in the liver can occur because of:
• Increased delivery of free fatty acids (FFA) to the liver
• Increased synthesis of fatty acids in the liver
• Decreased α-oxidation of FFA
• Decreased synthesis or secretion of very-low-density lipoprotein.

8. What conditions are associated with NASH?

Morbid obesity is the most common. Jejunoileal and gastric bypass for obesity are also associated with NASH. Non–insulin-dependent diabetes mellitus occurs in 20–75% of patients with NASH. Hyperlipidemia is seen in 20–80% of patients. Less commonly, short bowel syndrome and long-term use of total parenteral nutrition are associated with NASH. Jejunal diverticulosis with bacterial overgrowth can cause NASH. In children, galactosemia, abetalipoproteinemia, Weber-Christian disease, fructose intolerance, and cholesterol ester storage disease are associated with fatty infiltration.

9. Describe the clinical features of NASH.

Most patients with primary NASH are women (65–83%), and most are obese (69–100%). The majority of patients are 10–40% heavier than ideal body weight. Non–insulin-dependent diabetes mellitus is present in 25–75% of patients. The mean age at diagnosis is 50 years, but ages range from 16 to 80 years. A high proportion of patients (48–100%) have no symptoms of liver disease. A small proportion may have right upper quadrant discomfort. Many patients come to light when liver tests are done as part of the management of other conditions associated with NASH (e.g., dyslipidemia). Although patients may not have any signs of liver disease, some may have hepatomegaly. A few patients may present with signs and symptoms of decompensated cirrhosis.

10. What is the most common laboratory abnormality in patients with NASH?

A 2–3-fold elevation of serum levels of ALT and AST. The AST/ALT ratio appears to be a useful index for distinguishing nonalcoholic steatohepatitis from alcoholic liver disease. Although values < 1 suggest NASH, a ratio of ≤ 2 is strongly suggestive of alcoholic liver disease.

11. What other laboratory abnormalities may be found?

Bilirubin levels are usually normal. In 12–17% of patients, the bilirubin barely exceeds 1.5–2.0 mg/dl. Alkaline phosphatase levels are modestly elevated in 39–59% of patients. Hypoalbuminemia and hypoprothrombinemia are less common. Hemosiderosis with elevated iron saturations may be seen.

Immunoserologic findings compatible with autoimmune hepatitis are commonly present with primary NASH. Hypergammaglobulinemia is present in 13–30% of patients with primary NASH. Although smooth muscle antibodies are absent, antinuclear antibodies, ranging in titer from 1:40 to 1:320, are observed in 40% of patients.

Hyperlipidemia (hypertriglyceridemia and hypercholesterolemia) is found in about 20% of patients. In a group of overweight patients (150–300% of ideal weight for height), lipoprotein abnormalities, particularly type IV hyperlipidemia, are common (54%). The lipoprotein abnormalities are mostly found in patients with less fibrotic NASH. Abnormal results of iron tests (elevated levels of serum ferritin and transferrin saturation) were seen in 58% of a series of patients. Elevations in serum ferritin levels as great as fivefold have been reported in the absence of histologic evidence of idiopathic genetic hemochromatosis.

The lack of specificity of standard liver tests limits their usefulness in diagnosing NASH and differentiating it from fatty liver without inflammation. If all of the serologic tests for other causes of liver disease are negative and the patient has a risk factor for NASH (e.g., obesity, diabetes mellitus, a diagnosis of fatty liver or NASH as a cause of the elevated liver tests can usually be made with some degree of certainty.

12. List the four types of biopsy findings in patients with fatty liver disease, and give the prevalence of each.

Type 1: fatty liver alone (37%)
Type 2: fat accumulation and lobular inflammation (7.5%)
Type 3: fat accumulation and ballooning degeneration (14%)
Type 4: fat accumulation, ballooning degeneration, and either Mallory hyaline or fibrosis (41%; highest proportion of cirrhosis and liver-related death)

13. What medications are associated with NASH?

Chloroquine, diltiazem, nifedipine, amiodarone, glucocorticoids, tamoxifen, and estrogens.

14. Summarize the classification of NASH.

Classification of Nonalcoholic Steatohepatitis

Primary NASH	**Secondary NASH** *(cont'd)*
• Obesity	*Other metabolic factors*
• Diabetes	• Total parenteral nutrition
• Hyperlipidemia	• Acute starvation
Secondary NASH	• Rapid weight loss
Drug treatments	*Miscellaneous*
• Amiodarone	• Bacterial overgrowth (jejunal diverticulosis)
• Glucocorticoids	• Limb lipodystrophy
• Synthetic estrogens	• Abetalipoproteinemia
• Tamoxifen	• Weber-Christian disease
Surgical procedures	
• Jejunal bypass	
• Gastroplasty for morbid obesity	
• Biliopancreatic diversion	
• Extensive small bowel resection	

15. Describe the typical radiologic features of NASH.

The most specific tests for the diagnosis of fatty liver and therefore NASH appear to be imaging techniques. Ultrasound is a relatively specific method for the identification of fat in the liver (a hyperechoic or bright liver). The sensitivity of ultrasound in diagnosing small amounts of fat is unclear. On CT scan the liver appears less dense than the spleen with a ratio of densities < 0.9. On MRI, the changes of NASH are most pronounced on T1 weighted images; the liver appears very hypointense (dark). Neither MR nor CT imaging is more sensitive than ultrasound in the diagnosis of fatty liver, nor does either help in distinguishing fatty liver from NASH. Tumors of the liver can have the appearance of focal fat, especially on ultrasound. Additional imaging by either CT or MRI may be necessary in this group of patients to be certain that the findings represent focal fat and not a malignancy.

16. Is liver biopsy necessary to establish the diagnosis and what are the pathologic features of NASH?

The definitive diagnosis of steatohepatitis can be made only by liver biopsy. Sonography may suggest the presence of a fatty liver, but it cannot detect hepatitis. The histologic stage (prefibrotic vs. fibrotic vs. cirrhotic) also can be definitively identified only by liver biopsy. Staging is useful in assessing prognosis and potential therapeutic interventions.

17. What histologic changes are associated with NASH?

Histologic changes of NASH may mirror those of alcoholic steatohepatitis. The main findings are macrovesicular and microvesicular fatty changes within the centrilobular hepatocytes (zone 3). Polymorphonuclear and mononuclear leukocyte and lymphocyte infiltration of portal tracts and parenchyma also is present. Although the changes are most often seen in zone 3, fatty changes within the hepatocytes and inflammatory changes may occur in all zones of the hepatic lobule. Histologic exam may show focal necrosis of centrilobular hepatocytes and hyaline (Mallory bodies) within these hepatocytes. The hyaline bodies are usually sparse, small, and centrilobular. The ultrastructure of Mallory bodies in patients with NASH is similar to those in patients with alcoholic hepatitis. The wide spectrum of fibrosis ranges from mild to cirrhotic. Typically, the fibrosis begins in the centrilobular region and is pericellular or perivenular but may develop along the sinusoids. The prevalence of mild-to-moderate fibrosis is 76–100%; of severe fibrosis, 15–50%. Cirrhosis is described less frequently in adults (7–16%) and is absent in children. Approximately 10–20% of patients may have cirrhosis. Iron may be found within hepatocytes and Kupffer cells, but the hepatic iron index is < 1.9.

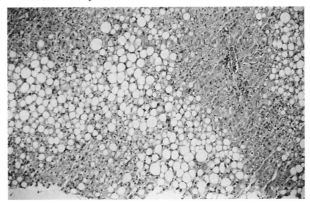

Nonalcoholic steatohepatitis with inflammatory cells, fat cells and necrosis (hematoxylyn-eosin stain).

18. What grading and staging system is used to describe the histologic features of NASH?

Grading and Staging of NASH

Necroinflammatory activity

Grade 1   Steatosis (predominantly macrovesicular) involving up to 66% of biopsy; occasional ballooned zone 3 hepatocytes; scattered rate of intra-acinar PMNs with or without intra-acinar lymphocytes; no or mild portal chronic inflammation.

Grade 2   Steatosis of any degree; obvious ballooning of hepatocytes (predominantly zone 3); intra-acinar PMNs; may be associated with zone 3 pericellular fibrosis; portal and intra-acinar chronic inflammation (mild to moderate).

Grade 3   Panacinar steatosis; obvious ballooning and disarray, predominantly in zone 3; intra-acinar inflammation noted as scattered PMNs; PMNs associated with ballooned hepatocytes with or without mild chronic inflammation; portal chronic inflammation mild or moderate, not marked.

Grading and Staging of NASH (Continued)

Fibrosis

Stage 1	Zone 3 perisinusoidal/pericellular fibrosis; focally or extensively present.
Stage 2	Zone 3 perisinusoidal/pericellular fibrosis with focal or extensive periportal fibrosis.
Stage 3	Zone 3 perisinusoidal/pericellular fibrosis and portal fibrosis with focal or extensive bridging fibrosis.
Stage 4	Cirrhosis

PMN = polymorphonuclear neutrophil.
From Brunt EM, Janney CG, Di Bisceglie AM, et al: Nonalcoholic steatohepatitis: A proposal for grading and staging the histological lesions. Am J Gastroenterol 94:2467–2474, 1999, with permission.

19. How is NASH treated?

Although there are no established treatments for NASH, empirical treatment strategies have been proposed. Gradual weight reduction can improve laboratory abnormalities, histologic changes, and hepatomegaly. However, improvements can be achieved even if the patient remains obese. On the other hand, striking weight losses also have been associated with progression of NASH. The long-term benefit of weight loss is difficult to evaluate because patients with NASH would have to maintain sustained reductions in weight. Obese patients with NASH rarely achieve or maintain sustained reductions in weight. Moreover, the effect of weight loss on liver disease is not consistent. For patients with significant obesity (75% overweight) who are not successful at dieting, gastric bypass or gastroplasty may significantly reduce steatosis.

Ursodeoxycholic acid may have a membrane-stabilizing and cytoprotective effect, although some studies have failed to demonstrate a significant benefit. Despite its lipid-lowering properties, clofibrate therapy for 1 year in patients with NASH and hypertriglyceridemia was not found to be beneficial.

A small trial suggests that gemfibrazole improves transaminases and serum lipids after 1 month's treatment, possibly by inhibiting free fatty acid mobilization from adipose tissue. Small, short-duration studies suggest that α-tocopherol, vitamin E, and combinations of lecithin, vitamin C, low-dose vitamin E, β-carotene, selenium, and vitamin B complex can produce some improvements in liver tests. Some of these studies failed to show an improvement in histology. No evidence indicates that treatment of non–insulin-dependent diabetes associated with NASH has an effect on liver disease. Future therapies may be directed at cytokine-triggered mechanisms, including COX-2 inhibitors and measures to reduce accumulation of visceral fat.

Patients with decompensated cirrhosis from NASH can undergo successful liver transplantation, but it is possible for NASH to recur in the graft after transplantation. The weight gain and dyslipidemias seen after successful liver transplantation may contribute to the recurrence of NASH.

20. What proportion of patients with NASH undergo liver transplantation?

Although the vast majority of patients with NASH exhibit a benign course, progressive disease has been reported in 15–20% of patients. However, few patients with NASH develop cirrhosis and liver failure and require transplantation.

Follow-up of patients transplanted for NASH has been limited, but recurrence has been noted as early as 6–10 weeks after transplantation. Rapid weight gain and the presence of a functioning jejunoileal bypass seem to be the most reliable predictors of recurrent NASH. No therapy has been reported to be of value in treating recurrent NASH after transplantation with the exception of reversing a jejunoileal bypass. Weight loss in obese patients transplanted for primary NASH has been proposed as important in preventing recurrent disease.

21. Are there any other liver diseases, besides alcoholic liver disease, in which fat is seen on biopsy?

Microvesicular fatty changes can be seen in hepatitis C and Wilson's disease.

BIBLIOGRAPHY

1. Angulo P, Keach JC, Batts KP, Lindor KD: Independent predictors of liver fibrosis in patients with nonalcoholic steatohepatitis. Hepatology 30:1356–1362, 1999.
2. Bacon BR, Farahvash MJ, Janney CG, et al: Nonalcoholic steatohepatitis: An expanded clinical entity. Gastroenterology
107:1103–1109, 1994.
3. Brunt EM, Janney CG, Di Bisceglie AM, et al: Nonalcoholic steatohepatitis: A proposal for grading and staging the histological lesions. Am J Gastroenterol 94:2467–2474, 1999.
4. Caldwell SH, Oelsner DH, Iezzoni JC, et al: Cryptogenic cirrhosis: Clinical characterization and risk factors for underlying disease. Hepatology 29:664–669, 1999.
5. Diehl AM: Nonalcoholic steatohepatitis. Semin Liver Dis 10:221–229, 1999.
6. Kim WR, Poterucha JJ, Porayko MK et al: Recurrence of nonalcoholic steatohepatitis following liver transplantation.
Transplantation 62:1802–1805, 1996.
7. Matteoni CA, Younossi ZM, Gramlich T, et al: Nonalcoholic fatty liver disease: A spectrum of clinical and pathological
severity. Gastroenterology 116:1413–1419, 1999.
8. Powell EE, Cooksley WGE, Hanson R, et al: The natural history of nonalcoholic steatohepatitis: A follow-up study of
forty-two patients for up to 21 years. Hepatology 11:74–80, 1990.
9. Sheth SG, Gordon FD, Chopra S: Nonalcoholic steatohepatitis. Ann Intern Med 126:137–145, 1997.
10. Sorbi D, Boynton J, Lindor KD: The ratio of aspartate aminotransferase to alanine aminotransferase: Potential value in
differentiating nonalcoholic steatohepatitis from alcoholic liver disease. Am J Gastroenterol 94:1018–1022, 1999.
11. Teli MR, James OFW, Burt AD, et al: The natural history of nonalcoholic fatty liver: A follow-up study. Hepatology
22:1714–1719, 1995.
12. Tilg H, Diehl AM: Cytokines in alcoholic and nonalcoholic steatohepatitis. N Engl J Med 343:1467–1476, 2000.
13. Wanless IR, Lentz JS: Fatty liver hepatitis (steatohepatitis) and obesity: An autopsy study with analysis of risk factors.
Hepatology 12:1106–1110, 1990.

29. LIVER TRANSPLANTATION

Andrew J. Muir, M.D., and James F. Trotter, M.D.

PATIENT REFERRAL AND SELECTION

1. For patients with chronic liver disease, when is the appropriate time to refer for liver transplantation?

The decision to list a patient for transplantation ultimately rests with the transplant center. Minimal listing criteria have been developed by consensus of members of the United Network for Organ Sharing (UNOS) to identify patients with < 90% 1-year anticipated survival without transplant. The current minimal listing UNOS criteria require a Child-Turcotte-Pugh (CTP) score of at least seven. All patients with a CTP score > 7 should be referred for transplant evaluation. Other indications for transplant referral include ascites, encephalopathy, portal hypertensive bleeding, or depressed hepatic function. Coexistent medical disorders such as coronary artery disease or chronic obstructive lung disease may jeopardize successful liver transplant, especially in the elderly. Most transplant centers do not list patients older than 65 years with significant comorbities.

2. How is the CTP score determined?

Child-Turcotte-Pugh Criteria

PARAMETER	POINTS		
	1	2	3
Ascites	Absent/slight	Moderate/controlled by diuretics	Severe
Bilirubin (mg/dl)	< 2.0	2.0–3.0	> 3.0
For PSC or PBC	< 4	4–10	> 10
Albumin (gm/dl)	> 3.5	2.8–3.5	< 2.8
PT (sec > control; INR)	1–3 (< 1.7)	4–6 (1.8–2.3)	> 6 (> 2.3)
Encephalopathy	None	Grade 1–2	Grade 3–4
Total score Class A 5–6 Class B 7–9 Class C 10–15			

PSC = primary sclerosing cholangitis, PBC = primary biliary cirrhosis, PT = prothrombin time, INR = international normalized ratio.

3. On what basis are donor livers allocated?

Donor livers are allocated on the basis of UNOS status, ABO blood group, recipient body size, and donor liver size. At most transplant centers in the United States, the median waiting time for a liver transplant is 1–3 years. Therefore, early referral should be considered before the onset of complications that may affect either the patient's surgical candidacy or survival on the waiting list.

4. How is UNOS status determined?

1   Fulminant liver failure

2a   In ICU with a life expectancy < 7 days; CTP score ≥ 10; meets at least one of the medical criteria (documented unresponsive active variceal hemorrhage, portal gastropathy, hepatorenal syndrome, refractory ascites/hepatohydrothorax, or stage III or IV encephalopathy unresponsive to medical therapy)

2b   CTP score ≥ 10 or CTP score ≥ 7 and one of the medical criteria (listed with 2a status).
3   Requires continuous care and has CTP > 7.
7   Temporarily inactive.

5. What can be done to improve the availability of donor organs?

A recent report estimated that only 15–20% of potential donors in the United States donated their organs. Although logistic issues undoubtedly contribute to this low rate, many families refuse consent for donation. Reports have found that rates of consent for donation are significantly lower among minority groups. A Howard University survey of the African-American community found five principal reasons for refusal of donation:
1. Lack of awareness of the status of organ transplantation
2. Religious beliefs and misconceptions about transplantation
3. Distrust of the medical establishment
4. Fear of premature death among potential organ donors
5. Desire for recipients to be African-American.

Public Education Programs conducted by African American organ procurement coordinators have decreased apprehension about organ donation and increased minority participation.

6. Given the long waiting period for liver transplant, is living donor liver transplantation (LDLT) an option?

Approximately 10% of patients listed for liver transplantation in the United States die each year awaiting a suitable donor organ. To help reduce this high mortality rate, several transplant centers now offer LDLT for selected patients. Most adult–adult LDLTs in the United States utilize the right hepatic lobe from the donor. The key advantage of LDLT is reduction in waiting time for the recipient. Disadvantages of LDLT include risk to the donor and lack of long-term viability data for the LDLT. Among the 300 adult–adult right hepatic lobe LDLTs performed in the United States since 1997, there has been 1 reported death of a donor. Morbidity, including bile leaks and infections, occurs in approximately 5% of donors. A recent series found the procedure effective and safe for both donor and recipient when performed at an experienced transplant center.

7. What factors are considered in donor selection for LDLT?

Donor selection requires a thorough medical and psychological evaluation to ensure that the patient can tolerate the procedure and understands the risks. Donors should be similar in size to the recipient and 18– 60 years of age; they should have an identical or compatible blood type. The discovery of significant medical problems in the donor may preclude organ donation.

8. List the diseases for which transplant is performed.

Indications for transplant, with the percent of total transplants for the years 1996–1998:
Acute liver failure (7%)
• Cryptogenic
• Viral hepatitis (A, B, other)
• Drug-induced (acetaminophen, isoniazid, disulfiram, halothane, ecstasy, other)
• Metabolic liver disease (Wilson's disease, Reye's syndrome)
• Vascular (ischemic liver failure)
• Toxin (*Amanita* sp. mushroom)
Chronic liver failure (75%)
• Alcoholic liver disease
• Chronic viral hepatitis (B, B+D, C)
• Autoimmune hepatitis
• Primary biliary cirrhosis
• Primary sclerosing cholangitis
• Nonalcoholic steatohepatitis
• Budd-Chiari syndrome
• Drug-induced cirrhosis (methotrexate, amiodarone)
• Sarcoidosis
• Graft-vs.-host disease
• Polycystic liver disease
• Cryptogenic cirrhosis

Congenital/metabolic liver disease (9%)
- Hemochromatosis
- Wilson's disease
- Alpha-1 antitrypsin deficiency

- Cystic fibrosis
- Amyloidosis

Hepatic tumors (2%)
- Hepatocellular carcinoma (for tumors < 5 cm)
- Hepatic adenoma
- Carcinoid tumor

9. What dose of acetaminophen is hepatotoxic?

Acetaminophen is the most common cause of drug-induced liver failure. Acute ingestion of > 12 gm of acetaminophen is predictive of hepatic injury. Its toxic metabolite, N-acetyl-p-benzo-quinoneimine, results from metabolism by the cytochrome P450 system. Chronic alcohol ingestion and use of many medications (e.g., phenytoin, carbamazepine, isoniazid, rifampin) may induce the cytochrome P450 system, which reduces the amount of acetaminophen required to induce hepatotoxicity. The acetaminophen level is highly predictive of hepatotoxicity. Without treatment, an acetaminophen level > 300 µg/ml at 4 hours or > 45 µg/ml at 15 hours is associated with a 90% risk of hepatotoxicity.

10. How can acetaminophen hepatotoxicity be treated?

All patients with elevated liver enzymes and a history consistent with acetaminophen overdose should be considered for treatment. If patients present within 4 hours of ingestion, activated charcoal can reduce acetaminophen absorption. N-acetylcysteine (Mucomyst), a glutathione precursor, remains the treatment of choice for acetaminophen-induced hepatotoxicity. The loading dose is 150 mg/kg, followed by 70 mg/kg every 4 hours for 17 doses. Although more effective when given within 10 hours of ingestion, benefits may occur with administration up to 24 hours.

11. A 21-year-old woman is admitted after an overdose of acetaminophen. How do you determine whether she should be referred for liver transplantation?

Although hepatotoxicity resolves in many patients with acetaminophen intoxication, the King's College Criteria identified two groups of patients unlikely to recover. Patients with an arterial blood pH < 7.30 had a 90% mortality rate without liver transplantation. In patients with a combination of prothrombin time (PT) > 100 seconds, serum creatinine > 3.3 mg/dl, and grade III or IV encephalopathy, the mortality rate was 81%. Patients with worsening liver function or any of these signs need prompt transfer to a liver transplant center.

12. Define fulminant hepatic failure.

Fulminant hepatic failure is defined as the onset of encephalopathy within 8 weeks of the development of symptoms in a patient with no preexisting liver disease. Patients typically present with a history of progressive lethargy and jaundice over the course of several days.

13. What are the common causes of fulminant hepatic failure?

Possible causes include viral hepatitis, drugs or toxins, Wilson's disease, Budd Chiari syndrome, and hepatic ischemia. Hepatitis C is a rare cause of fulminant hepatic failure. The largest series of fulminant hepatitis patients (n = 295) reported in the United States, identified the following causes:
- Acetaminophen (20%)
- Cryptogenic (15%)
- Drug reactions (12%)

- Hepatitis B (10%)
- Hepatitis A (7%)

14. How should patients with fulminant hepatic failure be managed?

Patients with fulminant hepatic failure require prompt referral to a liver transplant center. Patients may progress from stage II encephalopathy to full coma within a matter of hours. The

King's College Criteria also address fulminant hepatic failure from causes other than acetaminophen. Patients fulfilling the following criteria have a > 90% risk of mortality and will benefit from liver transplantation:
1. PT > 100 seconds *or*
2. Any three of the following:
   • Age < 10 years or > 40 years
   • Etiology: non-A, non-B hepatitis; halothane; drug reaction
   • Duration of jaundice before onset of encephalopathy > 7 days
   • PT > 50 seconds
   • Serum bilirubin > 18 mg/dl

15. What other options are available to support a patient with fulminant hepatic failure?
Several versions of bioartificial livers are currently in clinical trials to examine their ability to support patients with fulminant hepatic failure until a donor liver is available or regeneration occurs. The artificial livers use either porcine or hepatoblastoma-derived hepatocytes as a biofilter over which either plasma or whole blood is perfused.

16. What conditions are considered contraindications to liver transplantation?
Absolute contraindications
• Extrahepatic malignancy
• Uncontrolled sepsis/infection
• Active alcohol or drug use
• Inadequate social support
• Hepatocellular carcinoma (lesions > 5 cm)
• Advanced cardiopulmonary disease (including coronary artery disease, congestive heart failure, and severe chronic obstructive pulmonary disease)
• Human immunodeficiency virus (HIV) infection
Relative contraindications
These conditions vary according to severity of disease and experience of the center:
• Portal vein thrombosis
• Cholangiocarcinoma (previous experience reveals a high rate of recurrence and poor survival)
• Advanced age (> 65 years)
• Pulmonary hypertension (uncontrolled)

17. Which features of the psychosocial profile connote a good prognosis for continued abstinence from alcohol?
For patients with a history of alcohol abuse, most centers require a period of abstinence (usually 6–12 months) and evaluation with a substance abuse professional before transplantation is considered. The length of abstinence may not be a good predictor of recidivism. If the onset of symptoms of liver disease led to abstinence, the patient may use alcohol when feeling well again. Recognition of alcoholism by the patient and family members is especially important, as demonstrated through adherence to an alcohol rehabilitation program. Other features associated with a low rate of recidivism include lack of comorbid substance abuse, social function, and lack of family history.

18. What is the prognosis for alcoholic patients who undergo liver transplantation?
Properly selected alcoholics usually do well after transplantation. The long-term posttransplant survival rate of appropriately selected alcoholics is higher than that of comparable nonalcoholic patients.

19. Which factors measured before transplant correlate with reduced survival rates after liver transplantation?
Early experience with liver transplantation found that cholangiocarcinoma and hepatitis B infection were associated with poor outcome. As a result, cholangiocarcinoma has become a

contraindication for transplant. The outcomes with hepatitis B have improved with the introduction of hepatitis B immunoglobulin and lamivudine. Previous reports suggested that clinical factors, including CTP score, are not good predictors of survival after transplantation. However, poor renal function before transplant predicts poorer survival rates. Repeat transplant is also associated with worse outcome.

20. How does the quality of the graft affect survival rates?

Fatty infiltration is associated with increased primary nonfunction and decreased survival rates. Although older donor age (> 50 years) led to decreased survival at 3 months in one study, many of the donor livers were assessed as fair or poor by the harvesting surgeon. Recipients of older donor livers with a good assessment had survival rates similar to those for recipients of younger donor livers.

EARLY POSTTRANSPLANT PERIOD (1–4 WEEKS)

21. How do cyclosporine and tacrolimus (FK506) prevent allograft rejection?

Cyclosporine and tacrolimus have different binding sites but a similar mechanism of action. Cyclosporine binds to cyclophyllin, whereas tacrolimus binds to the FK-binding protein to create an active complex. The active complex inhibits calcineurin, a calcium-dependent phosphatase, which prevents T-cell activation through inhibition of several critical transcription factors and cytokines, including interleukin-2 (IL-2).

22. Describe the typical immunosuppressive regimen.

The specific immunosuppressive regimen varies from center to center. Current immunosuppressive therapy involves multiple agents that operate through different mechanisms to increase the immunosuppressive effect while minimizing the side effects of any one agent. The two most common regimens at this time are as follows:

1. Cyclosporine (Sandimmune or Neoral), prednisone and azathioprine (Imuran) or mycophenolate mofetil (Cellcept)

2. Tacrolimus (Prograf) and prednisone

23. How do azathioprine and mycophenolate mofetil work?

Azathioprine is a derivative of 6-mercaptopurine and inhibits purine biosynthesis. It is the prodrug for 6-mercaptopurine, which is metabolized by hypoxanthine guanine phosphoribosyltransferase to thioinosinic and thioguanylic acid. These compounds suppress inosinic acid synthesis and therefore interfere with purine biosynthesis. **Mycophenolate mofetil** impairs lymphocyte function by blocking purine biosynthesis through inhibition of the enzyme inosine monophosphate dehydrogenase. Neither azathioprine nor mycophenolate causes nephrotoxicity, but both may cause bone marrow suppression and dyspepsia.

24. What is the role of long-term maintenance corticosteroids?

Increasing evidence indicates that long-term maintenance corticosteroids may not be necessary to prevent rejection. Liver transplantation may be performed successfully without corticosteroids or with a rapid (14-day) steroid taper. In addition, many centers wean patients from corticosteroids within 1–2 years after transplantation.

25. What other antirejection drugs are available? How do they work?

Sirolimus is a macrolide antibiotic recently approved by the Food and Drug Administration (FDA) for prevention of acute renal transplant rejection. Ongoing studies should provide more information about sirolimus, and its role may increase in liver transplantation. Sirolimus is related structurally to tacrolimus and shares the same binding site. However, sirolimus possesses a distinct mechanism of action and does not affect calcineurin activity. Instead, it blocks signals transduced from IL-2 receptors and other growth factors to the nucleus, thus inhibiting T- and B-cell proliferation.

Antithymocyte globulin (Atgam, Thymoglobulin) is a purified immunoglobulin prepared from hyperimmune serum of horse, rabbit, sheep, or goat after immunization with human thymic lymphocytes. Antithymocyte globulin binds to the surface of T lymphocytes in the circulation, resulting in lymphopenia and impaired T lymphocyte immune responses. Antithymocyte globulin is given for steroid-resistant rejection and administered parenterally at a daily dose of 10–30 mg/kg over several hours.

Muromonab-CD3 (OKT3) was the first monoclonal antibody approved by the FDA for use in humans. OKT3 is directed to the ε chain of CD3, a three-chain molecule associated with the T-cell antigen receptor (TCR). CD3 is necessary for CD4-positive T-cell activation by alloantigens and for CD8-positive T-cell direct cellular cytotoxicity. The main indication of OKT3 is control of acute rejection. OKT3 is administered intravenously. After administration, a cytokine-release syndrome with flu-like symptoms is evident within 30–60 minutes. OKT3 also may lead to pulmonary edema and exacerbate congestive heart failure or coronary artery disease.

Daclizumab (Zenapax) and **basiliximab** (Simulect) are chimeric (murine/human) monoclonal antibodies that block the IL-2 receptor on T lymphocytes, thus interfering with the signal that activates T cells. When used as part of induction therapy in combination with corticosteroids and cyclosporine, both daclizumab and basiliximab reduced rejection episodes in renal transplantation.

26. A patient sustains a grand mal seizure 36 hours after liver transplant. The cyclosporine level is within acceptable limits. The patient is in a postictal state but has no obvious focal neurologic deficits. Which factors contribute to an increased risk of seizures after transplant?

Both cyclosporine and tacrolimus (FK506) have been associated with neurotoxicity, including seizures, paresthesias, ataxia, and delirium. Tremor is common with both medications and may improve with time. In general, these side effects were more common with intravenous preparations and elevated drug levels. In addition, they are usually reversible by reduction in dosage or discontinuation.

27. Three weeks after transplant a patient receives erythromycin for atypical pneumonia. Does this action affect immunosuppresive therapy?

Cyclosporine and tacrolimus are metabolized by the cytochrome P450 system, specifically P450-IIIA. Medications that inhibit P450-IIIA raise cyclosporine and tacrolimus levels and place the patient at risk for toxicity or excessive immunosuppression. Medications that induce P450-IIIA lower levels and increase the risk of rejection or require higher doses (with increased costs) of the immunosuppressant. If these medications are necessary, dose adjustment and monitoring of cyclosporine and tacrolimus may be necessary. Medications that commonly interact with cyclosporine and tacrolimus include:

Increased drug levels		Reduced drug levels
Erythromycin	Itraconazole	Phenytoin
Clarithromycin	Verapamil	Carbamazepine
Ketoconazole	Diltiazem	Phenobarbital
Fluconazole	Amiodarone	Rifampin

28. A patient who had an uncomplicated operation has rising liver enzymes on day 10 after transplantation. What is the differential diagnosis? Which tests should be obtained?

Elevated liver enzymes within the first 7–14 days may be the first indication of a significant problem with the hepatic allograft. A common cause of elevated liver enzymes is acute allograft rejection. Approximately 30–60 % of all liver transplant recipients experience acute cellular rejection within the first 3 months after transplant. Early diagnosis is critical to ensure prompt initiation of immunosuppressive therapy (corticosteroid pulse or OKT3) to prevent graft loss. Liver biopsy remains the gold standard for the diagnosis of cellular rejection. The differential diagnosis should include thrombus of the hepatic artery or portal vein, biliary leak, cholangitis, drug toxicity, recurrent viral hepatitis, and opportunistic infection. In general, opportunistic infections and recurrent viral hepatitis appear later than day 10. Appropriate tests may include cyclosporine or tacrolimus level, Doppler ultrasound, cholangiogram, and liver biopsy. If these tests are unrevealing, infectious etiologies should be considered.

29. A patient with cirrhosis from chronic hepatitis C undergoes liver transplantation. Ten days later, his liver enzymes increase. What are the histologic findings of acute rejection vs. posttransplant hepatitis C on liver biopsy?

The histologic features of acute cellular rejection include (1) mixed cellular infiltrate (including eosinophils) in the portal triad; (2) inflammation of the bile ducts presenting as either apoptosis or intraepithelial lymphocytes; and (3) endothelialitis of the central or portal veins. Recurrent hepatitis C can be difficult to distinguish from rejection. The histology may demonstrate a predominantly lymphocytic infiltrate in the portal areas rather than the mixed cellular infiltrate of rejection. Early in the course, steatosis may be the only finding of recurrent hepatitis C. Other signs include spotty parenchymal inflammation and vacuolization of the biliary epithelium.

30. List the other posttransplant complications manifested by elevated liver enzymes.

- Hepatic artery thrombosis
- Portal vein thrombosis
- Biliary leaks

- Medications
- Opportunistic infection
- Recurrent hepatic disease

31. How does artery thrombosis present? How is it managed?

Hepatic artery thrombosis remains a serious complication following transplant. The clinical presentation may be variable, but it usually is associated with elevated transaminases. Other signs include decreased bile output, persistent elevation of PT or bilirubin, and bacteremia. Cessation of hepatic artery blood flow preferentially causes ischemic damage to the extrahepatic biliary tree, resulting in breakdown of the biliary tree and development of bilomas, bile leaks, and eventually strictures. Early hepatic artery thrombosis may be amenable to interventional radiologic intervention but usually warrants reoperation. In hepatic artery thrombosis, retransplantation is usually required for successful long-term outcome.

32. How does portal vein thrombosis present? How is it managed?

In the early posttransplant period, portal vein thrombosis may present with signs of graft dysfunction and require immediate revascularization or retransplantation. Late thrombosis may be well tolerated or lead to graft dysfunction and portal hypertension. Balloon angioplasty, stent placement, and thrombolytic infusion have been used to reestablish the portal circulation.

33. Where do biliary leaks occur?

Biliary leaks may be asymptomatic but can lead to peritonitis. Biliary leaks can occur at the biliary anastomosis, at the T-tube exit site, at the time of T-tube removal, and within the liver as a result of bile duct destruction. Ischemic damage from hepatic artery thrombosis may be a contributing factor.

34. What patterns may characterize elevated liver enzymes due to medications?

A cholestatic pattern may occur with cyclosporine, tacrolimus, azathioprine, sulfa drugs, and various antibiotics. A hepatocellular pattern may occur with azathioprine, nonsteroidal anti-inflammatory drugs, and some antibiotics.

35. What is the most common opportunistic infection?

The most common opportunistic infection of the hepatic allograft is cytomegalovirus (CMV) infection. The infection may present as elevated liver enzymes. However, CMV infection is uncommon in the first month after transplant.

36. Which liver diseases are likely to recur?

Almost all patients with hepatitis C have recurrence of HCV infection. Most patients have mild-to-moderate transaminase elevations and mild-to-moderate inflammation on biopsy. In a minority of patients, both hepatitis B and C infection may lead to fibrosing cholestatic hepatitis, which can lead to cirrhosis and graft loss during the first year. Recurrent disease may also occur with autoimmune hepatitis, primary biliary cirrhosis, and sclerosing cholangitis.

LONG-TERM TRANSPLANT PERIOD (> 4 WEEKS)

37. A patient with early allograft rejection is treated with a 7-day course of OKT3 and returns 1 week later with headache, mild fatigue, low-grade fever, and increased liver enzymes. Is OKT3 toxicity the cause?

This scenario is unlikely to be due to OKT3 toxicity. Most reactions occur during the initial few days of OKT3 therapy and include rigors, flash pulmonary edema, bronchospasm, arthralgias, nausea, vomiting, and diarrhea. One concern is aseptic meningitis, which can present during or after OKT3 toxicity with headache, fever, fatigue, and meningismus.

38. If it is not OKT3 toxicity, what is the most likely diagnosis?

The differential diagnosis includes CMV infection, incomplete treatment of rejection, post-surgical complications (hepatic artery thrombosis, hepatic abscess, biliary leak), cyclosporine or tacrolimus toxicity, and other opportunistic infections, including Epstein-Barr virus and fungal infections. CMV is the most likely diagnosis in the patient described in question 37.

39. What are the risk factors for CMV infection? How can it be prevented?

Most CMV infections occur within 1–4 months after liver transplantation. Patients who were initially seronegative for CMV and received a graft from a seropositive donor are at greatest risk. Other risk factors include the use of antilymphocyte antibodies and acute cellular rejection. Patients at high risk for CMV infection should receive prophylaxis with ganciclovir. Patients at lower risk for CMV infection, including those who are seropositive for CMV before transplant, may receive ganciclovir or acyclovir for prophylaxis.

40. What are the signs of CMV infection? How is it diagnosed and treated?

Signs of CMV infection include fever, malaise, leukopenia, thrombocytopenia, and organ involvement (e.g., hepatitis, gastroenteritis, pancreatitis, pneumonia, retinitis). The CMV DNA assay correlates well with viremia and has gained wide acceptance as a diagnostic tool. In addition, the liver biopsy is diagnostic if the viral inclusions are present in the hepatic parenchyma or if the immunohistochemical stains are positive. Treatment requires a 2–4 week course of intravenous ganciclovir.

41. What are the clinical, biochemical, and histologic features of chronic rejection?

Chronic allograft rejection is characterized by an insidious but progressive rise in alkaline phosphatase and bilirubin. Patients are usually asymptomatic, and synthetic function remains intact until the late stages. The pathogenesis of this syndrome remains unclear, but the evidence favors an impressive loss of bile ducts and development of obliterative arteriopathy in the small hepatic arteries. The histologic exam usually reveals a normal-appearing parenchyma with few mononuclear infiltrates in the portal areas but absence of bile ducts in almost all of the portal triads. Later in the course, patients develop strictures and dilations in the larger bile ducts, resembling primary sclerosing cholangitis. In such cases, the clinical course may be complicated by recurrent attacks of biliary sepsis. The differential diagnosis at this stage includes hepatic artery thrombosis, CMV cholangitis, anastomotic strictures of the biliary tree, and recurrent primary sclerosing cholangitis.

42. How do you treat chronic rejection?

The process frequently progresses to graft failure, but recent reports indicate that 20–30% of patients may respond to additional immunosuppressive therapy. Patients with chronic rejection also may need evaluation for retransplantation.

43. How often is it necessary to perform a second liver transplant? For what reasons are repeat transplants performed?

Approximately 10% of the liver transplants performed in the United States are retransplants. Early retransplants are usually performed for primary nonfunction and hepatic artery thrombosis. Improved immunosuppression and improved surgical techniques have reduced the early retransplant rate. Late retransplants may be necessary for recurrence of the original disease (e.g., viral hepatitis, autoimmune hepatitis, primary biliary cirrhosis, primary sclerosing cholangitis) or chronic rejection.

44. Describe the long-term metabolic complications in liver transplant recipients.

Although patients experience a dramatic improvement in quality of life after liver transplant, they are at risk for complications associated with the use of immunosuppressive regimens:

- Weight gain may result from corticosteroid use and liberation from the pretransplant diet.
- Hyperglycemia may result from corticosteroids, and patients with diabetes may experience poor glucose control.
- Hypertension is common with cyclosporine and tacrolimus, and associated renal insufficiency may exacerbate this problem.
- Hyperlipidemia may result from use of corticosteroids and cyclosporine. Although it may improve as immunosuppression is lowered, persistent hyperlipidemia needs aggressive treatment.

All of these factors may place patients at greater risk for cardiovascular or cerebrovascular disease, and patients should receive counseling about appropriate diet, exercise, and smoking cessation.

45. Why is osteoporosis a concern after liver transplant?

Patients may be at risk for osteoporosis associated with corticosteroid use, particularly if they received significant steroids before transplant. A low threshold for measurement of bone density before transplantation may be appropriate in certain populations. In addition, patients at risk should receive calcium and vitamin D supplementation.

46. Are liver transplant recipients at increased risk to develop cancer?

Immunosuppression significantly increases the risk of malignancy and complicates approximately 2% of liver transplants. Patients appear especially at risk for skin cancers, including squamous cell carcinoma and melanoma. They should avoid exposure to ultraviolet light.

47. What is posttransplant lymphoproliferative disorder (PTLD)? How is it managed?

Most cases of PTLD are B-cell types, and the pathogenesis is related to Epstein-Barr virus (EBV) infection. The risk also appears related to the degree of immunosuppression (including OKT3 use). The clinical presentation includes fever, lymphadenopathy, and symptoms related to the involved organ. Extranodal masses are common, and organs typically involved include the gastrointestinal tract, liver, lung, skin, and central nervous system. Excisional biopsy is often necessary to make the diagnosis. First-line treatment involves reduction in immunosuppression. Referral for oncology consultation is also necessary for consideration of chemotherapy or radiation.

48. A liver transplant patient complains in the emergency department of cough and shortness of breath. How does one suspect, diagnose, and treat *Pneumocystis carinii* infection?

P. carinii pneumonia (PCP) is an opportunistic infection. The clinical presentation is variable, but typical symptoms include fever, shortness of breath, and nonproductive cough. If left untreated, PCP may progress rapidly to respiratory failure. As a result, patients typically receive prophylaxis with trimethoprim/sulfamethoxazole (TMP/SMX). In the event of noncompliance, a high index of suspicion remains appropriate. Definitive diagnosis often requires bronchoscopy or bronchoalveolar lavage and should not delay treatment in the appropriate setting. Fortunately, PCP is a relatively rare complication after liver transplantation, probably because of prophylaxis with TMP/SMX and the reduction in immunosuppression compared with 10 years ago. Most transplant centers recommend at least 1 year of TMP/SMX prophylaxis for PCP.

49. What factors contribute to metabolic bone disease after transplantation?

Chronic liver diseases, particularly cholestatic liver diseases, are associated with osteopenia. The pathogenesis originally was thought to be related to decreased bile salt flow and vitamin D malabsorption, but plasma vitamin D levels are normal. Instead, patients appear to have inhibition of bone formation and low or normal bone resorption. Before transplant, therefore, these patients may already have significant bone loss. After transplant, glucocorticoids worsen the condition and place patients at risk for fractures. One study measured the bone density of 20 women with primary biliary cirrhosis. At 3 months after transplant, bone density declined at a mean rate of 18.1% per year. The nadir in bone density appeared to occur within the first 6 months. As glucocorticoid use decreased, bone density improved and ultimately surpassed the pretransplant density at 2 years.

50. A patient who underwent liver transplantation for cirrhosis due to hepatitis C returns with persistently elevated liver enzymes. Liver biopsy reveals chronic active hepatitis but no cirrhosis. Should he be treated with interferon-alpha?

Virtually all patients who receive a liver transplant for hepatitis C have recurrent disease. Diagnosis of recurrence requires identification of the HCV RNA and biopsy findings consistent with hepatitis C. A small minority of patients have fibrosing cholestatic hepatitis, which may have an aggressive course and lead to graft loss within 1 year. Most patients have mild-to-moderate elevations in transaminases and mild-to-moderate fibrosis on biopsy. Optimal management is less clear. Five-year survival rates appear comparable to those of other patients. However, hepatitis C infection after transplantation may have a more aggressive course with faster development of cirrhosis. The current concern is that survival may be poorer when more 10-year data are available.

Treatment of recurrent hepatitis C involves interferon-alpha and ribavirin. Experience in the post-transplant setting is limited, and trials are ongoing. Many transplant centers avoid treatment within the first 6 months because of concern that interferon-alpha may promote rejection. Current experience suggests that the viral eradication may be difficult after transplantation, but treatment may decrease inflammation and improve histology. Consequently, patients with biochemical and histologic evidence of aggressive hepatitis C are considered for treatment at most transplant centers 6 months after transplantation. Given the side effects of interferon-alpha and ribavirin, lower doses may be adequate.

51. Can recurrent hepatitis C be prevented?

At this time, no prophylactic treatment is available for recurrent hepatitis C. Studies are in progress to examine the role of interferon-alpha and ribavirin in preventing recurrent disease. Aggressive early treatment may have a role in preventing or blunting infection. However, the concern remains of increasing the risk of rejection. Ongoing trials should provide more information.

BIBLIOGRAPHY

1. Beresford TP, Turcotte JG, Merion R, et al: A rational approach to liver transplantation for the alcoholic. Psychosomatics 31:241–254, 1990.
2. Bray GP, Harrison PM, O'Grady JG, et al: Long-term anticonvulsant therapy worsens paracetamol-induced fulminant hepatic failure. Hum Exp Toxicol 11:265–270, 1992.
3. Clipston NA, Crabtree GR: Identification of calcineurin as a key signalling enzyme in T-lymphocyte activation. Nature 357:695–697, 1993.
4. Deschenes M, Villeneuve JP, Dagenais M, et al: Lack of relationship between the severity of cirrhosis and short-term survival after transplantation. Liver Transpl Surg 3:532–537, 1997.
5. Eastell R, Dickson ER, Hodgson SF, et al: Rates of vertebral bone loss before and after liver transplantation in women with primary biliary cirrhosis. Hepatology 14:819–827, 1996.
6. Eckhoff DE, Pirsch JD, D'Alessandro AM, et al: Pretransplant status and patient survival following liver transplantation. Transplantation 60:920–925, 1995.
7. Eidelman BH, Abu-Elmagd K, Wilson J, et al: Neurologic complications of FK 506. Transplant Proc 23: 3175–3178, 1991.
8. European FK506 Multicenter Study Group: Randomized trial comparing tacrolimus (FK 506) and cyclosporin in prevention of liver allograft rejection. Lancet 344:423–428, 1994.
9. Foster PF, Fabrega F, Karademir S, et al: Prediction of abstinence from ethanol in alcoholic recipients following liver transplantation. Hepatology 25:1469–1477, 1997.
10. Golling M, Safer A, Kriesche B, et al: Transplant survival following liver transplant: A multivariate analysis. Transplant Proc 30: 3239–3240, 1998.

11. Gonzalez E, Rimola A, Navasa M, et al: Liver transplantation in patients with non-biliary cirrhosis: Prognostic value of preoperative factors. J Hepatol 28:320–328, 1998.
12. Gralnek IM, Liu H, Shapiro MF, Martin P: The United States liver donor population in the 1990s. Transplantation 67:1019–1023, 1999.
13. Hoofnagle JH, Lombardero M, Zetterman RK, et al: Donor age and outcome of liver transplantation. Hepatology 24:89–96, 1996.
14. Makin AJ, Wendon J, Williams R: A 7-year experience of severe acetaminophen-induced hepatotoxicity (1987–1993). Gastroenterology 109:1907–1916, 1995.
15. Marcos A, Fisher RA, Ham JM, et al: Right lobe living donor liver transplantation. Transplantation 68:798–903, 1999.
16. Marsman WA, Wiesner RH, Rodriguez L, et al: Use of fatty donor liver is associated with diminished early patient and graft survival. Transplantation 62:1246–1251, 1996.
17. Nolan CM, Sandblom RE, Thummel KE, et al: Hepatotoxicity associated with acetaminophen usage in patients receiving multiple drug therapy for tuberculosis. Chest 105:408–411, 1994.
18. O'Grady JG, Alexander GJM, Hayllar KM, Williams R: Early indicators of prognosis in fulminant hepatic failure. Gastroenterology 97:439–445, 1989.
19. O'Keefe SJ, Tamura J, Kincaid RL, et al: FK-506- and CsA-sensitive activation of the interleukin-2 promoter by calcineurin. Nature 357:692–694, 1992.
20. Ortho Multicenter Study Group: A randomized clinical trial of OKT3 monoclonal antibody for acute rejection of cadaveric renal transplants. N Engl J Med 313:337–342, 1985.
21. Prescott LF: Paracetamol overdosage: Pharmacological consideration and clinical management. Drugs 25:290–314, 1983.
22. Prottas JM, Batten HL: The willingness to give: The public and the supply of transplantable organs. J Health Polit Policy Law 16:121–124, 1991.
23. Ringe B, Wittekind C, Bechstein WO, et al: The role of liver transplantation in hepatobiliary surgery. Ann Surg 209:88–89, 1989.
24. Schiodt FV, Atillasoy V: Etiology and outcome for 295 patients with acute liver failure in the United States. Liver Transpl Surg 5: 29–34, 1999.
25. Shafer T, Wood RP, Van Buren CT et al: A success story in minority donation: The LifeGift/Ben Taub General Hospital In-House Coordinator Program. Transpl Proc 29:3753–3755, 1997.
26. Sheil AGR, Disney APS, Mathew TH, et al: Lymphoma incidence, cyclosporine, and the evolution and major impact of malignancy following organ transplantation. Transpl Proc 29:825–827, 1997.
27. Stegall MD, Wachs M, Everson G, et al: Prednisone withdrawal 14 days after liver transplantation with mycophenolate: A prospective trial of cyclosporine and tacrolimus. Transplantation 64:1755–1760, 1997.
28. Stegall MD, Everson GT, Schroter G, et al: Prednisone withdrawal late after adult liver transplantation reduces diabetes, hypertension, hypercholesterolemia without causing graft loss. Hepatology 25: 173–177, 1997.
29. Vale JA, Proudfoot AT. Paracetamol (acetaminophen) poisoning. Lancet 346:547–552, 1995.
30. Vincenti F, Kirkman R, Light S, et al: Interleukin-2-receptor blockade with daclizumab to prevent acute rejection in renal transplantation. Daclizumab Triple Therapy Study Group. N Engl J Med 338:161–165, 1998.
31. Wiesner RH, Batts KP, Krom RA: Evolving concepts in the diagnosis, pathogenesis, and treatment of chronic hepatic allograft rejection. Liver Transpl Surg 5:388–400, 1999.
32. Wong T, Devlin J, Rolando N, et al: Clinical characteristics affecting the outcome of liver retransplantation. Transplantation 64:878–882, 1997.

30. FULMINANT HEPATIC FAILURE

Satheesh Nair, M.D., and Paul J. Thuluvath, M.D., FRCP

1. Define fulminant hepatic failure.

Fulminant hepatic failure (FHF) describes rapidly progressive liver failure with onset of encephalopathy within 8 weeks of onset of symptoms in patients without previous history of liver disease. When the onset of encephalopathy is delayed more than 8 weeks but less than 6 months, the term late-onset hepatic failure (LOHF) is used. Despite suggestions that these definitions should be revised, so far no consensus has been reached.

2. Define hyperacute FHF. What is its prognosis in comparison with acute FHF?

Hyperacute FHF is defined as onset of encephalopathy within 2 weeks of onset of jaundice. It has a better prognosis than acute FHF. Without liver transplantation, the survival of patients with hyperacute FHF is 30% compared with 7–10% for acute FHF.

3. What are the differences between FHF and LOHF?

LOHF is associated with ascites more often than FHF. Cerebral edema is less common in LOHF. In addition, the cause of FHF and LOHF may be different as described later. Patients with FHF patients need liver transplantation more urgently than patients with LOHF.

4. What are the common causes of FHF and LOHF?

The causes depend on the country and the nature of the referral center. Acute viral hepatitis is by far the most common cause (62–68%) in the United States and many European countries (72% in France), but in England paracetamol (acetaminophen) overdose is the most common cause (45–54%) of acute liver failure. Hepatitis A, B, D, and E viruses cause predominantly FHF, whereas hepatitis C and non-A, non-B, non-C viruses cause LOHF. Acetaminophen and halothane usually result in hyperacute FHF, but other drug-induced liver diseases usually result in LOHF.

5. What other causes should be considered in the differential diagnosis? How often is the cause not identified?

The rare causes of acute liver failure include Wilson's disease, autoimmune chronic active hepatitis, Budd-Chiari syndrome, acute fatty liver of pregnancy, diffuse malignant infiltration of liver (hepatoma, lymphoma and metastases), reactivation of hepatitis B virus (HBV), and hyperthermia. Wilson's disease and autoimmune chronic active hepatitis usually present as LOHF. In a significant number of patients (19–41%), the cause of acute liver failure remains undetermined and usually presents as LOHF. It is presumed that most of these patients have acute non-ABCDE viral hepatitis. Some may have HBV-DNA in the liver when carefully tested; however, the causative agent remains unidentified in a significant proportion of patients with FHF and LOHF.

6. What diagnostic clues suggest fulminant Wilson's disease as the cause of FHF? What is the treatment?

Very high bilirubin levels (high levels of unconjugated bilirubin due to hemolysis) with low alkaline phosphatase levels and hemolytic anemia should raise suspicion of Wilson's disease. Even in the absence of these features, Wilson's disease should be ruled out in any young patient presenting with FHF. High serum and urine copper levels with low serum ceruloplasmin levels are highly suggestive of Wilson's disease. Ceruloplasmin may be normal in fulminant Wilson's disease, because it is an acute-phase reactant. Kayser-Fleischer rings, if present, are highly suggestive. The treatment of fulminant Wilson's disease is liver transplantation because D-penicillamine takes time and is not effective in this setting.

7. **A 24-year old woman is brought to the emergency department after taking 16 tablets of acetaminophen (500 mg each) over the course of 12 hours. She has a history of seizure disorder and is taking phenytoin and carbamazepine. She is asymptomatic, but her husband, who is a paramedic, is concerned about the hepatotoxicty of acetaminophen. Her liver function tests are normal. Is she at risk of acetaminophen toxicity? Should she receive N-acetyl cysteine?**

Both phenytoin and carbamazepine are potent inducers of cytochrome P450. Because acetaminophen toxicity is due to a metabolite generated by cytochrome P450, drugs that induce this enzyme enhance the toxicity of acetaminophen. Alcoholics (enzyme induction by alcohol + depleted glutathione stores) and malnourished or fasting peoples (low glutathione stores) are also at a high risk even from a low-dose exposure. Although the patient's liver function tests are normal, she should receive n-acetyl cysteine (NAC), especially since she is at a high risk. Use of the "normogram" to decide treatment has not been validated in patients with accelerated acetaminophen metabolism. Normal levels of aspartate aminotransferase (AST) and alanine aminotransferase (ALT) do not rule out hepatotoxicity because acetaminophen hepatotoxicity usually manifests 24–48 hours after ingestion. The typical dose of NAC is 140 mg/kg followed by 17 doses of 70 mg/kg.

8. **What antidotes are used for mushroom poisoning** *(Amanita phalloides)***?**

Penicillin at doses of 300,000–1,000,000 million units/kg/day and silibinin at 20–50 mg/kg/day are given simultaneously. Penicillin is an antagonist of amatoxin, and silibinin prevents the hepatocellular uptake of amatoxin.

9. **A woman at 37 weeks of pregnancy is admitted with jaundice and mild encephalopathy. She has no known liver disease in the past. Platelet count is 60,000 and prothrombin time is 18 seconds. Hematocrit is within normal limits. Hepatitis viral serologies are negative. What is the best treatment? What is the likely finding on liver biopsy? What other causes of FHF have a similar histologic picture?**

FHF in the third trimester may be due to acute fatty liver of pregnancy (AFLP) or HELLP syndrome (hemolysis, elevated liver enzymes, and low platelets). Other causes of FHF also should be considered in the differential diagnosis. Clinical distinction between AFLP and HELLP is not always easy. Thrombocytopenia may be seen in AFLP because of associated disseminated intravascular coagulation (DIC). A shrunken liver and persistent hypoglycemia suggest AFLP. AFLP has a worse prognosis than HELLP. Immediate delivery is the best option for either condition. Close monitoring of liver function is essential because some patients continue to deteriorate even after delivery. Hepatic rupture complicates pregnancy in rare patients and should be suspected in any patient presenting with abdominal pain and shock. Liver biopsy in AFLP shows microvescicular steatosis. Other causes of microvescicular steatosis that can present as FHF are Reye's syndrome and valproic acid toxicity.

10. **A 42-year-old woman is admitted with jaundice that she developed 6–8 weeks earlier. For the past few days she has become more drowsy and confused. She has no previous history of liver disease, alcoholism or drug use. Liver biochemistry showed albumin 2.2 g/dl, total protein 8.9 g/dl, ALT 900 U/L, AST 780 U/L, ALP 200 U/L and bilirubin 18 mg/dL; prothrombin time was 28 seconds. Viral serology studies for hepatitis A, B C, and E were negative. CT scan of the abdomen was unrevealing. What is the best course of action?**

Autoimmune hepatitis is an important consideration. A high globulin fraction should alert the physician to such a possibility, although patients with FHF due to autoimmune hepatitis may present without hyperglobulinemia. Wilson's disease is unlikely but should be ruled out. In addition to antinuclear antibodies (ANAs) and anti-smooth muscle antibodies (ASMAs), a transjugular liver biopsy should be considered. The diagnosis of autoimmune hepatitis is important so that a therapeutic trial with steroids can be initiated. Many patients respond well to steroids. Liver transplant evaluation and intensive care should be initiated while the efficacy of steroid treatment is assessed.

11. Does the prognosis of FHF vary with the cause? How does one predict the prognosis?

The prognosis is better for patients with hepatitis A and acetaminophen-induced liver failure. This survival advantage is seen even in patients with coma and severe coagulopathy. The prognostic variables are similar for all causes of fulminant hepatic failure except acetaminophen toxicity. In patients with acetaminophen toxicity, severe acidosis (arterial pH < 7.3) is associated with a mortality rate of approximately 95%. In the absence of severe acidosis, presence of all three adverse factors (creatinine >3.4, international normalized ratio [INR] > 6.5, and stage III and IV encephalopathy) are necessary to identify patients with a 95% mortality rate.

Prognostic indicators for non–acetaminophen-induced FHF are given in the table below. With one adverse factor, the mortality rate is around 80%; the rate increases to 95% with three or more adverse factors. However, prothrombin time > 100 seconds is an absolute indication (even in the absence of other adverse factors) for liver transplantation in patients with non-acetaminophen-induced liver failure. Factor V level is an important predictor of mortality in FHF. In patients with stage III or IV coma, the chance of survival without liver transplantation is < 10% if factor V level is < 15–20%.

Prognosis of LOHF can be determined by the Childs-Pugh grading system, which uses albumin, bilirubin, prothrombin time, ascites and encephalopathy as prognostic variables.

Prognostic Indicators Associated with Poor Outcome in Fulminant Hepatic Failure

ACETAMINOPHEN-INDUCED	NON–ACETAMINOPHEN-INDUCED
Arterial pH < 7.3	Non-A, non-B, non-C hepatitis, drugs, toxins
INR > 6.5 or PT >100 sec	INR > 3.5 or PT > 50 sec
Creatinine > 3.4 mg/dl	Creatinine > 3.4 mg/dl
Stage III or IV encephalopathy	Jaundice > 7 days before onset of encephalopathy
	Bilirubin >18 mg/dl
	Age <10 or >40 years

INR = international normalized ratio, PT = prothrombin time.
Adapted from O'Grady JG, Alexander GJ, Hayllar KM, Williams R: Early indicators of prognosis in fulminant hepatic failure. Gastroenterology 97:439–445, 1989.

12. What is the natural course of fulminant and subfulminant hepatic failure without liver transplantation?

The overall mortality rate, including all causes, without liver transplantation is about 70%. The mortality rate is around 50% for hepatitis A and acetaminophen-induced FHF. In patients with coma (stage IV hepatic encephalopathy) and severe coagulopathy or factor V level < 15%, the chance of survival without liver transplantation is < 10%.

13. What complications are common in patients with FHF?

Although liver failure results in numerous metabolic changes, patients usually die because of increased intracranial pressure (ICP), infectious complications, or multiorgan failure. Other common complications are coagulopathy, renal failure, lactic acidosis, hypoglycemia, hypophosphatemia, hypoxemia, and hypotension, all of which are interrelated and ultimately lead to multiorgan failure.

14. What causes coagulopathy, hypoglycemia, and lactic acidosis in FHF?

Coagulopathy is due to a combination of reduced synthesis of clotting factors and increased peripheral consumption as a result of low-grade DIC. Hypoglycemia is due to impaired gluconeogenesis, reduced mobilization of glycogen, and increase in circulating insulin. Lactic acidosis results from a combination of tissue hypoxia and poor hepatic uptake and metabolism of lactate.

15. What causes hypotension and hypoxemia in FHF?

Hypotension, in the presence of adequate fluid intake, is due to high cardiac output and lowered peripheral vascular resistance. Arterial hypoxemia is seen in the presence of infection, alveolar hemorrhage, arteriovenous shunting, and adult respiratory distress syndrome.

16. Why are patients with FHF prone to infections?

Because of suppression of immune function, impaired neutrophil and Kupffer cell functions, and deficiency of opsonins, patients are prone to both bacterial (gram-negative and gram-positive) and fungal (candidal) infection.

17. How common is cerebral edema in FHF? What causes it?

Approximately 80% of patients with FHF and coma develop cerebral edema, which is perhaps the most common cause of death (brainstem or cerebellar coning is seen in 80% of patients at autopsy). The pathogenesis of cerebral edema remains poorly explained. It is presumed to be due to a combination of swelling of astrocytes (perhaps mediated by toxins) and extravasation of fluids (disruption of blood-brain barrier).

18. Can one make a definite diagnosis of raised intracranial tension in patients with FHF on clinical grounds alone?

Although arterial hypertension, bradycardia, and decorticate posturing are seen in patients with raised ICP, a clinical diagnosis is not always reliable. Many patients also have associated hepatic encephalopathy. Moreover, rapid fluctuations in ICP occur frequently but are impossible to detect clinically. Hence, direct measurement of ICP by placing extradural/subdural transducers is recommended. Raised ICP is defined as pressure > 25 mmHg.

19. What is the therapeutic goal in treating raised ICP in FHF? What are the therapeutic options?

The therapeutic goal is to maintain the cerebral perfusion pressure > 50–60 mmHg:

Cerebral perfusion pressure = mean arterial pressure – intracranial pressure

To achieve this goal, ICP should be reduced to < 20 mmHg. Three options are available. The most commonly used treatment is mannitol infusion. Hyperventilation, which lowers the partial pressure of carbon dioxide (PCO_2), can also decrease ICP. If both options are unsuccessful, thiopental infusion is recommended to induce coma. Elevation of the head also is recommended. Precipitating factors such as hypoxia, hypercapnia, cough, vomiting, frequent suction (while off respirator), and fever should be avoided or corrected.

20. Does ICP monitoring improve the prognosis of patients with FHF? What are the complications of ICP monitoring?

ICP monitoring and orthotopic liver transplantation (OLT) are the two major advances in the management of FHF in the past decade. Proper management of ICP has improved the outcome in FHF. ICP monitoring may be associated with intracranial hemorrhage and infection. However, such complications are higher during the learning phase and seem to decrease with experience. Epidural transducers are the most commonly used devices (61%) in the U.S. and have the lowest complication rate (3.8%). Subdural bolts and parenchymal monitors (fiberoptic pressure transducers in direct contact with brain parenchyma and intraventricular catheters) are associated with complication rates of 20% and 22%, respectively. Fatal hemorrhages occur in 1% of patients with epidural monitoring, 5% with subdural bolts, and 4% with parenchymal monitoring.

21. What are the classic hemodynamic features of FHF?

The classical features are increased cardiac output (2–3 times normal), low vascular resistance, and arterial hypotension. The most likely mediator is a vasodilator, perhaps nitric oxide, released from the hepatocyte. As a result, hypotension is resistant to vasopressors.

22. How do you differentiate DIC related to sepsis from coagulopathy due to FHF?

Elevated prothrombin time (PT) and partial thromboplastin time (PTT) and low platelets are seen in both DIC and hepatic failure. In this setting, factor VIII levels are useful. Factor VIII, which is synthesized in the vascular endothelium, is normal in coagulopathy due to liver failure, whereas it is low in a consumptive coagulopathy such as DIC. However, in FHF low-grade DIC is also common, making a distinction impossible and probably clinically irrelevant.

23. What causes renal failure in FHF?

Renal failure (defined as urine output < 300 ml/24 hours and serum creatinine > 3.4 mg/dl) is seen in about 70% of patients with acetaminophen-induced FHF and about 30% with non–acetaminophen-induced FHF. The cause is often multifactorial:

- Hypovolemia secondary to vomiting, poor oral intake, diarrhea and/or GI bleeding.
- Hepatorenal syndrome.
- Acute tubular necrosis from nephrotoxic drugs (antibiotics such as gentamicin and amphotericin) and contrast agents.
- Direct nephrotoxicity from toxin (e.g., acetaminophen, carbon tetrachloride [CCl_4)].

Blood urea nitrogen is not reliable indicator of renal function as urea synthesis is reduced in FHF and may be normal despite severe renal dysfunction.

24. A patient with FHF is admitted to intensive care for close observation. He is awaiting liver transplantation, but his PT continues to rise and he is becoming more encephalopathic. He is on assisted ventilation. The nurse tells you that his systolic blood pressure is 70 mmHg. What should be your response?

Although patients with FHF tend to have some degree of hypotension due to intense peripheral vasodilatation, look for a treatable cause. The first step is to ensure adequate intravascular volume, which is best assessed by pulmonary capillary wedge pressure (PCWP). A potential cause of hypovolemia is GI bleeding. If PCWP is low, nasogastric aspiration should be performed until bile is drained to rule out upper GI bleeding. If PCWP is acceptable (10–12 mmHg), other causes should be sought. Because the patient is on assisted ventilation, pneumothorax should be ruled out by chest radiograph. Also look for cardiac tamponade on echocardiogram. If these causes are ruled out, the hypotension should be considered to be due to sepsis, and empiric antibiotics should be started. Fungal infections are common in patients with prolonged ICU stay, especially if they had previous antibiotics. Because cerebral perfusion pressure depends on arterial pressure, hypotension should be treated with a vasopressor (after correcting hypovolemia), preferably norepinephrine.

25. Is it necessary to refer patients with FHF to a tertiary center? How does one manage patients with FHF?

It is important to refer patients at an early stage to a center where they can be managed by a team with expertise. Early referral also provides adequate time to evaluate the patient for liver transplantation. Patients with FHF should be managed in an ICU by an experienced team. The cause of liver failure should be determined and treated if possible (e.g., acetaminophen toxicity). The patient's head should be elevated to minimize positional influence on ICP. Sedation should be avoided if possible. Patients should have central venous pressure monitoring (Swan-Ganz catheter if necessary), and careful attention should be given to fluid replacement and correction of acidosis, electrolyte imbalances, and hypoglycemia. Arterial oxygen saturation should be monitored, and airways should be protected by endotracheal intubation in patients with stage III–IV hepatic encephalopathy. Patients should be treated with H_2 receptor antagonists (or proton pump inhibitors) as a prophylaxis against stress ulcers. Although prophylactic replacement of fresh frozen plasma does not reduce morbidity or mortality and makes it difficult to interpret the most valuable prognostic indicator, it should not be withheld in the presence of bleeding or for placement of an ICP monitor. Platelets should be transfused in patients with severe thrombocytopenia.

26. How is hypotension treated?

Hypotension should be treated with adequate fluid replacement and vasopressors; however, care should be taken to avoid pulmonary edema in patients with renal failure. Continuous arteriovenous hemofiltration should be instituted in patients with uncorrected acidosis, fluid overload, hyperkalemia, and worsening creatinine levels.

27. Should prophylactic antibiotics be used?

No convincing evidence supports prophylactic antibacterial or antifungal treatment, but treatment should be started at the slightest suspicion of infection. It is important to culture all body fluids and catheter tips for bacteria and fungi on a daily basis. Patients with evidence of infection should be treated with antifungal agents if there is no immediate response to antibacterial treatment, especially if they had previous antibiotics or have renal failure.

28. What is the basis for use of prostaglandins in the management of FHF? How successful is the treatment?

The use of prostaglandin E_1 (PGE_1) is based on an uncontrolled study by investigators in Toronto, in which 12 of 14 patients with grade III or IV hepatic encephalopathy survived. The authors attributed the high survival rate to continuous infusion of PGE_1. The rationale for this treatment in FHF remains poorly explained. Immunomodulation, improvements in tissue perfusion, and direct antiviral effects may explain the increase in survival rates. However, a controlled study by the same group and a few other small studies have failed to show any benefit with PGE_1 therapy. Current evidence indicates no role for the routine use of PGE_1 in patients with FHF.

29. Do hepatotrophic agents have a role in the management of FHF?

Various hepatotrophic agents have been identified, but so far the clinical experience is limited to insulin and glucagon therapy. In controlled trials, insulin and glucagon therapy have failed to improve survival rates in patients with severe acute hepatitis. In the future, other growth factors, such as transforming growth factor alpha and hepatocyte growth factor, may become available for clinical trials.

30. How successful is liver transplantation in FHF?

The experience from major centers suggests that a significant number of patients with FHF (30–40%) die without receiving liver transplantation because of unavailability of a suitable donor or complications that prevent OLT, such as sepsis, neurologic damage, and multiorgan failure. The results of OLT in patients with FHF have improved significantly over the past decade, mainly because of better selection criteria and better management in intensive care. The 1-year survival rate of patients after liver transplantation for FHF is around 70% (some centers have reported survival rates as high as 90%), which is lower than the rate for non-FHF recipients. A recent study showed that FHF recipients are less likely to be matched for ABO blood type than non-FHF counterparts, which may partly explain the survival difference. ABO mismatch and abnormal kidney function are independent predictors of adverse outcome in patients receiving liver transplantation for FHF.

31. What is auxiliary liver transplantation?

Patients with FHF die from complications due to hepatic dysfunction rather than from failure of the liver to regenerate. Given sufficient time, the liver will regenerate in most patients. Thus, it may be possible to support patients with a liver temporarily so that the native liver regenerates and regains function. In auxiliary liver transplanation, a donor liver (few segments) is placed in a heterotropic position without recipient hepatectomy. Once the native liver regenerates, the allograft can be removed or left to atrophy (by rejection). Thus patients are spared the necessity of lifelong immunosuppression. The two positions in which the auxiliary liver is placed are right upper quadrant just inferior to the native liver or lower abdomen near the distal aorta.

32. Does artificial liver support have a role in the management of acute liver failure?

Artificial liver support is one of the most exciting areas in hepatology. OLT is a drastic and expensive procedure, but it improves survival in patients with FHF. However, many patients die because of the unavailability of a suitable donor. Liver assist devices may be useful in patients as a bridge to emergency OLT; such devices may help to stabilize patients with uncontrolled ICP or even negate the need for OLT if the liver is able to regenerate. Numerous such devices are currently tested in small clinical studies. Results appear promising, but controlled studies are needed.

33. Are there any other promising therapies that may be used as a bridge to OLT?

Charcoal hemoperfusion and other perusion devices are of no proven value and have not improved survival rates. In bioartificial livers, hepatocyte-lined membranes or microcarriers are used to perform synthetic and biotransformation functions; the hepatoctyes are derived from porcine or human hepatoblastoma. These devices however, are still in experimental stages and the results, although encouraging, remain unproved.

Reports of heterotropic auxiliary liver transplantation are not encouraging, but further studies are needed. Despite anecdotal reports of successful use, xenografts must be considered as an experimental procedure. In the future, better immunologic manipulation may improve the results of xenotransplantation. Transplantation of hepatocytes is a promising field. Harvested hepatocytes (from a portion of the liver of a donor) are injected into the spleen, from where they migrate to populate the liver. Currently, the only proven treatment for FHF is liver transplantation. However, organ shortage is a major problem in the U.S., and many patients die waiting for a liver transplantation. Although living donor transplantation has been used successfully in children, experience in adults is limited. This option may become more common in the future unless there is a breakthrough in xenotransplantation or bioartificial liver.

BIBLIOGRAPHY

1. Bernuau J, Goudeau A, Poynard T, et al: Multivariate analysis of prognostic factors in fulminant hepatitis B. Hepatology 6:648–651, 1986.
2. Detre K, Belle S, Beringer K, Daily OP: Liver transplantation for fulminant hepatic failure in the United States: October 1987 through December 1991. Clin Transplant 8:274–280, 1994.
3. Gimson AE, O'Grady J, Ede RJ, et al: Late onset of hepatic failure: Clinical, serological and histological features. Hepatology 6:288–294, 1986.
4. Harrison, PM, Keays R, Bray GP, et al: Improved outcome of paracetamol induced fulminant hepatic failure by late administration of acetylcysteine. Lancet i:1572–1573, 1990.
5. Keays R, Harrison PM, Wendon JA, et al: Intravenous acetylcysteine in paracetamol induced fulminant hepatic failure: A prospective controlled trial. BMJ 303:1026–1029, 1991.
6. Lidofsky SD: Liver transplantation for fulminant hepatic failure. Gastroenterol Clin North Am 22:257–269, 1993.
7. Lidofsky SD, Bass NM, Pager MC, et al: Intracranial pressure monitoring and liver transplantation for fulminant hepatic failure. Hepatology 16:1–7, 1992.
8. Mortimer DJ, Elias E: Liver transplantation for fulminant hepatic failure. Prog Liver Dis 10:349–367, 1992.
9. Munoz SJ: Difficult management problems in fulminant hepatic failure. Semin Liver Dis 13:395–413, 1993.
10. O'Grady JG, Alexander GJ, Hayllar KM, Williams R: Early indicators of prognosis in fulminant hepatic failure. Gastroenterology 97:439–445, 1989.
11. Sussman NL, Gislason GT, Kelly JH: Extracorporeal liver support: Application to fulminant hepatic failure. J Clin Gastroenterol 18:320–324, 1994.
12. Lee WM: Management of acute liver failure. Semin Liver Dis 16:369–378, 1996
13. Mas A, Rodes J: Fulminant hepatic failure. Lancet 1349:1081–1085, 1997

31. ASCITES

Carlos Guarner, M.D., and Bruce A. Runyon, M.D.

1. What are the most common causes of ascites?

Ascites is the accumulation of fluid within the peritoneal cavity. More than 80% of patients with ascites have decompensated chronic liver disease. However, it is important to know the other possible causes of ascites, because treatment and prognosis may be quite different. Peritoneal carcinomatosis is the second most common cause of ascites, followed by acute alcoholic hepatitis, heart failure, fulminant or subacute hepatic failure, pancreatic disease, dialysis ascites, nephrotic syndrome, hepatic vein obstruction, chylous ascites, bile ascites, and miscellaneous disorders of the peritoneum.

2. Should a diagnostic tap be performed routinely on all patients with ascites at the time of admission to the hospital?

Ascites is readily diagnosed when large amounts of fluid are present in the peritoneal cavity. If clinical examination is not definitive in detecting or excluding ascites, ultrasonography may be helpful. In addition, ultrasonography may provide information about the cause of ascites, e.g., by documenting parenchymal liver disease, splenomegaly, and an enlarged portal vein. Abdominal tap may be performed easily and safely, and analysis of ascitic fluid provides useful data for differentiating causes of ascites. Moreover, more than 30% of patients with cirrhosis and ascites have ascitic fluid infection at the time of admission to the hospital or develop it during hospitalization. As a rule, therefore, diagnostic abdominal tap should be performed routinely (1) in all patients with new-onset ascites and (2) at the time of admission in patients with ascites. In addition, it should be repeated in patients whose clinical condition deteriorates during hospitalization, especially when they develop signs or symptoms of bacterial infection, hepatic encephalopathy, gastrointestinal hemorrhage, or deterioration of renal function.

3. How should a diagnostic paracentesis be performed?

Although paracentesis is a simple and safe procedure, precautions should be taken to avoid complications. Paracentesis should be performed under sterile conditions. The abdomen should be cleaned and disinfected with an iodine solution, and the physician should wear sterile gloves during the entire procedure. The needle should be inserted in an area that is dull to percussion. The midline between the umbilicus and symphysis pubis was the preferable site of needle insertion in the past. However, three factors have changed this philosophy: (1) the frequency of therapeutic paracentesis, (2) the thickness of the panniculus in the midline in the obese patient, and (3) the frequency of obesity in patients with cirrhosis. Now the left lower quadrant appears to be the best site for needle insertion. Because the panniculus is less thick in this area, the needle traverses less tissue. Occasionally even a 3.5-inch needle will not reach ascitic fluid in the midline in obese patients. Therapeutic taps in the lower quadrants drain more fluid than midline taps. Patients on lactulose tend to have a distended cecum. Therefore, the left lower quadrant is chosen over the right lower quadrant. A site is chosen in the left lower quadrant two finger breadths cephalad from the anterior superior iliac spine and two finger-breadths medial to this landmark.

Scars should be avoided, because they are often sites of collateral vessels and adherent bowel. Between 30 and 50 ml of ascitic fluid should be withdrawn for analysis. After paracentesis patients should recline for 30 minutes on the opposite side of the paracentesis to avoid leakage of ascitic fluid.

4. What tests should be routinely ordered on ascitic fluid?

Analysis of ascitic fluid is useful for the differential diagnosis of ascites. However, it is not necessary to order all tests on every specimen. The most important tests are cell count, bacterial culture, albumin, and total protein.

The **white blood cell count** is probably the single most important test performed on ascitic fluid, because it provides immediate information about possible bacterial infection. An absolute neutrophil count ≥ 250 cells/mm^3 provides presumptive evidence of bacterial infection of ascitic fluid and warrants initiation of empirical antibiotics. An elevated white blood cell count with a predominance of lymphocytes strongly suggests peritoneal carcinomatosis or tuberculous peritonitis.

Albumin concentration of ascitic fluid allows calculation of the serum-ascites albumin gradient to classify specimens into high- or low-gradient categories (see question 5).

Ascitic fluid should be cultured by inoculating **blood culture** bottles at the bedside. The sensitivity of this method is higher than that of the conventional technique in detecting bacterial growth. Automated systems for bacterial growth culture such as BacT/ALERT provide an earlier microbiologic diagnosis of ascitic fluid infection (usually less than 12 hours). Specific culture for tuberculosis should be ordered when tuberculous peritonitis is suspected on clinical grounds and the ascitic fluid white cell count is elevated with a predominance of lymphocytic cells.

Total protein concentration of ascitic fluid has been used to classify ascitic fluid into transudates and exudates. Presently, this classification is not particularly helpful, because > 30% of cirrhotic ascites samples are exudates. Nevertheless, total protein concentration of ascitic fluid should be ordered routinely, because it is useful for determining which patients are at high risk of developing spontaneous bacterial peritonitis (SBP) (total protein < 1.0 gm/dl) and for differentiating spontaneous from secondary bacterial peritonitis. Measurement of glucose and lactate dehydrogenase (LDH) in ascitic fluid also has been found to be helpful in making this distinction (see question 9).

Amylase activity of ascitic fluid is markedly elevated in pancreatic ascites and gut perforation into ascites.

Gram stain of ascitic fluid is usually negative in cirrhotic patients with early SBP, but it may be helpful in identifying patients with gut perforation, in whom multiple types of bacteria are seen.

Cytology of ascitic fluid is useful in detecting malignant ascites when the peritoneum is involved with the malignant process. Unfortunately, ascitic fluid cytology is not useful in detecting hepatocellular carcinoma, which seldom metastasizes to the peritoneum

Other tests proposed as helpful in detecting malignant ascites, such as fibronectin, cholesterol, and carcinoembryonic antigen, have limited, if any, value in ascitic fluid analysis.

5. Why is it useful to measure serum-ascites albumin gradient?

Serum-ascites albumin gradient (SAAG) is more useful than the total protein concentration of ascitic fluid in the classification of ascites. This gradient is physiologically based on oncotic-hydrostatic balance and is related directly to portal pressure. The serum-ascites albumin gradient is calculated by subtracting the albumin concentration of ascitic fluid from the albumin concentration of serum obtained on the same day:

$$SAAG = albumin_{serum} - albumin_{ascites}$$

Patients with gradients ≥ 1.1 gm/dl have portal hypertension, whereas patients with gradients <1.1 gm/dl do not:

Serum–ascites albumin gradient ≥ 1.1 gm/dl $\downarrow$ Portal hypertension	Serum–ascites albumin gradient < 1.1 gm/dl $\downarrow$ Normal portal pressure

6. What are the causes of high (i.e., ≥ 1.1 gm/dl) serum-ascites albumin gradients?

The most common cause of a high serum-ascites albumin gradient is cirrhosis, but any cause of portal hypertension leads to a high gradient (e.g., alcoholic hepatitis, cardiac ascites, massive liver metastases, fulminant hepatic failure, Budd-Chiari syndrome, portal vein thrombosis, venoocclusive disease, myxedema, fatty liver of pregnancy, "mixed" ascites). Mixed ascites is due to two different causes, including one that causes portal hypertension (e.g., cirrhosis and tuberculous peritonitis).

7. What are the causes of low (i.e., < 1.1 gm/dl) serum-ascites albumin gradients?

Low-gradient ascites is found in the absense of portal hypertension and is usually due to peritoneal disease. The most common cause is peritoneal carcinomatosis. Other causes are tuberculous peritonitis, pancreatic disease, biliary ascites, nephrotic syndrome, serositis, and bowel obstruction or infarction.

8. What are the variants of ascitic fluid infection?

Ascitic fluid infection can be spontaneous or secondary to an intraabdominal, surgically treatable source of infection. More than 90% of ascitic fluid infections in cirrhotic patients are spontaneous. According to the characteristics of ascitic fluid culture and polymorphonuclear cell (PMN) count, four different variants of ascitic fluid infection have been described in cirrhotic patients. SBP is defined as an ascitic fluid infection with PMN count ≥ 250 cells/mm^3 and positive culture (usually for a single organism). Culture-negative neutrocytic ascites (CNNA) is defined as an ascitic fluid PMN count ≥ 250 cells/mm^3 with a negative culture. Bacterascites is defined as an ascitic fluid PMN count < 250 cells/mm^3 with a positive culture for a single organism. Polymicrobial bacterascites is defined as an ascitic fluid with PMN count < 250 cells/mm^3 with a positive culture for more than one organism. This condition usually is caused by gut puncture by the needle during attempted paracentesis.

9. How do you differentiate spontaneous from secondary peritonitis?

It is important to differentiate spontaneous from secondary peritonitis in cirrhotic patients, because treatment for SBP is medical, whereas treatment for secondary peritonitis is usually surgical. Although secondary peritonitis represents $< 10\%$ of ascitic fluid infections, it should be considered in any patient with neutrocytic ascites. Analysis of ascitic fluid is helpful in differentiating the two entities. Secondary bacterial peritonitis should be suspected when ascitic fluid analysis shows two or three of the following criteria: total protein > 1 gm/dl, glucose < 50 mg/dl, and LDH > 225 mU/ml (or higher than the upper limit of normal for serum). Most of the ascitic fluid cultures in such patients are polymicrobial, whereas in patients with SBP the infection is usually monomicrobial. Patients with suspected secondary peritonitis must be evaluated by emergency radiologic techniques to confirm and localize the possible visceral perforation. In patients with nonperforation secondary peritonitis, these criteria are not as useful; however, PMN cell count after 48 hours of treatment increases beyond the pretreatment value and ascitic fluid culture remains positive. Conversely, ascitic fluid PMN cell count decreases rapidly in appropriately treated patients with SBP, and ascitic fluid culture becomes negative.

10. Who is at high risk of developing SBP?
- Cirrhotic patients with gastrointestinal hemorrhage
- Cirrhotic patients with ascitic fluid total protein < 1gm/dl, especially those with high bilirubin (> 3.2 mg/dl) or low platelet count ($< 98,000$ cells/mm^3)
- Cirrhotics who have survived an episode of SBP
- Patients with fulminant hepatic failure

11. What is the pathogenesis of SBP?

Gram-negative bacteria are the most common causative agents isolated in bacterial infections in cirrhotic patients. Therefore, it has been suggested that the gut may be the source of the bacteria. Direct passage of intestinal bacteria to portal blood or ascitic fluid has not been documented in cirrhotic patients, if the gut mucosa has not lost its integrity. Bacterial translocation, defined as the passage of viable bacteria from gastrointestinal tract to mesenteric lymph nodes, has been demonstrated in an experimental model of cirrhotic rats with ascites and in cirrhotic patients submitted to a laparotomy. In fact, genetic identity has been observed between bacteria isolated in the gut, mesenteric lymph nodes, and ascitic fluid in cirrhotic rats. Intestinal baterial overgrowth seems to be the main mechanism of bacterial translocation in cirrhotic rats. Reducing the quantity of intestinal flora has been shown to decrease the incidence of bacterial translocation and SBP. Several immune deficiencies, especially decreased activity of the reticuloendothelial system and low serum complement levels, lead to frequent and prolonged bacteremia in cirrhotic patients and to colonization of body fluids, such as ascitic fluid. The development of a bacterial infection depends on the capacity of ascitic fluid to kill the bacteria. In vitro, the capacity of ascitic fluid to kill bacteria (i.e., opsonic activity) is related directly to total protein and C3 concentration of ascitic fluid. Cirrhotic patients with low ascitic fluid opsonic activity have low C3, low total protein, and thus a higher incidence of SBP. In contrast, patients with high ascitic fluid opsonic activity have high C3 and high total protein; thus bacterial colonization may resolve spontaneously.

12. What single test provides early information about possible ascitic fluid infection?

The decision to start empirical antibiotic treatment must be made as soon as possible, because the survival rate depends in part on early diagnosis and treatment. Gram stain is positive in only 5–10% of patients, and bacterial culture of ascitic fluid takes at least 12 hours to demonstrate growth. The ascitic fluid neutrophil count is highly sensitive in detecting bacterial infection of peritoneal fluid, and the result should be available in a matter of minutes. An absolute neutrophil count ≥ 250 cells/mm^3 warrants empiric antibiotic treatment. Ascitic fluid for cell count should be immediately injected into a tube containing an anticoagulant (i.e., "purple top" tube) to avoid clotting of the specimen. Other tests, such as ascitic fluid pH or lactate or arterial-ascitic fluid gradient of pH or lactate, are significantly less sensitive than ascitic fluid neutrophil count and are currently not used in clinical practice.

13. What is the treatment of choice for suspected SBP?

A relatively broad-spectrum antibiotic combination, such as an aminoglycoside plus ampicillin, was routinely used in the past for treatment of suspected SBP. However, most cirrhotic patients treated with an aminoglycoside developed nephrotoxicity, even if serum levels were controlled. Third-generation cephalosporins cover most of the flora responsible for SBP; they are more effective than the combination of ampicillin and aminoglycoside and lack nephrotoxicity. Cefotaxime or a similar cephalosporin should be started when SBP is suspected. Recently, it was demonstrated that 2.0 gm of cefotaxime, given intravenously every 8–12 hours, is as effective as dosing every 6 hours. A short course of therapy (5 days) has been shown to be as effective as a long course (10 days). Amoxicillin-clavulanic acid, initially intravenously (1–0.2 gm/8 hr) and then orally (500 mg–125 mg/8 hr), has been shown to be as effective as cefotaxime but less expensive. Unfortuantely, intravenous amoxicillin-clavulanic acid is not available in the U.S.

Patients with uncomplicated SBP (i.e., those without shock, ileus, gastrointestinal hemorrhage, or hepatic encephalopathy) can be safely treated with oral ofloxacin (400 mg/12 hr). Patients on prophylaxis for SBP with quinolones develop infections caused by gram-negative cocci or quinolone-resistant gram-negative bacilli. Empiric cefotaxime or amoxicillin-clavulanic acid are also effective in such patients. One recent study has shown that intravenous albumin administration, at a dose of 1.5 gm/kg at the time of diagnosis of SBP and 1 gm/kg on day 3 of treatment, reduces the incidence of renal impairment and death. Albumin should be considered especially in patients with SBP and blood urea nitrogen (BUN) > 30 mg/dl and/or serum bilirubin > 4 mg/dl (Fig. 1).

14. When should antibiotic treatment be started in a patient with cirrhosis and suspected ascitic fluid infection?

Empirical antibiotic treatment must be started as soon as possible to improve survival rates. Therefore, it is important to perform routine bacterial cultures of ascitic fluid, blood, urine, and sputum as well as an ascitic fluid cell count and differential when a hospitalized patient with ascites develops clinical signs of possible infection (fever, abdominal pain, encephalopathy) or shows deterioration in clinical or laboratory parameters. In addition, ascitic fluid and urine should be analyzed when cirrhotic patients with ascites are admitted to the hospital; about 20% are infected at this time. A high level of suspicion for bacterial infection is appropriate, because it is a reversible cause of deterioration and a frequent cause of death in patients with cirrhosis. Empirical antibiotics should be started immediately after performing cultures and ascitic fluid analysis whenever (1) bacterial infection is suspected based on abdominal pain or fever or (2) ascitic fluid neutrophils are ≥ 250 cells/mm^3 (see Fig. 1).

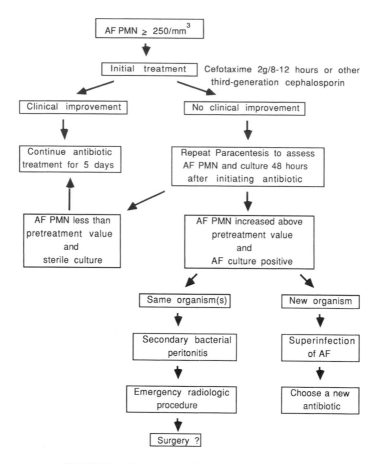

FIGURE 1.   Management of spontaneous bacterial peritonitis.

15. Should the PMN cell count in ascitic fluid be monitored during treatment of SBP?

Ascitic fluid culture becomes negative after a single 2-gm dose of cefotaxime in 86% of patients with SBP. The neutrophil count also decreases rapidly to normal values during therapy in 90%. Superinfection or early recurrence after treatment with third-generation cephalosporins is uncommon. Repeat paracentesis is not necessary, if the setting (advanced cirrhosis) is typical, one orgainsm is cultured, and the patient has the usual dramatic response to treatment. However, 2 or 3 days after starting antibiotic treatment, repeat paracentesis can be considered to confirm the decrease in PMNs in the fluid and sterility of the fluid.

16. Does bacterascites represent a real peritoneal infection? Should it be treated?

Recent studies have documented the short-term natural history of monomicrobial nonneutrocytic bacterascites. A repeat paracentesis of patients with bacterascites before starting antibiotic therapy showed that in 62–86% the episode of bacterascites resolved spontaneously. Of interest, all patients who progressed to SBP had symptoms of bacterial infection at the time of the first tap. Such data demonstrate that bacterascites is a dynamic process; its evolution may depend on several factors, including systemic and ascitic fluid defenses as well as organism virulence. According to these studies, symptomatic patients with bacterascites should be treated with antibiotics. Asymptomatic patients need not receive antibiotic treatment but should be reevaluated with a second tap. If the PMN count is $\geq 250/mm^3$, antibiotics should be started.

17. Which subgroups of patients with liver disease should receive treatment to prevent bacterial infection?

Because enteric aerobic gram-negative bacteria are the most frequent causative agents isolated in bacterial infections in cirrhosis and because bacterial translocation seems to be an important step in pathogenesis, inhibition of intestinal gram-negative bacteria should be an effective method of preventing bacterial infections. Patients with liver disease who are at high risk of developing bacterial infection and/or SBP should be considered for selective intestinal decontamination (SID). SID consists of the inhibition of the gram-negative flora of the gut with preservation of gram-positive cocci and anaerobic bacteria. Preservation of the anaerobes is important in preventing intestinal colonization, overgrowth, and subsequent translocation of pathogenic bacteria. Several trials have shown that SID with oral norfloxacin is highly effective in preventing bacterial infections and/or SBP in cirrhotic inpatients with (1) gastrointestinal hemorrhage (400 mg twice daily) or (2) low ascitic fluid protein (400 mg/day) and (3) in patients with fulminant hepatic failure (400 mg/day). Long-term antibiotic therapy has been used in preventing the first episode of SBP as well as recurrences. Long-term prophylactic treatment decreases the incidence of SBP in both conditions, but increases the appearance of quinolone-resistant bacteria and infections. Secondary prophylaxis is generally well accepted, especially in patients awaiting liver transplantation. Long-term primary prophylaxis is currently being evaluated in more restrictive groups of patients, such as those with low ascitic fluid total protein and high serum bilirubin (> 3.2 mg/dl) or low platelet count (< 98,000 cells/mm^3).

18. Why is it important to know the sodium balance in patients with cirrhosis and ascites?

Ascites formation in cirrhosis is due to renal retention of sodium and water. The aim of medical treatment of ascites in patients with cirrhosis is to mobilize the ascitic fluid by creating a net negative balance of sodium. This goal is accomplished by reducing sodium intake in the diet and increasing urinary sodium excretion. Therefore, knowledge of urinary excretion of sodium allows the clinician to plan initial treatment. In addition, urinary sodium excretion is an easily determined prognostic indicator. Patients with cirrhosis and a urinary sodium excretion < 10 mEq/day have a 2-year survival rate of 20%, whereas those with sodium excretion > 10 mEq/day have a 2-year survival rate of 60%.

19. Describe the initial treatment of patients with cirrhosis and ascites.

Cirrhotic patients with ascites should be treated initially by dietary sodium restriction (50–88 mEq/day) and diuretics. A more severe restriction of sodium intake may worsen anorexia and malnutrition. Water restriction is usually not necessary, if serum sodium concentration is above 120 mEq/L. In 15–20% of patients a negative sodium balance may be obtained with dietary sodium restriction in the absence of diuretics. However, because 80–85% of patients need diuretics, it is reasonable to start diuretics in all patients. The initial dose of diuretics should be 100 mg of spironolactone and 40 mg of furosemide—both drugs are given orally in a single morning dose. If the body weight does not decrease or the urinary sodium excretion does not increase after 2–3 days of treatment, the dose of both diuretics should be progressively increased, usually in simultaneous increments of 100 mg/day and 40 mg/day, respectively. Serial monitoring of urinary sodium excretion and daily weight is the best way to determine the optimal dose of diuretics. Doses should be increased until a negative sodium balance is obtained (i.e., urinary excretion is greater than dietary intake) with corresponding weight loss. The ceiling doses of spironolactone and furosemide are 400 mg and 160 mg per day, respectively. Once ascites has been mobilized, diuretic dosage should be adjusted individually to keep the patient free of ascites. Patients with tense ascites should be treated initially with a therapeutic paracentesis of 4 or more liters (Fig. 2).

20. What is refractory ascites?

Refractory ascites is an inadequate response to sodium-restricted diet and high-dose diuretic treatment. This inadequate response is manifested by the absence of weight loss or the development of complications of diuretics. Excessive sodium intake, bacterial infection, occult gastrointestinal hemorrhage, and intake of prostaglandin inhibitors (e.g., aspirin or nonsteroidal anti-inflammatory drugs) should be excluded before labeling patients as refractory. Less than 10% of cirrhotic patients

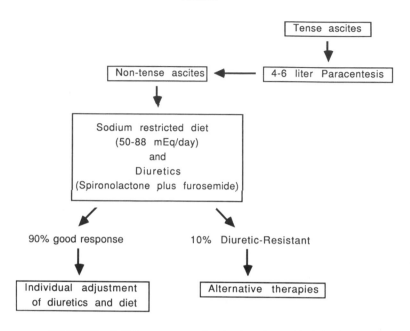

FIGURE 2.   Initial management of ascites in patients with cirrhosis.

are refractory to standard medical therapy. This small group should be evaluated for other therapeutic options, such as liver transplantation, chronic outpatient paracenteses (usually every 2 weeks), peritoneovenous shunt, or transjugular intrahepatic portosystemic stent-shunt (TIPS).

21. Which patients should be treated with large-volume paracentesis?

Large-volume paracentesis is an old but safe and effective procedure to mobilize ascitic fluid in cirrhotic patients. Interest in this procedure has been renewed in the past decade. Recently, it has been shown that therapeutic paracentesis not only is safe but also may have additional beneficial effects on the hemodynamic status of patients with tense ascites. However, repeated large-volume paracenteses cause depletion of proteins and, theoretically, may predispose to SBP. Therefore, therapeutic paracentesis should not be used as a routine treatment of all cirrhotic patients with ascites and should be reserved for treating patients with tense and/or refractory ascites.

22. Is there currently any indication for peritoneovenous shunt?

Peritoneovenous shunt was introduced for the treatment of cirrhotics with refractory ascites in 1974 by LeVeen and associates. After initial enthusiasm, many complications were reported and the enthusiasm decreased progressively. The number of complications is especially high in patients with severe hepatocellular insufficiency. Peritoneovenous shunt does not reduce mortality during the initial hospitalization and does not improve long-term survival in cirrhotic patients. Therefore, peritoneovenous shunts should be considered in cirrhotic patients with refractory ascites who are not candidates for liver transplantation and in whom large-volume paracentesis is difficult.

23. Which patients with cirrhosis and ascites should be considered for TIPS?

TIPS is an interventional radiologic technique that consists of creating a fistula between a hepatic vein and a portal vein and then placing an expandable metal stent in the balloon-dilated fistula to maintain patency. This technique was introduced to treat patients with recurrent variceal hemorrhage by decreasing portal pressure. Initial results show that TIPS could be useful in the treatment of cirrhotics with refractory ascites. However, the incidence of shunt dysfunction is still quite high. A recently published controlled trial has reported a survival advantage after TIPS in treatment of cirrhotic patients with refractory ascites.

24. Which patients with cirrhosis and ascites should be evaluated for liver transplantation?

The probability of survival after the first onset of ascites has been estimated at 50% and 20% after 1 and 5 years of follow-up, respectively. The prognosis is even worse in patients with diuretic-resistant ascites; the 1-year survival rate is 25%. Because the 1-year survival rate after liver transplantation is > 75%, patients with cirrhosis who develop ascites should be considered for liver transplantation. Once the fluid becomes diuretic-resistant, consideration for transplantation becomes even more urgent. However, some alcoholic patients with diuretic-resistant ascites may become diuretic-sensitive after months of alcohol abstinence.

25. What is the hepatorenal syndrome?

The hepatorenal syndrome occurs in patients with advanced liver failure and portal hypertension. It is characterized by impaired renal function due to arterial vasodilatation and reflex activation of the endogenous vasoconstrictive systems. According to clinical outcome, hepatorenal syndrome can be divided into two types:

Type I is characterized by a rapid and progressive reduction of renal function defined by a doubling of the initial serum creatinine to a level > 2.5 mg/dl or a 50% reduction of the initial 24-hour creatinine clearance to a level < 20 ml/min in less than 2 weeks.

In **type II**, renal failure does not have such a rapidly progressive course.

26. What are the criteria for hepatorenal syndrome?

1. Chronic or acute liver disease with advanced hepatic failure and portal hypertension.
2. Low glomerular filtration rate, as indicated by serum creatinine > 1.5 mg/dl or 24-hour creatinine clearance < 40 ml/min.
3. Absence of shock, ongoing bacterial infection, current or recent treatment with nephrotoxic drugs, and absence of gastrointestinal fluid losses by repeated vomiting or intense diarrhea or renal fluid losses.
4. No sustained improvement in renal function following diuretic withdrawal and expansion of plasma volume with 1.5 L of isotonic saline.
5. Proteinuria < 500 mg/dl and no ultrasonographic evidence of obstructive uropathy or parenchymal disease.

27. Derscribe the treatment of patients with hepatorenal syndrome.

Liver transplantation is currently the treatment of choice in patients with hepatorenal syndrome. Unfortunately, patients with hepatorenal syndrome type I usually die before an organ is available. The mortality rate of patients with hepatorenal syndrome type I is almost 100% in less than 2 months. Treatments such as hemodialysis, peritoneovenous shunt, albumin infusion, and dopamine infusion have been evaluated and found to be of only transient benefit or without benefit. Recent prospective but uncontrolled studies have shown that hepatorenal syndrome can be reversed by the administration of vasoconstrictive drugs, such as ornipressin, associated with albumin expansion. Randomized controlled trials are needed. Perhaps these agents will allow some patients to survive long enough to undergo liver transplantation.

28. Should volume expanders be infused after large-volume paracentesis?

Plasma volume expansion after large-volume paracentesis is controversial. Volume expanders were introduced to avoid theoretical hemodynamic disturbances that may develop in cirrhotic patients after therapeutic paracentesis of 5 or more liters of ascitic fluid. One study reported that patients receiving albumin infusion after large-volume paracentesis had less hyponatremia and azotemia than patients who did not receive albumin. However, albumin infusion did not decrease symptomatic complications or hospital readmissions or increase survival rates. Because albumin infusion is expensive, less costly volume expanders have been tried. Additional studies are needed.

At this time, volume expanders should be viewed as optional until it is demonstrated that volume expansion after therapeutic paracentesis has a beneficial effect on morbidity or survival.

BIBLIOGRAPHY

1. Akriviadis EA, Runyon BA: The value of an algorithm in differentiating spontaneous from secondary bacterial peritonitis. Gastroenterology 98:127–133, 1990.
2. Arroyo V, Ginés P, Gerbes AL, et al: Definition and diagnostic criteria of refractory ascites and hepatorenal syndrome in cirrhosis. Hepatology 23:164–176, 1996.
3. Felisart J, Rimola A, Arroyo V, et al: Cefotaxime is more effective than is ampicillin-tobramycin in cirrhotics with severe infections. Hepatology 5:457–462, 1985.
4. Gines P, Rimola A, Planas R, et al: Norfloxacin prevents spontaneous bacterial peritonitis recurrence in cirrhosis: Results of a double-blind, placebo-controlled trial. Hepatology 12:716–724, 1990.
5. Gines P, Tito L, Arroyo V, et al: Randomized comparative study of therapeutic paracentesis with and without intravenous albumin in cirrhosis. Gastroenterology 94:1493–1502, 1998.
6. Guarner C, Runyon BA, Young S, et al: Intestinal bacterial overgrowth and bacterial translocation in an experimental model of cirrhosis in rats. J Hepatol 26:1372–1378, 1997.
7. Guarner C, Solá R, Soriano G, Andreu M, et al: Risk of a first community-acquired spontaneous bacterial peritonitis in cirrhotics with low ascitic fluid protein levels. Gastroenterology 117:414–419, 1999.
8. Guarner C, Soriano G: Spontaneous bacterial peritonitis. Semin Liver Dis 17:203–217, 1997.
9. McHutchison JG, Runyon BA: Spontaneous bacterial peritonitis. In Surawicz CM, Owen RL (eds): Gastrointestinal and Hepatic Infections. Philadelphia, W.B. Saunders, 1994, pp 455–475.
10. Navasa M, Follo A, Llovet JM, et al: Randomized, comparative study of oral ofloxacin versus intravenous cefotaxime in spontaneous bacterial peritonitis. Gastroenterology 111:1011–1017, 1996.
11. Novella MT, Solá R, Soriano G, et al: Continuous vs inpatient prophylaxis of the first episode of spontaneous bacterial peritonitis with norfloxacin. Hepatology 25:532–536, 1997.
12. Ortiz J, Soriano G, Coll P, Novella MT, et al: Early microbiologic diagnosis of spontaneous bacterial peritonitis with BacT/ALERT. J Hepatol 26:839–844, 1997.
13. Ortiz J, Vila MC, Soriano G, et al: Infections caused by *Escherichia coli* resistant to norfloxacin in hospitalized cirrhotic patients. Hepatology 29:1064–1069, 1999.
14. Ricart E, Soriano G, Novella MT, et al: Amoxicillin-clavulanic acid versus cefotaxime in the therapy of bacterial infections in cirrhotic patients. J Hepatol 32:596–602, 2000.
15. Rimola A, Garcia-Tsao G, Navasa M, et al, for the International Ascites Club: Diagnosis, treatment and prophylaxis of spontaneous bacterial peritonitis: A consensus document. J Hepatol 32:142–153, 2000.
15a. Rossle M, Ochs A, Gulberg V, et al: A comparison of paracentesis and transjugular intrahepatic portosystemic shunting in patients with ascites. N Engl J Med 342:1701–1707, 2000.
16. Runyon BA: Low-protein-concentration ascitic fluid is predisposed to spontaneous bacterial peritonitis. Gastroenterology 191:1343–1346, 1986.
17. Runyon BA: Ascites. In Schiff E, Schiff L (eds): Diseases of the Liver, 7th ed. Philadelphia, J.B. Lippincott, 1993, pp 990–1015.
18. Runyon BA: Refractory ascites. Semin Liver Dis 13:343–351, 1993.
19. Runyon BA: Care of patients with ascites. N Engl J Med 330:337–342, 1994.
20. Runyon BA: Malignancy-related ascites and ascitic fluid humoral tests of malignancy [editorial]. J Clin Gastoenterol 18:94–98, 1994.
21. Runyon BA, Canawati HN, Akriviadis EA: Optimization of ascitic fluid culture technique. Gastroenterology 95:1351–1355, 1988.
22. Runyon BA, McHutchison JG, Antillon MR, et al: Short-course vs long-course antibiotic treatment of spontaneous bacterial peritonitis: A randomized controlled study of 100 patients. Gastroenterology 100:1737–1742, 1991.
23. Runyon BA, Montano AA, Akriviadis EA, et al: The serum-ascites albumin gradient is superior to the exudate-transudate concept in the differential diagnosis of ascites. Ann Intern Med 117:215–220, 1992.
24. Soriano G, Guarner C, Teixido M, et al: Selective intestinal decontamination prevents spontaneous bacterial peritonitis. Gastroenterology 100:477–481, 1991.
25. Soriano G, Guarner C, Tomas A, et al: Norfloxacin prevents bacterial infection in cirrhotics with gastrointestinal hemorrhage. Gastroenterology 103:1267–1272, 1992.
26. Sort P, Navasa M, Arroyo V, Aldeguer X, et al: Effect of intravenous albumin on renal impairment and mortality in patients with cirrhosis and spontaneous bacterial peritonitis. N Engl J Med 341:403–409, 1999.
27. Stanley MM, Ochi S, Lee KK, et al: Peritoneovenous shunting as compared with medical treatment in patients with alcoholic cirrhosis and massive ascites. N Engl J Med 321:1632–1638, 1989.
28. Such J, Runyon BA. Spontaneous bacterial peritonitis. Clin Infect Dis 27:669–704, 1998.

32. LIVER ABSCESS

Jorge L. Herrera, M.D.

1. What are the two major categories of liver abscess?

The two types of liver abscess are pyogenic and amebic. Pyogenic abscesses usually arise from intraabdominal infections, whereas amebic abscesses arise from colonic infection with invasive *Entamoeba histolytica*. This differentiation is important because diagnostic approach and management differ for the two conditions.

2. Describe the clinical features of pyogenic liver abscess.

Most patients are middle-aged or older, with a recent shift in age toward younger patients. The median age is 51 years, according to a recent series. The condition is equally prevalent in both sexes. The clinical findings are nonspecific but may include fever, chills, right-upper-quadrant pain, malaise, and weight loss. Fever may be absent in up to 30% of cases. Abdominal pain is present in only 45% of cases. Only 37% present with the classic findings of fever and right-upper-quadrant tenderness, reinforcing the often nonspecific nature of signs and symptoms. In many patients, the clinical presentation may be dominated by the underlying cause, such as appendicitis, diverticulitis, or biliary disease.

Comorbidities are common, including diabetes mellitus, malignancy, alcoholism, cardiovascular disease, and chronic renal failure. The mean duration of symptoms before hospital admission is 26 days, with a range of 1–200 days and a median of 14 days.

3. What are the clinical features of amebic liver abscess?

Patients tend to be younger (30–40 years), are more often male, have more severe right-upper-quadrant pain, and are febrile in 90% of cases. A history of travel to endemic areas is common, although it may be remote. Prior symptoms suggestive of previous colonic amebiasis are present in only 5–15% of patients. Concurrent hepatic abscess and amebic dysentery are unusual.

4. What laboratory features are distinctive in patients with liver abscess?

Results of routine laboratory tests are not diagnostic for pyogenic or amebic liver abscess. Leukocytosis is often present but may be absent in a significant number of patients. Normochromic normocytic anemia is present in over 70% of patients. Eosinophilia is characteristically absent in patients with amebic cysts. The erythrocyte sedimentation rate is invariably raised. Liver test abnormalities are not specific. Over 90% of patients have elevation of alkaline phosphatase (AP), but aspartate aminotransferase (AST) and alanine aminostranferase (ALT) are elevated to lesser degrees. If significant hyperbilirubinemia is present, the biliary tree is the likely source of the abscess; bilirubin levels are lowest in patients with cryptogenic liver abscess. Hypoalbuminemia is frequently described, and a level < 2 gm/dl carries a poor prognosis. Blood cultures are positive in 50% of patients with pyogenic abscess, and 75–90% of aspirates from the abscesses are positive for bacteria.

5. What are the most common sources of pyogenic liver abscess?

Biliary tract disease is the most common known source of pyogenic liver abscess, accounting for 35% of cases. In most cases the cause cannot be identified, and the disease is therefore termed cryptogenic. Most abscesses related to biliary disease result from cholangitis or acute cholecystitis. Malignant tumors of the pancreas, common bile duct, and ampulla account for 10–20% of hepatic abscesses originating in the biliary tree. Endoscopic or surgical intervention in the biliary tree also may result in hepatic abscess formation. Parasitic invasion of the biliary tree by roundworms or flukes leads to biliary infection and possible hepatic abscess.

Another common source of pyogenic liver abscesses is intraabdominal infections with bacterial seeding through the portal vein. Diverticulitis, Crohn's disease, ulcerative colitis, and bowel perforation account for 30% of pyogenic liver abscesses. Appendicitis is a rare cause of liver abscess except in older or immunocompromised patients, in whom the diagnosis of appendicitis may be delayed. About 15% of liver abscesses arise by direct extension from a contiguous source, such as a subphrenic abscess or empyema of the gallbladder. Pyogenic infection may be carried to the liver in hepatic arterial blood flow from distant localized infections, such as endocarditis or severe dental disease.

6. List the organisms that commonly cause pyogenic liver abscess.

Gram-negative organisms are implicated in 50–70% cases. *Escherichia coli* is the most common aerobic gram-negative organism cultured. Aerobic gram-positive organisms account for approximately 25% of infections, and up to 50% of cases are caused by anaerobes. Recent reports suggest that aerobes are becoming a more common cause of abscess than anaerobes.

Bacteriology of Pyogenic Liver Abscess

GRAM-NEGATIVE AEROBES (50–70%)	GRAM-POSITIVE AEROBES (25%)	ANAEROBES (40–50%)
Escherichia coli (35–45%)	*Streptococcus faecalis*	*Fusobacterium nucleatum*
Klebsiella sp.	β Streptococci	*Bacteroides* sp.
Proteus sp.	α Streptococci	*Bacteroides fragilis*
Enterobacter sp.	Staphylococci	*Peptostreptococcus* sp.
Serratia sp.		*Actinomyces* sp.
Morganella sp.		*Clostridium* sp.
Actinobacter sp.		

From Frey CF, Zhu Y, Suzuki M, Isaji S: Liver abscess. Surg Clin North Am 69:259–271, 1989, with permission.

7. Do negative cultures from an abscess aspirate indicate a nonpyogenic abscess?

No. Although most cultures are positive, a negative culture may reflect improper handling of the specimen or prior antibiotic therapy. Proper collection and culture techniques are of critical importance for growing anaerobic organisms. Culture material should be transported to the laboratory immediately in the syringe used for aspiration to avoid exposure to air. Never submit swabs for culture of liver abscess. Anaerobic organisms may require at least several days and up to 1 week or more for sufficient growth to establish a diagnosis. For this reason, a Gram stain of the aspirate is of paramount importance. A Gram stain that demonstrates organisms with no growth in cultures after 2 or 3 days suggests an anaerobic pathogen. All aspirated material should be cultured for aerobic, anaerobic, and microaerophilic organisms.

8. What abnormalities can be detected on standard radiologic studies of patients with liver abscess?

A chest radiograph may be abnormal in 50–80% of patients with liver abscess. Right-lower-lobe atelectasis, right pleural effusion, and an elevated right hemidiaphragm may be clues to the presence of a liver abscess. Perforation of a pyogenic liver abscess into the thoracic cavity may result in empyema. In plain abdominal films, air can be seen in the abscess cavities in 10–20% of cases. Gastric displacement due to enlargement of the liver also may be seen. These features are not sensitive for the diagnosis of liver abscess.

9. Which imaging studies should be obtained in evaluating a suspected liver abscess?

Ultrasonography is the initial procedure of choice. It is noninvasive and highly accurate, with a sensitivity of 80–90%. It is the preferred modality to distinguish cystic from solid lesions and in most patients is more accurate than computed tomographic (CT) scanning for visualizing the biliary tree.

Ultrasonography, however, is operator-dependent, and its accuracy may be affected by the patient's habitus or overlying gas. CT with intravenous contrast aids in the identification of smaller abscesses that may be missed on ultrasound examination; it is especially useful in the detection of microabscesses. CT scanning provides an assessment not only of the liver but also of the entire peritoneal cavity, which may provide information about the primary lesions causing the liver abscess.

Magnetic resonance imaging (MRI) does not add much to the sensitivity of CT scanning. Scintigraphy with technetium sulfur colloid is sensitive for detecting lesions > 2 cm in diameter. Gallium scanning may add to the sensitivity of technetium scanning, because pyogenic liver abscess avidly takes up gallium. Amebic abscesses, however, tend to concentrate gallium only in the periphery of the abscess cavity. In general, scintigraphy is the least helpful of the scanning modalities.

10. What areas of the liver are usually affected by hepatic abscess?

Right lobe only	65% of patients
Both lobes	30%
Left lobe only	5%

11. How can the location, size, and number of liver abscesses help to determine the source?

Pyogenic liver abscesses arising from a biliary source tend to be multiple and of small size and involve both lobes of the liver. Septic emboli from the portal vein may be solitary and tend to be more common in the right lobe of the liver because most of the portal vein flow goes to the right lobe. Abscesses arising from a contiguous source tend to be solitary and localized to one lobe only.

Amebic liver abscesses tend to be solitary and large. Most commonly they are located in the right lobe of the liver. The right lobe receives a major part of the venous drainage from the cecum and ascending colon, which are the parts of the bowel most commonly affected by amebiasis. Abscesses located in the dome of the liver or complicated by a bronchopleural fistula are typically amebic in origin.

12. When should a hepatic abscess be aspirated?

Hepatic abscesses should be aspirated if they are thought to be pyogenic and not amebic. Patients with multiple abscesses, coexistent biliary disease, or an intraabdominal inflammatory process are more likely to have pyogenic abscess. In such patients, aspiration under ultrasound guidance with Gram stain and culture helps to guide antibiotic selection. Aspiration of amebic abscesses should be considered under the following circumstances: (1) when pyogenic abscess or secondary infection of an amebic abscess cannot be excluded; (2) when the patient does not respond to adequate therapy for amebic liver abscess; or (3) when the abscess is very large and causes severe pain.

13. In what situation should an amebic liver abscess be treated by open surgical drainage?

When the amebic abscess is located in the left lobe of the liver and response to therapy is not dramatic within the first 24–48 hours, open surgical drainage should be performed. Complications of left-lobe amebic abscess, such as cardiac tamponade, are associated with high mortality and require prompt intervention to prevent their occurrence.

14. Does aspiration of an amebic hepatic abscess yield diagnostic material in most patients?

No. Trophozoites are found in < 20% of aspirates. Although classically the contents of amebic abscess are described as "anchovy paste" in appearance, in practice most aspirated material does not conform to this description. The contents of an amebic abscess are typically odorless. Foul-smelling aspirates or a positive Gram stain should suggest a pyogenic abscess or secondarily infected amebic abscess.

15. How often is the biliary tree involved in patients with amebic liver abscess?

Bile is lethal to amebas; thus, infection of the gallbladder and bile ducts does not occur. In patients with a large amebic or pyogenic abscess, compression of the biliary system may result in jaundice, but cholangitis occurs only with secondary bacterial infection.

16. How can the diagnosis of an amebic abscess be confirmed?

Amebic abscesses are best differentiated from pyogenic abscesses by serologic tests:

Hemagglutination (IHA)	Gel diffusion precipitin (GDP)
Indirect immunofluorescence (IF)	Complement fixation (CF)
Counterimmunoelectrophoresis (CIE)	Latex agglutination (LA)
Immunoelectrophoresis (IEP)	Enzyme-linked immunosorbent assay (ELISA)

Serologic tests are positive only in patients with invasive amebiasis, such as hepatic abscess or amebic colitis. They are negative in asymptomatic carriers. With the exception of CF, these tests are highly sensitive (95–99%). The IHA is extremely sensitive, and a negative test excludes the diagnosis; a titer > 1:512 is present in almost all patients with invasive disease. IHA, however, remains positive for many years, and a positive titer may indicate prior infection. GDP titers usually become negative 6 months after the infection, and this is the test of choice for patients from endemic areas with prior exposure to amebiasis. A high GDP titer in a patient with hepatic abscess suggests an amebic abscess, even if the patient has a prior history of invasive amebiasis. In general, the choice of serologic tests depends on availability and epidemiologic considerations.

17. Describe the treatment for pyogenic liver abscess.

For single abscess or several large abscesses, treatment consists of antibiotics and appropriate drainage. Drainage should be performed percutaneously whenever possible. The combination of percutaneous drainage with intravenous antibiotics results in a 76% cure rate, compared with 65% for antibiotic alone and 61% for surgery alone.

It is not clear whether percutaneous catheter drainage is superior to aspiration without catheter placement. Most centers favor catheter drainage over simple aspiration. Surgical drainage should be performed only if more conservative measures do not result in complete resolution or if surgery is needed to treat a primary intraabdominal lesion. For multiple microabscesses, antibiotic therapy and correction of the underlying biliary abnormality may suffice.

Antibiotic coverage involves a combination of antibiotics directed against anaerobes, gram-negative aerobes, and enterococci. Thus, the combination of an aminoglycoside or cephalosporin for aerobic gram-negative organisms, clindamycin or metronidazole for anaerobes, and penicillin or ampicillin for enterococci is commonly used. The antibiotic regimen may be altered as needed, depending on culture results or clinical response. Intravenous treatment should be continued for 10–14 days or longer if drains are still in place. Two weeks of oral therapy may be added.

18. Describe the treatment for amebic liver abscess.

Metronidazole is the only drug active against the extraintestinal form of amebiasis. A dose of 750 mg 3 times/day for 10 days is recommended. Even at this dose, metronidazole is somewhat less effective in the intestinal form of the disease; thus, a luminal amebicide such as iodoquinol (diiodohydroxyquin), 650 mg 3 times/day for 20 days, should be prescribed to eradicate the intestinal form and prevent recurrence. Uncomplicated amebic abscess should be managed conservatively with metronidazole. Needle aspiration should be considered for large (> 7cm) abscesses and for patients who fail to respond after 7 days of metronidazole. Operative intervention should be performed only for complications or when conservative therapy fails.

19. List the potential complications of pyogenic liver abscess.

Untreated, pyogenic liver abscesses have a mortality rate of 100%. Other complications include rupture into the peritoneal cavity, which may form subphrenic, perihepatic, or subhepatic abscess or peritonitis. Rupture into the pleural space may cause empyema. Rupture into the pericardial sac may result in pericarditis and pericardial tamponade. Metastatic septic emboli involving the lungs, brain, or eyes also may occur.

20. List the potential complications of amebic liver abscess.

The complications of amebic liver abscess are similar to those of pyogenic liver abscess. Rupture into the pleural space results in amebic empyema. Rupture into the lung parenchyma may produce a lung abscess or bronchopleural fistula. Pericardial extension occurs in 1–2% of patients and is associated with amebic abscesses in the left lobe of the liver. A serous pericardial effusion may indicate impending rupture. Constrictive pericarditis occasionally follows suppurative amebic pericarditis. Brain abscess from hematogenous spread of the infection also has been reported.

21. What is the prognosis for patients with liver abscess?
The prognosis depends on the rapidity of diagnosis and the underlying illness. Patients with amebic liver abscess generally do well with appropriate treatment; morbidity and mortality rates are 4.5% and 2.2%, respectively, in recent series. Response to treatment is prompt and dramatic. Healing of the abscess leads to residual scar tissue associated with subcapsular retraction. Occasionally, in patients with large abscess, a residual cavity surrounded by fibroconnective tissue may persist.

The mortality rate associated with pyogenic liver abscess has been reduced to 5–10% with prompt recognition and adequate antibiotic therapy; it is highest in patients with multiple abscesses. Mortality is highly dependent on the underlying disease process. Morbidity remains high at 50%, primarily because of the complexity of therapy and the need for prolonged drainage.

BIBLIOGRAPHY

1. Block MA: Abscesses of the liver (other than amebic). In Haubrich WS, Schaffner F, Berk JE (eds): Bockus Gastroenterology, 5th ed. Philadelphia, W.B. Saunders, 1995, pp 2405–2427.
2. Crippin JS, Wang KK: A unrecognized etiology for pyogenic hepatic abscesses in normal hosts: Dental disease. Am J Gastroenterol 87:1740–1742, 1992.
3. DeCock KM, Reynolds TB: Amebic and pyogenic liver abscess. In Schitt L, Schiff ER (eds): Diseases of the Liver, 7th ed. Philadelphia, J.B. Lippincott, 1993, pp 1320–1337.
4. Filice C, Di Perri G, Strosselli M, et al: Outcome of hepatic amebic abscesses managed with three different therapeutic strategies. Dig Dis Sci 37:240–247, 1992.
5. Frey CF, Zhu Y, Suzuki M, Isaji S: Liver abscesses. Surg Clin North Am 69:259–271, 1989.
6. Kandel G, Marcon NE: Pyogenic liver abscess: New concepts of an old disease. Am J Gastroenterol 79:65–71, 1984.
7. Knight R: Hepatic amebiasis. Semin Liver Dis 4:277–292, 1984.
8. Monroe LS: Gastrointestinal parasites. In Haubrich WS, Schaffner F, Berk JE (eds): Bockus Gastroenterology, 5th ed. Philadelphia, W.D. Saunders, 1995, pp 3123–3134.
9. Ralls PW, Barnes PF, Johnson MB, et al: Medical treatment of hepatic amoebic abscess: Rare need for percutaneous drainage. Radiology 165:805–807, 1987.
10. Teague M, Baddour LM, Wruble LD: Liver abscess: A harbinger of Crohn's disease. Am J Gastroenterol 83:1412–1414, 1988.
11. Vukmir RB: Pyogenic hepatic abscess. Ann Emerg Med 20:421–423, 1991.
12. Chou FF, Sheen-chen SM, Chen YS, Chen MC: Single and multiple pyogenic liver abscesses: Clinical course, etiology and results of treatment. World J Surg 21:384–389, 1997.
13. Akgun Y, Tacyildiz IH, Celik Y: Amebic liver abscess: Changing trends over 20 years. World J Surg 23:102–106, 1999.
14. Rajak CL, Gupta S, Jain S, et al: Percutaneous treatment of liver abscesses: Needle aspiration versus catheter drainage. AJR 170:1035–1039, 1998.
15. Seeto RK, Rockey DC: Pyogenic liver abscess: Changes in etiology, management and outcome. Medicine 75:99–113, 1996.

33. INHERITABLE FORMS OF LIVER DISEASE

Bruce R. Bacon, M.D.

HEMOCHROMATOSIS

1. How are the various iron-loading disorders in humans classified?

The usual way to classify iron-overload syndromes is to distinguish among hereditary hemochromatosis, secondary iron overload, and parenteral iron overload. **Hereditary hemochromatosis** (HH) results in increased iron absorption from the gut, with preferential deposition of iron in the parenchymal cells of the liver, heart, pancreas, and other endocrine glands.

In **secondary iron overload**, some other stimulus causes the gastrointestinal tract to absorb increased amounts of iron. Increased absorption of iron is caused by an underlying disorder. Examples include various anemias due to ineffective erythropoiesis, chronic liver disease, and, rarely, excessive intake of medicinal iron.

In **parenteral iron overload**, patients have received excessive amounts of iron as either red blood cell transfusions or iron-dextran given parenterally. In patients with severe hypoplastic anemias, red blood cell transfusion may be necessary. Over time patients become significantly iron-loaded. Unfortunately, some physicians give iron-dextran injections to patients with anemia that is not due to iron deficiency; such patients also become iron-loaded. Parenteral iron overload is always iatrogenic and should be avoided or minimized. In patients who truly need repeated red blood cell transfusions (in the absence of blood loss), a chelation program with deferoxamine should be initiated to prevent toxic accumulation of excessive iron.

2. What are neonatal iron overload and African iron overload?

Neonatal iron overload is a rare condition that is most likely related to an intrauterine viral infection. Infants are born with increased amounts of hepatic iron. They do very poorly and, in general, die without liver transplantation.

African iron overload, previously called Bantu hemosiderosis, was thought to be a disorder in which excessive amounts of iron were ingested from alcoholic beverages brewed in iron drums. Recent studies have suggested that this disorder may have a genetic component distinct from the genetic disorder found in HH (i.e., it is not *HFE*-linked). African-Americans may be at risk for developing iron overload from a genetic disease.

3. How much iron is usually absorbed per day?

A typical Western diet contains approximately 10–20 mg of iron, which usually is found in heme-containing compounds. Normal daily iron absorption is approximately 1–2 mg, representing about a 10% efficiency of absorption. Patients with iron deficiency, HH, or ineffective erythropoiesis absorb increased amounts of iron (up to 3–6 mg/day).

4. Where is iron normally found in the body?

The normal adult male contains about 4 gm of total body iron, which is roughly divided between the 2.5 gm of iron in the hemoglobin of circulating red blood cells, 1 gm of iron in storage sites in the reticuloendothelial system of the spleen and bone marrow and the parenchymal and reticuloendothelial system of the liver, and 200–400 mg in the myoglobin of skeletal muscle. In addition, all cells contain some iron because mitochondria contain iron both in heme, which is the central portion of cytochromes involved in electron transport, and in iron sulfur clusters, which also are involved in electron transport. Iron is bound to transferrin in both the intra- and extravascular compartments. Storage iron within cells is found in ferritin and, as this amount increases, in hemosiderin. Serum ferritin is proportional to total body iron stores in patients with iron deficiency or uncomplicated HH and is biochemically different from tissue ferritin.

5. Discuss the genetic defect in patients with HH.

In 1996, the gene responsible for hemochromatosis was identified and named *HFE*. *HFE* codes for a major histocompatibility complex (MHC) type 1-like protein that is membrane-spanning with a short intracytoplasmic tail, a transmembrane region, and three extracellular alpha loops. A single missense mutation results in loss of a cysteine at amino acid position 282 with replacement by a tyrosine (C282Y), which leads to disruption of a disulfide bridge and thus to the lack of a critical fold in the alpha$_1$ loop. As a result, *HFE* fails to interact with beta$_2$ microglobulin (β_2M), which is necessary to the function of MHC class 1 proteins.

In 1997, it was demonstrated that the *HFE*/β_2M complex binds to transferrin receptor and is necessary for transferrin receptor-mediated iron uptake into cells. This observation linked *HFE* with a protein of iron metabolism. C282Y homozygosity is found in approximately 85–90% of patients with hemochromatosis. A second mutation, whereby a histidine at amino acid position 63 is replaced by an aspartate (H63D), is common but less important in cellular iron homeostasis. Cell and molecular biologic studies have demonstrated that when C282Y-mutant *HFE* is transfected into cells, a decrease in intracellular iron (due either to a decrease in cellular uptake or a decrease in transferrin receptor cycling within the cell) leads to upregulation of the divalent metal transporter-1 (DMT-1), which is responsible for iron absorption in the villus cells of the intestine. It is presumed that the crypt cells of the intestine are involved in whole-body iron sensing. If these cells sense iron deficiency because of the C282Y mutation in *HFE*, upregulation of DMT-1 as cells mature to migrate up the villus results in an increase in absorption of iron and the ultimate development of hemochromatosis.

6. What are the usual toxic manifestations of iron overload?

In chronic iron overload, an increase in oxidant stress results in lipid peroxidation to lipid-containing components of the cell, such as organelle membranes. This process causes organelle damage. Hepatocellular injury and/or death ensues with phagocytosis by Kupffer cells. Iron loaded Kupffer cells become activated, producing profibrogenic cytokines such as transforming growth factor beta$_1$ (TGF-β1), which, in turn, activates hepatic stellate cells. Hepatic stellate cells are responsible for increased collagen synthesis and hepatic fibrogenesis.

7. What are the most common symptoms in patients with HH?

Currently, most patients are identified by abnormal iron studies on routine screening chemistry panels or by screening family members of a known patient. When identified in this manner, patients typically have no symptoms or physical findings. Nonetheless, it is useful to be aware of the symptoms that patients with more established HH can exhibit. Typically they are nonspecific and include fatigue, malaise, and lethargy. Other more organ-specific symptoms are arthralgias and symptoms related to complications of chronic liver disease, diabetes, and congestive heart failure.

8. Describe the most common physical findings in patients with HH.

The way in which patients come to medical attention determines whether they have physical findings. Thus, patients identified by screening tests have no abnormal physical findings. In contrast, physical findings in patients with advanced disease may include grayish or "bronzed" skin pigmentation, typically in sun-exposed areas; hepatomegaly with or without cirrhosis; arthropathy with swelling and tenderness over the second and third metacarpophalangeal joints; and other findings related to complications of chronic liver disease.

9. How is the diagnosis of hemochromatosis established?

Patients with abnormal iron studies on screening blood work, any of the symptoms and physical findings of hemochromatosis, or a positive family history of hemochromatosis should have blood studies of iron metabolism either repeated or performed for the first time. These studies include serum iron, total iron-binding capacity (TIBC) or transferrin, and serum ferritin. The transferrin saturation (TS) should be calculated from the ratio of iron to TIBC or transferrin. Blood samples for these studies are drawn in the fasting state to minimize the possibility of false-positive results. If the TS is > 45% or if the serum ferritin is elevated, hemochromatosis should be strongly considered, especially in patients without evidence of other liver disease (e.g., chronic viral hepatitis, alcoholic liver disease, nonalcoholic steatohepatitis) known to have abnormal iron studies in the absence of significant iron overload.

If iron studies are abnormal, mutation analysis of *HFE* should be performed. If patients are homozygous for the C282Y mutation, or compound heterozygotes (C282Y/H63D) and under the age of 40 years with normal liver enzymes (alanine aminostranferase and aspartate aminotransferase), no further evaluation is necessary. Plans for therapeutic phlebotomy can be initiated. In patients over the age of 40 years, or with abnormal liver enzymes or markedly elevated ferritin (> 1,000 ng/ml), the next step is to perform a percutaneous liver biopsy to obtain tissue for routine histology, including Perls' Prussian blue staining for storage iron, and biochemical determination of hepatic iron concentration (HIC). From the HIC, the hepatic iron index (HII) can be calculated and a specific recommendation about the presence or absence of HH can be made.

10. How commonly do abnormal iron studies occur in other types of liver disease?

In various studies, approximately 30–50% of patients with chronic viral hepatitis, alcoholic liver disease, and nonalcoholic steatohepatitis have abnormal serum iron studies. Usually, the serum ferritin is abnormal. In general, an elevation in transferrin saturation is much more specific for HH. Thus, if the serum ferritin is elevated and the transferrin saturation is normal, another form of liver disease may be responsible. In contrast, if the serum ferritin is normal and the transferrin saturation is elevated, the likely diagnosis is hemochromatosis, particularly in young patients. Differentiation of HH in the presence of other liver diseases is now much easier with the use of genetic testing (*HFE* mutation analysis for C282Y and H63D).

11. Is computed tomography (CT) or magnetic resonance imaging (MRI) useful in diagnosing hemochromatosis?

In massively iron-loaded patients, CT and MRI show the liver to be white or black, respectively, consistent with the kinds of changes associated with increased iron deposition. In more subtle and earlier cases, overlap is tremendous, and imaging studies are not useful. Thus, in heavily iron-loaded patients, the diagnosis is usually apparent without imaging tests, and in mild or subtler cases, they are unhelpful. CT or MRI is useful only in the patient who is likely to have severe iron overload but for whom a liver biopsy is either unsafe or refused. Again, this problem is less common with the advent of genetic testing.

12. On liver biopsy, what is the typical cellular and lobular distribution of iron in HH?

In early HH in young people, iron is found entirely in hepatocytes and a periportal (zone 1) distribution. In heavier iron-loading in older patients, iron is still predominantly hepatocellular, but some iron may be found in Kupffer cells and bile ductular cells. The periportal-to-pericentral (zone 1-to-zone 3) gradient is maintained but may be less distinct in more heavily loaded patients. When patients develop cirrhosis, the pattern is typically micronodular, and regenerative nodules may show less intense iron staining.

13. How useful is hepatic iron concentration?

Since genetic testing has become readily available, liver biopsy and determinations of HIC and HII are less important. Nonetheless, whenever a liver biopsy is performed in a patient with suspected HH, the quantitative HIC should be obtained. In symptomatic patients, HIC is typically > 10,000 µg/gm. The iron concentration threshold for the development of fibrosis is approximately 22,000 µg/gm. Lower iron concentrations can be found in cirrhotic HH with a coexistent toxin, such as alcohol or hepatitis C or B virus. Young people with early HH may have only moderate increases in HIC. In the past, discrepancies in HIC concentration with age were clarified by use of the HII.

14. How is the HII used in diagnosing HH?

The HII, introduced in 1986, is based on the observation that HIC increases progressively with age in patients with homozygous HH. In contrast, in patients with secondary iron overload or in heterozygotes, there is no progressive increase in iron over time. Therefore, the HII can distinguish patients with homozygous HH from patients with secondary iron overload and heterozygotes. The HII is calculated by dividing the HIC (in μmol/gm) by the patient's age (in years). A value > 1.9 is consistent with homozygous HH. With the advent of genetic testing, about 15% of patients with HH have an HII < 1.9, with some as low as 1.0. Thus, the HII is no longer the gold standard for diagnosis of HH. The HII is not useful in parenteral iron overload.

15. How do you treat a patient with HH?

Treatment of HH is relatively straightforward and includes weekly or twice-weekly phlebotomy of 1 unit of whole blood. Each unit of blood contains about 200–250 mg of iron, depending on the hemoglobin. Therefore, a patient who presents with symptomatic HH and who has up to 20 gm of excessive storage iron requires removal of over 80 units of blood, which takes close to 2 years at a rate of 1 unit of blood per week. Patients need to be aware that this treatment can be tedious and prolonged. Some patients cannot tolerate removal of 1 unit of blood per week, and occasionally schedules are adjusted to remove only one-half unit every other week. In contrast, in young patients who are only mildly iron-loaded, iron stores may be depleted quickly with only 10–20 phlebotomies. The goal of initial phlebotomy treatment is to reduce tissue iron stores, not to create iron deficiency. Once the ferritin is < 50 ng/ml and the transferrin saturation is < 50%, the majority of excessive iron stores have been successfully depleted, and most patients can go into a maintenance phlebotomy regimen (1 unit of blood removed every 2–3 months).

16. What kind of a response to treatment can you expect?

Many patients feel better after phlebotomy therapy has begun, even if they were asymptomatic before treatment. Energy level may improve, with less fatigue and less abdominal pain. Liver enzymes typically improve once iron stores have been depleted. Increased hepatic size diminishes. Cardiac function may improve, and about 50% of patients with glucose intolerance are more easily managed. Unfortunately, advanced cirrhosis, arthropathy, and hypogonadism do not improve with phlebotomy.

17. What is the prognosis for a patient with hemochromatosis?

Patients who are diagnosed and treated before the development of cirrhosis can expect a normal lifespan. The most common causes of death in hemochromatosis are complications of chronic liver disease and hepatocellular cancer. Patients who are diagnosed and treated early should not experience any of these complications.

18. Because hemochromatosis is an inherited disorder, what is my responsibility to family members once a patient has been identified?

Once a patient has been fully identified, all first-degree relatives should be offered screening with genetic testing (*HFE* mutation analysis for C282Y and H63D) and tests for transferrin saturation and ferritin. If genetic testing shows that the relative is a C282Y homozygote or a compound heterozygote (C282Y/H63D) and has abnormal iron studies, HH is confirmed. A liver biopsy may not be necessary. HLA studies are no longer performed.

ALPHA$_1$-ANTITRYPSIN DEFICIENCY

19. What is the function of alpha$_1$-antitrypsin in healthy people?

Alpha$_1$-antitrypsin (α_1-AT) is a protease inhibitor synthesized in the liver. It is responsible for inhibiting trypsin, collagenase, elastase, and proteases of polymorphonuclear neutrophils. In patients deficient in α_1-AT, the function of these proteases is unopposed. In the lung, this can lead to a progressive decrease in elastin and development of premature emphysema. The liver fails to secrete α_1-AT, and aggregates of the defective protein are found, leading by unclear means to the development of cirrhosis. Over 75 different protease inhibitor (Pi) alleles have been identified. Pi MM is normal, and Pi ZZ results in the lowest levels of α_1-AT.

20. How common is α_1-AT deficiency?

Alpha$_1$-AT deficiency occurs in approximately 1 in 2,000 people.

21. Where is the abnormal gene located?

The gene is located on chromosome 14 and results in a single amino acid substitution (replacement of glutamic acid by lysine at the 342 position), which causes a deficiency in sialic acid.

22. What is the nature of the defect that causes α_1-AT deficiency?

Alpha$_1$-AT deficiency is a protein-secretory defect. Normally this protein is translocated into the lumen of the endoplasmic reticulum, interacts with chaperone proteins, folds properly, is transported to the Golgi complex, and then is exported out of the cell. In patients with α_1-AT deficiency, the protein structure is abnormal because of the deficiency of sialic acid, and the proper folding in the endoplasmic reticulum occurs for only 10–20% of the molecules, with resultant failure to export via the Golgi complex and accumulation within the hepatocyte. In one detailed Swedish study, α_1-AT deficiency of the Pi ZZ type caused cirrhosis in only about 12% of patients. Chronic obstructive pulmonary disease (COPD) was present in 75% of patients, and of these, 59% were classified as having primary emphysema. It is not known why some patients with low levels of α_1-AT develop liver or lung disease and others do not.

23. Describe the common symptoms and physical findings of α_1-AT deficiency.

Adults with liver involvement may have no symptoms until they develop signs and symptoms of chronic liver disease. Similarly, children may have no specific problems until they develop complications from chronic liver disease. In adults with lung disease, typical findings include premature emphysema, which can be markedly exacerbated by smoking.

24. How is the diagnosis of α_1-AT deficiency established?

It is useful to order α_1-AT levels and phenotype in all patients evaluated for chronic liver disease because no clinical presentation suggests the diagnosis (apart from premature emphysema). Certain heterozygous states can result in chronic liver disease; for example, SZ as well as ZZ patients can develop cirrhosis. MZ heterozygotes usually do not develop disease unless they have some other liver condition, such as alcoholic liver disease or chronic viral hepatitis. Liver disease due to other causes may progress more rapidly in people who have an MZ phenotype.

25. What histopathologic stain is used to diagnose α_1-AT deficiency?

Periodic acid-Schiff-diastase. Periodic acid-Schiff (PAS) stains both glycogen and α_1-AT globules a dark, reddish-purple, and diastase digests the glycogen. Thus, when a PAS-diastase stain is used, the glycogen has been removed by the diastase, and the only positively staining globules are those due to α_1-AT. In cirrhosis, these globules characteristically occur at the periphery of the nodules and can be seen in multiple sizes within the hepatocyte. Immunohistochemical staining also can be used to detect α_1-AT globules, and electron microscopy can show characteristic globules trapped in the Golgi apparatus.

26. How is α_1-AT deficiency treated?

The only treatment for α_1-AT–related liver disease is symptomatic management of complications and liver transplantation. With liver transplantation, the phenotype becomes that of the transplanted liver.

27. What is the prognosis for patients with α_1-antitrypsin deficiency? Should family screening be performed?

The prognosis depends entirely on the severity of the underlying lung or liver disease. Typically, patients who have lung disease do not have liver disease, and those who have liver disease do not have lung disease, although in some patients both organs are severely involved. In patients with decompensated cirrhosis, the prognosis relates largely to the availability of organs for liver transplantation. Patients with transplants typically do fine. Family screening should be performed with α_1-AT levels and phenotype. This screening is largely for prognostic information; definitive therapy for liver disease, other than liver transplantation, is not available.

WILSON'S DISEASE

28. How common is Wilson's disease?

Wilson's disease has an estimated prevalence of 1 in 30,000 people.

29. Where is the Wilson's disease gene located?

The abnormal gene responsible for Wilson's disease, an autosomal recessive disorder, is located on chromosome 13 and recently has been cloned. The gene has homology for the Menke's disease gene, which also results in a disorder of copper metabolism. The Wilson's disease gene (called *ATP7B*) codes for a P-type adenosine triphosphatase, which is a membrane-spanning copper-transport protein. The exact location of this protein within hepatocytes is not definite, but it most likely causes a defect in transfer of hepatocellular lysosomal copper into bile. This defect results in the gradual accumulation of tissue copper with subsequent hepatotoxicity. Unfortunately, there are over 60 mutations in the Wilson's disease gene, and genetic testing has limited usefulness.

30. What is the usual age of onset of Wilson's disease?

Wilson's disease is characteristically a disease of adolescents and young adults. Clinical manifestations have not been seen before the age of 5 years. By 15 years of age, almost one-half of the patients have some clinical manifestations of the disease. Rare cases of Wilson's disease have been identified in patients in their 40s or 50s.

31. Which organ systems are involved in Wilson's disease?

The liver is uniformly involved. All patients with neurologic abnormalities due to Wilson's disease have liver involvement. Wilson's disease also can affect the eyes, kidneys, joints, and red blood cells. Thus, patients can have cirrhosis, neurologic deficits with tremor and choreic movements, ophthalmologic manifestations such as Kayser-Fleischer rings, psychiatric problems, nephrolithiasis, arthropathy, and hemolytic anemia.

32. What are the different types of hepatic manifestations in Wilson's disease?

The typical patient who presents with symptoms from Wilson's disease already has cirrhosis. However, patients can present with chronic hepatitis, and in all young people with chronic hepatitis a serum ceruloplasmin level should be performed as a screening test for Wilson's disease. Rarely, patients present with fulminant hepatic failure, which is uniformly fatal without successful liver transplantation. Finally, patients can present early in the disease with hepatic steatosis. As with chronic hepatitis, young patients with fatty liver should be screened for Wilson's disease.

33. How is the diagnosis of Wilson's disease established?

Initial evaluation should include measurement of serum ceruloplasmin and, if abnormal, a 24-hour urinary copper level. About 85–90% of patients have depressed serum ceruloplasmin levels, but a normal level does not rule out the disorder. If the ceruloplasmin is decreased or the 24-hour urinary copper level is elevated, a liver biopsy should be performed for histologic interpretation and quantitative copper determination. Histologic changes include hepatic steatosis, chronic hepatitis, or cirrhosis. Histochemical staining for copper with rhodamine is not particularly sensitive. Usually, in established Wilson's disease, hepatic copper concentrations are > 250 µg/gm (dry weight) and can be as high as 3,000 µg/gm. Although elevated hepatic copper concentrations can occur in other cholestatic liver diseases, the clinical presentation allows an easy differentiation between Wilson's disease and primary biliary cirrhosis, extrahepatic biliary obstruction, and intrahepatic cholestasis of childhood.

34. What forms of treatment are available for patients with Wilson's disease?

The mainstay of treatment has been the copper-chelating drug D-penicillamine. Because D-penicillamine is frequently associated with side effects, trientine also has been used. Trientine is equally efficacious and probably has fewer side effects. Maintenance therapy with dietary zinc supplementation also has been used. Neurologic disorders can improve with therapy. Patients who present with complications of chronic liver disease or with fulminant hepatic failure should be quickly considered for orthotopic liver transplantation.

35. Is it necessary to perform family screening in Wilson's disease?

Wilson's disease is an autosomal recessive disorder, and all first-degree relatives of the patient should be screened. If the ceruloplasmin level is reduced, a 24-hour urinary copper level should be obtained, followed by a liver biopsy for histology and quantitative copper determination. Genetic testing can be valuable for family screening if genotyping has been done on the proband and is available to family members.

36. Compare Wilson's disease and hereditary hemochromatosis.

Both disorders involve abnormal metal metabolism and are inherited as autosomal recessive disorders. The mechanism of tissue damage is probably related to metal-induced oxidant stress for both disorders. In HH, the gene is on chromosome 6, whereas in Wilson's disease the abnormal gene is on chromosome 13. HH occurs in approximately 1 in 250 people, but Wilson's disease occurs in only about 1 in 30,000. The inherited defect in HH causes an increased absorption of iron by the intestine, with the liver a passive recipient of the excessive iron; in contrast, the inherited defect in Wilson's disease is in the liver, resulting in decreased hepatic excretion of copper with excessive deposition and subsequent toxicity. Although the liver is affected in both Wilson's disease and HH, the other affected organs are quite variable. In hemochromatosis, the heart, pancreas, joints, skin, and endocrine organs are affected; in Wilson's disease, the brain, eyes, red blood cells, kidneys, and bone are affected. Both disorders are fully treatable if diagnosis is made promptly before the development of end-stage complications.

BIBLIOGRAPHY

1. Bacon BR: Causes of iron overload. N Engl J Med 326:126–127, 1992.
2. Bacon BR, Britton RS: The pathology of hepatic iron overload: A free radical-mediated process? Hepatology 11:127–137, 1990.
3. Bacon BR, Powell LW, Adams PC, et al: Molecular medicine and hemochromatosis: At the crossroads. Gastroenterology 116:193–207, 1999.
4. Bacon BR, Olynyk JK, Brunt EM, et al: *HFE* genotype in patients with hemochromatosis and other liver diseases. Ann Intern Med 130:953–962, 1999.
5. Bassett ML, Halliday JW, Powell LW: Value of hepatic iron measurements in early hemochromatosis and determination of the critical iron level associated with fibrosis. Hepatology 6:24–29, 1986.
6. Crystal RG: a1-Antitrypsin deficiency, emphysema, and liver disease: Genetics and strategies for therapy. J Clin Invest 85:1343–1352, 1990.
7. Edwards CQ, Griffen LM, Goldgar D, et al: Prevalence of hemochromatosis among 11,065 presumably healthy blood donors. N Engl J Med 318:1355–1362, 1988.
8. Eriksson S, Calson J, Veley R: Risk of cirrhosis and primary liver cancer in alpha$_1$-antitrypsin deficiency. N Engl J Med 314:736–739, 1986.
9. Feder JN, Gnirke A, Thomas W: A novel MHC class I-like gene is mutated in patients with hereditary haemochromatosis. Nature Genet 13:399–408, 1996.
10. Hill GM, Brewer GJ, Prasad AS, et al: Treatment of Wilson's disease with zinc. I: Oral zinc therapy regimens. Hepatology 7:522–528, 1987.
11. Hodges JR, Millward-Sadler GH, Barbatis C, Wright R: Heterozygous MZ alpha$_1$-antitrypsin deficiency in adults with chronic active hepatitis and cryptogenic cirrhosis. N Engl J Med 304:557–560, 1981.
12. Larsson C: Natural history and life expectancy in severe alpha$_1$-antitrypsin deficiency, Pi Z. Acta Med Scand 204:345–351, 1978.
13. Niederau C, Fischer R, Sonnenberg A, et al: Survival and causes of death in cirrhotic and noncirrhotic patients with primary hemochromatosis. N Engl J Med 313:1256–1262, 1985.
14. Perlmutter DH: The cellular basis for liver injury in α_1-antitrypsin deficiency. Hepatology 13:172–185, 1991.
15. Powell LW, Jazwinska E, Halliday JW: Primary iron overload. In Brock JH, Halliday JW, Powell LW (eds): Iron Metabolism in Health and Disease. London, W.B. Saunders, 1994, pp 227–270.
16. Scheinberg IH, Jaffe ME, Sternlieb I: The use of trientine in preventing the effects of interrupting penicillamine therapy in Wilson's disease. N Engl J Med 317:209–213, 1987.
17. Schilsky ML: Identification of the Wilson's disease gene: Clues for disease pathogenesis and the potential for molecular diagnosis. Hepatology 20:529–533, 1994.
18. Sternlieb I: Perspectives on Wilson's disease. Hepatology 12:1234–1239, 1990.
19. Stremmel W, Meyerrose KW, Niederau C, et al: Wilson's disease: Clinical presentation, treatment, and survival. Ann Intern Med 15:720–726, 1991.

34. LIVER HISTOPATHOLOGY

Janet K. Stephens, M.D., Ph.D., and George H. Warren, M.D.

LIVER MICROANATOMY AND INJURY PATTERNS

1. Explain the role of liver biopsy.

Liver biopsies play an important role in patient care. They may confirm or advance a diagnosis, guide additional studies, help to evaluate therapeutic efficacy, and gauge prognosis. The liver biopsy must be of adequate size and contain an appropriate number of portal tracts and central veins to allow proper assessment. However, the liver has a limited pattern of pathologic response to injury, especially for inflammatory diseases, and, as in other organs, biopsy represents a static look at an ongoing dynamic process.

2. Many liver biopsy reports say that the basic architecture is intact and then list a string of abnormalities. What is the basic architecture?

Histologically, the liver has three functional components: hepatocytes, central veins and sinusoids, and portal tracts (triads). The basic liver architecture is formed by cords of hepatocytes, which, in adults, are one cell layer thick. The liver cells are separated by vascular sinusoids lined by endothelial cells and Kupffer cells; the latter are part of the reticuloendothelial system and have macrophage function. Central veins, also called terminal hepatic venules, collect the circulating blood after it percolates through the sinusoids and then carry the blood to larger hepatic veins. Distributed at regular intervals are portal tracts, which contain interlobular bile ducts, small hepatic arteries, small portal veins, and fibrous stroma with scant numbers of mononuclear cells. The row of hepatocytes immediately adjacent to the portal tract is termed the limiting plate.

3. What are the geographic differences in pathology between portions of hepatic acini?

The functional unit of the liver is represented by hepatic acini, which are three-dimensional units built around a central axis containing a portal tract and its blood vessels. From the portal area, plates of hepatocytes radiate out toward central veins, located at the periphery of the acinus. The acinus can be divided into three zones: zone 1 is closest to the portal tracts, zone 3 is closest to the central veins, and zone 2 lies between. A gradient exists between zone 1 and zone 3; zone 1 is the best supplied with oxygen and various nutrients.

4. What is meant by distortion of the hepatic architecture?

Usually it indicates fibrosis and perhaps formation of regenerative nodules of hepatocytes. These changes can alter the relationships of central veins, portal tracts, and hepatic cords.

5. How are degrees of fibrosis designated?

The pathologist indicates how generalized scarring is, how much collagen is present, whether anatomic structures such as portal tracts and central veins are connected by scar (bridging fibrosis), and whether the scarring has altered the architecture into nodules of hepatocytes (cirrhosis).

6. What criteria are used to define the presence of cirrhosis?

Cirrhosis is the end stage of all chronic liver disease. By definition, it is a process that diffusely involves the liver with progressive fibrosis, resulting in the formation of nodules. Therefore, focal scarring, even if significant and associated with nodules, is not cirrhosis because the process is not diffuse.

7. Can the presence of cirrhosis be proved by a needle biopsy specimen?

Not always. **Micronodular cirrhosis** (nodules ≤ 3 mm), most often due to ethanol injury (also biliary tract disease, hemochromatosis) is highly uniform throughout the liver, and usually nodules are clearly defined on a needle specimen. **Macronodular cirrhosis** (nodules > 3mm), due most commonly to chronic viral hepatitis, is less uniform. One sometimes sees relatively sparse fibrosis in a needle specimen, with some fairly normal lobules noted, even when cirrhosis is suspected clinically. By nature of the biopsy technique, the softer lobular tissue may come out in the needle more easily than the fibrous tissue, or the needle may pass through large nodules and appear relatively uninvolved. The end result is that scarring can be underrepresented.

8. What types of liver cell injury are seen on needle specimens? What causes each type?

It may be difficult to determine a specific cause for liver injury seen on needle biopsy, because both hepatocytes and bile ducts have a limited pattern of response. Histopathologic features may overlap in many disease processes.

Types of Liver Cell Injury

TYPE	CAUSES
Fatty change	Ethanol, obesity, diabetes, drugs
Councilman bodies (acidophilic bodies)	Viral hepatitis, drugs, nonspecific reaction
Mallory bodies (hyaline)	Ethanol, obesity, diabetes, drugs, Wilson's disease, biliary tract, disease, hepatocellular carcinoma
Hydropic change (ballooning degeneration)	Viral hepatitis, drugs, cholestasis
Cholestasis	Duct obstruction or injury, drugs, viral hepatitis
Interlobular duct injury	Primary biliary cirrhosis, primary sclerosing cholangitis, hepatitis C
Piecemeal necrosis	Viral hepatitis, primary biliary cirrhosis, drugs, Wilson's disease
Increased iron stores	Hemochromatosis, transfusions, hemolysis
Granulomas	Tuberculosis, fungi, drugs

9. In addition to biopsy findings, what is needed to determine the cause of an injury?

A thorough clinical history is important in the evaluation of any liver biopsy. Laboratory evaluations should include aspartate aminotransferase (AST), alanine aminotransferase (ALT), alkaline phosphatase, serum gamma-glutamyl transferase (GGT), protein, bilirubin, iron, total iron-binding capacity, ferritin, and, if indicated, infectious serologies, autoimmune serologies, and cultures. Special laboratory tests may include quantitative liver iron or copper, ceruloplasmin, and α_1-antitrypsin levels. Radiologic changes should be assessed by endoscopic retrograde cholangiopancreatography (ERCP), ultrasound, and computed tomography (CT). Liver biopsies cannot be interpreted in a clinical vacuum.

FATTY CHANGE AND STEATOHEPATITIS

10. Injury from either acute or chronic ethanol ingestion is one of the most common insults to the liver. Describe the major characteristics of mild and severe injury.

Alcoholic liver disease results in a spectrum of changes, including fatty liver, alcoholic hepatitis, and alcoholic cirrhosis. In fatty liver, as the name implies, the hepatocytes contain globules of fat, usually larger than and compressing the hepatocyte nucleus (referred to as macrovesicular steatosis). Initially this change occurs around central veins but may extend to involve the entire acinus. Biopsies from patients with alcoholic hepatitis also may show fatty change. In addition, hepatocytes are swollen, with areas of necrosis, associated with acute inflammation (polymorphs, polymorphonuclear neutrophils [PMNs]). Hepatocytes may contain perinuclear Mallory hyaline. Hyaline represents aggregates of the intermediate filament cytokeratin. However, hyaline also may be found in a number of other conditions (nonalcoholic steatohepatitis [NASH], Wilson's disease, hepatocellular carcinoma, primary biliary cirrhosis). Alcoholic cirrhosis, which is micronodular, may have superimposed fatty change and/or hepatitis.

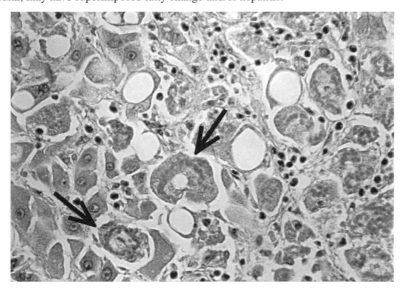

Alcoholic hepatitis with prominent hyaline (hematoxylin-eosin stain).

11. What is hyaline?

Hyaline is composed of irregular, ropelike strings of eosinophilic material in the cytoplasm, which represent aggregates of microfilaments. Although the fat and neutrophils can resolve relatively quickly after alcohol abstinence, hyaline can take up to 6 weeks to disappear.

12. How does scarring progress with alcohol injury?

Many patients with ethanol injury show initial scarring around central veins with delicate, spider web-like fibrosis along the sinusoids. Eventually, bridging fibrosis connects central veins and portal tracts and adjacent portal tracts. When cirrhosis is fully developed, most of the native central veins have been obliterated.

13. Is alcoholic cirrhosis micronodular or macronodular?

Micronodular, because the scarring is relatively uniform throughout the liver. These small or "micro" nodules have become subdivided by the portal-central bridging fibrosis. With complete alcohol abstinence, the nodules can regenerate to a size > 3 mm, but the central veins are decreased in number and the nodules lack multiple portal tracts. One usually sees central veins and portal tracts in some nodules of macronodular cirrhosis (e.g., those from viral hepatitis).

14. Sometimes a biopsy shows "alcoholic hepatitis," but the patient denies drinking ethanol at all. Is the pathologist's diagnosis incorrect, or is there a differential diagnosis for alcoholic hepatitis?

Steatohepatitis is the better term to describe the pattern of liver cell injury known as alcoholic hepatitis. Over 20 conditions can show hyaline on biopsy, and several of these can show full-blown steatohepatitis. Clinicopathologic correlation is required to determine the cause. A partial list of disorders resembling alcohol-related liver injury includes obesity, Wilson's disease, diabetes mellitus, vitamin A toxicity, dugs (e.g., glucocorticoids, amiodarone), prolonged cholestasis (e.g., primary biliary cirrhosis), and jejunal-ileal bypass or gastric stapling.

15. How are the diseases resembling alcoholic hepatitis differentiated?

Most of these conditions can be detected by history taking. The common ones are obesity and diabetes mellitus. Obese or diabetic patients occasionally show pathologic changes quite similar to alcoholic liver disease, including fat, hyaline, and sinusoidal scarring. In patients younger than 40 years, particularly those under 30 years old, Wilson's disease should be excluded by multiple laboratory tests and quantitative liver copper analysis. Hyaline can be present in primary biliary cirrhosis (PBC), but it is characteristically limited to the periportal zone. Of the important drugs, the antiarrhythmic amiodarone may have a half-life up to 3 months, and ongoing injury may lead to death from liver failure. Clinical history of drug and toxin exposure is critical in liver disease. When all choices in the differential are exhausted, you should recognize that many alcoholics are exquisitely good at keeping their drinking a secret. The biopsy may confirm the nature and degree of injury, but the history-taker solves the case.

VIRAL HEPATITIS

16. How can a liver biopsy help in patients with viral hepatitis?

A biopsy is helpful in assessing the amount of inflammatory activity (grade), its chronicity, and the degree of irreversible fibrosis or cirrhosis (stage). It can help to predict and evaluate response to medication. It is also useful in determining the presence of a second process in addition to the serologically established hepatitides A, B, B and D coinfection, and C.

17. When, if ever, is a biopsy ordered for patients with hepatitis A? With hepatitis B and C?

Because hepatitis A does not cause chronic liver disease, biopsy is rarely needed. Biopsies may be ordered to distinguish severe cholestasis in hepatitis A from large duct obstruction or to determine if bridging necrosis or the rare fulminant necrosis is present. Usually, if a patient is positive for antihepatitis A, IgM type, there is no need for biopsy. Hepatitis B, hepatitis B and D coinfection, and hepatitis C can cause chronic hepatitis leading to cirrhosis in addition to acute and/or fulminant disease. Liver biopsy helps to determine the severity of liver injury with regard to inflammatory activity and fibrosis. The histologic features may help to determine both treatment and prognosis.

18. Does chronic hepatitis have unique histopathologic features?

No. Chronic hepatitis is a clinical and pathologic syndrome that may have a variety of causes. It is a chronic necroinflammatory process in which hepatocytes are preferentially injured compared with bile ducts. In addition to viral infection, chronic hepatitis may be autoimmune or drug-related. Histologic features of chronic cholestatic disease, including PBC, primary sclerosing cholangitis (PSC), and autoimmune cholangitis, as well as metabolic diseases, including Wilson's disease and alpha-1-antitrypsin (α_1AT) deficiency, may overlap with those of chronic hepatitis.

19. What features are typical of chronic hepatitis?

Whereas parenchymal inflammation predominates in acute hepatitis, chronic hepatitis usually is associated with varying degrees of portal and periportal inflammation, parenchymal hepatitis. and fibrosis. The inflammatory cell infiltrate is typically mononuclear and includes lymphocytes, plasma cells, and macrophages. Once the inflammatory infiltrate crosses the limiting plate, it usually is associated with local hepatocyte damage, piecemeal necrosis, and inflammation. Lobular inflammation is accompanied by some hepatocellular necrosis (acidophilic or Councilman bodies). With time, chronic hepatitis leads to progressive fibrosis and, without treatment, to cirrhosis. The fibrosis begins in portal areas, extends to periportal areas, and begins bridging to other portal tracts and central veins. (See figure on following page.)

20. How is chronic hepatitis graded and staged?

Vaarious systems are used to evaluate chronic hepatitis, the simplest of which was proposed by Batts and Ludwig. A four-point grading system is used for both inflammatory activity and degree of fibrosis:

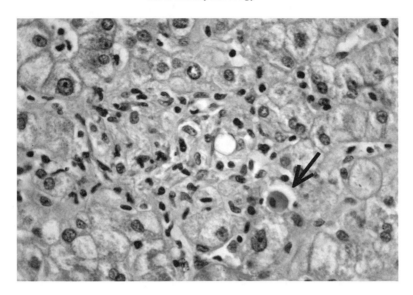

Biopsy, ordered to investigate fever of unknown origin, shows hepatitis with disorganized hepatocytes, lymphocytic infiltrate, and Councilman body *(arrow)* (hematoxylin-eosin stain).

Inflammatory activity

Grade 1   Minimal patchy, piecemeal necrosis and lobular inflammation/necrosis.

Grade 2   Mild portal inflammation with piecemeal necrosis involving some or all portal tracts with focal hepatocellular damage.

Grade 3   Moderate piecemeal necrosis involving all portal tracts with increased hepatocellular damage.

Grade 4   Severe portal inflammation with piecemeal necrosis; bridging fibrosis and diffuse hepatocellular damage may be present.

Fibrosis

Stage 1   Portal fibrosis (fibrous portal expansion)

Stage 2   Periportal fibrosis (periportal fibrosis with rare portal-portal septa)

Stage 3   Septal fibrosis (fibrous septa with architectural distortion)

Stage 4   Cirrhosis

Example. A liver biopsy from a patient with hepatitis C, which shows mild portal inflammation with piecemeal necrosis in most of the portal tracts and periportal expansion with a few fibrous septa, is characterized as chronic hepatitis C with mild activity (grade 2) and portal and focal bridging fibrosis (stage 2).

21. What features in the liver biopsy help to predict etiology?

Biopsies from patients with chronic hepatitis B may show some of the changes described above as well as a "ground-glass" change to the cell cytoplasm. This change reflects accumulation of hepatitis B surface antigen within the endoplasmic reticulum of the hepatocytes. Chronic hepatitis C may be associated with prominent lymphoid aggregates within portal tracts, sometimes including germinal centers and occasionally bile duct damage, although not to the degree seen in primary biliary disorders. In addition, biopsies may show focal, nonzonal macrovesicular steatosis. The inflammatory infiltrate in patients with autoimmune hepatitis typically shows a predominance of plasma cells.

22. Can chronic viral hepatitis be confused with other injuries?

Autoimmune hepatitis looks quite similar to chronic viral hepatitis, but plasma cells are more prominent in autoimmune injury, and various confirmatory serologic tests are available.

Some drug injuries, PBC, PSC and other disorders can pose difficult diagnostic problems. Some cases of α_1AT deficiency show piecemeal necrosis, but a periodic acid–Schiff–diastase stain reveals numerous magenta cytoplasmic globules in hepatocytes.

CHOLESTASIS

23. In patients with acute or chronic cholestasis, can the liver biopsy distinguish among the various differential diagnoses?
Maybe. Diagnosing cholestasis requires evaluation of the many causes in a systematic fashion: increased production of bilirubin, decreased excretion of bilirubin, and liver cell injuries. Hemolysis typically causes only mild hyperbilirubinemia. Extrahepatic obstruction is typically diagnosed by tests other than liver biopsy. Therefore, cases coming to liver biopsy are the difficult ones to solve; clinical and radiologic findings have solved the easy cases. The pathologist must ask whether the specimen shows associated inflammation or noninflammatory, "bland" cholestasis. The pathologist also must look for clues that suggest large duct obstruction or interlobular duct inflammatory injury. Subtle lesions in the head of the pancreas and ampulla of Vater can be missed. A stone may be missed. Other questions include the following: (1) Does the patient have hepatitis? (2) Has viral injury been excluded? (3) What are the patient's toxic exposures at work, home, or play? (4) Has every drug been sought and disclosed? (5) Have granulomatous causes been excluded?

DRUG INJURY

24. What histologic changes suggest drug- or toxin-related liver injury?
Three findings should make a pathologist press the clinician to "find the drug":
1. Significant fatty change, which most often is related to toxic ethanol injury.
2. A liver biopsy that shows features of a hypersensitivity reaction. Such cases resemble viral hepatitis, with an abundance of eosinophils. Eosinophils also may be present nonspecifically with viral hepatitis, connective tissue disorders, and some neoplasms (usually an infiltrate of Hodgkin's disease), but when eosinophils are a striking feature, the clinician should search for a drug or toxin.

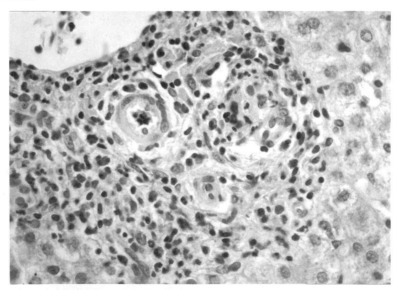

Nitrofurantoin hepatitis with prominent eosinophils (hematoxylin-eosin stain).

3. A liver that looks like it is recovering from a point-in-time injury, with numerous liver cell mitotic figures. These findings suggest that a single or short episode of drug or toxin exposure may be to blame.

Finally, in the absence of other obvious causes, granulomas should be added to the list. Otherwise, the answer lies in a good history, repeatedly taken, to generate a list of possible agents. This list is supplied to the pathologist, who evaluates whether the observed changes can be caused by one of these exposures. Then you need a good literature source.

BILE DUCT DISORDERS

25. In a patient with large duct obstruction, conjugated hyperbilirubinemia, an ultrasound showing bile duct stones, and clinical cholangitis, what would a biopsy show?

In this clinical situation, it is unusual that a liver biopsy would be necessary. If done, such a biopsy would show centrilobular cholestasis, portal tract edema, and neutrophils within portal tract stroma and within bile duct epithelium and lumens. One needs to remember that neutrophils within edematous portal stroma are a feature of large duct obstruction, even when frank cholangitis is not present.

26. When is primary biliary cirrhosis (PBC) diagnosed?

PBC is chronic progressive cholestatic liver disease that occurs in middle-aged patients, usually women, and often is associated with other autoimmune diseases. Patients may present with jaundice and pruritus. Laboratory testing reveals an elevated serum antimitochondrial antibody as well as increased alkaline phosphatase, bilirubin, and GGT.

27. How is PBC staged?

Stage depends on the degree of bile duct damage and fibrosis. **Stage I** (early changes) consists of damage to septal and larger interlobular bile ducts, characterized by biliary epithelial damage with infiltration of the duct by lymphocytes, plasma cells, eosinophils, and rare polymorphs. The inflammatory infiltrate may include granulomas and lymphoid follicles (florid duct lesion). At this point, the process is confined within the portal tract.

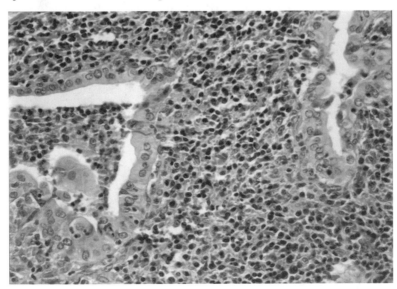

Primary biliary cirrhosis, with a florid duct lesion (hematoxylin-eosin stain).

In **stage II** disease, the inflammatory process extends beyond the portal tract, and piecemeal necrosis may be seen. Bile ducts begin to disappear. Associated with this scenario may be bile ductular (cholangiolar) proliferation (along the edges of the portal tracts) and evidence of chronic cholestasis, including feathery degeneration within the cytoplasm of hepatocytes, accumulation of bile pigment, periportal accumulation of copper (not generalized as in Wilson's disease), and, occasionally, Mallory bodies.

Stage III is associated with increasing fibrosis and bridging between portal areas, with decreased amounts of inflammation.

Stage IV represents "biliary" (micronodular) cirrhosis.

28. When is primary sclerosing cholangitis (PSC) diagnosed?

PSC shares many clinical biochemical and pathologic features with PBC, although it can affect both intra- and extrahepatic ducts. PSC is strongly associated with inflammatory bowel disease, particularly ulcerative colitis. Patients may present with increased alkaline phosphatase, IgG, and/or IgM and positive perinuclear antineutrophil cytoplasmic antibodies (p-ANCAs). The classic lesion of PSC is "onionskin" or concentric periductular fibrosis, with damage to the ductal epithelium.

29. How is PSC staged?

Like PBC, PSC is staged according to bile duct changes and fibrosis. **Stage I** (early disease) is associated with bile duct damage and inflammation and is largely confined within portal tracts. In **stage II** disease, the fibroinflammatory process is periportal. In **stage III**, bridging fibrosis is present, and bile ducts are decreased in numbers. **Stage IV** represents end-stage disease (cirrhosis).

30. What are the most common biopsy findings in patients with PSC?

The onionskin lesion is *rarely* seen on percutaneous biopsy. The most common findings on biopsy are nonspecific fibrosis with inflammation of portal tracts and paucity of normal bile ducts. In addition, in patients with extrahepatic disease, it may be hard to separate intrahepatic PSC from the effects of obstruction. Obstruction causes proliferation and dilatation of interlobular ducts and an increased number of periportal PMNs. A major goal of the biopsy interpretation is to consider PSC and then to suggest ERCP to confirm the diagnosis.

GRANULOMATOUS INFLAMMATION

31. What is a granuloma?

A granuloma is a sharply (or fairly sharply) defined aggregate of histiocytes.

32. How common are granulomas in liver biopsies?

Most systemic granulomatous diseases involve the liver to some extent. Granulomas may be identified in 10% of routine liver biopsies, probably in relation to the liver's large population of phagocytic cells, including Kupffer cells and other macrophages.

33. What causes granulomas in the liver?

The differential list is long and varied. Tuberculosis and sarcoidosis are the most common causes. Other infectious agents include viruses (cytomegalovirus, Epstein-Barr virus), bacteria (brucellosis, nocardiosis, tularemia), *Richettsia* spp. (Q fever [*Coxiella burnetii*]), spirochetes, various fungi, and protozoa. Noninfectious causes, in addition to sarcoidosis, include PBC, drug reaction, extrahepatic inflammatory disease (chronic granulomatous disease of childhood, chronic inflammatory bowel disease, rheumatoid arthritis), neoplasms (Hodgkin's disease), and foreign substances (talc, mineral oil).

34. In patients with fever of unknown origin, do negative stains for fungi and acid-fast bacilli exclude infection?

Not at all. Cultures for these organisms are more sensitive than special histologic stains. If infection is a possibility, a core of liver should be submitted with sterile precautions and without fixative to the microbiology laboratory. In addition, tissue in formalin should be sent to the surgical pathology laboratory for microscopic sections. Tissue also may be sent for molecular analysis to determine whether an infectious agent is present.

35. Are acid-fast bacilli hard to identify on biopsy?

In *Mycobacterium tuberculosis* infection, few organisms may be detected in the sections. Usually, stains are negative but cultures are positive.

36. What are the different types of granulomas? Is the distinction of diagnostic use?

Epithelioid granulomas are nodular aggregates of plump macrophages, often associated with multinucleated giant cells, lymphocytes, and plasma cells. They are typically seen in sarcoidosis and central caseating necrosis or tuberculosis.

Fibrin-ring granulomas are formed by a fibrin band encircling a lipid droplet, with associated inflammation. They were first described with Q fever but also may be seen after infection with cytomegalovirus or Epstein-Barr virus as well as with drug (allopurinol) toxicity and in association with systemic lupus erythematosus.

Lipogranulomas are composed of lipid deposits and vaculoated macrophages. They are formed in the presence of exogenous or endogenous fat accumulation.

Microgranulomas are composed of small, round clusters of plump Kupffer cells. They are a relatively nonspecific finding.

37. How often are liver granulomas secondary to a drug reaction?

Perhaps one-third of granulomatous liver reactions are caused by drugs, including allopurinol, nitrofurantoin, alpha-methyldopa, phenylbutazone, carbamazepine, procainamide, diphenylhydantoin, quinidine, isoniazid, and sulfanilamide

INHERITED LIVER DISEASE

38. If the ratio of serum iron to total iron-binding capacity (TIBC) and serum ferritin levels are significantly elevated, is a liver biopsy indicated?

Yes. The biopsy can tell you where the iron is stored (hepatocytes vs. Kupffer cells), the amount of iron can be graded, the complications of iron storage (fibrosis, cirrhosis, hepatocellular carcinoma) can be assessed, and the biopsy can be sent for quantitative iron determination.

39. What is hematochromatosis? Can it be diagnosed by histologic findings?

Hemochromatosis is an autosomal recessive disorder characterized by massive deposits of iron in many organs, including liver, pancreas, heart, joints, and skin. Untreated, it leads to the development of micronodular cirrhosis. In genetic hemochromatosis, hepatocytes and biliary epithelium contain increased stainable iron. The biopsy may be relatively normal or show bridging fibrosis or even micronodular cirrhosis. Hepatocyte iron is deposited in a graded fashion, from periportal areas to central veins, and can be scored on a 4-point system. Recently, a new major histocompatibility complex class I-like candidate gene (HFE) for hereditary hemochromatosis was identified on chromosome 6. Two mutations have been identified, C282Y and H63D. Testing is currently available for both sites.

40. If the laboratory tests are supported by 4+-iron deposition, is this sufficient evidence to diagnose genetic hemochromatosis?

The diagnosis of genetic hemochromatosis can be established with liver biopsy, quantitative iron determination performed on liver tissue, and genetic testing for the C282Y or H63D mutation.

41. What disorders are problematic in the clinical differential diagnosis of hemochromatosis?

The list of disorders associated with increased hepatic iron is long. The pattern of distribution of the iron may be of some help in establishing the diagnosis:

Predominantly hepatocellular distribution
Genetic hemochromatosis
Alcoholic liver disease
Porphyria cutanea tarda
Distributed predominantly in Kupffer cells
Multiple transfusion
Hemolytic anemias
Mixed hepatocellular and Kupffer cell distribution
Megaloblastic anemia
Anemia secondary to chronic infection

42. How does age affect the interpretation of quantitative iron results?

Among patients with hemochromatosis, young patients will have accumulated less iron than older patients, and menstruating women will have less iron than men of the same age. The hepatic iron index (HII) takes these factors into account:

$$HII = \text{Hepatic iron concentration (mg/gm liver dry wt)}/[56 \times age]$$

Patients with genetic homozygous hemochromatosis characteristically show an $HII > 1.9$, whereas patients with other causes of iron overload, including chronic alcoholic liver disease, show an $HII < 1.9$.

43. What is Wilson's disease? Can liver biopsy help to establish the diagnosis?

Wilson's disease is an autosomal recessive disorder of copper metabolism, characterized by excessive accumulation of copper in the liver and other organs. The gene for Wilson's disease has been localized to chromosome 13 (13q14-q21). The disease can show a range of appearances on liver biopsy, depending to some extent on the patient's age. In children and young adolescents, the most common appearance may be fatty change. In older adolescents and young adults, a liver biopsy may show chronic hepatitis with piecemeal necrosis. Adults tend to show cirrhosis, and Mallory's hyaline may be part of this change. In either adolescents or adults, confluent necrosis leading to fulminant hepatic failure may supervene.

44. What other tests are helpful in patient's with Wilson's disease?

Quantitative copper testing of the liver is useful; in patients with Wilson disease, levels typically are > 250 µg/gm dry weight liver (normal level $= 38$ µg/gm). The levels may be much higher in the absence of cirrhosis. Conditions associated with chronic cholestasis (PBC, PSC) also have elevated liver copper levels (range $= 150$–350 µg/gm). Other helpful measurements include serum ceruloplasmin (< 20 mg/dl in patients with Wilson's disease; normal levels $= 23$–50 mg/dl) and 24-hour urinary copper (> 100 µg/dl; normal $= < 30$ µg/dl).

45. What are the features of α_1AT deficiency on liver biopsy?

Alpha$_1$ AT is the major circulating inhibitor of serine proteases (Pi). Its primary target is the potent elastase found in PMNs. It thus acts to protect tissues against injury during active, acute inflammation. It is a 52-kd glycoprotein synthesized in the liver under the control of codominant alleles at a locus on the long arm of chromosome 14. These genes are highly polymorphic, with more than 75 known alleles. Many of the Pi variants are associated with fairly normal serum concentration and function and are thus of little clinical significance. However a few result in low circulating levels of α_1AT (i.e., PiZZ) and are of pathologic significance. Liver biopsies show classic PAS-positive, diastase-resistant globules with periportal hepatocytes. Portal fibrosis and chronic hepatitis also may be present. Liver cell dysplasia may be seen, and patients older than 50 years, especially men, are at risk of developing hepatocellular carcinoma.

46. Is the presence of PAS-positive, diastase-resistant globules diagnostic for α_1AT deficiency?

No. Various inflammatory conditions may be associated with overproduction of the enzyme, as may congestion or hypoxia. Clinical correlation with electrophoretic analysis is key.

NEOPLASMS

47. Discuss the role of liver biopsy in diagnosing metastatic neoplasms.

First, an adequate sample of the neoplasm must be obtained. Biopsy can confirm metastasis to the liver from a known primary tumor. Most metastatic disease is not curable, and it is appropriate to make the diagnosis with the minimally invasive technique of liver needle biopsy. Some biopsies show tumor that is probably metastatic but for which no primary tumor is known. In such cases, biopsy findings can guide further work-up, but it may not be possible to identify the primary tumor from the needle specimen. A needle specimen may be used to diagnose or stage malignant lymphoma.

48. Discuss the role of biopsy in diagnosing primary liver tumors.

For vascular tumors, radiologic methods may be used rather than biopsy, but three types of liver masses deserve special consideration: hepatocellular carcinoma, liver cell adenoma, and focal nodular hyperplasia. Each of these diagnoses may be suggested by needle biopsy samples, but definitive diagnosis frequently is difficult and, in some cases, impossible without larger samples or complete resection of the mass.

Higher-grade **hepatocellular carcinomas** are usually straightforward, but low-grade hepatocellular carcinomas can be difficult to distinguish from normal tissue or a regenerative nodule in the setting of cirrhosis.

Liver cell adenomas in women taking oral contraceptives may show characteristic features, but occasionally well-differentiated hepatocellular carcinomas can resemble liver cell adenomas.

Focal nodular hyperplasia is a localized lobulated nodule of hyperplastic liver cells surrounding a central scar. This condition can be confused with macronodular cirrhosis on a needle biopsy specimen (or even a wedge biopsy specimen). Definitive classification may require excision of the nodule.

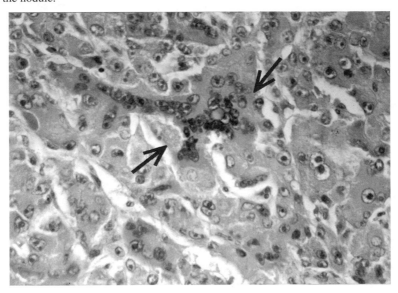

Hepatocellular carcinoma with prominent giant cell *(arrows)* (hematoxylin-eosin stain).

49. Can the clinical laboratory help in classifying tumors?

Marked elevation of serum alpha-fetoprotein levels in hepatocellular carcinomas or similar markers for other tumors can be a great help.

TRANSPLANTATION

50. Describe the role of liver biopsy in the evaluation of transplant patients with abnormal liver function tests in the early postoperative period.

Liver transplantation is a well-accepted treatment for patients with advanced liver disease that is unresponsive to conventional therapy. In the first few weeks and months after transplant, the major causes of abnormal liver function tests (LFTs) include preservation injury, acute rejection, opportunistic infections (e.g., cytomegalovirus hepatitis), vascular compromise, and/or biliary stricture. Acute allograft rejection is perhaps the most common and results from direct alloantigenic stimulation of recipient T cells by donor dendritic cells (antigen-presenting cells). The effector T cells can then preferentially injure biliary epithelial cells of both interlobular and septal bile ducts as well as endothelial cells of intrahepatic arteries and veins. Hepatocytes and sinusoidal lining cells are not prime targets.

51. What are the three main features of acute rejection?

1. Predominantly mononuclear with mixed portal inflammation (lymphocytes, macrophages, plasma cells, PMNs, eosinophils)
2. Subendothelial inflammation (endothelialitis), which may involve both portal and central veins and even the hepatic artery
3. Bile duct infiltration by inflammatory cells with associated damage

52. What criteria help to distinguish recurrent hepatitis C after transplant from allograft rejection?

Hepatitis C recurs in virtually all patients transplanted for that disease. The distinction of recurrent hepatitis from acute allograft rejection can be difficult. In general, however, recurrent hepatitis C is characterized by a mononuclear rather than a mixed portal infiltrate. Bile duct damage, although it may occur, is focal and mild. Hepatitis C usually is associated with a lobular hepatitis and perhaps hepatocyte necrosis. These findings are unusual in allograft rejection, unless it is severe. As with any disease process, correlation with clinical findings is key.

53. Describe the role of liver biopsy in the evaluation of abnormal LFTs in the first year after transplant (and beyond).

Common causes of abnormal LFTs in the first year after transplant include acute rejection (usually due to inadequate immunosuppression), opportunistic infection, recurrent viral hepatitis, chronic rejection, steatohepatitis, and various recurrent diseases (e.g., PBC, PSC, autoimmune hepatitis). Chronic rejection is characterized histologically by either loss of small bile ducts ("ductopenic" rejection) or obliterative vasculopathy (affecting hilar structures). The former can be diagnosed by liver biopsy, whereas the latter may require examination of the explanted liver. Chronic rejection on liver biopsy is characterized classically by bile duct loss in more than 50% of portal tracts, either in a single biopsy or a series of biopsies. It is probably irreversible. Chronic rejection may first manifest as prominent bile duct abnormalities or damage with some degree of bile duct loss. Unlike acute allograft rejection, the amount of bile duct damage is typically out of proportion to the degree of inflammation.

54. How can a liver biopsy help in the evaluation of a bone marrow transplant patient with elevated LFTs?

Complications of bone marrow transplant include veno-occlusive disease (VOD) and graft vs. host disease (GVHD). VOD is characterized by liver dysfunction and is due to the use of high-dose cytoreductive therapy. It develops within 1–4 weeks after transplantation. On biopsy it is characterized by occlusion of central veins, sinusoidal fibrosis, and pericentral hepatocyte necrosis. Acute GVHD develops within 6 weeks after transplant and affects the skin, gastrointestinal tract, and liver. It is characterized by degenerative bile duct lesions with some degree of mononuclear inflammation. Cholestasis may be present. Chronic GVHD is a multiorgan process that develops 80–400 days after transplant and often is preceded by acute GVHD. The changes in the liver are similar to those in acute disease, but the ducts show more prominent changes and are likely to be reduced in number or destroyed. A prominent periportal mononuclear infiltrate or even piecemeal necrosis may be seen.

BIBLIOGRAPHY

1. Andrews NC: Disorder of iron metabolism. N Engl J Med 341:1986–1995, 1999.
2. Batts KP, Ludwig J: Chronic hepatitis: An update on terminology and reporting. Am J Surg Pathol 19:1409–1417, 1995.
3. DeMetris AJ, Batts KP, Dhillon AP, et al: Banff schema for grading liver allograft rejection: An international consensus document. Hepatology 25:658–663, 1997.
4. Gerber JA, Thung SN: Histology of the liver. Am J Surg Pathol 11:709–722, 1987.
5. Kanel GC, Korula J: Developmental, familial and metabolic disorders. In Atlas of Liver Pathology. Philadelphia, W. B. Saunders, 1992, pp 135–174.
6. Krawitt EL: Autoimmune hepatitis. N Engl J Med 334:897–903, 1996.
7. Lee RG: General principles. In Diagnostic Liver Pathology. St. Louis, Mosby, 1994, pp 1–22.
8. Olynyk JK, Cullen DJ, Aquillia S et al: A population-based study of the clinical expression of the hemochromoatosis gene. N Engl J Med 341:718–724, 1999.
9. Scheuer PJ: Pathologic features and evoluation of primary biliary cirrhosis and primary sclerosing cholangitis. Mayo Clin Proc 73:179–183, 1998.
10. Shulman HM, Sharma P, Amos D et al: A coded histologic study of hepatic graft-versus-host-disease after human bone marrow transplantation. Hepatology 8:463–470, 1988.
11. Shulman HM, Fisher LB, Schoch HG, et al: Venoocclusive disease of the liver after marrow transplantation: Histological correlates of clinical signs and symptoms. Hepatology 19:1171–1180, 1994.
12. Snover DC, Freese DK, Sharp HL, et al: Liver allograft rejection: An analysis of the use of biopsy in determining outcome of rejection. Am J Surg Pathol 11:1–10, 1987.
13. Zimmerman HJ, Maddrey WE: Toxic and drug-induced hepatitis. In Schiff L, Schiff ER (eds): Diseases of the Liver. Philadelphia, J.B. Lippincott, 1993, pp 707–783.

35. HEPATOBILIARY CYSTIC DISEASE

Randall E. Lee, M.D.

1. **Describe the five major classes and subtypes of bile duct cysts.**
   Type Ia: choledochal cyst
   Type Ib: segmental choledochal dilation
   Type Ic: diffuse or cylindrical duct dilation
   Type II: extrahepatic duct diverticula
   Type III: choledochocele
   Type IVa: multiple intra- and extrahepatic duct cysts
   Type IVb: multiple extrahepatic duct cysts
   Type V: intrahepatic duct cysts

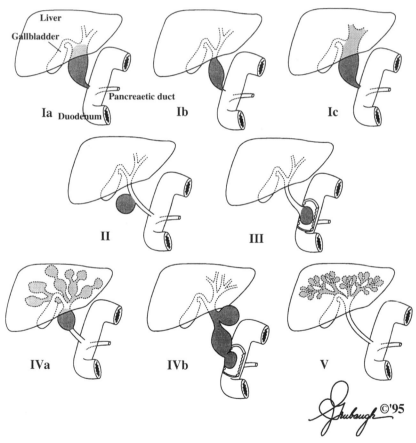

Classification of bile duct cysts.

2. **What is the incidence of cancer within a bile duct cyst?**
   The incidence of cancer within a bile duct cyst is about 2–15%. Many cases occurred in patients who had undergone an internal drainage procedure rather than excision of the cyst.

3. Describe the typical clinical presentation of a bile duct cyst.

The classic clinical presentation of a bile duct cyst is the triad of abdominal pain, jaundice, and abdominal mass. Typically, however, only one or two of these symptoms are present at any one time. Many reports describe fever as a presenting symptom. Most cases are diagnosed in childhood.

4. Describe the preferred treatment for patients with bile duct cyst disease.

The preferred treatment is complete surgical excision of the cyst rather than internal drainage. Postoperative complications, such as stricture formation, recurrent jaundice, and cholangitis, occur in about 8% of patients undergoing complete excision. The corresponding complication rate for patients undergoing internal drainage is about 50%. The risk of bile duct cancer is reduced but not eliminated by complete excision. Symptomatic unilobar intrahepatic bile duct cyst disease may be treated by resection of the affected lobe. Patients who have recurrent symptoms may be candidates for liver transplantation if there is no evidence of cholangiocarcinoma.

5. What is the role of cholangiopancreatography in patients with bile duct cyst disease?

Patients with extrahepatic bile duct cysts have an increased incidence of anomalous pancreaticobiliary junction. Cholangiopancreatography—percutaneously, endoscopically, or intraoperatively—allows definitive identification of the pancreatic duct insertion, which is critical to the planning of excision. In addition, cholangiography can distinguish multiple intrahepatic bile duct cysts from multiple hepatic cysts, which appear similar on CT. With refinement, the noninvasive technique of magnetic resonance cholangiopancreatography (MRCP) may be the preferred imaging modality. ERCP should be performed with caution in patients with suspected Caroli's disease or Caroli's syndrome because of the increased risk of recurrent cholangitis and sepsis. Nevertheless, therapeutic ERCP remains a useful tool for the management of acute cholangitis due to bile duct stones.

6. Compare the main features of Caroli's disease and Caroli's syndrome.

Initially described by Caroli in 1958, both entities are characterized by congenital dilations of the intrahepatic bile ducts. Patients usually become symptomatic as children or young adults, presenting with abdominal pain and hepatomegaly. Patients with the rare **Caroli's disease** have cystic dilations limited to the larger intrahepatic bile ducts. Some reports of Caroli's disease describe lesions in only one of the hepatic lobes. The cystic dilations of the larger intrahepatic ducts predispose to recurrent intrahepatic calculi and cholangitis. The mode of inheritance is uncertain.

In the more common **Caroli's syndrome**, the cystic dilations are distributed along the portal tract. This distribution is believed to result from a ductal plate malformation that affects the bile ducts at all levels, including the smaller interlobular ducts. Caroli's syndrome is associated with congenital hepatic fibrosis. Consequently, patients often have manifestations of portal hypertension, such as splenomegaly and esophageal varices. The mode of inheritance is autosomal recessive. Caroli's syndrome also is referred to as Caroli's disease type 2.

7. What disease commonly is associated with polycystic liver disease (PLD)?

PLD is characterized by numerous cysts scattered throughout the liver parenchyma. Most commonly it is associated with autosomal dominant polycystic kidney disease (ADPKD). There are also strong associations between ADPKD and intracranial saccular aneurysms (berry aneurysms), mitral valve prolapse, and colonic diverticula. In Caucasians, ADPKD occurs in about 1 in 400 to 1 in 1,000 people. Most families affected by ADPKD have a genetic defect located on chromosome 16 (ADPKD1) or chromosome 4 (ADPKD2). Slightly less than one-half of ADPKD patients develop end-stage renal disease. Polycystic liver disease also exists as a rare autosomal dominant disorder that is genetically distinct from ADPKD. Patients with isolated PLD have no kidney disease but may have an increased risk for intracranial aneurysms.

8. What are the risk factors for polycystic liver disease in patients with ADPKD?

Polycystic liver disease is the most common extrarenal manifestation of ADPKD. The presence and severity of polycystic liver disease in patients with ADPKD increases with age, female gender, number and frequency of pregnancies, and severity of renal disease.

9. **Describe the clinical manifestations of complicated polycystic liver disease.**

The common complications of polycystic liver disease include mass effect and cyst infection. Compression of adjacent structures by large cysts or by massive involvement may be manifest by chronic pain, anorexia, or obstructive jaundice. Clinical clues to the presence of a cyst infection include fever, right upper quadrant abdominal pain, and leukocytosis. A definitive diagnosis of cyst infection usually requires percutaneous CT or ultrasound-guided fine-needle aspiration.

10. **How does the presence of liver cysts affect hepatic function?**

Hepatic function usually is not affected by liver cysts. In the absence of complications, the serum aminotransferase, bilirubin, and alkaline phosphatase typically are within normal range or only slightly elevated. In patients with ADPKD, serum chemistry abnormalities generally reflect the degree of renal dysfunction.

11. **What are the treatment options for patients with symptomatic polycystic liver disease?**

Symptomatic liver cysts may be treated either percutaneously or surgically. Simple ultrasound- or CT-guided percutaneous aspiration results in rapid reaccumulation of the cyst fluid. The rate of cyst recurrence is greatly reduced by instilling a sclerosing agent, such as absolute ethanol, at the time of aspiration. Patients treated in this manner may experience a low-grade fever and transient pain as well as ethanol intoxication. Percutaneous sclerosis of a liver cyst is contraindicated when the cyst communicates with either the biliary system or peritoneal cavity.

Infected cysts do not resolve with systemic antibiotic therapy alone. Administration of antibiotics should be combined with either percutaneous or surgical drainage. Patients with intractable pain or anorexia due to massive polycystic hepatomegaly may be candidates for either isolated orthotopic liver transplant or combined liver and kidney transplant (if they are dialysis-dependent).

12. **What is the significance of a simple hepatic cyst?**

Simple hepatic cysts (often called solitary hepatic cysts) are benign fluid collections usually surrounded by a thin columnar epithelium. They frequently are noted as an incidental finding on hepatic ultrasonography or CT scanning. Simple hepatic cysts are not associated with cystic disease in other organs, and there is no genetic transmission. Many, but not all, simple hepatic cysts are solitary, and most are asymptomatic. Treatment is indicated if symptoms develop. Cyst-related symptoms include abdominal pain, increasing abdominal girth, and obstructive jaundice.

13. **Describe the ultrasonographic characteristics of a simple hepatic cyst.**

On ultrasound examinations, a simple hepatic cyst has no internal echoes, a smooth margin with the surrounding parenchyma, and no appreciable wall. The absence of any of these characteristics should make one suspect a complication, such as a cyst infection, or another diagnosis, such as hydatid cyst.

14. **What are the characteristics of a simple hepatic cyst on CT and magnetic resonance imaging (MRI)?**

A simple hepatic cyst appears on CT as a thin-walled lesion that does not enhance with iodinated intravenous contrast agents. The density of the lesion is that of water. On MRI, a simple hepatic cyst is a homogeneous, very-low-intensity lesion on T1-weighted scans and a discrete high-intensity lesion on T2-weighted scans.

15. **What is *Echinococcus granulosus*?**

E. granulosus is the small tapeworm responsible for unilocular hydatid cyst disease. The adult worm is 2–8 mm long and consists of a bulbous scolex with four suckers and a coronet of hooklets, followed by three or four body segments called proglottids. The last proglottid typically is gravid with hundreds of eggs. Each egg measures only about 0.03 mm in diameter.

16. **Describe the life cycle of *E. granulosus*.**

The adult worm lives in the intestinal lumen of the definitive host, usually a predator such as a dog, fox, or cat. Eggs discharged from the gravid proglottid segment leave the definitive host in the feces. The eggs are ingested through contaminated food or water by an intermediate host such as a rabbit or sheep. Ingested eggs hatch in the duodenum, and the larvae penetrate the intestinal mucosa to be carried by the circulatory system to the capillary beds of distant organs. As a defense mechanism, the intermediate host lays down layers of connective tissue around each larva, thus forming the hydatid cyst. New scolices bud from the inner wall of the cyst. Over time, daughter cysts may form within the original cyst. When infected viscera are eaten by a predator, the scolices develop into adult worms.

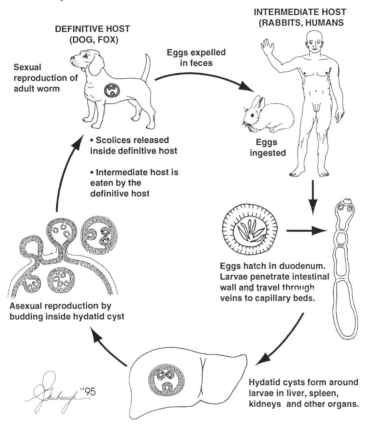

Life cycle of *Echinococcus granulosus.*

17. Where and how does *E. granulosus* infect humans?

Human infection by *E. granulosus* occurs throughout the world, including Alaska, Canada, and the western United States. Infections occur most commonly in sheep- and cattle-raising areas where dogs assist in herding. Humans usually are infected as intermediate hosts when they ingest egg-contaminated food or water or allow infected dogs to lick them in the mouth. Over one-half of all human infections involve the liver. Additional common sites for hydatid cysts are the lungs, spleen, kidneys, heart, bones, and brain.

18. Describe the typical clinical presentation of hepatic hydatid cyst disease.

Hydatid cysts grow at a rate of about 1–5 cm/ year. Many patients unsuspectingly harbor the infection until they present with a palpable abdominal mass or other symptoms. The symptoms of hydatid cyst disease are related primarily to the mass effect of the slowly enlarging cyst: abdominal pain from the stretching hepatic capsule, jaundice from compression of the bile duct, or portal hypertension from portal vein obstruction. Approximately 20% of patients have cysts that communicate with the biliary tree and may have symptoms similar to those of choledocholithiasis. Leakage of a cyst into the peritoneal cavity may cause an intense antigenic response, resulting in eosinophilia, bronchial spasm, or anaphylactic shock.

19. How is echinococcosis diagnosed?

Confirming a diagnosis of echinococcosis usually requires a combination of diagnostic imaging and serologic tests. CT scans may show the hydatid cyst as a sharply defined, low-density lesion with spoke-like septations. The presence of a calcified rim of daughter cysts greatly enhances the specificity of the CT findings. When imaged by ultrasound, the hydatid cyst appears as a complex mass with multiple internal echoes from debris and septations. Enzyme-linked immunosorbent assay or indirect hemagglutinin serologic assays for echinococcal antibodies are positive in about 85–90% of patients. Recovery of scolices from a suspected hydatid cyst by percutaneous needle aspiration is diagnostic, but this technique must be used with caution because of the risk of spilling scolices into the peritoneal cavity.

20. What are the treatment options for hepatic hydatid cyst disease?

Open surgical drainage of the hydatid cysts has been the preferred method of therapy. However, a prospective randomized trial of 50 patients found that medical therapy with albendazole combined with percutaneous drainage and hypertonic saline irrigation of the cysts is as effective as surgical drainage, with fewer complications and shorter durations of hospitalization.

BIBLIOGRAPHY

1. Asselah T, Ernst O, Sergent G, et al: Caroli's disease: A magnetic resonance cholangiopancreatography diagnosis. Am J Gastroenterol 93:109–110, 1998.
2. Bernardino ME, Galamobs JT: Computed tomography and magnetic resonance imaging of the liver. Semin Liver Dis 9:32–49, 1998.
3. Caroli-Bosc FX, Demarquay JF, Conio M, et al: The role of therapeutic endoscopy associated with extracorporeal shockwave lithotripsy and bile acid treatment in the management of Caroli's disease. Endoscopy 30:559–563., 1998.
4. Cheng TC, Bogitsh BJ: Extraintestinal tapeworms: Human hydatidosis. In Bogitsh B, Cheng TC (eds): Human Parasitology, 2nd ed. San Diego, Academic Press, 1998, pp 298–307.
5. D'Agata IDA, Jonas MM, Perez-Atayde AR, Guay-Woodford LM: Combined cystic disease of the liver and kidney. Semin Liver Dis 14:215–227, 1994.
6. Gabow PA: Autosomal dominant polycystic kidney disease. N Engl J Med 1993;329:332–342, 1993.
7. Khuroo MS, Wani NA, Javid G, et al: Percutaneous drainage compared with surgery for hepatic hydatid cysts. N Engl J Med 337:881–887, 1997.
8. Iglesias DM, Palmitano JA, Arrizurieta E, et al: Isolated polycystic liver disease not linked to polycystic kidney disease 1 and 2. Dig Dis Sci 44:385–388, 1999.
9. Jacobs JE, Birnbaum BA: Computed tomography imaging of focal hepatic lesions. Semin Roentgenol 30:308–323, 1995.
10. Jeyarajah DR, Gonwa TA, Testa G, et al: Liver and kidney transplantation for polycystic disease. Transplantation 66:529–544, 1998.
11. Larssen TB, Jensen DK, Viste A, Horn A: Single-session alcohol sclerotherapy in symptomatic benign hepatic cysts. Long term results. Acta Radiol 40:636–638, 1999.
12. Mergo PJ, Ros PR. Benign lesions of the liver. Radiol Clin North Am 36:319–331, 1998.
13. Nisenbaum HL, Rowling SE: Ultrasound of focal hepatic lesions. Semin Roentgenol 30:324–346, 1995.
14. Pirson Y, Lannoy N, Peters D, et al: Isolated polycystic liver disease as a distinct genetic disease, unlinked to polycystic kidney disease 1 and polycystic kidney disease 2. Hepatology 23:249–252, 1996.
15. Que F, Nagorney DM, Gross JB, Torres VE: Liver resection and cyst fenestration in the treatment of severe polycystic liver disease. Gastroenterology 108:487–494, 1995.
16. Schievink WI, Spetzler RF: Screening for intracranial aneurysms in patients with isolated polycystic liver disease. J Neurosurg 89:719–721, 1998.
17. Schiano TD, Fiel MI, Miller CM, et al: Adult presentation of Caroli's syndrome treated with orthotopic liver transplantation. Am J Gastroenterol 92:1938–1940, 1997.
18. Swenson K, Seu P, Kinkhabwala M, et al: Liver transplantation for adult polycystic liver disease. Hepatology 28:412–415, 1998.
19. Todani T, Watanabe Y, Narusue M, et al: Congenital bile duct cysts: Classification, operative procedures, and review of thirty-seven cases including cancer arising from choledochal cyst. Am J Surg 134:263–269, 1977.

36. GALLBLADDER: STONES, CRYSTALS, SLUDGE, AND POLYPS

Leslie H. Bernstein, M.D., MACG

1. What is the magnitude of gallstone disease in western populations?

In studies performed in the United States and Italy, about 10–15% of adults have gallstones. Only about 20% of persons identified to have gallstones develop symptoms (roughly 1–2% chance per year).

2. What populations are at greatest risk for gallstones?

- Women are twice as likely as men to develop gallstones.
- Female Pima Indians of the western United States carry the highest risk; about 75% develop gallstones by the fourth decade of life.
- Scandinavian women also are highly predisposed to gallstones (50% by age 50 years).

3. What are the three principal factors involved in gallstone formation?

- Cholesterol supersaturation
- Accelerated nucleation
- Gallbladder hypomotility

4. What is the first step in gallstone formation?

Nucleation, which involves the formation of insoluble deposits from supersaturated bile within the biliary system. Factors that influence nucleation include bile transit time; gallbladder contraction (frequency and completeness); bile composition and concentrations of cholesterol, phospholipid, and bile salts; pigment concentration; and presence of bacteria, mucin, and glycoproteins such as IgA.

5. What drugs and medical therapy are associated with gallstone/sludge formation?

- Ceftriaxone is an antibiotic with a proclivity to concentrate and crystallize with calcium in the biliary tree.
- Total parenteral nutrition (TPN) and fasting promote gallbladder atony and sludge formation.
- Progestins, oral contraceptives, and octreotide (somatostatin) impair gallbladder emptying and promote sludge and stone formation.

6. What is gallbladder sludge?

A super concentrated mixture of bile acids, bilirubin, cholesterol, mucus, and proteins that exhibits variable degrees of fluidity and is prone to precipitate into solid or semisolid form.

7. Can gallbladder sludge cause acute medical problems?

Yes. Gallbladder contraction and discharge of sludge into the cystic duct and common bile duct can cause acalculous cholecystitis or "idiopathic pancreatitis." Acalculous cholecystitis often is seen among intensive care patients who are fed after prolonged fasting—especially when blood transfusions and TPN are needed, because they promote bile pigment accumulation and "gelfaction" of sludge.

8. How are sludge-induced acalculous cholecystitis and idiopathic pancreatitis diagnosed?

Fortunately, hepato-iminodiacetic acid (HIDA) scans are often positive when no stones can be seen on routine sonogram. Endoscopic ultrasound (EUS) exam of the common bile duct and gallbladder has detected sludge and/or small stones in 30% of patients deemed to have idiopathic pancreatitis.

9. Why is rapid weight reduction a risk factor for development of gallstones? Can such gallstones be prevented?

During strict caloric restriction hepatic cholesterol secretion increases. Prolonged fasting leads to supersaturation of bile with cholesterol, increased mucus production, and decreased gallbladder motility, all of which promote gallstone formation. About 25% of obese patients who undergo strict caloric restriction develop gallstones. In experimental animals, aspirin decreases nucleation by lowering mucin synthesis, and both aspirin and ursodeoxycholic acid (UDCA) help to prevent stone formation in morbidly obese patients undergoing rapid weight loss.

10. How do yellow, black, and brown biliary stones differ clinically?

Yellow stones are almost pure cholesterol monohydrate. They account for over 80% of gallstones in western populations. The major excretory route of cholesterol is into bile, and a number of factors lead to its precipitation and accretion. In Asian rim populations, cholesterol stones have replaced pigment stones as the most frequent cause of cholelithiasis. This change may reflect westernization of the their diet and a decrease in the incidence of biliary parasites.

Black stones are associated with chronic hemolysis and cirrhosis. They form in the gallbladder from bilirubin precipitation and are usually quite soft; however, they may contain some calcium salts and be radiopaque. They rarely cause obstruction and usually are not responsible for cholestatic syndromes associated with sickle cell disease.

Brown stones are universally associated with colonization of bile with enteric bacteria and/or parasites. The bacteria produce beta-glucoronidase, phospholipase A, and hydrolases, which promote formation of calcium-bile salt and bilirubin complexes. Brown stones have a soft, clay-like consistency and are found in the intra- and extrahepatic ducts, *not* the gallbladder. They are more common among Asian populations and usually present as acute pyogenic cholangitis.

11. Discuss the migration of gallstones.

Large gallstones occasionally escape the gallbladder and produce obstructive symptoms elsewhere in the GI tract. Most often the obstruction is to the small bowel and occurs with impaction of the stone in a normal ileum. This **gallstone ileus** is the second most common cause of small bowel obstruction in adults without a history of previous surgery. Escape of the stone is usually by way of fistula formation between the inflamed gallbladder and the duodenum (cholecystoduodenal fistula). Stones escaping the small bowel may impact in the colon if it is narrowed by previous diverticular disease. Rarely, stones may enter the stomach by way of a fistula and obstruct the pylorus (**Bouveret's syndrome**). Cholecystocolonic fistula also may occur, leading in some cases to diarrhea provoked by the entry of bile salts into the colon. Fistulous connection between the duodenum and the common duct may be due to either peptic ulcer or gallstone disease, but the former is more common. Plain films frequently demonstrate air in the gallbladder or biliary tree, and occasionally a stone may be seen in the bowel.

12. What causes cholecystitis in patients with stone disease?

Impaction of stone(s) within the neck of the gallbladder or cystic duct results in distention and ischemia of the gallbladder wall (cholecystitis). Cultures of bile during the early phase of the disease are usually sterile. Secondary bacterial infection and even gangrene may ensue after prolonged cholecystitis.

13. What rheumatologic disease may cause acute cholecystitis?

In polyarteritis nodosa, vasculitis of the cystic duct artery can cause acute cholecystitis.

14. What are the two types of therapy for biliary stones?

Dissolution therapy and stone destruction.

15. Describe the two types of dissolution therapy.

Oral therapy is limited to small stones (usually < 1 cm), which are composed of cholesterol and are not calcified. Both dihydroxy bile salts have been used, but UDCA is associated with less hepatotoxicity than chenodiol, probably because gut bacteria can convert UDCA to the toxic lithocholic acid. Oral dissolution therapy is slow and costly and requires continuation for life to prevent recurrence.

Contact dissolution uses solvents that rapidly solubilize pigment and cholesterol. They must be administered by a catheter placed by the invasive radiologist or endoscopist. Methyl tertiary butyl ether or propyl acetate may be used, but leakage into the duodenum may cause sedation, and leakage from gallbladder puncture may necessitate cholecystectomy. Rapid reformation is also common unless oral therapy is added.

16. What methods are used for stone destruction?

Common bile duct stones may be crushed with an endoscopically placed mechanical lithotriptor. Laser destruction and acoustic destruction have been used experimentally within the common bile duct but remain impractical because of ductal injury. Endoscopic papillotomy and basket or balloon extraction remain the procedure of choice. For **gallbladder stones**, focused extracorporeal shock wave lithotripsy has been used with some success. Hepatic damage, complications induced by fragmented stones, and high cost of equipment are the major drawbacks. A functioning gallbladder is necessary to expel the fragments into the duodenum during the months after therapy.

17. How accurate is ultrasonography for detection of cholecystolithiasis? Of choledocholithiasis?

Because of the shadowing that results from stones and the ease with which the gallbladder is discerned by transabdominal sonography, cholecystolithiasis can be diagnosed with a sensitivity and specificity of over 90%. Sludge usually can be seen as movable echogenic material without shadowing. Transabdominal sonography has become the procedure of choice for diagnosing gallbladder disease, replacing the oral cholecystogram, which is subject to the additional vagaries of compliance, absorption, uptake, conjugation, excretion, and concentration. Unfortunately, ultrasound accuracy drops to about 20% for imaging of stones within the common duct. Dilated intrahepatic and common ducts can be visualized, but utility is decreased by previous obstructive disease, which leaves ducts dilated, and failure of diagnostic dilation to occur regularly in stone disease of the ductal system.

18. What is the role of EUS in detection of choledocholithiasis?

The loss of accuracy in ultrasound detection of choledocholithiasis can be regained by substitution of EUS. EUS detects over 90% of common bile duct stones compared with the gold standard of endoscopic retrograde cholangiopancreatography. Although stones cannot be treated by EUS, fine-needle aspiration of paraduodenal masses can be performed if lesions of the head of the pancreas are seen.

19. A polypoid lesion of the gallbladder 1 cm in diameter is seen on transabdominal sonography in a 65-year-old woman with postprandial distress. What is the differential diagnosis?

Polypoid lesions of the gallbladder wall include cholesterol polyps, adenomyomatous lesions, hamartomas (a fairly common site in Peutz-Jeghers syndrome), carcinoid, tubular or villous adenoma, adenocarcinoma, and metastatic disease, particularly melanoma. The differentiation of neoplastic and benign lesions is a primary problem. Malignant lesions are more likely to be sessile and larger than 1 cm. Polyps > 1.5 cm have about a 95% chance of being malignant. Differentiation is far better with enhanced CT or EUS than with simple transabdominal ultrasound. On EUS cholesterol and adenomyomatous lesions show characteristic patterns.

20. If the lesion is benign, should the gallbladder be removed?

All lesions > 1 cm should be removed to be absolutely certain of benignity. Other lesions may be followed by ultrasound for a change in size or the appearance of new lesions. If biliary dyskinetic symptoms are present, as in the case above, surgery is indicated in the absence of medical contraindication.

21. What is a porcelain gallbladder?

The porcelain gallbladder is characterized by intramural calcification of the gallbladder wall. The diagnosis can be made by plain abdominal radiographs or abdominal CT. Prophylactic cholecystectomy is recommended to prevent development of carcinoma, which may occur in over 20% of cases.

22. What is Mirizzi's syndrome?

Mirizzi's syndrome occurs when a stone impacts in the neck of the gallbladder or cystic duct and causes extrinsic compression of the common bile duct. The diagnosis should be considered when cases of cholecystitis are associated with higher than usual bilirubin levels (> 5 mg/dl) or dilation of the intrahepatic or common hepatic duct (but *not* the common bile duct).

BIBLIOGRAPHY

1. Angelico M, Della Guardia P: Review article: Hepatobiliary complication associated with total parenteral nutrition. Aliment Pharmacol Ther 14(Suppl 2):54–57, 2000.
2. Carey MC: Pathogenesis of gallstones: Recent Prog Med 83:379–391, 1992.
3. dela Porte PL, Lafont H, Domingo N, et al: Composition of biliary "sludge" in patients with cholesterol or mixed gallstones. J Hepatol 125:352–360, 2000.
4. Donovan JM: Physical and metabolic factors in gallstone pathogenesis. Gastroenterol Clin North Am 28:75–97, 1999.
5. Erlinger S, Chanson P, Dumont M, et al: Effect of octreotide on biliary lipid composition and occurrence of cholesterol crystals in patients with acromegaly. A prospective study. Dig Dis Sci 39:2384–2388, 1994.
6. Fest D, Larocca A, Villanova N, et al: Review: Low caloric intake and gallbladder motor function. Aliment Pharmacol Ther 14(Suppl 2):51–53, 2000.
7. Frossard JL, Sosa-Valencia L, Amouyal G, et al: Usefulness of endoscopic ultrasonography in patients with "idiopathic" acute pancreatitis. Am J Med 109:196–200, 2000.
8. Lee SP: Pathophysiology of gallstone formation. Clin Ther 12:194–199, 1990.
9. Mainprize KS, Gould SW, Gilbert JM: Surgical management of polypoid lesions of the gallbladder. Br J Surg 87:414–417, 2000.
10. Smith JL, Roach PD, Wittenberg LN, et al: Effects of simvastatin on hepatic cholesterol metabolism bile lithogenicity and bile acid hydrophobicity in patients with gallstones. J Gastroenterol Hepatol 15:871–879, 2000.
11. Sugiyama M, Atomi Y, Yammamoto T: Endoscopic ultrasonography for differential diagnosis of polypoid gallbladder lesions: Analysis in surgical and follow-up series. Gut 46:250–254, 2000.
12. Tudka J, Wechsler JG, Mason R, et al: The effect of ursodeoxycholic acid on nulceation time in patients with solitary or multiple gallbladder stones. Am J Gastroenterol 89:1206–1210, 1994.

37. SPHINCTER OF ODDI DYSFUNCTION

Milton T. Smith, M.D.

1. What is the sphincter of Oddi?

The sphincter of Oddi is a fibromuscular sheath that encircles the terminal portion of the common bile duct, pancreatic duct, and common channel as they traverse the wall of the duodenum. Smooth muscle fibers in the sphincter are arranged in both a circular and longitudinal fashion. Although the choledochal sphincter was recognized in 1681 by Francis Glisson, it was named after Ruggero Oddi, who published his morphologic observations of the sphincter in 1887 as a medical student at the University of Perugia, Italy.

2. Name the major components of the sphincter of Oddi.

The sphincter of Oddi is composed of three contiguous segments:
1. The sphincter choledochus, which surrounds the distal common bile duct
2. The sphincter pancreaticus around the duct of Wirsung
3. The sphincter ampulla, which encircles the common channel.

Manometric studies have shown that the length of the physiologic sphincter zone is approximately 8–10 mm, which may be shorter than its actual anatomic length.

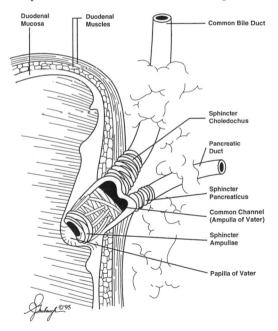

3. What are the normal functions of the sphincter of Oddi?

There are three major functions: (1) regulation of bile flow (and pancreatic juice) into the duodenum, (2) prevention of reflux of duodenal contents into the bile ducts and pancreas, and (3) promotion of gallbladder filling with hepatic bile. All three functions appear to be related to the sphincter's ability to regulate the pressure gradient between the ductal systems and duodenum. Reciprocal contractile activity between the gallbladder and sphincter of Oddi promotes gallbladder filling during the interdigestive period.

259

4. Describe the physiologic characteristics of the sphincter of Oddi.

The physiologic control of the sphincter of Oddi appears to be multifactorial. Motor activity of the sphincter is coordinated with motility of the remainder of the GI tract and with the migrating motor complex during fasting. The sphincter is also responsive to multiple neurologic and hormonal stimuli and may be modulated, via reflex mechanisms, by other areas in the pancreaticobiliary tree. The sphincter receives both sympathetic and parasympathetic innervation, and its activity is increased by cholinergic stimulation. Cholecystokinin appears to be the major hormonal regulator and causes sphincter of Oddi inhibition with a reciprocal effect (i.e., contraction) on the gallbladder. The physiologic role of other GI hormones, such as gastrin and secretin, is less clear.

5. What is sphincter of Oddi dysfunction (SOD)?

Sphincter of Oddi dysfunction is a benign, noncalculous obstruction to the flow of bile or pancreatic juice at the level of the pancreaticobiliary junction. Patients typically present with unexplained abdominal pain, with or without associated elevations in liver enzymes. SOD is found in approximately 50% of patients with "idiopathic" pancreatitis. When the cause of symptoms is thought to be at the level of the sphincter of Oddi, the term *sphincter of Oddi dysfunction* is preferred over other terms (e.g., papillary stenosis, biliary dyskinesia, postcholecystectomy syndrome).

6. What causes sphincter of Oddi dysfunction?

Partial obstruction of the sphincter segment on either an organic (i.e., structural) or functional (i.e., dysmotility) basis. Patients may be subdivided into those with sphincter stenosis vs. sphincter dyskinesia. True structural stenosis of the sphincter and papillary orifice is believed to be due to inflammation and fibrosis or possibly mucosal hyperplasia. Conditions that may contribute to the inflammatory/fibrotic process include the passage of small common bile duct stones and, possibly, recurrent episodes of pancreatitis. The cause of functional SOD is unknown. It is usually difficult to separate patients who have organic vs. functional stenosis, and overlap in etiologies is almost certain.

7. When should a diagnosis of SOD be considered?

A sphincter motility disturbance should be considered in three main clinical settings:

1. **Postcholecystectomy abdominal pain.** Most studies have focused on SOD in this setting. Patients typically say, "I feel like my gallbladder is still in." The differential diagnosis of postcholecystectomy pain is extensive (see table).

2. **Idiopathic recurrent pancreatitis.** Thorough sphincter evaluations show abnormal basal sphincter pressure in 50–60% of such patients.

3. **Episodic gallbladder-like pain with negative diagnostic tests** (including abdominal ultrasound and gallbladder ejection fraction). In patients with in-situ gallbladders and biliary-type pain, the gallbladder is usually the focus of evaluation. Recent studies suggest that some of these patients also may have SOD and abnormal SO manometry. Optimal management awaits further study.

Potential Causes of Postcholecystectomy Abdominal Pain

Musculoskeletal origin: secondary to trauma, muscular spasm/strain

Esophageal origin: esophageal spasm, gastroesophageal reflux

Pleural/pulmonary origin: pleural effusion, lower lobe pneumonia

Cardiac origin: coronary artery disease, pericarditis

Luminal GI tract origin: peptic ulcer disease, gastritis, duodenitis, obstruction, irritable bowel syndrome

Neoplasm: esophageal, gastric, pulmonary, biliary, pancreatic, papillary, other intra-abdominal tumors

Nonneoplastic intra-abdominal processes: Fitz-Hugh-Curtis syndrome, endometriosis

Narcotic withdrawal

Pancreaticobiliary origin: residual or recurrent stones, strictures, tumors, chronic pancreatitis, pseudocyst, expanding hepatic cyst/mass, sphincter of Oddi dysfunction

8. Describe the clinical classification used for patients with SOD.

Two broad categories are based on clinical presentation. Most patients have biliary-type abdominal pain, and a smaller group has symptoms referable to the pancreas. To deal with the different causes and overlap in clinical presentations, a classification system was developed based on clinical history, laboratory evaluation, and the results of diagnostic ERCP that subdivides patients with the biliary-type pain into three groups:

Criteria
   a. Typical biliary-type pain
   b. Abnormal liver enzymes (aspartate aminostransferase [AST] and/or alkaline phosphatase > 2–3 times normal on at least two occasions)
   c. Delayed drainage of ERCP contrast (> 45 min)
   d. Dilated common bile duct (> 12 mm)

Milwaukee classification
   Biliary type I: meets all criteria above (a, b, c, and d)
   Biliary type II: typical biliary-type pain (1) plus one or two of b, c, and d
   Biliary type III: biliary-type pain only (a)

Type I patients are likely to have a true structural stenosis of the sphincter, type II may be structural or functional, and type III is usually functional. Some experts have found this classification system useful in determining which patients are likely to have abnormal findings on SO manometry as well as predicting which patients will respond to endoscopic sphincterotomy. A similar classification scheme has been described for patients with SOD and predominant pancreatic symptoms.

9. Describe the nature of the pain episodes experienced by patients with suspected SOD.

Most patients have undergone a prior cholecystectomy; they experience improvement in pain after cholecystectomy but develop recurrent abdominal pain after surgery. Others do not benefit or are made even worse by cholecystectomy, presumably relating to removal of a volume reservoir. Recurrent attacks of pain often develop within 3–5 years postoperatively. The pain is usually similar in character to the pain prior to cholecystectomy. It is typically located in the right upper quadrant of the abdomen or epigastrium, with or without radiation toward the right shoulder, scapula, or back and is usually steady and noncolicky.

In most patients, episodes of pain initially occur infrequently, lasting several hours, followed by pain-free intervals. In some patients, the frequency and severity of attacks progress over time so that a chronic baseline pain syndrome develops with intermittent acute episodes.

The relationship of pain episodes to meals is also variable. The onset of pain within 1–3 hours postprandially is common, and many patients can identify certain foods (such as fatty or spicy foods) that seem to precipitate attacks. Unfortunately, other attacks of pain seem to have no consistent relationship to meals or types of food. A subset of patients have a sensitivity to opiate-containing medications, which cause exacerbations of abdominal pain.

10. Describe the physical and laboratory findings in patients with suspected SOD.

Most patients are women, typically aged 30–50, who have undergone a prior cholecystectomy. The reason for the female predominance is unclear but may simply reflect the higher incidence of gallstones and subsequent cholecystectomy in women.

The physical examination between pain episodes is normal. During an attack of pain, the patient is distressed but afebrile. The abdominal examination is usually significant only for nonspecific tenderness. The absence of fever, palpable organomegaly, and definite signs of peritonitis excludes patients with pancreatitis.

Laboratory tests during or immediately after a pain episode may be helpful. During an acute attack, some patients have transient elevations of liver (AST, alkaline phosphatase) and/or pancreatic enzymes (amylase, lipase). Repeated evaluation of enzymes may be helpful because elevations are characteristically episodic. In most patients seen for suspected SOD, these tests as well as the white blood cell count are normal.

11. How is a diagnosis of sphincter of Oddi dysfunction established?

The diagnosis of SOD is initially based on clinical suspicion. Several diagnostic tests have been reported to be helpful in defining SOD, but none is ideal and their value is controversial.

Noninvasive diagnostic tests
Liver and/or pancreatic enzymes during pain
Pain provocation tests (Nardi test)
Fatty-meal ultrasonography
Secretin ultrasonography
Quantitative hepatobiliary scintigraphy

Invasive diagnostic tests
Endoscopic retrograde cholangio-
    pancreatography (ERCP)
Endoscopic sphincter of Oddi manometry

12. Does SOD occur in association with other conditions?

An interesting feature of SOD is the common association with other smooth muscle disorders of the gut, including nonspecific esophageal dysmotility, delayed gastric emptying, and irritable bowel-type complaints. These associations suggest that some patients with SOD may have a more generalized dysmotility syndrome and that therapy directed solely at the sphincter of Oddi may not totally alleviate the symptoms.

13. Describe the usefulness of the noninvasive diagnostic tests.

Transient elevation of **liver or pancreatitic enzymes** (> 2 times upper limits of normal) during an attack of pain supports the presence of ductal outflow obstruction but is not specific for SOD. Other causes of obstruction, such as choledocholithiasis, should be ruled out.

Pain provocation tests, such as the morphine-neostigmine (Nardi test), have been used to support the diagnosis of SOD. After administration of these drugs, patients are observed for provocation of pain development of enzyme (liver and/or pancreatic) abnormalities. Morphine increases sphincter resistance, and neostigmine (Prostigmin), an anticholinesterase inhibitor, increases pancreatic juice flow. Unfortunately, the test is not sufficiently sensitive or specific.

Other noninvasive tests involve the use of **ultrasound** to determine common bile duct and/or pancreatic duct diameter before and after administration of a provocative agent. **Fatty-meal ultrasonography** involves administering fat (Lipomul, 1.5 ml/kg; Mead-Johnson Laboratories, Evansville, IN) to stimulate endogenous cholecystokinin release and enhance biliary flow. Bile duct diameter is measured at 15-minute intervals for 60 minutes. A normal response is either no change or a decrease in duct diameter. An increase by > 2 mm from baseline suggests partial biliary obstruction but does not distinguish SOD from other causes of obstruction (e.g., stones, stricture, tumor).

Secretin ultrasonography involves measuring the pancreatic duct diameter before and after administering secretin (1 mg/kg) to stimulate pancreatic juice flow. The ductal diameter may increase normally due to enhanced flow but returns to baseline within 30 minutes. An exaggeration of this response suggests outflow obstruction (e.g., pancreatic duct dilation to 2 mm above baseline that persists after 30 minutes). Both transabdominal and endoscopic ultrasound have been used to measure pancreatic ductal diameter after secretin stimulation. The sensitivity and specificity of these tests are uncertain. They may be influenced by the presence of chronic pancreatitis due to low pancreatic juice flow. Magnetic resonance cholangiopancreatography (MRCP) also can be used to determine pancreatic ductal diameter.

Quantitative hepatobiliary scintigraphy involves determining hepatic uptake and hepatobiliary clearance of an injected isotope. Although delayed uptake and clearance may be found in patients with SOD, this technique is also nonspecific and may be abnormal in patients with mechanical common duct obstruction or parenchymal liver disease. Quantitative criteria are inaccurate if the gallbladder is still present.

14. How is ERCP used in diagnosing SOD?

ERCP is helpful in ruling out other pancreaticobiliary conditions that may cause similar pain, such as retained stones, strictures, papillary tumors, and chronic pancreatitis. It also allows accurate measurement of ductal diameters and biliary and/or pancreatic drainage times. Reproduction of the patient's pain during contrast injection into the biliary tree and difficulty achieving cannulation are not reliable markers of SOD.

15. How is endoscopic SO manometry performed?

Endoscopic SO manometry is considered by many to be the most reliable method of studying sphincter function. It involves directly measuring sphincter pressure with a triple-lumen, water-perfused catheter that is passed through the duodenoscope into the bile duct or pancreas. The proximal end of the catheter is connected to external transducers and a paper recording device. The technology is virtually identical to systems used for esophageal manometry, except that the catheter is miniaturized to permit passage through the operating channel of the duodenoscope and papillary orifice. Sphincter pressures are recorded as the catheter is slowly withdrawn from the duct and stationed within the sphincter zone (station pull-through technique). Duodenal pressure is taken as the zero reference point when measuring ductal and sphincter pressures.

Several aspects of sphincter motor activity can be measured with endoscopic manometry. First, the sphincter exhibits a resting basal tone that is usually 10–40 mm Hg above duodenal pressure. Superimposed phasic pressure waves are also seen. The amplitude, frequency, and propagation direction of phasic waves are recorded.

SO motor activity is influenced by several pharmacologic and hormonal agents. The endoscopist must avoid using agents during manometry that are known to affect the sphincter (e.g., glucagon, atropine, morphine). Similarly, medications affecting the sphincter should be discontinued prior to manometric study, if possible (e.g., opiate analgesics, smooth muscle relaxants). The usual narcotics and antiperistaltic agents (e.g., glucagon, atropine) used for routine ERCP are withheld if SO manometry is to be performed, and only diazepam or midazolam is used for sedation. This often makes the procedure quite demanding for patient and physician because of suboptimal sedation and movement of the papilla during attempts to cannulate. Recent studies have shown that meperidine (Demerol) does not affect SO basal pressure, as previously assumed.

16. What manometric abnormalities are used to diagnose SOD?

1. Elevated basal sphincter pressure
2. Increased frequency or amplitude of phasic waves
3. Increased proportion of phasic waves propagated in the retrograde direction
4. Paradoxical sphincter response to cholecystokinin-octapeptide (CCK-OP) injection.

Some patients have more than one of these findings, although no evidence indicates that multiple abnormalities increase the specificity of the test. Elevated basal sphincter pressure is the most widely agreed upon abnormality and the finding most often used to make clinical decisions. Studies vary in defining the normal range for basal sphincter pressure, but values exceeding 40 mmHg (using duodenal pressure as the zero reference) are generally considered abnormal. Elevated basal pressure may be seen in both structural stenosis of the sphincter and dyskinesia. Some investigators have attempted to distinguish these entities based on the response to pharmacologic agents such as amyl nitrite or CCK-OP; these agents have no effect on elevated pressure in patients with stenosis but may transiently lower basal pressure and abolish phasic waves in patients with dyskinesia.

Although increased frequency of phasic waves (tachyoddia) and excessive retrograde propagation of phasic waves (i.e., > 50%) are observed in some patients, most experts consider the basal sphincter pressure to be more important. These abnormalities are usually seen in patients with abnormal basal sphincter pressure.

CCK-OP can be given to patients whose baseline manometric study is normal to create a situation that more closely resembles the fed state. Some patients with SOD appear to have a paradoxical response to intravenously administered CCK-OP with elevation of basal sphincter pressure. Although conceptually attractive, the paradoxical response to CCK-OP is infrequently observed and thus has limited usefulness.

Elevated basal pancreatic sphincter pressure (> 40 mmHg) is considered the gold standard for the diagnosis of pancreatic sphincter dysfunction.

17. What are the major problems associated with SO manometry?

(1) Requires deep cannulation, (2) may be poorly tolerated by patients, (3) short duration of study, and (4) risk of postmanometry pancreatitis.

18. **What steps can be taken to minimize the risk of post-SO manometry pancreatitis?**

1. Avoidance of trauma to the papilla by using gentle cannulation techniques

2. Limiting the time of pancreatic manometry when performed

3. Recannulation and drainage of the pancreatic duct after manometry (shown to be effective in one study but awaiting confirmation)

4. Limiting catheter perfusion rate to 0.25 ml/lumen/min or less

5. Sterilization of accessories and periodic culturing of ERCP endoscopes and manometry equipment

6. Use of aspiration-type manometry catheter for measuring pancreatic sphincter pressure. The aspiration catheter uses two channels for pressure measurements while aspirating infused fluid and pancreatic juice from the third channel. This device can significantly reduce the frequency of postmanometry pancreatitis.

19. **Should patients with suspected SOD be evaluated for microlithiasis (subtle gallbladder disease)?**

Patients with biliary-type pain and intact gallbladder but no demonstrable gallstones on ultrasound or ERCP may have a more subtle form of gallbladder disease. Two tests may be helpful: (1) hepatobiliary cholescintigraphy with cholecystokinin administration to determine gallbladder ejection fraction (GB-EF%) and (2) microscopic examination of gallbladder bile for the presence of cholesterol or calcium bilirubinate crystals.

An abnormally low GB-EF% (<40%) implies impaired gallbladder emptying of bile and has been used to identify patients with acalculous biliary pain who may respond to cholecystectomy. Gallbladders removed from such patients often show chronic cholecystitis and/or a narrowed cystic duct. Microscopic examination of gallbladder bile for the presence of crystals is most useful in patients with idiopathic recurrent pancreatitis (IRP). Bile is aspirated from the duodenum or directly from the bile duct at ERCP after cholecystokinin administration to induce gallbladder contraction. The presence of cholesterol or bile pigment crystals is generally accepted as evidence of gallstone disease (i.e., microlithiasis). Patients with microlithiasis and IRP frequently respond to standard therapy, such as cholecystectomy or an oral dissolution agent (Actigall), if cholesterol crystals are found.

20. **Describe the relationship between SOD and pancreatitis.**

SOD has been implicated in the pathogenesis of both IRP and chronic pancreatitis. When studying the biliary sphincter, investigators have reported elevated basal sphincter pressure in 15–57% of patients with IRP, although the significance of this finding is controversial. When the pancreatic sphincter also is studied, abnormalities are found in 50–60%. Most studies report favorable results of sphincter ablation in such patients, although additional outcome studies are needed. Medical therapy for SOD in this setting has not been sufficiently evaluated. Abnormal SO manometry studies are common in patients with chronic pancreatitis. Whether this finding is a cause or result of the chronic fibrosis and inflammatory process is unclear.

21. **Is SO manometry necessary to confirm a diagnosis of SOD before treatment?**

No. The decision to perform SO manometry is usually based on the severity of the patient's symptoms, response to conservative therapy, and classification (see question 8).

Virtually all patients, including those with more severe symptoms, should first be given a trial of medical therapy to determine response. Prospective, randomized, controlled trials show that calcium channel blockers decrease pain in most patients. Patients with more severe symptoms, particularly if unresponsive to conservative treatment, are potential candidates for SO manometry to confirm the diagnosis prior to more aggressive therapies. Classification of patients with suspected biliary pain into biliary groups I, II, and III may predict the likelihood of an abnormal manometric study and response to sphincter ablation.

SO manometry is considered unnecessary for patients who meet the criteria for biliary type I SOD. Approximataely 80–90% have abnormal manometry, and over 90% have a favorable response to biliary sphincterotomy, even if SO manometry results are normal. By contrast, SO manometry is considered by some experts to be helpful for type II patients, because basal sphincter pressure is elevated in only about 50%. In a prospective, randomized trial by Geenen et al., the response rate to endoscopic sphincterotomy was significantly higher (94% at 4 years) in type II patients with elevated sphincter pressure compared with only a 30% response in patients with normal manometry. The decision to perform ERCP and SO manometry in type III patients with abdominal pain but no objective evidence of partial biliary obstruction is more difficult. They are less likely to have abnormal manometry and have a lower response rate to endoscopic therapy.

22. Is manometry of both biliary and pancreatic duct sphincters necessary?

This question is important because evidence suggests that the incidence of pancreatitis with biliary manometry alone is minimal compared with studies involving the pancreatic sphincter. However, if only biliary manometry is performed, no information is obtained about the pancreatic portion of the sphincter. Studies have shown that elevated sphincter pressure may indeed be isolated to one portion of the sphincter. An acceptable approach is to attempt to study the bile duct sphincter first; if the study is abnormal, proceed with therapy. If the bile duct sphincter is normal and the patient has IRP, or if the pancreas is cannulated first, the pancreatic sphincter can be evaluated with an aspiration catheter. Studying both sphincters is necessary for full evaluation.

23. Are the results of SO manometry reproducible?

Most studies indicate that SO manometry results are reproducible on separate measurements.

24. What are the treatment options for SOD?

Noninvasive treatments	Invasive treatments
Low-fat diet	Endoscopic balloon dilation
Analgesics	Injection of botulinum toxin
Nitrates	Temporary stenting (biliary or pancreatic)
Calcium channel antagonists	Sphincter ablation
Anticholinergics (e.g., dicyclomine)	Endoscopic sphincterotomy
	Surgical sphincteroplasty

Surprisingly few data are available about the efficacy of medical therapies in patients with manometrically documented SOD. As an initial approach, patients should be given a course of medical therapy, including a trial of a low-fat diet, antispasmodics, and nonaddictive analgesics. Sublingual nitroglycerin, nifedipine, and dicyclomine are variably effective and appear to work best for patients with mild, infrequent symptoms. None of these agents is specific for the sphincter of Oddi, and their use is often limited by side effects.

Invasive treatment modalities are appropriate for patients with more severe symptoms who fail conservative measures. Endoscopic balloon dilation and temporary stenting are too hazardous because of excessive pancreatitis. Intrasphincteric injection of botulinum toxin (Botox), a potent inhibitor of acetylcholine release from nerve endings, has recently been proposed as a method of lowering sphincter pressure in patients with SOD. Wehrmann et al. recently reported a 55% short-term symptomatic response to Botox injection in manometrically proven type III biliary SOD. Botox response predicts subsequent sphincterotomy response in patients with recurrent symptoms. Unfortunately, two ERCPs are required.

25. When is sphincterotomy indicated in biliary SOD?

Most patients failing noninvasive measures are considered for endoscopic sphincterotomy. Stratification of patients according to the Milwaukee classification (see question 8) is helpful, because over 90% of type I patients have a favorable response to endoscopic sphincterotomy. Type II patients have a good response to sphincterotomy (92%) when elevated basal sphincter pressure is documented by SO manometry. Limited data suggest that only about one-half of type III patients are improved after biliary sphincterotomy. Surgical ablation of the sphincter of Oddi (sphincterotomy or sphincteroplasty) is mostly of historic value. Rarely is a surgical procedure required for endoscopic failures.

26. What is the risk of pancreatitis after biliary sphincterotomy for SOD?

Pancreatitis is the most common complication (up to 25–30% in some series). Pancreatic duct stenting decreased the risk of pancreatitis from 26% to 7% in patients with pancreatic sphincter hypertension who underwent biliary sphincterotomy.

27. How is pancreatic SOD treated?

Some patients improve after biliary sphincterotomy alone, most likely due to severing the fibers in the common channel or fibers in a figure-of-8 and overlapping configuration. Patients with documented pancreatic sphincter hypertension and recurrent pancreatitis or disabling pain (unresponsive to other measures) generally are considered candidates for endoscopic pancreatic sphincterotomy. The exact depth, type of current, and landmarks for pancreatic sphincterotomy are uncertain. Two endosocopic techniques have been used: (1) placement of a short pancreatic stent is used as a guide for needle-knife pancreatic sphincterotomy, and (2) a standard pull-type sphincterotome is placed in the pancreatic orifice and a cephalad incision is made up to 5–8 mm in length. Whether it is necessary to place a pancreatic stent after the second technique has not been proved in randomized trials but seems appropriate. Some endoscopists also perform a concomitant biliary sphincterotomy to lessen the potential risk of transient cholestasis or cholangitis.

28. What complications are associated with endoscopic pancreatic sphincterotomy?

Potential early complications include pancreatitis, bleeding, perforation, and biliary obstruction. Complication rates appear to be higher when sphincterotomy is performed for indications other than chronic pancreatitis (e.g., SOD associated with pain or recurrent pancreatitis). The risk of complications is independent of technique (pull-type sphincterotome vs. needle-knife). Delayed complications include sphincter restenosis and complications associated with concomitant pancreatic stent placement, such as stent migration or pancreatic ductal changes. The latter finding is reversible in most cases. The reported frequency of pancreatitis after major papilla endoscopic pancreatic sphincterotomy in recent selected series is 3–14%.

29. What is the risk of restenosis after endoscopic biliary sphincterotomy?

The overall risk of restenosis after endoscopic sphincterotomy appears to be low.

30. Why do some patients with suspected SOD not respond to biliary sphincter ablation?

The finding of abnormal SO manometric results in a symptomatic patient does not prove a cause-effect relationship. In some patients, elevated sphincter pressure may be the consequence rather than the cause of disease. Potential reasons for residual or recurrent symptoms after biliary sphincterotomy include undetected stones, residual pancreatic sphincter hypertension, restenosis, incomplete sphincterotomy, strictures, pancreatic parenchymal disease or pseudocyst, or another disease accounting for the patient's symptoms that is unrelated to the biliary tree or pancreas.

ACKNOWLEDGMENT

The author is grateful to Dr. Glen A. Lehman for reviewing the sphincter of Oddi dysfunction chapter from the first edition of *GI/Liver Secrets* and for his suggestions for the preparation of this manuscript.

BIBLIOGRAPHY

 1. Cotton PB: Unexplained RUQ abdominal pain: Possible biliary dyskinesia? Contemp Gastroenterol (May/June):23–28, 1990.
 2. Elta GH, Barnett JL: Meperidine need not be proscribed during sphincter of Oddi manometry. Gastrointest Endosc 40:7–9, 1994.
 3. Eversman D, Fogel EL, Rusche M, et al: Frquency of abnormal pancreatic and biliary sphincter manometry compared with clinical suspicion of sphincter of Oddi dysfunction. Gastrointest Endosc 50:637–641, 1999.
 4. Freeman ML, Nelson DB, Sherman S, et al: Complications of endoscopic biliary sphincterotomy. N Engl J Med 335:909–918, 1996.
 5. Goff JS: Common bile duct sphincter of Oddi stenting in patients with suspected sphincter dysfunction. Am J Gastroenterol 90:586–589, 1995.

6. Hawes RH, Lehman GA: Complications of sphincter of Oddi manometry and their prevention. Gastrointest Endosc Clin North Am 3:107–118, 1993.
7. Hogan WJ (ed): The sphincter of Oddi primer for the pancreaticobiliary endoscopist. Gastrointest Endosc Clin North Am 3:1–178, 1993.
8. Hogan WJ, Geenen JE: Biliary dyskinesia. Endoscopy 20:179–183, 1988.
9. Hogan WJ, Geenen JE, Dodds WJ: Dysmotility disturbances of the biliary tract: Classification, diagnosis, and treatment. Semin Liver Dis 7:302–310, 1987.
10. Kalayci C, Choudari CP, Sherman S, et al: Correlation of secretin stimulated MRCP findings with sphincter of oddi manometry. Gastrointest Endosc 49: AB79, 1999.
11. Komorowski RA: Anatomy and histopathology of the human sphincter of Oddi. Gastrointest Endosc Clin North Am 3:1–11, 1993.
12. Kozarek RA: Biliary dyskinesia: Are we any closer to defining the entity? Gastrointest Endosc Clin North Am 3:167–178, 1993.
13. Lans JL, Parikh NP, Geenen JE: Application of sphincter of Oddi manometry in routine clinical investigations. Endoscopy 23:139–143, 1991.
14. Manoukian AV, Schmalz MJ, Geenen JE, et al: The incidence of post-sphincterotomy stenosis in group II patients with sphincter of Oddi dysfunction. Gastrointest Endosc 39:496–498, 1993.
15. Rolny P, Geenen JE, Hogan WJ: Post-cholecystectomy patients with "objective signs" of partial bile outflow obstruction: Clinical characteristics, sphincter of Oddi manometry findings, and results of therapy. Gastrointest Endosc 39:778–781, 1993.
16. Sand J, Nordback I, Koskinen M, et al: Nifedipine for suspected type II sphincter of Oddi dyskinesia. Am J Gastroenterol 4:530–535, 1993.
17. Schmalz MJ, Geenen JE, Hogan WJ, et al: Pain on common bile duct injection during ERCP: Does it indicate sphincter of Oddi dysfunction? Gastrointest Endosc 36:458–461, 1990.
18. Sherman S, Troiano FP, Hawes RH, et al: Sphincter of Oddi manometry: Decreased risk of clinical pancreatitis with use of a modified aspirating catheter. Gastrointest Endosc 36:462–466, 1990.
19. Sostre S, Kalloo AN, Spiegler EJ, et al: A noninvasive test of sphincter of Oddi dysfunction in postcholecystectomy patients: The scintigraphic score. J Nucl Med 33:1216–1222, 1992.
20. Steinberg WM: Sphincter of Oddi dysfunction: A clinical controversy. Gastroenterology 95:1409–1415, 1988.
21. Tarnasky PR, Palesch YY, Cunningham JT, et al: Pancreatic stenting prevents pancreatitis after biliary sphincterotomy in patients with sphincter of Oddi dysfunction. Gastroenterology 115:1518–1524, 1998.
22. Toouli J, Roberts-Thomson IC, Dent J, Lee J: Manometric disorders in patients with suspected sphincter of Oddi dysfunction. Gastroenterology 88:1243–1250, 1985.
23. Venu RP: The role of the endoscopist in sphincter of Oddi manometry. Gastrointest Endosc Clin North Am 3:67–80, 1993.
24. Venu RP, Geenen JE, Hogan WJ, et al: Idiopathic recurrent pancreatitis: An approach to diagnosis and treatment. Dig Dis Sci 34:56–60, 1989.
25. Wehrmann T, Seifert H, Seipp M, et al: Endoscoopic injection of Botulinum toxin for biliary sphincter of Oddi dysfunction. Endoscopy 30:702–707, 1998.
26. Wiedmeyer DA, Stewart ET, Taylor AJ: Radiologic evaluation of structure and function of the sphincter of Oddi. Gastrointest Endosc Clin North Am 3:13–40, 1993.

IV. Pancreatic Disorders

38. ACUTE PANCREATITIS

Ramona M. Lim, M.D., and Jamie S. Barkin, M.D., FACP, MACG

1. What are the most common causes of acute pancreatitis (AP)?

Gallstones (30–50%) and alcohol abuse (up to 66% of first episodes) account for most cases. So-called idiopathic AP, in which a source is not identified, accounts for 8–25% of cases; in up to two-thirds of these patients, however, microlithiasis may be identified by repeat ultrasound or collection of bile.

2. What is the mortality rate of gallstone-associated pancreatitis?

Twelve percent during the first attack. Mortality tends to decrease with subsequent attacks.

3. Is pregnancy associated with AP?

Yes. Most episodes occur in the third trimester or postpartum period. Coexisting cholelithiasis with stones or microlithiasis is present in about 90% of cases. The overall prognosis is good. Other causes include hyperlipidemia and medications. Ectopic pregnancy can simulate the presentation of acute pancreatitis with abdominal pain and elevated serum amylase.

4. Which is seen more commonly with hyperparathyroidism—acute or chronic pancreatitis?

Chronic pancreatitis. AP accounts for one-third of cases; the rest are chronic.

5. What percentage of AP is caused by drugs? Which drugs?

Five percent. Drugs for which the association is definite include azathioprine, 6-mercaptopurine, sulfonamides, thiazide diuretics, furosemide, estrogens, tetracyclines, valproic acid, pentamidine, intravenous lipid infusion, and L-asparaginase. Drugs for which the association is probable include chlorthalidone, ethacrynic acid, phenformin, nonsteroidal anti-inflammatory agents, nitrofurantoin, methyldopa, corticosteroids, didanosine, angiotensin-converting enzyme inhibitors, 5-ASA compounds, cimetidine, ranitidine, acetaminophen, metronidazole, and salicylates. Drug-induced pancreatitis can occur immediately on initiation of a drug or be delayed by years.

6. Which compounds have a dose-related effect in drug- and poison-induced pancreatitis?

Ethyl alcohol, organophosphorus insecticides, and IV lipid infusions.

7. What etiologies must be considered in post-transplant patients with AP?

Secondary hyperparathyroidism, hyperlipidemia, viral infections, vasculitis, and immunosuppressive therapy, particularly with corticosteroids, azathioprine, and L-asparaginase.

8. What infections cause AP in immunocompetent hosts?

Overall, infection-associated pancreatitis is uncommon. However, several viruses have been implicated, including mumps, coxsackie, and hepatitis A and B. Bacterial causes, including *Mycoplasma* spp., *Salmonella* spp., and *Mycobacterium tuberculosis*, as well as intraductal parasitic infections, particularly ascaris and clonorchis, also have been cited.

9. What are the two most common causes of the increased incidence of AP in patients with AIDS?

Drugs and infections. Frequently used drugs, such as pentamidine, trimethoprim-sulfamethoxazole, and didanosine, can result in AP. The incidence of infection-associated pancreatitis is also higher, with cytomegalovirus accounting for most cases. Other agents include *Cryptococcus neoformans, M. tuberculosis*, and herpes simplex virus. Disseminated infections with *Mycobacterium avium* complex, *Toxoplasma gondii, Pneumocystis carinii, Leishmania* spp., and *Candida* spp. may involve the pancreas but rarely cause clinical symptoms. Pancreatic neoplasms, including Kaposi's sarcoma and lymphoma, may develop in about 5% of patients with AIDS.

10. What types of trauma may cause AP?

Blunt rather than penetrating trauma may induce pancreatitis, usually involving the body of the pancreas at the point where it is compressed against the spine. In adults, frequently mechanisms include steering wheel or seat-belt injury. Trauma is the most common cause of AP in children, frequently resulting from bicycle handle-bar injury. Sequelae of trauma are pseudocyst formation as well as pancreatic duct strictures, which may result in recurrent and chronic pancreatitis.

11. Is pancreas divisum associated with an increased incidence of recurrent AP?

Controversial. Pancreas divisum is congenital failure of fusion of the ventral and dorsal pancreatic anlagen. It is the most common congenital anatomic variant (5–10%) of the human pancreas. Most patients are not predisposed to development of pancreatitis. However, the combination of pancreas divisum with a small accessory ampullary orifice leading to dorsal pancreatic duct obstruction may result in pancreatitis; therefore, endoscopic or surgical decompression of the dorsal pancreatic duct may be offered to patients with changes of chronic pancreatitis (i.e., duct dilation) in the dorsal pancreatic duct.

12. Should patients with so-called idiopathic AP undergo pancreatic duct visualization?

Yes. In approximately 35–40% of such patients, surgically or endoscopically remediable abnormalities are detected by endoscopic retrograde cholangiopancreatography (ERCP). Conditions include ultrasound-negative choledocholithiasis and cholelithiasis; choledochoceles; obstructions of pancreatic duct by calculi, strictures, small pseudocysts, annular pancreas, carcinoma, intraductal mucin secreting tumors, or ampullary tumors; sphincter of Oddi dysfunction; and (more controversial) pancreas divisum. Magnetic resonance cholangiopancreatography (MRCP) allows noninvasive, direct visualization of the pancreaticobiliary system without intrapancreatic ductal contrast medium injection and thus avoids the most frequent complication of ERCP, which is acute pancreatitis. Preliminary evidence suggests that its diagnostic accuracy in centers of expertise rivals that of conventional ERCP, but additional randomized trials and greater experience at the local level are necessary before this technique is used routinely. With improved sensitivity, it may become a screening test to identify patients needing ERCP.

13. Does the magnitude of hyperamylasemia correlate with the severity of pancreatitis?

No. The serum amylase level typically rises 2–12 hours after onset of symptoms, then slowly declines over 3–5 days. Conversely, elevations of serum lipase levels tend to persist longer. The magnitude of hyperamylasemia has no prognostic value in acute pancreatitis; levels may remain normal in up to 10% of cases of lethal pancreatitis.

14. What are the nonpancreatic sources of hyperamylasemia?

Diseases of the salivary glands, lungs, fallopian tubes, ovarian cysts, gallbladder, and small bowel may result in elevations of serum amylase. Tumors of the colon, lung, and ovary may cause hyperamylasemia. Any condition associated with increased small bowel permeability (perforation, infarction, and obstruction) or diminished renal clearance of pancreatic enzymes (renal failure) may cause elevations in both amylase and lipase in the absence of clinical pancreatitis.

15. Define macroamylasemia and macrolipasemia.

In **macroamylasemia**, amylase complexes with immunoglobulin A, and the large molecules do not undergo glomerular filtration. Therefore, serum amylase activity is increased, but urinary amylase levels or amylase-creatinine clearance ratio is low. **Macrolipasemia**, in which lipase is complexed with immunoglobulin A, also has been documented in patients with cirrhosis or non-Hodgkin's lymphoma. Knowledge of these entities may prevent unnecessary evaluation and treatment in patients with elevated serum amylase or lipase secondary to macroamylasemia and/or macrolipasemia.

16. What etiology of acute AP should be suspected in patients without measurable elevations in serum amylase levels?

Hypertriglyceridemia results in false-negative serum values of amylase and lipase that can be detected by dilution of the serum. Of note, although measured serum amylase activity is frequently normal, urinary amylase concentration is markedly elevated. Fredickson type I, IV, and V hyperlipoproteinemias often are associated with severe pancreatitis, usually with triglyceride levels > 1000 mg/dl. Recurrences may be prevented by treatment aimed at avoiding elevations in serum triglycerides (usually > 750 mg/dl).

17. What prognostic scoring systems are used to assess the severity of AP?

Ranson's criteria, frequently used to assess the severity of ethanol-associated pancreatitis, can be applied only at 48 hours. Eleven indices are assessed over 48 hours—5 on admission and 6 at 48 hours. Mild pancreatitis (score < 3) can be distinguished from complicated pancreatitis (≥ 3) in 90% of cases. The Ranson's score correlates with morbidity and mortality. Mortality rates are negligible in mild cases but increase with scores ≥ 3 (score of 3–4 = 15%, score of 5–6 = 40%). In severe cases (score > 6), mortality rates approach 100%.

The **simplified Glasgow criteria**, which can be applied to nonalcoholic pancreatitis, measure 8 parameters at any time within the first 48 hours.

The **APACHE-II** (Acute Physiology and Chronic Health Evaluation) score can be applied at time of admission and is based on a point system depending on patient age, chronic illness, and various physiologic variables. APACHE-II points ≥ 8 portend an unfavorable prognosis. It is, however, a cumbersome and clinically impractical system.

Prognostic Scoring Criteria in Acute Pancreatitis

ETHANOL-ASSOCIATED (RANSON'S CRITERIA)		BILIARY ORIGIN (SIMPLIFIED GLASGOW CRITERIA)
At admission	**Within 48 hr of admission**	**During initial 48 hr**
Age > 55 yr	Hct drop > 10%	Age > 55 yr
WBC > 16,000/mm^3	BUN rise > 5 mg/dl	WBC > 15,000/mm^3
Glucose > 200 mg/dl	Calcium < 8 mg/dl	LDH > 600 IU/L
LDH > 350 IU/L	PaO$_2$ < 60 mmHg	Glucose > 180 mg/dl
AST > 250 U/L	Base deficit > 4 mEq/L	Albumin < 3.2 g/dl
	Fluid sequestration > 6 L	Calcium < 8 mg/dl
		PaO$_2$ < 60 mmHg
		BUN > 45 mg/dl

WBC = white blood cell count, LDH = lactate dehydrogenase, AST = aspartate aminotransferase, Hct - hematocrit, BUN = blood urea nigrogen, PaO$_2$ = partial pressure of oxygen in arterial blood.

APACHE-II Scoring System for Severity of Acute Pancreatitis

Age: ≥ 45 yr assigned ascending points to age 75 (6 points maximum)
Acute physiology score (points assigned for abnormal values; 50 points maximum)
    Vital signs
    Arterial blood gases
    Serum electrolytes
    Glasgow coma score (15 minus actual GCS)
Chronic health score (points assigned for severe organ system dysfunction or immunocompromise)
    Liver: cirrhosis, portal hypertension, encephalopathy/coma
    Cardiovascular: New York Heart Association class IV
    Respiratory : severe chronic obstructive, restrictive, or vascular disease

Renal: chronic dialysis
Immunocompromise: leukemia, lymphoma, AIDS, or immunosuppressive therapy

18. Explain the role of serum markers in assessing the severity of AP.

Serum markers help to distinguish mild from severe disease. Proposed values include neutrophil elastase, interleukin (IL)-6 and IL-8, C-reactive protein, platelet activating factor, and urinary trypsinogen activation peptide, but most are not routinely used in clinical practice.

19. What is most accurate predictor of severe pancreatitis and poor outcome?

Extrapancreatic organ failure (i.e., shock, renal failure, respiratory insufficiency, gastrointestinal bleeding) portends a poor prognosis. The clinical presence of (1) hypotension with shock, (2) organ system failure, and (3) peritoneal sepsis is as accurate as any scoring system for prediction of severity in AP. Obesity appears to be an independent risk factor.

20. Can CT scan provide prognostic information in AP?

Yes. The CT Severity Index, as characterized by Balthazar, uses the presence of peripancreatic inflammation or phlegmon combined with the degree of pancreatic necrosis at initial CT study. This technique, which correlates with Ranson criteria in prognostic assessment, involves injection of rapid-bolus administration of intravenous contrast for assessment of necrosis. Necrosis is defined as lack of enhancement of all or a portion of the gland during scanning.

Computed Tomography Severity Index

		POINTS
Grade of acute pancreatitis		
A	Normal pancreas	0
B	Pancreatic enlargement	1
C	Pancreatic or peripancreatic inflammation	2
D	Single peripancreatic fluid collection	3
E	Multiple fluid collections	4
Degree of necrosis		
No necrosis		0
Necrosis in one-third of pancreas		2
Necrosis in one-half of pancreas		4
Necrosis in more than one-half of pancreas		6
AP grade (0–4) + necrosis (0–6) = CT Severity Index		

The presence of necrosis increases the likelihood of infection and portends a less favorable outcome. Patients with pancreatic necrosis have a 30–50% chance of developing infection of the necrosis; higher degrees of necrosis worsen the prognosis. Mortality and disease severity are low with scores up to 2, but scores of 7–10 are associated with 17% mortality and 92% morbidity rates. CT findings are generally not helpful in differentiating sterile from infected necrosis, although the presence of gas bubbles suggests infected necrosis. CT-guided needle aspiration with Gram stain and culture of the aspirate allows diagnosis of suspected infected necrosis.

21. When and why should a CT scan be obtained in patients with AP?

CT scan with rapid bolus IV contrast should be obtained whenever severe pancreatitis is clinically suspected based on: (1) failure of the patient to improve clinically, (2) presence of organ failure, or (3) suspicion of infected necrosis with fever > 101°F or leukocytosis. Its purpose is to determine whether necrosis is present, and, if present, to guide a needle for aspiration to determine whether the necrosis is secondarily infected. Because other intra-abdominal conditions can mimic AP, CT scan also confirms that AP is the cause of the problem.

Inflammation resulting from sterile necrosis cannot be distinguished clinically from infection of necrosis. Pancreatic infection usually occurs 5 or more days after onset of pancreatitis. CT with IV contrast should not be performed until volume status is repleted and renal function is accurately assessed.

22. Should patients with coexisting alcoholism and cholelithiasis have cholecystectomy to prevent further attacks of AP?
    No. Cholecystectomy does not prevent recurrent attacks in patients with coexisting alcoholism because the disease almost always follows the pattern of alcohol-related pancreatitis.

23. What is the most common cause of so-called idiopathic AP?
    Biliary sludge (microlithiasis) is identified in approximately 70% of patients with idiopathic AP. Sonography may not be sensitive in detecting sludge; the most sensitive test is microscopic examination of bile obtained either at ERCP or during duodenal aspiration after CCK administration. The theory that many cases of idiopathic AP are caused by gallstones too small to be visualized by conventional imaging is supported by the reduction of recurrences of AP in patients treated with endoscopic sphincterotomy or cholecystectomy compared with untreated patients (10% vs. 73%, p < 0.01). Chemical dissolution with ursodeoxycholic acid also can prevent recurrences.

24. What is the most reliable marker for diagnosing biliary AP?
    A greater than threefold elevation of **serum levels of alanine aminostranferase** (ALT) has a positive predictive value of 95%. Bilirubin and alkaline phosphatase levels are not specific for biliary tract origin. Amylase-lipase ratios also are not helpful.

25. When should ERCP be performed in acute biliary pancreatitis?
    Early ERCP with endoscopic sphincterotomy for stone extraction and biliary decompression has proved beneficial for patients with predicted severe biliary pancreatitis and evidence of persistent or progressive biliary obstruction (i.e., cholangitis or jaundice). Of note, the best clinical predictor of persistent common bile duct stones is an elevated **total serum bilirubin level** (> 1.35 mg/dl) on hospital day 2 (sensitivity of 90% and specificity of 63%). However, the routine use of prelaparoscopic cholecystectomy ERCP in all patients with presumed gallstone pancreatitis is no longer justified. Patients without evidence of ongoing biliary obstruction or suspicion of stones should have intraoperative cholangiogram at time of laparoscopic cholecystectomy, with bile duct exploration or postoperative ERCP as indicated.

26. Overall, what is the mortality rate of patients who develop infected pancreatic necrosis?
    Thirty-eight percent compared with 9% in patients with sterile necrosis. Blood cultures are neither sensitive for isolation of microorganisms nor specific for site of infection. Sonographic or CT-guided percutaneous aspirates of suspected areas of necrosis are the procedures of choice.

27. What is the most common organism isolated in infected pancreatic necrosis?
    Escherichia coli is isolated in 51% of percutaneous aspirates. Gram stain or culture of pancreatic aspirates may identify a single microorganism or a polymicrobial infection. Other common infections result from *Enterococcus* spp. (19%), *Staphylococcus* spp. (18%), *Proteus* spp. (10%), *Klebsiella* spp. (10%), *Pseudomonas* spp. (10%), *Streptococcus faecalis* (7%), and *Bacteroides* (6%) spp. These organisms probably reach the pancreas by translocation across the bowel wall. Infection also can result from local lymphatic, hematogenous, or biliary spread.

28. Discuss the role of prophylactic antibiotics in AP.
    Evidence supports use of prophylactic antibiotics in patients with acute necrotizing pancreatitis. Septic complications may be avoided if the antibiotic penetrates pancreatic tissue in levels sufficient to prevent colonization of the inflamed pancreas after bacterial translocation from the gut. Empirical use of **imipenem** in patients with acute necrotizing pancreatitis may significantly reduce the incidence of septic events, including possible pancreatic sepsis. There is no consensus

about antibiotic prophylaxis in prognostically severe AP without demonstrable necrosis. Fluoro-quinolones, third-generation cephalosporins, or ureidopenicillins, combined with metronidazole, are an acceptable alternative. Regimens composed of first- and second-generation cephalosporins or aminoglycosides are inadequate because of poor tissue penetration. Although septic events can be decreased, the effect of antibiotic prophylaxis on mortality is unclear.

29. Does fungal infection of the pancreas occur in AP?
Yes. Fungal infection is uncommon, but increased antibiotic use may modify its prevalence. Clinicians should be aware of this entity, particularly in patients with suspected infected pancreatic necrosis, so that appropriate fungal smear and culture of percutaneous aspirates are obtained. Documentation of infected pancreatic necrosis, either bacterial or fungal, requires prompt surgical debridement.

30. When and by what route should nutritional support be initiated in patients with AP?
Oral feeding should be initiated as soon as possible when the patient is hungry and without nausea, vomiting, or evidence of gastrointestinal ileus. It is irrelevant in the presence of pain or elevation of serum pancreatic enzymes. If oral feedings are not tolerated, nutritional supplementation should be considered. The decision to use parenteral or enteral nutrition is controversial, although mounting evidence suggests that enteral feeding is more beneficial. **Enteral nutrition**, by a jejunal feeding tube placed beyond the ligament of Treitz, has the advantage of preserving bowel function and integrity, thus reducing bacterial translocation and theoretically decreasing the incidence of pancreatic infection. Enteral nutrition is also less expensive than parenteral nutrition, has fewer problems with stress-induced hyperglycemia, and has a lower incidence of septic complications (e.g., catheter sepsis). A recent study showed that while enteral infusions of elemental diets did not rest the pancreas in healthy subjects, the enzyme secretory responses to elemental diets were suppressed in all patients with AP.

31. Should all acute fluid collections that develop in the course of AP be drained?
No. Acute fluid collections commonly occur in more than 50% of patients with moderate-to-severe acute pancreatitis, but most regress spontaneously within 6 weeks. They are irregular in shape, lack a clear wall of granulation tissue, and represent a serous or exudative reaction to pancreatic injury. They do not directly communicate with the pancreatic duct and, therefore, do not have high pancreatic enzyme concentration, as do pseudocysts. Nearly 65% resolve spontaneously; 10–15% may develop a capsule and progress to pseudocyst formation. Intervention may be considered when the collection persists beyond 6 weeks after the onset of pancreatitis and results in symptoms (e.g., pain), when obstructive symptoms result from mass effect, or when infection or malignancy is suspected.

32. What are pseudocysts?
They are localized fluid collections containing necrotic tissue, debris, pancreatic enzymes, and blood. They develop 1–4 weeks after onset of AP and represent extravasated pancreatic secretions with inflammatory response, often in communication with the pancreatic duct. They lack a true epithelial lining but are surrounded by granulation tissue and collagen. They appear round or oval in shape; 85% are located in the body or tail and 15% in the head of the pancreas. They also may occur in the lesser sac or extend to the neck, mediastinum, retroperitoneum, pelvis, and scrotum.

33. When should a pseudocyst be suspected?
When (1) serum amylase levels remain persistently high, (2) an episode of pancreatitis fails to resolve, (3) a patient has persistent abdominal pain after clinical resolution of AP, or (4) an epigastric mass is felt after an episode of AP.

34. What are the indications for drainage of pancreatic pseudocysts?
(1) Presence of symptoms, (2) enlargement of cyst, (3) presence of complications (infection, hemorrhage, rupture, and obstruction), and (4) suspicion of malignancy.

35. How are pseudocysts drained?

Percutaneous or endoscopic drainage is successful in 85% of cases, but surgical drainage is sometimes necessary. **Percutaneous catheter drainage** is preferred for poor-risk patients, immature cysts, and infected pseudocysts. It should not be used in the presence of a known main pancreatic duct stricture close to the ampulla because of the risk of developing a permanent external fistula. ERCP or MRCP may be helpful to see ductal anatomy. For mature cysts that are symptomatic, especially when they are smaller or located in the pancreatic head, **endoscopic drainage** is an excellent modality. Endoscopic expertise is required to perform transenteric (endoscopic cysto-gastrostomy or endoscopic cystoduodenostomy) or transpapillary drainage, which are associated with improved success rates and lower recurrence rates. **Surgical drainage** is warranted when percutaneous or endoscopic drainage fails and in the presence of multiple or giant pseudocysts and/or other complications related to chronic pancreatitis. Suspected malignancy probably is best managed surgically to obtain excisional histopathology.

36. Discuss the complications of an untreated pancreatic pseudocyst.

Secondary infection occurs in approximately 10% of pseudocysts. CT scan may suggest infection by demonstrating gas bubbles within the pseudocyst, but percutaneous aspiration with Gram stain and/or culture is the usual diagnostic modality.

Pseudocyst rupture occurs in < 3% of patients. Clinical presentation varies widely from acute abdominal catastrophe to a silent event producing pancreatic ascites or pleural effusion.

Pancreatic ascites, secondary to leakage from a pseudocyst (70%) or pancreatic duct (10–20%), is characterized by ascitic fluid with high amylase levels (usually > 1000 μ/dl) and protein (usually > 2.5 gm/dl). Medical management consists of TPN and octreotide. ERCP can demonstrate the site of leakage, and endoscopic stenting of the main pancreatic duct may allow resolution of the ascites.

Pancreatic fistulas usually develop from external drainage of a pseudocyst. They may close spontaneously or with the aid of octreotide, which decreases fistula output. Surgical intervention may be necessary for persistent high output (> 200 ml/day) fistulae.

Obstruction of the GI tract, urinary system, vena cava, or portal vein by a pseudocyst necessitates drainage.

Jaundice (seen in approximately 10% of pseudocysts) is due to hepatic dysfunction, extrahepatic biliary obstruction, stenosis of the intrapancreatic portion of the distal common bile duct from pancreatitis, and choledocholithiasis.

Pseudoaneurysm occurs when the pseudocyst erodes into an adjacent vessel (5–10% of patients).Clinical signs include an expanding pseudocyst with pain, hypotension, and falling hematocrit. If the pseudocyst is in communication with the pancreatic duct, massive GI bleeding (hematemesis or melena) results from bleeding directly in the pancreatic duct (hemosuccus pancreaticus). Intra-abdominal bleeding results from rupture of the pseudoaneurysm.

37. What triad of clinical findings suggests intrapseudocyst hemorrhage?

(1) Increase in the size of the mass, (2) localized bruit over the mass, and (3) sudden decrease in hemoglobin and hematocrit without obvious external blood loss.

38. What complications of AP can result in acute massive upper GI bleed?

Isolated **gastric varices** may result from splenic vein thrombosis. Splenectomy with gastric devascularization is curative. **Hemosuccus pancreaticus**, a rare event, is bleeding through the pancreatic duct into the duodenum due to erosion of a pseudocyst into adjacent vasculature (see question 36). Blood emanating from the ampulla may be visualized endoscopically and can arise from hemosuccus pancreaticus or hemobilia. Bolus dynamic CT scan is the most useful initial diagnostic test to detect the presence of hemorrhage (attenuation > 30 HU) and pseudoaneurysms. Selective mesenteric arteriography during active bleeding distinguishes hemosuccus pancreaticus from hemobilia, identifies the source of arterial or venous bleeding, and determines whether the blood traverses a pancreatic pseudocyst or abscess before drainage into the pancreatic duct. Selective arterial embolization during angiography also may control bleeding.

39. What are the pulmonary manifestations of AP?

Pulmonary abnormalities are found in approximately 10–20% of patients with AP. **Pleural effusions** are common; most are left-sided (although bilateral and right-sided effusion occur) and exudative (high fluid amylase level). Physical examination may reveal basilar rales and atelectasis. Early arterial hypoxia is due to a right-to-left shunt from microthrombi of the pulmonary vasculature, and **adult respiratory distress syndrome** (ARDS) is seen in up to 20% of patients with severe AP. It is important to assess oxygenation early in the course of AP.

40. What are the causes of early mortality in AP?

Cardiovascular collapse mediated by circulating vasoactive kinins, ARDS, intra-abdominal hemorrhage, acute renal failure, and acute cholangitis. Acute renal failure in the setting of prolonged hypovolemia and shock leads to acute tubular necrosis, and the mortality rate approaches 50%.

41. What are the causes of late mortality in AP?

Septic complications, particularly infected pancreatic necrosis and abscess, and pneumonitis tend to occur after the first week of illness and account for most instances of late mortality.

42. What other organ system lesions are associated with AP?

Polyserositis of articular synovium, pleura, or pericardium may occur. Subcutaneous fat necrosis may cause a skin rash resembling erythema nodosum. Fat necrosis adjacent to synovium may result in arthritis, revealing synovial fluid with many leukocytes and high lipase concentration. Distant fat necrosis, while clinically evident in only 1% of cases of AP, may be seen in up to 10% of patients on autopsy. Purtscher's retinopathy, a rare complication of AP, leads to sudden blindness due to occlusion of the posterior retinal artery with aggregated granulocytes.

BIBLIOGRAPHY

1. Balthazar EJ, Robinson DL, Megibow AJ, Ranson JH: Acute pancreatitis: Value of CT in establishing prognosis. Radiology 174:331–336, 1990.
2. Banks PA: Predictors of severity in acute pancreatitis. Pancreas 6(Suppl 1):S7–S12, 1991.
3. Banks PA, Gerzof SG, Langevin RE, et al. CT-guided aspiration of suspected pancreatic infection: Bacteriology and clinical outcome. Int J Pancreatol 18:265–270, 1995.
4. Banks PA: Practice guidelines in acute pancreatitis. Am J Gastroenterol 92:377–386, 1997.
5. Banks PA: Acute and chronic pancreatitis. In Sleisenger MH (ed): Sleisenger and Fordtran's Gastrointestinal and Liver Disease, 6th ed. Philadelphia, W.B. Saunders, 1998, pp 809–862.
6. Blamey SL, Imrie CW, O'Neill J, et al: Prognostic factors in acute pancreatitis. Gut 25:1340–1346, 1984.
7. Bonacini M: Pancreatic involvement in human immunodeficiency virus infection. J Clin Gastroenterol 13:58–64, 1991.
8. Bradley EL: A clinically based classification system for acute pancreatitis. Arch Surg 128:586–590, 1993.
9. Buscail L, Escourrou J, Delvaux M, et al: Microscopic examination of bile directly collected during endoscopic cannulation of the papilla: Utility in patients with suspected microlithiasis. Dig Dis Sci 37:116–120, 1992.
10. Chang L, Lo SK, Stabile BE, et al: Gallstone pancreatitis: A prospective study on the incidence of cholangitis and clinical predictors of retained common bile duct stones. Am J Gastroenterol 93:527–531, 1998.
11. Fan ST, Lai EC, Mok FP, et al: Early treatment of acute biliary pancreatitis by endoscopic papillotomy. N Engl J Med 328:228–232, 1993.
12. Kalfarentzos F, Kehagias J, Mead N, et al: Enteral nutrition is superior to parenteral nutrition in severe acute pancreatitis: Results of a randomized prospective trial. Br J Surg 84:1665–1669, 1997.
13. Karimgani I, Porter KA, Langevin RE, Banks PA: Prognostic factors in sterile pancreatic necrosis. Gastroenterology 103:1636–1640, 1992.
14. Lans JI, Geenen JE, Johanson JF, Hogan WJ: Endoscopic therapy in patients with pancreas divisum and acute pancreatitis: A prospective, randomized, controlled clinical trial. Gastrointest Endosc 38:430–434, 1992.
15. Lee SP, Nicholls JF, Park HZ: Biliary sludge as a cause of acute pancreatitis. N Engl J Med 326:589–593, 1992.
16. Mergener K, Baillie J: Endoscopic treatment for acute biliary pancreatitis: When and whom? Gastroenterol Clin North Am 28:601–613, 1999.
17. Neoptolemos JP, Carr-Locke DL, London NJ, et al: Controlled trial of urgent endoscopic retrograde cholangiopancreatography and endoscopic sphincterotomy versus conservative treatment for acute pancreatitis due to gallstones. Lancet ii:979–983, 1988.
18. Neoptolemos JP, Kemppainen EA, Mayer JM, et al: Early prediction of severity of acute pancreatitis by urinary trypsinogen activation peptide: A multicentre study. Lancet 355:1955–1960, 2000.
19. O'Keefe SJ, Abou-Assi SG, Lee RB, Anderson FP: Enteral infusions of elemental diets stimulate pancreatic enzyme secretion in normal subjects but not in patients with acute pancreatitis [abstract]. In Proceedings of the American College of Gastroenterology 2000 Annual Scientific Meeting, New York, 2000, p 163.
20. Pederzoli P, Bassi C, Vesenteni S, Campedelli A: A randomized multicenter clinical trial of antibiotic prophylaxis of septic complications in acute necrotizing pancreatitis with imipenem. Surg Gynecol Obstet 176:480–483, 1993.

21. Pitchumoni CS, Agarwal N: Pancreatic pseudocysts: When and how should drainage be performed? Gastroenterol Clin North Am 28:615–639, 1999.
22. Powell JJ, Miles R, Siriwardena AK: Antibiotic prophylaxis in the initial management of severe acute pancreatitis. Br J Surg 85:582–587, 1998.
23. Ranson JH: Etiologic and prognostic factors in human acute pancreatitis: A review. Am J Gastroenterol 77:633–638, 1982.
24. Ratschko M, Fenner T, Lankisch PG: The role of antibiotic prophylaxis in the treatment of acute pancreatitis. Gastroenterol Clin North Am 28:641–659, 1999.
25. Ros E, Navarro S, Bru C, et al: Occult microlithiasis in 'idiopathic' acute pancreatitis: Prevention of relapses by chole-cystectomy or ursodeoxycholic acid therapy. Gastroenterology 101:1701–1709, 1991.
26. Scolapio JS, Malhi-Chowla N, Ukleja A: Nutrition supplementation in patients with acute and chronic pancreatitis. Gastroenterol Clin North Am 28:695–707, 1999.
27. Steinberg W, Tenner S: Acute pancreatitis. N Engl J Med 330:1198–1210, 1994.
28. Tenner S, Dubner H, Steinberg W: Predicting gallstone pancreatitis with laboratory parameters: A meta analysis. Am J Gastroenterol 89:1863–1866, 1994.
29. Topazian M, Gorelick FS. Acute pancreatitis. In Yamada T (ed): Textbook of Gastroenterology, 3rd ed. Philadelphia, Lippincott Williams & Wilkins, 1999, pp 2121–2150.

39. CHRONIC PANCREATITIS

Ramona M. Lim, M.D., and Jamie S. Barkin, M.D., FACP, MACG

1. What classification system is used for chronic pancreatitis (CP)?

The Marseilles-Rome classification of CP was modified by Sarles into four groups based on morphology, molecular biology, and epidemiology:

1. **Lithogenic CP** (chronic calcifying pancreatitis), the largest group, is characterized by irregular fibrosis of the pancreas with intraductal protein plugs, ductal injury, and intraductal stones. Alcohol is the leading cause.

2. **Obstructive CP** demonstrates glandular changes, including uniform fibrosis, ductal changes with dilation, and acinar atrophy, all of which may improve when the obstruction of the pancreatic duct (often by intraductal tumor or benign ductal stricture) is removed.

3. **Inflammatory CP** is characterized histologically by mononuclear cell infiltration with associated exocrine parenchyma destruction, diffuse fibrosis, and atrophy. It is associated with autoimmune diseases such as Sjögren's syndrome, primary sclerosing cholangitis, and autoimmune pancreatitis.

4. **Pancreatic fibrosis** is characterized by silent, diffuse perilobular fibrosis, as seen in so-called idiopathic senile CP.

2. What is the most common cause of chronic pancreatitis in adults?

In western societies, chronic alcohol abuse accounts for 70% of cases of CP. The type of alcohol and pattern of drinking have no influence on the risk of developing CP. It may be influenced by genetic predisposition in the host, although experimental and epidemiologic studies also suggest that diets high in fat and protein may increase the risk for alcohol-induced pancreatitis.

3. How is idiopathic CP diagnosed?

By exclusion of known causes of CP, including nutritional or hereditary causes, hypercalcemia, trauma with residual duct injury, hyperlipidemia, autoimmunity, pancreas divisum, ampullary and duodenal diseases causing obstructive CP, and primary pancreatic tumors causing obstructive pancreatitis.

4. What is nutritional CP?

Tropical (or nutritional) pancreatitis, seen in southern India, Indonesia, and sub-Saharan Africa, is believed to result from severe protein-calorie malnutrition. It is characterized by hypoalbuminemia, marked emaciation, bilateral parotid gland enlargement, and hair and skin changes resembling kwashiorkor.

5. What genetic factors influence the development of CP?

Hereditary pancreatitis is found in different areas of the world (United States, New Zealand, Ireland, and France) and is inherited through an autosomal dominant gene of incomplete penetrance (80%) and variable expression. It affects both sexes equally and typically presents as episodes of acute pancreatitis in childhood by age 10–12. These patients have a predisposition to pancreatic cancer.

Exocrine pancreatic insufficiency also afflicts approximately 85% of patients with **cystic fibrosis**, the most common autosomal recessive defect in whites. Although painful, clinically apparent bouts of pancreatitis are less common, this defect causes reduced pancreatic ductal chloride secretions with the production of less alkaline and less hydrated pancreatic juice. Protein-rich acinar secretions become inspissated, with proximal duct obstruction and acinar cell destruction with fibrosis. Mutations in the cystic fibrosis transmembrane conductance regulator (CFTR) gene lead to the development of pancreatic insufficiency.

6. Can the diagnosis of CP be excluded in patients without abdominal pain?

No. Although pain is the most common presenting symptom of CP, it may be absent in up to 15% of patients with alcohol-related CP and in up to 23% of patients with nonalcoholic CP. A minority of patients with CP are pain-free and present solely with exocrine and/or endocrine insufficiency, so-called idiopathic senile CP.

7. What causes weight loss in patients with CP?

(1) Decreased caloric intake due to fear of aggravation of abdominal pain (sitophobia), (2) malabsorption, and (3) uncontrolled diabetes.

8. Are measurements of serum pancreatic enzymes helpful in the diagnosis of CP?

Serum amylase and lipase levels are not typically helpful in the diagnosis of CP, because they lack sufficient sensitivity or specificity. Levels may be elevated, normal, or low despite attacks of pain. No serologic test is sensitive or specific for diagnosis of CP; however, low levels of trypsin may be suggestive of CP.

9. What specialized test directly measures pancreatic exocrine function?

The secretin stimulation test, with or without concomitant CCK administration, measures the volume of secretion and the concentration of output of bicarbonate (via aspiration of duodenal contents) in response to injection of secretin. Bicarbonate levels < 50 mEq/L are consistent with CP; levels > 50 mEq/L but below 75 mEq/L are indeterminate; levels > 75 mEq/L are normal. The test is invasive, requiring duodenal tube insertion for collection of secretions, but has a reported sensitivity of 75–95%.

10. What conditions may be associated with a false-positive secretin stimulation test?

Primary diabetes mellitus, Billroth II gastrectomy, celiac sprue, and cirrhosis.

11. Is steatorrhea an early symptom of chronic pancreatitis?

No, because 90% of exocrine function must be lost before steatorrhea develops. A secretin test may be abnormal when 60% of the exocrine function is lost. Patients can have symptoms of bloating discomfort, abdominal pain, or change in bowel habits when 60–90% of the pancreatic function is lost. It is important to keep in mind this subset of patients with so-called early CP.

12. What indirect tests of pancreatic secretory function are used?

The bentiromide and pancreolauryl tests are noninvasive methods of assessing pancreatic secretory function but are no longer available in the United States. Most indirect tests of pancreatic function measure the absorption of some compound that first requires digestion by pancreatic enzymes, thereby indirectly assessing pancreatic function. The **bentiromide test** exploits the lack of the digestive enzyme chymotrypsin in CP. It involves the ingestion of bentiromide, a tripeptide digested by pancreatic chymotrypsin with subsequent release of paraaminobenzoic acid (PABA). Free PABA is absorbed in the small intestine, conjugated in the liver, then excreted in the urine. Recovery of ≥ 50% of the administered dosage in a 6-hour urine collection is considered normal. False-positive results may be seen in patients with diabetes mellitus, renal insufficiency, liver disease, or malabsorptive states other than CP. The **pancreolauryl test** exploits the reduced secretion of arylesterases from the pancreas. After ingestion of fluorescein dilaurate (with a standard breakfast), arylesterases release fluorescein from the dilaurate. Free fluorescein is absorbed in the small intestine, conjugated in the liver, then excreted in the urine. False-positive results may be seen in patients with chronic inflammatory bowel disease, severe biliary diseases, and Billroth II gastrectomy.

Other indirect tests of pancreatic function include the **fecal chymotrypsin** and **fecal elastase tests**, [^{14}C]olein test, and 72-hour quantitative **fecal fat determination** (with subsequent correction after pancreatic enzyme replacement). The limitation of most indirect tests of pancreatic function is their lack of sensitivity except in cases of advanced CP, when patients typically already develop steatorrhea.

13. Are plain abdominal radiographs helpful in the diagnosis of CP?

Yes. Although plain abdominal radiographs cannot exclude the diagnosis, the presence of focal or diffuse pancreatic calcification (seen in 30–40% of cases) makes the diagnosis of advanced CP almost certain and obviates the need for additional testing. However, calcification is not found in early CP. In addition, one must be certain that the calcifications are within the pancreas and do not simply represent vascular calcifications.

14. What osseous abnormalities may be seen in patients with CP?

Approximately 5% of patients demonstrate medullary infarcts or aseptic necrosis of the femoral or humeral head. Long bones of the hands and feet are affected most often. These abnormalities result from medullary fat necrosis during episodes of acute pancreatitis.

15. What other imaging modalities are used in establishing the diagnosis of CP?

Ultrasound findings of CP include pancreatic duct dilation, calcifications, cavities, and, in milder disease, reduction in parenchymal echogenicity or irregular gland contour. This test has a reported sensitivity of 70% and specificity of 90% in the diagnosis of CP. **CT** findings of CP include pancreatic duct dilation, calcifications, and cystic lesions. Other significant findings include heterogeneous density of the pancreatic gland with atrophy or enlargement. CT is as specific as ultrasound but more sensitive (80%).

16. When is ERCP useful in the diagnosis of CP?

Changes of early CP may not be seen on ERCP. ERCP may assess ductular changes that occur in advanced CP, such as irregularity, dilatation, tortuosity, stenosis, cysts, and ductal calculi. These findings may culminate in a "chain of lakes" appearance in the main pancreatic duct with intermittent points of obstruction in a dilated pancreatic duct. ERCP is the gold standard against which all other imaging tests are evaluated, because it has 90% sensitivity and 100% specificity in diagnosing CP (see Cambridge grading).

In general, there is good correlation between the changes observed on ERCP and results of secretin-pancreozymin test. ERCP may be useful in distinguishing CP from pancreatic cancer. A dominant stricture, as opposed to ductular ectasia (with multiple stenosis, irregular branching ducts, and intraductular calculi), is highly suggestive of pancreatic cancer instead of CP.

17. Summarize the Cambridge grading system of CP based on ERCP findings.

Normal	Main duct normal; side branches normal
Equivocal	Main duct normal; > 3 abnormal side branches
Mild	Main duct normal; ≥ 3 abnormal side branches
Moderate	Main duct abnormal; ≥ 3 abnormal side branches
Marked	Main duct abnormal; ≥ 3 abnormal side branches
	and one or more of the following additional changes:
	Large cavities (> 10 mm)
	Intraductal filling defects or calculi
	Duct obstruction
	Severe duct dilation or irregularities

18. Discuss the role of endoscopic ultrasound (EUS) in the diagnosis of CP.

EUS features of CP include ductal and parenchymal changes such as echotexture of the gland, calcifications, lobulations, and bands of fibrosis. A prospective evaluation comparing EUS with ERCP and secretin stimulation test in the diagnosis of CP showed good correlation in normal subjects as well as patients with moderate (3–4 features) or severe disease (> 5 features). The agreement was poor for mild EUS changes (1–2 features) compared with ERCP and secretin stimulation test; moderate EUS criteria (3–4 features) for CP also correlated poorly with secretin test results but had a 92% concordance with ERCP in moderate disease. In summary, compared with ERCP, EUS is accurate and at least as sensitive for detection of moderate-to-severe CP.

19. Summarize the EUS features of CP and their implications.

EUS FEATURE	IMPLICATION
Ductal changes	
Duct size > 3 mm	Ductal dilation
Tortuous pancreatic duct	Ductal irregularity
Intraductal echogenic foci	Stones/calcification
Echogenic duct wall	Ductal fibrosis
Side-branch ectasia	Periductal fibrosis
Parenchymal changes	
Inhomogeneous echo-pattern	Edema
Reduced echogenic foci (1–3 mm)	Edema
Enhanced echogenic foci	Calcifications
Prominent interlobular septae	Fibrosis
Lobular outer gland margin	Fibrosis, glandular atrophy
Large echo-poor cavities (> 5 mm)	Pseudocyst

20. Discuss the role of magnetic resonance cholangiopancreatography (MRCP).

Preliminary experience with MRCP shows close correlation with ERCP in CP with ductal dilation, ductal narrowing, and filling defects, but MRCP cannot directly visualize calculi. Its potential benefit over ERCP is its ability to evaluate concomitantly both pancreatic parenchyma and ducts, especially to visualize areas proximal to obstruction. Additional studies are necessary to assess more fully the role of EUS and MRCP in CP.

21. What is the most common complication of CP?

Pseudocysts occur in up to 25% of patients with CP. Pseudocyst formation should be suspected in any patient with stable CP who experiences worsening of abdominal pain. In contrast to acute pseudocysts (defined as being present for < 6 weeks), chronic pseudocysts, especially those > 6 cm, almost never resolve spontaneously; overall, they are less prone to serious complications. However, most cases of pseudoaneurysm have been associated with CP in patients with a pseudocyst. An asymptomatic pseudocyst should be observed, regardless of its size.

22. How are pseudocysts treated?

Effective treatment includes surgical excision for pseudocysts localized to the tail of the pancreas and internal or external drainage (surgical, endoscopic, or radiographic). **Octreotide**, a long-acting somatostatin analog, may decrease pseudocyst size when used alone or in combination with catheter drainage. Surgical or endoscopic **internal drainage** is usually the treatment of choice. The pseudocyst should be mature (i.e., present for longer than 6 weeks with a formed cyst wall). Surgical cystogastrostomy, cystoduodenostomy, or cystojejunostomy is the procedure of choice. Endoscopic cystogastrostomy or cystoduodenostomy requires abutment onto adjacent viscera. EUS can aid the endoscopist in determining the distance of a pseudocyst from the GI lumen, assessing cyst contents, and avoiding adjacent vasculature during drainage. **External drainage** is necessary for immature or infected pseudocysts. This method is associated with a higher recurrence and superinfection rate (particularly when CT-guided percutaneous rather than surgical drainage is performed) that probably is related to debris in the cyst that is not removed by catheter drainage alone.

23. What extrapancreatic complications can be caused by CP?

Distal common bile duct (CBD) and duodenal obstruction may result from extrinsic obstruction of these structures by edema or fibrosis at the head of the pancreas or an adjacent pseudocyst. External pancreatic fistulas are rare but occur most frequently after operative or percutaneous drainage of a pseudocyst. Internal pancreatic fistulas typically occur spontaneously from main pancreatic duct rupture or pseudocyst leakage, almost always in cases of alcoholic pancreatitis.

24. How is distal CBD obstruction diagnosed and treated?

In distal CBD obstruction (5–10% of cases), ERCP may demonstrate the narrowing of the distal CBD in the form of gradual tapering, bird's beak stenosis, or "hourglass" stricture. Complications of biliary obstruction include jaundice, pain, ascending cholangitis, and secondary biliary cirrhosis. Other causes of jaundice, such as associated hepatocellular disease (from toxins, alcohol, or viral hepatitis) should be excluded. Treatment options include close observation with serial liver function tests vs. endoscopic or surgical decompression procedures. If abnormal LFTs persist secondary to obstruction, decompression is advised to prevent secondary biliary cirrhosis. Endoscopic biliary stent drainage may provide temporary benefit, although series have demonstrated that this approach is problematic as long-term therapy because of stent blockage. Particularly for younger patients, surgical bypass by surgical choledochoduodenostomy is preferred. When associated with concomitant pseudocyst or dilated pancreatic duct, surgical biliary decompression may be combined with lateral pancreaticojejunostomy.

25. What are the symptoms of duodenal obstruction? How is it treated?

Presenting symptoms of duodenal obstruction (5% of cases) include vomiting and abdominal pain. Jaundice is present with associated CBD stenosis. Treatment includes supportive medical management initially, but with persistent stenosis surgery is warranted. Gastroenterostomy may be performed alone or in combination with either biliary drainage (if jaundice is due to CBD stenosis) or lateral pancreaticojejunostomy (if pain results from pancreatic duct obstruction). A Whipple procedure or duodenum-preserving resection of the head of the pancreas is indicated in the presence of an associated mass at the head of the pancreas.

26. How are external and internal pancreatic fistulas treated?

Treatment strategies for **external pancreatic fistulas** include long acting somatostatin analogs (octreotide, 50–100 μg SQ every 8 hours) to decrease pancreatic secretion and maintenance of oral nutrition. Endoscopic stenting of the main pancreatic duct may be indicated if ERCP demonstrates the site of ductal disruption. Time is usually the healer. **Internal pancreatic fistulas** typically result in intractable pancreatic ascites or pleural effusions. Treatment options include total parenteral nutrition, large-volume paracentesis or thoracentesis, octreotide administration, and endoscopic stenting of the main pancreatic duct. Surgical decompression or resection may be required if ERCP demonstrates a pancreatic duct leak or a blocked pancreatic duct without visualizing the source of ductal disruption or pseudocyst.

27. What is pancreatic ascites?

Pancreatic ascites results from persistent leakage of pancreatic fluid from a pseudocyst or a disrupted pancreatic duct. Its incidence in CP is < 1%, but it may occur in up to 15% of patients with pseudocysts. Pancreatic ascites may be distinguished from ascites secondary to cirrhosis by the finding of high ascitic fluid amylase levels greater than serum levels and high fluid protein or albumin levels. The initial approach includes supportive measures to improve nutrition, administration of octreotide (100–250 μg SQ every 4 hours) to suppress pancreatic secretion, and large-volume paracentesis. Recently endoscopic therapy with stent placement in the pancreatic duct to bridge the ductal disruption has been extremely beneficial in resolving ascites and obviating the need for surgery. If ERCP shows a blocked duct so that the source of ductal disruption cannot be visualized, surgical intervention usually is required.

28. Why is the presence of gastric varices in the absence of esophageal varices suggestive of CP?

Isolated gastric varices resulting from splenic vein thrombosis occur in approximately 5% of patients with CP. Thrombosis of the splenic vein results from its close proximity to an inflamed or fibrotic pancreas, leading to intrasplenic venous hypertension, splenomegaly, and collateral circulation through the short gastric veins. Massive GI hemorrhage may occur. The treatment of choice is splenectomy with gastric devascularization.

29. Is the presence of signs of fat-soluble vitamin deficiencies highly suggestive of CP?

No. Although absorption of fat-soluble vitamins (A, D, E, and K) is diminished, marked deficiency is relatively uncommon. The clinical presence of easy bruisability, bone pain, and decreased night vision resulting from deficiencies of vitamins K, D, and A, respectively, is more suggestive of small intestinal disease with malabsorption, such as celiac sprue.

30. Are patients with CP predisposed to nephrolithiasis?

Yes. Hyperoxaluria and resultant oxalate stone formation may develop. Patients with untreated steatorrhea have high concentrations of long-chain fatty acids in the colon, which bind intraluminal calcium by formation of insoluble calcium soaps. Consequently, less calcium is available to bind to and precipitate unabsorbed dietary oxalate as calcium oxalate; therefore, more free oxalate is absorbed and excreted in the urine.

31. How should hyperoxaluria be treated in patients with CP?

One of four approaches can be used: low dietary oxalate intake, low dietary long-chain triglycerides, pancreatic enzyme substitution, and increased intake of either calcium (3 gm/day) or aluminum in the form of antacids (3.5 gm/day). Obviously the initial approach is adequate pancreatic enzyme replacement.

32. Can patients with CP develop vitamin B12 malabsorption?

Yes. The probable mechanism is competitive binding of cobalamin by cobalamin-binding proteins (rather than intrinsic factor), which usually are destroyed by pancreatic proteases. It is correctable with administration of pancreatic enzymes and occurs in 40% of patients with advanced CP.

33. Does retinopathy occur in patients with CP?

Nondiabetic retinopathy results from deficiency of vitamin A and/or zinc. Diabetic retinopathy and other microvascular complications of diabetes are less common. However, the prevalence of diabetic retinopathy and neuropathy in patients with CP is comparable to that in patients with idiopathic diabetes mellitus if corrected for the duration of diabetes.

34. How much lipase is necessary in the form of pancreatic enzyme supplementation for treatment of steatorrhea?

Malassimilation occurs if < 5–10% of normal maximal enzyme output is delivered to the duodenum. To prevent malabsortion, 28,000 IU of lipase should be delivered to the duodenum during a 4-hour postprandial period. Pancreatic enzyme replacement is a mainstay of treatment in patients with pancreatic insufficiency, such as occurs with CP or subsequent to gastric surgery with Billroth II anastamosis and vagotomy, and in patients with duodenal obstruction with bypass. Adequate pancreatic enzyme replacement for steatorrhea requires preparations with high lipase content. Pancreatic enzymes are also available in enteric- and non–enteric-coated preparations. The advantage of enteric-coated compounds is that they do not dissolve in the stomach and are less susceptible to acid pepsin inactivation of pancreatic enzymes, a major limiting factor for effective therapy. Pancreatic enzyme supplementation decreases postprandial symptoms of bloating and fullness. The usual dose is at least 30,000 units with each meal, given as 10,000 units before eating and 20,000 units during the meal to ensure adequate mixing. Adjuvant therapy, with the addition of an H_2-receptor antagonist or proton pump inhibitor, may be considered with non–enteric-coated preparations to counteract the acid inactivation (low gastric and duodenal pH < 4) of lipase. They are not necessary with enteric-coated compounds; the resultant increase in intragastric pH may cause premature release of enzymes into the stomach rather than the small intestine.

35. What are nonsurgical modalities of pain control in chronic pancreatitis?

In escalating order: cessation of alcohol intake, non-narcotic analgesics, and celiac plexus block. In severe cases, narcotic analgesics may be needed to control pain, and secondary addiction is a risk. Celiac plexus block, placed under radiologic guidance into the celiac ganglion, has mixed results in alleviation of pain due to CP. The occasional benefits usually last only for ≤ 3 months, with less effective pain relief with repeated treatments. Correctable causes of pain, such as presence of pseudocyst, duodenal or bile duct obstruction, should be sought.

36. Does pancreatic enzyme supplementation decrease pain?

Pancreatic enzymes should be supplemented in all patients with CP to correct exocrine insufficiency. They may decrease pain by reducing the abdominal distention and diarrhea associated with malassimilation. Pancreatic enzymes are also useful in decreasing chronic pain in patients with mild disease (non–alcohol-induced CP, especially women and patients with pancreas divisum and small duct disease). Conversely, male patients with alcohol-associated CP are much less likely to respond to such treatment. Whereas pancreatic enzyme preparations with enteric coating and high lipase content are preferred in treatment of steatorrhea due to CP, the treatment of chronic pain in CP is facilitated by the use of high-protease content preparations, preferably non–enteric-coated.

37. Does endoscopy have a therapeutic as well as diagnostic role?

The role of endoscopy is less well defined in the treatment of pain in patients with CP. The endoscopic drainage of pancreatic pseudocysts is well established, whereas the treatment of pancreatic duct stenoses and pancreatic duct stones is still controversial. Numerous reports suggest that endoscopic sphincterotomy with pancreatic stricture dilation and pancreatic duct stent placement relieves recurrent or persistent pain associated with CP. Several studies also have reported marked improvement in pain after endoscopic techniques for removal of intraductal pancreatic stones, such as lithotripsy and pancreatic duct sphincterotomy with stone extraction. Although endoscopic techniques show promise for pain management in CP, substantiation is needed in the form of randomized, blinded, prospective trials.

38. Discuss the role of surgical decompression in pain control.

Surgical decompression procedures remain technically difficult but may offer longer-lasting pain control. Lateral pancreaticojejunostomy (modified Puestow procedure) is preferred in patients with ductal obstruction in the head of the pancreas and distal duct dilatation, whereas partial pancreatic resection should be considered in patients without ductal dilatation, so-called small-duct disease, or localized distal (tail) disease. Pain relief can be achieved with surgery in up to 50–80% of patients with CP.

BIBLIOGRAPHY

1. Ammann RW: Chronic pancreatitis in the elderly. Gastroenterol Clin North Am 19:905–914, 1990.
2. Banks PA: Acute and chronic pancreatitis. In Sleisenger MH (ed): Sleisenger and Fordtran's Gastrointestinal and Liver Disease, 6th ed. Philadelphia, W.B. Saunders, 809–862, 1998.
3. Barkin JS, Reiner DK, Deutch E: Sandostatin for control of catheter drainage of pancreatic pseudocyst. Pancreas 16:245–248, 1991.
4. Barnes SM, Kontny BG, Prinz RA: Somatostatin analog treatment of pancreatic fistulas. Int J Pancreatol 14:181–188, 1993.
5. Bhutani M: Endoscopic ultrasound in pancreatic diseases: Indications, limitations, and the future. Gastroenterol Clin North Am 28:747–770, 1999.
6. Catalano MF, Lahoti S, Geenen JE, Hogan WJ: Prospective evaluation of endoscopic ultrasonography, endoscopic retrograde pancreatography, and secretin test in the diagnosis of chronic pancreatitis. Gastrointest Endosc 48:11–17, 1998.
7. Choudari CP, Lehman GA, Sherman S: Pancreatitis and cystic fibrosis gene mutations. Gastroenterol Clin North Am 28:543–549, 1999.
8. Cohn JA, Friedman KJ, Noone PG, et al: Relation between mutations of the cystic fibrosis gene and idiopathic pancreatitis. N Engl J Med 339:653–658, 1998.
9. Comfort M, Steinberg A: Pedigree of a family with hereditary chronic relapsing pancreatitis. Gastroenterology 21:54–63, 1952.
10. Greenberger NJ: Enzymatic therapy in patients with chronic pancreatitis. Gastroenterol Clin North Am 28:687–693, 1999.
11. Gullo L, Barbara L: Treatment of pancreatic pseudocysts with octreotide. Lancet 338:540–541, 1991.
12. Huibregtse K, Smits ME: Endoscopic management of diseases of the pancreas. Am J Gastroenterol 89(Suppl 8):S66–S77, 1994.
13. Jakobs R, Riemann J: The role of endoscopy in acute recurrent and chronic pancreatitis and pancreatic cancer. Gastroenterol Clin North Am 28:783–800, 1999.
14. Korazek RA, Ball TJ, Patterson DJ, et al: Endoscopic pancreatic duct sphincterotomy: indications, technique, and analysis of results. Gastrointest Endosc 40:592–598, 1994.

15. Kozarek RA, Jiranek GC, Traverso LW: Endoscopic treatment of pancreatic ascites. Am J Surg 168:223–226, 1994.
16. Lankisch PG, Seidensticker F, Otto J, et al: Secretin-pancreozymin test (SPT) and endoscopic retrograde cholangiopancreatography (ERCP): Both are necessary for diagnosing or excluding chronic pancreatitis. Pancreas 12:149–152, 1996.
17. Lowenfels AB, Maisonneuve P, Lankisch PG: Chronic pancreatitis and other risk factors for pancreatic cancer. Gastroenterol Clin North Am 28:673–685, 1999.
18. Owyang C: Chronic pancreatitis. In Yamada T (ed): Textbook of Gastroenterology, 3rd ed. Philadelphia, Lippincott Williams & Wilkins, 1999, pp 2151–2177.
19. Saeed ZA, Ramirez FC, Hepps KS: Endoscopic stent placement for internal and external pancreatic fistulas. Gastroenterology 105:1213–1217, 1993.
20. Sahai AV, Zimmerman M, Aabakken L, et al: Prospective assessment of the ability of endoscopic ultrasound to diagnose, exclude, or establish the severity of chronic pancreatitis found by endoscopic retrograde cholangiopancreatography. Gastrointest Endosc 48:18–25, 1998.
21. Sarles H: Definition and classifications of pancreatitis. Pancreas 6:470–474, 1991.
22. Scolapio JS, Malhi-Chowla N, Ukleja A: Nutritional supplementation in patients with acute and chronic pancreatitis. Gastroenterol Clin North Am 28:695–707, 1999.
23. Segal I, Parekh D, Lipschitz J, et al: Treatment of pancreatic ascites and external pancreatic fistulas with a long-acting somatostatin analogue (Sandostatin). Digestion 54(Suppl 1):53–58, 1993.
24. Smits ME, Badiga SM, Rauws EA, et al: Long-term results of pancreatic stents in chronic pancreatitis. Gastrointest Endosc 42:461–467, 1995.
25. Steer ML, Waxman I, Freedman S: Chronic pancreatitis. N Engl J Med 332:1482–1490, 1995.
26. Warshaw AL, Banks PA, Fernandez-Del Castillo C: AGA technical review: Treatment of pain in chronic pancreatitis. Gastroenterology 115:765–776, 1998.
27. Whitcomb DC: The spectrum of complications of hereditary pancreatitis: Is this a model for future gene therapy? Gastroenterol Clin North Am 28:525–541, 1999.

40. PANCREATIC CANCER

Sergey V. Kantsevoy, M.D., Ph.D., and Anthony N. Kalloo, M.D.

1. What are the most common histologic forms of malignant tumors of the pancreas?

Almost 90% of pancreatic cancers are moderately well-differentiated adenocarcinomas, derived from the pancreatic ductal epithelium. About 5% of pancreatic cancers originate from the pancreatic islet cells. Other rare types of pancreatic cancer include sarcomas, lymphomas, and cystadenocarcinomas.

2. Define intraductal papillary-mucinous tumors of the pancreas.

Intraductal papillary-mucinous tumors (IPMT) of the pancreas (also called mucinous ductal ectasia, mucin-producing tumors, ductectatic mucinous cystadenomas, intraductal cystadenomas, intraductal papillary tumors) are characterized by intraductal papillary growth and production of mucin. These tumors usually grow slowly and cause dilatation of the main pancreatic duct and its branches with potential development of cellular hyperplasia, atypia, and malignancy.

3. What is the most common location of the pancreatic adenocarcinoma?

Eighty percent of pancreatic adenocarcinomas are located in the head of the pancreas. This location may lead to obstruction of the distal common bile duct with development of obstructive jaundice.

4. What is Courvoisier's sign?

A palpable, distended gallbladder in the right upper quadrant in a patient with jaundice is called Courvoisier's sign. Usually it results from a malignant bile duct obstruction such as pancreatic cancer with complete obstruction of the distal common bile duct and accumulation of bile in the gallbladder. This finding is not specific for pancreatic cancer. Patients with distal cholangiocarcinoma or an ampullary mass may also present with Courvoisier's sign.

5. What is the survival rate for patients with pancreatic cancer?

Less than 20% of patients with pancreatic cancer are alive 1 year after diagnosis and less than 3% survive longer than 5 years. Surgical resection of the tumor is the only curative treatment. At the time of diagnosis 40% of patients already have locally advanced disease, and more than 40% have visceral metastasis. The stage of the disease at presentation and the surgeon's ability to remove the tumor completely are the most important determinants of treatment outcome and long-term survival.

6. What are the risk factors for development of pancreatic cancer?

Smokers are twice as likely to develop pancreatic cancer as nonsmokers. Pancreatic cancer is more common in countries where the diet contains a large amount of fat and meat products. In contrast, high intake of dietary fiber appears to be protective. Extensive studies have failed to prove a definitive link between coffee intake and development of pancreatic cancer. Recent studies indicated that diabetes mellitus (especially recent onset of diabetes in an older patient) may be a risk factor. Chronic pancreatitis increases the risk. Some patients may have genetic (familial) predisposition. Patients with pernicious anemia and patients who have undergone partial gastrectomy have an elevated risk. Predisposing environmental hazards include oil refining, paper manufacturing, and chemical manufacturing.

7. Is alcohol consumption an important risk factor for development of pancreatic cancer?

Many epidemiologic studies in Europe and the United States have failed to find a consistent direct association between alcohol intake and development of pancreatic cancer.

8. What are the most common symptoms in patients with pancreatic cancer?

Patients with pancreatic cancer usually present with abdominal pain, frequently radiating to the back; weight loss; nausea; anorexia; generalized weakness; and easy fatigability. Obstructive jaundice may develop early in the disease in patients with a mass in the head of the pancreas. Jaundice may never develop or develop late in patients with a tumor in the body or tail of the pancreas; in such patients, jaundice indicates the presence of liver metastases.

9. What imaging modalities are used to diagnose pancreatic cancer?

Transabdominal ultrasound is usually the first diagnostic test. Its sensitivity in the detection of pancreatic tumors is around 70%. CT and MRI are more sensitive than transabdominal ultrasound, especially for detection of regional and distal metastases. Endoscopic ultrasonography is the most accurate (sensitivity: 77–100%) diagnostic modality to detect small tumors and to evaluate the local spread of tumor into surrounding organs and blood vessels. Endoscopic retrograde cholangiopancreatography (ERCP) is sensitive (78–95%) and specific (88–95%) for pancreatic cancer and frequently is used to perform palliative drainage of the biliary ducts.

10. What is the "double-duct sign" in patients with pancreatic cancer?

The double-duct sign, noted on ERCP, demonstrates the presence of stenosis of the common bile duct and pancreatic duct in the head of the pancreas. In patients with obstructive jaundice or a pancreatic mass, the double-duct sign has a specificity of 85% in predicting pancreatic cancer.

11. Can serum markers diagnose pancreatic cancer?

Many potential serum markers are currently under evaluation to facilitate the early detection of pancreatic cancer. The carbohydrate antigen CA 19-9 is highly sensitive (> 90%) in diagnosing pancreatic cancer but has low specificity (75%) and is often normal in early stages of the disease (tumor < 1 cm in diameter). Many conditions can lead to elevation of CA 19-9: chronic pancreatitis, biliary diseases, and other types of GI cancer. After complete resection of pancreatic cancer, the serum level of CA 19-9 usually falls. Persistently elevated serum levels of CA 19-9 after surgery may indicate inadequate resection or metastatic lesions. Recurrence of pancreatic cancer can manifest with elevation of CA 19-9 levels following a decline after surgical resection.

12. What are the common biochemical abnormalities in patients with pancreatic cancer?

Patients with biliary tract obstruction can present with elevated serum bilirubin and alkaline phosphatase (obstructive pattern). Serum amylase is elevated in only 5% of patients.

13. Is chemotherapy effective for patients with advanced pancreatic cancer?

Traditional chemotherapy with 5-fluorouracil has an overall response rate below 10% with no effect on quality of life or survival. Gemcitabine, which in one study demonstrated improvement in disease-related symptoms and survival in advanced pancreatic cancer, is now under clinical evaluation as a single agent and in combination with 5-fluorouracil and cisplatin.

14. What is the median survival after the diagnosis of advanced pancreatic cancer?

Pancreatic cancer has the poorest prognosis among other GI tumors. It is the fifth leading cause of death in the United States. The median survival of patients with advanced pancreatic carcinoma is approximately 4 months.

15. Describe the role of celiac blockade in patients with pancreatic cancer.

Celiac blockade (chemical splanchnicectomy) is injection of 50% alcohol on each side of the aorta at the level of celiac axis. This procedure has been shown prospectively to improve preexisting pain significantly and to delay onset of pain in asymptomatic patients. Celiac blockade can be done at laparotomy, under radiologic guidance, or at the time of endoscopic ultrasound.

16. What is a Whipple resection?

Whipple resection (pancreaticoduodenectomy) is the most common surgical procedure for resectable cancer located in the head of the pancreas. It involves a partial gastrectomy (resection of the antrum), cholecystectomy, and removal of the distal common bile duct, duodenum, head of the pancreas, proximal jejunum and regional lymphatic nodes. The procedure usually includes pancreaticojejunostomy, hepaticojejunostomy, and gastrojejunostomy.

17. What surgical procedures are used for cancer in the body and tail of the pancreas?

Surgical resection usually consists of distal pancreatectomy and splenectomy. This operation is technically easier than the Whipple procedure.

18. When do patients with pancreatic cancer need palliative procedures?

Patients with unresectable cancer in the head of the pancreas can develop obstructive jaundice, pruritus, or cholangitis. These conditions can be palliated by endoscopic placement of plastic or self-expending metal stents (Wallstent). If endoscopic stent placement is not possible, transhepatic transcutaneous stents can be inserted by an interventional radiologist. When placement of stents by an endoscopist or radiologist fails, bypass surgical procedure (cholecystojejunostomy or hepaticojejunostomy) may be indicated. In patients with duodenal obstruction by a large pancreatic mass, endoscopy with palliative placement of an expandable stent into the duodenum is indicated to relieve the obstruction. If endoscopy is not possible, surgical bypass procedure (gastrojejunostomy) may be performed.

BIBLIOGRAPHY

 1. Alonso Casado O, Hernandez Gallardo D, Moreno Gonzalez E, et al: Intraductal papillary-mucinous tumors: An entity which is infrequent and difficult to diagnose. Hepatogastroenterology 47:275–284, 2000.
 2. Cello JP: Pancreatic cancer. In Feldman M, Scharschmidt BF, Sleisenger MH (eds): Sleisenger & Fordtran's Gastrointestinal and Liver Disease: Pathophysiology/Diagnosis/Management, vol. 1. Philadelphia: W. B. Saunders, 1998, pp 863–870.
 3. Lee JH, Whittington R, Williams NN, et al: Outcome of pancreaticoduodenectomy and impact of adjuvant therapy for ampullary carcinomas. Int J Radiat Oncol Biol Phys 47:945–953, 2000.
 4. Lillemoe KD: Current management of pancreatic carcinoma. Ann Surg 221:133–148, 1995.
 5. Lorenz M, Heinrich S, Staib-Sebler E, et al: Regional chemotherapy in the treatment of advanced pancreatic cancer—is it relevant? Eur J Cancer 36:957–965, 2000.
 6. Menges M, Lerch MM, Zeitz M: The double duct sign in patients with malignant and benign pancreatic lesions. Gastrointest Endosc 52:74–77, 2000.
 7. Parker SL, Tong T, Bolden S, Wingo PA: Cancer statistics, 1997. CA Cancer J Clin 47:5–27, 1997.
 8. Parks RW, Garden OJ: Ensuring early diagnosis in pancreatic cancer. Practitioner 244:336–338, 340–341, 343, 2000.
 9. Rice D, Geller A, Bender CE, et al: Surgical and interventional palliative treatment of upper gastrointestinal malignancies. Eur J Gastroenterol Hepatol 12:403–408, 2000.
10. Todd KE, Gloor B, Reber HA: Pancreatic Adenocarcinoma. In Yamada T (ed): Textbook of Gastroenterology, vol. 2. Philadelphia, Lippincott Williams & Wilkins, 1999. pp 2178–2192.
11. van Riel JM, van Groeningen CJ: Palliative chemotherapy in advanced gastrointestinal cancer. Eur J Gastroenterol Hepatol 12:391–396, 2000.
12. Watanapa P, Williamson RC: Surgical palliation for pancreatic cancer: Developments during the past two decades. Br J Surg 79:8–20, 1992.

41. CYSTIC DISEASE OF THE PANCREAS

Randall E. Lee, M.D.

1. Provide a differential diagnosis for a cystic pancreatic lesion.
Pancreatic pseudocyst
Serous cystic neoplasm
Intraductal papillary mucinous neoplasm (IPMN)
Mucinous cystic neoplasm
Benign cysts associated with von Hippel-Lindau disease
Retention cyst
Cystic necrosis of pancreatic ductal adenocarcinoma

2. What is the difference between a true pancreatic cyst and a pancreatic pseudocyst?
A true pancreatic cyst has an epithelial cell lining. A pancreatic pseudocyst is lined only by inflammatory tissue; it has no epithelium. True pancreatic cysts account for only 10–15% of all cystic lesions of the pancreas.

3. What is the difference between an acute fluid collection and a pseudocyst?
Within the first 4 weeks of an acute attack of pancreatitis, areas of necrosis appear as **acute fluid collections** on computed tomography (CT) scans. These acute fluid collections do not have a well-defined wall and are often irregularly shaped. They do not communicate with the pancreatic duct, and the fluid contained within does not have a high amylase content. The rate of spontaneous resolution is about 65%.

A pancreatic **pseudocyst** is a localized collection of amylase-rich fluid enclosed by a well-defined wall of inflammatory tissue. Pseudocysts are rounded or ovoid and frequently communicate with the pancreatic duct. The rate of spontaneous resolution is about 30%.

4. Describe the pathogenesis and characteristics of a pancreatic pseudocyst.
A pseudocyst develops from necrosis of pancreatic and peripancreatic tissue due to leakage of pancreatic enzymes from a disrupted pancreatic duct. The most common condition associated with pseudocysts is alcoholic pancreatitis, which accounts for about 60% of all pseudocysts. Other associated conditions include pancreatitis due to biliary stones, trauma, medications, and hyperlipidemia.

5. Describe the typical clinical presentation of a pancreatic pseudocyst.
Formation of a pancreatic pseudocyst should be suspected if a patient with acute pancreatitis develops any of the following:
- Failure of acute pancreatitis symptoms to resolve after about 7–10 days
- Recurrence of acute pancreatitis symptoms after initial improvement
- Epigastric abdominal mass
- Persistently elevated serum amylase
- Obstructive jaundice

6. What criteria suggest that a pseudocyst will not resolve spontaneously?
A pancreatic pseudocyst has a low probability of spontaneous resolution if there is concurrent evidence of chronic pancreatitis, such as pancreatic calcifications, or if the pseudocyst is a consequence of traumatic pancreatitis. The strict criteria of pseudocyst diameter > 6 cm or persistence for > 6 weeks are no longer accepted as absolute.

7. When should a pseudocyst be drained?

A pseudocyst should be drained if it causes symptoms, increases in size, shows evidence of infection, causes critical compression of an adjacent structure such as the bile duct, or is complicated by internal hemorrhage. Asymptomatic pseudocysts may be observed carefully, regardless of size or duration.

8. List three methods for draining a pancreatic pseudocyst.

1. Surgical drainage
2. CT- or ultrasound-guided percutaneous catheter drainage
3. Transpapillary, transgastric, or transduodenal endoscopic drainage

9. Compare the three methods for draining a pancreatic pseudocyst.

Surgical drainage is the procedure of choice for patients in whom a cystic neoplasm cannot be ruled out. An intraoperative biopsy of the cyst wall can confirm the presence or absence of a malignant epithelial cell lining. Surgical drainage also is indicated for patients who have multiple or recurrent pseudocysts or concurrent pancreatic duct stricture. Surgical drainage of a thin-walled pseudocyst should be delayed for 4–6 weeks. This delay allows thickening and maturation of the pseudocyst wall, thus increasing the holding power of sutures. The surgical mortality rate is about 3%, and the recurrence rate is about 8%.

Percutaneous catheter drainage is preferred for high-risk patients with symptomatic thin-walled or expanding pseudocysts or infected pseudocysts. This method should not be used in patients who have a main pancreatic duct stricture because of the high risk of creating a pancreaticocutaneous fistula. The reported mortality rate is about 2%; the recurrence rate is about 7%.

Endoscopic drainage may be performed in selected patients. The reported mortality rate is less than 1%, and the recurrence rate is about 16%. The outcome of endoscopic drainage is highly dependent on the skill and expertise of the endoscopist.

10. What criteria suggest that a pancreatic pseudocyst may undergo successful endoscopic drainage?

1. Endoscopic retrograde cholangiopancreatography (ERCP) demonstrates a communication between the pseudocyst and the main pancreatic duct.

2. The pseudocyst impinges on and is adherent to the wall of the stomach or duodenum, creating an endoluminal bulge. Imaging with endoscopic ultrasonography (EUS) and CT is recommended to confirm close contact between the pseudocyst and adjacent gastric or duodenal wall, to avoid puncturing large submucosal blood vessels and to rule out the presence of a pseudoaneurysm.

A pseudocyst with a wall > 1 cm thick is a poor candidate for endoscopic drainage because of the difficulty in puncturing the pseudocyst wall.

11. How does a pancreatic abscess appear on CT scan?

A pancreatic abscess may appear as an ill-defined, nonenhancing fluid collection of mixed densities. Unfortunately, this CT appearance may be confused with a noninfected pseudocyst. The presence of gas within the cystic area strongly suggests infection by gas-forming organisms.

12. What clinical criteria suggest the development of a pancreatic abscess?

A pancreatic abscess typically develops from secondary bacterial infection of necrotic pancreatic tissue during an episode of acute pancreatitis. The abscess often causes temperatures > 38.5°C, leukocytosis > 10,000 cells/mm^3, and increasing abdominal pain. All of these signs also may be found in noninfected patients with severe pancreatitis. Percutaneous needle aspiration of the area and Gram stain of the fluid may help to confirm the diagnosis of pancreatic abscess.

13. Define hemosuccus pancreaticus.

Hemosuccus pancreaticus describes the rare phenomenon of major bleeding into the main pancreatic duct from a pseudoaneurysm. Massive gastrointestinal or intraabdominal bleeding from pseudocyst erosion into a pancreatic or peripancreatic blood vessel occurs in about 5–10% of patients with pseudocysts. Patients with hemosuccus pancreaticus form a subset of this group. Clinical signs suggestive of pseudoaneurysm hemorrhage include an enlarging pulsatile abdominal mass with or without a bruit, recurrent gastrointestinal bleeding, and increasing abdominal pain. For patients suspected of having pseudoaneurysm hemorrhage, obtain a bolus contrast helical CT scan to confirm the diagnosis, followed by angiography for further localization and embolization or immediate surgical exploration.

14. What is a serous cystadenoma?

A serous cystadenoma (SCA) is an uncommon pancreatic neoplasm characterized by numerous cysts filled with a glycogen-rich, low-viscosity serous fluid and lined by flat or cuboidal epithelium. Imaging by CT, EUS, or magnetic resonance imaging (MRI) classically shows a honeycomb of small cysts with a sunburst calcification in a central scar. SCAs are benign, and conservative observation may be appropriate for an elderly or high-surgical risk patient. Complete surgical resection is indicated if the patient is symptomatic or if the diagnosis is uncertain.

15. What disease commonly is manifest by retinal angiomatosis, central nervous system (CNS) hemangioblastomas, and pancreatic serous cystadenomas?

Retinal angiomatosis and CNS hemangioblastomas in association with multiple pancreatic serous cystadenomas are the common manifestations of von Hippel-Lindau disease (VHL). VHL also is associated with renal cell carcinoma, islet cell tumors, pheochromocytomas, and benign cysts of the liver, lung, spleen, adrenal gland, and kidney. VHL is caused by a mutation of a tumor suppressor gene on chromosome 3p25. The mode of inheritance is autosomal dominant with variable penetrance. The pancreatic cysts may precede other manifestations of the disease by several years and may be the only abdominal manifestation. An evaluation for VHL is recommended for patients who have both pancreatic cysts and cysts in other organ systems.

16. Describe the characteristics of a mucinous cystic neoplasm (MCN).

MCN is an uncommon pancreatic tumor characterized by large cysts filled with mucin and lined by a columnar epithelium. Many MCNs have an ovarian-like stroma surrounding the epithelial cells. MCNs typically form in the pancreas tail or body and are much more common in women than in men. The most frequent presenting symptoms are epigastric pain and an enlarging abdominal mass. Obstructive jaundice is rare. Radiologic images usually show larger and less numerous cysts compared with serous cystadenomas. ERCP generally shows no communication between the pancreatic ducts and the neoplasm.

Although MCNs may be subclassified as benign mucinous cystadenomas, borderline mucinous cystic neoplasms, and malignant mucinous cystadenocarcinomas, a single MCN may contain both benign and malignant epithelium. Most clinicians consider all MCNs as potentially malignant. The treatment of choice is complete surgical resection with highly detailed histologic examination. The 2- and 5-year survival rate for patients with invasive mucinous cystadenocarcinoma is about 65% and 30%, respectively, which is much higher than that for patients with pancreatic ductal adenocarcinoma.

17. What is an IPMN? How does it differ from a MCN?

An intraductal papillary mucinous neoplasm is an intraductal pancreatic neoplasm that may appear cystic because of dilations of the ducts. IPMN encompasses the pancreatic neoplasms previously known as villous adenoma, papillary carcinoma, and ductectatic mucinous cystadenoma. Unlike mucinous cystic neoplasms, IPMNs afflict both genders equally and tend to arise in the head of the pancreas. An ovarian-like stroma is not found around the epithelial cells. Obstructive jaundice, abdominal pain, and weight loss are common presenting symptoms. ERCP demonstrates direct communication between the pancreatic ducts and the neoplasm. The finding of mucin extruding from the ampulla of Vater is considered highly specific for an IPMN.

18. What conditions are most commonly associated with a pancreatic retention cyst?
Pancreatic retention cysts are dilated areas of the pancreatic duct that result from an obstruction of the duct. Retention cysts usually are < 1 cm in diameter and commonly are associated with chronic pancreatitis, advanced cystic fibrosis, or a duct-obstructing carcinoma.

BIBLIOGRAPHY

 1. Adsay NV, Longnecker DS, Klimstra DS: Pancreatic tumors with cystic dilatation of the ducts: Intraductal papillary mucinous neoplasms and intraductal oncocytic papillary neoplasms. Semin Diagn Pathol 17:16–30, 2000.
 2. Beckingham IJ, Krige JE, Bornman PC, Terblanche J: Long term outcome of endoscopic drainage of pancreatic pseudocysts. Am J Gastroenterol 94:71–74, 1999.
 3. Clark LA, Pappas TN: Comment on: Long term outcome of endoscopic drainage of pancreatic pseudocysts. Am J Gastroenterol 94:8–9, 1999.
 4. Compton C. Serous cystic tumors of the pancreas. Semin Diagn Pathol 17:43–55, 2000.
 5. Elton E, Howell DA, Amberson SM, Dykes TA: Combined angiographic and endoscopic management of bleeding pancreatic pseudoaneurysms. Gastrointest Endosc 46:544–549, 1997.
 6. Godil A, Chen YK: Endoscopic management of benign pancreatic disease. Pancreas 20:1–13, 2000.
 7. Howell DA, Elton E, Parsons WG. Endoscopic management of pseudocysts of the pancreas. Gastrointest Endosc Clin North Am 8:143–162, 1998.
 8. Kloppel G: Pseudocysts and other non-neoplastic cysts of the pancreas. Semin Diagn Pathol 17:7–15, 2000.
 9. Pitchumoni CS, Agarwal N: Pancreatic pseudocysts: When and how should drainage be performed? Gastroenterol Clin North Am 28:615–639, 1999.
10. Ratschko M, Fenner T, Lankisch PG: The role of antibiotic prophylaxis in the treatment of acute pancreatitis. Gastroenterol Clin North Am 28:641–659, 1999.
11. Wilentz RE, Albores-Saavedra J, Hruban RH: Mucinous cystic neoplasms of the pancreas. Semin Diagn Pathol 17:31–42, 2000.

V. Small and Large Bowel Disorders

42. CELIAC DISEASE, TROPICAL SPRUE, WHIPPLE'S DISEASE, LYMPHANGIECTASIA, AND NSAIDS

Shams Tabrez, M.D., and Ingram M. Roberts, M.D.

1. What is the best screening test for fat malabsorption?

Microscopic examination of stool using Sudan stain to detect fat is the best screening test for fat malabsorption. This test has a 100% sensitivity and 96% specificity. A stool sample is smeared on a microscope slide and mixed with ethanolic Sudan III and glacial acetic acid. The slide is covered, heated just until boiling, and then examined for the presence of fatty acid globules. The presence of more than 100 globules > 6 um in diameter per high-powered field ($\times 430$) indicates a definite increase in fecal fat excretion. The number of globules correlates well with the quantitative amount of fecal fat present.

2. What is the best quantitative test for fat malabsorption?

The 72-hour stool fat collection. The patient is given a diet consisting of 100 gm of fat per day. Stool is collected, usually for 72 hours. The normal coefficient for absorption is approximately 93% of ingested fat. Consequently, if 100 gm of fat is digested, 7 gm or less of fat should appear in stool over a 24-hour period. If > 7 gm of fecal fat is present, steatorrhea secondary to malabsorption is confirmed.

3. Under what physiologic conditions is fecal fat excretion increased?
- Diet high in fiber (> 100 gm/day)
- Ingestion of solid-form dietary fat (e.g., whole peanuts)
- In the neonatal period, when intraluminal levels of pancreatic lipase and bile salts are low
- When olestra is consumed

4. What is the best test to differentiate malabsorption caused by small bowel enteropathy vs. pancreatic insufficiency?

d-Xylose is one of the best tests to differentiate mucosal disease from pancreatic insufficiency as the cause of malabsorption. Normally, d-xylose is absorbed completely in the small bowel and excreted unchanged in the urine.

5. How is the d-xylose test performed?

A 25-gm dose of d-xylose is given orally after an overnight fast, and urine is collected for 5 hours. Normal urine excretion should be > 5 gm of d-xylose. One-hour serum collection is also helpful but not as sensitive as urine collection. Normal serum levels 1 hour after ingestion are > 20 mg/dl.

6. What conditions may cause a false-positive d-xylose test?
- Delayed gastric emptying
- Vomiting
- Renal insufficiency
- Myxedema
- Ascites

7. What is the GSE panel?

A panel of serologic tests used to detect celiac disease or gluten-sensitive enteropathy (GSE). Three antibodies are directed against the connective tissue (reticulin-like structures) or surface component of smooth muscle fibrils:

A-EmA   Antiendomysial antibody (IgA)
AGA   Antigliadin antibody (IgG or pooled Ig)
R1-ARA   Antireticulin antibody (IgA)

A-EmA has 100% specificity for celiac disease, whereas its sensitivity is 85% and 90%, respectively, for untreated adult and childhood celiac disease. It can persist in low titers in 10–25% of patients on a gluten-free diet, despite normal histology. AGA has fairly good sensitivity (68–76%), but it also may be found in 10–20% of patients with other diseases that affect the small intestinal mucosa. AGA is a helpful test in monitoring GSE, because it always becomes negative with the regrowth of jejunal villi in celiac patients after a gluten-free diet. RI-ARA has a higher specificity than AGA in celiac children but a relatively low sensitivity (< 40–50%).

8. What is tissue transglutaminase?

Recently, tissue transglutaminase has been touted as the most sensitive and specific marker for celiac disease. Tissue transglutaminase is believed to be the autoantigen to which the endomysial antibodies react. Studies have shown that specificity for antitransglutaminase is comparable to that for antiendomysial antibodies; however, some investigators have observed that the antibody to transglutaminase is a more sensitive test, detecting 98-100% of patients with celiac sprue.

9. Name the conditions to consider in previously responsive patients with celiac sprue who begin to deteriorate.

Noncompliance with gluten-free diet is the most common cause of deterioration in a previously responsive patient.

Lymphoma is the most common malignancy complicating celiac disease, especially that of mucosal T-cell origin. Diagnosis of lymphoma requires a high index of suspicion because onset can be insidious or abrupt, and the histologic appearance can be indistinguishable from that of celiac sprue. A careful search for lymphoma is needed in patients with celiac sprue who do not respond to gluten withdrawal and patients with recurrent weight loss and malabsorption despite strict adherence to a gluten-free diet. Computed tomographic (CT) scan and exploratory laparotomy may be necessary to establish the diagnosis.

Refractory sprue has clinical features and mucosal lesions indistinguishable from celiac sprue, but patients do not respond to a gluten-free diet, either at the onset of diagnosis or after becoming refractory to dietary therapy. Some patients may respond to corticosteroids or other immunosuppressive drugs, such as azathioprine, cyclophosphamide, or cyclosporine. Other patients do not respond to any treatment and face a dismal prognosis. The absence of Paneth cells on small bowel biopsy is a poor prognostic sign.

Collagenous sprue is a subset of refractory sprue characterized by the progressive development of a thick band of collagen-like material beneath the basement membrane of epithelial cells. It is usually refractory to all forms of treatment other than parenteral alimentation.

10. Describe the manifestations of Whipple's disease.

Whipple's disease is a chronic systemic illness with various potential manifestations. The most common presentation includes weight loss (90%), diarrhea (> 70%), and arthralgias (> 70%). Arthralgias may exist for many years before the diagnosis of Whipple's disease. Cardiac involvement includes congestive heart failure, pericarditis, and valvular heart disease (30%). Lymphadenopathy and hyperpigmentation are frequent findings on physical examination. Hematochezia is rare, but occult bleeding has been detected in up to 80% of patients with Whipple's disease. The most common central nervous system manifestations (5%) are dementia, ocular disturbances, meningoencephalitis, and cerebellar symptoms, including ataxia and mild clonus.

11. What is the differential diagnosis of a macrophage infiltrate of the small bowel lamina propria?

Whipple's disease: inclusions are rounded or sickle-shaped.

Mycobacterium avium-intracellulare: inclusions contain acid-fast bacilli. This condition is commonly seen in AIDS patients with small bowel involvement.

Histoplasmosis or cryptococcosis: inclusions contain large, round, encapsulated organisms.

Macroglobulinemia: no inclusions are seen, and there are only faintly staining, homogeneously periodic acid–Schiff (PAS)-positive macrophages.

Miscellaneous disease: PAS-positive macrophages are frequently present in the normal gastric and rectal mucosa and may contain lipids or mucin, respectively.

12. What causes Whipple's disease?

Tropheryma whippelii causes the disease in humans but has been cultured only recently. The organism was identified by direct amplification of a 16S-rRNA sequence from a microbial pathogen in tissue. According to phylogenetic analysis, this bacterium is a gram-positive actinomycete that is not closely related to any known genus. Prolonged treatment with antibiotics (up to 6 months) is often required to eradicate the organism. Measurements of *T. whippelii* DNA concentration in tissue by polymerase chain reaction is the most sensitive marker of patient response to antibiotic therapy. Of interest, *T. whippelii* DNA has been found in the small intestine of asymptomatic patients, suggesting that host factors play a role in disease penetration, just as in *Helicobacter pylori* infection.

13. What are the complications of the enteropathy induced by nonsteroidal anti-inflammatory drugs (NSAIDs)?

NSAID-induced enteropathy is associated with intestinal bleeding, protein loss, ileal dysfunction, and malabsorption. There is no close relationship between upper endoscopic findings and evidence of intestinal bleeding among NSAID-treated patients, even when blood loss has led to iron-deficiency anemia. Chronic blood loss and protein loss seem to occur from the inflammatory site. Protein loss can result in significant hypoalbuminemia. Ileal dysfunction can lead to bile acid malabsorption and, in rare cases, mild vitamin B12 malabsorption. Mefenamic acid (Postel) and sulindac (Clinoril) have been implicated as causes of severe malabsorption with subtotal villus atrophy that resembles celiac disease.

14. Does scleroderma produce any manifestations in the small bowel?

Patients with scleroderma may have small bowel dysfunction due to absent cycling of the normal contractile pattern, known as the migrating motor complex. Small bowel motility studies reveal markedly diminished amplitude in all phasic pressure waves. This finding may manifest clinically as intestinal pseudoobstruction and bacterial overgrowth. Patients may suffer from nausea, vomiting, abdominal pain, diarrhea, and malabsorption. Small bowel radiographic series may show megaduodenum and dilated loops of jejunum.

15. How does octreotide affect intestinal motility and bacterial overgrowth in scleroderma?

Octreotide evokes alternating phase-1 and phase-3 activity in normal people and patients with scleroderma. In patients with scleroderma, these complexes propagate at the same velocity and have two-thirds the amplitude of spontaneous complexes in normal people. This effect is independent of motilin because octreotide inhibits motilin release. Octreotide may retard gastric antral motility—unlike erythromycin, which markedly stimulates gastric antral motor activity.

16. Describe the different forms of lymphangiectasia.

Congenital intestinal lymphangiectasia (Milroy's disease) results from a malformation of the lymphatic system. Many areas in the body can be affected. Patients with congenital disease may present at any time from childhood to adulthood and usually have asymmetric lymphedema.

Secondary lymphangiectasia results from a disease that blocks intestinal lymph drainage. Causes of secondary lymphangiectasia include extensive abdominal or retroperitoneal carcinoma, lymphoma, retroperitoneal fibrosis, chronic pancreatitis, mesenteric tuberculosis or sarcoidosis, Crohn's disease, chronic congestive heart failure, and even constrictive pericarditis.

17. What are the clinical manifestations of abetalipoproteinemia?
Abetalipoproteinemia is an autosomal recessive condition characterized by the inability to form chylomicrons and very-low-density lipoprotein particles by the enterocytes because of abnormal apoprotein B. Most patients suffer severe fat malabsorption and retardation and rarely survive the third decade. The largest series of patients has been studied at the National Institutes of Health.

18. What are the different clinical presentations of eosinophilic gastroenteritis?
Eosinophilic gastroenteritis is characterized by eosinophilic infiltration in the gastrointestinal tract. Clinical features and severity depend on the layer and location of involvement. Mucosal involvement leads to protein-losing enteropathy, fecal blood loss, and malabsorption. Involvement of the muscle layer often causes obstruction of gastric or small bowel. Subserosal involvement causes ascites, pleural effusion, or, on occasion, pericarditis.

19. How are patients with eosinophilic gastroenteritis treated?
The mainstay of treatment for eosinophilic gastroenteritis is corticosteroids, even though no controlled trials have been performed. The recommended dosage of prednisone is usually 20–40 mg/day for treatment of the initial episode and relapses, with 5–10 mg/day for maintenance. Some patients respond to a short course of treatment but may suffer relapse. Others may require long-term maintenance therapy. The course of disease may wax and wane in severity but is rarely life-threatening. The therapeutic effect of oral sodium cromoglycate is controversial. Trial elimination diets have occasionally been successful, but relapse is common.

20. What are the common causes of diarrhea in a patient with Crohn's disease and ileal resection?
Ileal resection < 100 cm: bile salt diarrhea. Normally, conjugated bile acids are reabsorbed in the ileum. When < 100 cm ileum is resected, bile acids pass into the colon, causing direct irritation of the colonic epithelium and net water secretion by the colon. Bile-salt diarrhea is typically watery, may not start until a normal diet is resumed after surgery, is precipitated by a meal (typically after breakfast when a large amount of bile is stored in the gallbladder), and does not lead to weight loss. Patients benefit from an empirical trial of cholestyramine, a bile acid-binding agent.

Ileal resection >100 cm: steatorrhea. When > 100 cm of ileum is lost to surgical resection or disease, the daily loss of bile acids exceeds the ability of the liver to synthesize new bile acids; hence, the total circulation bile acid pool is diminished. Bile acid deficiency leads to impaired intraluminal micellar fat absorption or steatorrhea. Patients benefit from a low-fat diet or supplement of medium-chain triglycerides. The diminished circulating pool of bile acids also promotes formation of cholesterol gallstones.

21. Where are the endemic areas for tropical sprue?
Tropical sprue is endemic in Puerto Rico, Cuba, the Dominican Republic, and Haiti but not in Jamaica or the other West Indies islands. It is found in Central America, Venezuela, and Columbia. Sprue is common in the Indian subcontinent and Far East, although little information is available from China. Sprue has been reported among several visitors to countries in the Middle East. It is rare in Africa, although the occurrence of sprue among populations living in the central and southern parts is now well established.

22. How is tropical sprue treated?
The most effective therapy for tropical sprue in returning travelers or expatriates is a combination of folic acid and tetracycline. Folic acid should be given in a dosage of 5 mg/day orally and tetracycline in a dosage of 250 mg 4 times/day. Vitamin B12 should be given parenterally, in addition to the above combination, if a deficiency of this vitamin is discovered. Treatment should be continued for at least several months or until intestinal function returns to normal. Treatment

with folic acid alone may be effective in reversing small bowel abnormalities or even in curing the acute illness but not in curing the chronic form. On the other hand, long-term treatment with tetracycline alone may result in cure of both acute and chronic forms of sprue.

23. How is bacterial overgrowth diagnosed?

The gold standard for the diagnosis of bacterial overgrowth is demonstration of increased concentrations of bacteria (> 105 colony-forming units/ml) in fluid obtained from the intestine during duodenal intubation. If quantitative culture of the small bowel aspirate is not possible, the diagnosis can be made with various breath tests. With the lactulose-hydrogen breath test, a rise in breath hydrogen level of 12 ppm from baseline values is taken as diagnostic of bacterial overgrowth. The 14C-glycocholate and 14C-d-Xylose breath tests detect the release of the radiolabeled carbon dioxide as the result of bacterial deconjugation of bile acid and metabolism of Xylose. Normalization of the Schilling test after treatment with antibiotics is highly suggestive of bacterial overgrowth.

24. What is the mechanism of hyperoxaluria in short bowel syndrome?

Normally, intraluminal calcium binds to oxalate and prevents intestinal absorption of oxalate. With short bowel syndrome, malabsorption of fat leads to excessive luminal free fatty acids, which bind to calcium, allowing oxalate to pass unbound and become available for absorption. Excessive luminal free fatty acids and bile acids appear to increase colonic permeability to oxalate, further increasing its absorption. Therefore, hyperoxaluria appears to depend on the presence of an intact colon. To prevent calcium oxalate nephrolithiasis in patients with bowel disease, a low-oxalate and low-fat diet should be recommended.

BIBLIOGRAPHY

1. Bjarnason I, Hayllar J, Macpherson AJ, Russell AS: Side effects of nonsteroidal antiinflamatory drugs on the small and large intestine in humans. Gastroenterology 104:1832–1847, 1993.
2. Fleming JL, Wiesner RH, Shorter RG: Whipple's disease: Clinical, biochemical, and histopathologic features and assessment of treatment in 29 patients. Mayo Clin Proc 63:539–551, 1988.
3. Hofmann AF, Poley R: Role of bile acid malabsorption in pathogenesis of diarrhea and steatorrhea in patients with ileal resection: I. Response to cholestyramine or replacement of dietary long chain triglyceride by medium chain triglyceride. Gastroenterology 62:918–934, 1972.
4. Klipstein FA: Tropical sprue in travelers and expatriates living abroad. Gastroenterology 80:590–600, 1981.
5. Relman DA, Schmidt TM, MacDermott RP, Falkow S: Identification of the uncultured bacillus of Whipple's disease. N Engl J Med 327:293–301, 1992.
6. Roberts IM: Workup of the patient with malabsorption. Postgrad Med 81:32–42, 1987.
7. Soudah HC, Hasler WL, Owyang C: Effect of octreotide on intestinal motility and bacterial overgrowth in scleroderma. N Engl J Med 325:1461–1467, 1991.
8. Talley NJ, Shorter RG, Phillips SF, Zinsmeister AR: Eosinophilic gastroenteritis: A clinicopathological study of patients with disease of the mucosa, muscle layer, and subserosal tissues. Gut 31:54–58, 1990.
9. Trier JS: Celiac sprue. N Engl J Med 325:1709–1719, 1991.
10. Volta U, Molinaro N, Fusconi M, et al: IgA antiendomysial antibody test: A step forward in celiac disease screening. Dig Dis Sci 36:752–756, 1991.
11. Yamada T, Alpers DH, Owyang C, et al (eds): Textbook of Gastroenterology, 2nd ed. Philadelphia, J.B. Lippincott, 1995.
12. Balasekaran R, Porter JL, Santa Ana CA, Fordtran JS: Positive results on tests for steatorrha in persons consuming olestra potato chips. Ann Int Med 132: 279–282, 2000.
13. Raoult D, Birg ML, La Scola B: Cultivation of the bacillus of Whipple's disease. N Engl J Med 342: 620–625, 2000.
14. Street S, Donoghue HD, NeildGH: Tropheryma whippelii DNA in saliva of healthy people [letter]. Lancet 354:1178–1179, 1999.
15. Ramzan NN, Loftus E Jr, Burgart LJ: Diagnosis and monitoring of Whipple disease by polymerase chain reaction. Ann Intern Med 126:520–527, 1997.
16. Sollid LM: Molecular basis of celiac disease. Annu Rev Immunol 18:53–81, 2000.
17. Sblattero D, Berti I, Trevisol C, et al: Human recombinant tissue transglutaminase ELISA: An innovative diagnostic test for celiac disease. Am J Gastroenterol 95: 1253–1257, 2000.
18. Seissler J, Boms S, Wohlrab U, et al: Antibodies to human recombinant tissue transglutaminase measured by radioligand assay: Evidence for high diagnostic sensitivity for celiac disease. Horm Metab Res 31: 375–379, 1999.

43. CROHN'S DISEASE

Bret A. Lashner, M.D., and Aaron Brzezinski, M.D.

1. What is Crohn's disease?

Crohn's disease is the most commonly used term to describe a nonspecific inflammation of any segment of the intestine with discontinuous or skip areas of ulceration and granulomatous, fissuring, or transmural inflammation. Synonyms include regional enteritis, regional ileitis, granulomatous colitis, and granulomatous enteritis. Intestinal ulcerations can range from aphthous to deep and serpiginous. Although Crohn's disease is a heterogeneous entity, there are some common features related to the diagnosis, etiology, natural history, and treatment.

2. Who was Crohn?

Burrill B. Crohn was the first-listed author of the first description of the disease in U.S. medical literature in 1932. The other authors of the paper, Ginzburg and Oppenheimer, have fallen in historical importance because authorship order was determined alphabetically.

DIAGNOSIS

3. What symptoms and signs are suggestive of Crohn's disease?

Patients with Crohn's disease typically present with diarrhea and abdominal pain. The abdominal pain usually is insidious and located in the right lower quadrant; it occurs soon after eating and may be associated with a tender, inflammatory mass. Hematochezia may be present, but bleeding is much less common than in ulcerative colitis. Fever, weight loss, stomatitis, perianal fistulas and/or fissures, arthritis, and erythema nodosum are commonly seen. Although symptoms depend on site of involvement and behavior of disease, the most frequent presentation consists of diarrhea, abdominal pain, and weight loss.

4. Explain the Crohn's Disease Activity Index.

The Crohn's Disease Activity Index (CDAI) was developed for clinical trials. Calculation of the CDAI combines weighted scores of clinical and laboratory variables. CDAI scores < 150 indicate clinical remission, and scores > 450 indicate severely active disease. Although subjective and cumbersome, the CDAI is currently the standard measure of disease activity for all clinical trials.

Calculation of the Crohn's Disease Activity Index

VARIABLE	RANGE OF VALUES	WEIGHT
1. Liquid or soft stools summed over 7 days	0–70	2
2. Daily abdominal pain ratings summed over 7 days	0–21	6
3. General well-being ratings summed over 7 days	0–28	6
4. Number of extraintestinal manifestations	0–3	30
5. Use of opiates for diarrhea	0–1	4
6. Abdominal mass	0–5	10
7. 47 minus hematocrit in males, 42 minus hematocrit in females	—	6
8. Percent body weight below standard	—	1

CDAI equals the sum of each variable multiplied by its weight.

5. How is the diagnosis of Crohn's disease established?

The diagnosis of Crohn's disease is established by finding characteristic intestinal ulcerations and excluding alternative diagnoses. The ulcerations of Crohn's disease may appear aphthoid (Fig. 1) or deep and serpiginous along the longitudinal axis of the bowel (Fig. 2). Skip areas, cobblestoning, pseudopolyps, and rectal sparing are characteristic findings. Air contrast barium enema, small bowel series with a peroral pneumocolon, or colonoscopy may demonstrate typical lesions.

In a small bowel series, Crohn's disease often manifests by separation of bowel loops and a narrowed terminal ileal lumen, the so-called "string sign" (Fig. 3). Colonoscopic biopsy demonstrating granulomatous inflammation, a finding in about 10% of cases of Crohn's colitis, is diagnostic. Typical lesions of Crohn's disease also may be seen in the upper gastrointestinal tract. The inflammation is localized in the ileocecal region in approximately 50% of cases, the small bowel in approximately 25% of cases, the colon in 20% of cases, and the upper gastrointestinal tract or perirectum in 5%.

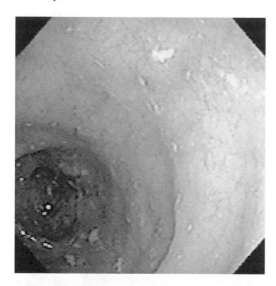

FIGURE 1.   Aphthoid ulcers in a patient with Crohn's colitis.

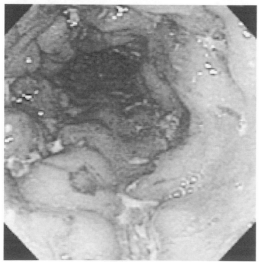

FIGURE 2.   Deep, serpiginous ulcers of Crohn's disease.

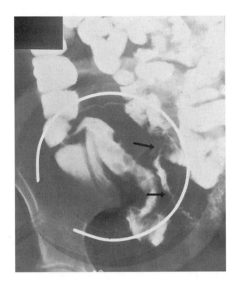

FIGURE 3.   String sign *(arrows)* from a small bowel series in a patient with Crohn's disease.

6. Which diseases can mimic the symptoms and signs of Crohn's disease?

The differential diagnosis of Crohn's disease is long. The most common mimics of Crohn's colitis are ischemic colitis, diverticulitis, and colorectal cancer. Infection with *Yersinia enterocolitica* or *Mycobacterium tuberculosis* may mimic Crohn's ileitis. Other important diseases in the differential diagnosis of Crohn's disease include irritable bowel syndrome, intestinal lymphoma, celiac sprue, radiation enteropathy, and nonsteroidal anti-inflammatory drug-induced enteropathy.

7. What serologic tests can help to establish the diagnosis?

Clinical, endoscopic, and histologic findings can establish the diagnosis and differentiate between Crohn's disease and ulcerative colitis in at least 90% of patients. In the 10% of patients with indeterminate colitis in whom the diagnosis is important to identify proper medical or surgical therapy, serologic testing may be helpful. Anti-*Saccharomyces cereviciae* antibody (ASCA) is seen in over 60% of patients with Crohn's disease and in less than 10% of patients with other gastrointestinal diseases such as ulcerative colitis and irritable bowel syndrome. *Saccharomyces cereviciae*, or baker's yeast, becomes antigenic when intestinal permeability is increased, as in Crohn's disease. The perinuclear antineutrophil cytoplasmic antibody (pANCA) has a 70% sensitivity for ulcerative colitis and a 10% sensitivity for Crohn's disease. ASCA and pANCA testing together have a sensitivity and specificity of over 90% for Crohn's disease.

Distinguishing Features of Ulcerative Colitis and Crohn's Disease

	ULCERATIVE COLITIS	CROHN'S DISEASE
Rectal bleeding	Usual	Sometimes
Abdominal mass	Rare	Often
Abdominal pain	Sometimes	Often
Perianal disease	Extremely rare	5–10%
Upper GI symptoms	Never	Occasional
Cigarette smoking	Very rare	Common
Malnutrition	Sometimes	Common
Low-grade fever	Sometimes	Often
Rectal disease	Usual	Sometimes

Table continued on following page

Distinguishing Features of Ulcerative Colitis and Crohn's Disease (Continued)

	ULCERATIVE COLITIS	CROHN'S DISEASE
Continuous disease	Usual	Sometimes
Granulomas	Never	10%
Crypt abscesses	Common	Rare
Discrete ulcers	Rare	Common
Aphthoid ulcers	Rare	Common
Cobblestone lesions	Never	Common
Skip lesions	Rare	Common
Ileal involvement	Rare; backwash ileitis	Usual
Fistulas	Never	Common
Cancer	Rare	Very rare
Microscopic skip lesions	Rare	Common
Transmural inflammation	Never	Common

ETIOLOGY

8. Is cigarette smoking associated with Crohn's disease?

Cigarette smokers are much more likely than nonsmokers to develop Crohn's disease. Over one-half of patients with Crohn's disease are cigarette smokers compared to about one-third of the U.S. adult population. Furthermore, patients with Crohn's disease are statistically significantly less likely to quit than controls. This finding is in direct contradistinction to the protective effect of cigarette smoking for ulcerative colitis. Although nicotine has been used to treat ulcerative colitis, it should be used in patients with Crohn's disease only as a means to quit smoking.

Evidence suggests that cigarette smokers with Crohn's disease have a worse prognosis than nonsmokers. Early recurrence, more severe complications, and a higher likelihood for repeat surgery are associated with cigarette smoking. Although it has not been shown that quitters can favorably change the course of their disease, it is reasonable to assume that they will have less severe complications and require surgery less often than smokers. For reasons related to their disease as well as cardiovascular health, patients with Crohn's disease *must quit smoking*.

9. What infectious agents may be responsible for Crohn's disease?

Mycobacterium paratuberculosis causes Johne's disease, a granulomatous inflammation of the terminal ileum and other parts of the intestine, in goats. In situ hybridization and culture of resected specimens in patients with Crohn's disease found *M. paratuberculosis* and other atypical mycobacteria in a small number of patients. A causal relationship has not been determined. Research concerning chronic infection with the measles virus and exposure to measles vaccine has been inconclusive and has not established an etiologic association.

10. Is there a genetic predisposition for developing Crohn's disease?

The principal theory about the pathogenesis of Crohn's disease is that in a genetically predisposed person, an environmental agent (i.e., infection, dietary substance that enters the blood stream through a permeable intestine, or nicotine) triggers an uncontrolled inflammatory response. The incidence of Crohn's disease ranges between 2 and 10 per 100,000 in the population. Crohn's disease occurs in more than one first- or second-degree family member in approximately 20% of cases. Children with a parent who has Crohn's disease have a lifetime risk of less than 3%. Spouses of patients with Crohn's disease rarely develop the disease. The genetic predisposition occurs from a number of important genetic mutations in key regulatory proteins of intestinal inflammation. Studies of genetic linkages among kindreds with inflammatory bowel disease suggests that mutations in chromosome 16 (IBD-1) and chromosome 12 (IBD-2) may be two of the implicated gene mutations in humans.

NATURAL HISTORY

11. Is the mortality rate increased in patients with Crohn's disease?

Patients with Crohn's disease, in general, do not have an increased mortality rate compared with age- and sex-matched controls. Some complications of Crohn's disease, such as malignancy, short bowel syndrome, and primary sclerosing cholangitis, are associated with an increased mortality rate. Fortunately, these complications are rare.

12. What factors predict a flare of Crohn's disease activity?

Cigarette smoking is the most important clinical risk factor for symptomatic recurrence. Smokers have a recurrence rate at least twice as high as nonsmokers. The effect of oral contraceptive use on recurrence rate is controversial. Although oral contraceptive use is not associated with an increased recurrence rate, there is a synergistic effect between smoking and oral contraceptive use. The combined effects are greater than the sum of the individual effects. Other risk factors for symptomatic recurrence are intestinal infections or nonsteroidal anti-inflammatory drug use.

13. Does the behavior of the disease predict its natural history?

Recently, Crohn's disease has been classified as inflammatory, stricturing, or fistulizing. **Inflammatory-type disease** is characterized by intestinal ulcerations with diarrhea, abdominal pain, an inflammatory mass, and possibly fever and weight loss. Inflammatory-type disease responds best to anti-inflammatory therapy, but recurrence is the rule rather than the exception. The natural history of inflammatory-type disease is aggressive with early recurrence.

Stricturing-type disease, on the other hand, has a more indolent course that does not respond well to anti-inflammatory therapy. Although all Crohn's disease begins as inflammation, the predominant pathology in patients with stricturing disease is extensive fibrosis in the lamina propria. Surgery is the best therapeutic option in patients with stricturing disease, and the need for a second surgery is much lower than with other types of Crohn's disease.

Fistulizing-type disease is characterized by enterocutaneous and/or enteroenteric fistulas. Fistulas occur in areas of inflammation, yet often originate in a segment of bowel proximal to a stricture. After successful medical or surgical therapy for fistulas, recurrence is common. Most patients with fistulas benefit from maintenance anti-inflammatory medical therapy to minimize the risk for recurrence.

14. Do patients with Crohn's disease have an increased risk for cancer?

Small bowel or large bowel cancer is a rarely reported phenomenon in patients with Crohn's disease; fewer than 100 cases have been reported in the literature. Epidemiologic studies, however, suggest that the risk of small bowel cancer is greatly elevated, whereas the risk of colorectal cancer is elevated only marginally above what is expected in the general population. Small bowel cancer in patients with Crohn's disease is distributed like Crohn's disease (ileum > jejunum > duodenum) which is exactly opposite to the distribution of sporadic small bowel cancer. Excluded loops and chronic fistulas also are risk factors for small bowel cancer in Crohn's disease. Colorectal cancer in Crohn's disease occurs near areas of inflammation. However, because the premalignant lesion of dysplasia, when present, is not as widespread in the colon of patients with Crohn's disease as it is in patients with ulcerative colitis, surveillance colonoscopy is less effective in decreasing mortality rates.

15. What are the extraintestinal manifestations of Crohn's disease?

The extraintestinal manifestations of Crohn's disease are similar to those of ulcerative colitis. A polyarticular, nondeforming arthritis is the most common extraintestinal manifestation, occurring in about 20% of patients. The arthritis responds to treatment of bowel symptoms. Primary sclerosing cholangitis is less common in Crohn's disease than in ulcerative colitis and does not respond to anti-inflammatory therapy directed to the bowel, including surgery. Erythema nodosum, pyoderma gangrenosum, iritis, uveitis, pancreatitis, nephrolithiasis, cholelithiasis, amyloidosis, osteoporosis, and ankylosing spondylitis are believed to be extraintestinal manifestations of Crohn's disease. Nephrolithiasis most often involves oxalate stones. Patients with Crohn's disease and fat malabsorption have preferential binding of luminal calcium to fatty acids rather than oxalate, and the subsequent increased absorption of dietary oxalate leads to stone formation.

TREATMENT

16. Which 5-aminosalicylic acid preparations are effective in treating Crohn's disease?

5-Aminosalicylic acid (5ASA) agents have been used for many years to treat inflammatory bowel disease, mostly ulcerative colitis. Sulfasalazine requires bacterial cleavage of the diazo bond between sulfapyradine and 5ASA for the 5ASA to have a local anti-inflammatory effect. Because bacteria are present in sufficient numbers only in the large bowel, sulfasalazine is effective only in patients with Crohn's colitis. Asacol, 5ASA coated with a compound that dissolves at pH 7 (terminal ileum), is commonly used for Crohn's patients with ileocolitis. Pentasa is 5ASA coated with ethylcellulose beads, which dissolve and release 5ASA throughout the small and large bowel. Theoretically, Pentasa should be most effective in patients with extensive small bowel disease. Of interest, all of these agents are approved for ulcerative colitis, but none is approved for use in Crohn's disease. 5ASA agents are used mostly in patients with mildly to moderately active disease. Their role in maintenance therapy is debatable.

17. Should steroids be used in Crohn's disease?

Steroids are effective in treating inflammatory-type Crohn's disease. Long-term use is not recommended because of the many serious adverse effects, such as osteoporosis, diabetes, and cataracts, to name a few. Steroids are not effective in stricturing Crohn's disease and in fact may worsen the condition of patients with fistulas, especially if localized infection is not adequately drained.

18. What is the role for immunosuppressive therapy in Crohn's disease?

Both azathioprine and 6-mercaptopurine are commonly used to treat Crohn's disease. Both are purine analogs that interfere with DNA synthesis of rapidly dividing cells such as lymphocytes and macrophages. These drugs are effective in both inducing and maintaining remission in inflammatory-type and fistulizing-type Crohn's disease and may be given for 4 years or longer. Important adverse effects include pancreatitis, allergy, and leukopenia. White blood cell counts and liver function tests need to be checked on a periodic basis. The onset of action may take as long as 6 months, but usually 2–3 months are required before a response is seen. In nonresponders, levels of the active metabolite, 6-thioguanine (6-TG), can be measured to determine whether the lack of response is due to lack of adherence to a medical regimen (6-TG level of 0), underdosing (6-TG level < 230 pmol/8×10^8 red blood cells), or true lack of response (6-TG level > 230 pmol/8×10^8 red blood cells).

19. Which biologic therapies are effective for Crohn's disease?

Infliximab is an IgG_1 chimeric mouse-human antibody to tumor necrosis factor (TNF) that, when infused intravenously, binds to soluble TNF and to the TNF on surface membranes of inflammatory cells, causing cell lysis. It has been approved for use in inflammatory-type Crohn's disease (a single infusion of 5 mg/kg) and fistulizing Crohn's disease (3 infusions of 5 mg/kg). In randomized clinical trials, 48% of patients with inflammatory-type disease and 55% of patients with fistulizing disease achieved complete remission—percentages that were significantly higher than in placebo-treated patients. Side effects during the infusion, such as nausea, headache, and pharyngitis, can be attenuated by slowing the infusion. The possible long-term side effect of lymphoma needs to be investigated further; 2 cases have been reported. No other biologic agents are available for Crohn's disease, but interleukin-10 and interleukin-11 are under study and show much promise.

20. Which medications are effective in maintaining remission?

Patients who have a high risk of recurrence after a medically or surgically induced remission should be considered for maintenance medications. Smokers, patients who have had more than one surgery, and patients with inflammatory-type or fistulizing disease have the highest risk of recurrence. Long-term therapy with azathioprine or 6-mercaptopurine has the best maintenance effect. 5ASA agents and enteric-coated fish oil preparations (eicosopentanoic acid) have a lesser maintenance effect.

21. What are the indications for surgery in Crohn's disease?

The adage "a chance to cut is a chance to cure" does not apply to Crohn's disease. Surgery is not a cure for Crohn's disease. The main goal of surgery is to treat the most important problem while preserving as much bowel as possible. Wide resection margins are not associated with decreased recurrence. The indications for surgery include active inflammatory-type disease refractory to medical therapy, prednisone dependence, intestinal strictures, fistulas, abscesses, growth retardation, bleeding, perforation, severe anorectal disease, and cancer. Besides resection and abscess drainage, there is considerable experience with strictureplasty (opening a stricture without removing bowel) and advancement flap surgery (removing a perirectal fistula by advancing normal mucosa over the internal os). A close working relationship between the internist/gastroenterologist and surgeon is extremely important for controlling disease and decreasing morbidity.

22. What therapeutic regimen is most often effective for stricturing-type Crohn's disease?

Stricturing-type Crohn's disease usually requires surgery. Anti-inflammatory therapy is not likely to relieve symptoms. The goals of surgery are to relieve symptoms and preserve bowel length. The surgery need not be a resection. Strictureplasties of strictured segments of small bowel or anastomoses can provide long-term relief of obstructive symptoms. In the most common type of strictureplasty, an incision is made on the longitudinal axis of a short stricture that is sutured along a perpendicular line. Before performing strictureplasty, the surgeon should send a frozen section to rule out carcinoma at the site of the stricture.

23. What therapeutic regimen is most often effective for inflammatory-type Crohn's disease?

Inflammatory-type Crohn's disease should respond to anti-inflammatory agents. 5-ASA agents usually are tried first because of their limited toxicity. Corticosteroids usually are tried next because of the relatively rapid onset of action. Azathioprine and 6-mercaptopurine usually are reserved for steroid-dependent inflammatory disease and maintenance of remission. Other anti-inflammatory medications shown to be effective include methotrexate and infliximab. Most often, these medications are used in steroid-refractory disease. Antibiotics, such as metronidazole and ciprofloxacin, have only marginal benefits and have not been shown to be consistently effective in clinical trials.

24. What therapeutic regimen is most often effective for fistulizing Crohn's disease?

An assessment of the degree of mucosal activity is an important determinant of therapy for fistulizing Crohn's disease. When active disease is present, anti-inflammatory therapy with 5-ASA agents, azathioprine, 6-mercaptopurine, or infliximab may be extremely helpful. In perianal fistulas, if mucosal disease is quiescent, surgical therapy with an advancement flap procedure may be the most appropriate treatment. Surgical drainage of any septic processes, especially in the perineum, and antibiotics also are needed. Placement of noncutting Seton sutures can facilitate continued drainage and promote healing (Fig. 4). Once remission is induced, azathioprine or 6-mercaptopurine can be used for maintenance.

25. When should nutritional support be used in patients with Crohn's disease?

Nutritional support can be used as primary or adjuvant therapy for Crohn's disease. Of interest, bowel rest and total parenteral nutrition (TPN) greatly improve most patients with inflammatory-type or fistulizing-type disease. Enteral nutrition is as effective as steroids in inducing remission in inflammatory-type Crohn's disease but has fewer side effects. Unfortunately, when food is introduced, symptoms and signs of active disease quickly return. Nutritional support also is effective

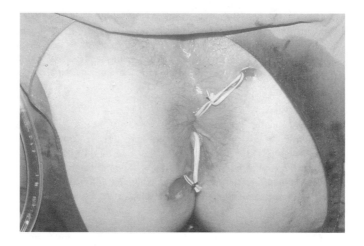

FIGURE 4.   Seton sutures placed in the perineum.

in children with Crohn's disease and growth retardation. Because of the expense and morbidity of TPN, long-term TPN should be reserved for patients with short bowel syndrome or extensive small bowel disease and patients who need nutritional support but do not tolerate enteral nutrition.

BIBLIOGRAPHY

 1. Belluzzi A, Brignola C, Campieri M, et al: Effect of an enteric-coated fish-oil preparation on relapses in Crohn's disease. N Engl J Med 334;1557–1560, 1996.
 2. Best WR, Becktel JM, Singleton JW. Rederived values of the eight coefficients of the Crohn's disease activity index (CDAI). Gastroenterology 1979;77:843–846, 1979.
 3. Crohn BB, Ginzburg L, Oppenheimer GD: Regional enteritis: A pathological and clinical entity. JAMA 99:1323–1329, 1932.
 4. Dubinsky MC, Lamothe S, Yang HY, et al: Pharmacogenomics and metabolite measurement for 6-mercaptopurine therapy in inflammatory bowel disease. Gastroenterology 118:705–713, 2000.
 5. Fazio VW, Marchetti F, Church JM, et al: Effect of resection margins on recurrence of Crohn's disease of the small bowel: A randomized controlled trial. Ann Surg 224:563–571, 1996.
 6. Feagan BG, Rochon J, Fedorak RN, et al: Methotrexate for the treatment of Crohn's disease. N Engl J Med 332:292–297, 1995.
 7. Fiocchi C. Inflammatory bowel disease: Etiology and pathogenesis. Gastroenterology 115:182–205, 1998.
 8. Lichtiger S, Present DH, Kornbluth A, et al: Cyclosporine in severe ulcerative colitis refractory to steroid therapy. N Engl J Med 330:1841–1845, 1994.
 9. Munkholm P, Langholz E, Davidsen M, Binder V: Intestinal cancer risk and mortality in patients with Crohn's disease. Gastroenterology 105:1716–1723, 1993.
10. Present DH, Rutgeerts P, Targan S, et al: Infliximab for the treatment of fistulas in patients with Crohn's disease. N Engl J Med 340:1398–1405, 1999.
11. Ruemmele FM, Targan SR, Levy G, et al: Diagnostic accuracy of serological assays in pediatric inflammatory bowel disease. Gastroenterology 115:822–829, 1998.
12. Silverstein MD, Loftus EV, Sandborn WJ, et al: Clinical course and costs of care for Crohn's disease: Markov model analysis of a population-based cohort. Gastroenterology 117:49–57, 1999.
13. Singleton JW, Law DH, Delly ML, et al: National Cooperative Crohn's Disease Study: Results of drug treatment. Gastroenterology 77:847–869, 1979.
14. Targan SR, Hoenir SB, Van Deventer SCH, et al: A short-term study of chimeric monoclonal antibody cA2 to TNF-alpha for Crohn's disease. N Engl J Med 337:1029–1035, 1997.
15. Timmer A, Sutherland LR, Martin F, et al: Oral contraceptive use and smoking are risk factors for relapse in Crohn's disease. Gastroenterology 114:1143–1150, 1998.
16. Valentine JF, Sninsky CA: Prevention and treatment of osteoporosis in patients with inflammatory bowel disease. Am J Gastroenterol 94:878–883, 1999.

44. ULCERATIVE COLITIS

Ramona O. Rajapakse, M.D., and Burton I. Korelitz, M.D.

1. What is ulcerative colitis?

Ulcerative colitis is a chronic inflammatory disease of the colon. It is distinct from Crohn's disease (CD) of the colon in that the inflammation is restricted mostly to the mucosa and involves only the colon.

2. Define backwash ileitis.

Backwash ileitis refers to unusual cases of ulcerative colitis that involve the terminal ileum. The endoscopic and radiologic appearance of backwash ileitis is the same as that of ulcerative colitis. When deep linear ulcers and strictures are seen in the ileum, Crohn's ileitis is the more likely diagnosis.

3. What is indeterminate colitis?

As more information is gathered about the pathogenesis of ulcerative colitis and CD, the distinction between them at times can be unclear. In about 7% of patients, endoscopic, histologic, or radiologic findings are insufficiently distinct to separate the two diseases. The colitis is then referred to as "indeterminate." Other patients carry the diagnosis of UC for many years until a change in signs and symptoms, consistent with CD, influences a change in diagnosis. In some patients the diagnosis of CD of the colon is recognized only after colectomy and the development of recurrent ileitis in the ileostomy or ileoanal pouch performed for what was thought to be ulcerative colitis.

4. Why is it important to distinguish between ulcerative colitis and Crohn's disease?

Medical treatment of the two diseases overlaps, but, unlike CD, ulcerative colitis is "curable" by total colectomy. Therefore, the correct diagnosis is of the utmost importance.

5. What causes ulcerative colitis?

The cause is unknown. The greatest risk factor is a positive family history. Approximately 15% of patients with inflammatory bowel disease (IBD) have a first-degree relative with the disease, but the familial association is less in ulcerative colitis than in CD. Similarly, the incidence of IBD in first-degree relatives of patients with IBD is 30–100 times higher than in the general population. The exact genetic link for ulcerative colitis has not been identified. Dietary antigens and bacteria have been proposed as possible triggers, but no evidence supports these theories. The incidence of ulcerative colitis is significantly higher in nonsmokers than in smokers and higher still in ex-smokers than in nonsmokers, supporting a protective effect of smoking. Whether this protective effect is secondary to nicotine or other constituents of cigarettes has not been fully established.

6. Who gets ulcerative colitis?

In most patients ulcerative colitis has its onset in the second or third decades of life. However, there may be a second peak in the fifth or sixth decades, although this peak may be false because of other types of colitis that mimic ulcerative colitis. The disease has been described in all nationalities and ethnic groups but is more common in whites than in nonwhites. It is also more common in Jews than non-Jews. The hereditary link is supported by population-based studies.

7. What are the signs and symptoms of ulcerative colitis?

The predominant symptom at onset of ulcerative colitis is diarrhea with or without blood in the stool. If inflammation is confined to the rectum, blood may be seen on the surface of the stool; other symptoms include tenesmus, urgency, rectal pain, and passage of mucus without diarrhea.

Other distributions of ulcerative colitis are proctosigmoiditis; left-sided disease, which extends more proximal to the descending colon, splenic flexure, or distal transverse colon; and universal colitis, which involves any length proximal to the mid-transverse colon and often the entire colon. The inflammation is almost always confluent in distribution and almost always involves the rectum when it is untreated with medication by enema.

More extensive colitis may be accompanied by systemic symptoms such as weight loss and malaise in addition to bloody diarrhea. Although pain is not a dominant feature, patients may complain of crampy abdominal discomfort relieved by a bowel movement and may have abdominal tenderness, usually localized to the left lower quadrant. Occasionally patients may present with "constipation" secondary to rectal spasm. Although patients may present with extraintestinal manifestations before bowel symptoms, more often they parallel the severity of the primary bowel disease.

8. How are patients with ulcerative colitis classified?

Truelove and Witts divided patients into those with severe, moderate, and mild disease based on symptoms, physical findings, and laboratory values. We add to this list the severity of endoscopic and radiologic appearances. A plain film of the abdomen showing any degree of dilation of the colon or ulceration and edema of the mucosa is indicative of a severe attack. Although endoscopic appearance does not always correlate well with clinical symptoms, the presence of severe mucosal disease indicates the need for more aggressive management.

Clinical Guide for Severity of Ulcerative Colitis

Mild	Fewer than 4 stools daily, with or without blood, with no systemic disturbance and a normal erythrocyte sedimentation rate (ESR).
Moderate	More than 4 stools daily but with minimal systemic disturbance.
Severe	More than 6 stools daily with blood and systemic disturbance as shown by fever, tachycardia, anemia, or ESR > 30.

9. How are the extraintestinal manifestations of ulcerative colitis classified?

Although ulcerative colitis involves primarily the bowel, it may be associated with manifestations in other organs. These manifestations are divided into those that coincide with the activity of bowel disease and those that occur independently of bowel disease.

EXTRA COLONIC MANIFESTATION	COINCIDES WITH COLITIS ACTIVITY
Colitic arthritis	Yes
Ankylosing spondylitis	No
Pyoderma gangrenosum	Yes
Erythema nodosum	Yes
Primary sclerosing cholangitis	No
Uveitis	Often, but not always
Episcleritis	Often, not always

10. What is colitic arthritis?

Colitic arthritis is a migratory arthritis affecting the knees, hips, ankles, wrists, and elbows. It responds well to corticosteroids.

11. Describe the association between ulcerative colitis and ankylosing spondylitis.

Patients with ulcerative colitis have a 30-fold increased risk of developing ankylosing spondylitis, which does not parallel disease activity. Many patients with early sacroiliitis alone are asymptomatic, and the diagnosis is made on radiographs.

12. Dsicuss the hepatic complications of ulcerative colitis.

Hepatic complications include fatty liver, pericholangitis, chronic active hepatitis, cirrhosis, and primary sclerosing cholangitis. Although most patients with sclerosing cholangitis have ulcerative colitis, only a minority of patients with ulcerative colitis develop sclerosing cholangitis. It is usually suspected with the finding of an abnormally elevated alkaline phosphatase or gamma glutamyl transferase (GGTP) enzyme. Sclerosing cholangitis is sometimes improved with ursodeoxycholic acid therapy (Actigall). Patients with sclerosing cholangitis and ulcerative colitis have a higher risk of developing colon cancer than those without. In addition, they are also at risk of developing cholangiocarcinoma. Cholestyramine may help in alleviating the pruritus associated with the disease, but the only cure is liver transplantation.

13. What are the ocular complications of ulcerative colitis?

Ocular complications include uveitis and episcleritis. Uveitis causes eye pain, photophobia, and blurred vision and requires prompt intervention to prevent permanent visual impairment.

14. Describe the association between ulcerative colitis and thromboembolic events.

Patients with IBD are at increased risk of thromboembolic events, most commonly deep venous thrombosis of the lower extremities. After a search for other causes of a hypercoagulable state, patients should receive standard therapy for the thrombosis.

15. How do I evaluate a patient with ulcerative colitis?

The management of ulcerative colitis depends on the severity and location of disease activity, which are best assessed by a careful clinical history, with emphasis on the duration and severity of symptoms, and physical examination, followed by endoscopic evaluation to determine the extent and severity of mucosal involvement. Although flexible sigmoidoscopy may indicate the severity of the disease, full colonoscopy is essential to determine the extent as well as the full severity. A plain radiograph of the abdomen also should be performed in flat and upright positions to recognize depth of ulceration and early or advanced toxic megacolon, which may be suspected by the presence of tympany in any of the segments of the abdomen.

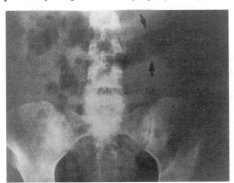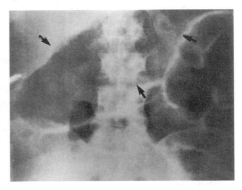

Toxic megacolon is a clue to imminent bowel perforation or worsening colitis. The condition is obvious when the width of the colon reaches 9 cm. *Left,* Early toxic dilation of the transverse colon with scalloped mucosa *(arrows).* The width of the colon was < 6 cm. In addition, a diseased segment of the sigmoid colon is outlined by air. *Right,* Late toxic megacolon involving primarily the transverse and descending colon *(arrows).* Inflammation has resulted in thickening of the bowel wall.

16. What are 5-ASA products?

Sulfasalazine, the first 5-ASA product, has been used successfully for many years in the treatment of mild-to-moderate ulcerative colitis. It is linked to sulfapyridine by a diazo bond that is cleaved by colonic bacteria. The active moiety is the 5-ASA. The side effects most commonly caused by sulfasalazine include nausea, vomiting, fever, and a rash, all of which are attributable primarily to the sulfapyridine, which is only a carrier. It also may cause agranulocytosis, autoimmune hemolytic anemia, folic acid deficiency, and infertility secondary to changes in sperm count and morphology. Newer preparations that contain only 5-ASA (mesalamine) are carried through or released in the small bowel. Mesalamine is currently available as a 4-gm enema (Rowasa), as a suppository, and in oral formulations (Asacol, Pentasa, Dipentum).

5-ASA	CARRIER MOLECULE	RELEASE	SITE OF ACTIVITY
Asacol	Eudragit-S	pH > 7.0	Terminal ileum and colon
Pentasa	Ethylcellulose beads, time release	pH > 6.0	Small bowel and colon
Olsalazine	Azo bond	Bacteria	Colon (ileum with bacterial overgrowth)
Sulfasalazine	Sulfapyridine	Bacteria	Colon (ileum with bacterial overgrowth)

17. How do I treat proctitis and proctosigmoiditis?

For mild-to-moderate ulcerative proctitis, topical therapy may suffice. If disease is limited to the anorectal region, a Rowasa suppository can be used once or twice daily. Hydrocortisone foam (cortifoam) or hydrocortisone enemas (cortenema) also may be used either alone or in alternation with the 5-ASA product. For proctosigmoiditis, the Rowasa enema, used alone or in alternation with a hydrocortisone enema, is effective. Only the Rowasa enema—not the Cortenema— has maintenance value. The patient must lie on the left side for at least 20 minutes after introducing the enema to ensure adequate delivery to the affected area. In some instances when tenesmus is severe, the enema is better introduced in the knee-chest position, taking advantage of the downhill gravity. Occasionally oral therapy may work better than suppositories; in other cases, a combination is required.

18. How do I treat an exacerbation of ulcerative colitis?

When the disease extends more proximally, oral therapies are required in addition to, or instead of, topical therapy. Choice of oral 5-ASA product is determined by the extent of involvement. Pentasa (4 gm) or Asacol (3.2 gm) can be used for universal colitis, and Dipentum (1 gm) for left-sided colitis. The dose of Asacol may be titrated within the limits of tolerability to a maximum of 4.8 gm/day. It is not yet known whether still higher doses of any of the three would have increased efficacy. If the disease fails to resolve with 5-ASA therapy or is moderately severe at presentation, a short course of oral corticosteroids should be prescribed to bring the disease under control. The maximal effective oral dose of prednisone is 60 mg daily. The dose may be tapered to 40 mg/day after 2–7 days, if the disease is brought under control. The formula for further tapering of prednisone is individualized. The 5-ASA drugs should be given concurrently with prednisone. Prednisone and other corticosteroids are not maintenance drugs.

19. What should I do if the disease is severe?

Severe disease requires admission to hospital for intravenous corticosteroids and fluids. Patients should be monitored carefully by serial physical examination, lab tests, and plain radiographs of the abdomen. Severe ulcerative colitis may progress to toxic megacolon. It is treated with intravenous corticosteroids, antibiotics, a small bowel tube attached to suction, "log rolling" from side to side and to the supine and prone positions, and sometimes by rectal tube. If these maneuvers are not successful, subtotal colectomy should be considered, preferably before a perforation occurs. If the colon is dilated and the mucosal surface is ragged on abdominal films, a surgical colleague should be involved in management decisions.

If there is no response to intravenous corticosteroids, intravenous cyclosporine should be considered. Rapid deterioration in clinical condition warrants early surgical intervention with ileostomy and subtotal colectomy. If there is time for a trial of cyclosporine, it should be administered only by physicians with extensive experience in its use. It is administered at a dose of 4 mg/kg/day intravenously by continuous infusion, with close monitoring of blood pressure, renal function, electrolytes, and drug blood levels. Cyclosporine should not be initiated if the serum cholesterol is low because it increases the risk of seizures. Bactrim is administered concurrently to prevent *Pneumocystis carinii* pneumonia. Failure to respond within 3 days portends a poor prognosis for medical therapy. Early medical intervention in expert hands can significantly reduce the number of severely ill patients who go to surgery.

20. Define toxic megacolon.

Toxic megacolon is defined as a severe attack of colitis with total or segmental dilation of the colon (diameter of transverse colon usually > 5–6 cm). Megacolon is considered toxic if 2 or more of the following criteria are positive in addition to the colon persistently outlined by air:

1. Tachycardia with a pulse rate > 100 beats/min
2. Temperature > 101.5°F
3. Leukocytosis > 10,000 cells/mm^3
4. Hypoalbuminemia < 3.0 gm/dl

21. How do I prevent a relapse?

Maintenance therapy should be initiated at the same time or soon after acute-phase therapy. For mild-to-moderate disease, a 5-ASA product may be all that is necessary. For more severe or recurrent disease, an immunosuppressive medication such as 6-mercaptopurine (6-MP) or azathioprine is more effective. 6-MP should be started at a dose of 50 mg/day, and the patient should be followed carefully with weekly blood counts for the first 3 weeks and less often thereafter. If the initial dose is tolerated well and the white cell count is normal, the dose may be gradually increased if clinically warranted. Early toxic reactions to these medications include pancreatitis (3%), hepatitis, rash, fever, and leukopenia. The occurrence of pancreatitis or hepatitis usually precludes further use of the same drug. Patients with allergic type reactions may be carefully desensitized to the same or the other immunosuppressive drug. High levels of the 6-MP metabolites 6-MMP (6 methyl mercaptopurine) and 6-TG (6-thioguanine) may predict which patients will develop toxicity. Although there is much ongoing research on anti-TNF agents and interleukins for the treatment of Crohn's disease, no evidence to date indicates that these medications are effective or useful in ulcerative colitis.

22. How often should patients have surveillance colonoscopy?

The current recommendations are as follows: for patients with left-sided colitis, surveillance should begin after 15 years of colitis. For patients with universal colitis, surveillance should begin after 8 years of colitis. Three biopsy specimens should be obtained every 10 cm throughout the colon. In addition, any strictured, raised, polypoid areas or those with unusual shapes or textures should be biopsied. Surveillance colonoscopy should be repeated annually for universal disease, perhaps less often for left-sided disease.

23. What should be done if a polyp or dysplasia is found?

Obvious polyps should be removed and the area surrounding the polyp biopsied. If the area is free of premalignant changes, nothing further need be done except for the usual surveillance. However, if dysplasia is found, colectomy is the treatment of choice. Dysplasia is a premalignant lesion classified as high-grade, low-grade, or indefinite. Although everyone agrees that high-grade dysplasia anywhere in the colon warrants proctocolectomy, there is less consensus about management of low-grade dysplasia. The diagnosis of low-grade dysplasia can be challenged when the biopsies are taken from areas of marked inflammation. Intensive treatment of the disease may lead to the recognition that the diagnosis of dysplasia was not accurate. Biopsies should be taken preferably from flat mucosa without inflammation. If a recommendation of colectomy depends on the diagnosis of dysplasia, a second expert gastrointestinal pathologist should review the biopsy slides before the final decision is made.

24. Define DALM.

DALM is a **d**ysplasia-**a**ssociated **l**esion or **m**ass and is an indication for total colectomy. If, however, the mass is a polyp and no dysplasia is present elsewhere in the colon, a simple polypectomy can be performed without colectomy and the surveillance routine continued.

25. Is surveillance effective?

Studies have shown that as many as 42% of patients with ulcerative colitis who are found to have high-grade dysplasia either already have cancer or develop it within a short time. The presence of low-grade dysplasia is also predictive of cancer: 19% of patients develop cancer of the colon or may even have cancer at the time of diagnosis. The finding of no dysplasia is predictive of a good short-term outcome. Outcome and case-controlled studies have shown that cancer in patients in a surveillance program is detected at an earlier and therefore more favorable stage. Patients who undergo screening have improved survival rates and lower cancer-related mortality rates.

26. Is diet important in the management of ulcerative colitis?

No evidence suggests that any one diet is beneficial in patients with ulcerative colitis. Apart from the advice that patients with lactose intolerance should avoid lactose-containing food, no dietary restrictions are necessary. Because chronically ill patients may be in a consistently negative caloric balance, maintaining a balanced diet is of the utmost importance.

27. Does stress exacerbate ulcerative colitis?

No studies to date support any role for psychological stresses, personality types, or overt psychiatric illness in the causation or exacerbation of ulcerative colitis. However, many physicians believe that psychosocial stress plays an important role not only in precipitating illness but also in preventing healing. This belief is validated by the fact that many patients experience exacerbations during times of emotional stress. When a patient remains ill despite maximal medical therapy, consideration should be given to psychological factors. A psychopharmocologist can be invaluable in this setting. Sometimes the addition of an anxiolytic agent or an antidepressant may be the final step required to bring ulcerative colitis under control.

As with any chronic illness, the approach to management should be multifaceted with expert medical and surgical teams, a psychopharmacologist, and knowledgeable ancillary staff.

28. How does menstruation affect ulcerative colitis?

Scattered information supplements our experience that the symptoms of both ulcerative colitis and Crohn's disease are aggravated or provoked coincidentally with the premenstrual period and in some cases throughout menstruation. Occasionally a 2–3-day course of steroids is warranted.

29. Do patients with ulcerative colitis have problems with fertility and pregnancy?

In considering the effects of ulcerative colitis on pregnancy and vice versa, two aspects are important: the effect of the disease itself and the effect of the medications used to treat the disease. Well-controlled disease appears to have no deleterious effects on fertility or pregnancy. However, if the disease is active at any time during pregnancy, the incidence of fetal loss may be increased. It is therefore important to maintain control of the disease before and during pregnancy.

Mesalamine (5-ASA) has a long record of safety in pregnancy. Corticosteroids have also proven to be safe during pregnancy. With regard to the immunosuppressants 6-MP and azathioprine, data from the transplant literature suggest safety during pregnancy. In our experience, however, these medications may cause fetal loss when used by women before pregnancy and an increased incidence of congenital abnormalities and spontaneous abortions when used by men within 3 months of conception. We therefore suggest that patients should discontinue these drugs, if clinically feasible, at least 3 months before planned conception. Sulfasalazine causes defects in sperm morphology and motility. It should be replaced with one of the newer 5-ASA products in male patients who are contemplating starting a family.

30. What medications are contraindicated in patients with ulcerative colitis?

Evidence suggests that nonsteroidal anti-inflammatory drugs may precipitate exacerbations of the disease and in some cases may even be implicated in the onset of disease. These drugs, including aspirin, should be avoided in patients with ulcerative colitis.

Anticoagulant therapy with warfarin may lead to increased bleeding in patients with active disease and bloody diarrhea. Ironically, heparin therapy has been reported to improve disease activity in some patients. Although heparin therapy is not the standard of care, it may be useful when anticoagulation is required for patients with active ulcerative colitis. Opioid derivatives should be avoided if possible in patients with any type of colitis because of their propensity to cause toxic dilatation of the colon.

31. What are the surgical options for management of ulcerative colitis?

When medical management fails or complications such as perforation or dysplasia occur, subtotal colectomy with ileostomy or ileoanal pouch is the procedure of choice. Many patients are frightened by the prospect of having an ileostomy, but education can do much to alleviate their fears. Fortunately, a large number of patients with ileostomies become accustomed to them and continue to lead normal lives.

The ileoanal pouch is a possible alternative. It consists of a double loop of ileum that is fashioned into a pouch and stapled to the rectal stump and stripped of its mucosa, thereby preserving the anal sphincter. Disadvantages of the pouch include recurrent inflammation or "pouchitis," frequent bowel movements, nocturnal incontinence, and the continued need for surveillance endoscopy. Pouchitis responds well to metronidazole, which can be used to treat the acute illness and also as a maintenance therapy to prevent recurrence. Some patients with refractory pouchitis may require excision of the pouch and substitution of an ileostomy at a later date.

BIBLIOGRAPHY

1. Adler DJ, Korelitz BI: The therapeutic efficacy of 6-mercaptopurine in refractory ulcerative colitis. Am J Gastroenterol 85:717–722, 1990.
2. Lichtiger S, Present DH, Kornbluth A, et al: Cyclosporine in severe ulcerative colitis refractory to steroid therapy. N Engl J Med 330:1841–1845, 1994.
3. Marshall JK, Irvine EJ: Rectal aminosalicylate therapy for distal ulcerative colitis: A meta-analysis. Aliment Pharmacol Ther 9:293–300, 1995.
4. Orholm M, Munkholm P, Langholz E, et al: Familial occurrence of inflammatory bowel disease. N Engl J Med 324:84–88, 1991.
5. Pemberton JH, Kelly KA, Beart RW, et al: Ileal pouch-anal anastomosis for chronic ulcerative colitis: Long-term results. Ann Surg 206:504–513, 1987.
6. Rajapakse RO, Korelitz BI, Zlatanic J, et al: Outcome of pregnancies when fathers are treated with 6-mercaptopurine for inflammatory bowel disease. Am J Gastroenterol 95:684–688, 2000.
7. Sandborn WJ: Pouchitis following ileal pouch-anal anastomosis: Definition, pathogenesis and treatment. Gastroenterology 107:1856 1860, 1994.
8. Sutherland LR, May GR, Shaffer EA: Sulfasalazine revisited: A meta-analysis of 5-aminosalicylic acid in the treatment of ulcerative colitis. Ann Intern Med 118:340–349, 1993.
9. Truelove SC, Witts LJ: Cortisone in ulcerative colitis. Final report on a therapeutic trial. BMJ 2:1041– 1048, 1955.
10. Winawer SJ, Fletcher RH, Miller L, et al: Colorectal cancer screening: Clinical guidelines and rationale. Gastroenterology 112:594–642, 1997.
11. Woolrich AJ, DaSilva MD, Korelitz BI: Surveillance in the routine management of ulcerative colitis: Predictive value of low-grade dysplasia. Gastroenterology 103:431–438, 1992.

45. SMALL BOWEL TUMORS

Yael Vin, M.D., and Jeffrey B. Matthews, M.D.

1. What is the incidence of small bowel tumors?

Although containing more than 75% of the length and 90% of the mucosal surface area of the gut, the small bowel is the least common site of primary cancer. It accounts for 3–6% of all GI tumors, two-thirds of which are malignant. Thus, cancer of the small bowel accounts for 1–2% of GI malignancies and 0.1–0.3% of all malignancies. Incidence varies among populations, ranging between 9.6 and 13 small bowel malignancies per million.

2. How is the low incidence of small bowel tumors explained?

- Products of bacterial metabolism in the large bowel (such as secondary bile acids) can be carcinogenic.
- The small bowel lumen is alkaline and therefore does not allow activation of certain carcinogens.
- The small bowel has well-developed lymphatic tissue, and large amounts of protective IgA are produced.
- Transit time is faster and exposure to carcinogens is shorter.
- Benzpyrene hydroxylase is present in higher concentrations in small bowel compared with colon and stomach. It converts benzpyrene, a known carcinogen in food, to less toxic metabolites.
- Relative dilution of carcinogens in the liquid contents of the small bowel as well as less irritation of the mucosa.
- Small bowel mucosa has a high cell turnover. Compared with the large bowel, it has fewer stem cells (carcinogen target cells), which are shielded within the crypts. Carcinogens induce programmed cell death (apoptosis) so that genetically mutant cells are removed.

3. List the primary small bowel tumors.

Primary small bowel tumors, benign and malignant, develop in all histologic components of the small bowel, as summarized in the table below:

TISSUE OF ORIGIN	BENIGN	MALIGNANT
Mucosa	Adenoma	Adenocarcinoma
Enterochromaffin		Carcinoid
Lymphoid		Lymphoma
Smooth muscle	Benign GIST (leiomyoma)	Malignant GIST (leiomyosarcoma)
Vascular	Hemangioma	Angiosarcoma
	Lymphangioma	Lymphangiosarcoma
		Kaposi's sarcoma
Connective tissue	Fibroma	Fibrosarcoma
Nerve	Neurofibroma	Neurofibrosarcoma
	Schwann cell tumor	Malignant schwannoma
Fat	Lipoma	Liposarcoma

GIST = gastrointestinal stromal tumor.

4. Which tumors are most common?

The most common tumors and their most frequent location are listed in the table below. Geographic and ethnic variations in histologic subtypes explain the large, overlapping ranges of percentiles.

SMALL BOWEL TUMOR	% BY HISTOLOGY*	COMMON SITE OF PRIMARY TUMOR
Adenocarcinoma	20–70	Duodenum (periampullary), jejunum
Carcinoid	1–4	Ileum (distal)
Lymphoma	3–50	Jejunum, ileum
Sarcoma	5–25	Jejunum, ileum

* Selected case series.

5. Which tumors commonly metastasize to the small bowel?

Despite the rarity of primary tumors, the small bowel is frequently involved in metastatic disease. Common primary malignancies, in order of frequency, include melanoma, ovarian cancer, bladder cancer, breast cancer, and lung cancer. Genitourinary and other GI tumors can involve the small bowel by direct extension.

6. Describe the common presenting signs and symptoms.

Presenting symptoms are often vague and nonspecific, leading to delayed diagnosis (mean duration of symptoms: 3–12 months). The number of small bowel tumors found on autopsies suggests that most tumors are asymptomatic. The most common presenting symptoms are abdominal pain, 67%; GI bleed (occult, melena or manifest bleeding), 41%; weight loss, 38%; nausea and vomiting, 33%. There is no clear difference in presentation between benign and malignant tumors.

7. List other, less frequent presentations.

- Bowel obstruction (13% of patients): usually a late sign due to liquid contents of the bowel
- Intussusception: in adults the common lead point is a small bowel tumor, usually benign (lipomas)
- Palpable mass: 7–18% of malignant cases (usually leiomyosarcomas)
- Painless jaundice in periampullary adenocarcinoma (it may be transient and resolve when the tumor undergoes necrosis and sloughing with free passage of bile)
- Perforation: almost always with lymphomas (25% of lymphomas present with perforation)

In addition, the presentation may mimick parasitic infection in immunoproliferative small intestinal disease (fever, diarrhea, abdominal pain) or carcinoid syndrome (flushing, hypotension, diarrhea) in metastatic carcinoid tumors. Intestinal ischemia has been reported sporadically with carcinoid tumors (vascular obstruction due to lymph node involvement and changes in vessel wall secondary to vasoactive factors secreted by the tumor).

8. What are the major risk factors for small bowel cancer?

- Age: incidence rises with age (mean age: 60 ± 10 years) across histologic subtypes.
- Sex: men have a higher incidence for all main histologic subgroups.
- Race: incidence of adenocarcinoma and carcinoid is slightly higher among blacks than whites.
- Diet: consumption of animal fat and protein as well as smoked or cured food is associated with a higher relative risk for developing adenocarcinoma.

9. Which heritable conditions increase the relative risk of small bowel cancer?

1. **Adenomatous polyposis coli** (familial adenomatous polyposis and Gardner's syndrome). Hereditary polyposis syndromes are associated with colorectal and duodenal adenomas. Patients are at risk for developing adenocarcinoma, especially around the ampulla of Vater, and should undergo endoscopic screening.

2. **Peutz-Jeghers syndrome** is associated with hamartomas of the GI tract. Although malignant degeneration is rare, patients have an increased incidence of small bowel adenocarcinoma.

3. **Hereditary nonpolyposis colon cancer** (Lynch II syndrome) is associated with a higher-than-expected incidence of small bowel adenocarcinoma.

4. **Von Recklinghausen's disease** (neurofibromatosis type 1) is associated with occasional schwannomas of the small bowel.

10. Which immunodepressed conditions increase the risk of small bowel cancer?

1. **HIV infection** will soon become the leading cause of primary GI lymphomas (usually high-grade B-cell non-Hodgkin's lymphoma). Although tumors are found more commonly in the colon and cecum, patients occasionally present with small bowel tumors (usually in the ileum). HIV is also associated with Kaposi's sarcoma, which usually involves the skin but can appear in any organ.

2. **Immunosuppresion** with cyclosporine is associated with an increased incidence of small bowel lymphomas in transplant patients.

3. **Congenital immunodeficiency syndromes** predispose to GI lymphoma.

11. Which conditions associated with an impaired mucosal barrier increase the risk of small bowel cancer?

1. **Crohn's disease** has a well-established association with small bowel adenocarcinoma. Severe disease (duration, fistulous disease, excluded loops of bowel) increases the risk of cancer. Prolonged treatment (especially with 6-mercaptopurine) has been suggested as another possible factor.

2. **Celiac disease** predisposes patients to the development of primary T-cell lymphoma. Control of the disease seems to decrease the risk for subsequent malignancy.

3. *Helicobacter pylori* **infection** may be a risk factor for gastric lymphoma. In addition, reports of regression of small bowel lymphomas (mucosa-associated lymphoid tissue [MALT]) after *H. pylori* treatment suggest a similar association.

12. What conditions associated with altered luminal contents increase the risk of small bowel cancer?

Previous cholecystectomy, ureterosigmoidostomy, and peptic ulcer disease.

13. How are small bowel tumors diagnosed?

1. **Plain radiographs** can show signs of obstruction but are not helpful in localizing and diagnosing the cause.

2. **Endoscopy** is the primary means of assessing the upper GI tract. Push enteroscopy (endoscope advanced into jejunum) and small bowel enteroscopy (flexible fiberoptic instrument with a balloon at the tip, propelled through the intestine by peristalsis) are also available. Disadvantages include incomplete view of the mucosa (because instruments are difficult to control) and limited instrument advancement (because of adhesions, strictures, and decreased motility).

3. **Barium studies** have an important role in the diagnosis of small bowel tumors. Sensitivity is lower with small bowel follow-through (61%) than with small bowel enteroclysis (95%). Small bowel enteroclysis is done by placing a tube in the duodenum and instilling a mixture of barium, air, and water or methyl cellulose.

4. **CT scan** has different sensitivities in identifying small bowel tumors, depending on location: almost 100% in the duodenum, 17% in the jejunum, and 70% in the ileum. Various small bowel neoplasms have characteristic features that make CT helpful for diagnosis. CT also can show the presence extensive metastatic disease.

5. **CT enteroclysis** (helical CT with enteroclysis) is a new method for detecting small bowel tumors and seems to be more sensitive than conventional barium studies.

6. **MRI** is effective in detecting small bowel tumors.

Other studies depend on presentation. For example, bleeding scan and angiography may be used to localize bleeding, whereas octreotide scan and levels of biologic markers are helpful when carcinoid syndrome is suspected.

14. What is the major cause of delay in diagnosis?

In some reported series, radiologic misinterpretation or false-negative exams.

15. List the different types of small bowel adenomas. How are they treated?

Adenomas may occur as part of a polyposis syndrome or sporadically.

• **Tubular adenoma:** usually a pedunculated lesion with low malignant potential. Although mostly asymptomatic, lesions may present with bleeding. Treatment should include endoscopic polypectomy or local surgical resection.

- **Villous adenoma:** sessile lesion with malignant potential (carcinoma is present in up to 30% of large periampullary tumors). Presentation may include bleeding, obstruction, or obstructive jaundice because of the common location in proximity to the ampulla of Vater. Treatment should include endoscopic polypectomy or surgical local resection. If invasive carcinoma is present in the specimen, major resection is required.
- **Brunner's gland adenomas:** hyperplasia of the glands in the first part of the duodenum with no malignant potential. Lesions are usually asymptomatic (incidental finding on endoscopy) but may mimic peptic ulcer disease or cause obstruction. Endoscopic resection of symptomatic lesions is adequate treatment.

16. How are adenocarcinomas treated?

With wide resection, including wide lymphadenectomy. Small bowel is resected with 5 cm of distal and proximal margins. For all tumors in the first and second and some in the third portion of the duodenum, pancreaticoduodenectomy is indicated. Because of the small number of patients, the role of adjuvant chemotherapy has not been clearly defined; there is no proof that it enhances survival in advanced disease. In practice, patients undergoing pancreaticoduodenectomy for duodenal tumors receive chemoradiation similar to that used for patients undergoing surgery for adenocarcinoma of the head of the pancreas. Patients with advanced-stage small bowel tumors receive chemotherapy regimens commonly used for colorectal tumors.

17. Describe the different types of primary intestinal lymphoma.

Small bowel lymphomas are non-Hodgkin's lymphomas, mainly of the B-cell type. The extranodal marginal zone B-cell MALT tumors are the most common type and are divided into two separate clinical and pathologic entities, as described in the table below.

MORPHOLOGY (WHO CLASSIFICATION)	MATURE (PERIPHERAL) B-CELL					MATURE T-CELL
	EXTRANODAL MARGINAL ZONE B-CELL LYMPHOMA (MALT TYPE)		DIFFUSE LARGE B-CELL	MANTLE CELL	BURKITT'S LYMPHOMA	ENTEROPATHY TYPE T-CELL (EATCL)
Subtypes	Adult western (non-IPSID)	IPSID	High-grade MALT type*		Usually nonendemic	
Population	No age predilection; slight female predominance	Low socioeconomic class, high rate of parasitic infections Median age: 25 yr Male predominance	HIV infection,-immuno--deficiency-related tumors	Rare Male predominance Median age: 63 yr	Children Peak incidence at age 8 yr Occasionally HIV- and immunosuppression-related Burkitt-like lymphoma	Celiac disease Malabsorption
Geographic distribution	Worldwide Most common type in developed nations	Middle East, Mediterranean	Worldwide	Worldwide	Worldwide	Common in Middle East
Common location in small bowel	Distal small bowel	Proximal small bowel	Ileum	Any region Multiple sites	Distal small bowel	Jejunum
Gross pathology	Usually single, ulcerated, protruding, or infiltrating mass	Diffuse infiltrating lesion		Multiple white, fleshy, nodular lesions (lymphomatous polyposis)	Often large mass	Large circumferential ulcer usually with no bulky infiltrating mass

IPSIP = immunoproliferative small intestinal disease
* High-grade transformation of low-grade MALT lymphoma should be classified as diffuse large B-cell lymphoma. The use of terms such as "high-grade MALT" or "high-grade IPSID" should be abandoned.

18. What defines a primary lymphoma of the gut?

Classic criteria (Dawson 1961) define primary lymphoma of the small bowel:
* Absence of peripheral lymphadenopathy on physical examination
* Absence of mediastinal lymphadenopathy on chest x-ray or CT
* Normal white blood cell count and peripheral smear
* Absence of bone marrow lymphoma
* Demonstration at laparotomy that disease is restricted to bowel and proximal lymph nodes with no involvement of liver or spleen

19. Describe the treatment of non-IPSID extranodal marginal B-cell lymphoma and Burkitt's lymphoma.

Treatment includes surgical resection or debulking for large tumors in stage III or IV. The goal of surgery may be curative in low-stage tumors (about 30% of tumors are resectable for cure at presentation). Surgery for more advanced disease prolongs survival by reducing complications (e.g., bleeding, obstruction, perforation, especially after chemotherapy) and tumor load before administration of adjuvant therapy. All patients receive chemotherapy, which is adjusted to tumor stage.

The role of radiation therapy is unclear. It may be effective for palliation in extensive nonresectable disease, but it does not prolong survival and carries a significant risk of acute morbidity from radiation enteritis.

Because of the increasing evidence connecting MALT lymphomas with *H. pylori*, patients with low-grade and low-stage (IE) disease are candidates for anti-*H. pylori* therapy as the initial treatment (in the stomach, complete regression was shown in 50–80% of patients). Very few patients actually fit into this category.

20. Describe the treatment of IPSID lymphoma, mantle cell lymphoma, and EATCL.

Because these tumors are more diffuse, surgery is not an option. Chemotherapy is the mainstay of management.

21. Define GI stromal tumor.

Traditionally leiomyoma and leiomyosarcoma were regarded as tumors originating from smooth muscle. In recent years this theory was questioned. With advanced immunohistochemistry and electron microscopy, it became evident that such tumors arise from different mesodermal components and differ from other smooth muscle tumors in the body. Therefore, the terms leiomyoma and leiomyosarcoma have been replaced by a more general term, gastrointestinal stromal tumor (GIST). The theory is that GISTs arise from the interstitial cell of Cajal, an intestinal pacemaker cell. GISTs may have myogenic features, neural features, or characteristics of both muscle and nerve (mixed GIST), or they may lack differentiation (GIST not otherwise specified). They can present with benign or malignant characteristics.

22. What features predict malignancy in small bowel stromal tumors?

Distinguishing between malignant and benign GISTs may present a challenge. **Clinical features** indicative of malignancy include tumors > 3 cm, rapid tumor growth on serial examination, and metastatic disease. **Histologic features** (in descending order of predictive value) include at least 5 mitoses per high power field, necrosis, hypercellularity, and cytologic atypia.

23. List the important markers of prognosis.

Tumor size, mitotic activity, spread of disease outside the bowel wall, poor histologic grade, short time from symptoms to diagnosis, and possibly DNA ploidy. Because it correlates with tumor size, DNA ploidy may not be an independent factor.

24. How are GISTs treated?

Surgical resection of the entire tumor, along with local extensions and localized peritoneal or liver metastasis, is the treatment of choice. Lymphatic spread is uncommon; therefore, resection of lymph nodes is not indicated. Because malignant GISTs are resistant to radiotherapy and chemotherapy, their role in adjuvant treatment is not defined.

25. What is carcinoid syndrome?

Systemic symptoms resulting from the secretion of humoral factors by the carcinoid tumor. Factors produced by GI carcinoids drain into the portal system and are metabolized by the liver with first passage. Therefore, the presence of carcinoid syndrome in patients with small bowel carcinoids is evidence of liver metastasis, which releases these factors into the systemic circulation.

26. Describe the clinical features of carcinoid syndrome.

1. **Episodic cutaneous flushing** of the face and upper trunk. Severe cases present with hypotension and tachycardia. Flushing episodes can be induced by stress, palpation of the liver, or anesthesia and last from seconds to minutes.

2. **Secretory watery diarrhea** occurs in 80% of patients with carcinoid syndrome.

3. **Bronchospasm** is seen in about 10% of patients with carcinoid syndrome. Treatment with bronchodilators can result in prolonged, intense vasodilatation.

Late manifestations of the disease include **venous telangectasias** (vascular lesions most often seen on the nose, lip, and malar areas) and **carcinoid heart disease**, which occurs in about one-half of patients and is characterized by plaques of fibrous tissue, most commonly on the endocardium of the valvular cusps, primarily of the right heart. This condition progresses with the development of tricuspid insufficiency and pulmonary stenosis and ultimately results in right heart failure.

27. What are the chemical mediators of carcinoid syndrome?

The chemical mediators of carcinoid syndrome are not completely understood. Significantly increased conversion of tryptophan to serotonin by the tumor seems to play a significant role. Serotonin is further metabolized to 5 hydroxyindolcacctic acid (HIAA). An increased level of HIAA in the urine is the diagnostic hallmark of carcinoid syndrome. Serotonin is the most likely cause of the diarrhea and also stimulates fibroblast growth, leading to carcinoid heart disease. Many other substances are produced by carcinoid tumors and may play a role in clinical manifestations, including histamine, kallikrein (both of which may contribute to flushing), bradykinin, somatostatin, and many other peptides as well as prostaglandins.

28. What is carcinoid crisis?

A dramatic and extreme manifestation of malignant carcinoid syndrome that includes an intense generalized flush, hypotension, bronchospasm, arrhythmias, and confusion or stupor that can last for hours or days. Carcinoid crisis can occur spontaneously, after palpation of tumor, or during physically stressful situations (particularly induction of anesthesia). Patients at risk of developing carcinoid crisis usually present with extensive disease or greatly elevated 5-HIAA levels (> 200 mg/day). This condition can be fatal.

29. How are patients with carcinoid syndrome evaluated?

The *first goal* is to confirm that symptoms are the result of a secreting tumor with biochemical testing: (1) urinary excretion of 5-HIAA and (2) blood serotonin levels, which are useful when urinary 5-HIAA is equivocal. Assays for other substances are not widely available. Provocative tests with epinephrine or pentagastrin occasionally are useful in patients with symptoms suggestive of carcinoid syndrome but normal or only marginally elevated biochemical markers. Patients are evaluated for flushing, hypotension, and tachycardia after intravenous injection of epinephrine or pentagastrin.

The *second goal* is to localize the tumor. Abdominal CT (with IV and oral contrast) often detects liver metastases but infrequently localizes the primary tumor. Because tumors contain a somatostatin receptor, indium-111 octreotide imaging is useful in localizing metastatic and primary tumors (60% sensitivity in identifying the primary site). Other studies, such as enteroclysis, endoscopic studies, MRI and angiography, are reserved for selected patients when the above modalities have failed.

Note: Multiple carcinoid tumors may occur in the small bowel.

30. How are carcinoid tumors treated?

The definitive treatment for carcinoid tumors of the small bowel is surgical resection with segmental lymphadenectomy. For patients with advanced metastatic disease, the following options are available:

- Surgery is reserved for the small group in whom metastases can be completely resected and local disease controlled. It prolongs survival or provides cure.
- Palliative surgery may be done for bowel obstruction or mesenteric ischemia.
- Reduction of tumor mass by resection of hepatic metastases palliates the symptoms of carcinoid syndrome, but because of the other therapies listed below, this approach has a limited role in the treatment of advanced disease.
- Chemotherapy is offered for metastatic disease only on an experimental basis. Previous studies showed limited response to multiple cytotoxic agents.
- In one study, immunotherapy with interferon alpha reduced urinary 5-HIAA in 42% of patients and led to tumor regression in 15%. The high rate of adverse reactions limits the use of this drug.
- Somatostatin analogs (such as octreotide) significantly decrease serotonin levels and are highly effective in controlling symptoms of the carcinoid syndrome. Octreotide can be life-saving in cases of carcinoid crisis. Occasionally octreotide treatment results in regression of the tumor.
- Liver-targeted strategies include hepatic artery occlusion/embolization, which has been shown to induce marked symptomatic improvement in 70% of patients and tumor regression in up to 50%. Response lasts 1–18 months. Eventually all patients have recurrences.

31. What is the prognosis of malignant small bowel tumors?

Overall survival of patients with small bowel malignancies is poor:

Adenocarcinoma: periampullary, 30–40% 5-year survival rate; elsewhere in the bowel, < 20%

Leiomyosarcoma: 30–40% 5-year survival rate

Lymphoma: 10–50% 5-year survival rate, with an average of 30%

Carcinoid: overall 5-year survival rate of 54%; 75% for local tumors, 19% for tumors with distant spread

BIBLIOGRAPHY

1. Abeloff MD: Clinical Oncology. 2nd ed. New York, Churchill Livingstone, 2000.
2. Bernstein D, Rogers A: Malignancy in Crohn's disease. Am J Gastroenterol 91:434–440, 1996.
3. Buckley JA, Jones B, Fishman EK: Small bowel cancer imaging features and staging. Radiol Clin North Am 35:381–402, 1997.
4. Cunningham JD, Aleali R, Aleali M, et al: Malignant Small bowel neoplasms: Histopathologic determinants of recurrence and survival. Ann Surg 225:300–306, 1997.
5. Feldman M: Sleisenger and Fordtran's Gastrointestinal and Liver Disease, 6th ed. Philadelphia, W.B.Saunders, 1998.
6. Gore RM: Small bowel cancer: Clinical and pathologic features. Radiol Clin North Am 35:351–360, 1997.
7. Maglinte DT, Reyes BL: Small bowel cancer radiologic diagnosis. Radiol Clin North Am 35:361–380, 1997.
8. Minardi AJ, Zibari GB, Aultman DF, et al: Small-bowel tumors. J Am Coll Surg 186:664–668, 1998.
9. Naef M, Buhlmann M, Baer HU: Small bowel tumors: Diagnosis, therapy and prognostic factors. Langenbeck's Arch Surg 384:176–180, 1999.
10. Neugut AI, Jacobson JS, Suh S, et al: The epidemiology of cancer of the small bowel. Cancer Epidemiol Biomark Prevent 7:243–251, 1998.
11. O'Boyle CJ, Kerin MJ, Feeley K, Given HF: Primary small intestinal tumors: Increased incidence of lymphoma and improved survival. Ann R Coll Surg 80:332–334, 1998.
12. Ojha A, Zacherl J, Scheuba C, Jakesz R, Wenzl E: Primary small bowel malignancies: single-center results of three decades. J Clin Gastroenterol 30:289–293, 2000.
13. Townsend CM: Sabiston Textbook of Surgery, 15th ed. Philadelphia, W.B. Saunders, 1997.

46. EOSINOPHILIC GASTROENTERITIS

Christian Jost, M.D., and Michael B. Wallace, M.D., M.P.H.

1. What is eosinophilic gastroenteritis?

Eosinophilic gastroenteritis is a rare, nonparasitic inflammatory disease of the GI tract with various degrees of eosinophilic infiltration anywhere in the tubular intestinal tract and biliary tree in the absence of vasculitis. Peripheral blood eosinophilia is present in 80% of cases.

2. Why should you know about this rare disease?

Although it is rare, eosinophilic gastroenteritis is treatable and mimics several more common GI diseases. It presents most often with abdominal pain, diarrhea, nausea, vomiting, dysphagia, and gastric outlet obstruction. One-third of patients report body weight loss of > 2.3 kg, especially if a malabsorptive complication is present. If bowel obstruction occurs, patients often require surgery. Spontaneous remission in untreated patients is rare.

3. What is the differential diagnosis of eosinophilic gastroenteritis?

Irritable bowel syndrome
Reflux esophagitis
Parasitic intestinal or extraintestinal disease
  • *Ancylostoma* spp. (hookworm)
  • *Anisakis* spp.
  • *Ascaris* spp.
  • *Capillaria* spp.
  • *Isospora belli* (immunocompromised patients)
  • *Strongyloides* spp.
  • *Toxocara* spp.
  • *Trichura* spp.
  • *Trichinella* spp.
Inflammatory bowel disease
  • Collagenous colitis
  • Ulcerative colitis
  • Crohn's disease
Allergies (food, dust, medication)
  • Celiac disease, cow's milk protein sensitivity, soybean protein sensitivity
  • Medications: gemfibrozil, clofazimine, gold salt azathioprine, sulfamethoxazole, carbamazepine, L-tryptophan

Eosinophilia-myalgia syndrome (L-tryptophan)
Idiopathic hypereosinophilic syndrome
Systemic vasculitis syndromes
  • Churg-Strauss granulomatous vasculitis
  • Polyarteritis nodosa
  • Dermatomyositis/polymyositis
  • Scleroderma
  • Eosinophilic fasciitis
Eosinophilic granuloma or histiocytosis X
Inflammatory fibroid GI polyps
Bowel obstruction
  • Intestinal primary tumors: gastric, colonic, extraintestinal malignancies
  • Extraintestinal tumors and inflammatory diseases
  • With peripheral blood eosinophilia: Hodgkin's lymphoma, mycosis fungoides, chronic myelogenous leukemia, and adenocarcinomas of the lung, stomach, pancreas, ovary, or uterus

4. What causes eosinophilic gastroenteritis?

This immune-mediated disease is most likely the result of several different factors affecting immunologic regulation (i.e., allergic, autoimmune). The initiating pathophysiologic steps are only partially understood. Although eosinophilic gastroenteritis is associated with allergic illnesses in almost one-half of patients, a specific allergic stimulus has not been identified.

5. Why does eosinophilic gastroenteritis have so many different clinical faces?

The anatomic location of the affected organs and the depth of the inflammatory infiltration of the intestinal wall layers and surrounding visceral structures determine the clinical manifestations.

1. **Mucosal eosinophilic infiltration without muscular involvement.** Intestinal eosinophilic mucositis presents as abdominal pain, vomiting, nausea, and diarrhea. It may be complicated by malabsorption with weight loss, protein-losing enteropathy, chronic intestinal blood loss (iron deficiency), or acute intestinal bleeding.

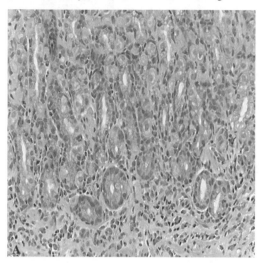
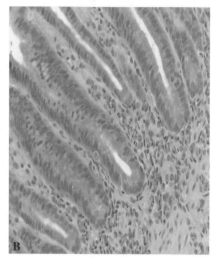

A, Endoscopic biopsy (H&E, 20 ×) from the gastric antrum. Histopathology shows eosinophilic mucosal and submucosal infiltration. *B,* Endoscopic biopsy from the duodenum (H&E, 20 ×) from the duodenum. Histopathology shows typical eosinophilic inflammatory infiltration of mucosa and submucosa.

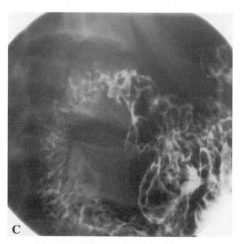
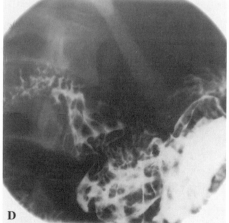

C, Barium double-contrast study. Cobblestone pattern is a typical sign of thickened mucosal folds. This patient has gastric and duodenal eosinophilic gastroenteritis. *D,* Barium double-contrast study of the gastric antrum and duodenum. Roughed mucosal folds are typical in eosinophilic gastroenteritis.

2. **Inflammation of the intestinal muscle layer (muscularis propria).** Muscle layer inflammation results in a rigid gut with symptoms of dysmotility, i.e., dysphagia with esophageal stricture or pseudoachalasia; vomiting and pain with obstruction of the gastric outlet, small intestine, or colon; or bacterial overgrowth. Recurrent acute cholangitis or pancreatitis can present in patients with ampullary infiltration, presumably due to ampullary stenosis.

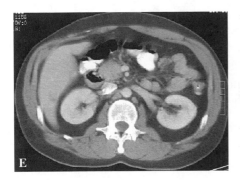 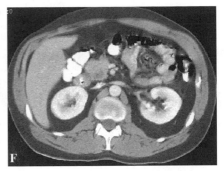

E, Early pancreatitis in duodenal eosinophilic gastroenteritis. *F,* Early pancreatitis in eosinophilic gastroenteritis with duodenal wall thickening.

3. **Subserosal/serosal inflammation**. Subserosal/serosal inflammation presents as eosinophilic peritonitis, ascites, pleural effusions (rare), or an inflammatory tumor with bowel obstruction. Ascitic eosinophil counts can reach more than 80%. The serosal involvement often is accompanied by muscular infiltration.

6. **What signs and symptoms suggest a probable diagnosis of eosinophilic gastroenteritis?**
   Depending on the anatomic structures involved, eosinophilic gastroenteritis presents as esophagitis, gastric outlet obstruction, diarrhea, malabsorption syndrome, protein-losing enteropathy, intestinal blood loss, enteritis syndrome, obstruction of the small or large intestine, peritoneal disease with ascites, biliary obstruction, periampullary tumor, or pancreatitis. Peripheral eosinophilia is present in most patients (80%) with eosinophilic gastroenteritis.

7. **What are the possible radiographic features of eosinophilic gastroenteritis?**
   Gastric retention or small intestinal hypomotility can be demonstrated by barium studies. Double-contrast barium enema or enteroclysis can show mucosal thickening with cobble-stoned or saw-tooth silhouette, nodular filling defects, or coarse folds in the small intestine (see Figs. C and D in question 5). It can mimic regional enteritis (Crohn's disease). Muscle layer disease presents with stiffened and narrowed tubular gut structures, complicated by obstruction of the esophagus, gastric outlet, duodenum, jejunum, ileum, or colon. CT imaging can reveal duodenal wall thickening, inflammatory tumors, or ascites.

8. **What steps should be taken to diagnose eosinophilic gastroenteritis?**
   1. Check the medical history for atopic diseases (present in 50% of patients).
   2. Exclude parasitic intestinal disease by history and three SAF stool samples.
   3. Perform eosinophil counts. Findings supportive of the diagnosis include the following:
      • In peripheral blood smear: eosinophils > 0.250 K/CUMM and 5–35%, respectively. Normal peripheral blood counts are found in 20% of patients.
      • In stool specimens: > 5% eosinophils in differential count of the leukocytes.
      • In deep mucosal biopsies: > 20 eosinophils/high-power (× 1000) field.
   4. When endoscopic biopsies are taken, large, deep specimens are recommended because inflammation spares the mucosal layer). Biopsies should be taken at up to 10 different locations, including the stomach and small bowel, because patchy distribution may lead to sampling error. The diagnosis of eosinophilic gastroenteritis should be proved by tissue biopsies. Endoscopic biopsies from abnormal- and normal-looking mucosa also are recommended. Although the colon and ileum are not often involved, colonic or ileal biopsies can prove the diagnosis.
   5. In deep muscular or peritoneal disease the diagnosis sometimes can be proved only with surgical resection or full-thickness surgical biopsy (open or laparoscopic surgery). Eosinophilic duodenitis with involvement of the duodenal papilla (Vater) can manifest as (recurrent) pancreatitis or cholangitis. ERCP draining of the pancreato-biliary system is indicated.

9. What do you want to exclude in patients with suspected eosinophilic gastroenteritis?
• Drug-induced intestinal disease (e.g., aspirin, gold therapy, gemfibrozil, clofazimine, L-tryptophan)
• Parasitic intestinal disease
• Inflammatory bowel disease, collagenous colitis
• Collagen-vascular disease (i.e., periarteritis nodosa, systemic lupus erythematosus, systemic sclerosis, dermatomyositis, Churg-Strauss syndrome)
• Malignant tumor infiltration
• Lymphoma (i.e., T-cell-lymphomas [Sezary syndrome], chronic myelogenous leukemia, Hodgkin's disease, intestinal lymphoma)

10. How is eosinophilic gastroenteritis treated?
Traditionally glucocorticoid therapy is recommended. Oral prednisone, 0.5 mg/kg day for 2 weeks, often induces remission, regardless of which gut layer is affected. Severe disease with impaired intestinal function should be treated with parenteral methylprednisolone (bolus of 125 mg followed by 0.5 mg/kg twice daily). A 2-week tapering period and complete withdrawal should be tried. Only a few patients need long-term corticosteroid therapy (up to several months). Nonglucocorticoid immune-modulatory therapies may be an alternative in the future:
• Montelukast, a leukotriene-1-receptor antagonist, was effective in several case reports.
• Cromolyn sodium showed efficacy in some case reports.
• Ketotifen, a mast cell stabilizer available in Europe, Canada, and Japan, showed efficacy in 6 patients.

In rare patients with suspected food allergy, a trial of elimination diets elucidates the individual pathogenesis and resolves the disease. Symptomatic treatment includes adequate pain relief, loperamide for diarrhea, and supplementation of deficiencies acquired by malabsorption. Recurrences can be treated with repeat short courses of prednisone. A few patients need long-term low-dose therapy to maintain remission.

BIBLIOGRAPHY

1. Anttila VJ, Valtonen M: Carbamazepine-induced eosinophilic colitis. Epilepsia 133:119–121, 1992.
2. Babb RR: Cromolyn sodium in the treatment of ulcerative colitis. J Clin Gastroenterol 2:229–231, 1980.
3. Bischoff SC, Mayer J, Nguyen QT, et al: Immunnohistological assessment of intestinal eosinophil activation in patients with eosinophilic gastroenteritis and inflammatory bowel disease [see comments]. Am J Gastroenterol 94:3521–3529, 1999.
4. Capron M, Spiegelberg HL, Prin L, et al: Role of IgE receptors in effector function of human eosinophils. J Immunol 132:462–468, 1984.
5. Cello JP: Eosinophilic gastroenteritis—a complex disease entity. Am J Med 67:1097–1104, 1979.
6. Desreumaux P, Bloget F, Seguy D, et al: Interleukin 3, granulocyte-macrophage colony-stimulating factor, and interleukin 5 in eosinophilic gastroenteritis. Gastroenterology 110:768–774, 1996.
7. Eliakim R, Karmeli F, Okon E, Rachmilewitz D: Ketotifen effectively prevents mucosal damage in experimental colitis. Gut 33:1498–1503, 1992.
8. Gallamini A, Carbone A, Lista P, et al: Intestinal T-cell lymphoma with massive tissue and blood eosinophilia mediated by IL-5. Leuk Lymphoma 17:155–161, 1995.
9. Gruber BL, Kaufman LD, Marchese MJ, et al: Anti-IgE autoantibodies in systemic lupus erythematosus. Prevalence and biologic activity. Arthritis Rheum 31:1000–1006, 1988.
10. Gruber BL, Baeza ML, Marchese MJ, et al: Prevalence and functional role of anti-IgE autoantibodies in urticarial syndromes. J Invest Dermatol 90:213–217, 1988.
11. Haberkern CM, Christie DL, Haas JE: Eosinophilic gastroenteritis presenting as ileocolitis. Gastroenterology 74:896–899, 1978.
12. Hertzman PA, Blevins WL, Mayer J, et al: Association of the eosinophilia-myalgia syndrome with the ingestion of tryptophan [see comments]. N Engl J Med 322:869–873, 1990
13. Heyman SN, Karmeli F, Brezis M, Rachmilewitz D: The effect of ketotifen on nitric oxide synthase activity. Br J Pharmacol 120:1545–1551, 1997.
14. Hogan SP, Mishra A, Brandt EB, et al: A critical role for eotaxin in experimental oral antigen-induced eosinophilic gastrointestinal allergy. Proc Natl Acad Sci USA 97:6681–6686, 2000.
15. Jones NL, Roifman CM, Griffiths AM, Sherman P: Ketotifen therapy for acute ulcerative colitis in children: A pilot study. Dig Dis Sci 43:609–615, 1998.
16. Kaijser R: Allergic diseases of the gut from the point of view of the surgeon. Arch Klin Chir 188:36–64, 1937.
17. Klein NC, Hargrove RL, Sleisenger MH, Jeffries GH: Eosinophilic gastroenteritis. Medicine (Baltimore) 49:299–319, 1970.

18. Lee CM, Changchien CS, Chen PC, et al: Eosinophilic gastroenteritis: 10 years experience. Am J Gastroenterol 88:70–74, 1993.
19. Lee M, Hodges WG, Huggins TL, Lee EL: Eosinophilic gastroenteritis. South Med J 89:189–194, 1996.
20. Lee JY, Medellin MV, Tumpkin C: Allergic reaction to gemfibrozil manifesting as eosinophilic gastroenteritis. South Med J 93:807–808, 2000.
21. MacCarty RL, Talley NJ: Barium studies in diffuse eosinophilic gastroenteritis. Gastrointest Radiol 15:183–187, 1990.
22. Martin DM, Goldman JA, Gilliam J, Nasrallah SM: Gold-induced eosinophilic enterocolitis: Response to oral cromolyn sodium. Gastroenterology 80:1567–1570, 1981.
23. Matsushita M, Hajiro K, Morita Y, et al: Eosinophilic gastroenteritis involving the entire digestive tract [see comments]. Am. J Gastroenterol 90:1868–1870, 1995.
24. Michet CJ Jr, Rakela J, Luthra HS: Auranofin-associated colitis and eosinophilia. Mayo Clin Proc 62:142–144, 1987.
25. Mishra A, Hogan SP, Brandt EB, Rothenberg ME: Peyer's patch eosinophils: Identification, characterization, and regulation by mucosal allergen exposure, interleukin-5, and eotaxin. Blood 96:1538–1444, 2000.
26. Moots RJ, Prouse P, Gumpel JM: Near fatal eosinophilic gastroenteritis responding to oral sodium chromoglycate. Gut 29:1282–1285, 1988.
27. Orenstein SR, Shalaby TM, Di Lorenzo C, et al: The spectrum of pediatric eosinophilic esophagitis beyond infancy: A clinical series of 30 children. Am J Gastroenterol 95:1422–1430, 2000.
28. Ravi S, Holubka J, Veneri R, et al: Clofazimine-induced eosinophilic gastroenteritis in AIDS [letter]. Am J Gastroenterol 88:612–613, 1993.
29. Riedel RR, de Jonge JP, Hartmann A: Gastrointestinal type 1 hypersensitivity to azathioprine. Klin Wochenschr 68:50–52, 1990.
30. Talley NJ, Shorter RG, Phillips SF, Zinsmeister AR: Eosinophilic gastroenteritis: A clinicopathological study of patients with disease of the mucosa, muscle layer, and subserosal tissues. Gut 31:54–58, 1990.
31. Sanderson CJ: Interleukin-5, eosinophils, and disease. Blood 79:3101–109, 1992.
32. Sanderson CJ: Pharmacological implications of interleukin-5 in the control of eosinophilia. Adv Pharmacol 23:163–177, 1992.
33. Schoonbroodt D, Horsmans Y, Laka A, et al: Eosinophilic gastroenteritis presenting with colitis and cholangitis. Dig Dis Sci 40:308–314, 1995.
34. Spiegelberg HL: Structure and function of Fc receptors for IgE on lymphocytes, monocytes, and macrophages. Adv Immunol 35:61–88, 1984.
35. Stahle-Backdahl M, Maim J, Veress B, et al: Increased presence of eosinophilic granulocytes expressing transforming growth factor-beta1 in collagenous colitis. Scand J Gastroenterol 35:742–746, 2000.
36. Stern M, Meagher L, Savill J, Haslett C: Apoptosis in human eosinophils. Programmed cell death in the eosinophil leads to phagocytosis by macrophages and is modulated by IL-5. J Immunol 148:3543 3549, 1992.
37. Tang S, Lo CY, Lo WK, Chan TM: Resolution of eosinophilic peritonitis with ketotifen. Am J Kidney Dis 30:433–436, 1997.
38. Vitellas KM, Bennett WF, Bova JG, et al: Idiopathic eosinophilic esophagitis [see comments]. Radiology 186:789–793, 1993.
39. Vo-Dinh T, Panjehpour M, Overholt BF, et al: In vivo cancer diagnosis of the esophagus using differential normalized fluorescence (DNF) indices. Lasers Surg Med 16:41–47, 1995.
40. Weller PF, Bubley GJ: The idiopathic hypereosinophilic syndrome. Blood 83:2759–2779, 1994.
41. Weller PF: Eosinophils: structure and functions. Curr Opin Immunol 6:85–90, 1994.
42. Weltman JK: Cytokines: regulators of eosinophilic inflammation. Allergy Asthma Proc. 21:203–207, 2000.
43. White MV, Baer H, Kubota Y, Kaliner M: Neutrophils and mast cells: characterization of cells responsive to neutrophil-derived histamine-releasing activity (HRA-N). JAllergy Clin.Immunol 84:773–780, 1989.
44. Wienand B, Sanner B, Liersch M: [Eosinophilic gastroenteritis as an allergic reaction to a trimethoprim- sulfonamide preparation]. Dtsch Med Wochenschr 116:371–374, 1991.
45. Zahavi I, Weizen T, Marcus H, et al: Ketotifen is protective against indomethacin-induced intestinal ulceration in the rat. Isr J Med Sci 32:312–315, 1996.

47. BACTERIAL OVERGROWTH

Jack A. DiPalma, M.D.

1. Define bacterial overgrowth.

Overgrowth is defined by an increased number of bacteria in areas of the gastrointestinal tract that usually do not provide the environment suitable for the colonization and proliferation of bacteria.

2. What is the usual bacterial presence in the gastrointesintal tract?

• Stomach	$< 10^4$/ml	• Ileum	$< 10^6$/ml
• Jejunum	$< 10^5$/ml	• Colon	$< 10^{10}$/ml

The type of species that colonize the small intestine is changed in bacterial overgrowth. In health, small bowel bacteria resemble oropharyngeal flora with gram-positive, aerobic organisms. In overgrowth, bacteria are mostly gram-negative, including *Escherichia coli*; anaerobic bacteria, including *Clostridia* and *Bacteroides* species, also predominate.

3. What factors influence small intestinal bacterial proliferation?

- Structural lesions
- Motility
- Excessive bacterial load
- Deficiency in host defenses

4. What kind of structural lesions predispose to overgrowth?

Obstruction to outflow of luminal contents can occur at the site of surgical anastomosis or with webs, adhesions, or strictures. Surgical diversions and blind loops or neoreservoirs, such as the continent ileostomy, predispose to small intestinal bacterial overgrowth. The jejunoileal bypass, once a popular surgical procedure for morbid obesity, created a long segment of diverted bowel and was often complicated by overgrowth. Diverticula and duplications are frequently colonized with colonic-type bacteria, leading to overgrowth.

5. How do motility disorders cause overgrowth?

Delayed transit of intestinal contents results in stasis. Overgrowth complicates intestinal pseudo-obstruction syndromes. The intestinal "house keeper" migratory motor complex, when disrupted, is associated with bacterial overgrowth. Paralytic ileus results in bacterial proliferation.

6. How can an excessive bacterial load be delivered to the small bowel?

Absence or incompetence of the ileocecal valve and enteric fistula can deliver bacteria to the small bowel in amounts that exceed clearing capacity.

7. Which impairments of host defenses are important?

- Acid suppression by surgery or medications
- Hypochlorhydric disorders such as pernicious anemia
- Immune deficiencies, particularly absence of secretory immunoglobulin A (IgA)
- Undernutrition, which can decrease gastric acidity and immune function

8. What conditions are associated with small intestinal bacterial overgrowth?
Reduced gastric acid

- Pernicious anemia
- Atrophic gastritis
- Gastric surgery
- Medications (H_2 receptor antagonists, proton-pump inhibitors)
- Neoreservoirs

Structural abnormalities
- Small bowel diverticula
- Surgical anastomosis and diversions
- Strictures
- Webs

- Adhesions
- Fistulas (colonteric, gastrocolic)
- Absent or incompetent ileocecal valves
- Neoreservoirs

Dysmotility syndromes
- Diabetes
- Scleroderma

- Acute enteric infection
- Intestinal pseudo-obstruction syndromes

9. What are the other risk factors for bacterial overgrowth?

Evidence indicates that overgrowth with colonic-type bacteria should be considered in patients over 75 years of age with chronic diarrhea, anorexia, or nausea, even if they have no apparent predisposition. Dysmotility is probably responsible. Additional data suggest that overgrowth may cause diarrhea or abdominal pain in children, especially those younger than 2 years. Recent data implicate bacterial overgrowth in some patients with irritable bowel syndrome.

10. What are the symptoms of overgrowth?

Clinical manifestations vary. Diarrhea, anorexia, nausea, weight loss, and anemia are cardinal symptoms, but the nature of the small bowel abnormality influences the presentation. Patients obstructed by stricture may have bloating and pain. Overgrowth in small intestinal diverticula may present insidiously with metabolic derangements. The eventual clinical consequence of overgrowth, regardless of cause, is steatorrhea, leading to weight loss. Malabsorption results in hypocalcemic disorders, night blindness, vitamin K deficiency, and osteomalacia. Cobalamin deficiency is common with severe overgrowth.

11. Why do patients with bacterial overgrowth develop anemia?

Anemia may be megaloblastic and macrocytic as a result of cobalamin deficiency. Microcytic anemia due to iron deficiency results mainly from blood loss, not bacterial overgrowth. Anaerobic bacteria compete for uptake of cobalamin–intrinsic factor complex. Whereas luminal bacteria consume cobalamin, folic acid is a product of bacterial substrate fermentation. Thus, an important clinical observation in small intestinal bacterial overgrowth is the finding of low B12 and high folate levels.

12. What other micronutrient deficiencies are clinically important?

In addition to iron and cobalamin deficiencies, other micronutrient deficiencies include deficiencies of water-soluble vitamins (e.g., thiamine and nicotinamide) and decreased absorption of fat-soluble vitamins (vitamins A, D, E, and K). Trace element malabsorption has not been carefully studied in overgrowth syndromes.

13. How is bacterial overgrowth diagnosed?

Small intestinal bacterial overgrowth is confirmed by the demonstration of elevated numbers of small bowel bacteria colonies and the replacement of oropharyngeal with predominantly colonic organisms. Because small bowel intubation and aspiration for microbial analysis are cumbersome, overgrowth is considered in patients with predisposing factors and appropriate history. Indirect testing may help to substantiate the diagnosis.

14. What indirect testing can be used?

Diagnosis of Bacterial Overgrowth

History	Prior surgery, medical conditions such as osteomalacia, night blindness, easy brusibility, tetany
Examination	Systemic disease: weight loss and malabsorption
Laboratory values	Hemoglobin (decreased), mean corpuscular volume (increased), vitamin B12 (decreased), folic acid (increased), fecal fat (increased)

Table continued on following page

Diagnosis of Bacterial Overgrowth (Continued)

Tests	Schilling test with intrinsic factor (decreased), ^{14}C-glycocholic acid (increased), ^{14}C-D-xylose (decreased), hydrogen testing with glucose or lactulose, jejunal aspirate for bacterial colony counts and strain identification.

15. What are the limitations of testing?

Jejunal intubation for aspiration with bacterial colony counts and stain identification can provide a definitive diagnosis by showing jejunal counts > 105 with colonic organisms. Because the test is cumbersome, some clinicians rely on indirect testing. Jejunal intubation can be performed endoscopically, and protected catheters can be used to obtain reliable aspirates.

Radiolabelled breath tests using glycocholic acid or xylose have been used for diagnosis of overgrowth. Glycocholic acid is released by bacterial deconjugation of radiolabelled bile acids. Xylose is catabolized by gram-negative aerobes and is absorbed in the proximal small bowel.

Fasting breath hydrogen is elevated in overgrowth patients, and early rises after glucose or lactulose challenge reflect small bowel fermentation of the substrate by abnormal concentrations of bacteria.

In general, **scintigraphic** and **hydrogen breath tests** are attractive alternatives to intubation tests for bacterial overgrowth. Hydrogen testing, although simple, inexpensive, and nonradioactive, does not have sufficient sensitivity or specificity.

16. What about other testing methods?

Quantification of urinary excretion of indican, drug metabolites, and conjugated para-aminobenzoic acid do not distinguish overgrowth from other types of malabsorption.

17. What is the treatment for bacterial overgrowth?

1. **Correction of the underlying condition**
   - Surgery
   - Prokinetic agents
2. **Nutrition**
   - Lactose-free, low-residue diet
   - Increase calories
   - Micronutrient supplementation (B12, fat soluble vitamins, trace elements)
3. **Antibiotics**

18. Do prokinetic agents help?

Surgery is often impractical or unacceptable, and prokinetic agents are tried to relieve stasis and improve outflow of small intestinal contents. However, standard stimulatory agents are not very effective. The long-acting somatostatin analog, octreotide, has been shown to stimulate motility in normal subjects and patients with scleroderma. It reduces overgrowth and improves symptoms in scleroderma.

19. Which antibiotics are preferred?

The optimal choice of antibiotic and dosage regimen has not been determined. Some investigators prefer broad-spectrum antibiotics such as cephalosporins, tetracyclines, or chloramphenicol. Others recommend narrower-spectrum drugs active against anaerobes, such as metronidazole, or against aeroanaerobes, such as fluoroquinolones. A recent study showed efficacy with either norfloxacin or amoxicillin-clavulanic acid.

20. How long should overgrowth be treated with antibiotics?

A single 7–10-day course usually suffices, but recurrence is frequent. Some patients require retreatment in weeks or months; others need continuous therapy. Prolonged antibiotic therapy poses significant risk, including resistance and enterocolitis.

21. What about probiotics?

Saccharomyces boulardi is a probiotic used in treatment of pseudomembranous colitis that has stated efficacy for bacterial overgrowth in children. Because antibiotics have potential side effects, probiotic therapy is attractive. A recent study in adults, however, showed no efficacy of *Saccharomyces boulardi* in treatment of overgrowth.

BIBLIOGRAPHY

1. Ahar A, Flourie B, Rambaud JC, et al: Antibiotic efficacy in small intestinal bacterial overgrowth-related chronic diarrhea: A cross-over, randomized trial. Gastroenterology 117:794–797, 1999.
2. de Boissieu D, Chaussain M, Badoual J, et al: Small-bowel bacterial overgrowth in children with chronic diarrhea, abdominal pain, or both. J Pediatr 128:203–207, 1996.
3. Pimentel M, Lin HC: Eradication of small bowel bacterial overgrowth decreases symptoms in irritable bowel syndrome [abstract]. Am J Gastroenterol 94:2652, 1999.
4. Riordan SM, McIver CJ, Wakefield D, et al: Small intestinal bacterial overgrowth in the symptomatic eldery. Am J Gastroenterol 92:47–51, 1997.
5. Riordan SM, McIver CK, Walker BM, et al: The lactulose breath hydrogen test and small intestinal bacterial overgrowth. Am J Gastroenterol 91:1795–1803, 1996.
6. Rose S, Young MA, Reynolds JC: Gastrointestinal manifestations of scleroderma. Gastroenterol Clin North Am 27:563–594, 1998.
7. Sherman PM: Bacterial overgrotwh. In Yamada T (ed): Textbook of Gastroenterology. Philadelphia, J.B. Lippincott , 1991, pp 1530–1539.
8. Soudah HC, Hasller WL, Owyang C: Effect of octreotide on intestinal motility and bacterial overgrowth in scleroderma. N Engl J Med 325:1461–1467, 1991.
9. Toskes PP, Kumar A: Enteric bacterial flora and bacterial overgrowth syndrome. In Feldman M (ed): Sleisenger and Fordtran's Gastrointestinal and Liver Disease, 6th ed. Philadelphia, W.B. Saunders, 1998, pp 1523–1535.

48. SHORT BOWEL SYNDROME

Jon A. Vanderhoof, M.D., and Rosemary J. Young, R.N., M.S.

1. Define short bowel syndrome.

Short bowel is a malabsorptive state that often follows massive resection of the small intestine. The definition is a functional one; the extent or location of resection is independent of the degree of malabsorption. In many patients, adequate caloric and macronutrient absorption is possible despite significant malabsorption of micronutrients and fluid. In other patients, malabsorption may be uncompensated despite aggressive therapy.

2. What are the most common causes of short bowel syndrome in infants and children?
- Necrotizing enterocolitis
- Intestinal atresia
- Gastroschisis
- Volvulus
- Meconium ileus
- Hirschsprung's disease

The largest number of patients are children who undergo resection due to necrotizing enterocolitis, which causes ischemic injury to the small intestine, most often in the ileum or proximal colon. Possible causes include milk protein allergy, abnormal immunologic response to bacteria, and ischemia.

3. List the most common causes of short bowel syndrome in older children.
- Crohn's disease with intestinal resection
- Intestinal tumors
- Radiation enteritis

4. List the most common causes of short bowel syndrome in adults.
- Crohn's disease with intestinal resections
- Radiation enteritis
- Trauma

5. What is the primary focus of therapy for short bowel syndrome?

Therapy is focused on replacing nutrients due to the loss of overall bowel absorptive surface. The inherent characteristics of the remaining small intestine are crucial in determining functional ability to adapt.

6. Explain the difference between the jejunal and ileal epithelium and how it affects nutrient absorption.

The jejunal epithelium differs significantly from the ileum because it is relatively porous, allowing free and rapid flux of water and electrolytes. Its characteristic long villi create a large absorptive surface area. Most carbohydrate, protein, and water-soluble vitamins are absorbed in the upper 200 cm of jejunum. Fat absorption, however, occurs over a larger area. The ileum is a site of significant reabsorption of fluid and electrolytes, and, because the porous structures between the cells in the ileum are much smaller, the potential for back diffusion of these substances is lower.

7. What is the goal of early therapy for short bowel syndrome?

Early therapy is directed toward stimulating intestinal adaptation, a process characterized by villus hyperplasia and resulting in increased length of villi, increased absorptive surface area, and a gradual increase in functional absorption.

8. How is the goal of early therapy achieved?

Enteral nutrition is necessary. Despite provision of adequate calories and nutrients by the parenteral route, enteral nutrition is key to stimulating adaptation. Direct contact of nutrients with intestinal epithelium stimulates increased work in the small intestine, resulting in mucosal cell proliferation, as well as stimulation of various trophic hormones that are secreted into the bloodstream and also stimulate adaptation.

9. What are the two main nutrients absorbed primarily from the ileum?

Vitamin B12 intrinsic factor and bile salts absorbed through site-specific receptors are the primary nutrients absorbed in the ileum. Therefore, loss of ileum may result in B12 deficiency and chronic bile acid malabsorption with eventual bile salt insufficiency and malabsorption of fat-soluble vitamins.

10. The initial phase of therapy for short bowel syndrome involves parenteral nutrition as the primary source of nutrition. Explain the focus of the therapy in relation to high-volume stool output.

Fluid and electrolyte balance is of primary importance in the immediate postoperative period. Standard solutions of total parenteral nutrition (TPN) can be used. Additional replacement fluid is prescribed by monitoring stool ostomy output for electrolyte content and replacing the amount of fluid loss on an ml-for-ml basis, according to losses accrued in the preceding 2 hours. Electrolyte concentration of the secreted fluid can be assessed on a daily basis to determine the appropriate replacement fluid. Replacing fluids with a solution separate from the parenteral nutrition and adjusting the rate of solution upward or downward, as needed, ensures metabolic stability and is more economical than frequent parenteral nutrition changes.

11. When is enteral nutrition initiated?

Enteral nutrition should begin as soon as fluid and electrolyte losses have diminished or been controlled.

12. Administration of what percentage of enteral feeding is necessary to prevent complications of parenteral nutrition and promote adaptation?

Even a small percentage of total required calories delivered to the GI tract stimulates intestinal adaptation. In general, the greater the amount of enteral nutrition, the better the adaptation response.

13. Enteral nutrients stimulate adaptation through two primary mechanisms. What are they?

Nutrients stimulate adaptation via direct contact with the mucosal epithelium. An increase in the workload of the epithelium stimulates autocrine or paracrine secretion of trophic substances, which in turn stimulates cell proliferation. Enteral nutrition also increases gastrointestinal secretions from the stomach, pancreas, and small intestine, which are also trophic to the small bowel.

14. What is the most beneficial formula type for continuous enteral fusion in infants < 1 year of age?

Elemental (amino acid) formulas are beneficial in reducing the risk of secondary protein intolerance (allergies) because many infants with short bowel syndrome are intolerant of hydrolyzed cow's milk protein. The transition to commercially available whole-protein formulas is often well tolerated after 1 year of age.

15. Oral feeding in patients with short bowel syndrome can markedly affect stool volume and nutrient malabsorption. What specific recommendations for the oral diet decrease nutrient losses?

High-carbohydrate diets can enhance bacterial growth by providing more substrate for bacterial fermentation and also increase osmotic load in the bowel, which contributes to diarrhea, especially in children. In adults, however, a low-fat, high-carbohydrate diet may be beneficial in decreasing oxylate absorption and calcium and magnesium losses, which are greater on a high-fat diet. In older children and adults, fiber-supplemented diets are well tolerated and may provide firmer stools with the beneficial effects of short-chain fatty acid production, which provides additional calories and enhances intestinal adaptation. Overall, a balanced diet of protein, fat, and carbohydrate is probably most beneficial.

16. The most critical time to monitor for micro- or macronutrient deficiency is during which phase of nutritional therapy?

During the later stages of therapy. As parenteral nutrition is weaned and enteral therapy constitutes the sole source of nutrition, it is critical to monitor for deficiencies. Fat-soluble vitamins, calcium, magnesium, zinc, and vitamin B12 deficiencies occur most commonly.

17. What is the function of cholestyramine?

Cholestyramine is beneficial in binding malabsorbed bile acids, especially after ileal resection, and may help to diminish the effects of secretory diarrhea.

18. Why must cholestyramine be used judiciously?

Patients may experience fat-soluble vitamin deficiency because cholestyramine binds all bile acids, which are necessary for fat absorption.

19. Frequent catheter line sepsis has been associated with what complication?

TPN-related liver disease may be more prominent, especially in children who experience frequent catheter sepsis on parenteral nutrition.

20. Why is small bowel bacterial overgrowth common in short bowel syndrome?

Because of dilatation of small intestine, poor motility, and lack of an ileocecal valve.

21. What are symptoms of small bowel bacterial overgrowth?

The most common symptoms include abdominal bloating, abdominal pain, exacerbation of diarrhea, and weight loss.

22. What are the most beneficial diagnostic studies to identify small bowel bacterial overgrowth?

- Glucose breath hydrogen test. Glucose is used rather than lactose because it is absorbed rapidly in the small bowel and usually is not malabsorbed into the colon. An increase > 20 ppm in the first hour after glucose consumption is considered diagnostic of small bowel bacterial overgrowth.
- Measurement of urine indicans (normal = nondetectable)
- Measurement of serum D-lactate levels (normal < 0.25 mmol/L)
- Empiric trial of antibiotic therapy

Small bowel dilatation, which occurs during adaptation of patients with short bowel syndrome, can become problematic with small bowel bacterial overgrowth. Surgical tapering and/or lengthening of the adapted bowel is sometimes beneficial.

23. Explain the mechanism of D-lactic acidosis. What are the symptoms? How is it treated?

D-lactic acidosis results from carbohydrate overload in the colon, which disturbs the normal pattern of colonic fermentation and leads to accumulation of D-lactate in the blood. Neurologic symptoms include headache, dizziness, seizure-like activity, and coma. D-lactic acidosis occurs more commonly in patients with short bowel syndrome and an intact colon; however, it also may occur in absence of the colon because bacterial overgrowth may occur in the remaining small bowel, which adapts by dilatation. Small bowel dilatation results in fluid stasis and promotes bacterial proliferation. A low-carbohydrate diet to decrease the substrate for bacterial fermentation and antibiotic therapy to decrease bacterial counts may be beneficial in less severe cases.

24. What is the primary complication of surgical procedures designed to slow intestinal transit via creation of intestinal valve-like areas?

Small bowel bacterial overgrowth.

25. List common methods to treat small bowel bacterial overgrowth.

• Rotation of broad-spectrum antibiotic therapy. Common medications initially utilized include Bactrim (4 mg TMP/kg/day and 20 mg SMZ/kg/day), gentamicin (5 mg/kg/day), and Flagyl (15-20 mg/kg/day). Some patients are best maintained on continuous antibiotic therapy rotating the type of antibiotic intermittently, whereas others may do well with a one-week course of antibiotics monthly.

• Low-carbohydrate, high-fat diet to reduce substrate for bacterial metabolism.

• Bowel cleansing with a polyethylene glycol (PEG) solution 1–2 times/week.

• Anti-inflammatory therapy for severe cases, including Azulfidine and/or prednisone therapy as indicated. Enteritis due to small bowel bacterial overgrowth is thought to result from similar mechanisms as inflammatory bowel disease, i.e., the body's immunologic reaction to numerous bacterial antigens. Suppression of the inflammation may be beneficial.

26. List dietary interventions and/or drugs that may stimulate intestinal adaptation.

• Glutamine therapy (the exact benefit is controversial, but it is believed to be safe)

• Growth hormone (currently under study)

• Long-chain fats (especially eicosapentaenoic acid and arachidonic acid, which have been shown in animal models to enhance adaptation)

27. What is the optimal time to consider small intestinal transplantation?

Small intestinal transplantation should be considered when the mortality risk of intravenous nutrition is significantly greater than it would be after transplantation. Because posttransplant mortality rates after 1 year are 40–60%, listing for transplantation should not be considered early in the course of therapy. However, when irreversible liver disease begins to appear, listing for transplantation should be considered.

28. What are the indications for liver/bowel or isolated bowel transplantation?

Liver/bowel transplantation should be considered when irreversible liver damage accompanies short bowel syndrome. Isolated small bowel transplants are indicated for progressive but reversible early TPN-related liver disease, loss of central venous access, or recurrent life-threatening episodes of sepsis.

29. What is the Bianchi procedure?

The Bianchi procedure involves narrowing a dilated intestinal segment.

30. When is the optimal time to consider the Bianchi procedure?

The Bianchi procedure may be effective if the dilated bowel segment is significantly impairing the patient's ability to digest and absorb nutrients because of symptoms of bacterial overgrowth. In addition, a dilated segment may contribute to poor motility of the bowel, which also enhances overgrowth and prevents enteral nutrition advancement.

31. What is the prognosis with small bowel, liver, and/or combined transplantation?

Results vary somewhat among centers. For liver transplantation, preliminary experience suggests a posttransplant survival rate at 1–2 years of approximately 70%. The 5-year survival rate of combined liver/bowel transplants is 60%; for isolated bowel transplant, it is approximately the same.

32. What problems slow or temporarily interrupt advancement of enteral nutrition?

• Increase in intestinal fluid losses > 25% above the usual level

• Stool that becomes watery and tests positive for reducing substances

• Visible (not occult) blood with loose stools

33. Describe the prognosis in patients on long-term home TPN.

The prognosis for patients with long-term home TPN is generally considered good. The long-term survival rate is 80–85% in centers structured to care for such patients.

34. What nutrient is the most beneficial in stimulating intestinal adaptation?

Fats, particularly long-chain fats, have been researched most thoroughly and found to be beneficial in intestinal adaptation. Malabsorption of fat occurs in patients with short bowel syndrome, but it is not associated with osmotic fluid loss.

35. What basic equation is used to wean patients from TPN as enteral nutrition is advanced?

During continuous enteral/parenteral therapy, for every increase in the enteral drip rate, the parenteral nutrition can be lowered by an isocalorically equivalent amount. Calculating the caloric exchanges must take into account malabsorption of some enteral nutrition; thus, isocaloric changes are not always possible. Weight gain and fluid and electrolyte balance also should be factored into changes in therapy.

36. Explain why oxalate kidney stones often complicate short bowel syndrome. What are the treatment options?

Increased fat malabsorption from an enteral diet binds calcium and frees oxalate, thus facilitating oxalate absorption and resulting in hyperoxaluria and calcium oxalate stones. Dietary restrictions in foods high in oxalate, such a rhubarb, cocoa, and tea, may be helpful in addition to lowering the fat content of the diet.

37. Explain the mechanism of the development of gallstones in patients with short bowel syndrome.

Gallstones develop because of gallbladder stasis due to lack of enteral feeding as well as cholesterol precipitation from the low concentration of bile salts in the bile, which are lost because of malabsorption. Early cholecystectomy may be advocated for some patients on long-term parenteral nutrition, but early enteral feeding is the best prevention. Use of ursodeoxycholic therapy also has been suggested.

38. Explain the loss of intestinal length and the portion of intestine lost in relationship to expected nutritional therapeutic interventions and complications.

The small intestine is approximately 275 cm in the newborn, growing to 5–6 meters in the adult. Most digestion and absorption of nutrients occur in the first 100 cm of the jejunum. Vitamin B12 and bile acids, however, are absorbed in the ileum. In adults, if < 200 cm of small bowel remain, TPN is required for a few months to allow adaptation. If < 60 cm of small intestine remain, lifetime TPN may be required. Probably because of greater adaptation, children with as little as 40 cm of small bowel are frequently weaned from TPN over time. Control of complications of bacterial overgrowth and associated enteritis also facilitates weaning from parenteral nutrition.

39. What two functions of the colon generally improve the prognosis for weaning from TPN in patients with short bowel syndrome?

Because the colon efficiently absorbs sodium, sodium depletion is unusual when > 50% of the colon is resected or not utilized. The colon also absorbs short-chain fatty acids, which can act as an energy source, salvaging calories from malabsorbed carbohydrates. Unfortunately, the presence of malabsorbed long-chain fatty acids and bile salts in the colon may result in watery diarrhea and increase oxylate absorption.

40. Explain briefly the essential functions of vitamin B12.

Vitamin B12 is an essential nutrient for all cells of the body. B12 deficiency causes failure of nuclear maturation and division and greatly inhibits the rate of red blood cell production. It is stored in large quantities in the liver (1000 µg), and the body requires about 1 µg/day to maintain normal red blood cell maturation. It may take several months for an adult to develop B12 deficiency.

41. Vitamin B12 deficiency is expected with the loss of how much intestine?

When > 60 cm of ileum is resected, B12 deficiency develops. Because B12 is poorly absorbed via the oral route, subcutaneous or intranasal delivery is often required when parenteral nutrition is discontinued.

42. What mechanism in short bowel syndrome often leads to the development of esophagitis, gastritis, and duodenitis? How are these disorders treated?

Loss of intestine probably results in the loss of the normal hormonal feedback loops that suppress gastrin secretion. People with short bowel syndrome have rapid intestinal transit due not only to significantly diminished bowel length but also to loss of enteroglucagon and peptide YY, which are vital in initiating the ileal brake. The standard treatment is acid suppression therapy.

BIBLIOGRAPHY

1. Buotos D, Pons S, Pernas JC, et al: Fecal lactate and short bowel syndrome. Dig Dis Sci 3:2315–2319, 1994.
2. Dahlquist NR, Perrault J, Callaway CW, Jones JD: D-lactic acidosis and Encephalopathy after jejunoileostomy: Response to overfeeding and to fasting in humans. Mayo Clin Proc 59:141–145, 1984.
3. Fanucci A, Cerro P, Fanucci E: Normal small bowel measurements by enteroclysis. Scand J Gastroenterol 23:574–576, 1988.
4. Feldman EJ, Dowling RH, McNaughton J, Peters TS: Effects of oral versus intravenous nutrition on intestinal adaptation after small bowel resection on the dog. Gastroenterology 70:712–719, 1976.
5. Jeejeebhoy KN: Therapy of the short gut syndrome. Lancet 1:1427–1430, 1983.
6. Lennard-Jones JE: Review article: Practical management of the short bowel. Aliment Pharmacol Ther 21:563–577, 1994.
7. Michail S, Vanderhoof JA: Parenteral nutrition in clinical practice. Ann Nestle 54:53–60, 1996.
8. Newton CR, Gonvers JJ, McIntyre PB, et al: Effect of different drinks on fluid and electrolyte losses from a jejunostomy. J R Soc Med 78:27–34, 1985.
9. Nightingale JMD, Kamm MA, van der Sijp JRM, et al: Gastrointestinal hormones in short bowel syndrome: Peptide YY may be the "colonic brake" to gastric emptying. Gut 39:267–272, 1996.
10. Nightingale JM, Lennard-Jones JE, Walker ER, Farthing MJG: Jejunal efflux in short bowel syndrome. Lancet 336:765–768, 1990.
11. Roslyn JJ, Pitt HA, Mann L, et al: Parenteral nutrition-induced gall bladder disease: A reason for early cholecystectomy. Am J Surg 148:58–63, 1984.
12. Simko V, Lin WG: Absorption of different elemental diets in short bowel syndrome lasting 15 years. Dig Dis 21:419–425, 1976.
13. Straus E, Gerson CD, Yalow RS: Hypersection of gastrin associated with short bowel syndrome. Gastroenterology 66:175–180, 1974.
14. Taylor SF, Sondheimer JM, Sokol RJ, et al: Noninfectious colitis associated with short gut syndrome in infants. J Pediatr 119:24–28, 1991.
15. Thompson JS: Management of the short bowel syndrome. Gastroenterol Clin North Am 23:403–420, 1994.
16. Underhill BML: Intestinal length in man. BMJ 2:1243–1246, 1955.
17. Vanderhoof JA: Short bowel syndrome. In Walker WA, Durie PR, Hamilton JR, et al (eds): Pediatric Gastrointestinal Disease, 2nd ed. St. Louis, Mosby, 1996, pp 830–840.
18. Vanderhoof JA: Short bowel syndrome: Parenteral nutrition versus intestinal transplantation. Pediatr Nutr ISPEN 1:8–15, 1999.
19. Vanderhoof JA: Short bowel syndrome. In Walker WA, Watkins JB (eds): Nutrition in Pediatrics, 2nd ed. Hamilton, B.C. Decker, 1996, pp 609–618.
20. Vanderhoof JA: Clinical management of the short bowel syndrome. In Balistreri WJ, Vanderhoof JA (eds): Pediatric Gastroenterology and Nutrition. London, Chapman & Hall, 1990, pp 24–33.
21. Vanderhoof JA, Kollman KA, Griffin SK, Adrian TE: Growth hormone and glutamine do not stimulate intestinal adaptation following massive small bowel resection in the rat. J Pediatr Gastroenterol Nutr 25:327–331, 1997.
22. Vanderhoof JA, Young RJ: Use of probiotics in childhood gastrointestinal disorders. J Pediatr Gastroenterol Nutr 27:323–332, 1998.
23. Vanderhoof JA, Young RJ, Murray N, Kaufman SS: Treatment strategies for small bowel bacterial overgrowth in short bowel syndrome. J Pediatr Gastroenterol Nutr 27:155–160, 1998.
24. Westergaard H, Spady DK: Short bowel syndrome. In Sleisenger MH, Fordtran JS (eds): Gastrointestinal Disease, 5th ed. Philadelphia, W.B. Saunders, 1993.
25. Williamson RCN: Intestinal adaptation: Mechanisms of control. N Engl J Med 298:1444–1450, 1978.

49. COLORECTAL CANCER

Neil Toribara, M.D., Ph.D.

1. What is colorectal cancer?

Colorectal cancer (CRC) includes both colon and rectal cancer. Over 95% of the primary cancers arising in the large bowel are adenocarcinomas; the remainder are lymphomas, malignant carcinoids, leiomyosarcomas, and Kaposi's sarcomas. Adenocarcinomas often are described by degree of differentiation, i.e., the degree to which the cells are organized into recognizable glands containing variable amounts of mucins (high-molecular-weight glycoproteins). Several variants of adenocarcinomas have been described. **Signet-ring carcinomas** are characterized by large, mucin-containing vacuoles, which displace the nucleus to one side of the cell. Occasionally islands of malignant cells are found in what appear to be "mucin lakes" (mucinous or colloid carcinomas). **Scirrhous carcinomas** have sparse gland formation accompanied by marked desmoplasia and dense fibrous tissue. As a general rule, poorly differentiated adenocarcinomas tend to be more aggressive, metastasize earlier, and have a poorer prognosis than well-differentiated tumors.

2. How does the pathophysiology of rectal cancer differ from cancer elsewhere in the colon?

The rectum is relatively immobile, lacks a serosal covering, and is located largely behind the peritoneal reflection, surrounded by perirectal fat. As a result, rectal cancers more commonly spread contiguously by direct extension into local structures, whereas colon cancer more commonly spreads via lymphatics and hematogenously. Thus, rectal cancers that have spread beyond the mucosa are treated with surgery and adjuvant radiation with or without chemotherapy, whereas colon cancers are treated with surgery and chemotherapy rather than radiation. Several observations suggest that the biologic behavior of the cecum and ascending colon may differ slightly from the biologic behavior of the rectum and sigmoid. Examples include different distributions of sporadic and hereditary nonpolyposis colon cancers and carbohydrate structures on surface glycoproteins.

3. How common is colorectal cancer?

Cancer is the second leading cause of death in the United States (after cardiovascular disease), and colorectal cancer is the second leading cause of death from malignancies (after lung cancer). The lifetime risk of developing CRC is 1 in 18 (5.5 %). The incidence is estimated at 130,000 new cases per year, with approximately 56,500 deaths in the year 2000. The incidence is lower in women, but because women live longer, the actual numbers of deaths in men and women are about equal. Of note, the mortality rate from colorectal cancer and breast cancer is approximately the same in women over the age of 60, although the incidence rate for breast cancer is substantially higher. The incidence of CRC peaked in the mid 1980s and has slowly declined since that time, reflecting the effects of increased availability of colonoscopy, gradual acceptance of CRC screening, and the lag time between polyp formation and malignant transformation.

4. What genetic mutations are involved in the genesis of CRC?

Cancer is caused by the accumulation of heritable mutations in cellular DNA, resulting in uncontrolled cell growth. The bowel mucosa is continually exposed to carcinogens, both of natural and man-made origin. Replicating linear DNA in actively dividing cells is more susceptible to the effects of mutagens than the condensed DNA of quiescent cells. Ordinarily, cells in the colonic mucosa replicate near the base of the colonic crypts, with terminal differentiation and eventually programmed cell death (apoptosis) as the cells migrate toward and onto the luminal surface of the bowel, thus minimizing contact between potential mutagens and vulnerable replicating DNA. Any process resulting in retention of replicative ability as cells migrate toward the colonic lumen, such as increased replication rate, abnormal differentiation, or decreased apoptosis, increases the risk of mutagenesis in the colonic mucosa.

5. Do the genetic defects leading to sporadic CRC differ from those in genetic syndromes associated with colon cancer?

Yes. In most sporadic CRC and familial adenomatous polyposis (FAP) syndrome, genetic abnormalities accumulate via loss of large pieces of DNA, known as loss of heterozygosity (LOH). The most common acquisition sequence of genetic abnormalities is thought to be APC, *ras*, p53, and DCC. The order of allelic deletion is not as important as the cumulative loss of DNA or LOH. In hereditary nonpolyposis colorectal cancer (HNPCC) and a small minority of sporadic CRCs, the abnormalities accrue through accumulation of point mutations, which cannot be corrected because of defects in the DNA repair system.

Comparison of Sporadic Colon Cancer with HNPCC and FAP

	SPORADIC CRC	HNPCC	FAP
Mean age at diagnosis	69	44	39
Arise from adenomas	Yes (< 10)*	Yes (< 10)	Yes (hundreds to thousands)†
Distribution	65% distal to splenic flexure	70% proximal to splenic flexure	Throughout entire colon and rectum
Genetic abnormalities	Polygenic‡	hMSH2, hMLH1, hMSH6, hPMS1, hPMS2	APC
Variants	—	Lynch II syndrome	Gardner's syndrome, AAPC
Malignancies at non-colonic sites	No	Yes	Yes
Mechanism for accumulating genetic abnormalities	Loss of heterozygosity: 85% / Failure of mismatch repair: 15%	Failure of mismatch repair	Loss of heterozygosity

* Individual adenomas in HNPCC are thought to have an increased risk of malignant transformation.
† A variant of FAP, attenuated adenomatous polyposis coli (AAPC), has 1–100 adenomas.
‡ 25% of "sporadic" CRCs are thought to have an inherited component; genetic abnormalities are not defined.

6. Describe the natural sequence from colon adenoma to colon cancer.

One of the major milestones in gastroenterology was the confirmation of the adenoma-carcinoma hypothesis that adenomatous polyps are premalignant lesions. The National Polyp Study showed that removal of colonic adenomas during colonoscopy prevented subsequent development of colorectal cancer, showing that colonic adenomas are a vital step, which can be interrupted, in the carcinogenic progression of sporadic CRC. The prevalence curves for adenomas and colorectal cancers parallel each other, with the adenoma curve shifted 5–10 years earlier than carcinomas. This suggests that the time needed for an adenoma to develop into cancer is 5–10 years, thus giving a significant window of time to discover and remove premalignant lesions.

7. How prevalent are colonic adenomas among the U.S. population?

The prevalence of adenomatous polyps appears to be highly dependent on the population studied, with rates as high as 50–60% in one series. Colonoscopic studies in asymptomatic populations have yielded somewhat lower rates. Two studies report 23–25% prevalence in male and female patients between the ages of 50 and 82 years; two other studies involving only males in Department of Veterans Affairs Medical Centers had prevalence rates of approximately 40%.

8. Where in the colon are polyps most commonly located?

Autopsy series have showed a relatively even distribution of adenomas throughout the colon, although larger polyps have a distal predominance, as expected from the distribution of CRCs.

9. How does the morphologic type of colon polyps influence endoscopic management?

Most adenomas appear to protrude into the bowel lumen either on a stalk (pedunculated) or directly from the bowel wall (sessile). Recently a "flat adenoma" has been described, which may be more difficult to diagnose even on colonoscopy, particularly in the setting of less-than-excellent bowel preparation. However, follow-up from the National Polyp Study and other smaller studies suggests that flat adenomas are not large contributors to the total number of CRC cases in the U.S. Even large sessile polyps often can be removed safely by lifting them away from the bowel wall, using submucosal injection of saline or saline with 1:10,000 dilution of epinephrine. Failure of submucosal injection to lift a sessile polyp may indicate invasive malignancy that fixes the adenoma to the bowel wall.

10. Give the mean age of onset and describe the anatomic distribution of CRC.

True sporadic CRCs occur at a mean age of 69; approximately 60% are distal to the splenic flexure (thus theoretically within the reach of a flexible sigmoidoscope). However, some studies have suggested that older patients and African-Americans appear to have an increased proportion of CRCs in the right colon. If this finding is supported by larger studies, it may have a profound effect on the choice of procedures for screening.

11. How are malignant polyps defined? How are they clinically managed?

Pathologists prefer the term *severe dysplasia* for adenomas with a focus of carcinoma in situ or intramucosal carcinoma, because complete endoscopic removal is curative. The term *malignant polyp* is reserved for the appoximately 5% of adenomas in which a focus of carcinoma has invaded beyond the muscularis mucosa into the submucosa, where lymphatic spread with metastasis is possible. A malignant polyp has at least one of the following characteristics: (1) poorly differentiated cancer, (2) invasion of veins or lymphatics, (3) extension of the carcinoma to < 2mm of the margin, or (4) invasion of submucosa of the bowel wall. Malignant polyps with any one of these characteristics should be surgically resected. Endoscopic removal of a malignant polyp is associated with a 10–25% relapse rate.

12. What determines prognosis?

Although the overall 5-year survival is about 62% in the U.S., there are significant differences among ethnic groups and in other countries. The best determinant of prognosis is stage at diagnosis. The two most widely used staging methods are the Dukes and TNM (tumor, node, metastasis) systems. Both give essentially equivalent information for prognostic purposes. The Dukes system is simpler and still widely used by gastroenterologists and surgeons, whereas TNM staging is used more widely among oncologists and pathologists. Other factors, such as aneuploidy (abnormal DNA content), poorly differentiated histology, invasion of venous or lymphatic structures, and mucinous or scirrhous histology, also predict poor prognosis. African-Americans appear to have a lower 5-year survival rate than Caucasians, probably because of decreased access to care. Cultural and genetic factors, however, cannot be ruled out entirely.

Dukes Classification vs. TNM Staging

DUKES CLASSIFICATION*	5-YR. SURVIVAL (%)	TNM STAGING[†]	5-YR. SURVIVAL (%)
		Stage 0	
		Carcinoma in situ Tis N0 M0	100
Stage A	95–100	**Stage I**	
Limited to mucosa		Tumor invades submucosa T1 N0 M0	95
		Tumor invades muscularis propria T2 N0 M0	80
Stage B1	80–85	**Stage II**	
Into muscularis propria		Tumor invades thorugh muscu-	
Stage B2	75	cularis propia into serosa or	
Through serosa		pericolonic, perirectal tissues T3 N0 M0	
		Tumor perforates or directly invades other organs T4 N0 M0	

Table continued on following page

Dukes Classification vs. TNM Staging (Continued)

DUKES CLASSIFICATION*	5-YR. SURVIVAL (%)	TNM STAGING†	5-YR. SURVIVAL (%)
Stage C1	65	**Stage III**	
1–4 regional nodes positive		Any perforation with nodal metas-	
Stage C2	42	tases	
> 4 regional nodes positive		N1: 1–3 nodes Any T N1 M0	
		N2: ≥ 4 nodes Any T N2 M0	
		N3: Any lymph node along any	
		named vascular trunk	
		Any T N3 M0	
Stage D‡	5	**Stage IV**	
Distant metastases		Any invasion of bowel wall with or	
		without lymph node metastasis	
		but with evidence of distant	
		metastasis Any T Any N M1	

* Gastrointestinal Tumor Study Group modification.
† American Joint Committee on Cancer.
‡ Stage D is included in only the Turnbull modification of Dukes classification.

13. Describe the work-up for colorectal cancer after initial diagnosis.

Surgical removal of the cancer remains the only curative therapy. Before surgery, visualization of the entire bowel, preferably by full colonoscopy, is indicated to exclude synchronous lesions (either adenomas or cancers) that may influence the operation. Preoperative laboratory tests should include complete blood count, blood chemistry panel-20, and carcinoembryonic antigen (CEA). If the CEA level is elevated at the time of diagnosis (approximately 60% of cases), it provides a convenient method for assessing effectiveness of the surgery and detecting early recurrences. Preoperative abdominal CT scan and chest radiograph are useful in looking for metastatic disease. MRI is useful as an adjunct if metastatic disease is suspected despite a negative CT (e.g., abnormal liver function tests or rising CEA after surgery). In rectal cancers, preoperative staging with transrectal ultrasound helps to determine the utility of adjunct radiation therapy. Recently, combined modality therapy (radiation + chemotherapy) has been used with some success to debulk large tumors before surgery.

14. What surgical margins are recommended?

Most surgeons attempt to include at least 5 cm on either side of the tumor within the resection block, although margins as small as 2 cm may be acceptable in the distal rectum to preserve sphincter function.

15. Describe the recommended schedule of colonoscopic follow-up after surgery.

If the margins are tumor-free, colonoscopy before 1–3 years after resection is probably not indicated, depending on the degree of presurgical visualization. The risk for developing metachronous neoplasms in a postresection patient is about the same as for a patient with an adenoma of unfavorable histology; therefore, intervals between colonoscopic screening exams should be similar.

16. What is the role of periodic colonosocpy and CEA testing in the long-term follow-up of patients with a history of CRC?

Use of colonoscopy and CEA to detect early recurrences of CRC is somewhat controversial because some studies indicate that detection of recurrent disease results in disease-free, long-term survival in only 3% of patients. Such surveillance should be undertaken only if the patient is willing to undergo repeat exploration based on the results. However, improved survival has been achieved in selected patients with isolated hepatic or pulmonary metastases, thus suggesting that in CEA-positive tumors, levels should be monitored for several years postoperatively, along with periodic repeat CT scans. The frequency is inversely proportional to the length of time since resection. *Caveat:* because CEA is excreted in the bile, elevated levels may be difficult to interpret in the presence of biliary obstruction or hepatic dysfunction. A reasonable approach is to check

CEA levels every 2 months for the first 6 months, every 4 months for up to 2 years, and then every 6 months for up to 5 years. CT scans every 6 months for 2 years and then yearly thereafter for up to 5 years may be valuable, particularly in CEA-negative tumors.

17. List the risk factors for developing CRC.

Age, diet, environment, personal history of neoplasm, family history of neoplasm, familial colon cancer syndromes, and inflammatory bowel disease.

18. How does age affect the risk for developing CRC?

The risk of developing colorectal cancer increases with age, starting at about age 40 and roughly doubling with each decade. Below age 40, the incidence of CRC is less than 6 in 100,000; however, by age 80 the incidence is approximately 500 per 100,000 in men and 400 per 100,000 in women. Because over 90% of colorectal cancers occur after age 50, most screening programs have arbitrarily chosen this as a starting age.

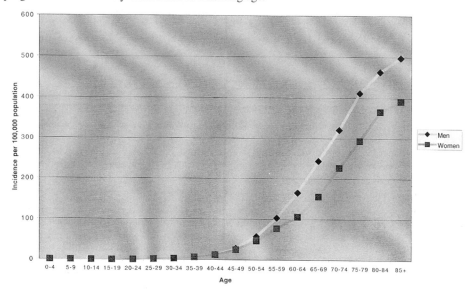

Age-specific incidence rates of colorectal cancer.

19. Discuss the effect of diet on the risk for developing CRC.

Diet is thought to account for the major differences in the incidence rates of CRC world-wide. Although epidemiologic studies and animal models suggest that a high-fat, low-fiber diet (typical of Western nations) increases the risk of developing CRC, prospective trials of low-fat, high-fiber diets have shown no effect. Similarly, other micronutrients, such as folate, reducing agents (vitamins C and E), and β-carotene, have shown promise in experimental conditions but failed to yield positive results in controlled trials. Calcium supplementation is the only dietary intervention which has shown a positive, albeit modest, effect in humans, using adenomas as a surrogate marker for the development of CRC. However, despite the failure of clinical trials to prove that dietary interventions can significantly reduce the risk of developing CRC, it is still prudent to advise a balanced low-fat, high-fiber diet for most patients.

20. What environmental factors affect the risk for developing CRC?

The risk of developing CRC is directly related to environmental factors. This effect is evident in comparing the rates of colorectal cancer in populations emigrating from a region with a low rate to a region with a high rate. For example, the incidence of colon cancer in the Japanese population shortly after World War II was about 10-fold less than in the U.S. Caucasian population in Hawaii (at age

60). The Issei (Japanese emigrants to the U.S.) had a higher rate than their Japanese counterparts, but it was still considerably lower than in the Caucasian population. However, the Nisei (the first generation to be born and raised in the U.S. but still ethnically of 100% Japanese ancestry) acquired essentially the same rate as indigenous Caucasians—a 10-fold increase over a single generation. In general, the U.S. and Western European nations have a higher rate of CRC than developing nations.

21. Discuss the effect of a personal history of neoplasm on the risk for developing CRC.

Adenomatous polyps are considered premalignant lesions, but the actual risk of neoplastic transformation is unknown. However several features are associated with a higher risk of finding carcinoma within a given polyp (advanced adenomas): large size, villous architecture, and dysplasia. The National Polyp Study showed that the risk of developing metachronous adenomas within 3 years increased from 20% in small adenomas to 33% in large adenomas and 50% in patients with multiple adenomas. In patients with a history of CRC, the risk of developing a subsequent CRC is higher than in the general population but approximately the same as in patients with an advanced adenoma.

22. How does a family history of neoplasm affect the risk of developing CRC?

The risk of developing CRC is increased approximately 2-fold if a first-degree relative has been diagnosed with CRC over age 65. The younger the age at which the relative was diagnosed, the higher the risk. The risk also rises if more than one first-degree relative has been diagnosed with CRC. Perhaps more significantly, the same risk seems to apply if first-degree relatives were found to have adenomatous polyps. Evidence suggests a slightly increased risk (approximately 1.5-fold) if third-degree relatives (e.g., cousins) have been diagnosed with CRC.

23. List the familial colon cancer syndromes.

Familial adenomatous polyposis (FAP)
Gardner's syndrome (FAP with extracolonic manifestations)
Hamartomatous polyp syndromes (e.g., Peutz-Jeghers syndrome and juvenile polyposis)
Hereditary nonpolyposis colorectal cancer (HNPCC)

24. How do FAP and Gardner's syndrome increase the risk of CRC?

FAP and Gardner's syndrome are inherited in an autosomal dominant manner. Their fully expressed forms are characterized by the development of hundreds to thousands of colonic adenomas, and 100% of patients expressing this phenotype develop CRC if colectomy is not performed. Most patients begin developing adenomas in their teens, and screening should start at that time. Members of FAP kindreds who have not developed adenomas by age 40 have not inherited the polyposis phenotype. The APC gene is responsible for both FAP and Gardner's syndrome. Most disease-causing mutations result in premature stop codons, which give rise to truncated proteins. Commercial tests are available to detect truncated proteins, and results can be used for accurate screening of affected kindreds. Mutations in the extreme beginning or end of the APC gene can cause an attenuated form of FAP, which is characterized by fewer adenomas (1–100) with a right-sided predominance. The increased risk of CRC is thought to be due to the sheer number of adenomatous polyps; each polyp has the same risk of malignant transformation as an "ordinary" sporadic adenoma. Both sulindac and celecoxib decrease the number of adenomas in patients with FAP, but neither is associated with complete regression and cannot be used in lieu of colectomy. Because 20% of patients with FAP subsequently develop ampullary adenocarcinomas, all patients with FAP should undergo periodic upper GI tract screening with both forward- and side-viewing endoscopes.

25. How do hamartomatous polyp syndromes affect the risk of developing CRC?

Hamartomatous polyp syndromes appear to be associated with a slightly increased risk of developing CRC, although nowhere near the risk associated with APC syndromes.

26. Describe the effect of HNPCC on the risk of developing CRC.

HNPCC, which is inherited in an autosomal dominant manner, is caused by inactivation of one of the proteins involved in DNA proofreading (usually hMSH2 or hMLH1), the so-called mismatch repair genes. As a result, errors that ordinarily occur at a frequency of about 1 per 1010 base pairs with intact proofreading occur at a frequency of about 1 per 107 base pairs (approximately 300 per cell per replication) and accumulate rapidly within the genome. Although most mutations are silent, occasionally a mutation gives one cell a growth advantage over adjacent cells, producing a clonal expansion containing the genetic change. One marker of this "mutator" phenotype is the inability to replicate accurately areas of mono-, di-, and trinucleotide repeats known as microsatellites (often slipping one or two repeat units). Many such areas are known within the human genome. Polymerase chain reaction provides a quick method of screening for microsatellite instability, which occurs in 90% of patients with HNPCC but only 15% of patients with sporadic CRC. Affected patients develop adenomas that, although few in number (hence the designation "nonpolyposis") are thought to have increased malignant potential because of their ability to accumulate mutations rapidly.

27. How is HNPCC diagnosed?

Patients with the HNPCC phenotype develop CRC at a mean age of 44. Seventy percent of cancers are proximal to the splenic flexure and would be missed during a flexible sigmoidoscopy. The original Amsterdam criteria required the "3-2-1 rules" for diagnosing HNPCC: (1) three relatives with CRC, one of whom is a first-degree relative of the other two; (2) involvement of two generations; and (3) one patient diagnosed under the age of 50. These criteria have been modified to include cancers at extracolonic sites (e.g., stomach, endometrium, ovaries, ureters, renal pelvis, small bowel, hepatobiliary tract, skin), for which patients with HNPCC have an increased risk. Mismatch repair genes probably are involved in a significant number of familial CRCs that do not fit the classic or modified HNPCC criteria. At present it is thought that 5–15% of CRCs are due to mismatch repair gene abnormalities, either inherited or acquired. Because these cancers acquire genetic abnormalities through accumulation of point mutations, they are largely diploid and therefore have a better prognosis than sporadic cancers, many of which are aneuploid. Second primaries are common, and screening should be performed for noncolonic as well as colonic malignancies.

28. How does inflammatory bowel disease affect the risk of developing CRC?

Patients with chronic inflammatory bowel disease (IBD) have an increased risk of developing colorectal cancer, particularly those with ulcerative colitis. In patients with ulcerative colitis, the risk begins to rise approximately 7 years after onset and increases with duration of the disease. In patients followed in tertiary care referral centers, the cumulative risk may be as high as 35% by 30 years. Several studies suggest that the risk in patients followed in the community may be much lower (11% at 32 years), perhaps because the patients followed in tertiary care centers have more severe and/or more difficult-to-control disease. Crohn's disease is also thought to be associated with an increased risk for developing CRC, although the magnitude of the risk is less than for ulcerative colitis, probably because the noncontiguous nature of the lesions puts less mucosa at risk. An excess of carcinomas of the small intestine, stomach, and anus as well as lymphomas has been reported in patients with Crohn's disease. It is thought that increased cell turnover due to inflammation is the important factor predisposing the colon to the development of malignancies in patients with IBD.

29. Describe the recommended screening protocol for patients with IBD.

Colonic dysplasia in IBD is thought to be a premalignant lesion, equivalent to adenomas in sporadic CRC. Because dysplastic epithelium has no gross morphologic characteristics that distinguish it from normal epithelium, current screening regimens rely on random biopsies taken during colonoscopies (usually 4 quadrant biopsies every 10 cm) to detect cellular abnormalities. Even the most aggressive screening regimens sample < 0.1% of the colonic mucosa, thus limiting the probability that a discrete focus of malignancy will be discovered. Paralleling the adenoma-carcinoma progression, most malignancies in IBD appear to arise within larger fields of dysplasia. The presence of even mild dysplasia, if confirmed, should be a cause for concern. Unfortunately, dysplasia is difficult to diagnose in the presence of inflammation. Because as many as 30% of patients with severe dysplasia already have CRC in colectomy specimens, the colon should be reexamined carefully with multiple biopsies, and total colectomy should be considered, particularly if the dysplasia is associated with a lesion or mass. Patients should undergo surveillance 8–10 years after onset of disease and, with negative examinations, probably every 2 years thereafter, at least in the community setting. After 25–30 years of disease, the frequency of surveillance colonoscopies should be increased to an annual basis. In an IBD clinic in a tertiary care center, annual colonoscopies beginning at 15–20 years of disease duration may be appropriate.

30. Can CRC be prevented?

Not completely. However, it is possible to reduce mortality by discovering and removing neoplasms at premalignant stages (e.g., polypectomy [secondary prevention]), discovering cancers at earlier, more curable stages (tertiary prevention), and using chemoprevention. Colonoscopy with removal of all adenomas is the most effective means of preventing colorectal cancers, as clearly shown in the National Polyp Study. Cost-effectiveness depends largely on the interval between screening examinations, cost of the procedures, and prevalence of adenomas and cancers within the target population. Analyses indicate that some strategies fall well below the benchmark figure of $40,000 per year of life saved, comparing favorably with mammography in women over the age of 50 (approximately $25,000 per year of life saved). Despite an increasing sentiment within the medical community that colonoscopy should be adopted as a primary screening method, third-party payers have yet to endorse its use in otherwise asymptomatic patients with a negative family history. However, with the recent announcement that the Health Care Financing Administration will fund colonoscopic screening every 10 years for Medicare beneficiaries, it seems likely that colonoscopic screening will become the standard of care in the not too distant future.

31. Which two clinical conditions should raise suspicion for the presence of colon cancer?

An unexplained iron deficiency anemia or sepsis with *Streptococcus bovis* as the pathogen should trigger investigation for colorectal cancer.

32. Is fecal occult blood testing (FOBT) effective in detecting colon polyps and cancer?

Yes. Even in the absence of iron deficiency anemia, FOBT has been shown to decrease mortality by 15–30% in three large randomized, controlled trials using guaiac-based methods. The higher figure was obtained by rehydrating the guaiac test cards, which doubled the sensitivity of the test but markedly decreased its specificity. Immunologic methods for testing human hemoglobin have shown some promise for increasing specificity but have not been widely used because of increased cost. Cost, convenience and lack of definitive markers has confined the use of stool testing for molecular markers of neoplastic transformation to research studies. Only large polyps (>1.5 cm in diameter) and cancers bleed enough to be detected routinely by FOBT. Thus, although FOBT screening can reduce mortality from CRC by discovering malignancies at earlier, curable stages, it is considerably less effective at detecting adenomas, whose removal prior to malignant transformation is a much more cost-effective strategy.

33. Does a program of periodic sigmoidoscopy decrease mortality from CRC?

Yes. The magnitude of this decrease is determined by a number of factors, including distribution of CRCs, extent of the exam, predictive value of the procedure for lesions beyond the extent of the exam, and number of patients undergoing screening. Over the past few decades, autopsy studies have confirmed that CRC distribution has moved proximally. If this trend continues, the value of screening by flexible sigmoidoscopy obviously will decrease. Colonoscopic studies have shown that patients with adenomas within the reach of the flexible sigmoidoscope have an increased risk of significant lesions (large adenomas, adenomas with villous histology and cancers) in the proximal colon and should have a full colonoscopy. With this strategy, one can detect approximately 80% of significant lesions with an examination to the splenic flexure and two-thirds of significant lesions if only the descending colon is reached. The same data suggest that one-half of significant lesions in the proximal colon have no sentinel lesions within the reach of a flexible sigmoidoscope and would be missed during screening.

34. Are there any effective blood tests to screen for CRC?

Serum tests to diagnose colorectal cancer are limited by the inherent problem that markers produced by malignant cells are hardest to detect in early, small tumors, which have the best prognosis. For example, the low sensitivity and specificity of CEA, particularly in stage A cancers, currently restricts its use to assessing the efficacy of surgery or monitoring for recurrent malignancies in cancers already known to be CEA-positive. To date, no putative serum markers of CRC have sufficient sensitivity or specificity to warrant use as primary screening modalities.

35. What radiologic tests have been suggested as screening methods for CRC?

Carefully performed air contrast barium enemas have sensitivities and specificities in the 90% range; however, in most centers the figures are considerably lower, perhaps because radiologic trainees tend to be less enthusiastic about classic techniques than more modern ultrasound-, CT-, or MRI-based procedures. Virtual colonoscopy using a helical CT scanner has shown promise, but high cost and dependence on excellent bowel preparations has limited its use.

36. Can CRC be prevented with medicines (chemoprevention)?

Because we cannot prevent CRCs by elimination of causative factors, the possibility of chemoprevention has generated considerable enthusiasm. Nonsteroidal anti-inflammatory drugs, including sulindac and aspirin, have shown promise in both experimental models and epidemiologic studies, although neither has shown effectiveness in prospective controlled trials. The epidemiologic studies strongly support an effect for aspirin, but GI tract toxicity and potential bleeding, along with the apparent lack of efficacy in short-term prospective trials (< 5 years), have prevented its widespread use for CRC prevention. Sulindac decreases the number and size of adenomas in patients with FAP but does not completely prevent progression to cancer. Its efficacy in sporadic adenomas is unclear. Selective cyclooxygenase-2 inhibitors, which have a much lower GI toxicity profile, are effective in animal models and patients with FAP, although they may be somewhat less effective than sulindac for FAP. Ongoing trials are examining their effects on sporadic adenoma recurrence.

BIBLIOGRAPHY

1. Bresalier RS, Kim YS: Malignant neoplasms of the large intestine. In Feldman M, Scharschmidt BF, Sleisenger MH (eds): Gastrointestinal and Liver Disease. Philadelphia, W.B. Saunders, 1998, pp 1906–1942.
2. Boland CR: Malignant tumors of the colon. In Yamada T, Alpers DH, Laine L, et al (eds): Textbook of Gastroenterology. Philadelphia, Lippincott Williams & Wilkins, 1999, pp 2023–2082.
3. Burt R: Colon cancer screening. Gastroenterology 119:837–853, 2000.
4. Fearon ER, Vogelstein B: A genetic model for colorectal tumorigenesis. Cell 61:759–767, 1990.
5. Giardiello FM, Hamilton SR, Krush AJ, et al: Treatment of colonic and rectal adenomas with sulindac in familial adenomatous polyposis. N Engl J Med 328:1313–1316, 1993.
6. Greenlee RT, Murray T, Bolden S, Wingo PA: Cancer statistics, 2000. CA Cancer J. Clin 50:7–33, 2000.
7. Lieberman DA, Weiss DG, Bond JH, et al: Use of colonoscopy to screen asymptomatic adults for colorectal cancer. Veterans Affairs Cooperative Study Group 380. N Engl J Med 343:162–168, 2000.
8. Lynch HT, Smyrk TC, Watson P, et al: Genetics, natural history, tumor spectrum and pathology of hereditary nonpolyposis colorectal cancer: An updated review. Gastroenterology 104:1535–1549, 1993.
9. Ries LA, Wingo PA, Miller DS, et al: The annual report to the nation on the status of cancer, 1973-1997, with a special section on colorectal cancer. Cancer 88:2398–2424, 2000.
10. Rustgi A: Hereditary gastrointestinal polyposis and non polyposis syndromes. N Engl J Med 331:1694–1702, 1994.
11. Selby JV, Friedman GD, Quesenberry CP, Weiss NS: A case-control study of screening sigmoidoscopy and mortality from colorectal cancer. N Engl J Med 326:653–657, 1992.
12. Steinbach G, Lynch PM, Phillips RK, et al: The effect of celecoxib, a cyclooxygenase-2 inhibitor, in familial adenomatous polyposis. N Engl J Med 342:1946–1952, 2000.
13. Toribara NW, Sleisenger MH: Screening for colorectal cancer. N Engl J Med 332:861–867, 1995.
14. Vasen HF, Watson P, Mecklin JP, Lynch HT: New clinical criteria for hereditary nonpolyposis colorectal cancer (HNPCC, Lynch syndrome) proposed by the International Collaborative group on HNPCC. Gastroenterology 1999; 116:1453–1456, 1999.
15. Winawer SJ, Zauber AG, Gerdes H, et al: Risk of colorectal cancer in the families of patients with adenomatous polyps. N Engl J Med 334:82–87, 1996.
16. Winawer SJ, Zauber AG, Ho MN, et al: Prevention of colorectal cancer by colonoscopic polypectomy. N Engl J Med 329:1977–1981, 1993.

50. ACUTE AND CHRONIC MEGACOLON

Michael F. Lyons, II, M.D.

1. What is Ogilvie's syndrome?

Ogilvie's syndrome is acute nontoxic megacolon. It was first described in 1948 in two patients with metastatic cancer who developed massive dilatation of the cecum and right colon without evidence of more distal colonic obstruction or inflammation. Since that time, numerous other clinical situations have been described and attributed to this syndrome. An alternative term for Ogilvie's syndrome is acute colonic pseudo-obstruction. A distinction must be made between toxic and nontoxic megacolon, however. No infection or inflammation is seen with nontoxic megacolon, unless the colon becomes dilated to the point of inducing ischemic changes in the colonic wall. In this setting, patients may show signs more consistent with a toxic megacolon.

2. Describe the clinical presentation of Ogilvie's syndrome.

The typical presentation of Ogilvie's syndrome is a postoperative patient who develops a distended abdomen. The patient is on, or recently weaned from, a ventilator. Although pain tends to be minimal in the early stages, nausea and vomiting occur in two-thirds of patients. The typical patient does not have bowel movements unless in the form of diarrhea. Of interest, one-half of patients continue to pass flatus. As the syndrome progresses, over 80% of patients develop a mild, steady pain related to the distention. Bowel sounds are universally present and are often high pitched and quite active during the early phase. Patients often have a low-grade fever and left-shifted leukocytosis. Although the condition can normalize at any point, patients can proceed to a silent, rigid abdomen, perforation, sepsis, and death. Perforation rates are under 10%, but death occurs in 15–30%. Of note, patients rarely die of perforation; death is related to multiorgan system failure.

3. What factors contribute to development of Ogilvie's syndrome?

The cause of Ogilvie's syndrome is not known, but Ogilvie theorized that colonic dilation was a physiologic response to an autonomic imbalance. More recently, investigators have shown that the excessive parasympathetic suppression in acute Ogilvie's syndrome can be pharmacologically reversed by parenteral administration of neostigmine.

Factors commonly associated with the evolution of Ogilvie's syndrome are listed below. In and of themselves, they do not cause Ogilvie's syndrome in the vast majority of patients. In the patients described by Ogilvie, tumor invasion of the celiac plexus led to interruption of the sympathetic innervation of the colon. This interruption was presumed to cause loss of peristalsis and dilatation of the right colon. Currently most patients with acute nontoxic megacolon do not have intraabdominal malignancy. Instead, most patients are in the immediate postoperative state, often have multiorgan system disease, often take numerous medications that significantly alter bowel function, or suffer multiple metabolic derangements that may be contributory.

Factors Associated with the Onset of Acute Nontoxic Megacolon (Ogilvie's Syndrome)

Recent surgery	Congestive heart failure
Chronic obstructive lung disease	Uremia
Recent general anesthesia	Underlying severe infections
Underlying neurologic disorders	Hip fracture
Medications	Electrolyte abnormalities
Diabetes	

4. Which medications may be associated with the development of Ogilvie's syndrome?

TYPE OF MEDICATION	EXAMPLES
Nonsteroidal analgesics	Fenoprofen, naproxen, sulindac
Opiate analgesics	Meperidine, propoxyphene, morphine
Antidepressants	Amitriptyline, protriptyline
Antipsychotics	Thioridazine, chlorpromazine, clozapine
Antiseizure drugs	Phenobarbital, phenytoin
Antacid agents	Sucralfate, aluminum/calcium antacids
Calcium antagonists	Nifedipine, verapamil, felodipine
Cationic agents	Iron/calcium supplements, barium sulfate, bismuth salts
Antiparkinson agents	Procyclidine, benztropine
Ganglionic blockers	Trimethaphan
MAO inhibitors	Sertraline, bupropion, phenelzine
Other agents	General anesthesia, heavy metals (intoxication)

MAO = monoamine oxidase.

5. Does cecal diameter predict perforation in Ogilvie's syndrome?

No. Cecal perforation correlates poorly with cecal diameter. The cecum routinely dilates to 9 or 10 cm in normal people undergoing air-contrast barium enema studies. Reported series of perforation in patients with obstructed colons reveal a mean cecal diameter of 11 cm. In patients with Ogilvie's syndrome, the cecum may perforate with diameters of < 12 cm, whereas others have an uncomplicated recovery with a cecal diameter up to 25 cm. One series showed an increase in cecal perforations with cecum dilatation > 14 cm in diameter in the setting of postoperative Ogilvie's syndrome. The rate and duration of cecal dilatation are important factors that suggest increased risk of perforation.

6. Describe the first step in the management of acute megacolon.

The first step in management of acute megacolon is to evaluate the cause:
• Ogilvie's syndrome: usually postoperative or after recent trauma
• Inflammatory causes: severe fulminant inflammatory bowel disease (Crohn's or ulcerative colitis), infectious colitis (bacillary or amebic dysentery), or pseudomembranous colitis
• Obstructive causes: mechanical obstruction from tumor, diverticular disease, or volvulus.
• Metabolic derangements and pharmacologic causes: electrolyte disturbances and medications listed in question 4

7. What elements of the history help to determine cause?

Inflammatory disease usually presents with an acute toxic picture. Patients often relate premonitory history of diarrhea, hematochezia, weight loss, or extraintestinal manifestations. Infectious colitis often is associated with consumption of improperly prepared food, raw meat, or recent foreign travel. Prior exposure to antibiotics should alert the clinician to the possibility of pseudomembranous colitis. Bloody diarrhea is not a typical feature of Ogilvie's syndrome; if it is present, think of inflammatory causes.

Obstructive disorders include luminal stenosis caused by neoplasm, diverticular strictures, and volvulus. Patients with colonic malignancy often have hypochromic microcytic anemia, history of hematochezia, guaiac-positive stool, or change in bowel habit. Patients with obstructing diverticular strictures usually have a history of recurrent episodes of lower abdominal pain and low-grade fever. Volvulus of the colon may occur at the sigmoid, cecum, transverse colon, or splenic flexure. Sigmoid volvulus is the most common cause, accounting for 70% of all cases of colonic volvulus. It is probably an acquired condition associated with diets high in vegetable fiber in developing countries and with chronic constipation and laxative abuse in Western Europe and the United States. Neurologic disorders such as Parkinson's disease, multiple sclerosis, Alzheimer's disease, and schizophrenia and use of neuropsychiatric drugs are strongly associated with the development of colonic volvulus. Large bowel volvulus is the underlying cause in 25% of pregnant women with bowel obstruction.

8. Describe the role of plain radiographs of the abdomen.

Inflammatory disease. Plain abdominal radiographs may reveal colonic wall thickening, ulceration, thumb printing, or loss of haustral folds.

Obstructive disorders. Obstructive sigmoid volvulus is suggested by a distended, ahaustral loop of bowel with an air-to-fluid ratio > 2:1 in the right lower quadrant. Cecal volvulus is characterized by dilated small bowel and a distended cecum in the left upper quadrant. Mechanical lower colonic obstruction may appear identical to fecal impaction or obstipation; radiographic enema or endoscopy is necessary to exclude mechanical obstruction.

9. How is Ogilvie's syndrome treated?
- Withhold oral feedings, give parenteral fluids, and place a functioning nasogastric tube.
- Correct electrolyte disturbances.
- Discontinue medicinal causes.
- Use mobilization techniques: bed to chair if possible; "log-roll" position change if the patient is confined to bed.
- Give enemas for elimination of obstructing stool; manual removal may be necessary if stool impaction is present.
- Order hypaque (water-soluble) enema radiograph or colonoscopy to exclude obstruction or volvulus.
- When obstruction and volvulus have been excluded and response to the above measures is incomplete, administration of neostigmine, 2.5 mg IV over 3 minutes, is highly effective. *Note:* Continuous cardiac monitoring during neostigmine administration is recommended because severe symptomatic bradycardia has been observed.
- Obtain serial abdominal radiographs (every 8–12 hr) to assess progression or resolution.
- Failure of conservative measures to decrease colonic dilation warrants colonic decompression, which can be achieved by colonoscopy, fluroscopic placement of a percutaneous-cecal decompression tube, or surgical cecostomy.

10. What causes acute toxic megacolon?

Acute megacolon is a serious, potentially life-threatening complication of ulcerative colitis or Crohn's colitis. The diagnosis of inflammatory bowel disease is rarely in question, because toxic megacolon tends to be a late manifestation of advanced inflammatory bowel disease. Another cause is pseudomembranous colitis. This presentation is usually seen in intensive care patients who have been taking antibiotics for several days. The patient is often on a ventilator or in a coma and is unable to relate intestinal symptoms. Typhlitis also can be associated with acute toxic megacolon. Other reported causes of acute toxic megacolon are rare but include amebic colitis, cytomegalovirus colitis, typhoid fever, and bacillary dysentery. Finally, colonic ischemia also can present with megacolon and may be catastrophic if not recognized.

11. Define typhlitis.

Typhlitis is a necrotizing process involving the cecum in the setting of neutropenia. Although it was originally described in children undergoing chemotherapy for leukemia, additional cases have been reported in adults undergoing chemotherapy for malignancy or immunosuppressive therapy for organ transplantation as well as in adults with drug-induced neutropenia (not associated with malignancy), aplastic anemia, and cyclic neutropenia. Typhlitis may involve the terminal ileum, right colon, and appendix. This necrotizing process can be devastating. Mucosal denudement (from unclear mechanisms) is followed by bacterial invasion with ensuing necrosis, colonic dilatation, and perforation. Death rates are high (averaging 40–50%). Death typically is due to perforation.

12. How can you distinguish between toxic and nontoxic acute megacolon?

The clinical situation is the best predictor of the various causes of toxic and nontoxic acute megacolon. Vigilant attention to history, medications, metabolism, and oxygenation status are key to establishing a diagnosis. Stool analysis positive for blood, leukocytes, and *Clostridium difficile* toxin are seen with various causes of acute toxic megacolon. In patients with neutropenia or leukemia, typhlitis must be considered. An abdominal radiograph distinguishes dilatation of the right colon and cecum from pancolonic dilatation. Acute toxic megacolon usually involves the entire colon in patients with ulcerative colitis. Thumbprinting on the colonic radiograph suggests ischemia. Likewise, loss of colonic haustral markings is typical of ulcerative colitis. Ulcerations on the colonic wall can be seen with cytomegalovirus, Crohn's disease, amebiasis, and bacillary infections.

13. Describe the clinical presentation of acute toxic megacolon related to inflammatory bowel disease.

Toxic megacolon is the most severe and potentially life-threatening complication of ulcerative colitis. Before the availability of aggressive diagnostic colonoscopy and medical therapy for ulcerative colitis, toxic megacolon was not infrequently the initial presentation. With a better understanding of diagnosis and treatment, it is now typically identified during progression of chronic disease. Patients usually present with a recent change in bowel pattern related to ulcerative colitis. Whereas some may have increased bleeding, the frequency of bowel movements may actually decrease in others. Patients complain of increased abdominal pain, bloating, and distention of the abdomen. They usually have a fever. Depending on the stage of toxicity, signs may include hypotension, hypovolemia, electrolyte abnormalities due to third-spacing of fluids, and even mental status changes. Other signs include tachycardia, left-shifted leukocytosis, anemia, and low serum albumin levels. An abdominal radiograph demonstrates dilatation, usually involving the entire colon, although in Crohn's disease and some cases of ulcerative colitis segmental dilatation has been reported. The isolated cecal dilatation of acute nontoxic megacolon is rarely seen with acute toxic megacolon of inflammatory bowel disease. Colonic perforation, septic shock, and death are not rare complications, and in the setting of a low serum albumin level (<1.9 gm/dl), the mortality rate after perforation approaches 90%.

14. Describe the treatment of acute toxic megacolon associated with inflammatory bowel disease.

Patients usually require a certain amount of resuscitation, including correction of fluid and electrolyte status. Blood transfusions may be required at the outset. Patients should be hospitalized and placed at bowel rest, initially including nasogastric suction. Colonic decompression may be required, but it should be done with patient positioning rather than colonoscopic decompression. Intravenous steroids and antibiotics should be initiated. Central line placement followed by the implementation of parenteral nutrition is required in patients who do not respond rapidly. Narcotic analgesics and anticholinergics should be avoided. Because steroids may mask a complication, close monitoring of the physical examination, daily laboratory values, and serial abdominal radiographs is vital to assess the need for early surgery.

15. Discuss the timing of surgical intervention.

The timing for surgical intervention is controversial. Data demonstrate that perforation is associated with a high mortality rate—up to 50% overall and up to 90% if profound hypoalbuminemia is present. Patients should undergo surgery immediately for colonic perforation, signs of peritonitis, signs of endotoxic shock, rapid clinical deterioration despite aggressive medical therapy, and massively dilated colon (as with acute nontoxic megacolon), especially in the setting of profound hypoalbuminemia (< 1.9 gm/dl). If the patient is stabilized with medical management, elective surgery may be considered, because most patients relapse within the next several weeks to months. Elective surgery should be scheduled between 1 and 4 weeks after medical stabilization, because surgical mortality rates are lowest during this period. There are no good clinical discriminators to predict relapse of megacolon.

16. How is chronic megacolon best classified?
  Congenital forms usually present in the neonatal period. Hirschsprung's disease is a familial disorder caused by an aganglionosis of the rectum, beginning at the dentate line of the anus and extending cephalad for variable lengths. The length of colonic involvement dictates the clinical presentation: longer segmental disease leads to presentation shortly after birth, whereas short segmental disease may present as late as adulthood. This finding led to classification of Hirschsprung's disease as short segment and ultra-short segment. Other variants involving more of the colon have been described.
  If patients with chronic nontoxic megacolon do not have one of the various forms of congenital megacolon, they are presumed to have an **acquired form**. Numerous causes have been reported. Some forms, such as idiopathic intestinal pseudo-obstruction, appear to be associated with familial clustering, although it is unclear whether the disease is genetically or environmentally acquired.

17. List the causes of chronic acquired megacolon.
  • Idiopathic (most common)
  • Amyloidosis
  • Parkinson's disease
  • Myopathic idiopathic intestinal pseudo-obstruction
  • Neuropathic idiopathic intestinal pseudo-obstruction
  • Muscular dystrophy
  • Chagas disease
  • Scleroderma
  • Diabetes
  • Psychogenic constipation
  • Porphyria
  • Pheochromocytoma
  • Hypothyroidism
  • Hypokalemia

18. Does a barium study of the colon help to sort out the various causes of acute and chronic megacolon?
  Yes. The following algorithm outlines the classic findings of the various forms of acute and chronic megacolon that may assist in evaluating patients with a dilated colon. The history usually helps to distinguish acute from chronic megacolon. Once history has been considered, the barium radiograph may be useful in developing a differential diagnosis. Remember that various types of mechanical obstruction can cause a dilated colon, including volvulus, intussusception, mass, stricture, inflammatory bowel disease, ischemia, and diverticulitis.

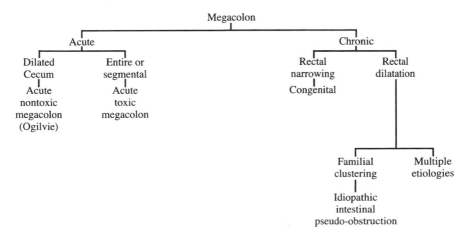

Algorithm for distinguishing nonobstructive types of megacolon.

BIBLIOGRAPHY

1. Amaro R, Rogers AI: Neostigmine infusion: New standard of care for acute colonic pseudo-obstruction. Am J Gastroenterol 95:304–305, 2000.
2. Barnes PRH, Lennard-Jones JE, Hawley PR, Todd IP: Hirschsprung's disease and idiopathic megacolon in adults and adolescents. Gut 27:534, 1986.
3. Faulk DL, Anuras S, Christensen J: Chronic intestinal pseudo-obstruction. Gastroenterology 74:922, 1978.
4. Fausel CS, Goff JS: Nonoperative management of acute idiopathic colonic pseudo-obstruction (Ogilvie's syndrome). West J Med 143:50, 1985.
5. Greenstein AJ, Sachar DB, Gibas A, et al: Outcome of toxic dilatation in ulcerative and Crohn's colitis. J Clin Gastroenterol 7:137, 1985.
6. Jalan KN, Sircus W, Card WI, et al: An experience of ulcerative colitis. I: Toxic dilation of 55 cases. Gastroenterology 57:68, 1969.
7. Nixon HH: Hirschsprung's disease: Progress in management and diagnostics. World J Surg 9:189, 1985.
8. Ponec RJ, Saunders MD, Kimmey MB: Neostigmine for the treatment of acute colonic pseudo-obstruction. N Engl J Med 341:137–141, 1999.
9. Preston DM, Lennard-Jones JE, Thomas BM: Towards a radiologic definition of idiopathic megacolon. Gastrointest Radiol 10:167, 1985.
10. Schuffler MD, Rohrmann CA, Chaffee RG, et al: Chronic intestinal pseudo-obstruction: A report of 27 cases and review of the literature. Medicine 60:173, 1981.
11. Trevisani GT, Hyman NH, Church JM: Neostigmine: Safe and effective treatment for acute colonic pseudo-obstruction. Dis Colon Rectum 43:599–603, 2000.
12. Vanek VW, Al-Salti M: Acute pseudo-obstruction of the colon (Ogilvie's syndrome): An analysis of 400 cases. Dis Colon Rectum 29:203, 1986.

51. CONSTIPATION AND FECAL INCONTINENCE

Peter E. Legnani, M.D., and Suzanne Rose, M.D., M.S.Ed.

1. What is constipation?

Infrequent bowel movements, painful passage of stool, hard consistency of stool, or difficulty in evacuating stool may be considered constipation by the patient. Population studies reveal that 5–30% of the population report these symptoms; prevalence increases with age. Complaints of constipation lead to an estimated 2.5 million doctor visits annually. Women outnumber men by 2:1.

2. Describe the normal mechanism of stool passage.

Defecation results from coordinated contraction and relaxation of both smooth and striated muscles. Normally, the first step is sensing that material is in the rectum. Stretch receptors in the muscularis propria of the rectum initiate a spinal reflex arc (rectoanal inhibitory reflex), stimulating inhibitory nerves that lead to relaxation of the internal anal sphincter. Next, the striated muscles of the pelvic floor (puborectalis and pubococcygeus) relax, resulting in perineal descent. The rectoanal angle is opened further from 90° to 130°, and the anal canal is stretched in the antero-posterior direction by flexure of the hips when the person assumes a sitting or squatting position. When the external anal sphincter relaxes, the final resistance to passage of stool is removed. Finally, rectal smooth muscle contraction, often with concomitant diaphragmatic and abdominal muscular contraction, results in expulsion of the rectal contents, followed by restoration of tone in the internal anal sphincter. Occasionally, fecal matter descends into the rectum at inconvenient moments. The defecatory mechanism may be interrupted by voluntary contraction of the pelvic floor muscles, which makes the anorectal angle more acute and stifles the passage of fecal matter

3. What are the major causes of constipation?

CAUSES	EXAMPLES
Metabolic disorders	Hypothyroidism, diabetes mellitus
Collagen vascular diseases	Scleroderma
Inherited muscular disorders	Familial visceral myopathy
Colonic disorders	Colonic inertia
Enteric neurologic disorders	Hirschsprung's disease, chronic intestinal pseudo-obstruction
Nonenteric neurologic disorders	Parkinson's disease, spinal cord injury, multiple sclerosis
Anorectal disorders	Anal stricture, rectocele
Medications	Opiates, antacids (calcium and aluminum), anticholinergics, anticonvulsants, antidepressants, parkinsonian agents, diuretics, iron, antihypertensive agents, calcium channel blockers

4. Describe the work-up for constipation.

A thorough history should focus on duration of constipation, presence of danger signs such as blood per rectum and weight loss, risk factors for colonic malignancy, signs of systemic illnesses, and direct questioning about both prescription and over-the-counter medications. Physical exam, including a detailed digital rectal exam and neurologic assessment, is supplemented by pertinent laboratory data to exclude underlying organic disease. It may be worthwhile to do a limited laboratory analysis of thyroid-stimulating hormone and calcium to exclude metabolic disorders. Colonoscopy or flexible sigmoidoscopy should be considered in all patients, and a decision about which (if either) study to perform should be based on the patient's age and clinical presentation. If this work-up is unrevealing, the patient is considered to have chronic idiopathic constipation.

5. **What tests are used in the evaluation of chronic constipation?**

Colonic marker studies with radiopaque plastic rings are used to measure gut transit time. This safe, effective technique involves swallowing inert rings in a capsule, followed by plain abdominal radiography on subsequent days. The markers can be commercially purchased or made in the office/hospital by sectioning a nasogastric tube into small rings. In normal patients, more than 80% of the rings should be passed by 5 days, and all of the markers should be passed by 1 week. Another method uses capsules with easily viewed markers of different shapes, which are swallowed on days 1, 2, and 3, followed by a plain abdominal film on day 5. The markers may be evenly distributed throughout the colon, suggesting colonic inertia, or localized to a single segment.

Anorectal manometry involves passing a pressure-recording catheter across the anal sphincter. Through techniques involving balloon distention within the rectum, rectal sensory thresholds and internal anal sphincter relaxation can be assessed directly. Manometry can be combined with surface EMG studies of the pelvic floor musculature and external anal sphincter to diagnose entities such as anismus (see below).

Defecography involves the placement of barium paste into the rectum, with radiography taken before and during evacuation of rectal contents. In addition to assessing the completeness of rectal expulsion, this test is also used to demonstrate anatomic abnormalities of the rectum (rectocele), prolapse, or pelvic floor dysfunction. New modalities using MRI to evaluate the function of the pelvic floor also may be considered, if available.

6. **What are the subsets of chronic idiopathic constipation?**

Based on assessment of colonic and anorectal function, chronic idiopathic constipation can be separated into the four major classes: (1) impaired colonic transit, (2) isolated anal sphincter dysfunction due to impaired rectoanal inhibitory reflex, (3) anorectal dysfunction due to physiologic abnormalities, and (4) constipation-predominant irritable bowel syndrome.

7. **What causes impaired colonic transit? How is it diagnosed?**

Delayed colonic transit may occur in isolated segments, in the entire colon, or as part of a diffuse GI motility disorder. **Colonic inertia** describes an isolated dysfunction of propulsive forces of the colon. Studies with radiopaque markers reveal persistence of markers throughout the left and right colon 5–7 days after ingestion, whereas other tests of upper GI motility are normal. Scintigraphic studies also may be done to evaluate colonic transit.

8. **What causes impaired rectoanal inhibitory reflex? How is it diagnosed?**

An impaired rectoanal inhibitory reflex is found in 8–10% of adults with severe idiopathic constipation. In children, it often is seen in conjunction with aganglionosis of the colon (**Hirschsprung's disease**). Adults may have a similar condition called short-segment Hirschsprung's disease. Aganglioniosis occurs within a very short segment of the distal colon, but ganglia are present in full-thickness biopsies of the remaining colon. The diagnostic finding on anal manometry is failure of the internal anal sphincter to relax with balloon distention. It is important to consider this syndrome, especially in young adults with long-standing severe constipation, because surgical posterior sphincterotomy often provides good symptomatic response.

9. **What physiologic abnormalities may lead to anorectal dysfunction? How are they diagnosed?**

Various physiologic abnormalities may lead to **dyschezia** (difficulty in defecating). Functional rectal obstruction may resul from dysfunction of the pelvic musculature, also termed **anismus, spastic pelvic floor syndrome**, or **anorectal dyssynergia**. Impaired relaxation during straining secondary to spasticity of the levator ani, failure of perineal descent, an abnormally angulated recto-anal axis, or a combination of these factors leads to functional obstruction of the anal outlet, terminating defecation. Measurement of the recto-anal angle and the change in the angle during defecography is necessary to make the diagnosis. Occasionally biofeedback ameliorates this condition.

Impaired rectal sensation leads to a decreased motor response and a decrease in the urge to defecate, as determined by balloon distention studies of the rectum. **Megarectum** usually occurs in the setting of fecal impaction and is seen most often in children and physically or mentally impaired elderly patients. Occasionally megarectum is associated with neurologic disease, such as lumbosacral spinal cord lesions, but most often it is due to longstanding fecal impaction. Increased rectal compliance, diminished rectal sensation, and impaired internal anal sphincter relaxation are noted on manometry. Finally, rectal contents can be directed away from the anal canal into a **rectocele** during increased abdominal pressure, leading to incomplete evacuation and retention of feces in the pouch. Endoscopy and barium enema often fail to diagnose a rectocele. Defecography remains the test of choice for diagnosing a rectocele.

10. What other symptoms may be associated with fecal impaction?
- Constipation
- Rectal discomfort
- Anorexia
- Nausea
- Vomiting
- Abdominal pain
- Paradoxical diarrhea
- Fecal incontinence
- Urinary frequency
- Urinary overflow incontinence

11. How is constipation due to irritable bowel syndrome diagnosed?
Constipation-predominant irritable bowel syndrome is diagnosed clinically. Usually it is seen in young or middle-aged adults, predominantly women. Constipation is noted along with abdominal pain, bloating, flatulence, straining, or incomplete evacuation (see Chapter 67).

12. Describe the general management of constipation.
Primary care physicians manage most patients who complain of constipation. Reassurance is beneficial to those who are concerned with less than daily stool patterns or weekly irregularities and may alleviate fears of severe disease. Dietary modifications, such as increasing fiber and daily fluid intake, may increase weekly bowel movements. In addition, increased exercise accelerates colonic transit time and may lead to an improvement in general well-being. Changes or substitutions of medications that alter colonic function may allow resumption of normal bowel pattern.

13. What medical agents can be used for treatment of chronic constipation?
Therapeutic agents fall into five major categories.
1. Bulk-forming agents and dietary fiber
2. Laxatives and cathartics
3. Prokinetic agents
4. Enemas
5. $5\text{-}HT_4$ agonists

14. Describe the proper use of bulk-forming laxatives and dietary fiber.
Bulk-forming laxatives and dietary fiber often benefit patients with mild constipation and should be initiated in every patient with chronic constipation once fecal impaction and obstruction have been ruled out. All patients should be encouraged to increase daily consumption of dietary fiber. A goal of 20–35 gm/day of cereals, fruits and vegetables, and bran is desirable but often requires specific dietary suggestions and relies on patient motivation. A variety of different compounds are available, all of which add to daily stool mass. **Psyllium**, derived from plant husks, has a very high water-binding capacity and is available over the counter. Psyllium is widely used, usually as a powder mixed with water. It is generally taken as one tablespoon mixed with water 1–3 times/day. **Wheat fiber** may be mixed with food and can double dietary fiber intake. **Methylcellulose**, a synthetic compound taken in either liquid or tablet form, is not absorbed and is generally not degraded by colonic bacteria. When any kind of bulk laxative is initiated, the starting dose should be low and gradually increased over 2–3 weeks to minimize the bloating and increased gas that often develop. Patients should be counseled to drink adequate fluids.

15. How should laxatives and cathartics be used?
Osmotic laxatives increase the water content of stools by trapping solute, inhibiting absorption, and stimulating intestinal secretion. **Lactulose** and **sorbitol** are nondigestible disaccharides

that are hydrolyzed in the small intestine, providing osmotically active solutes and stimulating intestinal fluid secretion. They are well tolerated but may lead to increased colonic gas production and abdominal distention. **Magnesium and phosphate sulfates** are poorly absorbed in the intestines and through osmotic action often lead to passage of liquid stool. They should not be used in patients with renal impairment, because hypermagnesemia and hyperphosphatemia have been reported. **Polyethelene glycol**, a nonabsorbable substance, can be used for severe cases of refractory constipation.

Cathartics stimulate intestinal motor activity and cause secretion of electrolytes. **Anthranoids** (aloe, cascara, and senna) are glycosides derived from plants; they are converted by bacteria in the colon to active forms that increase propulsive waves in the colon, leading to passage of stool. **Anthraquinones** are synthetic derivatives that also exert some action on the small intestine. They act reliably and quickly and usually produce soft, formed stools; high doses produce cramping and diarrhea. **Polyphenols** (bisacodyl and sodium picosulfonate) act via similar mechanisms and produce similar results as anthranoids. The safety of both classes for long-term daily use is not yet determined. Melanosis coli, a pigmentation of the colon noted in long-term users of laxatives, generally affects the proximal more than the distal colon and may persist for years after termination of laxative use.

Docusate sodium, a detergent widely used as a stool softener, stimulates mild fluid secretion by the small intestine and colon but has little effect on stool volume or colonic motility. It adds little to the treatment of constipation.

16. How do prokinetic agents work?

Prokinetic agents enhance the intrinsic motor function of the gut and have been used with varying success in the treatment of constipation. Cholinomimetics (e.g., **bethanecol**) stimulate muscarinic receptors and augment peristalsis but have frequent side effects. **Metoclopramide**, while useful in the treatment of gastroparesis through promotion of acetylcholine release and dopamine receptor blockade, is much less effective in stimulating colonic contractions. **Cisapride** carried great promise for many motility problems in the gut but is now available only on a highly regulated basis because of its association with torsade de pointes.

17. Describe the role of enemas.

Retention enemas provide direct and reliable results in fecal impaction, and are the mainstay of therapy for keeping the rectal vault clean in the setting of megarectum. Agents delivered via enema, including lukewarm tap water and water with soap suds, mineral oil, or phosphate sulfates, can be given on a daily or as-needed basis. In megarectum, prevention of recurrent impaction in conjunction with scheduled bowel training may allow resumption of a more normal bowel pattern. In this clinical setting, a low residue diet may be of benefit.

18. What are 5-HT$_4$ agonists?

A new class of agents targeting the 5-HT$_4$ receptor is under investigation in constipation-predominant irritable bowel disease. 5-HT$_4$ agonists stimulate GI transit and in animal studies have accelerated colonic and whole gut transit. Recent studies have demonstrated promise in patients with constipation-predominant IBS, but further investigation is needed.

19. Is surgery ever indicated for constipation?

Surgical treatment for constipation should be reserved for highly selected patients. Limited posterior myotomy in conjunction with a high-fiber diet can provide significant relief for patients in whom manometric testing demonstrates an absent rectoanal inhibitory reflex. In highly selected patients with disabling constipation due to proven colonic inertia, a subtotal colectomy with ileorectal anastamosis can provide good results.

20. Outline the approach to evaluation of patients with constipation.

See figure at top of facing page.

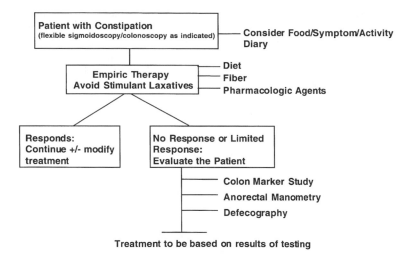

Treatment to be based on results of testing

21. What is fecal incontinence? Who is generally affected?

Fecal incontinence in adults is the involuntary loss of stool. In population-based studies involving all ages, the prevalence of incontinence ranges from 2–14%. This number may underestimate the problem because many patients do not report this embarrassing symptom to their physicians. In geriatric patients, the prevalence is even higher: 10–17% of nursing home residents and 13–47% of hospitalized elderly patients report incontinence. Women develop incontinence more often than men (in some studies up to 8 times more frequently).

22. How is continence normally maintained?

The pelvic floor muscles, including the internal and external anal sphincters and puborectalis muscle, are major contributors to maintenance of continence. The internal anal sphincter (IAS), an extension of the smooth muscle of the rectum, is controlled by the enteric nervous system, tonically contracted, and is largely responsible for the resting pressure in the anal canal. Sympathetic innervation by the hypogastric plexus initiates tonic contraction, whereas parasympathetic innervation from the sacral plexus mediates relaxation. The external anal sphincter (EAS) is a striated muscle, innervated by the pudendal nerve, and is partially contracted at rest. Contraction of the EAS is stimulated by rising external pressures (erect posture, coughing) via a spinal reflex. Scratching of the perineal skin elicits a similar contraction of the EAS known as the "anal wink." The puborectalis muscle, forming a U-shaped sling around the anorectal junction and connecting to the bony pelvis, may be the key muscle for maintaining continence. It maintains a sharp (90°) angle between the rectum and anal canal, thus obstructing the outlet and preventing the passage of solid stool. Much like the EAS, the puborectalis muscle is innervated by the pudendal nerve, is partially contracted at rest, and can voluntarily contract to further narrow the anorectal angle.

Another important component of the continence mechanism is the sampling reflex. When stool or flatus distends the rectum, a reflex relaxation of the IAS occurs, decreasing the length of the high-pressure zone of the anal canal and allowing contact of rectal contents with anal mucosa. If, during this "sampling" of rectal contents, liquid or solid feces is detected, the EAS contracts to prevent soiling. Other factors, such as stool volume and consistency, stool transit time, rectal sensation and compliance, and patient motivation play important roles in continence.

23. Describe the pathophysiology of fecal incontinence.

Normal functioning requires an intact neuromuscular system; the ability to sense impending defecation and to differentiate between gas, liquid, and solid; and the motivation to maintain continence. The major abnormalities of continence mechanisms involve impairments in rectal sensation, abnormal rectal compliance, and anal sphincter dysfunction secondary to muscle dysfunction or interruption and nerve damage.

Impaired proprioception in the levator ani, puborectalis, and sphincters can decrease the ability to sense rectal filling, leading to loss of the normal warning of imminent defecation. Because autonomic pathways remain intact, the IAS relaxes before the patient senses rectal distention, leading to incontinence. Longstanding diabetics may develop sensory abnormalities from neuoropathy with similar consequences.

Changes in **rectal compliance** can lead to incontinence. The rectum has elastic properties that allow it to maintain low intraluminal pressure in response to increasing volumes. If compliance is diminished, smaller volumes may lead to increased intraluminal pressures and incontinence, often associated with urgency and frequency. Conversely, incontinence also may result from increased rectal compliance and diminished sensation, as in fecal impaction and megarectum. In this setting, intact involuntary pathways relax the internal anal sphincter before the patient senses rectal distention, with resultant incontinence from "overflow" diarrhea.

Myopathic damage from disruption of the anal sphincters and sacral neuropathic disorders can diminish the high-pressure zone necessary to maintain continence, leading to soiling. A functional component also may lead to early muscle fatigue and incontinence. Rarely, massive diarrhea may overwhelm the normal continence mechanism.

24. What are the major causes of incontinence?

Anatomic defects	Obstetric injury (high birthweight infants, forceps-assisted deliveries)
	Surgical injury (fistula repair, hemorrhoidectomy)
	Trauma
Collagen vascular disease	Scleroderma
Congenital disorders	Spina bifida
Diarrheal conditions	Inflammatory bowel disease
	Infection
	Irritable bowel syndrome
	Laxatives
	Malabsorption
Neurologic disorders	Cerebrovascular accident
	Dementia
	Diabetes
	Multiple sclerosis
Overflow incontinence	Fecal impaction
Aging	May be multifactorial

25. Describe the work-up of incontinence.

A good history and physical exam are vital. The **history** should include general information about frequency, duration, and pattern of soilage; symptoms of diarrhea, constipation, urgency, or straining; and dietary intake. Prior anorectal surgery or trauma, diabetes mellitus or thyroid disease, neurologic events or illness, and progressive dementia may contribute to incontinence. A thorough obstetric history includes information about all deliveries, use of forceps for delivery, or significant perineal lacerations that may have affected the perineal floor. Finally, a comprehensive medication history must be obtained, including direct inquiry about over-the-counter medications, laxatives, and dietary substitutes such as sorbitol.

The **physical exam** must include careful inspection of the perineum, looking for scars, obvious lacerations, fissures, and hemorrhoids. Digital rectal exam detects distal rectal masses and fecal impaction. The resting tone and squeeze pressures of the anal sphincter should be noted and the strength of puborectalis contraction assessed. Neurologic evaluation should include a mental status examination, assessment of sacral reflexes (anal wink), checking the integrity of the spinal pathway, and evaluation of perineal sensation. Visualization of the anus with anoscopy, and flexible sigmoidoscopy or colonoscopy, as indicated, completes the exam.

26. What specialized tests are available for the evaluation of incontinence?

Anorectal manometry, which is performed with balloon catheters to test the function of the sphincters, enables measurement of the resting tone of the IAS, squeeze pressure of the EAS, and functional length of the high-pressure zone created by the sphincters. Certain manometric devices are also capable of measuring rectal sensation and rectal compliance.

Electromyography of the sphincters and puborectalis, performed with surface electrodes or needles, allows detection of denervation, conduction defects, and abnormalities in striated muscle function. This test may serve both a diagnostic and therapeutic function.

Pudendal nerve terminal motor assessment (PNTML) is performed by stimulating the right and/or left pudendal nerves at the ischial tuberosities and measuring the time to detect a muscular response (latency). This test is most useful in patients with obstetric injury, neurogenic incontinence, and rectal prolapse, all of which may have prolonged PNTML.

Defecography (described above) evaluates the anatomy and change in pelvic floor muscle position with defecation. Abnormalities often missed in endoscopic evaluation of the rectum, such as prolapse, perineal descent, and intussusception, are often detected with defecography.

Endoscopic ultrasound is a safe method for quick and easy evaluation of the structural integrity of the IAS and EAS.

27. How is incontinence treated?

The initial step is **correction of all modifiable factors**. Dietary changes, such as limiting sorbitol, lactose, and fructose ingestion and increasing dietary fiber, may firm the stool, allowing better rectal sensation and enhancing sphincter function. Over-the-counter medications that may cause diarrhea (e.g., magnesium-containing antacids) should be eliminated.

Biofeedback requires a patient who is able to understand the process, is sufficiently motivated, has some rectal sensation, and can generate a squeeze pressure through voluntary control of the EAS. Patients can be taught to recognize rectal distention and to increase the EAS pressure in response to balloon distention. In well-selected patients, good results may be noted after a single session.

Various surgical techniques have been used. Operative resuspension of rectal prolapse restores continence in up to two-thirds of patients. Repair of sphincteric defects, with removal of scar tissue and direct apposition of the sphincters, successfully relieves incontinence in approximately 50% of patients. Anterior plication of the levator ani, puborectalis, and EAS with restoration of the anorectal angle and tightening of the anal canal improves symptoms in approximately 62% of patients with idiopathic incontinence. Other techniques, such as anal encirclement with a wire or a silastic ring to tighten the anal canal mechanically, have been used, but frequent complications occur. Newer techniques using artificial sphincters are currently under study. Colostomy has been used for immobile patients suffering from recurrent bacteremia secondary to skin breakdown with fecal contamination of decubitus ulcers.

28. List the indications and contraindications for use of biofeedback.

INDICATIONS	CONTRAINDICATIONS
Anal sphincter weakness	Dementia
Anal sphincter muscle fatigue	Spinal cord injuries
Obstetric damage	Absent rectal sensation
Idiopathic fecal incontinence	Lack of motivation
Diabetes mellitus	Impaired rectal storage capacity
Meningomyelocele	

29. Outline the approach to evaluation of patients with fecal incontinence:

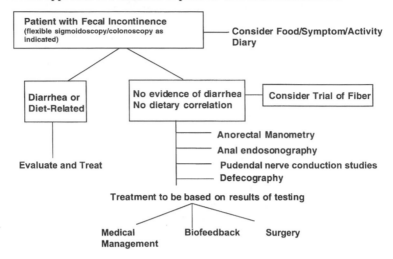

BIBLIOGRAPHY

1. Bishoff JT, Garrick M, Optenberg SAA, et al: Incidence of fecal and urinary incontinence following radical perineal and retropubic prostatectomy in a national population. J Urol 160:454–458, 1998.
2. Burkitt DP, Walker ARP, Painter NS: Effect of dietary fiber on stools and transit times, and its role in the causation of disease. Lancet 2:1408, 1972.
3. Camilleri M, Thompson WG, Fleshman JW, et al: Clinical management of intractable constipation. Ann Intern Med 121:520–528, 1994.
4. Caruana BJ. Wald A, Hinds JP, et al: Anorectal sensory and motor function in neurogenic fecal incontinence. Gastroenterology 100:465–470, 1991.
5. Cooper ZR, Rose S: Fecal incontinence: A clinical approach. Mount Sinai J Med 67:96–105, 2000.
6. De Lillo AR, Rose S: Functional bowel disorders in the geriatric patient: Constipation, fecal impaction, and incontinence. Am J Gastroenterol 9:901–905, 2000.
7. Enck P: Biofeedback training in disordered defecation: A critical review. Dig Dis Sci 38:1953–1960, 1993.
8. Freckner B, Von Euler C: Influence of pudendal block on the anal sphincters. Gut 16:482–489, 1975.
9. Gattuso JM, Kamm MA: Clinical features of idiopathic megarectum and idiopathic megacolon. Gut 41:93–99, 1997.
10. Goei R: Anorectal function in patients with defecation disorders and asymptomatic subjects: Evaluation with defecography. Radiology174:121, 1990.
11. Ho YH, Tan M, Goh HS: Clinical and physiologic effects of biofeedback in outlet obstruction constipation. Dis Colon Rectum 39:520–524, 1996.
12. Jost WH, Schrank B, Herold A, Leiss O: Functional outlet obstruction: Anismus, spastic pelvic floor syndrome, and dyscoordination of the voluntary sphincter muscles. Definition, diagnosis, and treatment from the neurologic point of view. Scand J Gastroenterol 34:449–453, 1999.
13. Kelvin FM, Maglinte DD, Benson JT: Evacuation proctography (defecography): An aid to investigation of pelvic floor disorders. Obstet Gynecol 83:307–314, 1994.
14. Metcalfe AM, Phillips SF, Zinmeister AR, et al: Simplified assessment of segmental colonic transit. Gastroenterology 92:40, 1987.
15. Miller R, Orrom WJ, Cornes H, et al: Anterior sphincter plication and levatorplasty in the treatment of fecal incontinence. Br J Surg 76:1058–1060, 1989.
16. Nelson R, Norton N, Cautley E, Furner S: Community based prevalence of anal incontinence. JAMA 274:559–561, 1995.
17. Prather CM, Camillieri M, Zinsmeister AR, et al: Tegaserod accelerates orocecal transit in patients with constipation predominant irritable bowel syndrome. Gastroenterology 118:463–468, 2000.
18. Rose S, Reynolds JC: Motility disorders of the colon. In Anuras S: Motility Disorders of the Gastrointestinal Tract: Principles and Practice. New York, Raven Press, 1992.
19. Sultan AH, Kamm MA, Hudson CN, et al: Anal sphincter disruption during vaginal delivery. N Engl J Med 329:1905–1911, 1993.
20. Sun WM, Read NW, Miner PB: Relation between rectal sensation and anal function in normal subjects and patients with fecal incontinence. Gut 1056–1061, 1990.
21. Wald A: Colonic transit and anorectal manometry in chronic idiopathic constipation. Arch Intern Med 146:1713, 1986.
22. You YT, Wang JY, Changchien CR: Segmental colectomy in the management of colonic inertia. Am Surg 64:775–777, 1998.

52. DIVERTICULITIS

Stephen R. Freeman, M.D.

1. How common is diverticular disease? What are the most frequent complications?

One-third of western populations have diverticulosis by age 50 and two-thirds by age 80. The majority remain asymptomatic; complications of bleeding or diverticulitis occur in 10–20%.

2. How do diverticula develop?

Although the cause is not known for certain, the presence of diverticula has been correlated with a decrease in dietary fiber; related factors are aging and increased intraluminal pressure. Decreased fiber in the colonic lumen leads to decreased stool volume, which results in more colonic segmentation during peristaltic activity in propelling contents aborally. Segmentation generates greater intraluminal pressures. The increased intraluminal pressure may predispose to diverticula formation. Each diverticulum is a result of herniation of mucosa through the muscular colonic wall at points of weakness, which correspond to sites of penetrating arteries.

3. Where are diverticula located?

In Western society, 85% of diverticula are located in the descending and sigmoid colon. The sigmoid colon is smaller in luminal diameter; therefore, wall tension pressure during segmentation is greater and probably responsible for predilection for diverticula formation in the sigmoid colon. In addition, use of Western style toilets results in increased intraluminal pressures compared with defecation performed in the knee-chest position, which is common in third-world countries where the incidence of diverticulosis is much less. Of interest, because diverticula are site-specific to the right colon in Asians, other factors must be important, such as genetics and other environmental factors. As western diet begins to permeate a nonwestern culture, the incidence of diverticulosis increases, as does the incidence of left-sided location.

4. How should symptomatic diverticulosis be managed?

Most clinicians emphasize the benefits of a high-fiber diet, regardless of the presence or absence of symptoms. Abdominal pain is thought to be related to spasm or distention of the colon, probably a factor in the pathogenesis of diverticula. There is no proven therapy. High-fiber diet is helpful, and antispasmodics often are used, although their benefit is unproven. Newer therapies for irritable bowel syndrome, a frequent underlying disorder in patients with diverticulosis, include 5-HT3 antagonists, 5-HT4 agonists, and other agents; this approach may offer more effective therapy in the future. A common recommendation for patients with diverticulosis, with or without symptoms, is avoidance of certain foods containing seeds and nuts. Little evidence supports this advice, which eliminates many nutritious and high-fiber foods. In a recent survey of colorectal surgeons, most respondents disagreed about the importance of avoiding seeds and nuts. A high-fiber diet without concern for avoiding nuts and seeds is probably the most appropriate advice.

5. What are the common signs and symptoms of diverticulitis?

The most common symptoms are abrupt onset of abdominal pain and an alteration in bowel pattern. Early acute diverticulitis is characterized by circumscribed abdominal pain and tenderness. The usual location of the pain is the left lower quadrant, but because diverticula, and hence diverticulitis, can develop at any site, inflammation may mimic other conditions. For example, transverse colon diverticulitis may mimic peptic ulcer disease, and right colon diverticulitis may mimic acute appendicitis. Signs of inflammation, such as fever and elevated white blood count, help to distinguish diverticulitis from the spasm of irritable bowel syndrome.

As the disease progresses in severity, localized abscess and phlegmonous reaction may develop. In addition to pain and tenderness, a mass may develop. Systemic signs of infection become more pronounced, i.e., fever and leukocytosis. In elderly patients and patients taking corticosteroids, the abdominal exam and usual signs are unreliable. Therefore, a high index of suspicion and use of imaging studies, such as CT scan, are quite important to avoid significant delay in diagnosis and increased operative mortality.

Obstipation has long been taught as a symptom of diverticulitis, but, in fact, diarrhea is not uncommon. Rectal bleeding is not a symptom of diverticulitis. Other causes, such as hemorrhoids, neoplasm, colitis, arteriovenous malformations, or arterial bleeding from diverticulosis, should be entertained if bleeding is the problem.

6. Outline the approach to the evaluation and diagnosis of acute diverticulitis, including physical exam and diagnostic procedures.

History and physical examination
  Usually > 60 years old
  Left lower quadrant tenderness and unremitting abdominal pain
  Fever
  Leukocytosis
Differential diagnosis

Elderly patients	*Middle-aged and young patients*
Ischemia	Appendicitis
Carcinoma	Salpingitis
Volvulus	Inflammatory bowel disease
Obstruction	Penetrating ulcer
Penetrating ulcer	Urosepsis
Nephrolithiasis/urosepsis	

Qualifiers
  Extremes of age (more virulent)
  Asian ancestry (right-sided symptoms)
  Corticosteroids
  Immunosuppression
  Chronic renal failure (abdominal examination insensitive)
Evaluations
  Plain x-rays: Good initial first step. May show ileus, obstruction, mass effect, ischemia, perforation
  Contrast enema: For mild-to-moderate cases when the diagnosis is in doubt, water-soluble contrast exam is safe and helpful; otherwise, delay the exam for 6–8 weeks.
  Endoscopy: Acute diverticulitis is a relative contraindication to endoscopy; must exclude perforation first. Examine only when the diagnosis is in doubt (rectal bleeding, anemia) to exclude ischemic bowel, Crohn's disease, carcinoma, and other possibilities.
  CT scan: Very helpful in staging the degree of complications and evaluating for other diseases. Should be considered in all cases of diverticulitis with a palpable mass or clinical toxicity, failure of medical therapy, orthopedic complications, and corticosteroid use.
  Ultrasound: Can be a safe and helpful noninvasive test to evaluate acute diverticulitis. Over 20% of exams are suboptimal because of intestinal gas; highly operator-dependent.

Adapted from Freeman SR, McNally PR: Diverticulitis. Med Clin North Am 77:1152, 1993.

7. List the common complications of diverticulitis.
Fistula, abscess, obstruction, and peritonitis from perforation.

8. Between what organs may fistulous communications develop?
Bowel, urinary bladder, skin, pelvic floor, and vagina may be involved in fistulous disease of diverticulitis. The most common is **colovesicular fistula** (colon to urinary bladder), which is seen almost exclusively in men and in women after hysterectomy. Pneumaturia is a pathognomonic sign of this fistula. Another clue is recurrent urinary tract infections, especially involving multiple

organisms. Demonstration of the fistulous connection is usually difficult. Reflux of contrast through the fistula via contrast enema or cystogram confirms the diagnosis, but such reflux is seen in a minority of patients. Colovesicular fistula is a strong indication for surgical correction.

Colovaginal fistulas occur almost exclusively in women with prior hysterectomies. The differential diagnosis includes Crohn's disease, previous pelvic irradiation, gynecologic surgery, and pelvic abscess from any cause. Diagnosis is suspected in the proper setting (recent diverticulitis) because of the presence of vaginal symptoms: vaginal discharge, severe vaginitis, flatus vaginalis, and feculent discharge (pathognomonic). Identification of the fistula can be difficult. Barium enema, oral charcoal, vaginography, and combined vaginoscopy and colonoscopy are various means of attempting to localize the fistula. Treatment is surgical resection of the diseased section of bowel.

9. How is diverticular stricture differentiated from strictures of other causes?

The signs favoring diverticular stricture are the presence of diverticula in the region of the colonic stricture, the suggestion of an extraluminal mass contributing to the stricture, and the suggestion of an intramural or extraluminal extravasation of contrast. The length of the stricture is helpful. Whereas a **malignant stricture** is usually < 3 cm in length and is associated with abrupt shoulders at either end, the **diverticular stricture** is longer (3–6 cm) with smoother contours. Very long strictures (6–10 cm) are more likely to be due to **Crohn's disease** or **ischemia**. Sometimes the location of the stricture is helpful. For example, the splenic flexure is an uncommon site for diverticulitis, but a common site for ischemia.

10. What extraintestinal complications are associated with diverticulitis?

Arthritis and pyoderma gangrenosum were reported in one study. Resection of the involved colon was effective in eliminating these problems. Initially all had been diagnosed incorrectly with inflammatory bowel disease.

Leg pain, possibly associated with thigh abscess or leg emphysema, may result from retroperitoneal perforation. The 70% mortality rate associated with this complication is probably due to delayed diagnosis and inadequate treatment. Treatment must include fecal diversion and wide surgical debridement as well as broad-spectrum antibiotics.

Renal disease has an association with diverticulosis. Patients with renal transplant and patients who undergo chronic hemodialysis and peritoneal dialysis are much more susceptible to life-threatening complications. Immunosuppression is part of the reason. In patients considered for renal transplant or continuous ambulatory peritoneal dialysis (CAPD), surgical resection of involved colon perhaps should be done beforehand if diverticulitis has been symptomatic. Patients with polycystic kidney disease and associated renal failure have a significantly higher incidence of diverticulitis, often complicated, than patients with renal failure due to other causes.

11. Which drugs are known to exacerbate diverticulitis?

Corticosteroids in high dose have been associated with development of acute diverticulitis. A cause-and-effect relationship is debatable, but inhibition of epithelial cell renewal has been hypothesized. Clearly, high-dose steroids may mask usual signs and symptoms of diverticulitis, leading to delay in diagnosis and more serious disease.

Nonsteroidal anti-inflammatory drugs also have been associated with more severe diverticulitis. The masking of early signs and symptoms has been hypothesized as the most likely reason.

12. What diagnostic tools are available to diagnose diverticulitis? What is the role of each?

Besides clinical and laboratory evaluation, imaging studies play an important role in diagnosis of diverticulitis. Although **contrast enema** may aggravate the disease and prove more harmful than helpful, experienced radiologists can perform this study safely and successfully. Because extravasation of barium may worsen peritonitis, many practitioners prefer water-soluble contrast.

CT is the test of choice for diagnostic evaluation of complicated diverticulitis, with a sensitivity of 90–95% and a specificity of 72%. It offers the added advantage of providing extraluminal information and helps to identify patients with nondiverticular causes of symptoms, such as ischemic colitis, mesenteric thrombosis, tubo-ovarian abscess, and pancreatitis. CT criteria for diagnosis of acute diverticulitis are localized colonic wall thickening (> 5 mm) and inflammation of pericolonic fat or the presence of pericolic abscess. The disadvantage of CT is the significantly higher cost.

Abdominal and pelvic **ultrasonography**, in the hands of interested and capable radiologists, is also a helpful test, with a sensitivity and specificity of 84% and 80%, respectively. Findings by ultrasound are similar to those on CT scan. Wall thickening, inflammation of pericolic fat, intramural and extraintestinal masses, and occasionally intramural fistula support the diagnosis of diverticulitis.

Endoscopy is generally thought to be contraindicated in acute diverticulitis because of the fear that scope manipulation and luminal air insufflation may worsen or enhance diverticular perforation and subsequent abscess or peritonitis. However, when the diagnosis is not clear and the differential includes obstructing carcinoma, ischemia, inflammatory bowel disease, and infectious colitis, endoscopy can be very helpful. The exam should be done carefully by an experienced endoscopist, with minimal air insufflation and no "slide-by" maneuvers of tight angulations. Findings suggestive of diverticulitis include peridiverticular erythema, edema, and pus.

13. How is mild diverticulitis defined and treated?

Mild diverticulitis is considered in patients with appropriately localized abdominal pain, usually in the left lower quadrant; fever and/or leukocytosis usually is present. The patient is nontoxic and able to take food and fluids orally without vomiting. Qualifying factors that may be imply more serious disease include age, underlying medical conditions, and concurrent medications. Diverticulitis tends to be more virulent in young (< 40 years) and very old patients. Immunocompromised patients, such as transplant recipients or patients with chronic renal failure or diabetes mellitus, are also at high risk for more virulent disease. Patients with right-sided diverticulitis tend to do less well. Mild disease is defined by lack of factors placing a patient at higher risk.

Treatment of mild disease is generally performed on an outpatient basis. Diet is commonly modified to include only clear liquids, more by convention than proof of efficacy. Antibiotic choice is commonly oral sulfa-trimethoprim (TMP/SMX) plus metronidazole. Ciprofloxacin or cephalexin may be substituted for TMP/SMX, clindamycin for metronidazole. Coverage is aimed at aerobic gram-negative organisms, and usually anaerobic coverage is added.

A Guide to Antimicrobial Therapy in Acute Diverticulitis

MODIFYING CIRCUMSTANCES	CAUSE	FIRST CHOICE	ALTERNATIVE	COMMENTS
Mild, nonperforating, with no high-risk factors	Aerobes *Escherichia coli* *Klebsiella* spp. Streptococci *Proteus* spp. *Enterobacter* spp. Anaerobes *Bacteroides fragilis* Peptostreptococci Peptococci *Clostridium* spp.	TMP/SMC + metronidazole	Ciprofloxacin or cephalexin for TMP/SMX Clindamycin for metronidazole	Outpatient, oral
Moderately ill, possible local abscess, ± high-risk factors	Same, including *Pseudomonas aeruginosa*	Ampicillin + aminoglycoside + metronidazole Imipenem/cilastatin Ampicillin/sulbactam Celoxitin Ticarcillin/clavulanate	Ciprofloxacin + metronidazole	Inpatient, IV + CT (catheter drainage of abscess) Consider surgery
Severly ill, toxic, peritonitis	Same, including *Pseudomonas aeruginosa*	Same	Same	Inpatient, IV + CT Consider early surgery

From Freeman SR, McNally PR: Diverticulitis. Med Clin North Am 77:1161, 1993, with permission.

14. What antibiotic regimen is appropriate for moderately severe disease? How is treatment otherwise different?

Antibiotics usually are given intravenously, most often on an inpatient basis. Many combinations are appropriate. Ampicillin, an aminoglycoside, and metronidazole may be used. Other choices include imipenum/cilastatin, or ampicillin/sulbactam, or a second generation cephalosporin (cefotetan or cefoxitin), or ticarcillin clavulanate. Ciprofloxacin plus metronidazole is a second choice. One goal for more severe disease is adequate coverage of *Pseudomonas aeruginosa*.

15. How is the management of severely ill patients different?

Severely ill patients usually are toxic with signs of peritonitis. The main difference in treatment from patients with less serious disease is the threshold for surgery. In toxic patients, an imaging study such as CT scan may be helpful in directing treatment, but early surgery is often the option most likely to result in favorable outcome.

16. What operations are available in the management of diverticulitis?

Surgical management involves resection of the diseased segment of colon. The surgery may involve abscess drainage and fecal diversion. Surgery, with those measures, may be done in one, two, or three stages (see figure on following page).

17. What are the indications for surgery for diverticulitis?

Surgery is indicated for complications such as sepsis, fistula formation, and obstruction. Patients with recurrent episodes of diverticulitis are candidates for surgery, as are those who fail medical therapy or deteriorate during original treatment. Occasionally, patients with a colonic stricture that cannot convincingly be shown not to be malignant are candidates for resection. The threshold for surgery is modified by the presence of high-risk factors: extremes of age, use of steroids, immunocompromise, and right-sided diverticulitis.

In the past decade, laparoscopic surgery has become applicable to an increasingly wider range of problems. This attractive technique has been used successfully for complicated diverticulitis. Several series demonstrate equal safety and effectiveness with laparoscopic surgery and the conventional approach with open laparotomy. The advantage of the laparoscopic approach is decreased morbidity and lower costs of hospitalization.

18. What are the preferred operations for diverticulitis?

The ideal solution is a **single operation**, during which the diseased bowel is resected and the remaining colon is anastomosed to maintain normal continuity. Examples of appropriate clinical scenarios include chronic obstruction, intractable pain, or recurrent episodes of medically responsive diverticulitis. In such cases, surgery is elective, allowing thorough preoperative bowel preparation.

Not uncommonly, a **two-stage procedure** is needed when bowel preparation cannot be performed beforehand—usually for medically unresponsive disease. A diverting colostomy is created as the diseased bowel segment is removed. Either a mucus fistula is created with the distal colonic segment, or it is oversewn and placed back in the abdomen (Hartman's pouch). Later (3–6 months), a second operation is performed to reestablish bowel continuity.

A **three-stage procedure** may be needed in severely ill patients. The initial operation is simple drainage of the pericolonic abscess and creation of a diverting colostomy. A second operation in 2–8 weeks is performed to resect the diseased bowel with reanastomosis of the bowel and maintenance of the colostomy to protect the anastomosis. A third surgery is performed in 2–4 weeks to take down the colostomy and restore bowel continuity.

The three-stage approach was standard management for much of the 20th century. Large reviews published in the past 20 years have pointed out the considerably reduced mortality and morbidity associated with the two-stage approach. The mortality rate for the two-stage procedure is 1–12%, whereas that for the three stage approach is 12–32%. The two-stage approach is now the procedure of choice for perforated diverticulitis.

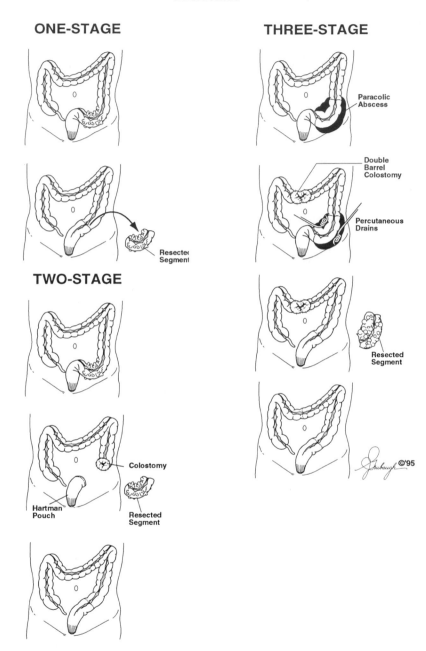

ONE-STAGE

TWO-STAGE

Colostomy

Hartman Pouch

Resected Segment

THREE-STAGE

Paracolic Abscess

Double Barrel Colostomy

Percutaneous Drains

Resected Segment

Resected Segment

Surgical options for treating complicated diverticulitis. **One-stage surgery** includes resection of diseased bowel and reanastomosis to reestablish normal bowel continuity. **Two-stage surgery** for more complicated disease involves fecal diversion via a proximal colostomy and resection of the diseased segment. The distal segment of the colon can be oversewn (Hartman pouch) or brought out as a mucous fistula. This is currently the most frequently performed operation for diverticulitis complicated by abscess. The first step in **three-stage surgery** involves fecal diversion and simple drainage of the involved area. Later the involved area is resected at a second operation and a reanastomosis of the segment is performed, leaving the suture line protected by the diverting colostomy. At a third surgery, the colostomy is taken down and bowel continuity is reestablished. (From Freeman SR, McNally PR: Diverticulitis. Med Clin North Am 77:1161, 1993, with permission.)

BIBIOGRAPHY

1. Almy TP, Howell DA: Medical progress: Diverticular disease of the colon. N Engl J Med 302:324–331, 1980.
2. Ferzoco LB, Raptopoulos V, Silen W: Acute diverticulitis (a clinical review). N Engl J Med 338:1521–1526, 1998.
3. Freeman SR, McNally PR, Diverticulitis: Med Clin North Am 77:1149–1167, 1993.
4. Greenall MJ, Levine AW, Nolan DT: Complications of diverticular disease: A review of the barium enema findings. Gastrointest Radiol 8:353–358, 1983
5. Klein S, Mayer L, Present DH et al: Extraintestinal manifestations in patients with diverticulitis. Ann Intern Med 108:700–702, 1988.
6. Mendeloff AI: Dietary fiber and gastrointestinal disease. Med Clin North Am 62:165–171, 1978.
7. Mendeloff AI: Thoughts on the epidemiology of divertivcular disease. Clin Gastroenterol 15:855–877, 1986.
8. Painter NS, Burkitt DP: Diverticular disease on the colon: A deficiency disease of western civilization. Br Med J 2:450–454, 1971.
9. Reve RV, Nahrwold DL: Diverticular disease. Curr Prob Surg 26:136, 1989.
10. Schechter S, Mulvey J, Eisenstat TE: Management of uncomplicated acute diverticulitis: Results of a survey. Dis Colon Rectum 42:470–475; discussion, 475–476, 1999.
11. Smith TR, Cho KC, Morehouse HT, et al: Comparison of computed tomography and contrast enema evaluation of diverticulitis. Dis Colon Rectum 33:1–6, 1990.
12. Stocchi L, Nelson H, Young-Fadok TM, et al: Safety and advantages of laparoscopic vs. open colectomy in the elderly: Matched-control study. Dis Colon Rectum 43:326–332, 2000.
13. Woods RJ, Lavery IC, Fazio VW, et al: Internal fistulas in diverticular disease. Dis Colon Rectum 31:591–596, 1988.
14. Wong WD, Wexner SD, Lowry A, et al: Practice parameters for the treatment of sigmoid diverticulitis—supporting documentation. The Standards Task Force, American Society of Colon and Rectal Surgeons. Dis Colon Rectum 43:290–297, 2000.
15. Younes Z, Johnson DA: New developments and concepts in antimicrobial therapy for intra-abdominal infections. Curr Gastroenterol Rep 2:277–282, 2000.

53. DISEASES OF THE APPENDIX

Frank H. Chae, M.D.

1. What is the first symptom of acute appendicitis?
Pain usually starts in the periumbilical area and later localizes to the right lower quadrant. Low-grade fever, anorexia, nausea, and vomiting may occur after the onset of pain.

2. What and where is McBurney's point?
The point of maximal tenderness elicited in the right lower quadrant during a physical exam, indicates an inflammation in the area. It is a point located two-thirds distally from the umbilicus along an axis drawn from the umbilicus to the anterior superior iliac spine.

3. Peak incidence of acute appendicitis occurs in what age group?
15–19 years of age.

4. The risk of perforation of the appendix is high in what age groups?
Children (< age 5 years) and elderly people (as high as 75%). Diabetics and immunosuppressed patients are also at risk.

5. What is the surgery mortality rate for nonperforated appendicitis? Perforated?
Less than 0.1% for nonperforated and as high as 4% for perforated appendicitis.

6. List the differential diagnoses for right lower quadrant pain.
Ectopic pregnancy, tubo-ovarian abscess, pelvic inflammatory disease, Mittelschmerz, torsion of ovary, incarcerated hernia, Crohn's disease, ulcerative colitis, diverticulitis, Meckel's diverticulitis, carcinoid tumor, infectious colitis, cholecystitis, and peptic ulcer disease.

7. How may acute cholecystitis and peptic ulcer disease present with right lower quadrant pain?
Perforation of gangrenous gallbladder or duodenal/gastric ulcer leads to collection of biliary and/or gastric fluid in the right lower quadrant.

8. What is a Meckel's diverticulum?
A congenital omphalomesenteric mucosa remnant that may contain ectopic gastric mucosa. Located on the antimesenteric side of the ileum, usually 2 feet from the ileocecal valve, it is found in 2% of the population, and 2% will develop diverticulitis. The gastric mucosa, if present, may lead to ileal ulcer and cause a small intestinal bleed.

9. In children, what two other conditions mimic acute appendicitis?
Gastroenteritis and mesenteric lymphadenitis (*Yersinia enterocolitica*).

10. What is an acceptable incidence rate for false-positive diagnosis of appendicitis?
A false-positive rate of 10–15% on appendectomy is within acceptable standards of surgical care. Lower false-positive rates may imply decreased vigilance for the diagnosis of appendicitis.

11. In older patients (age > 50 years), what condition may be indistinguishable from acute appendicitis?
Acute diverticulitis of either a redundant sigmoid colon or the cecum may present with right lower quadrant pain.

12. List the differentiating features of pelvic inflammatory disease (PID).

High fever, cervical motion tenderness, cervical discharge, and pain related to menses with tendency for bilateral onset.

13. Define Mittelschmerz.

Pain accompanying the rupture of ovarian follicle at mid-menstrual cycle. Although it is a common nonsurgical ailment, appendicitis should be ruled out.

14. What are the psoas and obturator signs?

Irritation of the retroperitoneal psoas muscle (pain on right hip extension) or internal obturator muscle (pain on internal rotation of the flexed right hip) by an inflamed retrocecal appendix.

15. What is Rovsing's sign?

Palpation of the left lower quadrant commonly leads to right lower quadrant pain in acute appendicitis.

16. How does appendicitis lead to Charcot's triad and gas in the portal vein?

Charcot's triad (fever/chills, right upper quadrant pain, and jaundice) and gas in the portal venous system may result from suppurative thrombosis of the portal vein due to appendiceal abscess. It should be rarely seen in the current setting of effective antibiotic coverage with early surgical removal of the infected appendix.

17. What is the most common tumor of the appendix? Describe its management.

Carcinoid. Appendectomy usually is performed, but if the tumor is infiltrating near the base or the cecum, right hemicolectomy is required. If metastatic disease is present, the tumor still should be removed for palliation.

18. When is CT-guided drainage of an appendiceal abscess an option?

An established abscess with an inaccessible appendix may be drained via CT-guided catheter placement, provided that the patient has no evidence of diffuse peritonitis or sepsis while taking antibiotics. An appendectomy is required after about 6–8 weeks of recovery because the rate of recurrent appendicitis may approach 20%.

19. What is the most common complication after appendectomy?

Subcutaneous wound infection. For perforated appendix or abscess, the fascia is closed and the skin is usually left open for delayed closure.

20. How does ultrasound help in the diagnosis of acute appendicitis?

Ultrasound helps when an active disease entity is identified, such as an appendiceal mass, tubo-ovarian abscess, or tubal ectopic pregnancy, but its usefulness is limited when the appendix appears "normal" or cannot be located.

21. When is laparoscopic appendectomy appropriate?

Laparoscopy helps as a minimally invasive evaluation tool when the diagnosis is uncertain, especially in young women or morbidly obese patients. If the appendix appears normal, it should be removed via laparoscope to narrow the differential diagnosis in the event of recurrent symptoms. Laparoscopy probably does not help in patients with a perforated appendix and abscess. Improved cosmesis, less wound infection, and pain are the benefits of laparoscopy, but the cost is greater and the length of hospitalization is equivalent to the open approach.

22. During an abdominal exploration for right lower quadrant pain, is removal of normal appendix appropriate in patients with Crohn's disease?

Yes. If the base of the appendix and the surrounding area of the cecum are free of inflammation despite active terminal ileal disease, an appendectomy still should be performed. If an enterocutaneous fistula develops postoperatively, it almost always results from the diseased ileum and not from the surgical site on the cecum.

23. Ovarian tumor is discovered during laparoscopic or open exploration. What steps should be taken?

The normal appendix should be removed after obtaining peritoneal washings with saline irrigation in the abdominal cavity. The washing is collected to look for free tumor cells. The ovarian mass should not be touched or biopsied. A strictly followed, elaborate ritual is performed for staging ovarian cancer. Patients should be brought back at a later time for surgical staging.

24. Does nonoperative therapy have any role in treating acute appendicitis?

In general, treating acute appendicitis with antibiotic therapy alone is not recommended in North America. The British have been known to treat uncomplicated acute appendicitis with antibiotics; however, their claims of success have been offset by high recurrence rates and high costs of delivery. This mode of therapy is controversial and not universally accepted. On the other hand, delayed appendectomy is appropriate after resolution of contained abscess or inflammation by antibiotic therapy (with or without catheter drainage) in patients with a perforated appendix— provided that the abscess does not spread systemically and is well-contained.

BIBLIOGRAPHY

1. Affleck DG, Handrahan DL, Egger MJ, Price RR: The laparoscopic management of appendicitis and cholelithiasis in pregnancy. Am J Surg 178:523–529, 1999.
2. Carr NJ: The pathology of acute appendicitis. Ann Diagn Pathol 4:46–58, 2000.
3. Khalili TM, Hiatt JR, Savar A, et al: Perforated appendicitis is not a contraindication to laparoscopy. Am Surg 65:965–967, 1999.
4. Lane JS, Sarkar R, Schmidt PJ, et al: Surgical approach to cecal diverticulitis. J Am Coll Surg 188: 629–634, 1999.
5. Martin JP, Connor PD, Charles K: Meckel's diverticulum. Am Fam Physician 61:1037–1042, 2000.
6. Meakins JL: Appendectomy and appendicitis. Can J Surg 42:90, 1999.
7. McKellar DP, Reiling RB, Eiseman B: Prognosis and Outcomes in Surgical Disease. St. Louis, Quality Medical Publishing, 1999.
8. Norton LW, Stiegmann GV, Eiseman B: Surgical Decision Making. Philadelphia, W.B. Saunders, 2000.
9. Schumpelick V, Dreuw B, Ophoff K, Prescher A: Appendix and cecum: Embryology, anatomy, and surgical approach. Surg Clin North Am 80:295–318, 2000.
10. Temple LK, Litwin DE, McLeod RS: A meta-analysis of laparoscopic versus open appendectomy in patients suspected of having acute appendicitis. Can J Surg 42:377–383, 1999.

54. COLITIS: PSEUDOMEMBRANOUS, MICROSCOPIC, COLLAGENOUS, AND RADIATION

Christina M. Surawicz, M.D.

PSEUDOMEMBRANOUS COLITIS

1. How common is *Clostridium difficile* disease?

Although 20–30% of persons who take antibiotics develop diarrhea, a smaller number develop the severe complication of *C. difficile* colitis. The frequency of *C. difficile* disease is not known, but it is estimated at 12/100,000 outpatients and 21/100 inpatients. The most severe complication, pseudomembranous colitis (PMC), occurs in about 5–8% of all cases of *C. difficile* infection.

2. What causes PMC?

Pseudomembranous colitis is due to overgrowth of the anaerobic gram-positive bacteria *C. difficile*, which causes disease by production of two toxins, A and B. It occurs most commonly as a result of antibiotic therapy, which disrupts the normal colonic flora and allows *C. difficile* to grow.

3. Is PMC always due to antibiotics?

No. Cases develop sporadically as well as in association with chemotherapy. The key factor appears to be an alteration in colon flora that allows the organism to grow and produce its toxins.

4. Which antibiotics are implicated most commonly?

Clindamycin, cephalosporins (especially third-generation), and ampicillin. But PMC can occur with any antibiotic, even single-dose preoperative antibiotics.

5. What are the risk factors for *C. difficile* disease?

Hospitalized patients, especially surgical patients, ICU patients, posttransplant patients, and elderly patients, are the most susceptible. Other risk factors include invasive procedures (especially gastrointestinal procedures), renal failure, cancer chemotherapy, residence in nursing home, severity of disease, and enteral feeding.

6. Why do some people develop *C. difficile* diarrhea while others are simply colonized?

A recent prospective study measured immune responses to toxin A and toxin B in hospitalized patients who became colonized with *C. difficile*. Those who did *not* develop diarrhea developed higher levels of IgG antibody to toxin A (but not to toxin B). Thus, immune response may explain why some people develop diarrhea and others are simply colonized. Obviously, further studies are needed.

7. How is the diagnosis made?

DIAGNOSTIC TEST	ACCURACY	COMMENTS
Cytotoxin B assay	Good sensitivity and specificity	Gold standard, but expensive. Results not ready for 24–48 hr
Enzyme immunoassays to detect toxin A or B	Good specificity. Sensitivity varies	EIAs are replacing toxin B assay in many labs because they are quick (hours) and less expensive
Stool cultures	Sensitive. Poor specificity	Carriers test positive
Latex agglutination test	Sensitive. Poor specificity	Not specific for *C. difficile*

8. What are the typical findings on colonoscopy?

Colonoscopy may be normal or show nonspecific colitis. With severe disease, the colon mucosa has creamy white-yellow plaques (pseudomembranes). Histologic studies show that the pseudomembrane usually arises from a point of superficial ulceration, accompanied by acute and chronic inflammation of the lamina propria.

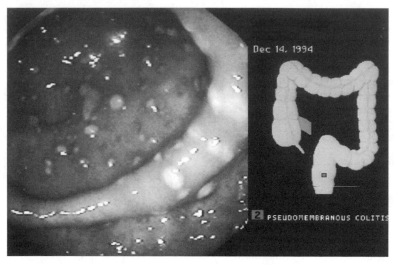

Endoscopic photograph of the white-yellow raised exudates seen in pseudomembranous colitis. (From Goff JS: Colitis:Radiation, microscopic, collagenous, and pseudomembranous. In McNally PR (ed): GI/Liver Secrets. Philadelphia, Hanley & Belfus, 1995, p 348, with permission.)

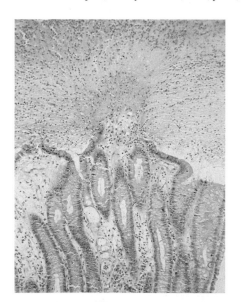

Pseudomembranous colitis. Microscopic section of colonic mucosa illustrates the pseudomembrane, composed of fibrin, polymorphonuclear cells, and debris, that emanates in a volcano-like fashion from the colon mucosa.

9. When is treatment indicated? What antibiotics are used?

The first step is to discontinue antibiotics, if possible. About 20% of cases, which are mild, resolve spontaneously. Treatment to eradicate *C. difficile* should be given in all but the mildest cases. The two most common antibiotics used to treat PMC are metronidazole and vancomycin.

Treatment for C. difficile *Disease*

DRUG	DOSE	COMMENT
Metronidazole	250–500 mg orally 4 times/day for 7–10 days	First line Avoid in first-trimester pregnancy Inexpensive
Vancomycin	125–500 mg orally 4 times/day for 7–10 days	Expensive ($600/10-day course)
Bacitracin	25,000 Units orally 4 times/day for 7–10 days	Expensive Does not taste good
Fusidic acid		Not available in US

10. What should be the first line choice of antibiotic?
Metronidazole is the first choice because it is less expensive and does not have the complication of development of vancomycin-resistant organisms.

11. When is vancomycin indicated?
When metronidazole cannot be used (i.e., first-trimester pregnancy, intolerable side effects) and when the patient fails to respond to metronidazole.

12. When should you expect a response to treatment?
Usually within 2–4 days, with resolution of diarrhea by 2 weeks.

13. When should you consult a surgeon?
When severe PMC is associated with toxic colon, increasing abdominal pain, or development of subserosal air in the colon on abdominal flat-plate radiographs.

14. What should you do if symptoms recur after therapy?
Although most patients respond to therapy, about 20% have recurrent symptoms after stopping the antibiotics, probably because continued abnormal fecal flora allows *C. difficile* to persist; perhaps spores germinate. One recurrence makes further recurrences even more likely (up to 40%).

15. What are the treatment options for recurrent *C. difficile* disease?
Patients need retreatment, with either metronidazole or vancomycin. Addition of a probiotic agent, such as the nonpathogenic yeast *Saccharomyces boulardii* (not yet available in the U.S), can decrease recurrences.

Treatment of Recurrent C. Difficile *Disease*

1. Retreat with antibiotic for 10–14 days
2. Reduce to 250–500 mg/day, and pulse or taper pulsed therapy to once daily, once every other day, and once every third day, with lengthening intervals.
3. Add probiotic agent if available.

16. How can we control *C. difficile* epidemics in hospitals?
Control mechanisms include handwashing, use of disposable equipment and vinyl gloves, limiting use of antibiotics, education programs, and infection control programs.

MICROSCOPIC COLITIDES

17. What are the microscopic colitides?
They are idiopathic colitides with mild inflammatory changes diagnosed only by colorectal biopsy and thus only microscopically. The microscopic colitides were first identified in 1976. A case of collagenous colitis was reported in a woman with chronic diarrhea and a normal GI evaluation.

Colorectal biopsy revealed unusual and specific histologic abnormalities of normal-appearing colon mucosa. The histology showed a thickened subepithelial collagen band and a slight increase in lymphocytes in the lamina propria. This entity was thus named collagenous colitis (CC). As more biopsies were taken from people with chronic diarrhea and normal colonic mucosa, the disease became more widely recognized. Several years later biopsy identified similar findings in other patients with chronic diarrhea but without the thickened collagen band. This clinical syndrome, initially named microscopic colitis, has been renamed lymphocytic colitis (LC) because of the mild increase in lymphocytes found in colon biopsies.

18. Compare collagenous colitis and lymphocytic colitis.

FEATURE	COLLAGENOUS COLITIS	LYMPHOCYTIC COLITIS
Gender incidence (female:male)	4–5:1	1:1
HLAB27-positive in some cases	No	Yes
Histology		
Increased in intraepithelial lymphocytes	Yes	Yes
Increased lymphocyte in lamina propria	Yes	Yes
Surface epithelial flattening	Yes	Yes
Thickened subepithelial collagen band (> 10 microns)	Yes	No

19. What is the diagnostic triad of collagenous colitis?
    An increase in intraepithelial lymphocytes (normal = 5/100 epithelial nuclei), a flattened surface epithelium, and a thickened subepithelial collagen band.

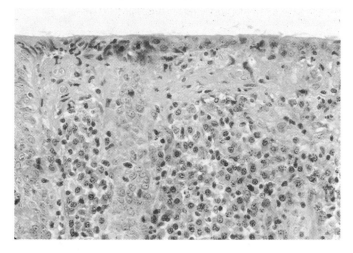

Collagenous colitis. Microscopic section of colonic mucosa shows flattened surface epithelium, thickened subepithelial collagen band, and slight increase in lamina propria lymphocytes.

20. How common are the microscopic colitides?
    The incidence of CC is 1.1 cases per 100,000 population. LC is more common at 3.1 cases per 100,000 population. Both are far less common than inflammatory bowel disease.

21. Which parts of the colon are most commonly affected?
    Microscopic colitides can be patchy. In one recent study, the highest yield was from biopsies of transverse colon. Most cases can be diagnosed by biopsies taken within the range of flexible sigmoidoscopy; sometimes colonoscopy with biopsy of the right colon is necessary.

22. What are the treatment options?

The natural history is not known, but spontaneous resolution may occur. Some patients do well on antidiarrheals or cholestyramine alone. Various treatment options have been tried because nothing is uniformly effective. Anti-inflammatory agents, such as sulfasalazine, 5-ASA preparations, and prednisone, have a response rate of about 70–80%. Some patients require stronger immunosuppressants such as methotrexate or azathioprine. Recent uncontrolled studies have shown some efficacy for budesonide, Pepto-Bismol, and pentoxyfylline. Further studies of treatment options are needed.

23. What is the role of nonsteroidal anti-inflammatory agents in the pathogenesis of microscopic colitides?

CC, which is more common in women, has been associated with use of nonsteroidal anti-inflammatory drugs (NSAIDs), which also is more common in women. A case-controlled study showed that patients with CC were 3 times more likely to take NSAIDS. If a patient with CC is taking NSAIDs, it is wise to discontinue them because the disease sometimes resolves when NSAIDs are stopped. However, there is no guarantee.

24. What are the associated conditions?

A wide variety of associated conditions is found in case reports, including rheumatologic conditions (e.g., rheumatoid arthritis, polyarthritis), thyroid disease, diabetes mellitus, systemic lupus erythematosus, sicca syndrome, atropic gastritis, and primary biliary cirrhosis. Although uncommon, celiac sprue and collagenous sprue also have been reported together.

RADIATION COLITIS

25. Which part of the gastrointestinal tract is most commonly injured by radiation?

The peristaltic movement of intestine in and out of the field of radiation decreases the degree of injury. The colon, especially the rectosigmoid, is highly susceptible to radiation injury because it is immobile. In addition, tumors in the pelvic area (e.g., cervix, uterus, prostate, testicles, bladder) often require high dosages of radiation.

26. What can be done to prevent radiation damage?

Limit the dosage and area of exposure, and shield adjacent tissues.

27. Which causes more damage, external beam or implant radiation therapy?

In general, implants cause less severe damage becaues of their smaller field of radiation.

28. What factors can aggravate radiation damage?

In addition to high doses of radiation given to fixed organs, which cannot shift during therapy, coadministration of chemotherapeutic agents enhances the damaging effects of radiation.

29. What symptoms are associated with total-body irradiation?

The initial symptoms are nausea and vomiting. Delayed symptoms are related to mucosal destruction, usually 5 days later (because cell turnover in the GI tract is typically 5 days), with diarrhea. Loss of mucosal defenses increases the chance of sepsis.

30. What are the early and late effects of localized radiation?

Early or acute changes are microscopic damage to mucosal and vascular epithelial cells. One typical histologic feature is the presence of atypical fibroblasts. Late or chronic changes more commonly involve fibrosis, which can cause strictures.

31. What are the acute symptoms of radiation colitis?

Diarrhea and tenesmus, usually occurring within 6 weeks. Rectal bleeding is less common.

32. What are the chronic symptoms of radiation colitis?
Diarrhea, rectal pain, and rectal bleeding, usually within 2 years of receiving radiation. Occasionally symptoms are delayed beyond this point.

33. Describe the colonoscopic findings.
Colonoscopy may be normal or may show telangiectasias or friable mucosa.

34. How can radiation colitis and proctitis be managed?
Various medications have been tried, including steroid enemas, systemic steroids, 5 ASA compounds, sulfasalazine, and sucralfate enemas.

35. What are the endoscopic therapies for chronic bleeding?
Argon laser photocoagulation, heater probe, and bipolar cautery have been used to treat localized bleeding from telangiectasias. Multiple treatment sessions often are needed. Patients should be transfused with blood as needed and take oral iron.

36. How are chronic radiation-induced bowel strictures managed?
Endoscopic dilation may be helpful. Surgery occasionally is needed.

BIBLIOGRAPHY

1. Alfa JM, Kabani A, Lyerly D, et al: Characterization of a toxin A-negative, toxin B-positive strain of Clostridium difficile responsible for a nosocomial outbreak of *Clostridium difficile*-associated diarrhea. J Clin Microbiol 38:2706–2714, 2000.
2. Brar HS, Surawicz CM: Pseudomembranous colitis: An update. Can J Gastroenterol 14:51–56, 2000.
3. Cleary RK: *Clostridium difficile*-associated diarrhea and colititis: Clinical manifestations, diagnosis, and treatment. Dis Colon Rectum 41:1435–1449, 1998.
4. Fine RD, Lee EL: Efficacy of open-label bismuth subsalicylate for the treatment of microscopic colitis. Gastroenterology 114:29–36, 1998.
5. Fine KD, Lee EL: Efficacy of open-label bismuth subsalicylate for the treatment of microscopic colitis. Gastroenterology 114:29–36, 1998.
6. Goff JS, Barnett JL, Pelke T, Appleman HD: Collagenous colitis: Histopathology and clinical course. Am J Gastroenterol 92:57–60, 1997.
7. Jackson BJ: Are collagenous colitis and lymphocytic colitis distinct syndromes? Dig Dis 13:301–311, 1995.
8. Jackson BK: Collagenous and lymphocytic colitis: Diagnosis and treatment. Clin Perspect Gastroenterol May/June:173–180, 1999.
9. Kochhar R, Sriram PV, Sharma SC, et al: Natural history of late radiation proctosigmoiditis treated with topical sucralfate suspension. Dig Dis Sci 44:973–978, 1999.
9a.. Kyne L, Warny M, Qamar A, Kelly C: Asymptomatic carriage of *Clostridium difficile* and serum levels of IgG antibody against toxin A. N Engl J Med 342:390–397, 2000.
10. Lindstrom CG: "Collagenous colitis" with watery diarrhea: A new entity? Pathol Eur 11:87–89, 1976.
11. McFarland LV: Epidemiology, risk factors and treatments for antibiotic-associated diarrhea. Dig Dis 16:292–307, 1998.
12. Nair S, Yadav D, Corpuz M, Pitchumoni CS: *Clostridium difficile* colitis: Factors influencing treatment failure and relapse—a prospective evaluation. Am J Gastroenerol 93:1873–1876, 1998.
13. Read NW, Krejs GJ, Read MG, et al: Chronic diarrhea of unknown origin. Gastroenterology 78:264–271, 1980.
14. Shiraishi M, Hiroyasu S, Ishimine T, Set al: Radiation enterocolitis: Overview of the past 15 years. World J Surg 22:491–493, 1998.
15. Surawicz CM, McFarland LV: Pseudomembranous colitis: Causes and cures. Digestion 60:91–100, 1999.
16. Surawicz CM, McFarland LV: Recurrent *Clostridium difficile* disease. Clin Perspect Gastroenterol March/April:24–26, 1999.
17. Williams CN: Collagenous colitis. Can J Gastroenterol 12:23–24, 1998.
18. Zins BJ, Sandborn WJ, Tremaine WJ: Collagenous and lymphocytic colitis: Subject review and therapeutic alternatives. Am J Gastroenterol 90:1394–1400, 1995.
20. Zins BJ, Tremaine WJ, Carpenter HA: Collagenous colitis: Mucosal biopsies and association with fecal leukocytes. Mayo Clin Proc 70:430–433, 1995.

55. UPPER GASTROINTESTINAL TRACT HEMORRHAGE

John S. Goff, M.D.

1. What are the signs and symptoms of upper gastrointestinal (UGI) bleeding?

Hematemesis can vary from material that looks like coffee grounds (blood darkened from acid exposure) to massive amounts of bright red blood. Melena (black, tarry stool) is usually found in patients with an UGI source of bleeding but may be seen in patients with a right colon bleed and slow transit. Brisker UGI bleeding results in maroon to red blood. Bright red blood per rectum, not associated with orthostatic blood pressure changes or syncope, is probably *not* from the UGI tract.

2. What historical facts help to determine the source of UGI bleeding?

Aspirin, other nonsteroidal anti-inflammatory drugs (NSAIDs), alcohol, and cigarettes are risk factors for gastric and duodenal lesions. Physical stress (e.g., trauma, central nervous system injury, burns) is commonly seen in patients with UGI bleeding. A history of heartburn and abdominal pain before onset of the bleeding strongly suggests a peptic source. A history of liver disease or suspected liver disease because of heavy alcohol use should raise the possibility of bleeding from varices. Vomiting before bleeding suggests a Mallory-Weiss tear as the possible cause. Inquiring about previous bleeding episodes is often useful.

3. How can the amount of acute blood lost be estimated clinically?

The acute loss of 500 ml of blood does not result in detectable physiologic changes; however, loss of 1000 ml produces orthostatic changes of 10–20 mmHg in systolic blood pressure and a pulse rise of 20 beats/minute or more. Loss of 2000 ml or more produces shock.

4. How can you distinguish an UGI bleed from a lower GI bleed in a patient who presents with blood per rectum?

The most obvious factor that points to an UGI source is a positive gastric aspirate for blood; however, this finding can be deceptive in patients with an oropharyngeal source of bleeding. Black stool per rectum (melena) suggests UGI bleeding but may be seen in some patients with cecal bleeding. Pepto-Bismol also produces black stool because it contains bismuth. Red blood per rectum is not likely to be from an upper source in the absence of associated syncope or orthostatic blood pressure changes. The presence of risk factors for UGI bleeding may be of some help (e.g., alcohol use, smoking, NSAID use, prior UGI bleed, UGI symptoms).

5. What are the first steps in managing a patient with UGI bleeding?

The first step is to establish intravenous access with one or two (if the bleed is major) large-bore catheters. Volume replacement should be initiated (see question 8) and vasopressors should be used if the patient is hypotensive and does not respond promptly to fluid resuscitation. Blood tests (hematocrit, platelet count, prothrombin time, partial thromboplastin time) should be done on blood obtained at the time of achieving intravenous access. A nasogastric tube, preferably of moderate to larger size, is placed next, followed by consultation with gastroenterology and surgery services.

6. How do you interpret the hematocrit values in a patient with acute UGI bleeding?

The hematocrit (Hct) falls over time with replacement of lost volume from extravascular fluid. In about 2 hours, ~ 25% of the final fall is achieved and ~ 50% is seen at 8 hours. The final

Hct value is seen at 72 hours after the initial acute loss of blood. Obviously, this timetable is accelerated if the patient is given intravenous fluid.

7. Why place a nasogastric (NG) tube?

The major reasons for placing an NG tube are to determine the source of bleeding and whether the patient is still actively bleeding. The finding of red blood when the NG tube is placed is associated with increased mortality rates, increased number of complications, and higher blood transfusion requirements. A secondary benefit is the clearing of blood from the stomach to aid in performing an urgent upper endoscopy (EGD). You need not worry about causing increased bleeding in patients with known liver disease (esophageal varices) when passing an NG tube.

8. What types of fluid should be used for resuscitation? When?

The fluid of choice for initial resuscitation is crystalloid (normal saline or Ringer's lactate). Packed red blood cells are the blood product of choice. Type-specific or universal donor blood (type O) can be given if the patient needs urgent replacement due to massive and ongoing losses. In elderly patients the Hct should be kept in the 30 range to help avoid cardiac complications. Fresh frozen plasma (FFP) should be considered if the patient is still bleeding and the international normalized ratio (INR) is > 1.5. Platelets should be used if the count is < 50,000 and bleeding is ongoing.

9. Does every patient with UGI bleeding need to be admitted to the intensive care unit or even hospitalized?

Patients are best treated by triage according to risk factors for further bleeding. Some can go home the same day as they present, and others need to go to the intensive care unit. The Rockall Score has been used successfully for triage. Risk factors for increased mortality are age > 65 years, comorbid illness, shock, and continued bleeding in the hospital. Patients with none of these risk factors and a clean-based, nonbleeding ulcer, mild gastritis, or low-grade esophagitis may be considered for discharge home.

10. What are the common causes of UGI bleeding? What are the uncommon causes?

Duodenal ulcers are the most common cause of acute UGI bleeding (30%), followed by gastric erosions (27%), gastric ulcers (22%), esophagitis (11%), duodenitis (10%), varices (5%), and Mallory-Weiss tears (5%). More unusual causes include (in no particular order) Dieulafoy's ulcers, gastric antral vascular ectasia (GAVE), cancer, portal hypertensive gastropathy, angiodysplasia, aortoenteric fistula, and hemobilia.

11. What is the role of NSAIDs in UGI bleeding?

An overall 2.74 increase in the relative risk for any GI complication is associated with the use of NSAIDs. If the patient is > 50 years old, the increase in relative risk is 5.57. If the patient has a history of a prior GI bleed, the increase in relative risk is 4.76, which is similar to the increase related to concomitant corticosteroid use. The increased relative risk is 12.7 for patients using NSAIDs and anticoagulants. NSAIDs probably have no additive effect in patients who also have *Helicobacter pylori*. Misoprostol given with NSAIDs prevents bleeding complication, but H_2RA drugs do not. Proton pump inhibitors have been shown to decrease the ulcer/bleed risk by fourfold. The new COX-2 selective prostaglandin inhibitors, celecoxib and rofecoxib, are associated with significantly fewer ulcers than traditional NSAIDs.

12. What are the possible sources of bleeding in a patient with cirrhosis who presents with UGI bleeding?

Cirrhosis is associated with only a 50% chance that the patient is bleeding from varices. The most common nonvariceal source of bleeding in cirrhotic patients is gastric erosions (~50%), followed by Mallory-Weiss tears (15%), duodenal and gastric ulcers (13.8% each), and esophagitis (11%). Portal hypertensive gastropathy (PHG) is also a nonvariceal source of bleeding in cirrhotic patients, but, unlike the other nonvariceal causes, it is related to portal pressure.

13. How is variceal bleeding diagnosed?

The easiest way is to see active bleeding from a varix. The next best criterion is to see a fibrin/platelet plug on a varix. The weakest criterion is finding no other identifiable source in the setting of moderate- to large-volume bleeding. Endoscopic ultrasound may be helpful in differentiating large gastric folds from gastric varices.

14. Which patients need endoscopy? When?

Ideally all patients with UGI bleeding need an EGD, but it is beneficial only if the results will affect patient management. Management changes include endoscopic therapy (see question 15) and triage, which may result in shorter or no hospital stay (see question 9). Clinical settings in which EGD often leads to interventions with a positive impact on outcome are advanced age (> 60 years old), liver disease, active bleeding, and rebleeding. EGD is best done within 12 hours of bleeding to maximize the chance of identifying the source.

15. What techniques are available to the endoscopist to control active bleeding?

The endoscopist usually relies heavily on cautery to control bleeding noted at the time of EGD. Available modalities include monopolar probes, bipolar probes, heater probes, argon plasma coagulator, and Nd-YAG lasers. There are various advantages and disadvantages to the use of each, but all are effective in controlling bleeding and preventing rebleeding except the monopolar technique. Frequently epinephrine (1:10,000) is used before cautery to slow or stop the bleeding, which allows more directed cautery treatment. Epinephrine alone is not as effective. Sclerosants (e.g., alcohol, ethanolamine) injected into the bleeding site have been used alone with some success. A newer technique is to use endoscopically placed clips to clamp off small bleeding vessels.

16. What therapy is available to control variceal hemorrhage?

Sclerotherapy (ES) and rubber-band ligation (EVL) are the main methods for controlling variceal bleeding via an endoscope. Both are reported to control active bleeding in up to 90% of cases. Rebleeding is less common with EVL than ES (26% vs. 44%). Patient mortality is reduced with use of endoscopic methods for treating varices. The mortality rate is lower with EVL than ES (24% vs 31%), and fewer complications are associated with EVL (11% vs 25%). It takes fewer sessions to obliterate the varices with EVL (3.7 vs 4.9 sessions). The major disadvantage of variceal ligation—required use of an overtube—has been overcome by the development of multiple ligation devices. EVL and ES can be used in combination, but this approach generally is reserved for gastric varices. The addition of intravenous infusions of octreotide enhances the beneficial effects of EVL and ES in prevention of rebleeding during the initial hospitalization. The Sengstaken-Blakemore tube, preferably with the Minnesota modification (a suction port above the esophageal balloon), is still a reasonable method for gaining initial control of massive bleeding from varices. If endoscopic therapy is ineffective, the clinician must choose between shunt surgery and a transjugular intrahepatic portosystemic shunt (TIPS) procedure, depending on availability.

17. Are all varices bad?

Only 25–40% of cirrhotic patients have a variceal hemorrhage. Portal pressure must exceed 12 mmHg to result in variceal development, and the pressure gradient is usually > 20 mmHg in patients with actual bleeding. Large varices, gastric varices, and varices with wale marks (dilated venules on the surface) are at higher risk of bleeding.

18. What special considerations need to be addressed in cirrhotic patients with acute UGI bleeding?

The likelihood of a serious coagulopathy that must be corrected is higher in cirrhotic patients. They are more prone to mental confusion from encephalopathy or alcohol withdrawal, which increases the risk of aspiration with its associated increase in mortality. Encephalopathy-related complications can be prevented by early endotracheal intubation and aggressive use of lactulose. Prophylactic antibiotics prevent complications and reduce mortality. Norfloxacin and ciprofloxacin, alone or in combination with amoxicillin and clavulanate (Augmentin), have been used successfully.

19. What is a visible vessel? What is its significance?

A visible vessel is the exposed side of a small vessel at the base of an ulcer. It may contain a fibrin/platelet plug or have an adherent clot over it. The finding is significant because of the increased risk for rebleeding. Other helpful endoscopic markers to predict the risk for ulcer rebleeding are outlined in the table below.

FINDING	RATE FOR REBLEEDING (%)
Spurting vessel	90
Visible vessel	~50
Adherent clot	20–30
Red dot ulcer base	10
Ulcer, clean base	5

20. What is the role of other diagnostic tests in evaluating UGI bleeding?

Radiolabeled red blood cell scans usually are not helpful for defining an UGI bleeding source unless it is beyond the reach of an endoscope. They may be useful for suggesting a proximal small bowel source for the bleeding, thus leading to small bowel endoscopy for further diagnosis and treatment. Barium studies have no place in the management of acute UGI bleeding. Angiography can be used to define an active bleeding site (the site needs to be bleeding at a rate of at least 0.5 ml/min) and possibly to treat it with either selective vasopressin infusion or embolization of the feeding blood vessel. *H. pylori* tests (antral biopsies for CLO test, Pyloritek test, or histologic examination) should be done in all patients with erosive lesions in the stomach or duodenum.

21. What medications can be used in the early management of acute UGI bleeding?

Vasopressin has been used for many years to reduce portal pressure in patients with bleeding varices. Unfortunately, it can produce ischemia in other organs (e.g., heart). This effect can be offset by simultaneous use of nitroglycerin. Prolonged use can cause fluid retention. Octreotide (Sandostatin, a somatostatin analog) lowers portal pressure without the side effects associated with vasopressin. It has been found useful for preventing variceal rebleeding by itself and in conjunction with sclerotherapy or variceal ligation. Tagamet (cimetidine) and proton pump inhibitors (omeprazole, lansoprazole, rebeprazole, and pantoprazole) have been shown to prevent rebleeding when given after an acute UGI bleed due to ulcers. Simple lansoprazole/omeprazole solution and intravenous pantoprazole are under evaluation for prevention of rebleeding. Factor replacement therapy is needed for patients with specific deficiencies, and desmopressin (DDAVP) is useful for transient correction of factor VIII deficiencies due to von Willebrand's disease, mild hemophilia A, or renal insufficiency.

22. Who should be treated with surgery for continued nonvariceal UGI bleeding? When?

Patients older than 60 years and patients with significant comorbid illness should be considered for surgery earlier because of the increased likelihood of a poor outcome with prolonged bleeding and multiple transfusions. Patients who have failed one attempt at endoscopic therapy—and certainly those who have failed two—should undergo surgery for rebleeding.

Giant ulcers (> 2 cm) are unlikely to be manageable with endoscopic methods, as are ulcers with bleeding from major arteries. On the other-hand, gastritis and esophagitis are poor candidates for surgical intervention in most acute settings.

23. What medications are used for patients who go home after a bleeding episode?

The main treatment after bleeding is acid suppression. Thus patients need histamine-2 receptor antagonists (cimetidine, ranitidine, famotidine, and nizatidine) or proton pump inhibitors. The latter are generally better at healing because of greater acid suppression. Antibiotics are added if the patient is positive for *H. pylori*. Oral iron supplementation is indicated for patients with a major bleed. Beta blockers should be considered for maintenance therapy in patients with bleeding due to portal hypertension. They can be discontinued once the varices are eradicated but may need to be continued if the source of bleeding is portal hypertensive gastropathy. Sucralfate

(Carafate) and misoprostol (Cytotec) may be useful in special cases. Selective COX-2 inhibitors should be substituted for standard NSAIDs in patients who need therapy for arthritic conditions.

24. What should patients receive by mouth after an UGI bleed? When?

Traditionally, patients are started on clear liquids once they are endoscoped or after several hours of observation without signs and symptoms of further bleeding. Some evidence indicates that this approach may not be necessary, but if the risk of rebleeding is substantial, it is best that there be no solid food in the stomach at the time of endoscopic or surgical intervention.

25. When should patients be sent home after an UGI bleed?

There is little need for prolonged hospital observation after a mild-to-moderate UGI bleed. Elderly patients who require blood transfusions need to be observed for a day or two after their last sign of bleeding or their last transfusion.

26. What should patients avoid once they have had an UGI bleed?

Patients need to be instructed to avoid all alcohol after having an acute UGI bleed. Smoking should be discouraged, as should the use of caffeine-containing beverages, especially on an empty stomach or in large quantities. NSAIDs should not be used unless accompanied by a drug that blocks their effect on GI bleeding (Cytotec or proton pump inhibitor).

27. How, when, and why should patients be followed after an episode of UGI bleeding?

An office visit is scheduled in 2–4 weeks to reenforce use of medications and to make long-term plans. A blood count is done to ensure that the patient is responding appropriately to therapy. Patients with signs of rebleeding or return of peptic symptoms should be seen promptly. Follow-up testing for residual *H. pylori* is indicated with return of symptoms (breath test, stool antigen test, or endoscopy with biopsy) and in selected asymptomatic patients. Endoscopy is repeated only in patients with major GI bleeding and no antecedent symptoms of peptic disease to confirm healing at 1–2 months after the bleed. Gastric ulcers should be followed to complete endoscopic healing to ensure that no cancer is present. Patients with varices are seen for repeat ES or EVL within 7–10 days of the first treatment and then every 2 weeks until the varices are eradicated.

BIBLIOGRAPHY

 1. CorleyDA, Stefan AM, Wolf M, et al: Early indicators of prognosis in upper gastrointestinal hemorrhage. Am J Gastroenterol 93:336, 1998.
 2. Laine L: Rolling review: Upper gastrointestinal bleeding. Aliment Pharmacol Ther 7:207, 1993.
 3. Lanza FA: A guideline for treatment and prevention of NSAID-induced ulcers. Am J Gastroenterol 93:2037, 1998.
 4. Lau JYW, Sung JJY, Lam YH, et al: Endoscopic treatment compared with surgery in patients with recurrent bleeding after initial endoscopic control of bleeding ulcers. N Engl J Med 340:751, 1999.
 5. Lee JG, Turnipseed S, Romano PS, et al: Endoscopy-based triage significantly reduces hospitalization rates and costs of treating upper gastrointestinal bleeding: A randomized controlled trial. Gastrointest Endosc 50:755, 1999.
 6. Lin HJ, Lo WC, Lee FY, et al: A prospective randomized comparative trial showing that omeprazole prevents rebleeding in patients with bleeding peptic ulcer after successful endoscopic therapy. Arch Intern Med 158:54, 1998.
 7. Nevens F, Bustami K, Scheys I, et al: Variceal pressure is a factor predicting the risk of first variceal bleeding: A prospective cohort study in cirrhotic patients. Hepatology 27:15, 1998.
 8. Rockall TA, Logan RF, Devlin,HB, et al: Selection of patients for early discharge or outpatient care after acute upper gastrointestinal haemorrhage: National audit of acute upper gastrointestinal haemorrhage. Lancet 347:1138, 1996.
 9. Stiegmann GV, Goff JS, Michalitz-Onody PA, et al: Endoscopic sclerotherapy as compared with endoscopic variceal ligation for bleeding esophageal varices. N Engl J Med 326:1527, 1992.
10. Wara P: Endoscopic prediction of major bleeding: A prospective study of stigmata of hemorrhage in bleeding ulcers. Gastroenterology 88:1209, 1985.

56. LOWER GASTROINTESTINAL TRACT BLEEDING

Ian M. Gralnek, M.D., M.S.H.S., and Dennis M. Jensen, M.D.

1. Define lower gastrointestinal (GI) bleeding.

Lower GI bleeding is bleeding from the colon. Bleeding between the ligament of Treitz and the ileocecal valve is considered small bowel bleeding. Bleeding from the esophagus, stomach, or duodenum is considered upper GI bleeding. Lower GI bleeding is further categorized as gross bleeding, in which red or maroon blood is visible in the stool, or occult bleeding, in which blood is not visible but discovered by chemical testing of the stool (i.e., guaiac-impregnated cards).

2. How common is lower GI bleeding?

In 1991, approximately 0.4% of people admitted to nonfederal, short-stay hospitals had a "first-listed" diagnosis of GI hemorrhage without hematemesis or melena. Although the causes of such hemorrhage were unspecified, many presumably were lower GI lesions. Survey studies have shown that 15% of adults report gross red blood on toilet paper after defecation, and 2–3% of apparently healthy people notice blood in the toilet or intermixed with stool.

3. Define hematochezia and melena.

Hematochezia is the passage of red or maroon blood per rectum. It may be pure blood, blood clots, blood intermixed with or coating formed stool, or bloody diarrhea. Hematochezia is usually a manifestation of bleeding from the lower GI tract. However, in approximately 10–20% of cases, it is seen with brisk upper GI (e.g., ulcers or varices) or small bowel bleeding (e.g., angiomas or tumors) with rapid transit of blood.

Melena is black-colored stool that is shiny, sticky, and foul-smelling. It results from conversion of hemoglobin to hematin by bacteria in the gut. Melena is almost always secondary to bleeding from an upper GI tract or small bowel source. In rare cases, it can be a manifestation of a right-sided colonic bleeding source with slow transit time.

4. Which "normal" conditions can masquerade as hematochezia?

Natural red pigments from beets may cause maroon-appearing stools. Patients who ingest laxatives to induce defecation and simultaneously drink cranberry juice or other red-colored drinks (such as Kool-Aid, soda pop, or fruit or vegetable juice) may have red or maroon stools. The stool is hemoccult-negative and easily distinguished from blood, even though it may alarm the patient.

5. Describe the different clinical presentations of patients with lower GI bleeding.

Patients usually present with hematochezia. However, a proximal colon lesion may present with melena or a combination of melena and hematochezia. In approximately 85% of patients, lower GI bleeding is acute, self-limited, and not hemodynamically significant (no resting tachycardia or postural hypotension). Such patients can be evaluated electively as outpatients. The remaining 15% of patients have more severe, ongoing, hemodynamically significant (resting tachycardia, postural hypotension) bleeding, and may require hospital admission, often to an ICU or monitored bed, and urgent evaluation.

6. How important is the history in assessing a patient with lower GI bleeding?

A complete history can help to identify a possible cause of the bleeding. The duration of bleeding should be determined. When did it start? Is this the first time that bleeding has been noticed, or is it a recurrent event? The quality of the blood should be determined. What color is the blood—red, maroon, or black? Is the blood coating formed stools or intermixed? Are blood clots being passed? A recent (within 30 days) colonoscopy with polypectomy indicates in most cases bleeding from the polypectomy site. Blood that drips or squirts after defecation usually indicates internal hemorrhoids. Does the patient have abdominal or perianal pain? Severe perianal pain or spasm (tenesmus) with bright red blood and formed stool usually indicates anal fissure.

Comorbid medical conditions and past medical history should be determined; prior surgeries may be relevant (e.g., for peptic ulcer disease). Surgery for an abdominal aortic aneurysm suggests possible aortoenteric fistula. Medication use, such as anticoagulants, aspirin, nonsteroidal anti-inflammatory drugs (NSAIDs), antiplatelet agents, over-the-counter cold medications containing aspirin or NSAIDs, and any "alternative medicine and vitamin preparations" (many containing salicylates), needs to be determined because it can cause any GI lesion to bleed.

7. What physical findings are important clues to the diagnosis?
- Orthostatic vital signs assessing hemodynamic status should be performed first.
- Examination of the lips and mucous membranes for telangectasias or pigmented macules may indicate Osler-Weber-Rendu disease, Peutz-Jeghers syndrome, or vascular ectasia in the gut.
- Cardiac auscultation should be performed with attention to a possible murmur of aortic stenosis. Some reports suggest an association between aortic stenosis and vascular ectasia of the GI tract.
- Abdominal examination should assess for bowel sounds, tenderness, masses, and surgical scars. Hepatosplenomegaly, ascites, and/or caput medusae may indicate chronic liver disease with portal hypertension, suggesting an esophageal, gastric, or colonic variceal bleed.
- Cutaneous purpura or petcchiae suggest a coagulopathy, and spider angiomata or jaundice may be another indicator of chronic liver disease.
- Joint swelling or deformity may indicate an arthritic condition and possible use of aspirin or NSAID products.
- Digital rectal exam to evaluate for prolapsed internal hemorrhoids or masses and stool examination for color and guaiac testing are mandatory.

8. Describe the role of anoscopy in the diagnosis of lower GI bleeding.
Anoscopy with a lighted, slotted anoscope determines whether there is active bleeding from internal hemorrhoids or a fissure. A visualized, nonbleeding hemorrhoid implies that bleeding is unlikely to be hemorrhoidal in origin. Anoscopy also helps to exclude an anal fissure as the source of bleeding. Neither internal hemorrhoids nor anal fissures can be adequately assessed by fiberoptic/video endoscopy.

9. Which laboratory tests are helpful for evaluation of lower GI bleeding?
All patients: hemoglobin, hematocrit, platelets, prothrombin time, partial thromboplastin time.
Acute severe bleeding: blood type and cross-matching.
Chronic GI blood loss: liver function tests, creatinine, reticulocyte count, serum iron, total iron-binding capacity, ferritin, red blood cell indices (mean cell volume, red blood cell distribution width).

10. When should a nasogastric (NG) tube be used for diagnostic evaluation of suspected lower GI bleeding?
Approximately 15% of patients with severe, ongoing hematochezia and severe anemia have an upper GI source of bleeding. To exclude this source, an NG or orogastric tube should be placed and gastric contents aspirated. An NG aspirate that is clear and nonbloody does not exclude an upper GI tract bleed unless bile is present. A bilious, nonbloody aspirate virtually excludes a bleeding site proximal to the ligament of Treitz when a patient has ongoing hematochezia. Guaiac testing of the NG aspirate is of no clinical utility, leads to many false-positive and false-negative results, and should not be performed.

11. Describe the initial management strategy.

The history, physical, and laboratory findings must be assessed to determine the severity of bleeding. **Severe lower GI bleeding** is persistent or recurrent bleeding that fails to stop spontaneously, with evidence of orthostatic hypotension and/or a decrease in baseline hematocrit of at least 8% after volume resuscitation. Such patients should be admitted directly to an ICU or monitored bed for volume resuscitation, cardiopulmonary monitoring, further diagnostic evaluation, and treatment. Volume resuscitation should include placing an intravenous line and administering crystalloid fluids (normal saline or lactated Ringer's solution) to correct the estimated volume depletion, packed red blood cells to correct anemia (hematocrit $\geq$ 30%), and fresh frozen plasma or platelets to correct any coagulopathy or thrombocytopenia. Intravenous access should include at least two peripheral catheter lines, one of at least 16 gauge. A general or GI surgeon should be consulted at the time of ICU admission. The importance of these initial resuscitative measures cannot be overemphasized.

Patients without persistent or recurrent bleeding or evidence of hemodynamic instability have a **self-limited lower GI bleed**. Such patients may be evaluated electively as outpatients or as inpatients if they are older (> 60 years) or have significant comorbid medical conditions.

12. What is the most common cause of lower GI bleeding in ambulatory adults?

Internal hemorrhoids. Hemorrhoidal disease is estimated to occur in 50–80% of the U.S. population. This rate is in sharp contrast to that in developing countries, where the lifetime prevalence is estimated to be < 5%. Hemorrhoidal disease is uncommon in adolescents and children.

13. How do hemorrhoids develop?

Many theories have been proposed. It is generally thought that chronic straining at defecation and a low-fiber diet predispose to hemorrhoidal disease. Over time, with increased colonic intraluminal pressure, submucosal and connective tissue support weakens and deteriorates with further enlargement of veins. As the anal lining descends, the hemorrhoids are more exposed to pressure from straining and/or direct trauma from stool. The results are stasis of blood, swelling, erosions, and subsequent bleeding.

14. How does hemorrhoidal bleeding present?

Bleeding from internal hemorrhoids is usually intermittent, sometimes massive, and often noted by patients at the time of defecation. Bright red blood is generally seen coating the stool or on toilet paper, or it may drip or squirt directly into the toilet water. Patients may have associated symptoms of anorectal discomfort or pain, pruritus, discharge, or prolapse. Bleeding internal hemorrhoids may simulate or mask other, more serious anorectal pathology, and a more complete endoscopic examination (flexible sigmoidoscopy or colonoscopy) of the colon is recommended before focusing on the internal hemorrhoids.

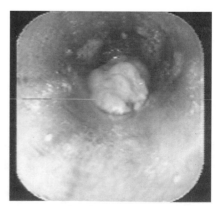

Internal hemorrhoid seen on slotted anoscopy. The patient was a 45-year-old white man with self-limited hematochezia and anemia.

15. List the other common causes of lower GI bleeding.
Diverticulosis, vascular ectasia, and neoplasms.

16. How common is diverticulosis?
Diverticulosis is an age-acquired condition that is usually asymptomatic and most often di-agnosed incidentally. The prevalence of diverticular disease of the colon increases with age and is > 50% in people older than 60 years. It is uncommon in persons < 40 years old.

17. What causes diverticulosis?
Dietary factors are theorized to play an important role. The high prevalence of diverticulosis in western countries is attributed to the consumption of a low-fiber diet, which presumably re-sults in decreased stool bulk, prolonged fecal transit time, increased colonic muscle contractions, elevated colonic intraluminal pressure, and eventual formation of diverticula.

18. Describe the complications of diverticulosis.
Complications, such as inflammation or bleeding, occur in about 20% of persons with colonic diverticular disease. Diverticular hemorrhage is reported in 3–5% of persons with colonic diverticulosis. Bleeding recurs in approximately 25% of patients. For patients with one recurrent bleed, the chance of a second recurrence is approximately 50%. Although colonic diverticula are predominantly left-sided, diverticular bleeding is most often right-sided in location. Men and women are equally affected.

19. How do patients with diverticulosis present? How are they treated?
Patients usually present with acute, massive, painless hematochezia. Although hospitaliza-tion and blood transfusions are usually required, diverticular bleeding is often self-limited and stops spontaneously or with medical therapy in 75–95% of patients. For patients with continued bleeding, surgical resection is the standard treatment. Diverticular bleeding is not chronic and does not cause chronic, occult blood loss.

20. Describe the vascular anatomy of bleeding diverticula.
The vasa recta, the intramural branches of the marginal artery supplying the colon, consis-tently penetrate the colonic wall from the serosa to the submucosa. A vas rectum intimately courses in the serosa over the dome of a diverticulum. Therefore, the vas rectum is separated from the diverticular lumen only by mucosa and a few muscle fibers. Histologic examination of bleeding colonic diverticula shows rupture of the underlying vas rectum, usually at the dome or neck of the diverticulum. The arterial defect is eccentric and faces the lumen of the diverticulum. With time, the arterial wall weakens and ruptures into the diverticulum. Arterial bleeding occurs through this communication.

21. Define vascular ectasias. Where are they most commonly located?
Vascular ectasias of the colon are a well-recognized, common cause of lower GI bleeding in older patients. They are age-acquired lesions, especially common in people > 50 years old, and occur with equal frequency in men and women. Sporadic vascular ectasias are also referred to as angiodysplasias, arteriovenous malformations, or angiomas. Vascular ectasias are located pre-dominantly in the cecum and proximal ascending colon, although they can occur throughout the rest of the colon, small bowel, and stomach. Twenty-five percent of patients have multiple le-sions. Endoscopically, the lesions are flat, bright red, and fern-like in appearance. Target irriga-tion of the lesion can precipitate bleeding, helping to confirm the diagnosis.

22. What causes vascular ectasias?
Histologically, vascular ectasias consist of ectatic, distorted, thin-walled veins, venules, and capillaries in the mucosa and/or submucosa. It is theorized that they develop secondary to re-peated episodes of colonic distention, resulting in increased colonic wall tension. This process

leads to obstruction of submucosal venous outflow where the vessels penetrate the colonic muscle layers. Over time, the submucosal veins, venules, and capillaries dilate and eventually form an arteriovenous communication.

23. Describe the clinical presentation of bleeding from colonic vascular ectasias.
  Bleeding is usually subacute and recurrent, although 15% of patients present with acute, massive hemorrhage. Another 10–15% present with occult blood loss and iron-deficiency anemia. Bleeding ceases spontaneously in > 90% of cases.

24. What is the association between colonic vascular ectasia and other vascular GI disorders?
  Sporadic colonic vascular ectasias are clinically and pathologically unrelated to other vascular anomalies that also can involve the GI tract, such as hereditary hemorrhagic telangiectasias (Osler-Weber-Rendu disease), congenital arteriovenous malformations, hemangiomas, or radiation telangiectasia.

25. What extrasystemic conditions are associated with colonic vascular ectasia?
  Controversy surrounds the association of vascular ectasia and aortic stenosis. Several reports describe cessation of GI bleeding after aortic valve replacement, but others have failed to corroborate this finding. Other conditions associated with colonic vascular ectasia are chronic renal failure, cirrhosis, and collagen vascular disease.

26. How often do colonic neoplasms cause lower GI bleeding?
  Colon cancer and colonic polyps more commonly present with occult GI blood loss and iron-deficiency anemia rather than gross hematochezia. In adults over age 40 with hematochezia, colon cancer must be excluded as a possible cause of bleeding because early detection improves survival. Unfortunately, colon cancer that presents with hematochezia is usually at an advanced tumor stage. Patients with colon cancer may report an associated change in bowel habits and/or weight loss. Physical examination may reveal a palpable abdominal or rectal mass.

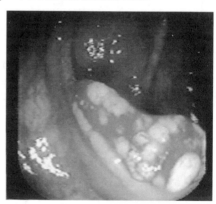

Bleeding sessile polyp (villous adenoma) of the right colon in a 57-year-old Hispanic woman. This polyp was resected endoscopically by piecemeal polypectomy.

27. Describe the presentation of ischemic colitis.
  Ischemic colitis can be classified as occlusive or nonocclusive. Most episodes have no identifiable cause. Patients usually present with acute onset of crampy, left lower quadrant abdominal pain and the urge to defecate, subsequently passing bloody diarrhea. Nausea, vomiting, fever, and tachycardia may be present. Abdominal examination is often unremarkable or reveals only mild- to-moderate tenderness. Rarely, patients present with peritoneal signs indicative of transmural damage and perforation. "Watershed areas" of the colon, such as the splenic flexure and sigmoid colon, are more commonly involved because of their poor collateral blood flow.

28. How is ischemic colitis diagnosed and treated?

Plain film abdominal radiographs may demonstrate "thumbprinting," caused by submucosal hemorrhage and edema in the colon wall. Flexible sigmoidoscopy or colonoscopy reveals segmental colonic involvement with erythema, friability, ulceration, and/or necrosis.

Treatment consists of supportive care with optimization of hemodynamic status and correction of any underlying medical condition that may have contributed to the ischemic event. If the patient has peritoneal signs or ongoing hemorrhage, laparotomy with surgical resection of the involved colon is indicated. There is no role for therapeutic endoscopy; patients often have diffuse, segmental colitis.

29. What are the other causes of of lower GI bleeding in an adult with hematochezia?

Literally dozens of obscure and rare causes of lower GI bleeding must be considered in the differential diagnosis. More common examples include radiation-induced protcitis/colitis, inflammatory bowel disease, infectious colitis, colonic varices, and intussusception of the colon. Less frequent causes of lower GI bleeding include the solitary rectal ulcer syndrome, portal colopathy, diversion colitis, mesenteric ischemia, aortoenteric fistula, vasculitis, colonic endometriosis, and runner's colitis.

30. Describe radiation-induced proctitis/colitis as a cause of lower GI bleeding.

Proctitis or colitis may be an acute or chronic complication of ionizing radiation for treatment of a gynecologic, prostatic, testicular, bladder, or rectal malignancy. Acute radiation injury occurs during or shortly after radiation therapy; chronic injury manifests clinically months to years later. Radiation-induced vascular damage causes ischemia, fibrosis, and mucosal ulcerations. Patients may complain of recurrent hematochezia, diarrhea, and tenesmus. Endoscopy reveals multiple, mucosal telangiectasias that are almost always the bleeding sites.

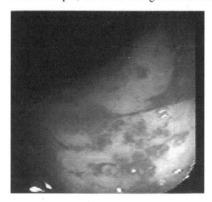

Bleeding radiation telangiectasia in a 72-year-old white man with anemia and recurrent hematochezia, occurring 1 year after radiation therapy for prostate cancer. The rectal telangiectasias were treated with a heater probe, which controlled the bleeding in three treatment sessions.

31. How is lower GI bleeding due to inflammatory bowel disease diagnosed and treated?

Hematochezia occurs more commonly in ulcerative colitis than in Crohn's disease. Endoscopic findings include mucosal erythema, edema, friability, and ulcerations. Infectious causes must be ruled out. There is no role for endoscopic therapy. Acute medical treatment includes systemic corticosteroids, 5-aminosalicylate products, and, more recently, cyclosporine. Surgery is reserved for patients not responding to medical therapy.

32. How is infectious colitis diagnosed and treated?

Bloody diarrhea can occur in colitis secondary to infection with *Shigella* spp., *Salmonella* spp., *Campylobacter jejuni*, enteroinvasive *Escherichia coli*, enterohemorrhagic *E. coli* serotype 0157:H7, *Clostridium difficile*, or *Entamoeba histolytica*. Diagnosis is made by stool culture, ova and parasite examination, and/or flexible sigmoidoscopy with biopsy. In patients with impaired immunity, cytomegalovirus or herpes simplex ulcerations and Kaposi's sarcoma lesions of the colon may cause bloody diarrhea. There is no role for therapeutic endoscopy, and antibiotic treatment is pathogen-specific.

33. Describe colonic varices as a cause of lower GI bleeding.

These portosystemic collaterals develop secondary to portal hypertension, usually in the rectosigmoid area. Hematochezia from colonic varices has been well documented and is usually intermittent, yet severe. Colonoscopy and arteriography are the primary methods for diagnosis. On colonoscopy, the varices appear as bluish, serpiginous columns. Bleeding colonic varices respond to protosystemic shunt surgery or segmental colonic resection. Selected cases of isolated colonic varices may be palliated with endoscopic sclerotherapy or band ligation.

34. How is intussusception of the colon diagnosed and treated?

Intussusception of the colon is rare in adults. Usually an underlying malignancy or polyp acts as the lead point for involution. Patients may present with crampy abdominal pain and hematochezia. Barium enema, ultrasonography, and abdominal CT have been used for diagnosis. Surgical resection of the involved bowel is the treatment of choice.

35. What is the most common cause of lower GI bleeding in children?

Meckel's diverticulum. Rarely, adults also may present with hemorrhage from this source. Meckel's diverticulum is the most common congenital anomaly of the gut (1–3% of the population) and is caused by failure of the vitelline duct to obliterate completely. It is located on the antimesenteric border of the ileum, within 100 cm of the ileocecal valve. Most Meckel's diverticula remain asymptomatic; however, GI bleeding is the most common complication. Almost all of those that bleed contain functioning heterotopic gastric mucosa (parietal cells), which secretes acid that causes ulceration within the diverticulum or the adjacent ileal mucosa, leading to eventual bleeding. Patients present with painless melena or hematochezia, commonly referred to as "currant jelly" stools.

36. How is Meckel's diverticulum diagnosed and treated?

Diagnosis can be made with a technetium-99m pertechnetate scintiscan (Meckel's scan), which demonstrates the heterotopic gastric mucosa by binding to the parietal cells. This test has a sensitivity of 75–100% in children but a lower rate in adults. There is a 15% false-positive and 25% false-negative rate. In actively bleeding Meckel's diverticula, arteriography may be diagnostic. In symptomatic patients, surgical resection of the diverticulum is the treatment of choice. Asymptomatic patients do not require treatment.

37. What are the other common causes of lower GI bleeding in adolescents and young adults?

1. Anal fissures related to constipation and rectal pain with bowel movements
2. Inflammatory bowel disease and infectious diarrhea in some families and travelers
3. Internal hemorrhoids in pregnant women and some young adults
4. Familial polyposis and juvenile polyps in patients with a positive family history

38. Can radiographic studies be used for diagnosis of severe lower GI bleeding?

Emergency barium enema has no role in a patient with severe lower GI bleeding. Barium enemas are rarely diagnostic and never therapeutic in such patients. In a critically ill patient, a technically adequate study is impossible to obtain because of the inability to prepare the patient, and barium remaining in the colon precludes emergency colonoscopy or visceral arteriography for several days.

Abdominal CT may be helpful in diagnosing aortoenteric fistula in a patient presenting with severe hematochezia. Prior abdominal vascular surgery (e.g., abdominal aortic aneurysm repair) should indicate the need for this diagnostic test. The limitation of CT is that patients are often too ill to be safely transported and monitored in the radiology department. Most patients with severe hematochezia do not require such diagnostic testing.

39. What is the role of radionuclide scanning for diagnosis of lower GI bleeding?

Two types of radionuclide "bleeding" scans are available: technetium-labeled sulfur colloid (99mTc sulfur colloid) and technetium-tagged autologous red blood cells (99mTc RBC scan). Each has a threshold rate of bleeding for localization by scanning of 0.05-0.1 ml/min. Sulfur colloid is cleared rapidly (within minutes) from the intravascular space by the reticuloendothelial system. The tagged RBCs have a longer half-life and allow imaging up to 24 hours after intravenous injection. Because of its limitations, sulfur colloid scanning has largely been replaced by tagged RBC scans.

40. How are tagged RBC scans performed?

Sequential images of the abdomen, using a gamma camera, are obtained. Images within the first 1–4 hours of radionuclide injection are often the most useful for localizing severe, active bleeding. Delayed RBC scans at 12 and 24 hours may detect intermittent GI bleeding. These scans may be useful for localizing colonic sites of actively bleeding diverticula, vascular ectasia, or tumors, particularly if early scans at 1–4 hours are positive. However, scintigraphy has a significant rate of incorrect localization of GI bleeding, and performing surgery on the basis of a positive RBC scan alone is not recommended. Radiologists usually prefer scintigraphy as the initial diagnostic test and, if it is positive, proceed with visceral arteriography. We recommend initial colonoscopy; if it is nondiagnostic, proceed to a tagged RBC scan (see algorithm with question 44). In many institutions, scintigraphy has replaced emergency visceral arteriography as an adjunct to colonoscopy because of its higher sensitivity, noninvasive technique, and lower cost.

41. When is visceral arteriography indicated for diagnosis and therapeutic intervention in patients with lower GI bleeding?

Selective visceral arteriography is potentially diagnostic as well as therapeutic. The **diagnostic yield** varies with patient selection, timing of the procedure, and skill of the angiographer from 12–72%. Extravasation of contrast material into the gut lumen may be seen with active bleeding at a rate of at least 1–1.5 ml/min. Selective arterial catheterization also can be used to diagnose abnormal vessels consistent with tumors or vascular ectasia as well as actively bleeding colonic diverticula.

Therapeutic interventions include vasopressin infusion and embolization techniques using autologous clots, absorbable gelatin (Gelfoam), metal coils, oxidized cellulose, and polyvinyl alcohol particles. Potential complications from visceral arteriography and transcatheter treatment are bowel ischemia and infarction, arterial thrombosis and embolization, hematoma formation, and contrast-induced renal failure.

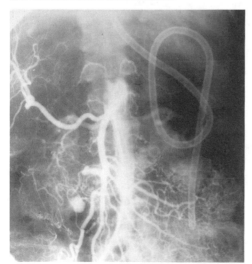

Positive emergency arteriogram in a patient with ongoing hematochezia and multiple diverticuli by colonoscopy. (Courtesy of Antoinette Gomes, M.D.)

42. When is flexible sigmoidoscopy indicated for diagnosis of lower GI bleeding?

Flexible sigmoidoscopy, performed with a 65-cm instrument, can diagnose lesions beyond the view of the anoscope and up to the descending colon. Enemas for clearance of stool and blood are important, although such clearance may not be possible in severely ill patients. Although diagnostic flexible sigmoidoscopy may obviate the need for other tests, a normal exam indicates the need for further studies. Turnaround exam (retroflexion) in the rectum allows visualization of lesions potentially missed by rigid sigmoidoscopy or anoscopy. Biopsies of involved colonic mucosa or suspicious lesions also may be obtained at the time of examination.

43. When is esophagogastroduodenoscopy (EGD) recommended in patients with the presumptive diagnosis of lower GI bleeding?

Exclusion by EGD of a bleeding lesion proximal to the ligament of Treitz is recommended if the nasogastric aspirate is grossly bloody, a nonbilious nonbloody aspirate returns, the history is suggestive of an upper GI source, or anoscopy and flexible sigmoidoscopy fail to identify a probable rectosigmoid bleeding source. A bile-containing, nonbloody gastric aspirate virtually excludes an upper GI source of bleeding. In our experience, 11% of patients presenting with severe hematochezia had an upper GI source of bleeding diagnosed at EGD (see table below), which is consistent with other published data. EGD should be performed before oral purge and urgent colonoscopy. Some authorities advocate EGD in all patients presenting with acute, severe hematochezia regardless of nasogastric aspirate results.

Causes of Severe Hematochezia in 100 Patients

LESION SITE	NO. OF PATIENTS
Colonic	74 (74%)
Vascular ectasia	30 (41%)
Diverticulosis	17 (23%)
Polyps or cancer	11 (15%)
Focal colitis	9 (12%)
Rectal lesions	4 (5%)
Other	3 (4%)
Upper GI	11 (11%)
Small bowel*	9 (9%)
No site found	6 (6%)

* A diagnosis of presumed small bowel site of bleeding was made when panendoscopy and colonoscopy were negative, but fresh blood or clots (or both) were coming through the ileocecal valve. (Courtesy of CURE Hemostasis Research Group.)

44. What is urgent colonoscopy? What is its role in diagnosing lower GI bleeding?

Urgent colonoscopy involves a full colonoscopic examination of the cecum and terminal ileum in a patient with severe hematochezia after the colon has been cleansed of stool and blood. In our experience, urgent colonoscopies are performed in the ICU with videocolonoscopes and necessary accessories for diagnosis and treatment. Until recently, urgent colonoscopy in patients with severe hematochezia was thought to be dangerous, often nondiagnostic, and impractical. However, this technique is feasible with adequate prior colonic cleansing. Colonoscopy also allows biopsies to be obtained and definitive endoscopic hemostasis (if clinically indicated).

At colonoscopy, diagnosis of a bleeding site can be made by visualization of active bleeding, a nonbleeding visible vessel, an adherent clot resistant to washing with an endoscopic catheter, or blood in an area around a clean lesion without other lesions in that segment of bowel. In our experience, initial colonoscopy and/or EGD can make a definitive diagnosis in approximately 90% of patients with ongoing hematochezia (see algorithm on following page).

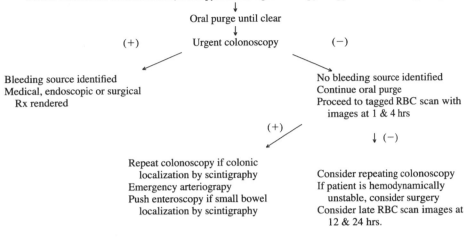

Patient with severe hematochezia (anoscopy/flexible sigmoidoscopy & upper GI source-negative)
↓
Oral purge until clear
↓
(+)   Urgent colonoscopy   (−)

Bleeding source identified
Medical, endoscopic or surgical
   Rx rendered

No bleeding source identified
Continue oral purge
Proceed to tagged RBC scan with
   images at 1 & 4 hrs

(+)   ↓ (−)

Repeat colonoscopy if colonic
   localization by scintigraphy
Emergency arteriograpy
Push enteroscopy if small bowel
   localization by scintigraphy

Consider repeating colonoscopy
If patient is hemodynamically
   unstable, consider surgery
Consider late RBC scan images at
   12 & 24 hrs.

Recommended approach to the patient with severe lower GI bleeding.

45. Describe colon cleansing as used prior to urgent colonoscopic evaluation.

Best results are achieved with an electrolyte-polyethylene glycol (PEG) solution, such as GoLytely, CoLyte, or NuLytely, performed simultaneously with resuscitation measures. The purge solution, administered orally or via nasogastric tube, is given at a rate of 1 liter every 30–45 minutes over 3–5 hours, until the rectal effluent is clear of stool and blood clots. Usually, 5–8 liters are sufficient to achieve this goal. Metoclopramide (10 mg intravenously before and then every 3–4 hours) helps to decrease the nausea and facilitate gastric emptying. The PEG solution should be administered at room temperature to maintain core body temperature. Once the rectal effluent is clear of stool and blood clots, colonoscopy can be performed safely and effectively.

46. What bleeding colonic lesions are amenable to endoscopic treatment?

Lower GI bleeding secondary to internal hemorrhoids, vascular ectasia, diverticula (with major stigmata of hemorrhage), colonic tumors or polyps, radiation telangiectasia, colonic varices, and colonic ulcers (with major stigmata of hemorrhage) are amenable to endoscopic hemostasis techniques.

47. List the main risks of endoscopic hemostasis performed via flexible sigmoidoscopy or colonoscopy. How can they be minimized?
- Perforation
- Postcoagulation syndrome (abdominal pain, focal rebound tenderness, fever, and leukocytosis without evidence of perforation)
- Delayed bleeding
- Rectal or colonic stenosis (rarely, due to repeated circumferential coagulation with Nd:YAG laser or argon plasma coagulator of radiation telangectasia or villous adenomas)

These risks are minimized if hemostasis procedures are performed by trained endoscopists.

48. When is emergency surgery indicated for acute lower GI bleeding?

A general or GI surgeon should be consulted on admitting the patient to the hospital. Emergency surgery is reserved for patients who have:
- Ongoing bleeding and persistent hypovolemic shock despite resuscitation efforts
- Ongoing bleeding and transfusion requirements (6 units of packed red blood cells and no diagnosis by emergency colonoscopy, scintigraphy, or arteriography)

• A specific segmental diagnosis made by colonoscopy and/or arteriography, in which surgery is determined to be the best mode of treatment.

Emergency surgery in the face of ongoing bleeding has a much higher mortality rate (25%) than elective surgery once bleeding has ceased (10%). The ability to accurately localize the bleeding site preoperatively allows segmental resection with decreased morbidity and mortality rates.

BIBLIOGRAPHY

1. Dennison AR, Wherry DC, Morris DL: Hemorrhoids: Nonoperative management. Surg Clin North Am 68:1401, 1988.
2. Freeman ML: The current endoscopic diagnosis and intensive care unit management of severe ulcer and other nonvariceal upper gastrointestinal hemorrhage. Gastrointest Endosc Clin North Am 1:209, 1991.
3. Hosking SW, Johnson AG, Smart HL: Anorectal varices, haemorrhoids, and portal hypertension. Lancet 1:349, 1989.
4. Jensen DM, Machicado GA: Colonoscopy for diagnosis and treatment of severe lower gastrointestinal bleeding. Routine outcomes and cost analysis. Gastrointest Endosc Clin North Am 7:477–498, 1997.
5. Jensen DM, Machicado GA, Jutabha R, Kovacs TOG: Urgent colonoscopy for the diagnosis and treatment of severe diverticular hemorrhage. N Engl J Med 342:78–82, 2000.
6. Jensen DM, Machicado GA: Diagnosis and treatment of severe hematochezia: The role of urgent colonoscopy after purge. Gastroenterology 95:1569, 1988.
7. Meyers MA, Alonso DR, Gray GF: Pathogenesis of bleeding colonic diverticulosis. Gastroenterology 71:577, 1976.
8. Miller LS, Barbarevech C, Friedman LS: Less frequent causes of lower gastrointestinal bleeding. Gastroenterol Clin North Am 23:21, 1994.
9. Randall GM, Jensen DM, Machicado GA: Prospective randomized comparative study of bipolar versus direct current electrocoagulation for treatment of bleeding internal hemorrhoids. Gastrointest Endosc 40:403, 1994.
10. Reinus JF, Brandt LJ: Vascular ectasias and diverticulosis: Common causes of lower intestinal bleeding. Gastroenterol Clin North Am 23:1, 1994.
11. Savides TJ, Jensen DM: Colonoscopic hemostasis for recurrent diverticular hemorrhage associated with a visible vessel: A report of three cases. Gastrointest Endosc 40:70, 1994.
12. Schrock TR: Colonoscopic diagnosis and treatment of lower gastrointestinal bleeding. Surg Clin North Am 69:1309, 1989.
13. Zuckerman DA, Bocchini TP, Birnbaum EH: Massive hemorrhage in the lower gastrointestinal tract in adults: Diagnostic imaging and intervention. AJR 161:703, 1993.

57. OCCULT AND OBSCURE GASTROINTESTINAL BLEEDING

John S. Goff, M.D.

1. What is occult gastrointestinal (GI) bleeding?
Bleeding that is not visible or hidden and is manifested by positive fecal occult blood (FOB) testing or iron deficiency anemia.

2. What physical examination findings may provide a clue to the source of bleeding?
Facial or oral telangiectasia can suggest hereditary telangiectasia (Osler-Weber-Rendu syndrome), whereas perioral pigmented spots may suggest Peutz-Jeghers syndrome (hereditary hamartomatous polyposis). Acanthosis nigricans in the axilla suggests possible malignancy. Purpura or ecchymoses implies a possible bleeding disorder.

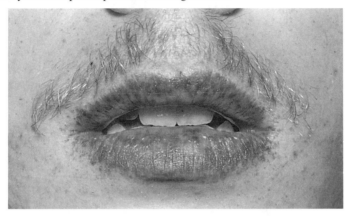

Photograph showing perioral hyperpigmentation seen with Peutz-Jeghers syndrome.

3. What tests are used to identify patients with occult GI bleeding? Which are best?
Hemoccult, Hemoccult II Sensa, HemeSelect, FECA, and Hemoquant are techniques for identifying nonvisible blood in stool. Hemoccult and Hemoccult II Sensa cards are impregnated with guaiac. They are developed by dropping on a solution of hydrogen peroxide and denatured alcohol. If blood is present, the spot turns blue. HemeSelect and FECA are immunologic tests for hemoglobin in stool samples. Hemoquant uses a fluorometric method for quantitative measurement of heme and heme-derived porphyrin in stool. The sensitivity and specificity are 0.67 and 0.90, respectively, for Hemoccult and 0.97 and 0.94 for Hemoquant. However, the Hemoquant is not a bedside test and is about 10 times more expensive.

4. What factors influence the results of FOB testing besides bleeding from the GI tract?
Pseudoperoxidase in various foods can result in a false-positive FOB test. Examples include rare red meat, raw broccoli, turnips, cauliflower, radishes, cantaloupe, and parsnips. Rehydrating Hemoccult cards also produces more false-positive results. A false-negative result can be caused by vitamin C ingestion, delayed development of the card (> 6 days), and testing when a lesion in the bowel is not actively bleeding. Iron ingestion probably does not cause false-positive results. Whether a stool specimen collected at digital rectal examination is more prone to produce false

positive results is controversial. Published studies seem to support the validity of a specimen collected at rectal examination.

5. What is the proper procedure for FOB testing?

For about three days before testing the patient should avoid the foods listed in question 4. They also should avoid aspirin and nonsteroidal anti-inflammatory drugs (NSAIDs). A sample of stool from three separate movements should be collected. The cards need to be developed in < 7 days and should not be rehydrated.

6. How much blood is needed to cause a positive FOB test?

As little as 2 ml of blood in the GI tract can produce a positive FOB test.

7. What effect does the use of the FOB test have on colon cancer mortality rates?

A 33% decrease in mortality rates has been reported in patients with positive FOB testing combined with endoscopic evaluation.

8. Who should be tested for occult blood? How often?

All patients $\geq$ 50 years old should have annual FOB testing.

9. What are the expected findings at colonoscopy in a patient over 50 years old who is not FOB positive? Who is FOB positive?

RESULT OF FOB	POLYP(S)	COLON CANCER
FOB negative	0.5–3%	7–35%
FOB positive	7–17%	20–43%

10. How should a patient with a positive FOB test be evaluated?

The patient needs a full colonoscopy. If the colonoscopy is negative, endoscopy (EGD) of the upper GI tract should be considered. The yield for EGD is increased by approximately 50% (13% vs 0.27%) if the patient is also iron deficient. Barium radiographs can be substituted, but their sensitivity for detecting causes of the positive FOB is lower.

11. What are the usual signs and symptoms of iron deficiency anemia?

Symptoms of iron deficiency include fatigue, tachycardia (anemia), pica (eating clay and other objects), and pagophagia (ice eating). Physical signs of iron deficiency are rare; they include cheilitis, glossitis, and koilonychia. Laboratory findings include high platelet counts, microcytosis, elevated total iron-binding capacity, and low ferritin values. Microcytosis also can be seen with thalassemia, anemia of chronic disease, and sideroblastic anemia.

12. How should a patient with a positive FOB and iron deficiency anemia be evaluated?

If the patient has no GI symptoms, as is usually the case, the evaluation should start with a colonoscopy. Otherwise, the symptomatic organ should be evaluated first. If the colon is normal, an upper EGD with biopsies of the proximal small bowel (duodenum) to look for sprue (celiac disease) is the next test. If both endoscopies are negative and the patient does not have sprue, a small bowel radiograph should be performed. A more involved evaluation is indicated for patients with negative results who have GI symptoms, do not respond to iron therapy, or have recurrent iron deficiency anemia (see questions 17 and 18).

13. How does the evaluation differ for patients who are only iron deficient?

The initial emphasis is plced on diagnosing sprue (celiac disease), non-GI tract sources of blood loss (e.g., menstrual bleeding, urinary tract), nutritional factors, and infectious causes (hookworm, *Strongyloidosis* sp., ascariasis). Ultimately a full GI tract evaluation may be required.

14. What is the yield for combined colonoscopy and EGD in patients who are FOB positive with or without iron deficiency?

Lesions can be found in 48–71% of such patients. Colonoscopy is positive in 20–30%; 5–11% have cancer. EGD is positive in 29–56% of cases. Synchronous lesions are found in 1–10% of patients.

15. How is sprue (celiac disease) diagnosed?

The best way to diagnose celiac disease is to demonstrate flattened small bowel villi in association with increased intraepithelial lymphocytes. The biopsies are usually obtained with EGD-directed jumbo biopsy forceps. Serologic testing is particularly helpful for following patients after treatment with a gluten-free diet because antibody titers should fall. The antibodies used are IgA endomysial antibodies, IgA antigliadin antibodies, and IgG antigliadin antibodies. The respective sensitivities for the three antibodies are 95%, 85%, and 80%; the respective specificities are 98%, 90%, and 92%. A positive antibody test should be confirmed with a small bowel biopsy.

16. What is meant by obscure GI bleeding?

Clinically observable bleeding with a negative standard evaluation, including such tests as an upper GI series, barium enema, upper EGD, and colonoscopy.

17. What tests are available for evaluating patients with obscure GI bleeding? How useful are they?

Several endoscopic and radiologic tests are available for further evaluation. Repeat standard upper and lower endoscopy should be considered early in the evaluation because the yield is approximately 35% (29% upper, 6% lower). Small bowel evaluation with enteroclysis is preferred over small bowel follow-through because of the increased yield (0–20% vs. 0–6%). Enteroscopy with a long scope (Sonde vs. push) has a yield of 30–75%, and also is helpful in evaluating the small bowel. Radiolabeled-red blood cell (RBC) scanning should be used when it is believed that the patient may be actively bleeding. If active bleeding is confirmed, the radiologist can proceed to an urgent angiogram. Elective angiography may have yields up to 40%, but data are limited. Pharmacological alteration of the coagulation system to enhance angiography is not encouraged because of high risk and poor yield. Intraoperative endoscopy is also moderately risky and is highly invasive, but the yield is high for finding a bleeding site (70–100%). Meckel scans are useful in young patients but rarely help in middle-aged or elderly patients.

18. How should you sequence the evaluation of patients with obscure GI bleeding?

The first step is to catch the patient in the act of bleeding. In patients with obvious findings of hematemesis or hematochezia, obtain a radiolabeled-RBC scan to confirm continued active bleeding. A positive scan may help to localize the bleeding to a specific part of the GI tract and indicates whether it is a good time to perform an angiogram to define the type and site of bleeding more accurately. If the patient does not have acute bleeding episodes, the sequence for evaluation begins with repeated upper and lower endoscopies, followed by small bowel enteroclysis, small bowel endoscopy, and elective angiography. Intraoperative endoscopy is a last resort.

19. Angiodysplasia (vascular malformations) are a common cause of obscure GI bleeding. How are they treated?

Endoscopic cautery (laser, bipolar, heater probe) is effective for reducing blood requirements if the lesions can be reached with the endoscope. Angiographic embolization is rarely useful unless the lesion is large and the feeding vessel can be selectively cannulated. Surgery may be useful for a localized lesion that is not otherwise accessible. Treatment for multiple vascular malformations (hereditary [Osler-Weber-Rendu syndrome] or nonhereditary) is use of estrogen-progesterone combinations; in difficult cases, octreotide may be helpful but is clearly more difficult to administer. Patients should avoid NSAIDs and anticoagulants.

20. What other lesions may cause obscure GI bleeding?

- Cameron's erosions (associated with large hiatal hernias)
- GAVE (gastric antral vascular ectasia or watermelon stomach)
- Portal hypertensive gastropathy
- Crohn's disease
- Nonesophageal varices
- Tumors (e.g., lymphoma, leiomyoma, carcinoid)
- Diverticula (particularly Meckel's diverticulum in younger patients)
- Small bowel or colonic ulcers
- Dieulafoy's ulcers
- Amyloidosis
- Hemorrhoids

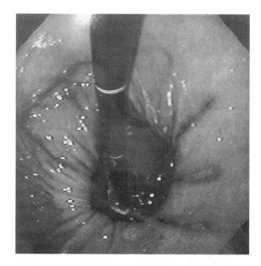

Endoscopic photograph of Cameron's (riding) erosions associated with large hiatal hernias illustrates the linear erosions running perpendicular to the gastric impression of the hiatus, characteristic of the Cameron erosions.

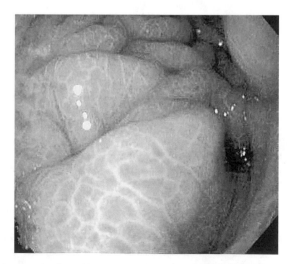

Endoscopic photograph of portal hypertensive gastropathy. (Courtesy of Mark Powis, M.D.)

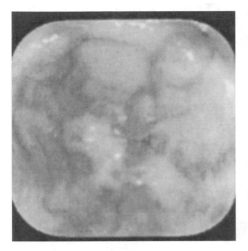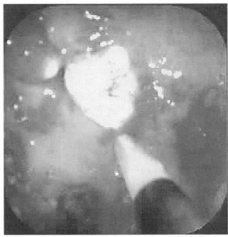

Left, Endoscopic photograph of gastric antral vascular ectasia (GAVE) or watermelon stomach. *Right*, Endoscopic photograph of GAVE after BiCAP therapy. (Courtesy of Mark Powis, M.D.)

BIBLIOGRAPHY

1. Ackerman Z, Eliakin R, Stalnikowicz R, Rachmilowitz: Role of small bowel biopsy in the endoscopic evaluation of adults with iron deficiency anemia. Am J Gastroenterol 91:2094, 1996.
2. Allison JE, Tekawa IS, Ranson CJ, Adrian AL: A comparison of fecal occult-blood tests for colorectal cancer. Lancet 348:1472, 1996.
3. Cave DR, Cooley JS: Intraoperative enteroscopy: Indications and techniques. Gastrointest Endosc Clin North Am 6:793, 1996.
4. Chen YK, Gladden DR, Kestenbaum DJ, Collen MJ: Is there a role of upper gastrointestinal endoscopy in the evaluation of patients with occult-positive stool and negative colonoscopy? Am J Gastroenterol 88:2026, 1993.
5. Kepczyk T, Kadakia SC: Prospective evaluation of the gastrointestinal tract in patients with iron deficiency anemia. Dig Dis Sci 40:1283, 1995.
6. Lewis BS, Waye JD: Chronic gastrointestinal bleeding of obscure origin: Role of small bowel enteroscopy. Gastroenterology 94:1117, 1998.
7. Ransohoff DF, Lang CA: Screening for colorectal cancer with fecal occult blood testing: A background paper. American College of Physicians. Ann Intern Med 126:811, 1997.
8. Rex DR, Lehman GA, Ulbright TM, et al: Colonic neoplasms in asymptomatic persons with negative fecal occult blood tests: Influence of age, gender, and family history. Am J Gastroenterol 88:825, 1993.
9. Rockey DC, Koch J, Cello JP, et al: Relative frequency of upper gastrointestinal and colonic lesions in patients with positive fecal occult-blood tests. N Engl J Med 339:153, 1998.
10. Rossini FP, Arrigoni A, Pennazio M: Octreotide in the management of bleeding due to angiodysplasia of the small intestine. Am J Gastroenterol 88:1424, 1993.
11. Rozen P, Knaani J, Samuel Z: Performance characteristics and comparison of two immunochemical and two guaiac fecal occult blood screening tests for colorectal neoplasia. Dig Dis Sci 42:2064, 1997.
12. Winawer SJ, Flectcher RH, Miller L: Colorectal cancer screening: Clinical guidelines and rationale. Gastroenterology 112:594, 1997.
13. Winawer SJ, Stewart ET, Zauber AG, et al: A comparison of colonoscopy and double-contrast barium enema for surveillance after polypectomy. N Engl J Med342:1766, 2000.
14. Zuckerman GR, Prakash C, Askin MP, Lewis BS: AGA technical review on the evaluation and management of occult and obscure gastrointestinal bleeding. Gastroenterology 118:201, 2000.

58. EVALUATION OF ACUTE ABDOMINAL PAIN

James E. Cremins, M.D., and Peter R. McNally, D.O.

1. Provide a useful clinical definition of an acute abdomen.

This clinical scenario is characterized by severe pain, often of rapid onset, that prevents bodily movement. When patients experience symptoms of pain for more than 6 hours, surgical intervention is usually necessary.

2. What are the four types of stimuli for abdominal pain?
1. Stretching or tension
2. Inflammation
3. Ischemia
4. Neoplasms

3. What are the three categories of abdominal pain?

1. **Visceral pain** occurs when noxious stimuli affect an abdominal viscus. The pain is usually dull (cramping, gnawing, or burning) and poorly localized to the ventral midline because the innervation to most viscera is multisegmental. Secondary autonomic effects such as diaphoresis, restlessness, nausea, vomiting, and pallor are common.

2. **Parietal pain** occurs when noxious stimuli irritate the parietal peritoneum. The pain is more intense and more precisely localized to the site of the lesion. Parietal pain is likely to be aggravated by coughing or movement.

3. **Referred pain** is experienced in areas remote from the site of injury. The remote site of pain referral is supplied by the same neurosegment as the involved organ; for example, gallbladder pain may be referred to the right scapula and pancreatic pain may radiate to the mid back.

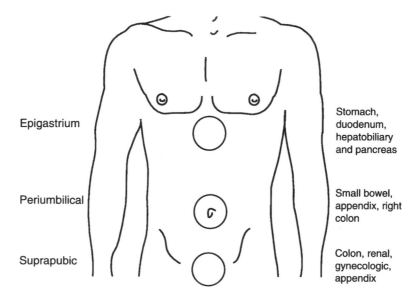

Location of visceral pain.

4. How does the character of the abdominal pain help in the evaluation?

Classification of Pain by the Rate of Development

Explosive and excruciating (instantaneous)	Myocardial infarction Perforated ulcer Ruptured aneurysm Biliary or renal colic (passage of a stone)
Rapid, severe, and constant (over minutes)	Acute pancreatitis Complete bowel obstruction Mesenteric thrombus
Gradual and steady pain (over hours)	Acute cholecystitis Diverticulitis Acute appendicitis
Intermittent and colicky pain (over hours)	Early subacute pancreatitis Mechanical small bowel obstruction

5. What are the important components of the physical examination for patients with acute abdominal pain?

General status	Is the patient hemodynamically unstable? Does he or she need immediate hemodynamic resuscitation and emergent laparotomy (e.g., ruptured spleen, hepatic tumor, aneurysm, ectopic pregnancy, or mesenteric apoplexy)?
Inspection	Visually evaluate for distention, hernias, scars, and hyperperistalsis.
Auscultation	Hyperperistalsis suggests obstruction; absence of peristalsis > 3 minutes suggests peritonitis (silent abdomen); bruits suggest presence of an aneurysm.
Percussion	Tympany suggests either intraluminal or free abdominal air.
Palpation	Start the examination away from the area of tenderness and be gentle. Abdominal pain with voluntary coughing suggests peritoneal signs. Deeply palpating the abdomen only diminishes patient trust and cooperation. The enlarged gallbladder will be missed on deep palpation. Inspiratory arrest during light palpation of the right hypochondrium suggests gallbladder pain (Murphy's sign). Localized pain suggests localized peritonitis (e.g., appendicitis, cholecystitis, diverticulitis). Findings on the abdominal examination of visceral ischemia or infarction are characteristically disproportionate to the degree of abdominal pain.
Pelvic and rectal exam	These exams should be done in any patient with abdominal pain. A painful examination may be the only sign of pelvic appendicitis, diverticulitis, or tuboovarian pathology. Bimanual examination is critical to exclude an obstetric or gynecologic cause.
Iliopsoas test	With the legs fully extended in a supine position, the patient is requested to raise the legs. Pain occurs when the psoas muscle is inflamed (e.g., appendicitis).
Obturator test	This test is performed by flexing the patient's thigh at right angles to the trunk and then rotating the leg externally. Inflammation of the obturator internus muscle causes pain (e.g., tuboovarian abscess or pelvic appendicitis).

6. Which laboratory tests should be obtained in patients with acute abdominal pain?

Although laboratory tests are helpful in confirming the evolution of a disease process, they are frequently not helpful in localizing the cause of abdominal pain.

- **Complete blood count (CBC).** Elevation of the white blood cell count suggests inflammation; however, absence of leukocytosis may be unhelpful early in the course of disease. A low hematocrit with a normal mean corpuscular volume (MCV) suggests acute blood loss, whereas a low hematocrit with a low MCV suggests iron deficiency from chronic GI blood loss or malabsorption.

- **Amylase elevations** (> 500 IU) suggest pancreatitis but are not specific. Lipase enzyme elevations are more specific for pancreatic origin.
- **Liver enzyme elevations** may be suggestive of hepatobiliary causes of pain. Elevations of aspartate or alanine aminotransferase suggest hepatocyte injury. Alkaline phosphatase or gamma glutamine transferase (GGT) elevations suggest canalicular or biliary injury. Total bilirubin elevations > 3 mg/dl suggest common bile duct obstruction or associated intrahepatic cholestasis.
- **Evidence of pyuria** on urinalysis suggests urinary tract infection but also may be seen in nephrolithiasis or even pelvic appendicitis.
- **Chemistry analysis** can be helpful in the global assessment of patient health, hyperglycemia, acidosis, and electrolyte disturbances.
- **Pregnancy tests** (beta human chorionic gonadotropin) should be ordered for all premenopausal women.
- **Stool examination** for occult blood is necessary.
- **Electrocardiography** is performed for all patients with possible myocardial infarction or > 50 years of age.

7. Which radiologic tests should be ordered to evaluate the patient with acute abdominal pain?

The selection of tests depends on the likelihood of the pretest clinical diagnosis and the ability of the radiologic test to confirm clinical suspicion.

- **Plain radiographs** of the abdomen are quick and readily available and can be done at the bedside. They reliably detect bowel obstruction and viscus perforation. Occasionally they may suggest stone disease (one-third of gallbladder and two-thirds of renal stones are calcified) or ruptured aortic aneurysm (separation of aortic wall calcium and mass effect). Free intraabdominal air is best detected with the patient in the left lateral decubitus position for 10 minutes (see chapter 73).
- **Ultrasound** of the abdomen is quick and noninvasive and can be performed at the bedside. The disadvantages of ultrasound include variable operator expertise and suboptimal examination in the obese or gaseous abdomen. Ultrasound is excellent for evaluating the gallbladder, bile ducts, liver, kidneys, and appendix (see chapter 75).
- **Computerized tomography (CT)** of the abdomen provides a detailed view of the anatomy. It is expensive, requires transportation of the patient, and is not always readily available. Oral and intravenous contrast agents are usually required. CT provides the best evaluation of the pancreas (see chapter 75).
- **Hepatoiminodiacetic (HIDA) scan** is the most accurate test for acute cholecystitis (see chapter 76).

8. Pain referred to the abdomen can be confusing. What are the common extraabdominal causes of referred abdominal pain?

Thoracic	Pneumonia, pulmonary embolism, pneumothorax, myocardial infarction or ischemia, esophageal spasm, or perforation
Neurogenic	Tabes dorsalis, radicular pain (spinal cord compression from tumor, abscess, compression, or varicella zoster infection)
Metabolic	Uremia, porphyria, acute adrenal insufficiency
Hematologic	Sickle cell anemia, hemolytic anemia, Henoch-Schönlein purpura
Toxins	Insect bites (scorpion bite-induced pancreatitis), lead poisoning

9. List the common causes of acute abdominal pain in gravid women.

- Appendicitis
- Ovarian cysts complicated by torsion, rupture, and hemorrhage
- Ectopic pregnancy
- Gallbladder problems

10. When the appendix is found to be entirely normal during a laparotomy performed for presumed appendicitis in a gravid woman, should the appendix be removed?

No. Removal of the normal appendix triples the risk of fetal loss.

11. What is the most common cause of acute abdominal pain in elderly patients?

Biliary tract disease is responsible for 25% of all cases of acute abdominal pain in elderly patients requiring hospitalization. Bowel obstruction and incarcerated hernia are the next most common, followed by appendicitis.

12. What symptoms are helpful in evaluating for appendicitis?

It is decidedly uncommon for acute appendicitis to present with nausea, vomiting, or diarrhea before abdominal pain. Usually acute appendicitis is heralded by pain and often followed by anorexia, nausea, and sometimes single-episode vomiting. Acute appendicitis should be first on the differential diagnosis list in any patient with acute abdominal pain without a prior history of appendectomy. The diagnosis of typical appendicitis requires only careful history and physical examination. Laboratory tests and radiographic studies are ancillary.

13. Discuss atypical forms of appendicitis.

When the appendix is retrocecal or retroileal in location, the inflamed appendix is often shielded from the anterior abdomen. The pain is often less pronounced, and localizing signs on physical examination are uncommon. Symptoms and signs of appendicitis in elderly patients are subtle. Pain is often minimal, fever only mild, and leukocytosis unreliable. A high index of suspicion is essential.

14. Describe the ultrasound findings of acute appendicitis.

The appendix appears as a round target with an anechoic lumen, surrounded by a hypoechoic and thickened (> 2 mm) appendiceal wall. This finding with reproduction of pain under the transducer has a diagnostic accuracy of 95% and a negative predictive value of 97%.

15. When laparotomy is performed for presumed appendicitis, what is the acceptable false-negative rate? How often is another cause identified in this setting?

A false-negative laparotomy rate of 10–20% is reported. In roughly 30% of these cases some other cause of abdominal pain is identified, such as mesenteric lymphadenitis, Meckel's diverticulum, cecal diverticulitis, pelvic inflammatory disease, ectopic pregnancy, or ileitis.

16. What is the single best test to evaluate patients infected with human immunodeficiency virus (HIV) who complain of acute abdominal pain?

Because of the variety of causes of abdominal pain in such patients, it has been argued that CT scan is the single best test.

17. What are the cardinal features of a ruptured tubal pregnancy?

• Amenorrhea (missed period or scant menses)
• Abdominal and pelvic pain
• Unilateral, tender adnexal mass
• Signs of blood loss

18. What are the characteristics of acute intestinal obstruction?

• Nausea and vomiting
• Failure to expel flatus
• Prior abdominal surgery or presence of hernia
• Peristaltic pain (colicky pain—every 10 minutes for jejunal obstruction and every 30 mintues for ileal obstruction)

19. List the clinical characteristics of large bowel obstruction.
- Most patients are over 50 years of age.
- Lower abdominal cramping pain is gradual in onset.
- Abdominal distention is a prominent feature.
- Dilated loops of bowel with haustra distinguish the colon from the small bowel.
- Sigmoidoscopy or single-column barium enema is important.
- Causes include obstructing neoplasm and cecal or sigmoid volvulus.

20. List the clinical characteristics of diverticulitis.
- Age > 50 years
- Localized left lower abdominal pain
- Palpable mass in the left lower quadrant

21. List the clinical hallmarks of acute cholecystitis.
- Patients often give a history of prior episodes of milder abdominal pain.
- Abdominal pain usually arises after a meal, especially in the evening after a large meal.
- Pain typically crescendos over 20–30 minutes and then plateaus.
- Pain lasting > 1–2 hours is usually accompanied by gallbladder wall inflammation.
- Associated nausea occurs in 90% of patients; vomiting may follow onset of pain in 50–80%.
- Radiation of pain to the back is common; pain radiates to the right scapula in 10% of cases.
- Low-grade fever is common.
- Right hypochondrium tenderness is generally present. Inspiratory arrest during gentle palpation of the right upper quadrant (Murphy's sign) suggests acute cholecystitis.
- Diagnostic tests include HIDA scan or ultrasound.

22. What is the differential diagnosis of acute cholecystitis?
- Liver: alcoholic hepatitis, liver metastasis, Fitz-Hugh-Curtis syndrome, congestive hepatopathy
- Pancreas: pancreatitis, pseudocyst
- GI tract: peptic ulcer disease with or without perforation, acute appendicitis (retrocecal)
- Kidney: pyelonephritis, renal colic
- Lung: pneumonia, pulmonary embolism, emphysema
- Heart: myocardial infarction, pericarditis
- Pre-eruptive varicella zoster

23. When should a patient undergo surgery for an acute abdomen?
When, in the judgment of the surgeon, a problem will be identifiable or treatable by surgical intervention. There is no substitute for good surgical judgment and intuition.

24. What conditions can result in an acute abdomen in HIV-infected patients?
Patients with HIV can have any of the usual causes of an acute abdomen; all non–HIV-specific diagnoses must be considered. Perforation is most often due to cytomegalovirus (CMV) infection in the distal small bowel or colon; this is the most common cause of the acute abdomen in late-stage HIV infection. CMV infection of the vascular endothelial cells leads to mucosal ischemic ulceration and perforation. HIV-associated lymphoma and Kaposi's sarcoma also can lead to perforation, but this finding is rare. AIDS cholangiopathy, papillitis and and drug-induced pancreatitis (e.g., pentamidine, bactrim, didanosine, ritonavir) are unique causes of abdominal pain in HIV-infected patients.

25. Are patients with systemic lupus erythematosus (SLE) at increased risk for intraabdominal catastrophe?
Approximately 2% of patients with SLE develop lupus vasculitis, one of the most devastating complications of SLE. The fatality rate is > 50%. Small vessels of the bowel wall are affected, leading to ulceration, hemorrhage, perforation, and infarction.

26. How common are severe GI manifestations of polyarteritis nodosa (PAN)?

PAN is a vasculitis that may have visceral involvement. GI bleeding from intestinal ischemia is seen in 6% of cases, bowel perforation in 5%, and bowel infarction in 1.4%. Acalculous chole-cystitis occurs in up to 17% because of direct vasculitic involvement of the gallbladder.

27. What causes of acute abdominal pain should be considered in illicit drug users?

Intravenous and smoked cocaine has been reported to cause acute mesenteric ischemia or "crack belly." Endocarditis in parenteral drug abusers may be associated with mesenteric emboli and bowel infarction.

BIBLIOGRAPHY

1. Brandt CP, Priebe PP, Eckhauser ML: Diagnostic laparoscopy in the intensive care patient: Avoiding the nontherapeutic laparotomy. Surg Endosc 7:168–172, 1993.
2. Clement DJ: Evaluation of the acute abdomen with CT: Is image everything? Am J Gastroenterol 88:1282–1283, 1993.
3. Connor TJ, Garcha IS, Ramshaw BJ, et al: Diagnostic laparoscopy for suspected appendicitis. Am Surg 61:187–189, 1995.
4. de Dombal FT: Acute abdominal pain in the elderly. J Clin Gastroenterol 19:331–335, 1994.
5. Epstein FB: Acute abdominal pain in pregnancy. Emerg Med Clin North Am 12:151–165, 1994.
6. Haubrich WS: Abdominal pain. In Haubrich WS, Schaffner, F, Berk JE (eds): Bockus Gastroenterology, 5th ed. Philadelphia, WB Saunders, 1995, pp 11–29.
7. Klein KB: Approach to the patient with abdominal pain. In Yamada T (ed): Textbook of Gastroenterology, 2nd ed. Philadelphia, J.B. Lippincott, 1995, pp 750–771.
8. Kovachev LS: "Cough sign": A reliable test in the diagnosis of intra-abdominal inflammation. Br J Surg 81:1542, 1994.
9. Linder JD, Monkemuller KE, Raijman I, et al: Cocaine-associated ischemic colitis. South Med J 93:909–913, 2000.
10. Mulholland MW: Approach to the patient with acute abdomen and fever of abdominal origin. In Yamada T (ed): Textbook of Gastroenterology, 2nd ed. Philadelphia, J.B. Lippincott, 1995, pp 783–796.
11. Nusair S, Nahir M, Almogy G, et al: Pancreatitis and chronic abdominal pain in patients with AIDS. Postgrad Med J 75:371–373, 1999.
12. Ridge JA, Way LW: Abdominal pain. In Sleisenger MH, Fordtran JS (eds): Gastrointestinal Disease: Pathophysiology, Diagnosis, Management, 5th ed. Philadelphia, W.B. Saunders, 1993, pp 150–162.
13. Sheikh RA, Prindiville TP, Yeramandra S, et al: Microsporidial AIDS cholangiopathy due to encephalitozoon intesti-nalis: Case report and review. Am J Gastroenterol 95:2364–2371, 2000.
14. Silen W: Cope's Early Diagnosis of the Abdomen. New York, Oxford University Press, 1979.
15. Taourel P, Baron MP, Pradel J, et al: Acute abdomen of unknown origin: Impact of CT on diagnosis and management. Gastrointest Radiol 17:287–291, 1992.
16. Wyatt SH, Fishman EK:The acute abdomen in individuals with AIDS. Radiol Clin North Am 32:1032–1043, 1994.
17. Wattoo MA, Osundeko O: Cocaine-induced intestinal ischemia. West J Med 170:47–49, 2000.

59. EVALUATION OF ACUTE DIARRHEA

Colonel Kent C. Holtzmuller, M.D.

1. What is the definition of acute diarrhea?

Diarrhea is defined by the passage of an increased number of stools of less-than-normal form and consistency. Acute diarrhea refers to acute onset of symptoms of < 14–30 days' duration. Diarrhea lasting longer than 1 month is considered chronic. American adults average about one episode of acute diarrhea annually.

2. Who should undergo medical evaluation for acute diarrhea?

Most cases of acute diarrhea are self-limited and require no medical evaluation. Evaluation should be reserved for patients with evidence of systemic toxicity (dehydration, bloody diarrhea, fever, severe abdominal pain), diarrhea of > 48 hours' duration, and elderly or immunocompromised patients.

3. What are the most common causes of acute bloody diarrhea?

Infectious dysentery, inflammatory bowel disease (ulcerative colitis and Crohn's disease), and ischemic colitis.

INFECTIOUS DYSENTERY

4. What is dysentery?

Dysentery is a disease process characterized by diarrhea that contains blood and polymorphonuclear cells. Dysentery results when an organism causes an inflammatory reaction, either by direct invasion of the colonic/ileal epithelium or by producing a toxin that causes cellular death and tissue damage. Symptoms associated with dysentery may include abdominal pain and cramping, tenesmus (painful urgency to evacuate stool), fever, and dehydration.

5. Name the common causes of infectious dysentery in the United States.

Campylobacter and *Salmonella* species are the principal causes of dysentery in the United States. *Shigella* species and certain strains of *Escherichia coli* (specifically O157H) are less common. Rarer causes include *Yersinia, Entamoeba, Aeromonas,* and *Plesiomonas* species.

6. What is the significance of stool leukocytes (white blood cells)?

The presence of fecal leukocytes helps to distinguish inflammatory from noninflammatory diarrhea. Normally, leukocytes are not present in stool. Fecal leukocytes are usually found in infectious diarrhea caused by *Campylobacter, Salmonella, Shigella,* and *Yersinia* species, *Clostridium difficile*, enterohemorrhagic and enteroinvasive strains of *E. coli*, and *Aeromonas* species. With ischemic colitis and inflammatory bowel disease, fecal leukocytes are due to mucosal bleeding. Diarrhea secondary to toxigenic bacteria (e.g., ETEC, *Vibrio cholerae*), viruses, and small bowel protozoan (e.g., *Giardia* sp.) do not contain stool leukocytes.

7. How do you evaluate a stool specimen for leukocytes?

The presence of white blood cells (WBCs) in the stool can be assayed by microscopic exam of the stool or a fecal lactoferrin assay. The fecal lactoferrin assay detects WBC enzymes. Microscopy is best performed on liquid stool or mucus:
1. Place a drop of liquid stool or mucus on a glass microscope slide.
2. Add several drops of methylene blue or Gram stain.
3. Mix the material thoroughly.

4. Place a coverslip over the mixture.

5. Wait several minutes to allow nuclear staining.

6. Scan the slide under high power to observe for leukocytes and red blood cells (positive result = > 3 leukocytes in four or more fields).

8. Which patients with diarrhea should be evaluated with a stool culture?

Stool culture should be obtained from patients with dysentery symptoms, immunocompromise, or persistent diarrhea (beyond 3–5 days). Patients with dysentery symptoms are much more likely to have a positive stool culture. The rate of bacterial isolation in patients hospitalized with dysentery is 40–60%.

9. By what mechanisms do toxigenic organisms produce diarrhea?

The toxins produced by organisms can be classified into two categories, cytotonic and cytotoxic. Cytotonic toxins cause a watery diarrhea by activation of intracellular enzymes, which cause net fluid secretion into the intestinal lumen. Cytotonic examples include toxins produced by *V. cholerae* and enterotoxigenic strains of *E. coli*. Cytotoxic toxins cause structural injury to the intestinal mucosa, which, in turn, causes inflammation and mucosal bleeding. Enterohemorrhagic *E. coli* produces a cytotoxin.

10. Which *Campylobacter* species are implicated as causes of dysentery? How is *Campylobacter* transmitted?

C. jejuni accounts for 98% of reported isolates. The less common isolates are *C. fetus* and *C. fecalis*. Direct contact with fecal matter from infected persons or animals and ingestion of contaminated food or water have been implicated in the transmission of *Campylobacter* infection.

11. Describe the clinical and endoscopic features of *Campylobacter* diarrhea.

The incubation period from ingestion until onset of symptoms is 1–7 days. Symptoms include diarrhea (often bloody), abdominal pain, malaise, headache, and fever (sometimes high). With or without antibiotic therapy, most patients recover within 7 days. Relapse may occur. The rectosigmoidoscopic findings may be indistinguishable from those of ulcerative colitis or Crohn's disease. Identification of comma-shaped, gram-negative bacteria on stool Gram stain suggests the diagnosis of *Campylobacter* infection. A rare extraintestinal complication of Campylobacter infection is Guillain-Barré syndrome.

12. How are *Salmonella* organisms classified?

Salmonella species are gram-negative, aerobic and facultative anaerobic bacteria of the Enterobacteriaceae family. Use of O and H antigens has identified 2200 different serotypes. The term **nontyphoidal salmonellosis** is used to denote disease caused by serotypes other than *S. typhi*.

13. List the types of illnesses that can be caused by *Salmonella*.

- Acute gastroenteritis: The degree of colonic involvement determines the extent of the dysentery-like symptoms.
- Bacteremia with or without gastrointestinal (GI) involvement
- Localized infection: Bacteremia can result in localized nonintestinal infections (e.g., bone, joints, meninges). Predisposing conditions for localized infection include abdominal aortic aneurysm, prosthetic heart valve, vascular grafts, and othopedic hardware.
- Typhoidal or enteric fever
- Asymptomatic carrier states: more common in older age, in women (3:1), and people with biliary disease)

14. What is typhoid fever?

Typhoid fever is a clinical syndrome characterized by marked hectic fever, persistent bacteremia, hepatosplenomegaly, and abdominal pain. The illness can be caused by any serotype of

Salmonella but results most commonly from *S. typhi* and less commonly from *S. paratyphi*. Because humans are the only known reservoir of *S. typhi*, transmission is primarily by the fecal-oral route. The illness usually lasts for 3–5 weeks. Up to 90% of patients may experience a "rose spot" rash on the upper anterior trunk within the first or second week of illness. Although diarrhea is unusual, ulceration of Peyer's patches in the intestinal wall may cause hemorrhage or perforation. A number of vaccines are successful against typhoid.

15. How is *Salmonella* infection treated?

Healthy patients with mild symptoms do not require antibiotic therapy. In fact, antibiotic therapy may prolong intestinal carriage of the organism. Antibiotic therapy is appropriate for patients at the extremes of age (very young or elderly), immunosuppressed patients, patients with evidence of bacteremia, and patients with severe cases of intestinal salmonellosis. A quinolone antibiotic is the treatment of choice.

16. Describe the characteristics of *Shigella* infection. How is it treated?

Shigella species is a gram-negative rod and member of the Enterobacteriaceae. Most infections (90–95%) are caused by four species: *S. sonnei*, *S. flexneri*, *S. dysenteriae*, and *S. boydii*. The organism is highly infectious, with a fecal-oral route of transmission. Infection can occur with the ingestion of as few as 10–100 organisms. Intestinal damage results primarily from direct invasion of the organism into the colonic epithelium and, to a lesser extent, from the production of an enterotoxin. The *Shigella* toxin is composed of an A subunit, which is catalytic, and a B subunit, which is responsible for binding. The endoscopic appearance of shigellosis shows intense involvement of the rectosigmoid with variable proximal involvement. Approximately 15% of cases involve pancolitis. In children, *Shigella* infection has been associated with seizures. Antimicrobial therapy is recommended for all cases of shigellosis: trimethoprim/sulfamethozazole for an infection acquired in North America and a fluoroquinolone for infections acquired in other areas.

17. What diarrheogenic illnesses are caused by *Escherichia coli*?

E. coli belongs to the family Enterobacteriaceae, a facultative anaerobic, gram-negative bacteria. The organisms are common inhabitants of the human GI tract, and most strains do not have the virulence factors necessary to cause disease. The four primary pathogenic strains of *E. coli* and the syndromes that they cause are listed below.

Enterotoxigenic *E. coli* (ETEC) accounts for most cases of traveler's diarrhea but is relatively rare in the United States. Fecal-oral transmission through the ingestion of contaminated food or water is the primary means of spread. Disease is produced by the adherence of ETEC to the mucosa, followed by the production of toxins (heat-labile "cholera-like" toxin). Invasion of the mucosa does not occur. The illness is usually self-limited, lasting 3–5-days. Symptoms include watery diarrhea and abdominal cramping. Occasionally, low-grade fever and, rarely, bloody diarrhea are associated with the illness.

Enteropathogenic *E. coli* (EPEC) lacks invasive properties. Dsease results from its enteroadherent properties. Illness caused by EPEC primarily affects young children (< 3 years of age) and must be considered as a probable cause of nursery and pediatric outbreaks of diarrhea. Profuse watery diarrhea, which may become chronic, is the usual presentation. As with ETEC, EPEC-caused illnesses rarely result in bloody diarrhea.

Enteroinvasive *E. coli* (EIEC) can invade the intestinal mucosa and cause acute dysentery. EIEC strains share characteristics with *Shigella* species and are not commonly found in the United States. Infants under the age of 1 year are most susceptible to EIEC strains in developed countries.

Enterohemorrhagic *E. coli* (EHEC) has a number of serotypes, but *E. coli* O157:H7 is the most important. *E. coli* O157:H7 is acquired primarily from the ingestion of contaminated beef, although outbreaks also have been associated with contaminated water, raw milk, unpasturized juices, and person-to-person transmission among household members. Drinking water contaminated by farm waste has been implicated in several recent large outbreaks. The typical clinical presentation begins with severe abdominal cramps and watery diarrhea followed by rapid progression to bloody diarrhea. The organism is not invasive but produces a Shiga-like toxin, cytotoxic to vascular endothelium. The disease can cause hemolytic uremic syndrome and thrombotic thrombocytopenia purpura (< 10% of cases). The very young and very old are the most susceptible to fatal complications. The most common cause of acute renal failure in North American children is O157:H7 infection.

18. What is the therapy for O157:H7–induced diarrhea?

Antibiotic therapy for O157:H7 is controversial. Early therapy with antibiotics may encourage development of hemolytic uremia syndrome. Supportive care, correction of fluid and electrolyte disturbances and hemodialysis for acute renal failure are the mainstays of therapy.

19. Describe the clinical presentation of infection with *Yersinia enterocolitica.*

The most common presentation of *Y. enterocolitica* infection includes diarrhea, abdominal pain, and low-grade fever. Microscopic examination of the stool usually shows red and white cells. Approximately 25% of the cases are grossly bloody. The clinical presentation of children and young adults may resemble that of appendicitis (right lower quadrant abdominal pain and tenderness, fever, and leukocytosis). Findings at surgery show mesenteric lymphadenitis and terminal ileitis. On rare occasions, a patient may progress to fulminant enterocolitis with intestinal perforation, peritonitis, and hemorrhage. Pharyngitis is common in children with Y. *enterocolitica* infection and is seen in up to 10% of adult cases. Patients with iron overload (hemochromatosis) are more susceptible to yersinial sepsis. Postinfectious manifestations of reactive arthritis, erythema nodosum, Reiter's syndrome, thyroiditis, myocarditis, and glomerulonephritis have been reported.

20. How is infection with *Y. enterocolitica* treated?

Most cases are self-limited and do not require antibiotic therapy. Severe cases can be treated with ceftriaxone, 1 gm/day intravenously for 5 days.

21. Which organisms are associated with seafood-induced dysentery?

Vibrio parahaemolyticus, a member of the Vibrionaceae family, is a halophilic organism (i.e., it grows only in media containing salt). It has been isolated in fish, crustaceans, and shellfish. The diarrhea is characteristically watery, but bloody diarrhea may be seen in up to 15% of patients. Other causes of seafood induced dysentery include *Plesiomonas shigelloides* (a member of the Vibrionaceae family) and *Campylobacter* species.

22. What parasites cause bloody diarrhea?

Entamoeba histolytica, Balantidium coli, Dientamoeba fragilis, and *Schistosoma* species. The most common cause of parasitic dysentery in the United States is amebiasis (*E. histolytica*). Although parasitic diarrhea is uncommon in the United States, it is a significant cause of morbidity and mortality worldwide.

23. Who is at risk for amebiasis? What are the potential complications of amebic dysentery?

Travelers to and immigrants from endemic areas, institutionalized patients, and homosexual men. Complications include toxic megacolon, intestinal perforation, peritonitis, ameboma, and liver abscess.

24. What is an ameboma?

An ameboma is a mass of granulation tissue and mucosal/submucosal inflammation in the cecum or right colon. The inflammatory process clinically manifests as a tender mass in the right lower abdomen. Approximately 0.5–1.5% of patients with amebic colitis have an ameboma. Barium enema may show an "apple-core" appearance. Diagnosis is confirmed with colonoscopy, and biopsy is necessary to rule out carcinoma or tuberculosis. Amebomas respond to antiamebic therapy; surgery generally is not required.

25. Which laboratory studies are useful in the diagnosis of amebic dysentery?

Microscopic examination of the stool for cysts and/or trophozoites or detection of circulating antibodies to *E. histolytica* by the indirect hemagglutination (IHAA) test. Approximately 80–90% of patients with amebic dysentery have a positive IHAA serology. A positive IHAA test in a patient with presumptive inflammatory bowel disease should raise the possibility of amebiasis.

26. Describe the treatment of amebic dysentery. What are the potential side effects?

Acute amebic dysentery is treated with metronidazole, 500–750 mg 3 times/day for 5–10 days. Consumption of alcohol during metronidazole therapy may induce an Antabuse effect (e.g., abdominal cramps, nausea, emesis, headache, flushing). Other drug interactions include potentiation of warfarin and lithium. Peripheral neuropathy is a potentially severe and chronic side effect of metronidazole. Other possible symptoms include a metallic taste and GI distress manifested by nausea, flatus, and diarrhea. Metronidazole is teratogenic and should not be taken during the first trimester of pregnancy.

27. Which parasites typically cause nonbloody diarrhea? What are the risks for acquisition?

Giardia, Cryptosporidiosis, and *Cyclospora* species typically cause nonbloody diarrhea. Contaminated water is the primary source for community outbreaks. *Giardia* species is a frequent culprit after consumption of water from mountainous lakes and streams. *Cyclospora* species should be considered in travelers to Nepal. Cryptosporidiosis is a significant cause of HIV-related diarrhea.

28. How do you obtain a stool specimen for ova and parasites exam?

An inverted, hat-like container is a convenient receptacle for collection of stool. The specimen should be free of contamination from urine and toilet water. Protozoan trophozoites degenerate rapidly with drying. The specimen should be fresh and processed expeditiously or preserved with a two-vial preservation technique. One vial contains a buffered formalin mixture; the other, a polyvinyl alcohol fixative. Erratic shedding of parasites requires stool collection for 3 consecutive days. Barium, antibiotics, mineral oil, antacids, bismuth, and enemas may interfere with parasite identification.

29. What is the most common cause of hospital-acquired diarrhea?

Diarrhea starting during or shortly after hospitalization is most commonly due to *C. difficile* infection. Other causes of hospital acquired diarrhea include enteral nutrition and hyperosmolar liquid medications (which commonly contain sorbitol). Other medications that can cause diarrhea include antacids, magnesium supplements, antibiotics, antineoplastics, cholinergics, theophylline, and prostaglandins.

30. What causes pseudomembranous colitis (PMC)? What are the risk factors?

PMC is caused by *C. difficile*, a gram-positive, spore-forming, anaerobic bacillus. The colitis induced by *C. difficile* is mediated by two toxins, enterotoxin A and cytotoxin B. Patients are susceptible to *C. difficile* diarrhea during and after the cessation of antibiotic therapy. The diarrhea typically presents 10 days after initiation of antibiotics but may begin within several days of initiation and up to 8 weeks after cessation. Clindamycin, penicillin, and cephalosporin antibiotics are the most frequent causes. Less frequently, tetracycline, erythromycin, and metronidazole may cause PMC. Rare causes are quinolone, parental aminoglycoside, and vancomycin. Other risk factors for PMC are chemotherapy, immunosuppression, and hospitalization. Improper hand washing by hospital personnel is a major route of in-hospital transmission of PMC.

31. How do you diagnose pseudomembranous colitis?

A stool assay for *C. difficile* toxin is the diagnostic test of choice. Stool culture is highly sensitive but not specific, because up to 20% of hospitalized patients are colonized with *C. difficile*. The endoscopic appearance ranges from normal to the classic yellow-white pseudomembrane that may appear as 1–3-mm plaques scattered or confluent over the colonic mucosa. The histologic appearance of the pseudomembrane shows a "summit" or "volcano" lesion on the surface of the colonic epithelium, which is composed of inflammatory cells, fibrin, and mucus. The absence of pseudomembranes on sigmoidoscopy does not exclude *C. difficile* colitis. Fifty percent of patients with PMC do not have characteristic pseudomembranes, and 10% of patients have mucosal changes confined to the right colon.

32. Describe the treatment of pseudomembranous colitis.

Antibiotic discontinuation results in complete cessation of symptoms in many patients. Consider drug therapy with oral vancomycin, metronidazole or Bacitracin in patients with moderate-to-severe symptoms. Vancomycin is expensive (up to $500 for a 5–10-day course). Intravenous **metronidazole** can be used in patients who cannot tolerate oral intake. Symptomatic relapse is seen in 15–20% of cases, regardless of which antibiotic is used.

An alternative to antibiotic therapy is oral **cholestyramine**. The cholestyramine resin binds *C. difficile* toxin while the colonic flora reconstitutes itself. Resin therapy has been advocated for use in mild cases and relapses.

Fecal enemas have been used experimentally to reestablish bacterial flora. The theoretical value of fecal enemas in clinical practice is diminished by limited patient acceptance.

33. What are the mechanisms of antibiotic-related diarrhea?

Antibiotics cause diarrhea by at least two mechanisms. The first is secondary to *C. difficile*, (see question 30). The second is due to osmotic diarrhea caused by impaired colonic fermentation of carbohydrates. Carbohydrates that are not absorbed in the small intestine normally undergo colonic bacterial fermentation to organic acids (acetic, propionic, butyric, and lactate acid). These organic acids are absorbed by the colon and provide energy for mucosal cells to absorb water and ions. Antibiotic reduction of colonic bacteria decreases the fermentation of organic acids and availability of "mucosal energy" to support net luminal water reabsorption. The unabsorbed carbohydrates also cause an osmotic diarrhea.

34. Outline the differential diagnosis of a patient with AIDS who presents with bloody diarrhea.

1. As with nonimmunosuppressed patients, colitis secondary to invasive bacteria (*Salmonella, Shigella, Campylobacter,* and *Yersinia* species), bacteria that produce cytotoxins (EHEC), and amebiasis must be considered.

2. Infections that can result in proctitis and bloody diarrhea include rectal gonorrhea, lymphogranuloma venereum (*Chlamydia trachomatis*), primary anorectal syphilis, and herpes simplex. The hallmark of herpes proctitis is severe rectal pain and tenesmus. In addition, a purulent rectal discharge is frequently present, and difficulty with urination, inguinal lymphadenopathy, and perianal ulcerations also may be noted.

3. Colitis characterized by abdominal pain, diarrhea, hematochezia, and fever is a common manifestation of cytomegalovirus (CMV) infection. Patchy involvement of the colonic mucosa is often seen on colonoscopy with CMV infection, and the diagnosis is aided by the identification of amphophilic intranuclear inclusion bodies.

4. Pseudomembranous colitis should be considered in AIDS patients with diarrhea, because often they are prescribed antibiotics.

5. Rarer causes of bloody diarrhea in AIDS are *Myocobacterium tuberculosis* and histoplasmosis. It should be noted that multiple concurrent causes of diarrhea can be present in this population.

6. *Cryptosporidium* sp., *Isospora belli, Cyclospora* sp., *Microsporidia* sp., *Giardia* sp., *Mycobacterium avium-intracellulare*, and lymphoma can affect the small bowel and cause nonbloody diarrhea.

7. AIDS patients with inflammatory bowel disease often exhibit amelioration of symptoms as the immune suppression worsens.

35. List the risk factors and therapy for infectious dysentery.

ORGANISM	RISK FACTORS/RESERVOIRS	THERAPY
Campylobacter sp.*	Contaminated food, water, raw milk, infected animals and humans	Erythromycin Quinolone
Salmonella sp.* (nontyphoidal)	Food (milk, eggs, poultry, meats), water, infected humans	Quinolone Ampicillin, TMP/SMX
Shigella sp.*	Food, water, infected humans	TMP/SMX Quinolone, ampicillin
Escherichia coli (EHEC)	Beef, raw milk, untreated water, direct contact	Supportive care
Aeromonas sp.*	Untreated water	TMP/SMX
Plesiomonas sp.	Uncooked shellfish	TMP/SMX
Yersinia sp.*	Food (milk products, tofu), water	TMP/SMX Ceftriaxone (severe)
Entamoeba histolytica	Travel to endemic areas (food, water, fruit)	Metronidazole
Clostridium difficile	Antibiotic use, hospitalization, chemo-therapy)	Metronidazole Vancomycin Cholestyramine

TMP/SMX = trimethroprim/sulfamethoxazole.
*Mild-to-moderate symptoms do not require antibiotic therapy.

36. Are antimotility agents contraindicated in patients with dysentery?

Historically, treatment of dysentery with antimotility agents, such as diphenoxylate-atropine (Lomotil) and loperamide (Imodium), has been contraindicated. It was believed that reduced intestinal motility would worsen dysentery by slowing pathogen clearance. Recent studies of patients with shigellosis dysentery given a combination of loperamide and antibiotic therapy had a shortened duration of diarrhea without adverse effects. Antimotility agents continue to be contraindicated in children with dysentery because of recurrent adverse case reports.

37. Several members of a family develop nausea, emesis, and watery diarrhea 2–6 hours after a picnic. Food at the picnic included ham, rice, and custard pie. What bacteria are likely to be the cause?

Enterotoxin-producing bacteria must be considered because the symptoms began soon after ingestion of the food. Two enterotoxin-producing bacteria that cause symptoms with such a short incubation are *Staphylococcus aureus* and *Bacillus cereus*. Coagulase-positive strains of *S. aureus* are responsible for many cases of food poisoning in the United States. *S. aureus* enterotoxin is heat-stable. The incubation period from ingestion to symptoms is approximately 3 hours (range = 1–6 hours). Growth of *S. aureus* is favored by foods with high sugar content (e.g., custard) and high salt intake (e.g., ham). Recovery is generally complete in 24–48 hours. *B. cereus* is a spore-forming, gram-positive rod that produces a diarrheogenic, heat-labile enterotoxin. Vomiting can occur within 2 hours of ingestion of contaminated food. Almost all cases of *B. cereus* develop diarrhea. Meat and rice are the most common food vehicles for infection.

38. What are the common causes of traveler's diarrhea?

More than 80% of diarrhea cases are secondary to a bacterial pathogen. *E. coli* (ETEC strains most common), *Campylobacter*, *Salmonella*, and *Shigella* species account for most traveler's diarrhea.

39. How can one avoid traveler's diarrhea?

"Safe" foods include steaming hot food and beverages, acidic foods such as citrus, dry foods, foods with high sugar content such as syrups and jellies, and carbonated drinks. Bottled uncarbonated water is not always safe. Avoid uncooked vegetables and unpeeled fruits. Also consume only safe foods on airplanes leaving high-risk areas. Chemoprophylaxis with bismuth salicylate (2 tablets with meals and at bedtime) is effective in reducing diarrhea. Chemoprophylaxis should be given to persons with prior gastric surgery, those taking acid blocking medicines (H-2 blockers and proton pump inhibitors), or those debilitated and immunosuppressed. Travelers who cannot risk or afford a short illness while traveling may opt for chemoprophylaxis.

40. Describe the treatment of traveler's diarrhea.

Patients with moderate-to-severe illness (e.g., activity restricted by diarrhea symptoms, fever, or bloody diarrhea) should be empirically treated with a quinolone antibiotic or TMP/SMX for 3–5 days to shorten the duration of symptoms. Bismuth subsalicylate is effective for mild-to-moderate diarrhea. Antimotility drugs can be used alone or with antibiotic therapy in adults but should be avoided in children.

41. What is cholera?

Cholera is a severe diarrheal disorder caused by the *V. cholera*, a gram-negative, comma-shaped bacteria. The illness is characterized by massive watery stool output, at times in excess of 1 L/hr. Dehydration, hypovolemic shock, and death occur rapidly if fluid replacement is not provided. The cholera organisms colonize the upper small bowel and release an enterotoxin that binds to and activates mucosal cyclic adenosine monophosphate (cAMP), which in turn activates chloride channels in mucosal crypts and leads to the massive secretory diarrhea. A second toxin, called the zonula occludens toxin (ZOT), increases intestinal permeability. The intestinal mucosa is not altered by the organism.

42. How is cholera treated?

Fluid replacement with either intravenous fluids or oral rehydration solution is the mainstay of therapy. A 2-day course of tetracycline is also beneficial.

43. What is oral rehydration solution? How does it work?

Oral rehydration solution (ORS) is composed primarily of water, salt, and glucose. The World Health Organization (WHO) ORS formula consists of 1 liter of purified water combined with 20 gm of glucose, 3.5 gm of sodium chloride, 5 gm of sodium bicarbonate, and 1.5 gm of potassium chloride. Glucose enhances sodium and water absorption across the small bowel villi, even in the presence of cholera enterotoxin. Rice starch can be substituted for glucose.

44. What viruses cause acute diarrhea?

Acute viral gastroenteritis can be caused by rotavirus, caliciviruses (includes Norwalk virus), enteric adenoviruses (types 40 and 41), and astrovirus. Rotavirus is a common cause of acute diarrhea in patients < 2 years of age. The Norwalk virus can cause widespread community outbreaks that affect persons of all ages. Fecal-oral transmission has been implicated as the transmission route for viral gastroenteritis. Raw shellfish have been implicated in outbreaks of Norwalk infection.

45. What are the clinical features of rotavirus gastroenteritis? What tests are available for diagnosis?

The clinical presentation of rotavirus can range from an asymptomatic carrier state to severe dehydration that can lead to death. Children under the age of 2 years are at greatest risk for infection. Following a 1–3-day incubation period, the rotavirus illness is characterized by vomiting and diarrhea for 5–7 days. Rotavirus accounts for 25% of acute diarrhea among U.S. children. Rotavirus is more prevalent during cooler months. Adults can develop mild infection with rotavirus. Commercial immunoassays are available to detect rotavirus in the stool.

46. What is Reiter's syndrome? Which enteric infections are associated with its development?

Reiter's syndrome is a triad of arthritis, urethritis, and conjunctivitis. Infections with *Salmonella* sp., *Shigella* sp., *Campylobacter jejuni*, and *Yersinia enterocolitica* have been associated with this syndrome. Approximately 80% of patients affected by Reiter's syndrome are HLA-B27 antigen-positive. The male-to-female ratio is 9:1.

INFLAMMATORY BOWEL DISEASE

47. How does one differentiate between acute infectious dysentery and acute onset of inflammatory bowel disease as the cause of bloody diarrhea?

The clinical symptoms and endoscopic findings of the colon are often similar in the two diagnoses. When evaluating a patient with bloody diarrhea, the clinician must use historical data, assess the patient's potential risk factors and associated symptoms, and evaluate endoscopic appearance, radiologic findings, and laboratory data to narrow the differential. Many of the infectious dysentery illnesses are self-limited in nature. Dysenteric illnesses that do not spontaneously resolve and are culture-negative should undergo investigation for inflammatory bowel disease.

48. Can a mucosal biopsy obtained on flexible sigmoidoscopy assist in differentiating among acute bacterial dysentery, ulcerative colitis, and Crohn's disease?

Yes. Biopsy findings are not 100% specific. However, there are distinguishing features among the three diseases:
- **Bacterial infection:** mucosal edema, neutrophilic infiltration of the superficial lamina propria, absence of plasmacytosis of the deep lamina propria, and preservation of the crypt architecture.
- **Ulcerative colitis:** crypt abscesses (clumps of neutrophils in the crypt lumen), chronic inflammation limited to the mucosa and submucosa, atrophy, and possibly dysplasia.
- **Crohn's disease:** the presence of granulomas is a hallmark finding. However, the absence of granulomas does not exclude Crohn's disease, because up to 50% of patients may not show granulomas on biopsy. Submucosal inflammation, focal ulceration, and patchy involvement in the biopsy specimen are also suggestive.

49. What is toxic megacolon? What are its risk factors?

Toxic megacolon is a complication of colitis manifested by acute dilatation of the colon, with associated fever, tachycardia, leukocytosis, anemia, and postural hypotension. Transmural inflammation interferes with colonic motility, leading to colonic dilation and risk for perforation. Severe idiopathic panulcerative colitis carries the highest risk for toxic megacolon, but it may occur with any severe colitis (e.g., amebiasis, shigellosis, EHEC, *C. difficile*, and *Campylobacter* sp.) Performance of barium enema or colonoscopy or the administration of antimotility agents (loperamide, diphenoxylate, anticholinergics, or opiates) in patients with severe colitis may precipitate toxic megacolon.

ISCHEMIC COLITIS

50. How is acute bacterial dysentery differentiated from acute onset of ischemic colitis?

The degree of bloody diarrhea is variable in patients with ischemic colitis, and it may be difficult to distinguish between the two diseases. Clinically, the patient with ischemic colitis complains of sudden-onset abdominal pain, and an acute abdominal series may show "thumbprinting" of the colonic mucosa.

Flexible sigmoidoscopy is the mainstay of diagnosis for ischemic colitis. The rectum usually is spared because of its collateral blood flow. Above the rectum, the mucosa becomes friable and edematous, and there may be hemorrhagic areas and ulcerations resembling those of Crohn's disease. Angiography generally is not helpful in the evaluation of ischemic colitis; ischemic colitis is a small-vessel disease (nonocclusive), as opposed to mesenteric midgut ischemia of the small bowel, which involves thrombosis or embolism in the superior mesenteric artery (occlusive). A barium enema is contraindicated in patients with suspected ischemic colitis, because colonic expansion during barium instillation may promote further ischemia.

51. Name the segment of colon most commonly affected by ischemia.

The left colon is the segment most commonly affected (75%). The next most common segments are the transverse colon (15%) and right colon (5%). Although any area of the colon can be affected by ischemia, the rectum is rarely involved because of its rich blood supply.

52. What are the predisposing factors for ischemic colitis?

Most patients with ischemic colitis are middle-aged or elderly and have a history of atherosclerotic heart disease and/or peripheral vascular disease. Medications implicated in colonic ischemia include digitalis, nonsteroidal anti-inflammatory drugs, diuretics, vasopressin, gold compounds, and some cancer chemotherapeutic agents. A common complication of surgical repair of an abdominal aortic aneurysm is colonic ischemia. During surgery, mucosal ischemia results from the prolonged low blood flow to the colon or from disruption of blood flow in the inferior mesenteric artery.

OTHER CAUSES

53. What is diversion colitis?

Diversion colitis is an inflammatory process in the portion of colon from which the fecal stream has been diverted. Usually it is seen in a Hartmann's pouch that is formed after a sigmoid resection. The endoscopic and histologic appearance of the mucosa is similar to that of ulcerative colitis. These changes resolve promptly after anastomosis of the bowel and restoration of the fecal stream. Proposed theories as to the cause of this inflammatory reaction include overgrowth of normal bowel flora and nutritional deficiency of short-chain fatty acids. Short-chain fatty acids are produced by anaerobic bacteria and are used as an energy source by the colonic epithelium cells.

54. List the rare or unusual causes of acute bloody diarrhea.

Unusual Causes of Bloody Diarrhea

Vasculitides	**Neoplastic diarrhea**
Behçet's disease	Chemotherapy
Henoch-Schönlein purpura	Graft-vs.-host disease (bone marrow transplantation)
Polyarteritis nodosa	Radiation therapy
Churg-Strauss disease	**Hematologic diarrhea**
Wegener's granulomatosis	Sickle cell disease
Cryoglobulinemia	**Iatrogenic diarrhea**
Systemic lupus erythematosus	Glutaraldehyde-sterilizing solution (residue on
Mechanical causes	equipment)
Intestinal intussusception	

55. *See next page.*

BIBLIOGRAPHY

1. American Academy of Pediatrics: Practice parameter: The management of acute gastroenteritis in young children. Pediatrics 97:424–435, 1996.
2. Cover TL, Aber RC: Yersinia enterocolitica. N Engl J Med 321:16–24, 1989.
3. DuPont HL: Guidelines on acute infectious diarrhea in adults. Am J Gastroenterol 92:1962–1975, 1997.
4. Goldberg MB, Rubin RH: The spectrum of Salmonella infection. Infect Dis Clin North Am 2:571–598, 1988.
5. Griffen PM, Ostroff SM, Tauxe RV, et al: Illnesses associated with *Escherichia coli* 0157:H7 infections. Ann Intern Med 109:705–712, 1988.
6. Farmer RG: Infectious causes of diarrhea in the differential diagnosis of inflammatory bowel disease. Med Clin North Am 74:29–38, 1990.
7. Finch MJ, Riley LW: *Campylobacter* infections in the United States. Arch Intern Med 144:1610–1612, 1984.
8. Hamer DH, Gorback SI: Infectious diarrhea and bacterial food poisoning. In Feldman M, Scharschmidt BF, Sleisenger MH (eds): Sleisenger and Fordtran's Gastrointestinal and Liver Disease, 6th ed. W.B. Saunders, 1998, pp 1594–1632.
9. Hogan DE: The emergency department approach to diarrhea. Emerg Clin North Am 14:673–694, 1996.
10. Greenberg SB: Serious waterborne and wilderness infections. Crit Care Clin 15:387–414, 1999.
11. Holmberg SD, Schell WL, Fanning GR, et al: *Aeromonas* intestinal infections in the United States. Ann Intern Med 105:683–689, 1986.

55. Describe the evaluation of a patient with acute bloody diarrhea.

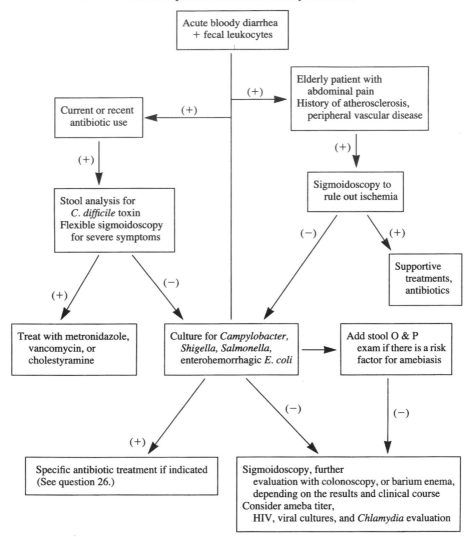

Evaluation of acute bloody diarrhea.

12. Krogstad DJ, Spencer HC, Healy GR: Amebiasis. N Engl J Med 298:262–265, 1978.
13. Lew EA, Poles MA, Dieterich DT: Diarrheal diseases associated with HIV infections. Gastroenterol Clin 26:259–290, 1997.
14. Murphy GS, Bodhidatta L, Echeverria P, et al: Ciprofloxacin and loperamide in the treatment of bacillary dysentery. Ann Intern Med 118:582–586, 1993.
15. Park SI, Giannella RA: Approach to the adult patient with acute diarrhea. Gastroenterol Clin North Am 22:483–497, 1993.
16. Smith PD: Infectious diarrheas in patients with AIDS. Gastroenterol Clin North Am 22:535–548, 1993.
17. Yaun SK, Liu FJ: Laboratory diagnosis of gastrointestinal tract and exocrine pancreatic diseases. In Henry JB (ed): Clinical and Diagnosis Management by Laboratory Methods. Philadelphia, W.B. Saunders, 1991, pp 536–549.

60. CHRONIC DIARRHEA

Lawrence R. Schiller, M.D.

1. Define chronic diarrhea.

Diarrhea is defined as an increase in the frequency and fluidity of stools. For most patients, diarrhea means the passage of loose stools. Although loose stool often is accompanied by an increase in the frequency of bowel movements, most patients do not classify the frequent passage of formed stools as diarrhea. Because stool consistency is difficult to quantitate, many investigators use frequency of defecation as a quantitative criterion for diarrhea. By this standard passage of more than two bowel movements per day is considered abnormal. Some authors also incorporate stool weight in the definition of diarrhea. Normal stool weight averages approximately 80 gm/day in women and 100 gm/day in men. The upper limit of normal stool weight (calculated as the mean plus two standard deviations) is approximately 200 gm/day. Normal stool weight depends on dietary intake, and some patients on high-fiber diets exceed 200 gm/day without reporting diarrhea. Thus, stool weight by itself is an imperfect criterion.

2. Summarize the criteria for diagnosis of diarrhea.

CRITERION	NORMAL RANGE	DIARRHEA, IF
Increased stool frequency	2–14 stools per week	> 2 stools per day
More liquid stool consistency	Soft—formed stools	Loose—unformed
Increased stool weight		
Men	0–240 gm/24 hr	> 240 gm/24 hr
Women	0–180 gm/24 hr	> 180 gm/24 hr

3. What other disorder may be described as "diarrhea"?

Occasionally patients with fecal incontinence describe the problem as "diarrhea," even when stools are formed. Physicians must be careful to distinguish fecal incontinence from diarrhea, because incontinence is usually due to problems with the muscles and nerves regulating continence.

4. What is the basic mechanism of all diarrheal diseases?

Diarrhea is due to the incomplete absorption of fluid from luminal contents. Normal stools are approximately 75% water and 25% solids. Normal fecal water output is approximately 60–80 ml/day. An increase in fecal water output of 50–100 ml is sufficient to cause loosening of the stool. This volume represents approximately 1% of the fluid load entering the upper intestine each day; thus malabsorption of only 1 or 2% of fluid entering the intestine may be sufficient to cause diarrhea (Fig. 1).

5. What pathologic processes can cause diarrhea?

Excessive stool water is due to the presence of some solute that osmotically obligates water retention within the lumen. This solute may be a poorly absorbed, osmotically active substance, such as magnesium ions, or an accumulation of ordinary electrolytes, such as sodium or potassium, that normally are absorbed easily by the intestine. When excessive stool water is due to ingestion of a poorly absorbed substance, the diarrhea is called **osmotic diarrhea**. Examples include lactose malabsorption and diarrhea induced by osmotic laxatives. When the excessive stool water results from the presence of excessive electrolytes due to reduction of electrolyte absorption or stimulation of electrolyte secretion, the diarrhea is known as **secretory diarrhea**. Causes of secretory diarrhea include infection, particularly infections that produce toxins that

411

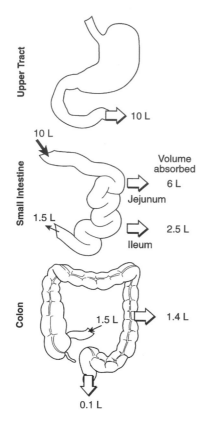

FIGURE 1. Fluid loads through the intestine. Each day approximately 9–10 L of fluid pass into the jejunum. This fluid consists of approximately 2 L of ingested food and drink, 1.5 L of saliva, 2.5 L of gastric juice, 1.5 L of bile, and 2.5 L of pancreatic juice. The jejunum absorbs most of this load as nutrients are taken up, and the ileum absorbs most of the rest. The colon absorbs more than 90% of the fluid load reaching it, leaving only 1% of the original fluid entering the jejunum to be excreted in stool. Substantial fluid malabsorption in the small bowel can overwhelm colonic absorptive capacity and may result in diarrhea. Less severe disruption of colonic absorption can lead to diarrhea because of the lack of a more distal absorbing segment. A reduction of absorptive efficiency of only 1% for the total intestine can result in diarrhea.

reduce intestinal fluid electrolyte absorption; reduction of mucosal surface area due to disease or surgery; absence of an ion transport mechanism; inflammation of the mucosa; ingestion of drugs or poisons; endogenous secretagogues such as bile acids; dysfunction due to abnormal regulation by nerves and hormones; and tumors producing circulating secretagogues.

6. List three classifications of diarrheal diseases.

Several schemes have been proposed, three of which can be useful clinically.

1. Differentiate between acute and chronic diarrheal diseases. Most cases of acute diarrhea are due to infections that are self-limited and run their courses over a few weeks. Diarrheas that last longer are probably due to some other mechanism. For practical purposes, a duration of 4 weeks can be used to differentiate acute and chronic diarrheas.

2. Categorize the diarrhea by epidemiologic characteristics (see question 7).

3. Divide diarrheal diseases by the characteristics of the stools produced. In this scheme diarrheas are classified as watery, fatty, or inflammatory (see questions 8–11). These distinctions are based on the gross characteristics of the stool and laboratory testing when appropriate. Watery stools are typically runny and lack blood, pus, or fat. Watery diarrhea is subdivided into secretory or osmotic, depending on stool electrolyte concentrations. Fatty stools have an excess of fat, which can be shown by qualitative testing with the Sudan stain or by quantitative analysis of a timed stool collection for fat. Inflammatory diarrheas typically contain blood or pus. If not grossly evident, these characteristics can be detected by a fecal occult blood test or by staining the stool for neutrophils. Classifying diarrheas by stool characteristics enables the physician to sort quickly through more likely and less likely diagnoses. This scheme is thus quite useful in chronic diarrheas in which construction of a reasonable differential diagnosis can lead to more appropriate testing and more rapid diagnosis.

7. **What are the likely causes of diarrhea according to epidemiologic characteristics?**
   Travelers
   > Bacterial infection (mostly acute)   Tropical sprue
   > Protozoal infections (e.g., amebiasis, giardiasis)
   Epidemics/outbreaks
   > Bacterial infection
   > Viral infection (e.g., rotavirus)
   > Protozoal infections (e.g., cryptosporidiosis)
   > Brainerd diarrhea (epidemic idiopathic secretory diarrhea)
   Patients with AIDS
   > Opportunistic infections (e.g., cryptosporidiosis, cytomegalovirus, herpes, *Mycobacterium avium* complex)
   > Drug side-effect
   > Lymphoma
   Institutionalized patients
   > *Clostridium difficile* toxin-mediated colitis   Drug side effect
   > Food poisoning   Fecal impaction with overflow
   > Tube feeding   diarrhea

8. **What are the likely causes of osmotic watery diarrhea?**
   Osmotic laxatives (e.g., Mg^{2+}, PO_{4-3}, SO_{4-2}) and carbohydrate malabsorption.

9. **List the likely causes of secretory watery diarrhea.**
   > Congenital syndromes (e.g., congenital   Endocrine diarrhea
   >   chloridorrhea)   Hyperthyroidism
   > Bacterial toxins   Addison's disease
   > Ileal bile acid malabsorption   Gastrinoma
   > Inflammatory bowel disease   VIPoma
   >   Ulcerative colitis   Somatostatinoma
   >   Crohn's disease   Carcinoid syndrome
   >   Microscopic colitis   Medullary carcinoma of the thyroid
   >   Lymphocytic colitis   Mastocytosis
   >   Collagenous colitis   Other tumors
   >   Diverticulitis   Colon carcinoma
   > Vasculitis   Lymphoma
   > Drugs and poisons   Villous adenoma
   > Laxative abuse (stimulant laxatives)   Idiopathic secretory diarrhea
   > Disordered motility/regulation   Epidemic secretory (Brainerd) diarrhea
   >   Postvagotomy diarrhea   Sporadic idiopathic secretory diarrhea
   >   Postsympathectomy diarrhea
   >   Diabetic autonomic neuropathy
   >   Irritable bowel syndrome

10. **List the likely causes of inflammatory diarrhea.**
    > Inflammatory bowel disease
    >   Ulcerative colitis   Diverticulitis
    >   Crohn's disease   Ulcerative jejunoileitis
    > Infectious diseases
    >   Pseudomembranous colitis
    >   Invasive bacterial infections (e.g., tuberculosis, yersinosis)
    >   Ulcerating viral infections (e.g., cytomegalovirus, herpes simplex)
    >   Invasive parasitic infections (e.g., amebiasis, strongyloides)
    > Ischemic colitis

Radiation colitis
Neoplasia: colon cancer, lymphoma

11. List the likely causes of fatty diarrhea.
Malabsorption syndromes

Mucosal diseases (e.g., celiac disease, Whipple's disease)

Small bowel bacterial overgrowth
Mesenteric ischemia

Short bowel syndrome
Maldigestion

Pancreatic exocrine insufficiency

Inadequate luminal bile acid concentration

12. Summarize the initial diagnostic scheme for patients with chronic diarrhea.
The scheme in Figure 2 is based on a careful history, looking for specific physical findings, and simple laboratory data to help classify the diarrhea as watery, fatty, or inflammatory. The value of obtaining a quantitative (as opposed to a spot) stool collection is debated among experts. A quantitative collection over 48 or 72 hours permits a better estimation of fluid, electrolyte, and fat excretion but is not absolutely necessary to the appropriate classification of diarrhea.

13. How do you distinguish secretory and osmotic watery diarrhea?
The most useful way to differentiate secretory and osmotic types of watery diarrhea is to measure fecal electrolytes and calculate the fecal osmotic gap. In many diarrheal conditions, sodium and potassium, with their accompanying anions, are the dominant electrolytes in stool water. Secretory diarrhea is characterized by failure to absorb electrolytes completely or actual electrolyte secretion by the intestine. Sodium, potassium, and their accompanying anions are responsible for the bulk of osmotic activity in stool water and the retention of water within the gut lumen. In contrast, in osmotic diarrheas ingestion of poorly absorbed osmotically active substances is responsible for holding water within the gut lumen. Electrolyte absorption is normal; thus, sodium and potassium concentrations may become quite low (Fig. 3). The fecal osmotic gap calculation takes advantage of these distinctions to differentiate the two conditions.

14. How is the fecal osmotic gap calculated?
First measure sodium and potassium in stool water. The sum of the concentrations of these two ions is multiplied by 2 to account for the anions that are also present. The product then is subtracted from 290 mosm/kg, the approximate osmolality of luminal contents within the intestine. This number is a constant because the relatively high permeability of the intestinal mucosa beyond the stomach means that osmotic equilibration has taken place by the time luminal contents reach the rectum. As an example, let us assume that a patient with watery diarrhea has a sodium concentration of 75 mmol/L and a potassium concentration of 65 mmol/L in stool water. Adding the two values yields a concentration of 140 mmol/L. Doubling this value to account for anions means that electrolytes account for 280 mosm/kg of stool water osmolality. Subtracting this value from 290 mosm/kg yields an osmotic gap of 10 mosm/kg.

15. How is the fecal osmotic gap interpreted?
Fecal osmotic gaps < 50 mosm/kg correlate well with diarrheas due to electrolyte secretion (or poor absorption). In contrast, if stool sodium is 10 mmol/L and potassium concentration is 20 mmol/L, the combined contribution of cations and anions in stool water is only 60 mosm/kg, yielding a fecal osmotic gap of 230 mosm/kg. This value represents the amount of some unmeasured substance that is contributing to fecal osmolality, presumably some poorly absorbed substance that is ingested but not absorbed. Fecal osmotic gaps > 50 mosm/kg are associated with osmotic diarrheas.

16. What precaution is necessary in measuring fecal osmotic gap?
Be certain that the stool has not been contaminated with either water or urine. Dilution by water or hypotonic urine falsely lowers fecal electrolyte concentrations and elevates the calculated

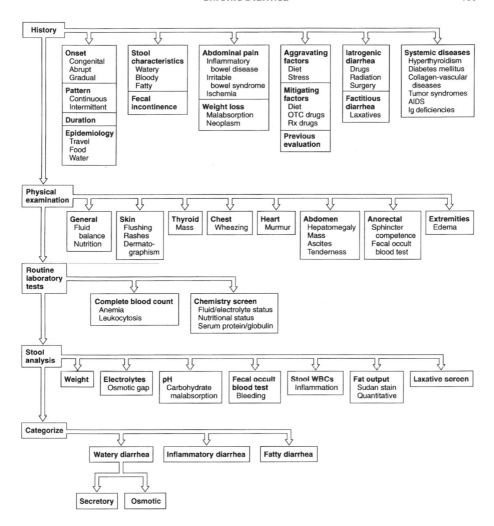

FIGURE 2. The initial evaluation plan for patients with chronic diarrhea is aimed at assessing the severity of the problem, looking for clues to etiology, and classifying the diarrhea as watery (with subtypes of osmotic and secretory diarrhea), inflammatory, or fatty. (From Fine KD, Schiller LR: AGA technical review on the evaluation and management of chronic diarrhea. Gastroenterology 116:1464–1486, 1999, with permission.)

osmotic gap. This problem can be detected by actually measuring fecal osmolality; values that are substantially < 290 mosm/kg indicate dilution. Contamination with hypertonic urine also may affect fecal electrolyte concentrations, but it is harder to detect unless the sum of measured cations and assumed anions is much greater than 290 mmol/L.

17. How do you evaluate osmotic diarrhea?

Osmotic diarrheas are typically due to ingestion of poorly absorbed cations, such as magnesium, or anions, such as sulfate. In addition, carbohydrate malabsorption, such as that due to ingestion of lactose in patients with lactase deficiency and ingestion of poorly absorbable sugar alcohols (e.g., sorbitol), can lead to osmotic diarrhea. Measuring stool pH can help to distinguish between osmotic diarrheas due to poorly absorbed cations and anions and those due to

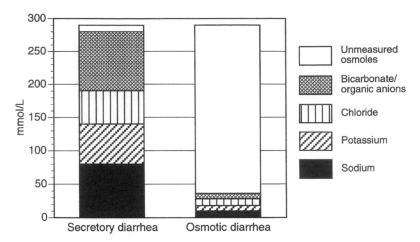

FIGURE 3.   Electrolyte patterns differ between osmotic and secretory diarrhea. In secretory diarrhea, electrolytes account for the bulk of the osmotic activity of stool water. In contrast, in osmotic diarrhea electrolyte
absorption is normal; therefore, electrolyte concentrations are very low. Most of the osmotic activity is due to
unmeasured osmoles. (Bicarbonate concentrations are "virtual" and are not directly measurable in most circumstances because of reaction with organic acids generated by fermentation by colonic bacteria.)

ingestion of poorly absorbed carbohydrates and sugar alcohols. Carbohydrates and sugar alcohols are fermented by colonic bacteria, reducing fecal pH below 5 due to production of short
chain fatty acids. In contrast, ingestion of poorly absorbed cations and anions does not have a
significant effect on stool pH, which is typically 7. Once acidic stools have been discovered,
check the diet and inquire about food additives and osmotic laxative ingestion. Specific testing
for magnesium and other ions in stool is readily available to confirm any suspicions (Fig. 4).

18. Describe the evaluation of chronic secretory diarrhea.

Because there are many causes of chronic secretory diarrhea, an extensive evaluation is possible (Fig. 5). Rare cases of infection should be excluded by bacterial culture and examination of
stool for parasites. Stimulant laxative abuse is best excluded by looking for laxatives in the urine
or stool. Structural disease and internal fistulas can be evaluated with small bowel radiography
and CT scanning of the abdomen and pelvis. Endoscopic examination of the upper gastrointestinal tract and colon is occasionally helpful and should include biopsy of even normal-appearing
mucosa, looking for microscopic evidence of disease. Systemic diseases, such as hyperthyroidism, adrenal insufficiency, and defective immunity, can be evaluated with appropriate tests
(see question 19).

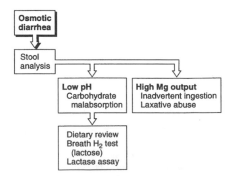

FIGURE 4.   Once a diagnosis of osmotic diarrhea
is made, evaluation is fairly straightforward. Only a
few etiologies are possible. (From Fine KD, Schiller
LR: AGA technical review on the evaluation and
management of chronic diarrhea. Gastroenterology
116:1464–1486, 1999, with permission.)

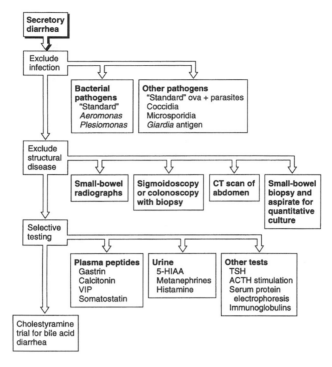

FIGURE 5. Evaluation of secretory diarrhea can be quite complex. This "mind map" can be used to guide the evaluation, depending on the specifics of each case. Not every test needs to be done in every patient. (From Fine KD, Schiller LR: AGA technical review on the evaluation and management of chronic diarrhea. Gastroenterology 116:1464–1486, 1999, with permission.)

19. Summarize the tests for evaluation of systemic diseases associated with chronic secretory diarrhea.

CONDITION	DIAGNOSTIC TESTS
Endocrine diseases	
Hyperthyroidism	Thyroid-stimulating hormone, T_4
Addison's disease	ACTH-stimulation test, cortisol
Panhypopituitarism	ACTH-stimulation test, TSH
Diabetes mellitus	Blood glucose, glycosylated hemoglobin
Endocrine tumor syndromes	
MEN-1 (Werner's syndrome)	
Hyperparathyroidism	Parathormone
Pancreatic endocrine tumors	Gastrin, VIP, insulin, glucagon
Pituitary tumors	Prolactin, growth hormone, ACTH
(Also may have adrenal cortical tumors, thyroid adenomas)	
MEN-2a (Sipple's syndrome)	
Medullary thyroid cancer	Calcitonin
Pheochromocytoma	Urine metanephrine
Hyperparathyroidism	Parathormone
MEN-2b (same as MEN-2a + neuromas, Marfanoid phenotype)	

Table continued on following page

CONDITION	DIAGNOSTIC TESTS
Hematologic diseases	
Leukemia, lymphoma	Complete blood count
Multiple myeloma	Serum protein electrophoresis
Immune system disorders	
AIDS	HIV serology
Amyloidosis	Mucosal biopsy
Common variable immunodeficiency, IgA deficiency	Immunoglobin levels
Heavy metal poisoning	Heavy metal screen

T_4 = thyroxine, ACTH = adrenocorticotropic hormone, TSH = thyroid-stimulating hormone, MEN = multiple endocrine neoplasia, VIP = vasoactive intestinal polypeptide, AIDS = acquired immunodeficiency syndrome, HIV = human immunodeficiency virus.

20. When should neuroendocrine tumors be suspected as a cause of chronic secretory diarrhea?

Neuroendocrine tumors are an uncommon cause of chronic secretory diarrhea. For example, one VIPoma may be expected per 10 million people per year. The table below lists these tumors and their markers. Because of their rarity as a cause for chronic diarrhea, other causes should be considered first. If tumor is visualized by CT scan or if systemic symptoms (e.g., flushing), are present, evaluation for neuroendocrine tumors may have a better yield. Blanket testing for tumor-associated peptides is likely to yield many more false-positives than true-positives and therefore can be quite misleading.

Neuroendocrine Tumors Causing Chronic Diarrhea and Their Markers

TUMOR	TYPICAL SYMPTOMS	MEDIATOR/TUMOR MARKER
Gastrinoma	Zollinger-Ellison syndrome: Pancreatic or duodenal tumor, peptic ulcer, steatorrhea, diarrhea	Gastrin
VIPoma	Verner-Morrison syndrome: Watery diarrhea, hypokalemia, achlorhydria, flushing	Vasoactive intestinal polypeptide
Medullary thyroid carcinoma	Thyroid mass, hypermotility	Calcitonin, prostaglandins
Pheochromocytoma	Adrenal mass, hypertension	Vasoactive intestinal polypeptide, norepinephrine, epinephrine
Carcinoid	Flushing, wheezing, right-sided cardiac valvular disease	Serotonin, kinins
Somatostatinoma	Nonketotic diabetes mellitus, steatorrhea, diabetes, gallstones	Somatostatin
Glucagonoma	Skin rash (migratory necrotizing erythema), mild diabetes	Glucagon
Mastocytosis	Flushing, dermatographism, nausea, vomiting, abdominal pain	Histamine

21. What is Bayes' theorem? How does it relate to peptide-secreting tumors?

Bayes' theorem links the prevalence of the diagnosis to the positive predictive value of a diagnostic test. The positive predictive value of a test depends on the likelihood of the condition in the population to be screened, not only the accuracy of the test. For example, peptide-secreting tumors are a rare cause of chronic diarrhea, with a prevalence of 1/5000 to 1/500,000 patients with chronic diarrhea, depending on tumor type. The following is a simplified formula for Bayes' theorem:

$$\text{Posttest odds} = \text{pretest odds} \times \text{likelihood ratio}$$

where the likelihood ratio = true-positive/true-negative result. Since the pretest odds of a peptide-secreting tumor are so long and the false-positive rate of serum peptide assays for peptide-secreting tumors is so high (~ 45%), the positive predictive value for serum peptide assays is substantially < 1%. An abnormal result would be misleading > 99% of the time.

22. What is the likely outcome in patients with chronic secretory diarrhea in whom a diagnosis cannot be reached?

Diagnostic testing may fail to reveal a cause for chronic diarrhea in up to 25% of patients with chronic diarrhea, depending on referral bias and extent of evaluation. Patients with continuous idiopathic secretory diarrhea have remarkably similar courses. In most cases, diarrhea begins suddenly, is associated with some initial weight loss, and resolves in 1–2 years without recurrence. It is therefore preferable to treat patients symptomatically rather than to repeat diagnostic testing once a thorough evaluation has been concluded.

23. Describe the evaluation of chronic fatty diarrhea.

Chronic fatty diarrhea is due to either maldigestion or malabsorption. Maldigestion can occur with pancreatic exocrine insufficiency or a bile acid deficiency that reduces fat emulsification. Malabsorption typically is due to mucosal diseases such as celiac disease, bacterial overgrowth, or small bowel fistula or resection.

Pancreatic exocrine insufficiency can be evaluated with a secretin test, bentiromide test, or stool chymotrypsin or elastase measurement. Because these tests are not widely available or have poor specificity and sensitivity, clinicians often resort to a therapeutic trial of pancreatic enzymes. The patient should be treated with a high dose of enzymes, and the effect of treatment on stool fat excretion as well as symptoms should be assessed.

Bile acid deficiency, a rare cause of maldigestion, is best assessed by measuring the bile acid concentration in duodenal contents postprandially. Tests showing excessive bile acid excretion in stool (radiolabeled bile acid excretion or total bile acid excretion tests) do not directly assess duodenal bile acid concentration, but if fecal bile acid excretion is high, reduced duodenal bile acid concentration can be inferred. Mucosal disease can be evaluated with small bowel biopsy and bacterial overgrowth can be assessed by breath hydrogen testing after an oral glucose load or by quantitative culture of intestinal contents (Fig. 6).

24. Describe the further evaluation of chronic inflammatory diarrhea.

Inflammatory diarrheas can be due to idiopathic inflammatory bowel diseases, such as ulcerative colitis or Crohn's disease; invasive chronic infectious diseases, such as tuberculosis or yersiniosis; ischemic colitis; radiation colitis; or some tumors. To sort through these diagnoses, the most appropriate tests include sigmoidoscopy or colonoscopy to inspect the colonic mucosa visually, colonic biopsy to look for microscopic evidence of inflammation, small bowel radiography or CT scanning of the abdomen, and special cultures for chronic infections, such as tuberculosis or yersiniosis. In most cases the diagnosis becomes apparent after these tests are completed (Fig. 7).

FIGURE 6. Evaluation of chronic fatty diarrhea is designed to determine whether malabsorption or maldigestion is the cause of excessive fecal fat excretion. (From Fine KD, Schiller LR: AGA technical review on the evaluation and management of chronic diarrhea. Gastroenterology 116: 1464–1486, 1999, with permission.)

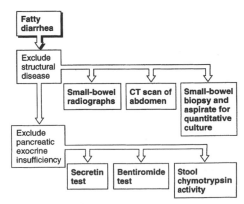

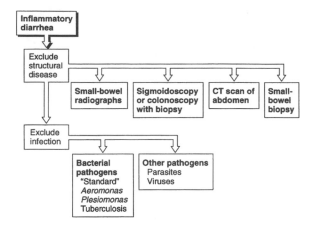

FIGURE 7. Chronic inflammatory diarrhea has a diverse differential diagnosis. Structural evaluation with endoscopic or radiographic techniques often yields a diagnosis. Mucosal biopsy may be needed to confirm the diagnosis. (From Fine KD, Schiller LR: AGA technical review on the evaluation and management of chronic diarrhea. Gastroenterology 116:1464–1486, 1999, with permission.)

25. How do you distinguish irritable bowel syndrome from chronic diarrhea?

The diagnosis of irritable bowel syndrome should be based on the presence of abdominal pain associated with defecation and abnormal bowel habits. Chronic continuous diarrhea in the absence of pain is not irritable bowel syndrome, although it may be functional in nature.

26. What causes of chronic diarrhea may be difficult to diagnose?

Fecal incontinence	Small bowel bacterial overgrowth
Iatrogenic diarrhea (drugs, surgery, radiation)	Pancreatic exocrine insufficiency
Surreptitious laxative ingestion	Carbohydrate malabsorption
Microscopic colitis syndrome	Peptide-secreting tumors
Bile acid-induced diarrhea	Chronic idiopathic secretory diarrhea

These conditions are seen in referral centers after routine evaluation has not disclosed a diagnosis. In general, the necessary tests are not difficult but have not been done because physicians have not considered these disorders in the differential diagnosis of chronic diarrhea.

27. What are common causes of iatrogenic diarrhea?

Most iatrogenic diarrheas are due to ingestion of drugs, some of which may not commonly cause diarrhea. About two-thirds of the drugs listed in the Physician's Desk Reference mention diarrhea as a possible side-effect. Therefore, the physician should obtain a history of all ingested drugs, including prescription medications, over-the-counter drugs, and herbal remedies. Other causes of iatrogenic diarrhea include operations, such as vagotomy, gastrectomy, and cholecystectomy, and radiation therapy during which the intestine is exposed to high doses of ionizing radiation.

Drugs Associated with Diarrhea

Antibiotics (most)	Antacids (e.g., containing magnesium)
Antineoplastic agents (many)	Acid-reducing agents (e.g., H_2-receptor
Anti-inflammatory agents (e.g., NSAIDs,	antagonists, proton pump inhibitors)
gold, 5-aminosalicylates)	Prostaglandin (e.g., misoprostol)
Antiarrhythmics (e.g., quinidine)	Vitamin/mineral supplements
Antihypertensives (e.g., beta-receptor blocking drugs)	Herbal products

28. What features should suggest surreptitious laxative ingestion?

Some patients who present with chronic diarrhea have diarrhea due to laxative abuse. In general, four groups of patients have this diagnosis:

Group	Characteristics
1. Patients with bulimia	Usually adolescent to young adult women; concerned about weight or manifesting an eating disorder
2. Secondary gain	May have disability claim pending, illness may induce concern or caring behavior in others
3. Munchausen's syndrome	Peripatetic patients who relish being diagnostic challenges; may undergo extensive testing repeatedly
4. Polle syndrome (Munchausen syndrome by proxy)	Dependent child or adult poisoned with laxatives by parent or caregiver to show effectiveness as caregiver; may have history of sibling who died with chronic diarrhea

Laxatives can be detected by chemical testing of stool or urine. The diagnosis should be confirmed before confronting the patient, and psychiatric consultation should be available to help with further management.

29. What is microscopic colitis syndrome?

Microscopic colitis is a syndrome characterized by chronic secretory diarrhea, a normal gross appearance of the colonic mucosa, and a typical pattern of inflammation in colon biopsy specimens. This pattern includes changes of the surface epithelium (flattening and irregularity), intraepithelial lymphocytosis, and an increased density of inflammatory cells in the lamina propria. There are two varieties: (1) collagenous colitis. in which the subepithelial collagen layer is thickened, and (2) lymphocytic colitis, in which the subepithelial collagen layer is of normal thickness. Microscopic colitis frequently occurs in older patients and often is associated with fecal incontinence. In many cases an actual or suspected rheumatological disease is present. Treatment is variably effective, but bismuth subsalicylate (Pepto-Bismol) has the greatest reported response rate.

30. Define bile acid diarrhea.

In patients with ileal resection or disease, the part of the small intestine with high-affinity bile acid transporters has been removed or is dysfunctional. Thus, excessive bile acid finds its way into the colon. If the bile acid concentration in colonic contents reaches a critical level of approximately 3–5 mmol/L, salt and water absorption by the colonic mucosa is inhibited and diarrhea results. Patients who have had extensive small bowel resections (>100 cm) often have so much fluid entering the colon that this critical bile acid level is not reached (Fig. 8).

In addition to this classical form of diarrhea due to bile acid malabsorption, some investigators have speculated that in many patients with an intact ileum bile acid malabsorption drives chronic diarrhea. Although tests of bile acid absorption frequently are abnormal in patients with idiopathic diarrhea, treatment with bile acid-sequestering resins, such as cholestyramine, is not often as effective in this group of patients as in those who have had surgical resection of the ileum.

31. What is the likely outcome in idiopathic secretory diarrhea?

Patients with chronic secretory diarrhea that evades a serious diagnostic evaluation often have a similar history of previous good health with sudden onset of diarrhea, often accompanied by acute but not progressive weight loss. Although acute onset suggests an acute infectious process, patients have negative microbiologic studies and do not respond to empiric antibiotics. Diarrhea usually persists for 12–30 months and then gradually subsides. This condition can be sporadic or occur in epidemics. The epidemic form (Brainerd diarrhea) seems to be associated with ingestion of potentially contaminated food or drink, but no organism has been implicated. Management consists of the effective use of nonspecific antidiarrheals until the process subsides.

32. What is the best nonspecific therapy for chronic diarrhea?

Because the evaluation of chronic diarrhea may extend over several weeks and the diagnosis is not always forthcoming, patients may need symptomatic therapy. The most effective agents are

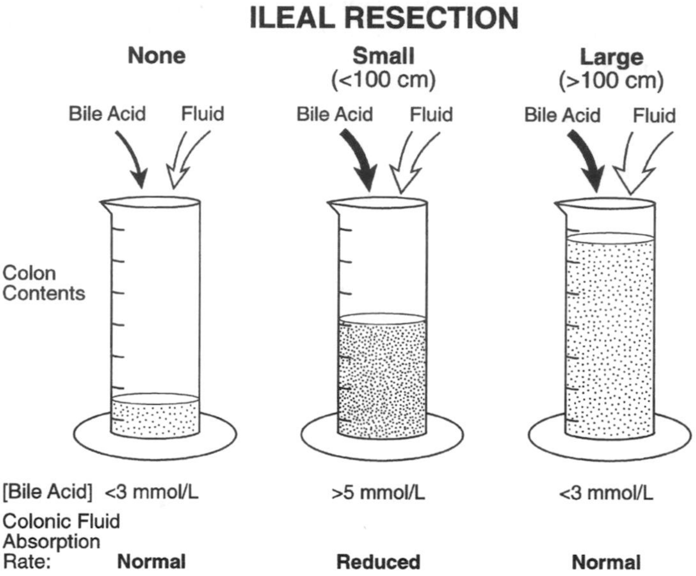

ILEAL RESECTION

FIGURE 8. Bile acid diarrhea occurs when bile acid malabsorption in the ileum is linked with relatively low fluid flows into the colon. As a result, the concentration of bile acid in colon contents is greater than the cathartic threshold of 3–5 mmol/L. If fluid flows are high (as with substantial small bowel resection), bile acid malabsorption may be just as severe, but bile acid concentrations are not high enough to impair absorption by the colon.

opiates. Traditional antidiarrheal agents, such as diphenoxylate and loperamide, work well in many patients but should be given on a routine schedule in patients with chronic diarrhea rather than on an as-needed basis. Typical doses of 1–2 tablets or capsules before meals and at bedtime improve symptoms in most people. When this therapy is ineffective, more potent opiates, such as codeine, opium, or morphine, can be used. With the stronger agents, doses should be low at first and increased gradually so that tolerance to the central nervous system effects can develop. Fortunately, the gut does not become tolerant to these agents; thus, one usually can find a dose that controls symptoms without producing severe side effects. Other agents sometimes used to manage chronic diarrhea include clonidine, octreotide, and cholestyramine, but they tend to be less effective than opiates and are often less well tolerated by patients, making them second-line agents in most circumstances.

Nonspecific Therapy for Chronic Diarrhea

AGENT	DOSE
Opiates	
μ-opiate receptor selective	
Diphenoxylate	2.5–5 mg 4 times/day
Loperamide	2–4 mg 4 times/day
Codeine	15–60 mg 4 times/day
Morphine	2–20 mg 4 times/day
Opium tincture	2–20 drops 4 times/day
δ-opiate receptor selective	
Racecadotril (acetorphan)	1.5 mg/kg 3 times/day*
Adrenergic agonist	
Clonidine	0.1–0.3 mg 3 times/day

Table continued on following page

Nonspecific Therapy for Chronic Diarrhea (Continued)

AGENT	DOSE
Somatostatin analog	
Octreotide	50–250 µg 3 times/day (subcutaneously)
Bile acid-binding resin	
Cholestyramine	4 gm 1–4 times/day

* Not yet approved in the United States

BIBLIOGRAPHY

1. Afzalpurkar RG, Schiller, LR, Little KH, et al: The self-limited nature of chronic idiopathic diarrhea. N Engl J Med 327:1849–1852, 1992.
2. Arrambide KA, Santa Ana CA, Schiller LR, et al: Loss of absorptive capacity for sodium chloride as a cause of diarrhea following partial ileal and right colon resection. Dig Dis Sci 34:193–201, 1989.
3. Bernstein CN, Riddell RH: Colonoscopy plus biopsy in the inflammatory bowel diseases. Gastrointest Endosc Clin North Am 10:755–774, 2000.
4. Bini EJ, Weinshel EH: Endoscopic evaluation of chronic human immunodeficiency virus-related diarrhea: Is colonoscopy superior to flexible sigmoidoscopy? Am J Gastroenterol 93:56–60, 1998.
5. Brandt LJ, Greenwald D (eds): Acute and Chronic Diarrhea: A Primer on Diagnosis and Treatment. Arlington, VA, American College of Gastroenterology, 1997.
6. Donowitz M, Kokke FT, Saidi R: Evaluation of patients with chronic diarrhea. N Engl J Med 332:725–729, 1995.
7. Eherer AJ, Fordtran JS: Fecal osmotic gap and pH in experimental diarrhea of various causes. Gastroenterology 103:545–551, 1992.
8. Farthing MJ: Oral rehydration therapy. Pharmacol Ther 64:477–492, 1994.
9. Farthing MJ: The role of somatostatin analogues in the treatment of refractory diarrhoea. Digestion 57 (Suppl 1):107–113, 1996.
10. Fine KD: Diarrhea. In Feldman M, Scharschmidt BF, Sleisenger MH (eds): Sleisenger and Fordtran's Gastrointestinal and Liver Disease: Pathophysiology, Diagnosis, Management, 6th ed. Philadelphia, W.B. Saunders, 1998, pp 128–152.
11. Fine KD, Schiller LR: AGA technical review on the evaluation and management of chronic diarrhea. Gastroenterology 116:1464–1486, 1999.
12. Freeman HJ: Small intestinal mucosal biopsy for investigation of diarrhea and malabsorption in adults. Gastrointest Endosc Clin North Am 10:739–753, 2000.
13. Giannella RA: Infections of the intestine. In Feldman M, Schiller LR (eds): Gastroenterology and Hepatology: The Comprehensive Visual Reference, vol. 7, Small Intestine. Philadelphia, Current Medicine, 1997, pp 12.1–12.19.
14. Powell DW: Approach to the patient with diarrhea. In Textbook of Gastroenterology, 3rd ed. Philadelphia, Lippincott Williams & Wilkins, 1999, pp 858–909.
15. Schiller LR: Diarrhea. Med Clin North Am 84:1259–1274, 2000.
16. Schiller LR: Secretory diarrhea. Curr Gastroenterol Rep 1:389–397, 1999.
17. Schiller LR: Review article: Anti-diarrhoeal pharmacology and therapeutics. Aliment Pharmacol Ther 9:87–106, 1995.
18. Simon DM, Cello JP, Valenzuela J, et al: Multicenter trial of octreotide in patients with refractory acquired immunodeficiency syndrome-associated diarrhea. Gastroenterology 108:1753–1760, 1995.
19. Schiller LR, Hogan RB, Morawski SG, et al: Studies of the prevalence and significance of radiolabeled bile acid malabsorption in a group of patients with idiopathic chronic diarrhea. Gastroenterology 92:151–160, 1987.
20. Schiller LR, Rivera LM, Santangelo WC, et al: Diagnostic value of fasting plasma peptide concentrations in patients with chronic diarrhea. Dig Dis Sci 39:2216–2222, 1994.
21. Schiller LR, Santa Ana CA, Morawski SG, et al: Studies of the antidiarrheal action of clonidine: Effects on motility and intestinal absorption. Gastroenterology 89:982–988, 1985.
22. Thillainayagam AV, Hunt JB, Farthing MJ: Enhancing clinical efficacy of oral rehydration therapy: Is low osmolality the key? Gastroenterology 114:197–210, 1998.
23. Wenzl HH, Fine KD, Schiller LR, Fordtran JS: Determinants of decreased fecal consistency in patients with diarrhea. Gastroenterology 108:1729–1738, 1995.

61. AIDS AND THE GASTROINTESTINAL TRACT

Klaus E. Mönkemüller, M.D., and C. Mel Wilcox, M.D.

1. **What are the two main esophageal symptoms in AIDS? Define each.**
   Odynophagia is pain on swallowing. **Dysphagia** is difficulty in swallowing, the sensation of "food stuck" in any part of the esophagus. Both are clearly associated with specific disorders.

2. **With which disorders is odynophagia associated?**
   Primarily esophageal ulceration, which is most commonly caused by cytomegalovirus (CMV), herpes simplex virus (HSV), or idiopathic esophageal ulceration (IEU). Less commonly, odynophagia can be observed with severe candidiasis.

3. **With which disorders is dysphagia associated?**
   Dysphagia most commonly results from candidiasis but also occurs in the presence of an obstructing neoplasm such as non-Hodgkin's lymphoma (NHL). In patients with a low CD4 cell count and esophageal symptoms, it may be appropriate to start empirical anticandidal therapy with fluconazole. If no improvement has occurred after 3 days of therapy, an upper endoscopy is indicated to evaluate for other disorders. Barium swallow does not play a role in the initial evaluation of esophageal disorders in AIDS, because it does not permit direct visualization and retrieval of mucosal specimens, which are required if ulceration or a mass is identified.

4. **What are the most common causes of solitary esophageal ulceration in AIDS?**
   The most common causes are CMV and IEU. On endoscopy CMV and idiopathic ulcers appear as large, well-circumscribed ulcerations, with normal-appearing surrounding mucosa. Antiretroviral medications such as didanosine (ddI) and zidovudine (AZT) also have been associated with pill-induced esophagitis. Ulcers caused by these drugs may be solitary, but multiple small, well-circumscribed ulcerations also occur. HSV usually is associated with multiple small, shallow esophageal ulcerations, often raised with a "volcano crater" appearance. Gastroesophageal reflux disease (GERD) also can present with ulcerations of the distal gastroesophageal junction, which generally are linear and superficial. Neoplasms (e.g., lymphoma), parasites (e.g., leishmania), and fungal infections (e.g.. histoplasmosis and *Candida* spp.) are rarely associated with solitary esophageal ulcers.

Causes of Esophageal Ulcers in AIDS

Viruses: cytomegalovirus, herpes simplex virus type II, Epstein-Barr virus, papovavirus, human herpes virus-6

Fungi: *Candida* spp., *Histoplasma capsulatum, Cryptococcus neoformans*, mucormycosis, aspergillosis, *Penicillium chrysogenum, Exophiala jeanselmani*

Bacteria: *Mycobacterium avium*-complex, *M. tuberculosis, Bartonella henselae, Nocardia asteroides, Actinomyces israelii*

Protozoa: cryptosporidia, *Leishmania donovanii, Pneumocystis carinii*

Tumors: non-Hodgkin's lymphoma, Kaposi's sarcoma, cancer (squamous cell and adenocarcinoma), lymphomatoid granulomatosis

Pill-induced: zalcitabine, zidovudine

Gastroesophageal disease

Idiopathic: idiopathic esophageal ulcer

5. **In general, how many biopsies should be obtained from an esophageal ulcer?**
   The exact number is not clearly established, but several studies suggest the range of 8–10. It is important to obtain biopsies from the ulcer margin to investigate for HSV and from the ulcer

base to investigate for CMV. If all biopsies are negative for viral, bacterial, fungal, and parasitic infections, a diagnosis of idiopathic esophageal ulcer can be made.

6. What is AIDS-cholangiopathy? How do patients present?

AIDS-cholangiopathy is a group of biliary tract abnormalities resembling sclerosing cholangitis that can be caused by a wide array of microorganisms and neoplasms, usually in patients with advanced immunodeficiency. Patients generally present with epigastric or right upper quadrant pain, fever and malaise. Although AIDS-cholangiopathy is a cholestatic disease, jaundice and pruritus are uncommon. The most common laboratory abnormality is a markedly elevated alkaline phosphatase. Bilirubin rarely exceeds 3 mg/dl, and transaminases are only mildly elevated. The diagnosis is best established by ERCP. Several cholangiographic patterns have been described, including papillary stenosis, sclerosing cholangitis, combined papillary stenosis and sclerosing cholangitis, isolated intrahepatic disease, and long extrahepatic bile duct strictures. Endoscopic sphincterotomy is appropriate only for the relief of pain in patients with papillary stenosis. Unfortunately, the disease is progressive, and medical therapy has no influence on its outcome.

7. What are the most common causes of AIDS-cholangiopathy? How are they diagnosed?

1. *Cryptosporidium parvum*
2. Microsporidia
   Enterocytozoon bieneusii
   Encephalocytozoon (formerly *Septata*) *intestinalis*
   Encephalocytozoon cuniculi
3. Cytomegalovirus
4. *Mycobacterium avium*-complex
5. *Cyclospora cayetanensis*
6. Non-Hodgkin's lymphoma
7. Kaposi's sarcoma

The diagnosis usually is established by obtaining biopsy specimens of the ampulla or duodenal mucosa, aspirated bile specimens, and biliary epithelial brush cytology. Despite its infectious origin, medical therapies aiming at the eradication of these organisms have not produced improvement in AIDS cholangiopathy, which is a gradually progressive disease.

8. What are the most common causes of pancreatitis in HIV-infected patients?

Several studies have documented chronic and/or recurrent elevation of serum amylase and lipase in up to 50% of patients with AIDS. Pancreatograms at the time of ERCP also have documented abnormalities of the pancreatic ducts consistent with chronic pancreatitis. These findings have led many investigators to hypothesize that pancreatic insufficiency from chronic pancreatitis is an important cause of chronic diarrhea in AIDS. Most cases of chronic pancreatitis are probably secondary to conditions such as alcohol abuse and medications. The most common medications associated with pancreatitis in AIDS are pentamidine, ddI, and zalcitabine (ddC). Infectious causes of pancreatitis include CMV, HSV and HIV itself.

9. How has highly active antiretroviral therapy (HAART) affected the incidence of opportunistic GI disorders?

Since the introduction of protease inhibitors and HAART in 1996, there has been a constant decline of GI opportunistic disorders in AIDS. It is postulated that improvement in the immune status, as reflected by an increase in CD4 cells, prevents the development of opportunistic disorders. In several case reports and studies, symptoms resolved even before any changes in the total CD4 cell count were apparent, suggesting that the antiretroviral medications promote elimination of the offending GI infection, probably secondary to immune-boosting mechanisms independent of the CD4 cell count and intrinsic antimicrobial activity.

10. Describe the clinical features and causes of enterocolitis in AIDS.

In evaluating an AIDS patient with diarrhea, careful attention should be directed to the history and physical exam. Enteritis (small bowel diarrhea) is associated with voluminous, watery bowel movements, abdominal bloating, cramping, borborygmi, and nausea. The abdominal pain tends to be periumbilical or diffuse. Abdominal exam reveals an increase in number and frequency of bowel sounds, which may be high-pitched. Conversely, colitis (large bowel diarrhea) is characterized by frequent, small bowel movements, with the presence of mucus, pus and/or blood ("dysentery"). Patients with prominent involvement of the distal colon also have "proctitis" symptoms, such as tenesmus, dyschezia (pain on defecation), and proctalgia (rectal pain). The most common causes of enteritis include cryptosporidiosis, microsporidiosis, giardiasis, cyclosporiasis, and viral infections. Colitis is generally secondary to CMV or bacteria such as *Shigella* spp., *Salmonella* spp., *Campylobacter jejuni*, and *Clostridium difficile*. *C. difficile* has become increasingly common because of the frequent use of antimicrobial medications.

11. Describe the clinical features of HSV proctitis in AIDS.

HSV proctitis is the most common cause of nongonococcal proctitis in sexually active gay men. HSV proctitis classically presents with tenesmus, purulent rectal discharge, severe proctalgia, fever, constipation, and anorectal bleeding. Painful inguinal lymphadenopathy is an almost universal finding. The pain tends to distribute in the region of the sacral roots (i.e., buttocks, perineal region, and posterior thigh). Because of the neural involvement by HSV and the presence of severe pain, patients also have impotence and difficulty in initiating micturition. Visual inspection and anoscopy commonly reveal the following lesions: vesicles, pustular rectal lesions, or diffuse ulcerations. HSV is a pathogen of the squamous mucosa, therefore, diffuse proctitis involving the entire rectum is rare. In severe cases, the columnar rectal and sigmoid mucosa has been involved. Differential diagnoses of HSV proctitis include lymphogranuloma venereum (*Chalymatobacterium granulomatis*), *Chlamydia trachomatis*, *Entamoeba histolytica*, *Salmonella* spp., and *Campylobacter jejuni*.

12. What is the recommended work-up for diarrhea in AIDS?

In general a stepwise approach is recommended. A thorough history and clinical exam are essential. It is also important to consider geographic location. For example, rotavirus is a common cause of diarrhea in Australian patients, microsporidiosis is virtually nonexistent in the south of the United States, and *Cyclospora cayetanensis* is a common cause of diarrhea in South America. Recent visit to a farm, contact with farm animals, or use of public swimming pools should raise the suspicion of cryptosporidiosis or microsporidiosis. Knowledge of the patient's immune status as reflected by CD4 cell count is also essential, because patients with more severe immunocompromise are predisposed to a wider array of opportunistic disorders. History of recently started or change in medications, such as antiretrovirals or antibacterials, is important, because many protease inhibitors are associated with diarrhea, and antibacterials are associated with *C. difficile* colitis.

The first step in the evaluation of diarrhea is to obtain at least three stool samples to investigate for ova and parasites and to culture for common bacteria such as *Shigella, Salmonella*, and *Campylobacter* spp. Stool samples also should be submitted for *C. difficile* toxin. In febrile patients, blood cultures should be obtained for common bacteria. If the CD4 count is below 50 cells/µl, cultures for *Mycobacerium avium*-complex should be obtained. If stool and blood culture studies are negative, the next step is endoscopic evaluation. In the presence of "colitis" symptoms, flexible sigmoidoscopy or colonoscopy is recommended. Because up to 40% of cases of CMV colitis may be isolated to the right colon, some authorities suggest the performance of a full colonoscopy. In the presence of "enteritis" symptoms or long-standing diarrhea, an EGD with duodenal biopsies is mandatory to evaluate for cryptosporidia, microsporidia, and giardiasis. The table below summarizes the studies and laboratory tests used in the evaluation of diarrhea in AIDS.

Studies and Laboratory Tests Used in the Evaluation of Diarrhea in AIDS

Stool
    Cultures (*Salmonella, Shigella, Campylobacter* spp.)
    Toxin (*Clostridium difficile*)
    Ova and parasites (*Giardia lamblia, Entamoeba histolytica, Cryptosporidium* spp.)
    Modified Kinyoun acid-fast (*Cryptosporidium* spp., *Isospora belli*)
    Concentrated stool (zinc sulfate, Shether sucrose flotation) (microsporidia)

Table continued on following page

Studies and Laboratory Tests Used in the Evaluation of Diarrhea in AIDS (Continued)

Blood
   Cultures (*Mycobacterium avium*-complex, *Salmonella, Campylobacter* spp.)
   Antibodies (*Entamoeba histolytica*, cytomegalovirus [CMV])

Gastrointestinal fluids
   Duodenal aspirate (*Giardia lamblia*, microsporidia)

Electron microscopy (*Cryptosporidium* spp., adenovirus)

Biopsy stains
   Hematoxylin-eosin
   Giemsa or methenamine silver (fungi)
   Methylene blue-azure II-basic fuchsin (microsporidia)
   Fite mycobacteria

Immunohistochemical stains (CMV)

Immunologic methods
   In-situ hybridization (CMV)
   DNA amplification (CMV)

Culture of tissue (colonic mucosal biopsy)
   CMV
   Herpes simplex virus
   Bacterial stool pathogens

13. How useful is endoscopy for the evaluation of diarrhea in AIDS?

The advantage of endoscopy is that it permits direct visualization and retrieval of tissue for histologic examination. The diagnostic yield of colonoscopy in HIV-infected patients with chronic diarrhea and negative stool studies ranges from 27–37%. CMV is the most common etiology identified. Because CMV disease is often located distally, sigmoidoscopy with biopsy may be sufficient work-up, but in 13–39% of cases of CMV enterocolitis, the virus can be detected only in the right colon. Therefore, if CMV is suspected as the cause of diarrhea, a full colonoscopy is warranted. However, it is still not clear whether colonoscopy has a higher yield than flexible sigmoidoscopy for the detection of organisms other than CMV. The value of upper endoscopy in the evaluation of chronic diarrhea has been demonstrated in several studies. The most commonly detected organisms include cryptosporidia and microsporidia.

14. What is the most common cause of viral diarrhea in AIDS?

CMV is one of the most common opportunistic infections in patients with AIDS, occurring late in the course of HIV infection when immunodeficiency is severe (CD4 lymphocyte count < 100/mm^3). CMV has been identified in mucosal biopsies in as many as 45% of patients with AIDS and diarrhea. CMV causes both enteritis and colitis. A number of other viral pathogens have been reported to involve the GI tract in patients with AIDS, but their clinical importance remains to be determined. Examples include adenovirus, rotavirus, astrovirus, picobirna virus, and coronavirus. There are also reports that HIV itself can be isolated from enterocytes and colonic cells. HIV may have a direct cytopathic effect in the intestinal mucosa, thus producing HIV enteropathy. HSV can cause proctitis that mimics diarrhea because of the rectal mucous discharge. However, HIV does not cause enterocolitis because it invades the squamous mucosa, not the columnar epithelium, such as the one lining the colonic and small bowel mucosa.

15. What is the most appropriate medical therapy for CMV enterocolitis?

The natural history of CMV colitis is variable. In untreated patients, it usually has a chronic course characterized by progressive diarrhea and weight loss, although occasionally symptoms and histologic abnormalities remit spontaneously. Unlike CMV retinitis, for which strong evidence supports induction therapy followed by lifelong maintenance therapy, the optimal duration of therapy and the need for maintenance therapy in CMV colitis are undefined. Two antivirals (foscarnet and ganciclovir) have been studied extensively in the therapy of CMV colitis and/or enteritis. Cidofovir, the newest agent, has been reported only in patients with retinal disease, but in our experience it is effective for GI disease. Fundoscopic examination at the time of diagnosis of CMV enterocolitis is mandatory, because duration of therapy is considerably longer for disseminated diseases than for disease limited to the GI tract.

A number of open-label trials of ganciclovir for HIV-infected patients with CMV GI disease have demonstrated clinical improvement in ~ 75% of patients. Open-label trials of foscarnet have yielded comparable results. The only placebo-controlled trial of ganciclovir in AIDS-associated CMV colitis found no clinically significant differences, probably because the treatment period was only 2 weeks. A randomized trial comparing ganciclovir with foscarnet in 48 AIDS patients with CMV GI disease found similar clinical efficacy (73%), regardless of the location of disease (esophagus vs. colon). Endoscopic improvement was documented in over 80% of patients.

16. Describe the epidemiologic and clinical features of cryptosporidiosis.

Cryposporidia are a common cause of chronic diarrhea in HIV-infected patients with severe immunodeficiency. There are at least 40 species of cryptosporidia, but the most common cause of human disease is *C. muri*. Cryptosporidia infect and than reproduce within the columnar small intestinal cells. Infection can occur from person-to-person, animal-to-person, or waterborne transmission (e.g., swimming pools, lakes). Therefore, a severely immunodeficient patient with AIDS who is not taking HAART is advised to abstain from contact with farm animals, public pools, and lakes. The life cycle is completed in a single host. Autoinfectious cycles follow ingestion of a few oocysts, leading to severe disease and persistent infection in severely immunodeficient hosts. The diarrhea is generally voluminous, watery, and yellow-green. The stool may contain mucus but rarely contains blood or leukocytes. The disease may wax and wane, but persistent and/or progressive disease generally presents with dehydration and electrolyte imbalances. Constitutional symptoms are prominent, including low-grade fever, malaise, anorexia, nausea, and vomiting.

17. Which bacteria most commonly cause diarrhea in AIDS?

Campylobacter, Salmonella, and *Shigella* spp. and *C. difficle. Yersinia enterocolitica, Staphylococcus aureus,* and *Aeromonas hydrophila* also have been associated with severe enterocolitis in HIV-infected patients. *C. difficile* colitis is a frequent cause of diarrhea in HIV-infected patients, most likely because of frequent exposure to antimicrobials and requirement for hospitalization. *Mycobacterium avium*-complex is a common pathogen in patients with advanced immunosuppression (i.e., CD4 count < 50/µl). An incidence of 39% has been described when the CD4 count remains < $10/mm^3$.

Causes of Diarrhea in AIDS

VIRUSES	BACTERIA	PARASITES	FUNGI
Cytomegalovirus	*Salmonella spp.*	*Giardia lamblia*	*Histoplasma capsulatum*
Astrovirus	*Shigella* spp.	*Entamoeba histolytica*	*Candida albicans*
Picornavirus	*Campylobacter jejuni*	Microsporidia	
Coronavirus	*Clostridium difficile*	*Enterocytozoon bieneusi*	
Rotavirus	*Mycobacterium avium*-	*Encephalocytozoon*	
Herpesvirus	complex	formerly *Septata*)	
Adenovirus	*Treponema pallidum*	*intestinalis*	
Small round virus	Spirochetes	*Cyclospora cayetanensis*	
HIV	*Neisseria gonorrhoeae*	*Cryptosporidium* spp.	
	Vibrio cholerae	*Isospora belli*	
	Aeromonas spp.	*Blastocytes hominis* (?)	
	Pseudomonas spp. (?)		
	Staphylococcus aureus		

18. Name the parasites that cause diarrhea in AIDS.

Among the protozoa, *Cryptosporidium parvum* is the most common parasite causing diarrhea in AIDS and has been identified in up to 11% of symptomatic patients. Although a cause of acute diarrhea, cryptosporidiosis is most commonly found in HIV-infected patients with chronic diarrhea. In some studies of HIV-infected patients with chronic diarrhea, microsporidia (*Enterocytozoon bieneusi* and *Encephalitozoon intestinalis*) are the most commonly identified pathogens. *Isospora belli* is a rare GI pathogen in HIV-infected patients in North America, whereas it is endemic in many developing countries such as Haiti.

19. What is bacillary peliosis hepatis (BPH)?

BPH produces multiple cystic blood-filled spaces in the liver. BPH is caused by an infection with the bacteria *Bartonella henselae* (formerly *Rochalimae*) and occurs in patients with advanced AIDS. Patients present with generalized and nonspecific symptoms, such as fever, weight loss, and malaise. Abdominal pain, nausea, vomiting, and diarrhea may be prominent. Skin manifestations include reddish vascular papules that can be confused with Kaposi's sarcoma. On abdominal exam hepatosplenomegaly and lymphadenopathy are the most prominent features. Histopathology of the liver lesions shows multiple cystic blood-filled spaces within fibromyxoid areas. The treatment of choice is erythromycin for at least 4–6 weeks, but doxycycline is a safe alternative.

ACKNOWLEDGMENT

To Ms. Denise Herrarte for her support in the preparation of this manuscript.

BIBLIOGRAPHY:

1. Blanshard C, Francis N, Gazzard BG: Investigation of chronic diarrhoea in acquired immunodeficiency syndrome. A prospective study in 155 patients. Gut 39:824–832, 1996.
2. Bonacini M. Pancreatic involvement in human immunodeficiency virus infection. J Clin Gastroenterol 13:58, 1991.
3. Cello JP: Acquired immunodeficiency syndrome cholangiopathy: Spectrum of disease. Am J Med 86:539, 1989.
4. Dieterich DT, Wilcox CM: Diagnosis and treatment of esophageal diseases associated with HIV-infection. Am J Gastroenterol 91:2265–2268, 1996.
5. Kotler DP, Reka S, Orenstein JM, Fox CH: Chronic idiopathic esophageal ulceration in the acquired immunodeficiency syndrome. J Clin Gastroenterol 15:284–290, 1992.
6. Mönkemüller KE, Wilcox CM: Diagnosis and treatment of colonic disease in AIDS. Gastrointest Endosc Clin North Am 8:889, 1998.
7. Mönkemüller KE, Wilcox CM: Diagnosis and treatment of esophageal ulcers in AIDS. Semin Gastroenterol 10:1, 1999.
8. Mönkemüller KE, Call SA, Lazenby AJ, Wilcox CM: Decline in the prevalence of opportunistic gastrointestinal disorders in the era of HAART. Am J Gastroenterol 95:457–462, 2000.
9. Mönkemüller KE, Bussian A, Lazenby A, Wilcox CM: Special histologic stains are rarely beneficial for the evaluation of HIV-related gastrointestinal infections. Am J Clin Pathol 114:387–394, 2000.
10. Smith PD, Quinn TC, Strober W, et al: Gastrointestinal infections in AIDS. Ann Intern Med 116:63, 1992.
11. Wilcox CM, Mönkemüller KE: Therapy of gastrointestinal infections in AIDS. Alim Pharmacol Ther 11:425–443, 1997.
12. Wilcox CM, Alexander LN, Clark WS, Thompson SE: Fluconazole compared with endoscopy for human immunodeficiency virus-infected patients with esophageal symptoms. Gastroenterology 110:1803–1808, 1996.
13. Wilcox CM, Straub RA, Schwartz DA: Prospective endoscopic characterization of cytomegalovirus esophagitis in patients with AIDS. Gastrointest Endosc 40:481–484, 1994.
14. Wilcox CM, Straub RF, Schwartz DA: Prospective evaluation of biopsy number for the diagnosis of viral esophagitis in patients with HIV infection and esophageal ulcer. Gastrointest Endosc 44:587–593, 1996.

62. INTESTINAL ISCHEMIA

Arvey I. Rogers, M.D., FACP, and Francisco Baigorri, M.D.

1. What is meant by ischemic bowel disease?

Ischemic bowel disease results from impaired organ perfusion by oxygen-carrying blood distributed via the mesenteric arterial circulation. A reduction in blood flow or reduced oxygen content of red blood cells results in tissue hypoxia. Ischemia affects principally the small and/or large intestine and is manifested clinically as acute or chronic abdominal pain, vomiting, sitophobia, weight loss, diarrhea, ileus, gastrointestinal (GI) bleeding, gut infarction, peritonitis, and fibrotic strictures.

2. What are the main components of the mesenteric circulation?

The mesenteric circulation consists of three major arteries (celiac axis, superior mesenteric, and inferior mesenteric) as inflow vessels and two major veins (superior and inferior mesenteric) as outflow vessels. This vascular system is referred to as the splanchnic circulation. Both arteries and veins course through the mesentery, providing blood to and draining it away from the digestive organs and spleen. The veins drain ultimately into the portal and hepatic veins.

The celiac axis provides blood to the stomach, duodenum, spleen, liver, and gallbladder. A portion of the duodenum, the entire small intestine, and half of the large intestine receive arterial blood via the superior mesenteric artery (SMA). The inferior mesenteric artery provides blood to the left colon and the rectum. The rectum is also perfused by branches of the internal iliac arteries.

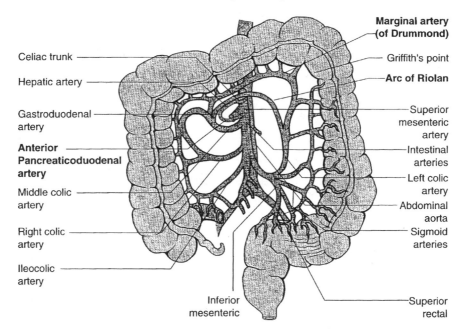

Mesenteric arterial anatomy. Three unpaired arterial branches of the aorta (celiac, superior mesenteric, and inferior mesenteric arteries) provide oxygenated blood to the small and large intestine. In most instances, veins parallel arteries. The superior mesenteric vein joins the splenic vein to form the portal vein, which enters the liver at its hilum. The inferior mesenteric vein joins the splenic vein near the juncture of the superior mesenteric and splenic veins. (Adapted from Rogers AI, Rosen CM: Mesenteric vascular insufficiency. In Schiller LR (ed): Small Intestine. Philadelphia, Current Medicine, 1997, with permission.)

3. Describe the collateral circulatory system between the systemic and splanchnic vascular networks.

Collateral channels exist between the three major mesenteric arteries. The major connections join the celiac axis and superior mesenteric vessels (pancreaticoduodenal cascade) and the superior and inferior mesenteric vessels via the marginal arteries (marginal artery of Drummond), which connect the middle colic (superior mesenteric) artery with the left colic (inferior mesenteric) artery. An additional vascular arcade connects the marginal artery of Drummond with a branch of the middle colic artery (arc of Riolan). Slowly developing occlusion of mesenteric arteries via atherosclerosis stimulates the enlargement of collateral channels to maintain arterial flow. As a result, chronic mesenteric arterial insufficiency (i.e., abdominal angina) is distinctly unusual unless two of the three major channels are occluded.

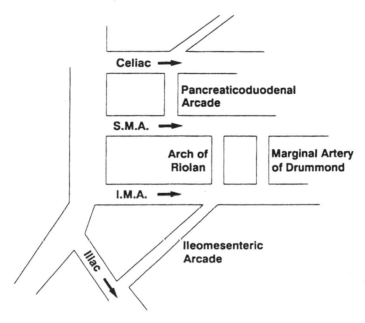

Schematic representation of collateral channels among the three major mesenteric arteries. The development of alternative anastomoses and collateral flow makes it theoretically possible that any single artery could supply all of the abdominal viscera with arterial blood given sufficient time and opportunity, i.e. gradual occlusion of one or two of the other major arterial vessels. One major anastomosis exists between the left branch of the middle colic artery (from the superior mesenteric artery [SMA]) and the left colic artery from the inferior mesenteric artery (IMA), forming the meandering mesenteric artery or the arc of Riolan. Its demonstration by angiography indicates occlusion of the SMA or IMA. The marginal artery of Drummond is an arterial connection that provides a continuous channel of collateral flow via the vasa recta to the small and large intestine. The ileomesenteric arcade establishes an important anastomosis between the mesenteric and systemic circulation between the superior hemorrhoidal artery, a branch of the IMA and the hypogastric artery, a branch of the iliac artery. (Adapted from Rogers AI, Rosen CM: Mesenteric vascular insufficiency. In. Schiller LR (ed): Small Intestine. Philadelphia, Current Medicine, 1997, with permission.)

4. A unique microcirculation functions to maintain oxygen delivery to the gut. Describe the components and how they respond to alterations in gut blood flow.

The microcirculation consists of arterioles, capillaries, and venules, all lined by endothelial cells. Arterioles resist and therefore regulate the flow of blood through the tissues. A steep gradient of pressure exists between the artery and terminal portion of the arteriole. The arterioles dilate when arterial perfusion pressure is reduced. Capillaries allow the exchange of materials between gut wall cells and blood vessels. When tissue hypoxia occurs, underperfused capillaries are recruited, increasing the density of perfused capillaries and thereby compensating for the steep gradient in tissue oxygen levels. The venules store blood for short periods before its mobilization to the heart after meals or in response to exercise. In the face of systemic hypotension, the tone of venous capacitance vessels is increased, enhancing venous return to the heart to ensure maintenance of cardiac output.

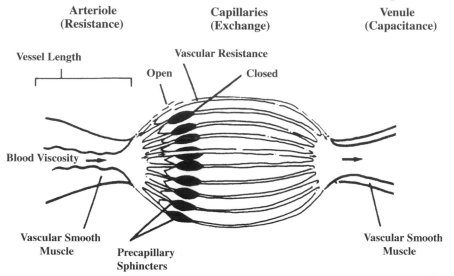

Intramural vascular anatomy. The assured delivery of oxygen-rich arterial blood to the various layers of the small and large intestinal wall during basal, meal-stimulated, and stress states of oxygen-rich arterial blood depends on the interplay between various anatomic and physiologic factors, i.e. blood viscosity, red blood cell oxygen saturation, arteriole length and resistance to flow, tone of precapillary sphincters, tone of vascular smooth muscle, and venous capacitance. See question 5 to gain a better understanding of the various factors influencing the regulation of blood flow. (Adapted from Rogers AI, Rosen CM: Mesenteric vascular insufficiency. In Schiller LR (ed): Small Intestine. Philadelphia, Current Medicine, 1997, with permission.)

5. What factors contribute to the regulation of gut blood flow?

Maintenance of gut blood flow depends on the interaction between factors that increase flow (vasodilators) and factors that reduce it (vasoconstrictors):

1. Cardiovascular factors (cardiac output, blood pressure, and blood volume)
2. Autonomic nervous system
   • Sympathetic nerves constrict, whereas parasympathetic nerves dilate vessels.
   • Nonadrenergic, noncholinergic (NANC) nerves dilate,whereas the intrinsic enteric nervous system constricts and dilates vessels.
3. Circulating hormones: norepinephrine, angiotensin II, and vasopressin constrict, whereas GI mucosal release of hormones dilates vessels.
4. Tissue substances released in response to ischemia, inflammation, or increased tissue metabolism (elaborated by endothelial cells lining the vessels of the microcirculation and by immunocytes such as mast cells and leukocytes).
5. Physical forces (transmural pressure and streaming velocity)

6. Does mesenteric ischemia always result from arterial occlusion?

No. Decreased perfusion of the gut secondary to prolonged vasoconstriction, in the absence of thrombotic or embolic occlusion, can produce ischemia of the bowel. Venous thrombosis also predisposes to gut ischemia.

7. What are the different varieties of ischemic bowel disease?

Arterial and venous, acute and chronic, occlusive and nonocclusive.

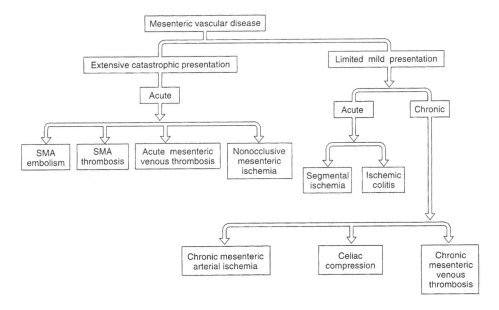

Classification of mesenteric vascular disease based on the extent of resulting ischemia. This particular classification, proposed by Williams et al., may facilitate more effective evaluation and management by focusing on extent of gut involvement.

8. Describe the pathophysiology of occlusive intestinal ischemia.

Intestinal ischemia results from tissue hypoxia. Hypoxia ensues when blood volume, its physical characteristics (red-cell mass), flow rate, or oxygen content is altered in the mesenteric arterial or venous circulation. Decreased flow affecting the arterial vasculature can result from an obstruction caused by a thrombus (acute or chronic), embolus (acute), or vasoconstriction. Thrombosis is usually secondary to rupture of an atherosclerotic plaque. The most common location for thrombotic or embolic occlusion is at the origin of the superior mesenteric artery; its angular branching off the aorta is a predisposing factor.

Patients can develop a syndrome of chronic, recurrent abdominal pain when the thrombosis or arterial wall thickening is complete enough to compromise luminal diameter by > 50%. With insufficient development of collateral circulation to provide compensated arterial flow to fulfill physiologic demands for increased delivery of oxygen to tissues (i.e., 30–90 minutes after a meal), ischemia and resulting tissue hypoxia lead to gut spasm and abdominal pain.

Less commonly patients develop mesenteric venous thrombosis that obstructs venous outflow from the gut and leads to congestion and ischemia. This condition may complicate inflammatory or neoplastic disease affecting the portal or mesenteric veins, polycythemia vera or thrombocytosis, profound dehydration, or hepatic cirrhosis.

9. Describe the pathophysiology of nonocclusive mesenteric ischemia.

Shock, profound hypovolemia, impaired cardiac output, or major thoracic or abdominal surgery are risk factors for gut hypoperfusion as a consequence of vasoconstriction of the mesenteric vasculature. This condition is known as nonocclusive mesenteric ischemia (NOMI).

Patients with NOMI have decreased perfusion of the mesenteric arteries due to vasoconstriction precipitated by an event resulting in hypotension or hypoperfusion (i.e., hypovolemia or cardiac failure). No occluding thrombus or embolus is present. NOMI is encountered most commonly in patients who have undergone major abdominal or thoracic surgery complicated by pulmonary edema, cardiac arrhythmias, or shock. Digoxin can worsen mesenteric vasoconstriction. Patients manifest the same symptoms and signs as patients with occlusive disease. Angiography reveals intense vasoconstriction and spasm that may persist even if the precipitating event is remedied. Selective (intraarterial) papaverine infusion can relieve the vasoconstriction.

10. What should I know about veno-occlusion as a cause of ischemic bowel?

Mesenteric venous thrombosis is a rare cause of ischemic bowel. Just as in mesenteric ischemia complicating arterial occlusion (or nonocclusion), most patients present with mid-abdominal pain that is severe and disproportionate to the minimal findings on physical examination of the abdomen. However, patients with veno-occlusive disease can present acutely or sub-acutely (weeks to months). Accurate diagnosis requires a high index of suspicion. Abdominal computed tomography (CT) with contrast is the diagnostic test of choice, revealing findings consistent with venous occlusion in more than 90% of patients: thickening and contrast enhancement of the bowel wall, enlarged superior mesenteric vein (SMV), thrombosis in the lumen of the SMV, and collateral vessels. If no signs of intestinal infarction are present, patients should be treated with anticoagulation and thrombolytics; otherwise, they should be operated immediately.

11. What is focal segmental ischemia?

The same pathophysiologic processes (embolus, thrombosis, venous occlusion, NOMI) capable of causing extensive bowel ischemia can also lead to a form of ischemia that is limited to a short segment of bowel. It is the result of the involvement of a few small arteries or, more rarely, veins and is known as focal segmental ischemia.

12. What clinical circumstances predispose to ischemic bowel disease?
Arterial
- Embolus: cardiac arrythmias, valvular heart disease (atrial fibrillation), myocardial infarction, mural thrombus, atrial myxoma, angiography.
- Thrombosis: atherosclerosis, hypercoagulable states (pregnancy, protein C or S deficiency, birth control pills, neoplasms, polycythemia vera, thrombocytosis), vascular aneurysms, vascular dissections, vasculitides.

Nonocclusive mesenteric ischemia: cardiogenic shock, hypovolemia, sepsis, vasoconstricting drugs.

Venous: hypercoagulable states, congestive heart failure, shock, portal hypertension, Budd-Chiari syndrome, carcinoma, trauma, sclerotherapy, peritonitis, diverticulitis, pancreatitis, inflammatory bowel disease, intestinal obstruction, postoperative states, trauma.

13. What are the common presenting complaints in patients with suspected gut ischemia?

Presenting complaints vary with the etiology of the ischemia. Most patients with intestinal ischemia complicating acute embolic or thrombotic occlusion of the SMA present with the sudden onset of acute, severe abdominal pain, usually mid-abdominal in location and of colicky character. Simultaneously, involuntary evacuation of bowel contents may occur because of the intense tonic contractions of gut smooth muscle provoked by ischemia. Abdominal pain resulting from smooth muscle spasm presents few abdominal physical findings.

Patients with acute mesenteric ischemia secondary to thrombotic occlusion may provide an antecedent history consistent with mesenteric angina, i.e. recurring postprandial mid- or diffuse abdominal pain, sometimes with a back-radiation component. Weight loss usually ensues because of sitophobia (fear of eating). Pain radiating to the back (possibly due to duodenal ischemia) and weight loss suggest pancreatic carcinoma. A negative abdominal CT mitigates against this consideration. Diarrhea, steatorrhea, and/or protein-losing enteropathy may complicate ischemia-induced atrophy of the small intestinal mucosa.

Veno-occlusive disease may have a more insidious onset characterized by vague abdominal pain, diarrhea, and vomiting. Acute occlusion may result in profound fluid sequestration and shock. It should be suspected in the appropriate clinical setting (see question 8).

Abdominal distention and a Hemoccult-positive stool may be the only presenting signs in the intensive or coronary care unit patient who develops NOMI and is incapable of complaining of abdominal pain.

14. What are the physical findings of gut ischemia?

Physical findings vary with the etiology and chronology of the ischemia. In the appropriate clinical setting, acute occlusion of the SMA via embolus or thrombosis should be suspected when a striking disparity exists between the subjective complaint of severe, diffuse abdominal pain and the minimal findings on abdominal examination. Early in the course of disease, only mild distention and normal or hyperactive bowel sounds are likely to be encountered. Abdominal arterial bruits are too nonspecific to be of value. Stools may be Hemoccult-positive. As the ischemia progresses to further bowel compromise, ileus develops, bowel sounds diminish, and abdominal distention ensues. Bloody diarrhea may occur. Hypotension and tachycardia signal volume sequestration, whereas fever and peritoneal signs indicate transmural injury and probable infarction.

Nonocclusive ischemia should be considered in the appropriate setting. Subjective complaints are less dramatic than with acute arterial occlusion. Physical findings vary with the duration of the arterial occlusion and may be similar to those described for acute arterial occlusion. Chronic, recurring abdominal pain on the basis of compromised flow through the SMA (i.e., mesenteric abdominal angina) is not associated with specific physical findings. Most patients have evidence of peripheral vascular disease; they also may exhibit findings associated with weight loss.

Physical findings in veno-occlusive disease depend on its etiology and severity (e.g., congestive heart failure, stigmata of chronic liver disease and portal hypertension, hepatomegaly, splenomegaly, evidence of hypercoagulability, abdominal mass). Tachycardia and hypotension are present if splanchnic volume has been sequestered.

15. What is a realistic differential diagnosis?

The differential diagnosis is broad and should include any cause of acute abdominal pain, unexplained ileus in the appropriate setting, and hypotension. Conditions usually considered include perforated viscus, small bowel obstruction, cecal volvulus, incarcerated hernia, dissecting aortic aneurysm, acute pancreatitis, and cholecystitis.

16. Do laboratory findings help at all?

Laboratory findings in gut ischemia are usually nonspecific and probably vary with the etiology, duration, severity, potential for reversing precipitating and complicating events, and extent of ischemic injury (i.e., which organs are involved). Early stages are associated with no abnormalities (other than those associated with a preexisting illness that may or may not have predisposed to gut ischemia). Abnormalities seen with gut ischemia and/or infarction are the consequence of volume sequestration and tissue hypoxia, inflammation, and necrosis (i.e., hemoconcentration, leukocytosis, and lactic acidosis). Increased levels of amylase, alkaline phosphatase, and creatine phosphokinase (CPK) are nonspecific findings. They may help to exclude mimicking etiologies, such as pancreatitis (increased levels of amylase and lipase) and choledocholithiasis (increased levels of alkaline phosphatase, alanine aminotransferanse [ALT], aspartate aminotransferase [AST], and bilirubin). Increased levels of CPK and alkaline phosphatase are nonspecific consequences of gut injury. The more abnormal the laboratory findings, the more severe the injury.

17. What studies are available to confirm a suspected diagnosis?

Conventional radiography, contrast-enhanced CT, Doppler ultrasound of mesenteric vessels, mesenteric angiography (magnetic resonance or invasive arteriography), laparoscopy, and enteroscopy are among the diagnostic techniques most frequently applied. Laparoscopy and enteroscopy are used less commonly. The clinical circumstances and findings dictate choices and sequence.

Unless dictated otherwise by clinical circumstances that point clearly to gut ischemia and/or infarction and away from mimicking etiologies, abdominal plain films (flat and upright) should be obtained first (see figure at top of following page). Helpful clues to the diagnosis of abdominal pain that may be seen on the plain radiographs of the abdomen include the following:

DISORDER	FINDING ON PLAIN ABDOMINAL RADIOGRAPHS
Small bowel obstruction	Dilated loops of bowel with or without air-fluid levels. Stair-step overlapping of loops of small bowel May see termination of luminal small bowel air at lead point of obstruction
Pancreatitis	Sentinel loop of jejunum or colon cut-off sign
Volvulus	Characteristic jejunual, sigmoid, or cecal bowel dilation
Pneumobilia	Air in the biliary tree, seen in emphysematous cholangitis or intraabdominal sepsis, caused by gas-forming bacteria
Pylephlebitis	Air in the hepatic/portal venous system suggests severe gut injury, infarction, advanced intraabdominal sepsis
Perforation	Free air under the diaphragm or air dissecting between loops of bowel
Bowel ischemia	Bowel wall thickening, loop separation, or thumb-printing
Pneumotosis cystoides intestinalis	Air in the bowel wall usually indicates pre- or actual bowel infarction

The administration of barium for a small bowel study should be avoided in anticipation that an abdominal CT or angiogram may be undertaken; the oral contrast interferes with the ability to perform and/or interpret findings of these studies. As mentioned earlier (see question 10), a dynamic, contrast-enhanced abdominal CT can be very valuable in diagnosing veno-occlusive disease.

18. Describe the role of Doppler ultrasound studies in diagnosis.

Fasting and meal-stimulated Duplex ultrasound is a noninvasive test that can be used to assess the patency of and blood flow through the major mesenteric vessels. Its greatest use is in diagnosing multivessel stenosis in cases of suspected mesenteric angina; findings include narrowing or occlusion at vessel origin and excessively turbulent flow. Its major limitations for diagnosing acute mesenteric arterial or venous occlusion include visualization limited to the proximal segment of the vessels and compromised visualization when ileus is present or the patient is obese. For these reasons, Duplex ultrasonographic scanning cannot be recommended in acutely ill patients.

19. What is the role of endoscopy (sigmoidoscopy, colonoscopy, and/or enteroscopy)?

Conventional enteroscopy should not be undertaken for purposes of diagnosing small bowel ischemic disease. Despite the fact that scattered case reports describe diagnostic findings in selected clinical settings, the technique using available endoscopic instruments and scope passage through the small intestine can be dangerous. Smaller scope diameter and improved technology to facilitate intestinal intubation may modify conventional wisdom. However, lower endoscopy (sigmoidoscopy or colonoscopy) is relatively safe and may be highly informative in patients with suspected ischemic colitis (see questions 27–31).

20. When should you undertake mesenteric arteriographic studies?

Early diagnosis and definitive nonsurgical or surgical therapy are important in patients with suspected ischemic bowel disease. The mortality rate is quite high when diagnosis and therapy are delayed and when peritoneal signs and acidosis ensue. Angiography is the gold standard for the diagnosis of mesenteric arterial occlusion and sometimes differentiates an embolic from a thrombotic event. The angiographic demonstration of an abrupt cut-off of a major (nonatherosclerotic) artery in the absence of collateral vessel enlargement suggests embolic occlusion, whereas associated vessel narrowing by atherosclerosis in association with the development of prominent collaterals is more consistent with thrombosis. The venous phase of the arteriogram may demonstrate veno-occlusive disease. The angiographic findings in nonocclusive mesenteric ischemia include vessel narrowing and beading and lack of arterial blush in the intestinal wall.

On occasion, angiography also can be therapeutic, allowing the selective infusion of vasodilating drugs such as papaverine to the affected spastic arteries or facilitating the performance of therapeutic angioplasty, balloon embolectomy, or stent placement. Angiography is not a benign procedure and carries definite risk, inasmuch as many affected patients have considerable atherosclerotic changes in femoral and mesenteric arteries. Infused contrast in association with hypovolemia, impaired cardiac output, and reduced renal blood flow increases the likelihood of renal damage. Nonetheless, angiography is the only definite way, short of exploratory surgery, to establish the diagnosis of mesenteric ischemia early in the disease when the patient still has a chance of surviving.

21. When should a patient with ischemic bowel disease be sent to the operating room?

A clinical picture compatible with acute ischemic bowel disease in which other diagnoses have been excluded should prompt angiography. If the findings are amenable to nonoperative management (i.e., NOMI treated with papaverine infusion, embolectomy) and there is no indication of bowel necrosis, the patient should be treated conservatively. Otherwise, patients should be taken to the operating room (1) to assess the degree and extent of gut injury, (2) to identify the site of and to relieve arterial obstruction, (3) to resect irreversibly damaged bowel, and (4) possibly to undergo revascularization. Bowel viability may be assessed by the injection of fluorescein dye.

22. Is there ever an indication for a "second-look" operation?

At the time of surgery there may be some doubt about the viability of a segment of bowel left intact, whether or not revascularization has been attempted. Under such circumstances, the patient may undergo a second operation to assess bowel viability 24–48 hours later. This is an area of ongoing, active controversy.

23. What is meant by reperfusion injury?

Reestablishing normal blood flow to the ischemic bowel does not always arrest injury to the bowel. Reperfusion of ischemic tissue can lead to paradoxical exaggeration of the injury. One of the prevailing theories to account for this observation is that reperfusion increases the number of active oxidants (free oxygen, H_2O_2, hydroxy radicals) that further injure the cells. The membranes of the enterocytes initially are damaged by the ischemic process, thereby making the intracellular components more vulnerable to injury. The enzyme xanthine dehydrogenase is abundantly present in cell cytoplasm and, when exposed to the pancreatic enzyme trypsin, undergoes conversion to xanthine oxidase. This enzyme is responsible for the formation of active oxidants during reperfusion. Some experimental data suggest that allopurinol, an inhibitor of xanthine oxidase, may reduce the risk of reperfusion injury.

24. What is abdominal angina? What is its clinical significance?

Abdominal angina refers to chronic, recurring abdominal pain due to diminished arterial flow through the mesenteric arteries. Affected patients are often hyperlipidemic or diabetic or chronic tobacco users and have associated peripheral vascular (arterial) disease. Abdominal angina can be viewed as claudication of the gut. Most often, the equivalent exercise stimulus is a meal; the pain is experienced 30–90 minutes postprandially and can last up to 4 hours. Some authorities believe that as food enters the stomach and the demand for blood increases, the flow of blood to the small intestine diminishes ("stealing blood"). Patients often complain of sitophobia (fear of eating) and experience weight loss due to decreased caloric intake. Profound and prolonged hypoxia of small intestinal mucosa may result in villous atrophy and diarrhea as well as protein-losing enteropathy and steatorrhea. The mesenteric arteries are severely atherosclerotic, and patients may develop an acute thrombotic occlusion with bowel ischemia. However, most patients experiencing thrombotic occlusion of a mesenteric artery have not had antecedent abdominal angina.

25. What is the role of angioplasty and stenting in the management of abdominal angina?

Angioplasty with or without stent placement may have a role in some patients with intestinal angina. Lesions located at the aortic orifices of the mesenteric arteries are not readily amenable to angioplasty because of their fixed diameter, but more distal lesions can be dilated without the morbidity and mortality of surgical intervention.

26. Which patients with abdominal angina should undergo surgical revascularization?

Surgical revascularization probably should be limited to a few patients. Indications include typical, disabling symptoms of abdominal angina (chronic postprandial abdominal pain, sitophobia, weight loss), angiographic evidence of occlusion of at least two major mesenteric arteries, inclusive of the SMA, and acceptable risk for surgery. Whether multiple vessels or only the SMA should be revascularized is controversial..

27. Can ischemia be isolated to the colon?

Yes. Ischemic colitis is the most common form of intestinal ischemia. Most patients are older than 60 years and have experienced nonoperative or postoperative reduction in blood flow to the large intestine, but the condition can be encountered in younger patients with risk factors (vasculitides, coagulopathies, sickle cell disease, cocaine use, long-distance runners). Psychotropic drugs, danazol, and estrogen have been implicated.

28. What are the most common symptoms of ischemic colitis?

The most common symptoms are sudden crampy, mild left lower abdominal pain and urgency to defecate. In the postoperative state, mild symptoms are often dismissed. Bright red blood per rectum or hematochezia may be seen. Tenderness can be elicited over the involved segment of bowel.

29. How is ischemic colitis diagnosed?

If ischemic colitis is suspected and no features suggest peritoneal irritation, a colonoscopy should be undertaken to confirm the diagnosis. Any region of the colon may be affected, but the key endoscopic feature of ischemic colitis is the tendency for *segmental* distribution. The rectosigmoid (20%), descending colon (20%), splenic flexure (11%), and all three in combination (14%) are affected most commonly. Changes may be isolated to the rectum (6%) or right colon (8%). Flexible sigmoidoscopy may not disclose changes consistent with ischemic colitis isolated to the splenic flexure. When the rectosigmoid region is involved with sparing of the rectum, the diagnosis is strongly suspected. The rectum is involved infrequently because of its dual blood supply. Barium enemas are less sensitive than colonoscopy for detecting mucosal changes but may reveal thumbprinting changes due to submucosal edema and hemorrhage. Angiography is not indicated in ischemic colitis, because the predisposing nonocclusive vascular factors are not demonstrable by angiography once ischemic injury has occurred.

30. Can endoscopic findings or histologic features establish a definitive diagnosis?

Neither endoscopic findings (edema, submucosal hemorrhage, friability, and/or ulcerations) nor histologic findings (nonspecific inflammation, epithelial sloughing, subepithelial hemorrhage, cell drop-out and hemosiderin deposition in muscle layers) are specific enough to make a definitive diagnosis. But in the right clinical setting (i.e., acute systemic hypotension, aortic bypass surgery), the diagnosis can be made with a high degree of certainty. Infectious colitis and inflammatory bowel disease should be considered in the differential diagnosis.

31. What are the sequelae of ischemic colitis? Can anything be done to modify the course of the disease?

Ischemic colitis is reversible in up to 50% of patients. Symptoms abate within 24–48 hours, and healing occurs without stricture in 1–2 weeks. The severely injured colon may require 1–6 months to heal completely. Irreversible damage occurs in the remaining 50% and includes the following courses: gangrene and perforation, segmental colitis, fulminant colitis, and ischemic stricture. The course cannot be predicted at the time of initial presentation.

Optimizing cardiac function is imperative; impaired cardiac output and cardiac arrhythmias should be corrected. Factors predisposing to vasoconstriction, digitalis therapy, vasopressor agents, and hypovolemia should be avoided when possible. Vasodilating agents are ineffective because low colonic blood flow has already returned to normal by the time the ischemia has occurred. The bowel should be placed at rest, broad-spectrum antibiotics should be administered, and a distended colon should be decompressed. Urgent surgery is necessary only in rare cases of rapid progression of ischemic injury to gangrene and infarction.

BIBLIOGRAPHY

1. Brandt LJ, Smithline AE: Ischemic lesions of the bowel. In Feldman M, Scharschmidt BF, Sleisenger MH (eds): Sleisenger's and Fordtran's Gastrointestinal and Liver Diseases, 6th ed. Philadelphia, W.B. Saunders, 1998, pp 2009–2024.
2. Jacobson E: Intestinal ischemia. In Mcnally PR (ed): GI/Liver Secrets. Philadelphia, Hanley & Belfus, 1996, pp 403–414.
3. Marston A: Vascular Disease of the Gastrointestinal Tract. Baltimore, Williams & Wilkins, 1986, pp 1–15.
4. Nicoloff AD, Williamson WK, Moneta GL, et al: Duplex ultrasonography in evaluation of splanchnic artery stenosis. Surg Clin North Am 77:339–356, 1997.
5. Shanley CJ, Ozaki K, Zelenock GB: Bypass grafting for chronic mesenteric ischemia. Surg Clin North Am 77:381–396, 1997.
6. Smithline AE, Brandt LJ, Boley SJ: Acute and chronic mesenteric ischemia. In Brandt LJ (ed): Clinical Practice of Gastroenterology, vol. 1, Philadelphia, Current Medicine, 1999, pp 574–586.

63. NUTRITIONAL ASSESSMENT AND THERAPY

LTC Jonathan P. Kushner, M.D., and Sandra E. Smith, R.D., M.S.

1. What is meant by nutritional status?

Nutritional status reflects how well nutrient intake contributes to body composition and function in the face of the existing metabolic needs. The four major body compartments are water, protein, mineral, and fat. The first three compose the lean body mass (LBM); functional capacity resides in a portion of the LBM called the body-cell mass. Nutritionists concentrate their efforts on preservation or restoration of this vital component.

2. Define malnutrition.

Malnutrition refers to states of overnutrition (obesity) or undernutrition relative to body requirements, resulting in dysfunction.

3. How do different types of malnutrition affect function and outcome?

Marasmus is protein-calorie undernutrition associated with significant physical wasting of energy stores (adipose tissue and somatic muscle protein) but preservation of visceral and serum proteins. Patients are not edematous and may have mild immune dysfunction. **Hypoalbuminemic malnutrition** occurs with stressed metabolism and is common in hospitalized patients. They may have adequate energy stores and body weight but have expanded extracellular space, depleted intracellular mass, edema, altered serum protein levels, and immune dysfunction. A similar state of relative protein deficiency occurs in classic **kwashiorkor**, in which caloric provision is adequate but quantity and quality of protein are not.

4. At what point does loss of body protein affect muscle and immune function?

Muscle and immune function are affected by a loss of 20% body protein. Patients with 10–20% weight loss may have lost 20% of body protein and are at higher risk for a poor clinical outcome. A 40% loss of LBM is generally incompatible with survival. Adequate recent intake may improve function before a noticeable change occurs in composition or weight.

5. Explain the differences between unstressed starvation and stressed metabolism.

In **unstressed starvation**, the body uses fat stores to preserve functioning tissue. Obligatory glucose-utilizing tissues, such as brain and red blood cells, derive energy from liver glycogen stores and gluconeogenesis. Gluconeogenic precursors include muscle amino acids, particularly alanine. Fortunately, after several days of starvation, the brain adapts to ketones and muscle protein is spared. Urinary nitrogen excretion, 12–15 gm/day initially, falls to 3–4 gm in the adapted state. Survival for months is possible.

In **stressed metabolism**, hormones and cytokines mobilize lean tissue amino acids for the synthesis of needed reactive proteins and glucose. Unlike unstressed starvation, gluconeogenesis and amino acid mobilization are not easily suppressed by exogenous energy provision, and nitrogen losses remain high. The lean mass catabolism supports the host response early on; when prolonged, however, it has deleterious consequences, including shortened survival.

6. How do you perform a simple nutritional assessment?

Simple bedside assessment may be as valuable for predicting nutrition-associated outcomes as sophisticated composition and function tests. One popular method, the Subjective Global Assessment, incorporates basic questions about weight history, intake, GI symptoms, disease state, functional level, and a physical examination to classify patients as well-nourished, mildly to moderately malnourished, or severely malnourished.

A weight history, estimate of recent intake, brief physical exam, consideration of disease stress/medications, and assessments of functional status and wound healing allow a good estimate of nutritional status. They predict the risk for malnutrition-associated complications as well as or better than laboratory data. Poor intake for longer than 1–2 weeks, a weight loss of more than 10%, or a weight less than 80% of desirable warrants closer nutritional assessment and follow-up.

7. List desirable weights for men and women according to the 1983 Metropolitan Life Tables.
Men: 135 lb for the first 5 feet, 3 inches of height plus 3 lb per additional inch (±10%)
Women: 119 lb for the first 5 feet, 0 inches of height plus 3 lb per additional inch (±10%).

8. What additional tools and techniques are available for nutritional assessment?
Low levels of certain serum proteins (e.g., albumin, prealbumin, transferrin) may suggest hypoalbuminemic malnutrition but are nonspecific nutritional markers and should not be used as the only component of a nutritional assessment. They may decline rapidly under stress or after surgery, but they are relatively preserved in unstressed starvation. Hydration, renal function, and medications may also affect serum protein levels.
Markers of immunity, such as lymphocyte count and delayed hypersensitivity reactions, are impaired by malnutrition but again are nonspecific.
Some laboratory tests for micronutrients (red cell folate, vitamin B12, ferritin) may help to interpret total body status. Others (zinc, copper) are less available, unreliable markers of whole body status. Urinary creatinine-height index estimates of muscle mass and anthropometric measures of skinfolds and circumferences are less reliable tools in the clinical setting and may not be predictive of outcome. Bedside bioelectric impedance analysis discerns fat from fat-free mass but needs further validation in patient populations. Isotopic body water determination, underwater densitometry, dual x-ray absorptiometry, neutron activation analysis, and assays of involuntary muscle function are research tools.

9. What are the components of energy expenditure? How are they affected clinically?
Energy is required for the maintenance of the living state, performance of work, repletion, and growth in children. Energy is derived largely from macronutrient oxidation of carbohydrate, fat, and protein.
Caloric equivalents

Carbohydrate	4.0 kcal/gm	IV dextrose	3.4 kcal/gm
Protein	4.0 kcal/gm	Fat	9.0 kcal/gm

Total energy expenditure (TEE)
TEE = resting energy expenditure (REE) + thermic effect of feeding (TEF) + energy expenditure of activity (EEA)
REE is estimated from the basal energy expenditure (BEE) modified for disease state/stress (REE is often 25–30 kcal/kg or 1.0–1.5 × BEE) or measured by indirect calorimetry.
TEF = 10% of REE if meals are taken in a typical bolus fashion; it is negligible with continuous feeds.
EEA is quite variable. An additional 5–30% of REE is needed in hospitalized patients.

10. How is basal energy expenditure (BEE) determined?
The BEE is determined primarily by the LBM. When energy expenditure is estimated from standard equations, such as the Harris-Benedict equation, the body weight used for the calculation is critical. Use of an edematous weight overrepresents the LBM; therefore, dry weight is estimated in the case of edema. In addition, standard equations do not accurately predict energy expenditure in obese patients.

11. What are the advantages of using a metabolic cart?
We can directly measure the REE using indirect calorimetry with a metabolic cart. The EEA must be estimated and added to the REE. Use of the cart also provides the respiratory quotient (RQ):

$$RQ = VCO_2/VO_2$$

where VCO_2 = carbon dioxide output and VO_2 = volume of oxygen utilization. An RQ of 0.7 reflects pure fat oxidation; an RQ of 1.0, pure carbohydrate oxidation; and values between, mixed fuel oxidation. An RQ > 1.0 suggests that lipogenesis from carbohydrate exceeds fat oxidation; i.e., overfeeding. Although use of the metabolic cart has not been demonstrated to improve outcome, direct measurement overcomes the significant individual variability of energy expenditure and the limitations of predictive formulas.

12. Describe the types of commonly prescribed oral diets.

The **clear liquid** diet supplies fluid and calories in a form that requires minimal digestion, stimulation, and elimination by the GI tract. It provides about 600 cal and 150 gm carbohydrate but inadequate protein, vitamins, and minerals. Clear liquids are hyperosmolar; diluting the beverages and eating slower may minimize GI symptoms. If clear liquids are needed for > 3 days, a dietitian can assist with supplementation.

The **full liquid** diet is used often in progressing from clear liquids to solid foods. It also may be used in patients with chewing problems, gastric stasis, or partial ileus. Typically, the diet provides > 2000 cal and 70 gm protein. It may be adequate in all nutrients (except fiber), especially if a high-protein supplement is added. Patients with lactose intolerance need special substitutions. Progression to solid foods should be accomplished with modifications or supplementation, as needed.

13. Why do patients recovering from recent gastrectomy pose a special challenge?

In addition to the anorexia that is common during illness, such patients may suffer from early satiety, slow recovery of GI function, delayed gastric emptying, or dumping syndrome. They are at increased risk for iron, calcium, vitamin D, magnesium, and vitamin B12 malabsorption. The typical postgastrectomy diet limits simple sugars, size of meals, and fluids with solids but encourages fluids and snacks between meals.

14. When should nutritional support be considered?

Situations that warrant potential intervention with nutritional support (forced feeding) include:
- Protein and calorie deprivation for 7–10 days in a previously well-nourished or mildly malnourished adult
- Hypermetabolism or hypercatabolism and protein-calorie deprivation for > 4 days
- Moderate-to-severe degree of malnutrition at presentation
- Starved or critically ill children who are not consuming adequate oral intake

Whether nutritional support contributes to improved patient outcomes continues to be debated on editorial pages. The guidelines of the American Society for Parenteral and Enteral Nutrition are under revision, and several of the references cited address this difficult question. Until the data become clear, the goal of nutritional support should be to avoid unnecessary starvation, support the host, and improve quality of life while avoiding potentially dangerous overfeeding that benefits inflammatory or infectious processes more than the host.

15. What types of enteral formulas may be prescribed?

Classification of Adult Enteral Formulas

CATEGORY	EXAMPLES	CHARACTERISTICS	INDICATIONS
Blenderized	Compleat Mod.	Contains some blenderized whole foods. 1 kcal/ml. 16% of kcal as protein. Expensive. Unpalatable.	Regulation of bowel function. Long-term feeding. Normal digestive and absorptive capacity.
Standard	Isocal (HN), Osmolite (HN), Ensure (HN)	Low residue. 1 kcal/ml. 13–17% of kcal as protein. May have MCT. May or may not be palatable.	General feeding. Fairly normal digestive and absorptive capacity. Low fecal residue.

Table continued on following page

Classification of Adult Enteral Formulas (Continued)

CATEGORY	EXAMPLES	CHARACTERISTICS	INDICATIONS
Fiber supplemented	Ultracal, Jevity, Fibersource	10–14 gm fiber/L. 1 kcal/ml. 14–18% of kcal as protein. Generally unpalatable.	Regulation of bowel function. Long-term feeding. Normal digestive and absorptive capacity.
High protein	Promote, Replete, IsoSource VHN	1 kcal/ml. 20–25% of kcal as protein. Elevated levels of some vitamins and zinc. Some contain added fiber.	Catabolism. Wound healing. Normal digestive and absorptive capacity.
Concentrated	Magnacal, Deliver 2.0, Nutren 2.0, Two-Cal HN	1.5–2.0 kcal/ml. 14–17% of kcal as protein. 69–77% water. Hyperosmolar.	Fluid/volume restriction. Normal digestive and absorptive capacity.
Hydrolyzed protein	Vital HN, Peptamen, Alitraq, Vivonex Plus, Subdue, Crucial	Peptides and/or amino acids. Some have added glutamine and/or arginine. Most low in LCT. May have added MCT. Expensive.	Limited digestive and absorptive capacity. Limited evidence of superiority over standard.
Immune	Impact, Immun-Aid	Enriched with arginine, omega-3 fats, Glutamine and/or RNA. Low omega-6.	Major stress, trauma, surgery, respiratory failure.
Renal	Suplena, Nepro, Magnacal Renal	Restricted in water, Na, K, P, Mg, and vitamin A.	Supplement or total feeding during renal failure, predialysis or with dialysis.
Hepatic	Hepatic-Aid II, NutriHep	Higher in branched-chain amino acids; reduced in aromatic amino acids and methionine. Expensive.	Hepatic encephalopathy, when standard formulas are not tolerated.
Modular additives	Casec, ProMod, Polycose, Microlipid, MCT	Protein powder, glucose polymers, vegetable oil, MCT oil	To modify kcal:N ratio of base formula.

All formulas are lactose-free except Compleat.
MCT = medium-chain triglyceride, LCT = long-chain triglyceride.

Specialty formulas are available for respiratory failure and diabetes; however, research demonstrating their superiority over other products is limited.

16. What is the most feared complication of forced enteral feeding? What precautions should be taken?

Aspiration. Incidence depends on definition. The risk is highest in patients with compromised airway protection or poor gastric emptying (gastric residual $\geq$ 200 ml). Precautions include elevation of the head of the bed, avoidance of bolus delivery, and monitoring of gastric residuals. Prokinetic medications may be considered. If gastric attempts fail, consider postpyloric or jejunal access.

17. List the potential mechanical complications of forced enteral feedings. What precautions are appropriate?

Complications: nasopharyngeal/labial irritation, sinusitis, esophageal/laryngeal ulceration, tube displacement, feeding tube obstruction.

Precautions: use small-bore (10-French) nasal or oral feeding tubes; tape tube securely; verify tube placement; flush tube (20–30 ml water) before and after administration of medications and feedings; declog with distilled water or pancreatic enzymes and bicarbonate.

18. List the potential GI complications along with appropriate precautions/response.

1. **For nausea, vomiting, distention,** and **pneumatosis intestinalis**, precautions include use of continuous vs. bolus feeding; initiation of feeding at a low rate (20–25 ml/hr) with gradual increases; use of isotonic and lower fat formulas; and avoidance of feeding during hemodynamic instability.

2. For **diarrhea** and **infectious complications**, the appropriate responses include a stool assay for *Clostridium difficile*; modification of medications (e.g., dilution of hyperosmolar medications); slow infusion rate with gradual increases; dilution of hypertonic formulas; avoidance of feeding contamination and boluses of cold formula; supplementation with pancreatic enzymes (if needed); possible change to a defined or fiber-containing formula (especially soluble fiber); gradual administration of MCTs; and correction of severe hypoalbuminemia (< 2.0–2.5 gm/dl).

19. What are the most common metabolic complications? How can they be avoided?

Dehydration and hyperglycemia are best avoided by use of the appropriate formula; gradual advancement of feeding; monitoring of fluids, weight, and lab values, especially potassium, phosphorus, magnesium, and glucose; avoidance of overfeeding; and water supplementation.

20. When should an enterostomy replace a nasoenteric tube for enteral access? Which enterostomies are preferable?

When forced enteral feedings are likely to exceed 4–6 weeks' duration, an enterostomy may be preferable to a nasal tube for patient comfort, tube stability and prevention of sinusitis. In many instances, the percutaneous endoscopic gastrostomy (PEG) has replaced surgically placed gastrostomies. Cost and operative time are reduced. Immediate and longer-term morbidities have been equal in controlled trials. Complications (about 5–10%) may include tube displacement, peristomal leaks and infections, peritonitis, or fasciitis, although major complications are rare. Jejunal feeding may reduce reflux and possibly aspiration compared with gastric or duodenal feeds in patients at highest risk of aspiration. Options include a jejunal extension through a PEG or surgical jejunostomy.

21. Discuss the two basic types of parenteral nutrition.

The two basic types of parenteral nutrition are defined by the site of administration. Either peripheral or central veins may be used. About 75–85% of the kilocalorie and protein needs of most patients can be met in 2.4–3.0 L/day of **peripheral parenteral nutrition** (PPN), which is lower in dextrose, amino acids, and thus osmolality (600–900 mOsm/L). The most common limitation is phlebitis. Patients with good peripheral access, good fluid tolerance, and anticipated therapy duration < 7–10 days may be candidates for PPN; otherwise, central venous access is needed for **total or central parenteral nutrition** (TPN/CPN). Peripherally inserted central catheters may be used for TPN.

22. How is fat delivered in parenteral nutrition?

Parenteral solutions can be delivered as total nutrient admixtures, in which fat is added to the TPN solution, or the fat can be given separately via a Y-catheter or peripheral vein. There are advantages and disadvantages to each method.

23. Discuss the vitamin and mineral content of parenteral solutions.

The standard multivitamin supplement for adult parenteral nutrition contains all known vitamins (except vitamin K, which is found in adequate amounts in the soybean oil lipid emulsions or can be added separately). The adult multitrace-5 mineral supplement contains zinc, copper, chromium, selenium, and manganese. The essential role of some trace minerals was first identified when patients receiving TPN without these minerals presented with clinical and laboratory abnormalities that resolved after supplementation. TPN usually does not contain iron; it is not compatible in lipid-containing parenteral solutions, and most people, especially men, do not require it during short-term support. Long-term patients, especially children, who cannot obtain sufficient iron enterally may need parenteral iron supplementation.

24. What are the potential complications of parenteral nutrition?

Potential complications include pneumothorax during line placement, thrombosis, embolism, improper tip location, catheter-related sepsis, metabolic abnormalities, GI atrophy, and hepatobiliary abnormalities. As the number of lumens increases (from single to triple), so may the incidence of infection.

25. What precautions may help to prevent complications?

Strict adherence to insertion and dressing change protocols, confirmation of line placement, gradual increase in nutrient delivery, and frequent monitoring of clinical (volume) and lab status.

26. Define refeeding syndrome. discuss overfeeding.

Because patients can easily be given large amounts of kcal in TPN, including IV dextrose from other sources, previously starved patients may exhibit refeeding syndrome, defined as salt/volume overload and an acute drop in serum levels of potassium, phosphorus, and possibly magnesium. Overfeeding calories, especially dextrose (> 4-6 mg/kg/min in stressed patients), may result in hyperglycemia, increased CO_2 production, and hepatic steatosis. Excessive long-chain, omega-6 fat (> 1.5 gm/kg/day or infusion rate > 0.1 gm/kg/hr) may exceed clearance capacity and interfere with the reticuloendothelial system.

27. Discuss the common hepatobiliary abnormalities in patients receiving TPN.

Biochemical abnormalities may be seen within 1 week but are considered reversible in patients on TPN for < month. Of patients receiving long-term TPN, 15% exhibit persistent abnormalities. Cholestasis is an early finding in TPN-fed infants, but steatosis is the most common early finding in adults. TPN-related hepatic dysfunction may be more common in patients with severe underlying illness, preexisting liver disease, renal insufficiency, extreme short-bowel, and sepsis. Contributing factors may include toxic TPN products (photo-oxidized amino acids), overfeeding with dextrose or fat, an elevated insulin-glucagon ratio, gut disuse with endotoxin permeation, bacterial overgrowth with production of cholestatic bile acids, reduced cholecystokinin secretion with biliary sludge and stones, and deficiencies of choline, carnitine, glutamine, glutathione, and other methionine pathway products. Prevention and therapy consist of avoidance of overfeeding, provision of adequate protein, cycling of TPN, and gut use when possible. Additional therapies require further research.

28. What is a "hidden" source of calories in the ICU?

Watch out for significant amounts of lipid calories from propofol, a sedative in 10% lipid emulsion (1.1 kcal/ml).

29. Is enteral nutrition preferable to parenteral nutrition?

Nutrients are metabolized (e.g., "first pass") and may be utilized more effectively via the enteral than the parenteral route. Production of secretory IgA is maintained by enteral nutrition and may prevent bacterial adherence to the intestinal mucosa. Unlike TPN, most enteral products contain glutamine. Fiber-containing enteral formulas result in the production of short-chain fatty acids that promote intestinal and colonic growth. Catabolic response may be lessened and gut mucosal proliferation enhanced with early enteral nutrition. Enteral nutrition may result in less infectious morbidity and multiorgan failure compared with TPN. Despite these theoretical benefits, early enteral nutrition (compared with parenteral nutrition) has resulted in significantly better outcome only in selected populations (e.g., patients with trauma, acute pancreatitis). Obviously, enteral feeding has no venous catheter-related risks and costs less than TPN. Long-term patients, especially those with a short gut, experience more hepatic failure when they are primarily TPN-dependent. Therefore, when the gut works and can be used safely, use it!

30. A 66-year-old man with gastric cancer is 5 feet, 6 inches tall and weighs 125 lbs (20 lb weight loss before admission). He has been on ventilator support for 2 days after surgery. He is sedated and febrile. Calculate his current nutrient requirements and feeding plan.

The estimated BEE is 1240 kcal/day. The patient's current postoperative, febrile state may warrant a 20–30% increase. No thermic effects of feeding are taking place. His activity is minimal, warranting perhaps the addition of 5% to the REE. Thus, his estimated total daily energy expenditure is as follows:

$$1240 \text{ (BEE)} + 300 \text{ (stress)} + 60 \text{ (activity)} = 1600 \text{ kcal}$$

Alternatively, his REE may be measured by indirect calorimetry. In unstressed patients, provision of at least 125–150 gm of carbohydrate per day (1.2-2.0 mg/kg/min) spares the gluconeogenic amino acids that otherwise would be used for obligatory glucose production. Above that level, fat and carbohydrate are equivalent energy sources for protein sparing.

31. Calculate the protein requirements of the same patient.

Most healthy people require no more than 0.8 gm of protein/kg/day to maintain protein (nitrogen) balance. The average hospitalized patient requires 1.0–1.5 gm of protein/kg. A highly stressed patient often requires 1.5–2.0 gm of protein/kg/day. More than 2.0–2.5 gm of protein/kg may exceed the body's capacity for net protein utilization. In our sample patient, the provision of 85 gm/day (1.5 gm/kg) is a good starting point. Whereas a nonprotein calorie-to-nitrogen ratio of 150:1 is thought to be optimal for patients with mild-to-moderate stress levels, a 100:1 ratio may be more appropriate with severe stress. Whether total or nonprotein calories are used to meet the estimated energy requirement, care should be taken to avoid gross overfeeding.

32. What are the patient's fluid requirements? Vitamin and mineral requirements?

For fluid requirements, a simple estimation is 30–35 ml/kg for most adults; hence, 1680–1960 ml/day for the sample patient. This estimate may need to be revised based on postoperative fluid status and sensible and insensible losses. Vitamin and mineral requirements for hospitalized patients are not known. It is general practice to provide 100–200% of the recommended daily allowances (RDAs) for enterally delivered micronutrients and the American Medical Association-recommended daily levels of vitamins and trace minerals for parenteral administration.

33. What is your nutritional prescription for the sample patient?

In patients with good nutritional status preoperatively, nutritional support is appropriate if adequate oral intake is not attained or anticipated by 7–10 days postoperatively. In the sample patient, who had a 13% weight loss before admission, nutritional support, if not started preoperatively, may be considered earlier in the postoperative course. His intubated status precludes oral diets. If the gut is functional and he has no absolute contraindications, enteral tube feeding should be considered. In addition, because of the potential harm of overfeeding carbohydrate or omega-6 fat in stressed patients, the concept of "permissive underfeeding" of calories, with adequate protein and micronutrients, has found favor with many practitioners. Thus, the patient should be prescribed no more than 1600 calories/day with perhaps a slight reduction in the nonprotein calorie component.

Enteral formula (for 1600 kcal and 85 gm protein/day with no fluid or renal limitations). A high-protein formula (e.g., 1 kcal/ml, 50–60 gm protein/L) should be used, starting at 20–25 ml/hr and advancing to a goal rate of 65–70 ml/hr. If a lower protein formula is used, he may need the addition of a protein module.

Parenteral formula (if the patient's gut is unusable). PPN may be tried, if peripheral veins are adequate and short-duration use is anticipated. However, it takes 2.5–3.0 L/day of PPN to meet 80% of kcal/protein needs. If CPN/TPN is indicated, the following format may be used:

Protein grams = gm/kg × kg   e.g., 1.5 × 56 = 85 gm = 340 kcal

Dextrose grams = (50–80% nonprotein kcal)/3.4   e.g., 70% × 1260/3.4 = 260 gm

Fat grams = (20–50% nonprotein kcal)/10   e.g., 30% × 1260/10 = 38 gm

Volume. Minimal volume for these nutrients is about 1400–1500 ml/day, which is 26 ml/kg in the sample patient. Order a higher volume if desired.

Minerals. For approximately 2 liters of volume or 2000 kcal, average requirements are:

Sodium	60–180 mEq	Potassium	80–120 mEq
Chloride	60–180 mEq	Magnesium	12–30 mEq
Calcium	10–15 mEq	Phosphorus	20–30 mmol

Typical order for 1500 ml:

24 mEq sodium chloride	55 mEq sodium acetate
30 mEq potassium chloride	8 mEq calcium gluconate
12 mEq magnesium sulfate	18 mmol potassium phosphate

Acetate: chloride ratios may be altered, if needed (e.g., more acetate, less chloride for metabolic acidosis). Other electrolytes may be increased or decreased, as needed, to correct preexisting abnormalities or to provide more salt if greater volume is ordered.

Micronutrients: Standard multivitamin/ multitrace mineral solutions should be ordered.

Medications: Regular insulin may be added at two-thirds of prior doses or sliding scale requirements. Other compatible medications also may be added.

34. How is nitrogen balance estimated?

After a patient has had a stable intake for at least 2 days, a 24-hour urine collection can be analyzed for urine urea nitrogen (UUN). To calculate nitrogen balance, subtract the grams of the 24-hour UUN (plus about 4 gm for nonurea urine, skin, and fecal nitrogen losses) from the intake of nitrogen over 24 hours (grams of dietary protein divided by 6.25). This formula is grossly accurate only if the collection is complete, if glomerular filtration rate is > 50 ml/min, and if the patient does not have large nonurea nitrogen losses.

35. How is nitrogen balance interpreted?

Although negative nitrogen balance is undesirable, bed rest, high-dose corticosteroids, and poorly controlled disease may maintain the patient in negative balance despite adequate delivery of calories and protein. Optimal efforts may only attenuate some of the losses. If balance remains unsatisfactory, check electrolytes, acid-base status, and blood glucose control. Increase protein delivery, if tolerated, and assess energy requirements with a metabolic cart. Initiate enteral or oral feeding when possible. Do not overfeed a stressed patient for the sole purpose of achieving a neutral or positive nitrogen balance. Once the patient's medical condition has stabilized and, if possible, some ambulation resumed, a positive 2–4-gm nitrogen balance may be attainable.

36. Summarize the typical findings in deficiency or excess of various micronutrients.

Vitamin and Mineral Deficiencies and Toxicities

MICRONUTRIENT	DEFICIENCY	TOXICITY
Vitamin A	Follicular hyperkeratosis, night blindness, corneal drying, keratomalacia	Dermatitis, xerosis, hair loss, joint pain, hyperostosis, edema, hypercalcemia, hepatomegaly, pseudotumor
Vitamin D	Rickets, osteomalacia, hypophosphatemia, muscle weakness	Fatigue, headache, hypercalcemia, bone decalcification
Vitamin E	Hemolytic anemia, myopathy, ataxia, ophthalmoplegia, retinopathy, areflexia	Rare: possible interference with vitamin K, arachidonic acid metabolism; headache, myopathy
Vitamin K	Bruisability, prolonged prothrombin time	Rapid IV infusion: possible flushing, cardiovascular collapse
Vitamin C	**Scurvy:** poor wound healing, perifollicular hemorrhage, gingivitis, dental defects, anemia, joint pain	Diarrhea; possible hyperoxaluria, uricosuria; interference with glucose, occult blood tests; dry mouth, dental erosion
Vitamin B1 (thiamine)	**Dry beriberi** (polyneuropathy): anorexia, low temperature **Wet beriberi** (high-output congestive heart failure): lactic acidosis **Wernicke-Korsakoff syndrome:** ataxia, nystagmus, memory loss, confabulation, ophthalmoplegia	Large dose IV: anorexia, ataxia, ileus, headache, irritability
Vitamin B2 (riboflavin)	Seborrheic dermatitis, stomatitis, cheilosis, geographic tongue, burning eyes, anemia	None
Vitamin B3 (niacin)	Anorexia, lethargy, burning sensations, glossitis, headache, stupor, seizures **Pellagra:** diarrhea, pigmented dermatitis, dementia	Hyperglycemia, hyperuricemia, GI symptoms, peptic ulcer, flushing, liver dysfunction

Table continued on following page

Vitamin and Mineral Deficiencies and Toxicities (Continued)

MICRONUTRIENT	DEFICIENCY	TOXICITY
Vitamin B6 (pyridoxine)	Peripheral neuritis, seborrhea, glossitis, stomatitis, anemia, CNS/EEG changes, seizures	Metabolic dependency, sensory neuropathy
Vitamin B12	Glossitis, paresthesias, CNS changes, megaloblastic anemia, depression, diarrhea	None
Folic acid	Glossitis, intestinal mucosal dysfunction, megaloblastic anemia	Antagonizes antiepileptic drugs, decreases zinc absorption
Biotin	Scaly dermatitis, hair loss, papillae atrophy, myalgia, paresthesias, hypercholesterolemia	None
Pantothenic acid	Malaise, GI symptoms, cramps, paresthesias	Diarrhea
Calcium	Paresthesias, tetany, seizures, osteopenia, arrhythmia	Hypercalciuria, GI symptoms, lethargy
Phosphorus	Hemolysis, muscle weakness, ophthalmoplegia, osteomalacia	Diarrhea
Magnesium	Paresthesias, tetany, seizures, arrhythymia	Diarrhea, muscle weakness, arrhythmia
Iron	Fatigue, dyspnea, glossitis, anemia, koilonychia	Iron overload (hepatic, cardiac), possible oxidation damage
Iodine	Goiter, hypothyroidism	Goiter, hypo/hyperthyroidism
Zinc	Lethargy, anorexia, loss of taste/smell, rash, hypogonadism, poor wound healing, immunosuppression	Impaired copper, iron metabolism, reduced HDL, immunosuppression
Copper	Anemia, neutropenia, lethargy, depigmentation, connective tissue weakness	GI symptoms, hepatic damage
Chromium	Glucose intolerance, neuropathy, hyperlipidemia	None
Selenium	Keshan's cardiomyopathy, muscle weakness	GI symptoms
Manganese	Possible weight loss, dermatitis, hair disturbances	Inhalation injury only
Molybdenum	Possible headache, vomiting, CNS changes	Interferes with copper metabolism, possible gout
Fluorine	Increased dental caries	Teeth mottling, possible bone integrity/fluorosis

37. What nutritional problems are encountered in patients with inflammatory bowel disease (IBD)?

Causes of malnutrition in IBD include anorexia, active inflammation, steroid use, bleeding, malabsorption, protein-losing enteropathy, surgical loss of bowel, infections, and fistulous losses. Besides protein loss, patients with Crohn's disease may have difficulty with the absorption of fat and fat-soluble vitamins, vitamin B12, magnesium, zinc, and other trace nutrients. Diarrhea may lead to salt, water, and potassium depletion.

38. What are the therapeutic options for nutritional problems in patients with IBD?

Caloric requirements for noninfected patients with IBD may be 30–50% above BEE. Consider 1.5 gm/kg/day protein, perhaps up to 2 gm/kg in patients taking steroids or with significant losses of gut protein, fistulas, or bleeds.

Mild or quiescent IBD may be treated with a standard oral diet. Fat, lactose, or fiber restrictions may benefit selected patients. Patients with more active disease present the challenge of maintaining or restoring the nutritional state while alleviating the disease. Studies suggest that neither enteral nor parenteral nutrition with bowel rest is superior to medical therapy for inducing remission. Large-scale randomized trials to compare bowel rest/TPN with enteral use have not been done, but existing data show no difference in short-term remission rates. Similarly, amino acid or peptide-based formulas are generally no more successful than whole-protein products. The use of omega 3 fish oils may reduce the inflammatory response in patients with Crohn's disease or ulcerative colitis but has not yet demonstrated clinically significant durable effects.

A reasonable approach may be to combine medical therapy with enteral usage; an elemental or semielemental formula may be tried if food or polymeric formulas are not tolerated. Bowel rest/TPN should be reserved for unresponsive cases or when gut use is contraindicated (obstruction, toxic megacolon, severe ileus, substantial GI bleed, or a high-output fistula).

39. What are the nutritional concerns in patients with short bowel syndrome?

Loss of bowel surface puts the patient at great risk for dehydration and malnutrition. The small bowel averages 600 cm in length and absorbs about 10 L/day of ingested and secreted fluids. A patient may tolerate substantial loss of small bowel, although preservation of < 2 ft with an intact colon and ileocecal valve or < 5 ft in the absence of the colon and ileocecal valve may make survival impossible with enteral use alone. In addition, the loss of the distal ileum precludes absorption of bile acids and vitamin B12. Remaining bowel, especially ileum, may adapt its absorptive ability over several years, but underlying disease may hamper this process.

40. Describe the management of nutritional problems in patients with short bowel syndrome.

Therapy in the acute postsurgical phase is aimed at intravenous fluid and electrolyte restoration. Parenteral nutrition may be required while the remaining gut function is assessed and adaptation takes place. Attempts at oral feeding should include frequent, small meals with initial limitations in fluid and fat consumption. Osmolar sugars (e.g., sorbitol), lactose, and high-oxalate foods are best avoided. In patients with small bowel-colon continuity, increased use of complex carbohydrates may allow the salvage of a few hundred calories from colonic production and absorption of short-chain fatty acids. Antimotility drugs and gastric acid suppression should be used if stool output remains high. Oral rehydration with glucose- and sodium-containing fluids (e.g., sports drinks) may help to prevent dehydration. Pancreatic enzymes, bile acid-binding resins (if bile acids are irritating the colon), and octreotide injections may play a role in selected cases. If oral diets fail, the use of elemental feedings may enhance absorption and nutritional state. Studies of gut rehabilitation with growth hormone and glutamine, as well as intestinal or combined intestinal-liver transplantation, are available at selected centers.

41. Describe the approach to nutritional support in patients with acute pancreatitis.

Pancreatitis can resemble other cases of stressed metabolism. If severe pancreatitis precludes the resumption of food intake beyond 4–5 days, consideration should be given to nutrition support. The route of feeding remains controversial; neither bowel/pancreatic rest nor nutritional support has been shown conclusively to alter the clinical course beyond improvement of the nutritional state. Several recent randomized trials suggest that distal (jejunal) enteral feeding may be tolerated as well as bowel rest/TPN, with fewer complications. The enteral route may be tried in the absence of GI dysfunction (e.g., ileus). Energy expenditure is variable, but most likely only 20–30% above basal. Use PPN or TPN if the enteral approach fails. Experiments suggest that parenteral nutrition, including intravenous fat, elicits little significant pancreatic secretion; however, all patients with pancreatitis should be monitored to exclude severe hypertriglyceridemia.

42. What are the nutritional considerations in patients with advanced liver disease?

Because the liver is the "first-pass" organ for nutrients delivered via the enteral route, both acute and chronic liver disease pose challenges to the nutritionist. Amino acids, except for the branched-chain group (BCAAs—leucine, isoleucine, valine), are metabolized by the liver. Excessive levels of the aromatic amino acids may gain access across the blood-brain barrier (they share a carrier with the BCAAs) and predispose to hepatic encephalopathy in the form of false neurotransmitters. Many patients with chronic liver disease show signs of malnutrition attributable to reduced intake and a stressed metabolic state; thus, adequate protein delivery is desirable. Several randomized trials suggest a better outcome in malnourished cirrhotics who receive enteral nutrition support. Malnourished transplant candidates should receive adequate nutrition preoperatively.

43. What forms of protein should be used in patients with advanced liver disease?
The dilemma centers on adequate protein delivery without precipitation of encephalopathy. Although enteral protein may be more encephalopathic than intravenously administered amino acids, the enteral route of feeding should be used when possible. Current recommendations suggest starting with 0.8–1.0 gm/kg protein in oral diets or enteral formulas, with monitoring of tolerance. Vegetable protein produces encephalopathy less often than animal-derived protein. If tolerated, advance toward 1.5 gm/kg in catabolic patients. Standard protein should be restricted or a specialized hepatic formulation used (with high BCAA levels and low levels of aromatics and methionine) *only* if encephalopathy ensues and and standard medical measures fail. Some controlled trials of hepatic formulas suggest improvement in mental status in encephalopathic patients. As in other diseases that require limited amino acid delivery, adequate calories must be provided to minimize endogenous protein breakdown.

44. Discuss the role of conditionally essential nutrients.
Glutamine has become the prototypical conditionally essential nutrient. Not needed from exogenous sources in healthy people and traditionally omitted from TPN solutions (instability), it remains a primary fuel for intestinal cells and the immune system. In stressed illness, it is redistributed and may be relatively deplete. Evidence of improved outcome has accumulated in several controlled trials in which glutamine was provided with TPN.

Arginine, like glutamine, is a nonessential amino acid in healthy people. In larger doses, however, it may stimulate growth hormone secretion, the immune system, and wound healing. **Nucleotides**, present in food but absent from parenteral and traditional enteral preparations, play an important role in the immune response.

45. Why is modification of dietary fat an area of intense interest?
The most commonly used polyunsaturates, the **ϖ-6 vegetable oils** (corn, safflower, sunflower), may prove deleterious in higher quantities. Although their major component, linoleic acid, is essential to humans at 2–3% of total calories, it serves as the precursor for arachidonic acid, prostaglandins, and leukotrienes that, at higher levels, are immunosuppressive and proinflammatory. Fats of the ϖ-3 variety (linolenic acid or eicosapentenoic and decosahexanoic acid, the "fish oils") competitively inhibit the formation of the arachidonic acid-derived cicosanoids and may improve immune parameters and outcome.

Medium-chain triglycerides are used enterally because of ease of transport and oxidation, with less tendency to immunosuppression and hyperlipidemia. Structured intravenous lipids, using combinations of long-, medium-, and short-chain fats, are under investigation.

46. Why is enteral use of viscous dietary fiber important?
Enteral use of viscous dietary fiber may be an important source of nutrition to colonocytes and perhaps other organs.

47. Discuss the role of antioxidants.
Oxidative damage plays a major role in aging, critical illness, tumorigenesis, and vascular disease. Nutrients may act as both prooxidants (e.g., iron) and antioxidants (vitamins A, C, and E, β-carotene, selenium) in a finely balanced system. Epidemiology suggests that people with lower iron stores and higher antioxidant intake suffer less from cancer and cardiovascular disease. Thus far, controlled trials using pharmacologic doses of a number of antioxidants have failed to reduce disease occurrence as hoped. Large-scale trials are still under way, but at present, intake of plant-based foods that also contain other chemically active substances appears more

beneficial than large doses of isolated antioxidants. As in other metabolic manipulations, we must find the right balance between benefit and harm to the host.

48. Discuss the role of growth hormones and immunomodulating factors.

Trials using anabolic agents such as growth hormone, insulin-like growth factor, or anabolic steroids, in conjunction with nutritional support, have demonstrated improvements in lean body composition or function, but significant improvement in clinical outcome must still be demonstrated.

A number of recent randomized trials suggest that immunomodulating formulas may be superior to standard nutritional prescriptions in critically ill patients or surgical patients with GI cancer. Which conditionally essential nutrients in these combination formulas provide the benefit is not yet clear. Further studies are awaited.

49. What guidelines help in deciding whether to use nutritional support in a terminally ill patient?

Recent court rulings and consensus opinions have treated nutritional support as a form of medical therapy rather than an unquestionable necessity for all patients. Decisions about nutritional support should be based on sound medical and nutritional principles. It is more difficult to determine how much improvement in quality of life is gained from adequate nutrition. Forced feeding can have adverse consequences. Each patient should be evaluated as an individual, and the principles of patient autonomy, beneficence, and integrity should be respected.

50. Who should take vitamin or mineral supplements?

Studies have documented inadequate intake of some trace minerals and vitamins as people age. Some evidence indicates that taking a multiple vitamin-mineral supplement that provides close to RDA levels of nutrients may decrease morbidity in the elderly. In response to findings that 10–30% of people over 50 years old have some degree of dietary vitamin B12 malabsorption (due to inadequate pepsin and gastric acid), it is recommended that people over 50 obtain the 1998 RDA of B12 (2.4 μg/day) from synthetic B12 in fortified foods or supplements. Supplemental B12 also may be considered in anyone taking long-term gastric acid suppression.

Vitamin and trace mineral supplementation is generally indicated for people with significantly inadequate food intake, malabsorption or other causes of nutrient losses. Calcium supplementation, in addition to RDA levels of vitamin D, may be required to meet the RDA for some adults. Supplementation of any nutrient over the tolerable upper intake limit established by the Institute of Medicine should be discouraged unless prescribed and monitored by a physician.

51. What adverse GI effects may be encountered in a patient using herbal supplements?

It is estimated that one-third to one-half of the U.S. population uses herbal products in supplementary form and that 60–75% do not inform health care providers. Because herbal products are not regulated and their composition not standardized, toxicity data are less clear than with regulated pharmaceuticals. However, popular products that may cause adverse GI effects include saw palmetto, ginkgo biloba (nonspecific GI upset), garlic (nausea, diarrhea), ginseng (nausea, diarrhea), aloe (diarrhea, abdominal pain), and guar gum (obstruction). In addition, hepatotoxicity (ranging from asymptomatic enzyme elevation to fulminant necrosis) has been documented with germander, chapparal, senna, atractylis, and callilepsis. Hepatotoxicity associated with the use of valerian, mistletoe, skullcap, and various Chinese herbal mixtures has been noted but awaits a cause-and-effect confirmation. The pyrrolizidine alkaloids in crotalaria, senecio, heliotropium, and comfrey have long been implicated in cases of veno-occlusive disease.

BIBLIOGRAPHY

1. ASPEN Board of Directors: Guidelines for the use of parenteral and enteral nutrition in adult and pediatric patients. J Parent Ent Nutr 17(Suppl 4):1SA–52SA, 1993.
2. Bulger E, Helton W: Nutrient antioxidants in gastrointestinal disease. Gastroenterol Clin North Am 27:403–419, 1998.
3. Detsky A, McGlaughlin J, Baker J, et al: What is subjective global assessment of nutritional status? J Parent Ent Nutr 11:8–13, 1987.

4. Heyland D, MacDonald S, Keefe L, et al: Total parenteral nutrition in the critically ill patient: A meta-analysis. JAMA 280:2013–2019, 1998.
5. Heys S, Walker L, Smith I, et al: Enteral nutritional supplementation with key nutrients in patients with critical illness and cancer: A meta-analysis of randomized controlled clinical trials. Ann Surg 229:467–477, 1999.
6. Hill G: Body composition research: Implications for the practice of clinical nutrition. J Parent Ent Nutr 16:197–218, 1992.
7. Hunter D, Jaksic T, Lewis D, et al: Resting energy expenditure in the critically ill: Estimation vs. measurement. Br J Surg 75:875–878, 1988.
8. Institute of Medicine: Dietary reference intakes for vitamin C, vitamin E, selenium, and carotenoids. Washington, DC, National Academy Press, 2000.
9. Institute of Medicine: Dietary reference intakes for thiamin, riboflavin, niacin, vitamin B6, folate, vitamin B12, pantothenic acid, biotin, and choline. Washington, DC, National Academy Press, 1998.
10. Institute of Medicine: Dietary reference intakes for calcium, phosphorous, magnesium, vitamin D, and fluoride. Washington, DC, National Academy Press, 1997.
11. Klein S, Kinney J, Jeejeebhoy K, et al: Nutrition support in clinical practice: Review of published data and recommendations for future research directions. J Parent Ent Nutr 21:133–156, 1997.
12. McClave S, Snider H: Use of indirect calorimetry in clinical nutrition. Nutr Clin Pract 7:207–221, 1992.
13. Moore F, Feliciano D, Andrassy R, et al: Early enteral feeding compared with parenteral reduces postoperative septic complications: Results of meta-analysis. Ann Surg 216:172–183, 1992.
14. Pomposelli J, Bistrian B: Is total parenteral nutrition immunosuppressive? N Horiz 2:224–229, 1994.
15. Rombeau J, Caldwell M (eds): Clinical Nutrition: Enteral and Tube Feeding, 3rd ed. Philadelphia, W.B. Saunders, 1997.
16. Rombeau J, Caldwell M (eds):Parenteral Nutrition, 3rd ed. Philadelphia, W.B. Saunders, 2000.
17. Sandstrom R, Drott C, Hyltander A, et al. The effect of postoperative intravenous feeding (TPN) on outcome following major surgery evaluated in a randomized study. Ann Surg 217:185–195, 1993.
18. Solomon S, Kirby D: The refeeding syndrome: A review. J Parent Ent Nutr 14:90–97, 1990.
19. Tripp F: The use of dietary supplements in the elderly: Current issues and recommendations. J Am Diet Assoc 97(10 Suppl 2):S181–S183, 1997.
20. Veterans' Administration TPN Cooperative Study Group: Perioperative total parenteral nutrition in surgical patients. N Engl J Med 325:525–532, 1991.

64. CRITICAL EVALUATION OF MEDICAL LITERATURE

Ronald L. Koretz, M.D.

1. Most physicians read journal articles by perusing the abstract and, if the topic seems interesting, reading the discussion. What is wrong with this approach?

Most of us become overwhelmed with the amount of information that we have to learn to take care of patients; the medical literature reflects this overload. Thus, we tend to confine our perusal of any particular article to the abstract and discussion to "cut to the quick." A problem arises when the "message" (or at least what we think the message is) cannot be supported by the data.

Conclusions are only as strong as the evidence used to formulate them. Not all studies are created equal. The two critical parts of an original article are the methods and results sections. If the methodology is inadequate to answer the question posed, there is no point in reading the article.

A "structured abstract" is more objective. It explicitly describes the methodology and results. This type of abstract is recognizable by the subheadings. Unfortunately, it is usually more boring to read.

2. Why is so much emphasis placed on the randomized clinical trial (RCT)?

Randomization into groups is not needed to assess the natural history of an illness, to develop hypotheses about the cause of a disease, or to determine the sensitivity and specificity of a diagnostic test. The RCT is an issue only for considering the efficacy of an intervention (either diagnostic or therapeutic).

We employ interventions to reduce subsequent morbidity or mortality. Because the word "reduce" implies a lower incidence of an adverse event than otherwise would occur, we require insight into what would have happened if no, or some other, intervention had been done instead.

In a few clinical conditions, the outcome for an individual patient can be absolutely predicted; if an intervention alters that outcome, its effect is established. (We do not need RCTs to assess cardiopulmonary resuscitation or long-term hemodialysis.) However, these situations are the exceptions; for most proposed interventions, control groups are needed for comparison.

In laboratory experiments, interventions are tightly controlled so that only one variable is altered. In so doing, any subsequent difference in outcome can be attributed to that isolated intervention. This same principle is true in clinical research.

A nonrandomized control group (retrospective or prospective) must differ from an interventional group in at least two ways: the receipt or nonreceipt of the intervention and the reason(s) why it was or was not received. The RCT begins with a homogeneous population; the allocation into a treatment or control arm occurs by chance so the intervention is the only variable that differentiates the two groups. As such, the RCT is the gold standard for assessing efficacy. The important principle about the RCT is that it is randomized, not that it is prospective.

3. What is the difference between sensitivity/specificity and positive/negative predictive value?

These terms are used when we consider diagnostic tests. Sensitivity and specificity are derived from populations in which the disease is known to be present or absent. Sensitivity refers to the percentage of people with the disease who have a positive test. Specificity refers to the percentage of people without the disease who have a negative test.

However, patients do not come to doctors with the diagnoses written on their foreheads. (If they did, we would not need any tests.) Unless the sensitivity is 100%, we cannot be sure that a negative test means that the disease is absent. Similarly, if the specificity is not 100%, we cannot be sure that

453

a positive test means that the disease is present. The positive and negative predictive values quantitate the probability that the disease is present if the test is positive or absent if the test is negative. The predictive values of a test depend on the prevalence of the disease in the tested population.

Let us consider the use of a screening test that is 95% sensitive and 95% specific. Let us further assume that, in the population we have chosen to screen, 0.1% have the disease. For every 100,000 people, 100 (0.1% of them) have the disease and 95 (95% of those 100) have a positive test. A 95% specificity means that 5% of the people without the disease will demonstrate test positivity; thus, 4995 of those 99,900 have "false-positive" tests. Of the 5090 (4995 + 95) positive tests, only 95 represent true positives; the positive predictive value is 1.90%. Only 5 of the 94,910 negative tests are false negatives; the negative predictive value is 99.9947%. (Of course, the predictive value of simply guessing a negative status for any person is 99.9%.) In contrast, if we were to use a test with the same sensitivity and specificity in a population in which the prevalence of the disease was 50%, the positive and negative predictive values would each be 95%.

This example makes an important point about testing strategy. Even a very good test can create problems in populations in which the pretest probability (equivalent to the prevalence) of the disease is low. If the likelihood that the disease is present is low, doing any test will have a high potential for a false-positive result.

4. Given the above discussion as well as the complex statistical tests used in many articles, do you need to know a lot about mathematics to be able to read critically?

It is a mistake to confuse critical reading with mathematical expertise. The statistical tests used in most papers are usually correct, and one does not have to be able to reproduce such calculations to read the paper. The important factors in critical reading are common sense and the knowledge of a few basic principles.

5. What are the basic principles of critical reading?

1. We have already discussed the first principle. The type of study that best establishes efficacy (or causation) is the RCT, because it is the only study design that changes a single variable.

2. You cannot assume that an improvement in a "surrogate" (also known as an "intermediate") outcome will translate into an improvement in clinical outcome. For example, the older trials of ulcer therapies almost universally showed that H2 blockers healed the crater. However, in a number of such studies, the improvement in mucosal appearance was not accompanied by a reduction in the amount of pain perceived by the patient. One aspect of common sense is to view the outcome from the perspective of the patient. In this way, you will be less impressed by improvements in surrogate markers.

3. Association cannot establish causation. This misinterpretation is commonly made.

6. Give an example of the third principle.

Let us consider the case-control study (patients with a particular condition matched to patients with similar demographic features but without the condition) reported by Selby et al. The investigators compared patients who had died from colorectal cancer to controls who had not died from this disease (because at least the large majority of them did not have colon cancer). They found a statistically significant association between previous sigmoidoscopy and not dying of distal colorectal cancer. Such an association could be explained by the hypothesis that the sigmoidoscopy prevented the colon cancer (or at least mortality due to colon cancer); in other words, factor A (sigmoidoscopy) caused factor B (not dying of distal cancer).

While such studies (characteristically found in the epidemiologic literature) are useful in developing hypotheses, they cannot prove them. Remembering that association cannot prove causation forces you to think about other possible explanations for the results. For instance, were the people who underwent sigmoidoscopy more health-conscious? Did they practice other good health habits (e.g., eating fruits and vegetables and avoiding red meat) that prevented the cancer? If so, factor C (good health habits) accounted for both A (undergoing sigmoidoscopy because of a belief that it was a good health practice) and B (not developing, and therefore not dying of, distal colon cancer).

When Selby et al. compared patients who did or did not die of more proximal colon cancer (cancers that were too far from the rectal orifice for the sigmoidoscope to visualize them), the association between lower cancer mortality and sigmoidoscopy was not present. For this reason, the investigators discounted the role of health habits, believing that good ones should have protected against proximal cancer mortality as well.

The principle that association cannot prove causation is always true (even if you cannot think of an alternative explanation). In this case, what if distal and proximal colon cancers have different etiologies and the cause(s) of the proximal lesions is (are) not correctable by good health habits? For example, what if the cause of distal cancer was diet, but the cause of proximal cancer was drinking water or inspired air? The fact that another hypothesis can explain the findings means that the first hypothesis does not have to be accepted as true. The important corollary is that a study using a non-randomized control group cannot prove that a particular intervention produced a certain outcome.

Many epidemiologic articles seem to assert causation from demonstration of association. However, if you look closely, you usually observe that the actual sentence contains some modifier, such as "may" or "might." A good reading habit to develop is to insert a negative modifying adverb whenever you see a positive modifier. If A "might"cause B, it also "might not."

7. **Explain the difference between relative and absolute rate reduction.**
    Viewing the world through the patient's eyes also sensitizes you to the difference between relative and absolute rate reduction differences. The absolute rate reduction refers to the arithmetical difference between the incidences of the event in the treated and control groups. The relative reduction expresses the difference between the two groups as a percentage of the rate in the control group. For example, an intervention that reduces the incidence of a particular complication from 0.50% to 0.25% can be truthfully said to lower the complication rate by 50%. However, 400 patients would have to be treated to prevent one complication. Because patients bear the expense and risk of an intervention, the absolute rate reduction is a more realistic way to describe an effect to them.

Definitions of Absolute Risk Difference, Relative Risk Difference, and Odds Ratio

	OUTCOME IN TWO GROUPS	
	TREATMENT	CONTROL
With outcome	A	B
Number		
Without outcome	C	D

$$\text{Absolute risk difference} = \frac{A}{A + C} - \frac{B}{B + D}$$

$$\text{Relative risk difference} = \frac{A/A + C}{B/B + D}$$

$$\text{Odds Ratio} = \frac{A/C}{B/D}$$

8. **What is meant by "getting out of the box"?**
    Another component of common sense is to "get out of the box;" in other words, to look at the data from a perspective that is different from that of the investigators. We did so when we applied the interpretation of association and causation to the Selby study. Getting out of the box is not as difficult as it might seem, but it does require some practice. Whenever you read any study, spend a few moments trying to create an alternative explanation to the one(s) provided by the investigators.

9. **Since there is so much literature, why not just read review articles?**
    The standard review article ("narrative review") is written by a putative expert viewing the topic from his or her personal perspective. No matter how objective the author attempts to be, the

review must reflect some degree of bias. To cite an example, data from RCTs in the early 1970s demonstrated the efficacy of thrombolytic therapy in acute myocardial infarction, but recommendations for this treatment did not appear in textbooks until the late 1980s.

The narrative review should be contrasted with the "systematic review." Systematic reviewing arrives at a conclusion only after making an objective assessment of available data. The author identifies a specific question and writes a protocol in which the entire methodology, including the planned analyses, is explicitly stated. A systematic search for pertinent literature (especially RCTs) is then undertaken. Predetermined endpoints are assessed; the conclusions are driven by the data. In many systematic reviews, different trials are combined by a statistical technique known as meta-analysis. The entire process is analogous to a research project.

10. If the RCT is the gold standard for deciding the efficacy of a particular intervention, can the results of such a trial be accepted without question?

A number of problems can arise even within the context of a randomized trial. Many of them are not unique to RCTs.

Problems that Arise in Randomized Controlled Trials

PROBLEM	EXPLANATION
Type I error	Although apparent statistical significance is demonstrated, no true difference exists between the treatment arms
Type II error	Although no statistically significant difference was observed, a true difference does exist between the treatment arms
Randomization breakdown	Differences exist between the treatment arms other than the receipt of the therapy in question
Extrapolation of data	The patient population studied is not representative of the patients encountered in clinical practice
Lack of blinding	The outcome being measured has some degree of subjectivity, and the investigator was aware of the treatment arm
Surrogate endpoints	Use of endpoints that do not directly reflect clinical outcome
Treatment of control group	Control group received some form of therapy (standard or nonstandard) not provided to treatment arm
Subgroup analysis	Prospective (or even retrospective) identification of subgroups of patients in which effect of intervention is assessed

11. How are type I errors reflected?

Type I errors are reflected by the p value. If $p = 0.04$, there is a 4% probability that the difference arose by chance. Although 0.04 is less than the traditionally accepted 0.05, such a chance difference will occur once every 25 times. The type I error is particularly likely to arise when a large number of comparisons are made. If 25 independent comparisons are undertaken, there is a 72% probability that at least one of them will have a p value $= 0.05$.

12. When do type II errors arise?

Type II errors arise when real differences are not identified. They are likely to occur when studies are "underpowered" (insufficient numbers of patients enrolled). Consider a disease that is fatal in 85% of cases and a treatment that is almost universally life-saving. A randomized trial finds that the survival rates in the treated and control groups are 100% and 0%, respectively. It is then concluded that the treatment is ineffective because the p value is > 0.05. This situation may occur if only one patient is entered into each treatment arm.

13. What causes randomization breakdown?

Tables containing the demographic features of the patients in each treatment arm usually are provided to demonstrate that the groups were comparable. In "quasi-randomized" trials, allocation is based on such factors as day of the week or record number. Such trials tend to show larger treatment effects, probably as a consequence of unconscious, or even conscious, bias that results in the assignment of better-risk patients to the treatment arm (i.e., randomization breakdown). In this case, the investigator knows into which arm allocation will occur at the time that the patient is evaluated for the study.

14. When does extrapolation of data pose a problem?

Data from RCTs are not always extrapolatable to your particular patient. For example, a study assessing the effect of antibiotics for *Helicobacter pylori* in treating ulcer disease is not necessarily applicable to patients in whom the disease is due to aspirin.

15. What problems may be involved with blinding?

Double blinding (both patient and investigator are unaware of the treatment employed) is an issue when subjective endpoints (e.g., pain or quality of life) are measured. This principle was elegantly demonstrated in two RCTs assessing the role of internal mammary artery ligation for treating cardiac angina. The use of sham surgery demonstrated that the placebo response rate to an invasive procedure may be very high, on the order of 75%. However, even apparently objective endpoints can have subjective components. For example, is the shadow on the chest radiograph pneumonia or only a confluence of interstitial markings? If the radiologist is not blinded, his or her bias may have an effect.

16. How may the control group pose a problem?

We usually envision a control group as one that is afforded no special treatment. However, this is not always the case. The ω-3 fatty acids found in fish oil are believed to be precursors of less proinflammatory cytokines than are the ω-6 fatty acids found in other foods. Trials comparing fish oils with placebos have suggested that the former reduces the inflammation of ulcerative colitis. However, the "placebo" was vegetable oil. If the original hypothesis is true, the difference may have been due to the fact that the controls were provided with excessive amounts of proinflammatory cytokine precursors (i.e., the controls received harmful therapy).

17. Discuss the problems involved in subgroup analyses.

It is difficult for most investigators to resist undertaking subgroup analyses. Such analyses assume that the randomization is still intact within the subgroups; this is not always the case. Bower et al. compared an experimental to a standard enteral feed in critically ill patients, using duration of stay in the hospital as an endpoint. The data were assessed only for the survivors, and duration of stay was allegedly shorter in those who received the experimental diet. However, the mortality rate in recipients was twice as high as in controls (p = 0.06). The authors justified this subgroup analysis because the mortality difference "was not statistically significant." Sicker patients are more likely to die and also to be hospitalized longer. Thus, fewer high-risk patients remained in the experimental group, and the randomization was no longer intact.

It is important to build any proposed subgroup analyses into the original protocol. It is too easy, after the fact, to scan the data and have your eye (or the computer) identify apparent differences. Such after-the-fact observations are not based on chance, and traditional p values have no meaning.

18. What is the difference between "per-protocol" and "intent-to-treat" analsyes?

A variant of subgroup analysis occurs when "per-protocol" rather than "intent-to-treat" analyses are used. In the former, only the patients who actually received the intervention are counted; in the latter, all patients are counted, even if they dropped out of the study.

19. What is the rationale for intent-to-treat analyses?

The randomization is most intact at the outset of the trial. Per-protocol analysis assumes that the remaining groups are still comparable. If patients drop out for some systematic reason, those who remain at the end are no longer representative of the entire group. Consider the trials that compared elemental diets to steroids in active Crohn's disease. Some RCTs excluded patients who could not tolerate the diet. Patients who could not tolerate the diet may have had more severe intestinal inflammation; there was no way to identify the comparable patients in the steroid arm. Hence, in the per-protocol analysis, sicker patients may have been selectively removed from only one arm, thereby creating a bias favoring that group. The per-protocol analyses showed no difference in outcome, and the investigators concluded that the two treatments were equivalent. However, trials that employed intent-to-treat analysis demonstrated that steroids produced remissions more often.

20. What is meta-analysis?

When several trials assess the same therapy and measure the same outcome, it is tempting to add the data together, a process known as "data-pooling." Meta-analysis combines data from similar trials, but only after each trial is weighted. The weighting factor is based on the **variance**; studies with lower variances (lower standard deviations or narrower confidence intervals) are weighted more heavily. Although meta-analysis is most commonly used to combine RCTs, the technique can be applied to other types of studies.

21. What are the advantages of data combination?

1. The first advantage relates to **precision**. A clinical study does not reveal absolute truth but rather a statistical approximation of truth. If one repeats a trial several times, the numbers vary each time, but they tend to group around the real truth. This concept can be appreciated by considering the process of coin flipping. If you flip an unloaded coin 10 times, in theory it should come up heads 5 times and tails 5 times. In reality, however, this theory usually does not apply. The coin may come up heads 6 times (60%) on the first occasion and tails 6 times on the second. If you flip the coin 100 times, it is less likely that heads or tails will appear 60% of the time; in other words, the variance from this larger experiment is lower, which is why meta-analysis usually weights larger trials more heavily. If you do this experiment many times and total the numbers, heads and tails will each appear about one-half of the time. Hence, the estimated effect calculated from meta-analysis (or even data-pooling) is better defined (more precise).

2. The second advantage relates to the **type II error**. Data combination provides a larger number of patients in the sample and thus increases the power of the observation. Meta-analysis formulas can report the result as the absolute risk difference, relative risk difference, or odds ratio (see table in question 7). The odds ratio is the most difficult of the three to comprehend intuitively. The number represents the odds that an event will occur in the treated group divided by the odds that it will occur in the control group. While an odds ratio is not the same as a relative risk difference, when the incidences in both groups are small, the two are very similar. (Assume that A and B are both small numbers in the formula in question 7.)

22. How is significance defined?

Significance traditionally is defined by the 95% confidence interval. The 95% confidence interval of a significant absolute risk difference does not overlap 0; a significant relative risk difference or odds ratio has a 95% confidence interval that does not overlap 1.

23. What are the problems with meta-analysis?

Meta-analysis is a **retrospective** process. One is limited to the trials and data that are available. It is also easy to make mistakes in abstracting the data; thus, provision should be made to do the abstraction at least twice and to resolve any differences that arise.

The most important drawback to data combination is that the trials are almost always different in some way, a phenomenon termed **heterogeneity**. If the trials are too heterogeneous, it makes no sense to try to combine them. For example, you would not combine survival data only from studies of emergent surgery for ruptured aneurysms and laparoscopic cholecystectomy to calculate postoperative mortality.

24. How can the problems associated with heterogeneity be addressed?

There are several ways to deal with heterogeneity. Its presence can be detected with a statistical test, although this approach is relatively insensitive. The **random effects model** is used to combine more heterogeneous data; this computation tends to produce the same risk difference or odds ratio but a wider confidence interval. Most often, one simply uses common sense to decide whether there is too much heterogeneity to attempt the combination.

Heterogeneity can be explored to look for potentially important confounding clinical variables, a process called **sensitivity** or **subgroup analysis**. The reviewer determines what factor(s) is (are) likely to account for the heterogeneity and then combines only those trials that contained that (those) particular factor(s). For example, if one is assessing the effect of beta blockers in preventing variceal bleeding, one may do subgroup analyses separating each cause of cirrhosis or type of beta blocker. It is important to decide on these factors beforehand. When the decision is made after the fact, the same issues that create problems with subgroup analyses of individual RCTs (e.g., unconscious identification of chance events) can arise.

25. What is evidence-based medicine?

Evidence based medicine (EBM) requires the incorporation of research data (especially high-quality data) into clinical decision making. However, although EBM requires consideration of the data, the ultimate decision does not rest solely on the results of published research. EBM is a multistep process that begins with a systematic review of the medical literature. A question is identified, the kind of data that will best answer the question is determined, and a search strategy is developed to find all of the pertinent publications.

Most commonly, such searches are conducted using a database known as MEDLINE, a collection of all articles published in the journals catalogued by the National Library of Medicine (the electronic equivalent of Index Medicus). MEDLINE can be accessed through the Internet by various addresses (e.g., National Library of Medicine [http://igm.nlm.nih.gov]). Because RCTs have been specifically labeled as such only recently, computer searches can miss large numbers of reports that were published before 1990. The data from the identified papers are critically reviewed, and a conclusion is derived. At times, the conclusion may be only that no reliable data are available.

The conclusion should be consistent with the known physiology and laboratory findings. If it is not, one needs to reexamine his or her conclusion as well as his or her understanding of the pathophysiology and laboratory research. If the conclusion does not agree with the prior knowledge, one, the other, or even both must be wrong.

Finally, the particular values and desires of the patient have to be incorporated. An EBM decision is a composite result of data-based conclusion, other knowledge, and the patient's values.

26. Does a source of systematic reviews or RCTs already exist so that I do not have to start from scratch each time?

A number of organizations are assembling collections of RCTs and/or systematic reviews. The Cochrane Collaboration is dedicated to the generation, maintenance, and dissemination of systematic reviews in all areas of health care. All of the systematic reviews produced by this group so far are available in a computer disc format called the Cochrane Library. The Cochrane Library also contains an index of all published RCTs and systematic reviews that the group has identified by hand-searching individual medical journals. It is updated every 3 months. The Cochrane Library is usually available in medical libraries; individual subscriptions can be purchased for about $300 per year. Abstracts of the systematic reviews are available free of charge on the Internet.

Other CD-ROM sources include Best Evidence and UpToDate. Best Evidence contains structured abstracts of articles believed to be methodologically sound and clinically relevant. UpToDate is another source of high-quality clinical trials.

27. Why do all of this work? Isn't it easier just to do what everyone else does or tells me to do?

The problem with doing what everybody else does is that many such practices have been encouraged by dogmatic pronouncement, are often not based on any evidence, and are even incorrect.

We live in a resource-limited medical environment, and we should prioritize those resources for activities for which available data establish efficacy.

28. Give an example by critically evaluating the literature advocating antiviral treatment of chronic hepatitis C.

The table below summarizes the arguments promoting antiviral treatment of chronic hepatitis C:

Observations Used to Support Antiviral Treatment of Hepatitis C*

Epidemiologic observations
1. There are 2,700,000 hepatitis C carriers in the United States, and there are 10,000 deaths or liver transplants annually due to hepatitis C. (Reference: Alter, 1999; Koretz, 1992.)
2. Retrospective and prospective natural history studies from tertiary liver centers indicate that a large percentage (?50%) of patients with chronic hepatitis C develop liver failure or cancer. (Reference: Tong, 1995.)
3. Hepatitis C is most common cause of liver failure requiring transplantation. (Reference: Koretz, 1992.)

Outcome after treatment
4. Using combination therapy (interferon and ribavirin), 30–40% of treatment-naive patients will develop a sustained virologic response (i.e., become and remain negative for hepatitis C-RNA in the serum). (Reference: Poynard, 1998.)
5. Patients who respond to treatment do not develop end-stage liver disease or cancer. (Reference: Marcellin, 1997.)
6. Data from retrospective studies suggest that patients who are treated with interferon have better long-term courses than do those who are not treated. (Reference: Brunetto, 1998.)
7. One RCT indicated that interferon therapy produced a reduction in the subsequent rate of development of hepatocellular cancer. (Reference: Nishiguchi, 1995.)
8. When calculated on a cost per year of life saved, analyses have suggested that the economic investment for antiviral therapy is comparable to other interventions undertaken in medicine. (Reference:Younossi, 1999.)

• See text below for discussion of the limitations of these observations.

Taking these claims at face value probably would lead to a decision to treat, even though the drugs are expensive and cause side effects universally. However, the decision is not as straightforward as it may seem.

There are a large number of carriers in the United States, and hepatitis C (often complicated by concomitant alcohol usage) is the single most common cause for the liver disease at transplant centers. However, the natural history as defined by tertiary referral centers does not reflect the natural history of all patients, primarily because sicker patients are included in the studies because of referral bias. These experiences overestimate the rate of progression of the disease and the subsequent incidence of bad outcomes.

Prospective studies of cohorts of patients identified at or near the time of infection with hepatitis C have painted a different picture. The incidence of liver failure has been about 10%, not 50%. Even 10% of a large number of patients will produce a burden for transplant centers. The existence of 2,700,000 carriers, but only 10,000 annual hepatic events, also tells us that the large majority of infected patients will never get into trouble. It would take 270 years to exhaust the supply of carriers if only 10,000 were removed each year.

The RCTs that have assessed the therapeutic value of antiviral treatment, with one exception, have used a surrogate endpoint, not a clinical one. We will return to this subject shortly, when we consider the true treatment effect.

The single RCT that addressed a clinical issue compared interferon with no interferon in patients with hepatitis C and cirrhosis. Nishiguchi et al. claimed that treatment reduced the subsequent incidence of hepatocellular carcinoma. However, the conclusion was based on a subgroup analysis. Patients in the treatment arm who failed the first course of therapy were supposed to be retreated; those who refused were dropped from the trial and lost to follow-up. Hence, the patients in the control arm were followed for a longer period on average; it should not be surprising that more cancers were identified in them. Furthermore, all treated patients who dropped out were nonresponders and probably at a higher risk of developing cancer. Thus, further bias was created in favor of the treated group, because the matching higher-risk patients were not dropped from the control arm.

The other data that evaluated long-term outcomes, especially cancer, were retrospective studies comparing patients who were treated with those who were not. Association cannot establish causation. If the untreated patients were not treated because they had more advanced disease, it would not be surprising that they subsequently had worse long-term courses.

What about the effect of treatment? We believe that 30–40% of treated patients will have a serologic response and that 10% of infected patients will get into trouble. Assuming that a serologic response is important, in order for the treatment to have any effect, those two minorities must overlap. If they do not, responders will have good long-term outcomes even if they are not treated, and all of those destined to develop end-stage liver disease will do so despite therapy.

Responders tend to have more recent infection, lower titers of virus in their blood stream, little if any evidence of fibrosis on liver biopsies, and infection with more benign genotypes. Thus, treatment response is not a random event. Responders appear less likely to develop end-stage liver disease in the first place. More importantly, patients destined to get into trouble are less likely (perhaps not likely at all) to respond to therapy.

The favorable conclusions of the cost analyses were based on a number of problematic assumptions. The natural history component of the models was based on data from tertiary referral centers. These models estimated that about one-half of infected patients would develop end-stage liver disease. This overestimation inflated the treatment effect. The analyses also assumed that a 30–40% response rate translated into a 30–40% reduction in the incidence of liver failure, a situation that is unlikely to be true.

Thus, critical evaluation of the data indicates that we do not know whether treatment is effective. The drug causes side effects (including occasional deaths) and is a drain on economic resources.

This exercise was an attempt to demonstrate why it is important to get out of the box and examine data critically. We must base therapeutic decisions on hard clinical data, not on unsubstantiated opinion or marketing programs. Because medicine will continue to be both resource-limited and filled with more interventional opportunities, critical reading and thinking are essential skills for all of us to develop and practice.

ANNOTATED BIBLIOGRAPHY

1. Alter MJ, Kruszon-Moran D, Nainan OV, et al: The prevalence of hepatitis C virus infection in the United States, 1988 through 1994. N Engl J Med 341:556–562, 1999. See question 28.
2. Antman EM, Lau J, Kupelnick B, et al: A comparison of results of meta-analyses of randomized control trials and recommendations of clinical experts. Treatments of myocardial infarction. JAMA 268:240–248, 1992. The delay in incorporating data from randomized controlled trials in review articles.
3. Bond JH, Koretz RL, Gitnick G: Colon cancer screening: Is it justified? Med Crossfire 1(2):31–41, 1999. Another explanation for the findings of Selby et al (reference 19).
4. Bower RH, Cerra FB, Bershadsky B, et al: Early enteral administration of a formula (Impact®) supplemented with arginine, nucleotides, and fish oil in intensive care unit patients: Results of a multicenter, prospective, randomized, clinical trial. Crit Care Med 23:436–449, 1995. Subgroup analysis in which randomization is no longer intact.
5. Brunetto MR, Oliveri F, Koehler M, et al: Effect of interferon-α on progression of cirrhosis to hepatocellular carcinoma: A retrospective cohort study. Lancet 351:1535–1539, 1998.
6. Cobb LA, Thomas GI, Dillard DH, et al: An evaluation of internal-mammary-artery ligation by a double-blind technique. N Engl J Med 260:1115–1118, 1959. Use of sham surgery to maintain blind.
7. Collen MJ, Hanan MR, Maher JA, et al: Cimetidine vs placebo in duodenal ulcer therapy. Six-week controlled double-blind investigation without any antacid therapy. Dig Dis Sci 25:744–749, 1980. Healing ulcer craters did not improve pain symptoms.
8. Dickersin K, Hewitt P, Mutch L, et al: Perusing the literature: Comparison of MEDLINE searching with a perinatal trials data base. Cont Clin Trials 6:306–317, 1985. Computer searching misses many randomized controlled trials.
9. Dimond FG, Kittle CF, Crockett JE: Comparison of internal mammary artery ligation and sham operation for angina pectoris. Am J Cardiol 5:483–486, 1960. Use of sham surgery to maintain blind.
10. Koretz RL: Acute hepatitis: Science and superstition. In Gitnick G (ed): Current Hepatology, vol 12. St. Louis, Mosby, 1992, pp 1–51.
11. Koretz RL: Decisions, decisions, decisions. Gastroenterology 118:1268–1269, 2000. Discussion of problems with assumptions in hepatitis C treatment cost analyses.

12. Lau J, Ioannidis JPA, Schmid CH: Quantitative synthesis in systematic reviews. Ann Intern Med 127:820–826, 1997. Basics of meta-analysis.
13. Malchow H, Steinhardt HJ, Lorenz-Meyer H, et al: Feasibility and effectiveness of a defined-formula diet regimen in treating active Crohn's disease. Scand J Gastroenterol 25:235–244, 1990. Use of intent-to-treat analysis led to correct conclusion.
14. Marcellin P, Boyer N, Gervais A, et al: Long term histologic improvement and loss of intrahepatic HCV RNA in patients with chronic hepatitis C and sustained response to interferon-a therapy. Ann Intern Med 127:875–881, 1997.
15. Nishiguchi S, Kuroki T, Nakatani S, et al: Randomised trial of effects of interferon-α on incidence of hepatocellular carcinoma in chronic active hepatitis C with cirrhosis. Lancet 346:1051–1055, 1995.
16. Poynard T, Marcellin P, Lee SS, et al: Randomised trial of interferon α2b plus ribavirin for 48 weeks or for 24 weeks versus interferon a2b plus placebo for 48 weeks for treatment of chronic infection with hepatitis C virus. Lancet 352:1426–1432, 1998.
17. Saverymuttu S, Hodgson HJF, Chadwick VS: Controlled trial comparing prednisolone with an elemental diet plus nonabsorbable antibiotics in active Crohn's disease. Gut 26:994–998, 1985. Failure to employ intent-to-treat analysis led to incorrect conclusion.
18. Schulz KF, Chalmers I, Hayes RJ, Altman DG: Empirical evidence of bias. Dimensions of methodological quality associated with estimates of treatment effects in controlled trials. JAMA 1995; 273:408–412, 1995. Non/quasirandomized controlled trials demonstrate larger treatment effects.
19. Selby JV, Friedman GD, Quesenberry CP, Weiss NS: A case-control study of screening sigmoidoscopy and mortality from colorectal cancer. N Engl J Med 326:653–657, 1992. A case-control study in which association is frequently misinterpreted as causation.
20. Stetson WF, Cort D, Rodgers J, et al: Dietary supplementation with fish oil in ulcerative colitis. Ann Intern Med 116:609–614, 1992. Randomized controlled trial in which control patients received potentially harmful "placebo."
21. Tong MJ, El-Farra NS, Reikes AR, et al: Clinical outcomes after transfusion-associated hepatitis. N Engl J Med 332:1463–1466, 1995.
22. Younossi AM, Singer ME, McHutchison JG, Shermock KM: Cost effectiveness of interferon α2b combined with ribavirin for the treatment of chronic hepatitis C. Hepatology 30:1318–1324, 1999.

65. POTPOURRI: NAUSEA AND VOMITING, HICCUPS, BULIMIA/ANOREXIA, RUMINATION

Steven S. Shay, M.D.

NAUSEA AND VOMITING

1. How is vomiting distinguished from regurgitation?

Vomiting is characterized by the presence of nausea and autonomic symptoms, such as salivation, followed by the forceful abdominal and thoracic muscle contractions associated with retching. In contrast, regurgitation is the sudden, effortless return of small volumes of gastric or esophageal contents into the pharynx and implies cricopharyngeal relaxation or insufficiency.

2. What disorders characteristically present with regurgitation?

Chronic regurgitation may result from oropharyngeal or esophageal disorders or gastroesophageal reflux. Patients with Zenker's diverticulum may accumulate secretions and food that empty into the pharynx, especially at night. Structural lesions, such as esophageal cancer, may obstruct the esophagus. Esophageal diverticula may cause accumulation of food particles and secretions and result in regurgitation when the contents are discharged into the esophageal lumen. Esophageal motility disorders, such as achalasia and primary esophageal spasm, also may be responsible for regurgitation.

3. What are the reflex pathways involved in the act of vomiting?

The vomiting center, located in the medulla, is composed of many efferent nuclei in serial communication with each other. When the entire circuit is activated by afferent stimuli, the complete act of vomiting occurs. However, some stimuli trigger only individual components of the vomiting act and result in nausea or salivation.

Three afferent limbs carry stimuli to the vomiting center: (1) vagal and sympathetic afferents from the GI tract, vestibular system, and heart; (2) the chemoreceptor trigger zone (CTZ) in the area postrema of the floor of the fourth ventricle, which can be stimulated by emetogenic toxins or drugs, such as digitalis and chemotherapeutic agents; and (3) loci high in the central nervous system (CNS).

4. What disorders must be considered in acute nausea and vomiting?

- Intraabdominal disorders
  Gastrointestinal
    Mechanical obstruction
      Stomach
      Small bowel
    Pseudo-obstruction
  Peritonitis
  Acute pancreatitis
  Acute cholecystitis
- Infections
  Epidemic (e.g., Norwalk agent)
  Viral hepatitis
- Toxins
  Staphylococcus aureus
  Bacillus cereus
  Clostridium perfringens
- Metabolic disorders
  Renal failure
  Ketoacidosis (e.g., diabetes)
  Addison's disease
- Central nervous system disorders
- Vestibular disorders
- Pregnancy
- Drugs
  Narcotics
  Digitalis
  Aminophylline
  Chemotherapeutic drugs

5. What specific symptoms or characteristics of acute nausea and vomiting should be sought to narrow the differential diagnosis?

The presence of abdominal pain strongly suggests an intraabdominal process as the cause of acute nausea and vomiting, and the character of the pain, physical findings, and initial routine diagnostic laboratory tests (e.g., amylase, liver tests, complete blood count) direct the subsequent diagnostic evaluation. Suspicion for peritonitis requires recumbent and upright abdominal radiographs, including the diaphragm, to exclude the presence of free air under the diaphragm. In contrast, the abdominal radiograph in patients with colicky pain may confirm the presence of obstruction (mechanical or pseudo-obstruction). Suspicion of biliary colic or acute cholecystitis requires ultrasound and/or hepato-iminoacetic acid (HIDA) scan, whereas pancreatitis is typically first suspected because of an increased amylase level.

The presence of systemic symptoms such as fever or diarrhea suggests the possibility of food poisoning with one of several toxins or an infection. Other systemic symptoms, such as polyuria and polydipsia, suggest a metabolic disorder. A chemistry screen should be obtained to exclude such disorders.

The presence of abnormal mental status, headache, meningismus, or a preceding head injury suggests the possibility of a CNS etiology and should prompt appropriate investigation. A history of vertigo or the presence of nystagmus suggests a motion disorder rather than CNS disease.

If there are no systemic symptoms, abdominal complaints, or CNS symptoms or signs, several other considerations should be entertained. The possibility of pregnancy should be considered early in any evaluation of nausea and vomiting. Serum and/or urine human chorionic gonadotropin levels should be obtained to avoid tests using radiation. All medications should be reviewed to exclude the possibility of drug-associated nausea and vomiting. Finally, Addison's disease needs to be considered.

6. What are the major etiologic considerations for chronic nausea and vomiting? How are they evaluated?

Disorders that typically present with chronic nausea and vomiting are (1) functional gastric outlet obstruction (gastroparesis), (2) small bowel dysmotility, and (3) psychogenic vomiting. One historical clue is that all of these disorders typically present with repeated postprandial vomiting.

7. Define gastroparesis. How is it diagnosed?

Gastroparesis is defined as an impairment in gastric emptying in the absence of mechanical obstruction in the stomach or small bowel. It may be seen with certain drugs (e.g., narcotics), after gastrectomy, in patients with diabetes, scleroderma, or amyloidosis, or for no apparent reason (idiopathic). It is often difficult to distinguish idiopathic gastroparesis from psychogenic vomiting. Radionuclide solid-food gastric emptying, most commonly using a radiolabeled fried-egg sandwich, is the most helpful test in making the diagnosis.

8. What may cause small bowel dysmotility? How are the causes distinguished?

In patients with intestinal pseudo-obstruction, no obstruction is found with appropriate diagnostic tests, especially small bowel follow-through, performed during recovery from an episode. Other signs, such as abdominal distention, pain, changes in bowel habits, orthostatic hypotension, or bladder symptoms, may be present. Intestinal pseudo-obstruction may be seen with certain medications or systemic disorders, most commonly scleroderma, diabetes, and amyloidosis. These systemic disorders, as well as jejunal diverticulosis, must be specifically excluded with appropriate diagnostic studies. When these diagnoses have been excluded, primary small bowel myopathy or neuropathy may be present. Esophageal motility may suggest the diagnosis when aperistalsis is found. If these disorders are suspected and esophageal motility is normal, consideration of small bowel motility and/or small bowel biopsy at laparotomy will need to be made on an individual basis. This is best done in a referral center with expertise in such disorders.

9. How is psychogenic vomiting diagnosed?

Psychogenic vomiting is a cause of recurring vomiting in patients, especially young women, with an underlying emotional disturbance. However, it is occasionally a manifestation of major depression or conversion reaction. Although psychogenic vomiting is a diagnosis of exclusion, certain characteristics suggest its presence, including vomiting that has been present for a long time, especially during emotional strain. Moreover, vomiting typically is seen after the meal rather than delayed, and it can be suppressed if necessary. Finally, the vomiting may be of surprisingly little concern to the patient and of more concern to family members. Abdominal pain may be a major associated symptom. The diagnosis needs to be considered to avoid extensive diagnostic procedures or abdominal surgery that may worsen and complicate the issue.

10. What consequences of vomiting should be anticipated and treated?

Be vigilant for metabolic derangements. Because of the loss of hydrogen ions in vomitus and contraction of extracellular fluid volume, alkalosis commonly develops. Secondly, potassium deficiency is common due to the loss of potassium in vomitus and wasting from the kidneys. Therefore, the clinical features of potassium deficiency, including muscle weakness, nocturia, and cardiac arrhythmias, may be present.

Another major consequence of vomiting is an emetogenic injury. With protracted or forceful vomiting, a Mallory-Weiss laceration or, rarely, Boerhaave's syndrome (transmural tear of the esophagus) may occur. These complications need to be considered in patients with vomiting who develop a subsequent gastrointestinal bleed, odynophagia, or catastrophic chest pain.

11. How do you treat the patient with nausea and vomiting?

In patients with severe acute nausea and vomiting, the metabolic derangements need to be sought as well as signs of dehydration. If present, they usually require hospitalization; initial therapy includes no intake by mouth and usually a nasogastric tube. The best therapy for nausea and vomiting is prompt diagnosis and treatment of the primary disorder. However, specific treatment of the nausea and vomiting is often required to control symptoms.

12. What drugs are used to treat nausea and vomiting?

Antihistamines (H1 antagonist)
   Dimenhydrinate (Dramamine)
   Promenthazine (Phenergan)
   Meclizine (Antivert)
   Cyclizine (Marezine)
Anticholinergic drugs
   Scopolamine
Phenothiazines
   Prochlorperazine (Compazine)
   Chlorpromazine (Thorazine)
Butyrophenone
   Haloperidol (Haldol)

Trimethobenzamide (Tigan)
Dopaminergic antagonists
   Metoclopramide (Reglan)
   Domperidone
Octreotide
Erythromycin
Cisapride (Propulsid; restricted use: see text)
Serotonin receptor antagonists
   Ondansetron (Zofran)

The antihistamines (H1 antagonists) and anticholinergics (scopolamine) are used primarily for patients with nausea and vomiting secondary to vestibular disorders or motion sickness. The anticholinergics commonly cause dry mouth as a side effect. The phenothiazines, haloperidol, and trimethobenzamide act primarily via the chemoreceptor trigger zone, although some information suggests that they decrease input via visceral afferents. A common side effect of these drugs is sedation. Rare but serious side effects include blood dyscrasias, jaundice, and extrapyramidal signs.

13. When are the prokinetic agents used in patients with nausea and vomiting?

Metoclopramide has a central dopamine antagonist effect; however, the peripheral dopamine antagonist effect is responsible for prokinetic activity. It has been used in gastroparesis and, in much larger doses, for prophylaxis against chemotherapy-associated nausea and vomiting.

Common side effects include anxiety, lethargy, and increased prolactin levels. Rare side effects include depression and dystonia, particularly in older patients. Domperidone has a prokinetic effect, but because it does not readily cross the blood-brain barrier, it has less CNS effect. Side effects are uncommon. Domperidone is not yet available in the United States.

14. What is the role of erythromycin, octreotide, and cisapride?

Erythromycin interacts with motilin receptors on gastrointestinal smooth muscle membranes in an action independent of its antibiotic effect. It is effective acutely in gastroparesis; less evidence indicates that it is effective on a prolonged basis.

Octreotide has been found to improve small bowel motility in patients with scleroderma and in combination with erythromycin often improves symptoms in patients with either idiopathic or scleroderma-associated psuedoobstruction.

Cisapride is available only via limited access protocol in patients with gastroparesis or pseudo-obstruction who cannot be treated with metoclopramide. Serious cardiac arrthymias have been reported, usually when cisapride is used in patients with risk factors for cardiac arrhythmias or drug interactions. Cisapride works by direct stimulation of the cholingeric nerves.

15. Discuss the use of serotonin receptor antagonists.

The newest agents for the treatment of nausea and vomiting are the serotonin antagonists. Ondansetron is an antagonist to the 5-HT3 receptor, which is one of three serotonin receptors that have been identified. This receptor is present in both the CNS and gastrointestinal tract. Ondansetron has been used primarily as prophylaxis against chemotherapy-associated nausea and vomiting. It appears to have only rare adverse effects.

16. What is the role of gastric pacing?

Gastric pacing for 2–3 months via electrodes implanted in gastric serosa improved gastric emptying and decreased symptoms with no adverse effects in a small number of patients with gastroparesis refractory to standard therapy. Controlled studies with more patients and longer follow-up are needed.

HICCUPS

17. What are hiccups?

Hiccups are spasmodic, involuntary contractions of the muscles of inspiration (not just the diaphragm) almost simultaneously with closure of the glottis. Closure of the glottis is responsible for the audible sound. Hiccups are usually short-lived, typically occur after meals or alcohol ingestion, and subside without treatment or with simple measures such as breath-holding, water ingestion, or Valsalva maneuvers.

18. When are hiccups pathologic? What are the consequences?

An episode of hiccups lasting 48 hours or recurring episodes of protracted hiccups are defined as chronic. Some unfortunate people have prolonged episodes of hiccups or constant hiccups for years. Chronic hiccups can be disabling, resulting in chronic fatigue, sleep deprivation, interference with normal eating, and depression. Thus, chronic hiccups, which occur predominantly in men, require diagnostic evaluation and prompt treatment. However, even acute hiccups, which also occur predominantly in men, can be devastating and require prompt treatment in certain settings, such as postoperatively or in the early period after myocardial infarction.

19. What causes chronic hiccups?

Because the afferent limb of the hiccup reflex includes the vagus and phrenic nerves as well as sympathetic fibers T6–12, a wide variety of intraabdominal and intrathoracic disorders have been associated with hiccups. In contrast, because hiccups result in physiologic changes (such as a decrease in lower esophageal sphincter pressure), some abnormalities, such as reflux esophagitis, usually are a result of hiccups rather than the cause. A variety of CNS disorders also have been found to cause chronic hiccups. Lastly, metabolic diseases, such as chronic renal failure and especially diabetes mellitus, are associated with chronic hiccups.

20. Describe the diagnostic evaluation for patients with chronic hiccups.

Fluoroscopy of the diaphragm should be performed. If the diaphragm shows unilateral involvement only (usually the left hemidiaphragm), the diagnostic evaluation should focus on the course of the phrenic nerve of the affected side. Bilateral diaphragmatic motion suggests an afferent or central origin.

Because a wide variety of intraabdominal and intrathoracic disorders are associated with chronic hiccups, unless associated symptoms point toward a specific organ system, one should begin with laboratory tests (complete blood count, chemistry screen), abdominal flat plate (mechanical obstruction), endoscopy (peptic ulcer disease, gastric cancer, infiltrating diseases), and chest radiograph. If these tests are negative, consider computed tomography (CT) scans of the abdomen and chest and magnetic resonance imaging (MRI) of the brain.

Unfortunately, a thorough evaluation may be negative or find only an abnormal condition that may be coexisting (gastritis) or secondary to the hiccups (esophagitis, for example).

21. What therapies are available for chronic hiccups?

The best therapy is directed toward the cause. Unfortunately, the diagnostic evaluation is often negative, and therapy may have to be directed toward the hiccups themselves. Simple measures, such as breath-holding, swallowing water, Valsalva maneuvers, or rebreathing into a bag, are rarely helpful for protracted hiccups. Instead, more vigorous mechanical approaches or drug therapy usually is necessary, and occasionally phrenic nerve ablation should be considered. In my experience, the best way to stop an episode of hiccups is firm digital stimulation of the posterior pharynx, often with a nasogastric tube in place and after removing gastric contents. This technique is unpleasant for patients and is useful primarily for patients with long intervals between isolated episodes of hiccups. For those whose hiccups recur a short time after cessation, this approach is not feasible.

22. Which drugs can improve or cure hiccups?

Various drugs have been proposed as effective therapy for hiccups, but experience with each is usually limited to a few cases. Chlorpromazine, metoclopramide, and nifedipine have advocates who proclaim their efficacy in chronic hiccups. In my experience and that of others, the single most effective medication is baclofen, a derivate of gamma-aminobutyric acid used as an antispasticity agent in patients with tics or dystonias. Occasionally, complete cessation of hiccups occurs, but most patients experience a variable decrease in the frequency of episodes. Nevertheless, for some unfortunate patients who suffer near-daily hiccups for a large proportion of their day, this partial response can be gratifying. Dosage begins at 5 mg 3 times/day and is increased in a stepwise fashion to a maximum dose of 25 mg 3 times/day. Side effects include somnolence and fatigue. Do not discontinue the medication suddenly, but taper it over time.

23. What invasive therapies have been used if drug therapy is ineffective?

When unilateral involvement is demonstrated at fluoroscopy and other measures have been exhausted, phrenic nerve intervention should be considered. Because respiratory function may be significantly impaired after diaphragmatic paralysis, pulmonary function tests should be obtained before intervention. Temporary diaphragmatic paralysis confirmed by fluoroscopy and concomitant cessation of hiccups should be demonstrated before permanent ablation of the phrenic nerve is considered. Initial results of phrenic nerve stimulation by surgical placement of electrodes on the phrenic nerve in the neck is a promising new approach.

EATING DISORDERS

24. If eating disorders are psychiatric illnesses, why should an internist be aware of them?

Anorexia nervosa and bulimia nervosa, the two major well-defined eating disorders, are relatively common. The American Psychiatric Association cited a prevalence rate of 0.5–1%. The internist or gastroenterologist needs to be aware of these disorders, because the family may bring the patient to the physician with concerns that profound weight loss, vomiting, or associated symptoms (e.g., constipation, abdominal pain, dyspepsia) suggest a gastrointestinal disorder. Successful management requires: (1) early suspicion that an eating disorder is present; (2) evaluation for complications; (3) exclusion of a gastrointestinal (e.g., Crohn's disease) or systemic (e.g., AIDS) disorder; and (4) prompt referral to a clinician experienced in treating eating disorders.

25. List the criteria required for the diagnosis of anorexia nervosa, according to the Diagnostic and Statistical Manual of Mental Disorders (DSM-IV).

1. Refusal to maintain body weight at or above a minimally normal weight for age and height.

2. Intense fear of gaining weight or becoming fat, even though underweight.

3. Disturbance in the way in which body weight or shape is experienced, undue influence of body weight or shape on self-evaluation, or denial of the seriousness of the current low body weight.

4. In postmenarcheal females, amenorrhea (i.e., absence of at least three consecutive menstrual cycles).

26. What other characteristics of anorexia nervosa may aid in its diagnosis?

Females are overwhelmingly affected; only 5–10% of patients are male. The onset in most patients is in late adolescence and early adulthood, at a mean age of 17 years. The onset is often associated with a stressful life event, such as going to college. There is a high incidence of sexual abuse among these patients. Associated symptoms include depressed mood, obsessive-compulsive acts (such as a preoccupation with food or food hoarding), and overcontrolling behavior resulting in a typically inflexible attitude in most life situations. Physical examination is dominated by the patient's emaciated state. Other clues include increased size of the salivary glands (especially the parotid gland) and signs of recurring vomiting, such as decreased dental enamel and calluses on the dorsum of the hand (Russell's sign).

27. Should any complications be anticipated in patients with anorexia nervosa?

Patients have findings related to degree of starvation. They may have mild leukopenia and normocytic anemia; moreover, endocrine evaluation may reveal hypoadrenocorticism and regression of the hypothalamic-pituitary-gonadal axis to a prepubertal pattern.

Vomiting and purging have sequelae. Repeated vomiting may cause an emetogenic injury. Electrolyte disturbances, especially hypokalemia, may be particularly profound in patients using large amounts of laxatives for purging. Rare patients who use Ipecac may have a cardiac and skeletal myopathy. Lastly, amylase may be elevated, although it is typically of the salivary isoamylase type.

28. What is the differential diagnosis for patients with suspected anorexia nervosa?

When the patient has many of the characteristic findings of an eating disorder, it should be the working diagnosis. Only a few disorders need to be considered and expeditiously excluded, including inflammatory bowel disease (especially Crohn's disease), celiac sprue, pancreatic insufficiency, or recurring mechanical obstruction. Nongastrointestinal problems include endocrine disorders (especially panhypopituitarism, Addison's disease, or hyperthyroidism), occult neoplasm, and AIDS.

Nutritional assessment should accompany consideration of the differential diagnoses, including transferrin, albumin, triceps skinfold, and an anergy panel. A prognostic nutritional index for patients with anorexia nervosa has been proposed to determine the need for aggressive nutritional support.

29. What is the natural history of anorexia nervosa?

The course of anorexia nervosa varies markedly, and the spectrum ranges from people with one episode and subsequent recovery to patients who have repeated relapses or an unremitting course leading to death. The early mortality rate is estimated at 5%; the late mortality rate may be as high as 13–20% because of suicide, arrhythmia, or emaciation.

30. How are patients with anorexia nervosa managed?

Because of the variable and serious nature of anorexia nervosa, treatment requires an experienced primary physician who can integrate a multiphasic treatment regimen. Medical management is required to restore weight and correct metabolic problems. In general, patients with moderate (65–80% of ideal body weight) and severe (< 65% of ideal body weight) weight loss or low prognostic nutritional index scores require nutrition supplementation. Hospitalization is required for the severely malnourished. A psychological approach also should be devised that uses one or a combination of the following:

1. Behavioral therapies, such as operant conditioning
2. Cognitive therapy, such as assessing and examining distortions in thought processes
3. Family counseling
4. Pharmacotherapy, such as chlorpromazine or antidepressants

31. What are the DSM-IV diagnostic criteria for bulimia nervosa?

1. Recurrent episodes of binge eating, characterized by both of the following:
   - Eating an amount of food that is definitely larger than most people would eat during a similar period and under similar circumstances.
   - A sense of lack of control over eating during the episode.

2. Recurrent inappropriate compensatory behavior to prevent weight gain, such as self-induced vomiting; misuse of laxatives, diuretics, enemas, or other medications; fasting; or excessive exercise.

3. Binge eating and compensatory behaviors both occur, on average, at least twice a week for 3 months.

4. Body shape and weight unduly influence self-evaluation.

5. The disturbance does not occur exclusively during episodes of anorexia nervosa.

Although some argue that bulimic patients are too similar to patients with anorexia nervosa to be differentiated, they have less body-image distortion and are more accepting of therapy.

32. What other characteristics of bulimia nervosa may aid in its diagnosis?

The vast predominance of females and age of onset mirror anorexia nervosa. However, bulimia nervosa is more common and, in various studies, has been reported in 1–3% of the adolescent and young adult female population.

Characteristically, patients try to conceal their binging or purging behavior, which tends to occur during periods of stress. Vomiting rarely occurs in public, as patients can control their vomiting until they are in a private location. Although vomiting is the most common compensatory behavior (80–90% of cases), approximately one-third of patients use laxatives. The vomiting initially may be forceful but later in the disease becomes nearly effortless. Rare patients use ipecac.

Bulimic patients characteristically have difficulty in developing personal relationships and, unlike patients with anorexia nervosa, may have chemical dependencies, especially alcohol. One-third have associated personality disorders.

Physical findings are not obvious. Because they are not malnourished, bulimics generally appear healthy, and other people who know the patient well, even family members, may not be aware of the disorder. The physical findings characteristic of patients with repeated vomiting may be present, as noted for anorexia nervosa. Complications are related to the compensatory vomiting and purging behavior and are the same as those for anorexia nervosa.

33. What is the natural history of bulimia nervosa?

The course of bulimia nervosa is variable. Approximately 40% of patients recover and remain well or have minor relapses. Another 15% have major relapses, and approximately 40% are ill most of the time or continuously.

34. What therapy is available for bulimic patients?

Bulimia nervosa can be managed on an outpatient basis. A program that includes both cognitive recognition of the patient's abnormal behavior and therapy directed at the abnormal behavior is the approach of choice. Antidepressants are useful as an adjunct but not as sole therapy.

35. What about patients with a suspected eating disorder who do not meet the strict criteria for anorexia nervosa or bulimia nervosa?

Certain patients have some, but not all, of the features of anorexia nervosa or bulimia nervosa. DSM-IV defines several other presentations as nonspecific eating disorders.

RUMINATION

36. What is rumination? How often does it occur?

Rumination is the regurgitation of mouthfuls of recently ingested food, with subsequent remastication and reswallowing, in the absence of apparent organic disease. Usually, rumination begins 15–20 minutes after a meal and continues until the stomach contents become sour as a result of acid (20–60 minutes later). As many as 20 episodes per meal are not uncommon. Patients do not describe it as distressful and often are embarrassed and attempt to hide the symptom. Eating large volumes of food quickly and with a lot of liquids facilitates rumination.

Rumination is uncommon in adults, although it is underreported because patients are unlikely to discuss a symptom that they consider embarrassing. Men predominate, and although no consistent intellectual or social characteristics are present, physicians and scientists are highly represented in various reviews.

37. What is the mechanism of rumination?

On observation, most people with rumination have abdominal and thoracic movements that precede and accompany the process. Gastroesophageal manometry performed postprandially has found that Valsalva maneuvers occur simultaneously with regurgitation. In one report, the Valsalva maneuver occurred repeatedly over a lower esophageal sphincter and with a pharyngeal maneuver that preceded the upper esophageal sphincter relaxation. Thus, a voluntary component is involved and has led to behavioral therapy and biofeedback as the therapy of choice. No case has been reported in which rumination was accompanied by reverse peristalsis, as described in ruminant animals.

38. Can complications occur with rumination?

Heartburn may start many years after the onset of rumination, suggesting that an acid-sensitive esophagus develops from repeated acid contact during ruminating. Rare reports of gastrointestinal bleeding and hemorrhagic esophagitis at endoscopy have been published.

39. What should be the therapeutic approach?

Behavioral therapy is the treatment of choice for adults. Changing the composition of food, slowing the speed of eating, and giving less water with the meal have been effective approaches in some reports. Biofeedback directed against the increased intraabdominal pressure that always precedes regurgitation episodes also has been effective. Aversive therapies, such as ingesting foods that are distasteful if regurgitated, should be avoided.

BIBLIOGRAPHY

1. Amarnath RP, Abell TL, Malagelada J: The rumination syndrome in adults. Ann Intern Med 105:513–518, 1986.
2. American Psychiatric Association: Eating disorders. In American Psychiatric Association: Diagnostic and Statistical Manual of Mental Disorders, 4th ed. Washington, DC, American Psychiatric Association, 1994, pp 539–550.
3. Dobelle H: Use of breathing pacemakers to suppress intractable hiccups of up to thirteen years duration. ASAIO 45:524–525, 1999.
4. Drossman DA: Anorexia: A comprehensive approach. Adv Intern Med 28:339, 1983.
5. Hanson JS, McCallum RW: The diagnosis and management of nausea and vomiting: A review. Am J Gastroenterol 80:210–218, 1985.
6. Katelaris PH, Jones DB: Chronic nausea and vomiting. Dig Dis 7:323–333, 1989.
7. King M: Update: Eating disorders. Compr Ther 17(3):35–40, 1991.
8. Launois S, Bizec JL, et al: Hiccup in adults: An overview. Eur Respir J 6:563–575, 1993.
9. Lewis JH: Hiccups: Causes and cures. J Clin Gastroenterol 7:539–552, 1985.
10. McCallum RW, Chen JDZ, Lin Z, et al: Gastric pacing improves emptying and symptoms in patients with gastroparesis. Gastroenterology 114:456–461, 1998.
11. Malagelada JR, Camilleri M: Unexplained vomiting: A diagnostic challenge. Ann Intern Med 101:211–218, 1984.
12. Malcolm MB, Thumshirn MB, Camilleri M, et al: Rumination syndrome. Mayo Clin Proc 72:646–652, 1997.
13. Ramirez FC, Graham DY: Treatment of intractable hiccup with baclofen. Am J Gastroenterol 87:1789–1791, 1992.
14. Shay SS: Regurgitation and rumination. In Castell DO (ed): The Esophagus. Boston, Little, Brown, 1992, pp 571–579.
15. Verne GN, Eaker EY, Hardy E, Sninsky CA: Effect of octreotide and erythromycin on idopathic and scleroderma-associated intestinal psuedoobstruction. Dig Dis Sci 40:1892–1901, 1995.
16. Woodside DB: A review of anorexia nervosa and bulimia nervosa. Curr Probl Pediatr 25:67–89, 1995.

66. FOREIGN BODIES AND THE GASTROINTESTINAL TRACT

George Triadafilopoulos, M.D.

1. How common are foreign bodies in the GI tract?

Every year, millions of foreign bodies enter the GI tract through the mouth or anus, and about 1500 to 3000 people die every year from ingestion of foreign objects. However, only about 10–20% of foreign bodies require removal through some form of therapeutic intervention; the rest pass through the GI tract without incident.

2. Which populations are at risk for foreign-body ingestion?

Eighty percent of foreign-body ingestions occur in children, whereas almost all foreign bodies inserted into the rectum are described in adults. Other groups at increased risk for foreign-body ingestion include psychiatric patients, inmates, and people who frequently use alcohol or sedative-hypnotic medications. Also at risk are elderly subjects, who may have poorly-fitting dentures, impaired cognitive function due to medications, or dementia and/or dysphagia after stroke. Intentional ingestion of foreign objects is well described in smugglers of illicit drugs, jewels, or other valuable items.

3. Which areas of the GI tract lead to problems in the passage of foreign bodies?

Several areas of anatomic or physiologic narrowing exist along the GI lumen and may compromise the spontaneous passage of foreign bodies: cricopharyngeal muscle, extrinsic compression of the middle esophagus from the aortic arch, lower esophageal sphincter, pylorus, ileocecal valve, rectal valves of Houston, and anal sphincters. In addition, numerous pathologic abnormalities, such as strictures or tumors, may impair spontaneous passage of foreign bodies (see question 12).

4. What objects are commonly ingested?

The object most commonly ingested by children is a coin. Meat boluses impacted above an esophageal stricture or ring account for most adult cases. Accidental loss of sex stimulant devices account for over one-half of foreign objects introduced through the anus.

5. Describe the typical clinical presentation of foreign-body ingestion.

Adults trace the onset of symptoms to the ingestion of a specific meal or foreign body. Mentally retarded, psychiatric patients or children may remain asymptomatic for months after ingestion, or they may not volunteer the history. Patients with impacted anorectal foreign bodies may relate a wide variety of medical histories to account for their predicament, ranging from accidents or assault to medical remedies.

6. What is suggested by respiratory symptoms related to foreign-body ingestion?

Patients presenting with wheezing, stridor, cough, or dyspnea after foreign-body ingestion may have foreign body entrapment in the hypopharynx, trachea, pyriform sinus, or Zenker's diverticulum.

7. Do ingested sharp objects perforate the intestine?

On rare occasions, sharp objects such as pins, needles, nails, and toothpicks may perforate the intestine but in 70–90% of cases they pass through the alimentary tract without complication. Two phenomena in the intestine allow safe passage: (1) foreign bodies pass with axial flow down the lumen, and (2) reflex relaxation and slowing of peristalsis cause sharp objects to turn around in the lumen so that the sharp end trails down the intestine. In the colon, the foreign object is centered in the fecal bolus, which further protects the bowel wall.

8. Why is it important to identify the type of foreign body ingested?

Although most foreign bodies traverse the GI tract without complication, specific exceptions re-quire special attention. Button alkaline batteries may cause coagulation necrosis in the esophagus, but once they reach the stomach, gastric acid neutralizes their risk. Sharp objects can perforate any part of the alimentary tract. Objects longer than 6 cm may become lodged in the C-loop of the duodenum.

9. How urgent is removal of a foreign body after ingestion?

Button batteries, typically ingested by small children, need to be removed urgently because of the severe trauma that they may cause in the esophagus. Any sharp object that carries a high risk for perforation should be removed as soon as possible before it passes to a level that is beyond the reach of an endoscope. For the same reasons, long objects (> 6 cm) should be re-moved when identified. Finally, objects lodged in the esophagus that compromise ability to handle oral secretions should be removed urgently to reduce the risk of aspiration.

10. Describe the signs and symptoms of a complication related to foreign-body ingestion.

Respiratory symptoms suggest entrapment of the foreign body in the hypopharynx, trachea, pyriform sinus, or Zenker's diverticulum (see question 6). Sharp objects may penetrate, obstruct, or perforate the esophagus or intestine, presenting with chest, neck, or abdominal pain that varies from mild discomfort to symptoms and signs of acute abdomen. Injury to the esophagus can lead to hematemesis, fever, tachycardia, neck swelling, and crepitus. Excessive drooling and inability to swallow saliva suggest esophageal obstruction. Abdominal distention, vomiting, and hyperac-tive bowel sounds suggest intestinal obstruction. Hypoactive or absent bowel sounds, guarding, rebound, and abdominal pain are seen with wall penetration or free perforation. Aortoenteric fis-tula due to ingestion of a sharp foreign body may cause massive hematemesis.

11. How should foreign bodies be removed?

Once identified, nearly all objects can be removed endoscopically. Other modalities have been used with variable success, although major complications have been reported. Consultation with a surgeon is appropriate for cases in which perforation or other major complications are probable.

12. Which anatomic/functional defects of the GI tract contribute to foreign body obstruction?

INTESTINAL SITE	ANATOMIC DEFECT	FUNCTIONAL DEFECT
Esophagus	Stenosis, atresia, rings, webs, benign/malignant-stricture, diverticula, vascular anomalies	Scleroderma, achalasia, Chagas disease
Stomach	Pyloric stenosis (congenital, malignancy, post-operative, gastroduodenal ulcer disease)	Gastroparesis (uremia, diabetes, hypothyroidism)
Intestine	Postoperative adhesion, Meckel's diverticulum, strictures (ischemic, anastomotic, Crohn's disease), malignancy	Idiopathic intestinal pseudo-obstruction, scleroderma
Colon	Strictures (ischemic, anastomotic, ulcerative colitis, Crohn's disease, radiation, trauma, infection, surgery), diverticular disease, malignancy	Cathartic colon, idiopathic constipa-tion, familial megacolon, idiopathic intestinal pseudo-obstruction
Anus	Stenosis (Crohn's disease, trauma, radiation, infection, surgery)	Hirschprung's disease

BIBLIOGRAPHY

1. American Society for Gastrointestinal Endoscopy: Guidelines for the Management of Ingested Foreign Bodies. Manchester, MA, ASGE publication 1026, 1995.
2. Barone JE, Yee J, Nealon TF Jr: Management of foreign bodies and trauma of the rectum. Surg Gynecol Obstet 156:453–457, 1983.
3. Busch DB, Starling JR: Rectal foreign bodies: Case reports and a comprehensive review of the world's literature. Surgery 100: 512–519, 1986.
4. Ginsberg GG: Management of ingested foreign objects and food bolus impactions. Gastrointest Endosc 41:33–38, 1995.
5. Lyons MF, Tsuchida AM: Foreign bodies of the gastrointestinal tract. Med Clin North Am 77:1101–1114, 1993.
6. Webb WA: Management of foreign bodies of the upper gastrointestinal tract: Update. Gastrointest Endosc 41:39–51, 1995.

67. IRRITABLE BOWEL SYNDROME

Arnold Wald, M.D.

1. What are functional gastrointestinal disorders?

Functional gastrointestinal (GI) disorders are defined as various combinations of chronic or recurrent GI symptoms that cannot be explained by structural or biochemical abnormalities. Their recognition as legitimate diagnostic entities has been delayed because western medicine historically defined illness based on the identification of histopathologic disease (biomedical model). The need for a framework to understand, categorize, and treat patients with functional GI symptoms has led to a broader concept of the biopsychosocial model of illness that legitimizes such symptoms and provides treatment rationales.

2. Define irritable bowel syndrome.

Irritable bowel syndrome (IBS) is defined broadly by the presence of chronic or recurrent abdominal pain and altered bowel habits in the absence of an organic disease that can produce similar symptoms. Altered bowel habits consist of diarrhea or constipation, either or both of which may occur in patients with IBS. Abdominal pain in the absence of altered bowel habits or vice versa does not fall under the diagnostic spectrum of IBS.

3. Discuss the epidemiology of functional GI disorders and IBS.

Large population surveys in the United States suggest that over two-thirds of the population has one or more functional GI complaints, although most do not seek medical attention. However, functional GI complaints are the most common digestive disorder encountered by gastroenterologists. Symptoms consistent with IBS occur in up to 22% of western adults. Although only a small percentage seek medical attention, IBS alone accounts for 12% of primary care visits and up to 28% of all referrals to gastroenterologists. It is the second leading cause of work absenteeism after the common cold.

4. What is the economic impact of IBS in the United States?

IBS accounts for an estimated 2.4–3.5 million physician visits per year in the U.S. and for an estimated 2.2 million prescriptions. One large study found that adults with IBS symptoms missed 3 times as many work days, were almost 3 times as likely to report that they were too sick to work, and incurred 70% higher medical costs than adults without IBS during the previous year.

5. Describe the pathophysiology of IBS symptoms.

Three major hypotheses, which are not mutually exclusive, have been proposed to explain IBS symptoms. The first and oldest theory is an underlying disorder of GI motility. Although little evidence substantiates this theory, some data indicate that many patients with IBS have an exaggerated GI motor response to meals and neurohumeral stimulants.

The second hypothesis is that emotional tension and psychological factors lead to IBS symptoms. Indeed, studies suggest that people who seek medical attention have more psychological distress than people with similar symptoms who do not. Thus, psychological and personality traits are not related to GI symptoms but may influence whether patients seek medical attention. However, psychological dysfunction is not found in the majority of patients with IBS seen in medical settings.

Finally, evidence suggests that about two-thirds of patients with IBS exhibit altered perception to bowel distention. The precise reasons are unclear but may include altered gut receptors or alterations in processing nociceptive impulses in the central nervous system.

6. Discuss the importance of symptom-based criteria for diagnosis of IBS.

Because they have no anatomic or biochemical basis for diagnosis, the functional GI disorders are diagnosed on the basis of symptoms. Working teams of acknowledged experts have reached a consensus regarding diagnostic criteria (although they are not universally accepted) termed the Rome criteria. Modifications were published in 1999 and are known as the Rome II criteria.

Research using symptom-based criteria allows investigators to test more homogenous populations, and the Rome criteria have been used in most if not all pharmaceutical studies of IBS conducted in the past 6 years. These symptoms also can be used as clinical guidelines to avoid misdiagnosis and to minimize clinical testing. Research studies emphasize the importance of the history in patients with suspected functional GI disorders and in making a "positive diagnosis" rather than a diagnosis of exclusion or a "wastebasket" diagnosis.

7. What are the symptom-based criteria for the diagnosis of IBS?

1. At least 12 weeks, which need not be consecutive, in the preceding 12 months of abdominal discomfort or pain with two of the following three features:
    • Relief with defecation
    • Onset associated with a change in frequency of stool
    • Onset associated with a change in form (appearance) of stool.
2. Abnormal stool form (lumpy, hard or loose, watery stool)
3. Abnormal stool passage (straining, urgency, or feeling of incomplete evacuation)
4. Passage of mucus
5. Bloating or feeling of abdominal distention

8. List the supportive symptoms of IBS.

1. < 3 bowel movements/week
2. > 3 bowel movements/day
3. Hard or lumpy stools
4. Loose (mushy) or watery stools
5. Straining during bowel movement
6. Urgency (having to rush to have a bowel movement)
7. Feeling of incomplete bowel movement
8. Passage of mucus (white material) during bowel movement
9. Abdominal fullness, bloating, or swelling

9. Distinguish between diarrhea-predominant and constipation-predominant IBS.

Diarrhea-predominant: 1 or more of criteria 2, 4, or 6 and none of criteria 1, 3, or 5 listed in question 8.

Constipation-predominant: 1 or more of criteria 1, 3, or 5 and none of criteria 2, 4, or 6 listed in queston 8.

10. Describe the various clinical presentations of IBS.

Universal to all patients with IBS is the presence of chronic or recurrent abdominal pain. The location and intensity of the pain is highly variable. It usually is described as crampy or as a generalized discomfort with superimposed periods of cramping. Many patients report exacerbation with eating or during periods of stress or emotional upset.

The various clinical presentations of IBS are defined by the pattern of altered bowel habits. Some patients have diarrhea predominance, whereas others have constipation predominance, each alternating with periods of normal bowel habits. A third group of patients has alternating constipation and diarrhea.

Constipation usually is characterized by passage of small, hard, pellet-like stools, often with defecatory straining, passage of mucus, and a sense of incomplete evacuation. Diarrhea usually is characterized by frequent passage of loose stools, often with great urgency but with normal daily stool volume. Invariably, symptoms of IBS occur during the daytime only and rarely, if ever, awaken the patient from sleep.

11. What symptoms are not typical of IBS and should prompt a thorough evaluation for organic disease?
- Nocturnal symptoms
- Onset in old age
- Weight loss (unless severe depression is present)
- Blood in stools or anemia

12. What diagnostic tests are appropriate in patients with suspected IBS?

The diagnosis of IBS is based on three steps: (1) identification of a symptom complex compatible with IBS, (2) frequent association of symptoms with factors that produce gut hyperactivity, and (3) exclusion of an organic cause of symptoms. The use of diagnostic studies to exclude organic disease should be prudent but not exhaustive, and tests should not be repeated after diagnosis. Testing should be based on presenting symptoms (diarrhea or constipation) and made in the context of the entire clinical picture, including recent or long-standing symptoms, psychological issues, and results of previous studies.

Sigmoidoscopy is helpful to exclude colitis and structural lesions and may reassure patients and physicians that no underlying organic disease is present. Mucosal biopsy specimens to look for microscopic or collagenous colitis are indicated only if diarrhea is a predominant symptom. Additional studies should include a complete blood count and may include laxative screening, examination of stool specimens for ova and parasites, and radiographic evaluation of the small bowel. Because IBS may coexist with other colonic disorders, full colonoscopy may be indicated.

13. Are food allergies or intolerances important in generating IBS symptoms? Is allergy testing or an elimination diet indicated?

Physicians should obtain a detailed dietary history to identify factors that may aggravate or cause symptoms, especially diarrhea and gas-bloat dyspepsia. Examples include lactose, fructose, and sorbitol; carbonated beverages; legumes and other gas-producing foods; and caffeinated beverages. Some authors suggest diagnostic tests for carbohydrate malabsorption, skin tests for particular foods, or exclusionary diets. Carbohydrate intolerance is unlikely to play a significant role in symptom generation for the following reasons:

1. The prevalence of carbohydrate intolerance is similar in patients with IBS and asymptomatic controls.

2. Patients with gas-bloat symptoms have no more gas in the GI tract than controls, but they have more symptoms when an equal amount of gas is infused into the intestines.

3. Patients with self-declared lactose intolerance respond to reduced lactose diets no better than they do to lactose-containing diets.

4. Exclusion diets generally do not produce improvement compared with placebo-controlled diets.

These observations extend to patients with positive skin testing to particular foods. Diagnostic studies for food intolerances add to health care costs and generally are unproven. However, exclusion diets are inexpensive and harmless and may produce improvement through placebo effects.

14. What are the four essential elements in the management of patients with IBS?

1. Establish a good physician-patient relationship.
2. Educate patients about their condition.
3. Emphasize the excellent prognosis and benign nature of the illness.
4. Employ therapeutic interventions centering on dietary modifications, pharmacotherapy, and behavior strategies tailored to the individual patient.

15. Elaborate on the four basic elements of management.

Initially, the physician should establish the diagnosis, exclude organic causes, educate patients about the disease, establish realistic expectations and consistent limits, and involve patients in disease management. It is critical to determine why the patient is seeking assistance (e.g., cancer phobia, disability, interpersonal distress, secondary gain, exacerbation of symptoms). Most patients can be treated by their primary care physician. However, specialty consultations may be needed to reinforce management strategies, perform additional diagnostic tests, or institute specialized treatment.

Psychological comorbidities do not cause symptoms, but they affect how patients respond to them and influence health care-seeking behavior. These issues are best explored over a series of visits when the physician-patient relationship has been established. It may be helpful to have patients fill out a self-administered test to identify psychological comorbidities. Such tests can be used as a basis for extended, more detailed inquiries and often lead to initiation of appropriate therapies.

16. What is the role of bulking agents in the treatment of IBS?

The most widely recommended agents for treating IBS are fiber preparations, which increase stool bulk, either by water retention or by serving as a substrate for microbial growth in the colon. Despite some physiologic basis for their use, efficacy is largely unproven. Although wheat bran may improve symptoms in patients with constipation-predominant IBS, patients often complain of increased bloating and cramps, especially if supplementation is too aggressive. As some patients experience improvement, a cautious trial of fiber is reasonable but probably not in patients with diarrhea or excessive bloating.

17. Are anticholinergics and antispasmodics useful in IBS?

Smooth muscle relaxants, also known as antispasmodics, are thought to relieve GI symptoms by inhibiting intestinal smooth muscle contractions, thereby decreasing colonic motor activity. Examples include the anticholinergics and calcium channel blockers. Most published trials have methodologic problems. However, a meta-analysis of 26 trials with 8 different drugs suggested efficacy for mebeverine, cimetropium, and dicyclomine, which are antimuscarinics, and octylonium, which has calcium-antagonist properties. It is uncertain whether these agents act peripherally on the GI tract or whether central nervous system effects such as sedation also play a role.

18. Discuss the role for psychotropic agents in treating patients with IBS and other functional GI disorders.

Tricyclic antidepressants in low doses have been advocated for chronic somatic or visceral pain. In one study of patients with noncardiac (functional) chest pain, imipramine, 50 mg/day, proved superior to placebo; however, the efficacy in patients with IBS remains unproven. In a recent retrospective review of the use of antidepressants in 138 patients with IBS over a 5-year period, improvement was particularly impressive in patients with pain predominance compared with diarrhea or constipation predominance. The presence of psychiatric comorbidity did not influence the clinical response. The mechanism of action when tricyclics are given in non-psychiatric dosages is hypothesized to involve effects on supraspinal structures. In addition, short-term administration of imipramine (up to 100 mg/day) prolonged mouth-to-cecum and whole-gut transit times in both the control group and patients with diarrhea-predominant IBS. This finding suggests the potential efficacy of heterocyclic antidepressants in patients with diarrhea and pain predominance. Although anecdotal reports suggest that selective serotonin re-uptake inhibitors (SSRIs) may be beneficial in the absence of psychiatric comorbidity, no published trials support their use. Thus, SSRIs are most appropriate for patients with a diagnosis of depression, obsessive compulsive disorder, or phobias.

19. How should antidiarrheal agents be prescribed for patients with IBS?

Synthetic opioids such as loperamide and diphenoxylate are effective treatments, especially in patients with diarrhea. These agents act on peripheral opioid receptors throughout the GI tract to decrease secretion and slow transit, allowing greater fluid reabsorption and improved stool consistency. For many patients, antidiarrheal agents should be used in anticipation of rather than in response to diarrhea. In patients who exhibit early morning symptoms on their way to work and patients who fear sudden urgent diarrhea in public places, 1–2 tablets of diphenoxylate or loperamide may minimize or eliminate symptoms and restore social confidence. Such bowel patterns can be identified by analyzing prospectively obtained bowel and food diaries.

20. What is the rationale for 5-hydroxytryptamine-3 antagonists? How should they be used in IBS?

5-hydroxytryptamine-3 antagonists (e.g., alosetron, ondansetron, granisetron) modulate visceral afferent activity from the GI tract and may improve abdominal pain. Alosetron was developed for use in IBS based upon its favorable effects on colonic motility and secretion and afferent neural systems. One controlled trial demonstrated that it was more effective than placebo for relieving abdominal pain and improving bowel function. The drug appeared to be most effective in female patients in whom diarrhea was predominant. The reason for the gender-specific benefit is unclear; further testing in men is ongoing. It is approved only for women whose predominant IBS symptom is diarrhea. The recommended dosage is 1 mg twice daily. Because of reports of severe constipation and ischemic colitis, alosetron should be used cautiously and only in women with diarrhea-predominant IBS who do not respond to other forms of therapy.

BIBLIOGRAPHY

 1. Camilleri M, Choi M-G: Review article: Irritable bowel syndrome. Aliment Pharmacol Ther 11:3–16, 1997.
 2. Camilleri M, Northcutt AR, Kong S, et al: Efficacy and safety of alosetron in women with irritable bowel syndrome. Lancet 355:1035–1040, 2000.
 3. Cannon RO, Quyyumi AA, Mincemover R, et al: Imipramine in patients in chest pain despite normal coronary angiograms. N Engl J Med 330:1411–1417, 1994.
 4. Clouse RE, et al: Antidepressant therapy in 138 patients with irritable bowel syndrome: A five year clinical experience. Aliment Pharmacol Ther 8:409–416, 1994
 5. Efskin PS, Baukler T, Vato MM: A double blind placebo controlled trial with loperamide in irritable bowel syndrome. Scand J Gastrol 31:463–468, 1996.
 6. Gorard DA, Libby GW, Farthing MJG: Influence of antidepressants on whole gut and orocaceal transit times in health and irritable bowel syndrome. Aliment Pharmacol Ther 8:159–166, 1994
 7. Jailwala J, Imperiale TF, Kroenke K: Pharmacologic treatment of the irritable bowel syndrome: A systematic review of randomized controlled trials. Ann Int Med 133:136–147, 2000.
 8. Klein KB: Controlled clinical trials in the irritable bowel syndrome: A critique. Gastroenterology 65:232–241, 1988.
 9. Longstreth GF: Irritable bowel syndrome: Diagnosis in the managed care era. Dig Dis Sci 42:1105– 1111, 1997.
10. Lucey MR, Clark ML, Loundes JO, Dawson AM: Is bran efficacious in irritable bowel syndrome: A double blind placebo controlled crossover study. Gut 28:221–225, 1987.
11. Lynn RB, Friedman LS: Irritable bowel syndrome: Managing the patient with abdominal pain and altered bowel habits. Med Clin North Am 79:373–390, 1995.
12. Mertz H, Naliboff B, Munakata J, Niazi N, Mayer EA: Altered rectal perception is a biological marker of patients with irritable bowel syndrome. Gastroenterology 109:40–52, 1995.
13. Poynard T, Naveau S, Mory B, et al: Meta-analysis of smooth muscle relaxants in the treatment of irritable bowel syndrome. Aliment Pharmacol Ther 8:499–510, 1994.
14. Suarez FL Savaiano DA, Levitt, MD: A comparison of symptoms after the consumption of milk or lactose-hydrolyzed milk by people with self-reported severe lactose intolerance. N Engl J Med 293:524–526, 1975.
15. Thompson WG, Longstreth GF, Drossman DA, et al: Functional bowel disorders, and functional abdominal pain. Gut 45(Suppl II):II43–II47, 1999.
16. Zwetchkenbaum J, Burakoff R: The irritable bowel syndrome and food hypersensitivity. Ann Allergy 61:47–49, 1988.

68. ENDOSCOPIC CANCER SCREENING AND SURVEILLANCE

Scot M. Lewey, D.O, and Peter R. McNally, D.O.

1. What is the difference between endoscopic cancer screening and surveillance?

Screening is the one-time application of a test in an asymptomatic person. Cancer screening is the search for cancer and precancerous lesions in asymptomatic persons.

Surveillance is repeated application of such tests over time. Cancer surveillance is the follow-up of persons with a known history of cancer or precancerous lesions.

Recommendations for cancer screening and surveillance are not based solely on medical data but also on patient expectations, state of medical technology, and prevailing medical-legal environment.

ESOPHAGUS

2. What is the risk of esophageal cancer in patients with achalasia?

2%. The pathogenesis is unknown, but chronic stasis is believed to play a role. The mean interval between diagnosis of achalasia and development of cancer is 17 years. Ninety percent of cancers are of the squamous cell type, and the remainder are adenocarcinomas. The risk for malignancy is not completely eliminated by medical or surgical treatment of achalasia. Esophageal cancer is usually far advanced before the dilated esophagus becomes obstructed and symptoms manifest; hence, the 5-year survival rate is poor (< 5%).

3. Can endoscopic surveillance detect early esophageal cancer among patients with long-standing achalasia?

Yes. There are examples of long term survival after surgery. Periodic endoscopic surveillance for all patients with achalasia is unlikely to be cost effective.

4. What are the surveillance recommendations for patients with esophageal achalasia?

No program is nationally recognized. A suggested schedule for endoscopic surveillance begins 15–20 years after initial symptoms or 10–15 years after medical or surgical treatment. The esophagus should be cleaned of debris before endoscopic examination. All surface abnormalities of the esophagus should be biopsied. Generally, endoscopic surveillance should not be conducted more frequently than every 1–3 years.

5. What is the malignant potential of Barrett's esophagus?

Barrett's esophagus is a premalignant condition with a reported cancer prevalence of 10–40%. Endoscopic surveillance studies suggest an incidence of 1 in 52–175 patient years. Surgical and medical treatment of gastroesophageal reflux has not been shown to reduce the incidence of cancer.

6. Should every patient with chronic gastroesophageal reflux disease (GERD) be screened for Barrett's esophagus?

No. A recent population-based study identified a clear association between chronic reflux symptoms and adenocarcinoma of the esophagus, which continues to exhibit a rising incidence. Because patients with GERD are at increased risk for Barrett's esophagus, some have suggested endoscopic screening for Barrett's esophagus among patients older than 50 years with longstanding GERD. Evidence-based studies are needed to determine whether this recommendation is worthwhile.

7. What are the screening recommendations for patients with GERD?

None. Unsedated upper endoscopy with "ultrathin" endoscopes may be cost effective.

8. What are the clinical determinants of relative risk for carcinoma among patients with Barrett's esophagus?

Only specialized, "intestinal-type" Barrett's epithelium is associated with risk for adenocarcinoma. Cancer may develop in Barrett's segments of any length, but patients with segments of metaplasia longer than 6 cm appear to be at greater risk. Histologic evidence of high-grade dysplasia is a good indicator for cancer risk.

9. How is Barrett's esophagus graded?

A histologic classification consisting of high-grade dysplasia (HGD), low-grade dysplasia (LGD)/indefinite, and no dysplasia is useful and reproducible, with an 86% interobserver agreement rate among expert pathologists for the diagnosis of HGD. Collective reports show a high correlation between HGD and carcinoma (32% of resected specimens). The significance of LGD is uncertain.

10. What techniques are available for surveillance of patients with Barrett's esophagus?

Because foci of HGD and cancer may be small and scattered throughout the Barrett's segment, their detection requires extensive surveillance biopsies. Quadrant sampling of the metaplastic segment at 1–2-cm intervals is recommended. The addition of exfoliative brush cytology may be especially helpful when less rigorous surveillance biopsies are obtained.

Changes in mucosal DNA content as detected by flow cytometry may provide useful information in the surveillance of Barrett's esophagus, but the technique is demanding, expensive, and still under evaluation. The utility of endoscopic ultrasound in Barrett's patients is unproven.

11. For which patients with Barrett's esophagus is endoscopic surveillance recommended?

An extensive endoscopic cancer surveillance program for Barrett's esophagus is most appropriate for patients considered candidates for surgical cure if HGD or cancer is found.

12. What is the first step in endoscopic surveillance of patients with Barrett's esophagus?

Index endoscopy. Aggressive antireflux therapy should be initiated before a surveillance program is begun because of the difficulty in distinguishing inflammatory dysplasia from neoplasia. Extensive sampling of the entire Barrett's segment should be performed, particularly of any areas with macroscopic abnormalities. A proven method involves quadrant biopsies with large-particle forceps at 1–2-cm intervals, starting 1 cm below the esophagogastric junction and extending to 1 cm above the squamocolumnar junction. Further management should be guided by the histologic findings (see questions 13–17).

13. What steps are recommended if cancer is found?

Review biopsies with an experienced pathologist. If the histologic diagnosis is confirmed and the patient is a surgical candidate, recommend operation after complete staging. If the histologic diagnosis is uncertain, urgent repeat biopsy is required.

14. Describe the management of high-grade dysplasia.

Review biopsies with an expert pathologist. If the diagnosis is confirmed and no endoscopic esophagitis or histologic inflammatory atypia is present, recommend surgery for the fit patient. If the surgical risk is considered excessive, frequent endoscopic surveillance should be performed. Some centers intensify endoscopic surveillance when HGD is present and recommend surgery only when cancer is detected. If esophagitis or inflammatory atypia is considered responsible for the dysplasia, institute aggressive proton-pump inhibitor therapy for 4–8 weeks and repeat surveillance biopsies.

15. What steps are recommended for patients with low-grade dysplasia or indefinite results?

Review biopsies with an expert pathologist. If the histologic diagnosis is confirmed and no endoscopic esophagitis or histologic inflammatory atypia is evident, surveillance biopsies should be performed every 12 months. If the result is indefinite because of extensive inflammatory atypia, institute aggressive antisecretory therapy for 8–12 weeks and repeat surveillance biopsies.

16. What surveillance is recommended if no dysplasia is found?

Begin serial endoscopy with surveillance biopsies every 24 months. A shorter surveillance period (12 months) is reasonable in patients with long-segment Barrett's esophagus (> 6 cm).

17. Should patients with short segment Barrett's esophagus (SSBE) undergo the same endoscopic surveillance?

Periodic surveillance of SSBE is probably necessary, but no guidelines are available.

18. Discuss the role of endoscopically applied vital staining of the esophagus for detection of dysplasia and cancer in patients with Barrett's esophagus.

Specialized columnar mucosa of Barrett's esophagus avidly stains with endoscopically applied methylene blue (MB). Barrett's segments with high-grade dysplasia or adenocarcinoma tend to exhibit a heterogeneous MB-staining pattern marked by variability of stain intensity. Some researchers suggest that MB-directed biopsies of Barrett's esophagus are a more accurate and cost effective technique than random biopsies for detection of Barrett's dysplasia and cancer.

19. What is the risk of esophageal cancer in patients with a history of caustic ingestion?

1000 times greater than the risk in the general population. The cumulative results of four series have characterized the findings associated with lye-related esophageal cancer:
- Mean age at onset of cancer: 47 years
- Interval from caustic ingestion to development of cancer: 14–47 years (mean = 40 years)
- Location of cancers: mostly in the mid-esophagus

Malignancy appears to develop after a shorter interval if the corrosive injury occurs later in life. Because the periesophageal fibrosis caused by the corrosive injury decreases esophageal compliance, cancer usually presents at an earlier stage. The resectability rate and 5-year survival rate for lye-associated esophageal carcinoma are 85% and 33%, respectively.

20. How often is endoscopic surveillance needed in patients with a history of caustic ingestion?

Begin endoscopic surveillance 15–20 years after the caustic ingestion. Generally, endoscopic examination should not be conducted more frequently than every 1–3 years. The threshold to evaluate swallowing problems with endoscopy should be low.

21. Define tylosis. What is the risk for esophageal malignancy?

Tylosis is an uncommon genetic disorder characterized by hyperkeratosis of the palms and soles. It is transmitted in an autosomal dominant pattern and associated with a predisposition for development of esophageal cancer. The prevalence of esophageal cancer in patients with tylosis can be > 90% by 65 years of age. Death from esophageal cancer has been reported in patients as young as 30 years. A prospective endoscopic surveillance program has been initiated for a large family cohort in England.

22. Outline the recommendations for endoscopic surveillance in patients with tylosis.

Start surveillance endoscopy at 30 years of age. Symptoms of dysphagia or swallowing difficulties should be evaluated promptly. Generally, endoscopic examination should not be conducted more frequently than every 1–3 years.

STOMACH AND SMALL BOWEL

23. What is the risk for malignancy among patients with gastric polyps?

In the U.S., gastric polyps are uncommon. The risk of malignant transformation of a gastric polyp depends on histology. Most gastric polyps (70–90%) are hyperplastic, and the risk for malignant transformation is low (< 4%). Adenomatous gastric polyps are a true neoplasm, and their risk for malignant transformation is as high as 75%. Fundic gland polyps have no malignant potential but may suggest the diagnosis of familial adenomatous polyposis syndrome (FAP) and the need for ampullary and lower GI endoscopic surveillance. (See Chapter 32.)

24. What are the recommendations for endoscopic surveillance in patients with adenomatous gastric polyps?

Begin surveillance endoscopy 1 year after removing all gastric polyps, evaluating for recurrence and new or previously missed polyps. If this exam is negative, surveillance endoscopy should be repeated no more frequently than every 3–5 years for patients with adenomatous polyps. The recurrence rate for gastric adenomas is 16%. When *Helicobacter pylori* gastritis is identified, eradication may inhibit progression of gastric adenoma to carcinoma.

25. Who is at risk for ampullary and small bowel adenomas and frank malignancy?

In patients with FAP, the relative risk of duodenal adenocarcinoma and ampullary carcinoma is increased. Adenomatous changes and carcinoma have been reported in the ampulla and lower pancreatic and bile ducts. Such changes may not be readily apparent at endoscopy. Periampullary adenomas have a high risk of dysplasia. Chemoprevention of ampullary adenomas with sulindac has been disappointing. Investigation of the new COX-II inhibitors and combination chemotherapy with sulindac and HMG-CoA reductase inhibitors (lovastatin) to inhibit apoptosis is under way.

26. What endoscopic surveillance of the upper GI tract is necessary in patients with FAP?

Once FAP is diagnosed, periodic surveillance endoscopy should be initiated with both end-viewing and side-viewing instruments. Antral and duodenal polyps should be biopsied. Endoscopic retrograde cholangiopancreatography should be performed when the ampulla appears deformed or abnormal. Recognition of high-grade dysplasia necessitates further therapy, although the type of therapy is not yet fully defined. Studies are needed to ascertain the effectiveness of chemoprevention, endoscopic ampullectomy/polypectomy, and, possibly, more extensive surgical procedures.

27. What is the risk for malignancy in the gastric remnant after gastrectomy surgery (gastric stump carcinoma)?

Gastric stump carcinoma is carcinoma arising from the gastric remnant at least 5 years after surgery for benign disease. Cumulative analysis of over 50 studies indicates a 2–4-fold increased incidence of gastric carcinoma beginning 15 years after the original surgery. Endoscopic surveillance studies have detected gastric stump carcinoma in 4–6% of patients, and the progression from dysplasia to cancer has been documented. Symptoms are an unreliable predictor of early gastric cancer, and multiple random biopsies are necessary to identify dysplasia, because the macroscopic abnormalities may not be apparent. The mean interval between gastric surgery and cancer is about 20 years. Variations in the reporting of gastric cancer risk among patients with pernicious anemia may be due to differences in dietary nitrosamines, genetics, *H. pylori* infection, and/or alcohol and tobacco use. Billroth II procedures are more commonly associated with gastric remnant carcinoma than Billroth I procedures, and dysplastic epithelium is most commonly found near and within the gastroenteric stoma.

28. How often should patients undergo endoscopic surveillance for stump carcinoma?

Initiate surveillance endoscopy 15–20 years after gastric surgery. Multiple biopsies should be taken and examined for dysplasia. Periodic endoscopic surveillance is reasonable, but the cost-effective frequency has not been determined. When mucosal dysplasia is identified, more frequent surveillance is indicated.

29. Are patients with pernicious anemia (PA) at risk for gastric carcinoma?

Yes. PA is associated with type A gastritis and is thought to arise from chronic autoimmune injury to the gastric mucosa. The reported incidence of gastric cancer in patients with PA ranges from 2–10%. The coincidence of gastric polyps and PA is common. A study of 152 Minnesota residents with PA documented only a single case of gastric cancer during a 30-year period and tempered the enthusiasm for surveillance endoscopy; however, a recent large population-based cohort study in Sweden and a retrospective study of over 30,000 veterans identified the subsequent risk of gastric malignancy after the diagnosis of PA to be increased by at least twofold. The gastric malignancy usually occurred within 1–2 years after initial diagnosis of PA.

30. Give the recommendations for endoscopic surveillance in patients with pernicious anemia.

Surveillance endoscopy is not currently recommended . However, index endoscopy at the time of the diagnosis of PA to evaluate other risk factors for gastric cancer (e.g., gastric polyps) seems reasonable.

COLON

31. What are the current guidelines for colorectal cancer screening in U.S. adults at "average" risk?

- Screening begins at age 50 years.
- Annual fecal occult blood test (FOBT)
- Annual FOBT plus flexible sigmoidoscopy every 5 years
- Double-contrast barium enema every 5–10 years
- Colonoscopy every 10 years

32. Give the current guidelines for surveillance colonoscopy in patients with a history of adenomatous polyps.

A periodic surveillance program should be customized according to adequacy of colon preparation and endoscopic findings.

Colonoscopy Findings	Next Colonoscopy
Single tubular adenoma	5 years
Numerous adenomas (around 5)	1–2 years
Large sessile (> 2 cm) adenoma, especially if it was removed piecemeal	3–6 months
Inadequate colon preparation	Repeat within 3–6 months
All other adenoma findings	3 years

33. Does a single first-degree relative with colon cancer increase the risk for colorectal cancer?

Yes. A positive family history for colon cancer approximately doubles the risk.

34. Outline the recommended surveillance for people with a family history of colon cancer.

Single first-degree relative with colorectal cancer diagnosed at age > 60 years: Begin surveillance at age 40 years. The preferred surveillance is colonoscopy every 10 years.

Single first-degree relative with colorectal cancer diagnosed at age < 60 years or multiple first-degree relatives with colorectal cancer: Begin surveillance at age 40 years or 10 years younger than the youngest affected relative (whichever is first). The preferred surveillance is colonoscopy every 3–5 years.

35. What is hereditary nonpolyposis colorectal cancer (HNPCC)?

HNPCC is disease of autosomal dominant inheritance in which colon cancer arises in discrete adenomas, but polyposis does not occur. The Amsterdam criteria are used for diagnosis:

1. At least three relatives with colorectal cancer (one must be a first-degree relative of the other two).
2. Colorectal cancer involving at least two generations.
3. One or more cases of colorectal cancer before age 50 years.

36. Outline the screening recommendation for patients with HNPCC.

Full colonoscopy should be performed for all members of the family. Examination begins at age 20–25 years and should be done every 2 years until age 40, when colonoscopy should be done annually.

37. What are the Lynch syndromes?

Lynch syndrome I (site-specific HNPCC type A) is characterized by predisposition to colorectal cancer. Lynch syndrome II (HNPCC type B), also known as cancer family syndrome, is characterized by an autosomal inherited risk for several cancers, including cancer of the female genital tract and colon. In both Lynch syndromes, colorectal cancer develops at a much younger age than sporadic colon cancers in the general population. Tumors also are commonly found in the right colon and are often mucinous carcinomas. The genetic defect in HNPCC is the loss of hMSH2 and hMLH1 genes.

38. Outline the recommendation for colonoscopic surveillance in patients who have undergone resection of colorectal cancer.

Before resection, the yields for synchronous colorectal cancer and adenomatous polyps at initial clearing colonoscopy are about 2% and 25%, respectively. If a well-prepared clearing colonoscopy was performed preoperatively, the yield of surveillance colonoscopy performed 6 months to 2 years after resection is 2–3% for anastomotic recurrence, 3–4% for metachronous cancer, and 25–33% for adenomas (similar to postadenoma removal). If preoperative clearing colonoscopy was not done or if the results were inadequate because of obstruction or bowel preparation, surveillance should be done 2–3 months postoperatively. After the clearing examination, colonoscopy should be done every 3–5 years.

39. Are patients with long-standing ulcerative colitis at increased risk for colorectal cancer?

Yes. Their risk is increased by 6–15-fold compared with the general population. The risk increases significantly after 8–10 years of pancolitis or > 14 years of left-sided colitis.

40. What are the current recommendations for colonoscopic surveillance of such patients?

The yield for cancer or high-grade dysplasia on initial colonoscopic surveillance in long-standing ulcerative colitis may be as high as 12% and 8%, respectively. Surveillance is recommended after 8–10 years of pancolitis and 15 years of left-sided colitis; colonoscopy should be performed every 1–2 years. Because neoplasia and dysplasia often are not evident endoscopically, random biopsies should be taken from the cecum to the rectum (> 4 biopsies for every 10-cm segment) and examined histologically. Any abnormal mucosa or mass lesions also should be biopsied. Approximately 64 biopsies are needed to detect the highest grade of dysplasia with a 95% probability. Weinstein recommends four biopsies every 10 cm to the sigmoid, then every 5 cm to the rectum.

41. Describe management strategy if cancer is found.

Review biopsies with an experienced pathologist. If the histologic diagnosis is confirmed and the patient is a surgical candidate, recommend proctocolectomy after complete staging. If the histologic diagnosis is uncertain, urgent repeat biopsy is required.

42. What strategy is recommended for high-grade dysplasia?

Review biopsies with an expert pathologist. If the diagnosis is confirmed, the likelihood that cancer will be identified in the resected specimen is 42%. Surgery is recommended.

43. Describe the recommended strategies for dysplasia-associated lesions and low-grade dysplasia.

For dysplasia-associated lesions, proctocolectomy is recommended, because the risk for malignancy is estimated at > 50%. For low-grade dysplasia or indefinite results, review biopsies with an expert pathologist. If the histologic diagnosis is confirmed and no endoscopic colitis or histologic inflammatory atypia is present, consider colectomy or more intensive surveillance biopsies every 3–6 months. Low-grade dysplasia carries a 19% likelihood of existing cancer.

44. What strategy is recommended if no dysplasia is found?

Serial endoscopy with surveillance biopsies every 12 months.

45. When a sporadic adenomatous colon polyp is identified in a patient with chronic ulcerative colitis (CUC), should colectomy be performed?

No. Although all adenomatous polyps of the colon are considered "dysplasia," the polyp itself does not connote the same risk as detecting mucosal dysplasia elsewhere in persons with CUC. The polyp should be removed endoscopically and the remainder of the colon sampled for mucosal dysplasia, as described above.

46. What is the risk of colorectal cancer in patients with Crohn's disease?

When Crohn's disease involves the colon, the risk of colorectal cancer is 6 times higher than in the general population. When Crohn's disease is confined to the ileum, the risk for colorectal cancer appears to be similar to that in the general population. Screening recommendations are less firmly established than for ulcerative colitis.

47. What surveillance schedule is appropriate for patients with Crohn's disease?

Biannual colonoscopy with multiple biopsies after 10 years of colitis is reasonable.

48. What are the surveillance recommendations for patients with FAP syndromes?

FAP is an autosomal dominant trait with universal penetrance. The colon is often "carpeted" with hundreds to thousands of polyps by the age of 10 years. Surveillance recommendations include annual sigmoidoscopic surveillance, initiated at age 10–12 years. When polyps are identified, full colonoscopy is recommended. Once multiple adenomas are documented, colectomy is recommended.

BIBLIOGRAPHY

1. Agarwal B, Rao CV, Bhendwal S, et al: Lovastatin augments sulindac-induced apoptosis in colon cancer cells and potentiates chemopreventive effects of sulindac. Gastroenterology 117:838–847, 1999.
2. Aggestrup S, Holm JC, Sorensen HR: Does achalasia predispose to cancer of the esophagus? Chest 102:1013–1016, 1992.
3. Appleqvist P, Salmo M: Lye corrosion carcinoma of the esophagus. Cancer 45:2655, 1980.
4. Armbrecht U, Stockbrugger RW, Rode J, et al: Development of gastric dysplasia in pernicious anemia: A clinical endoscopic follow up study of 80 patients. Gut 31:1105–1109, 1990.
5. Bond JH: Polyp guideline: Diagnosis, treatment, and surveillance for patients with nonfamilial colorectal polyps. Ann Intern Med 119:836–843, 1993.
6. Burt RW: Colon cancer screening. Gastroenterology 119:837–853, 2000.
7. Chuong JJH, DuBovik S, McCallum RW: Achalasia as a risk factor for esophageal carcinoma: A reappraisal. Dig Dis Sci 29:1105–1108, 1984.
8. Cooper GS, Yuang Z, Chak A, Rimm AA: Patterns of endoscopic follow-up after surgery for nonmetastatic coloretcal cancer. Gastrointest Endosc 52:33–38, 2000.
9. Dent J, Bremmer CG, Collen MJ, et al: Barrett's oesophagus: Working Party Reports of World Congress of Gastroenterology. Melbourne, Blackwell Scientific, 1990, pp 17–26.
10. Eckardt VF, Junginger T, Gabbert HE, Bettendorf U: Superficial esophageal carcinoma in achalasia, detected by endoscopic surveillance. Z Gastroenterol 30:411–414, 1992.
11. Ginsberg G, Al-kawas F, Fleischer D, et al: Should all gastric polyps be removed? Am J Gastroenterol 87:1268, 1992.
12. Hameeteman W, Tytgat GNJ, Houthoff HJ, Van Den Tweel JG: Barrett's esophagus: Development of dysplasia and adenocarcinoma. Gastroenterology 96:1249–1256, 1989.
13. Hsing AW, Hansson LE, McLaughlin JK, et al: Pernicious anemia and subsequent cancer: A population-based cohort study. Cancer 71:745–750, 1993.

14. Jagelman DG, Petras RE, Sivak MV, McGannon E: Gastric and duodenal polyps in familial adenomatous polyposis: A prospective study of the nature and prevalence of upper gastrointestinal polyps. Gut 28:306–314, 1987.
15. Johan G, Offerhaus A, Giardiello M, et al: The risk of upper gastrointestinal cancer in familial adenomatous polyposis. Gastroenterology 102:1980–1982, 1992.
16. Just-Viera JO, Haight C: Achalasia and carcinoma of the esophagus. Surg Gynecol Obstet 128:1081–1095, 1969.
17. Lagergren J, Bergstrom R, Lindgren A, et al: Symptomatic gastroesophageal reflux as a risk factor for esophageal adenocarcinoma. N Engl J Med 340:825–831, 1999.
18. Leape LL, Ashcraft KW, Scarpelli DG, et al: Hazard to health—liquid lye. N Engl J Med 248:232–235, 1971.
19. Levine DS, Haggitt RC, Blount PL, et al: An endoscopic biopsy protocol can differentiate high-grade dysplasia from early adenocarcinoma in Barrett's esophagus. Gastroenterology 105:40–50, 1993.
20. Marger RS, Marger D: Carcinoma of the esophagus and tylosis: A lethal genetic combination. Cancer 72:17–79, 1993.
21. Morson BC, Sobin LH, Grundmann E, et al: Precancerous conditions and epithelial dysplasia in the stomach. J Clin Pathol 33:711–721, 1980.
22. Peracchia A, Segalin A, Bardini R, et al: Esophageal carcinoma and achalasia: Prevalence, incidence and results of treatment. Hepatogastroenterology 38:514–516, 1991.
23. Rex DK, Johnson DA, Leiberman DA, et al: Colorectal cancer prevention 2000: Screening recommendations of the American College of Gastroneterology. Am J Gastroenterol 95:868–877, 2000.
24. Rubin PH, Friedman S, Harpazn, et al: Colonoscopic polypectomy in chronic colitis: Conservative management after endoscopic resection of dysplastic polyps. Gastroenterology 117:1295–1300, 1999.
25. Saito K, Arai K, Mori M, et al: Effect of *Helicobacter pylori* eradication on malignant transformation of gastric adenoma. Gastrointest Endosc 52:27–32, 2000.
26. Sandler RS, Nyren O, Ekbom A, et al: The risk of esophageal cancer in patients with achalasia: A population-based study. JAMA 274: 1359–1362, 1995.
27. Schafer LW, Larson DE, Melton LJ III, et al: Risk of development of gastric carcinoma in patients with pernicious anemia: A population based study in Rochester, Minnesota. Mayo Clin Proc 60:444–448, 1985.
28. Schnell T, Sontag SJ, Cheifec G, et al: High grade dysplasia is still not an indication for surgery in patients with Barrett's esophagus: An update. Gastroenterology 14:1149, 1998.
29. Sjoblom SM, Sipponen P, Jarvinen H: Gastroscopic follow up of pernicious anemia patients. Gut 34:28–32, 1993.
30. Sonnenberg A, Massey BT, McCarty DJ, Jacobsen SJ: Epidemiology of hospitalization for achalasia in the United States. Dig Dis Sci 38:233–244, 1993.
31. Stalnikowicz R, Benbassat J: Risk of gastric cancer after gastric surgery for benign disorders. Arch Intern Med 150:2022–2026, 1990.
32. Steinbach G, Lynch PM, Phillips RKS, et al: The effect of Celecoxib, a cyclooxygenase-2 inhibitor, in familial adenomatous polyposis. N Engl J Med 342:1946–1952, 2000.
33. Talley NJ, Zinsmeister AR, Weaver A, et al: Gastric adenocarcinoma and *Helicobacter pylori* infection. J Natl Cancer Inst 83:1734–1739, 1991.
34. Winawer SJ, Zauber AG, O'Brien MJ, et al: Randomized comparison of surveillance intervals after colonoscopic removal of newly diagnosed adenomatous polyps. N Engl J Med 328:901–906, 1993.

VI. *Multisystem Manifestations of GI Disease*

69. RHEUMATOLOGIC MANIFESTATIONS

Sterling G. West, M.D.

ENTEROPATHIC ARTHRITIS

1. What bowel diseases are associated with inflammatory arthritis?
- Idiopathic inflammatory bowel disease (ulcerative colitis, Crohn's disease), pouchitis
- Microscopic colitis and collagenous colitis
- Infectious gastroenteritis
- Whipple's disease
- Gluten-sensitive enteropathy (celiac disease)
- Intestinal bypass arthritis

2. How often does an inflammatory peripheral or spinal arthritis occur in patients with idiopathic inflammatory bowel disease?

	Ulcerative colitis	Crohn's Disease
Peripheral arthritis	10%	20%
Sacroiliitis	15%	15%
Sacroiliitis/spondylitis	5%	5%

3. What are the most common joints involved in inflammatory peripheral athritis in patients with ulcerative colitis and Crohn's disease?
Upper extremity and small joint involvement is more common in ulcerative colitis than Crohn's disease. Both affect the knee and ankle predominantly.

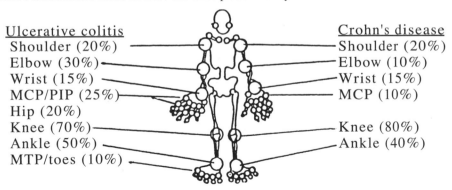

Ulcerative colitis		Crohn's disease
Shoulder (20%)		Shoulder (20%)
Elbow (30%)		Elbow (10%)
Wrist (15%)		Wrist (15%)
MCP/PIP (25%)		MCP (10%)
Hip (20%)		
Knee (70%)		Knee (80%)
Ankle (50%)		Ankle (40%)
MTP/toes (10%)		

4. Describe the clinical characteristics of the inflammatory peripheral arthritis associated with idiopathic inflammatory bowel disease (IBD).
The arthritis occurs equally in males and females, and children are affected as often as adults. The arthritis is typically acute in onset, migratory, and asymmetric, and it usually involves < 5 joints (i.e., pauciarticular). Synovial fluid analysis reveals an inflammatory fluid with up to 50,000 white blood cells/mm^3 (predominantly neutrophils) and negative findings on crystal examination

487

and cultures. Most arthritic episodes resolve in 1–2 months and do not result in radiographic changes or deformities.

5. What other extraintestinal manifestations are common in patients with idiopathic IBD and inflammatory peripheral arthritis?

The other extraintestinal manifestations are summarized by the mnemonic **PAIN**:

P = **P**yoderma gangrenosum (< 5%)
A = **A**phthous stomatitis (< 10%)
I = **I**nflammatory eye disease (acute anterior uveitis) (5–15%)
N = **N**odosum, erythema (< 10%)

6. What is the prevalence of perinuclear antineutrophil cytoplasmic antibody (pANCA) in patients with Crohn's disease and ulcerative colitis?

Between 25% (Crohn's disease) and 45% (ulcerative colitis) of patients can have pANCA, which is directed against bactericidal permeability-increasing (BPI) protein but not myeloperoxidase (MPO).

7. Do the extent and activity of IBD correlate with the activity of the peripheral inflammatory arthritis?

Patients with ulcerative colitis and Crohn's disease are more likely to develop peripheral arthritis if the colon is extensively involved. Most arthritic attacks occur during the first few years after onset of the bowel disease. The episodes coincide with flares of bowel disease in 60–70% of patients. Occasionally, the arthritis may precede symptoms of IBD, especially in children with Crohn's disease. Consequently, lack of GI symptoms and even a negative stool guaiac test do not exclude the possibility of occult Crohn's disease in a patient who presents with a characteristic arthritis.

8. What are the clinical characteristics of inflammatory spinal arthritis in idiopathic IBD?

The clinical characteristics and course of spinal arthritis in IBD are similar to those of ankylosing spondylitis. Inflammatory spinal arthritis occurs more commonly in males than females (3:1). Patients complain of back pain and prolonged stiffness, particularly at night and on waking. Pain and stiffness improve with exercise and movement. Physical examination reveals sacroiliac joint tenderness, global loss of spinal motion, and, in some patients, reduced chest expansion.

9. Which points in the history and physical examination are helpful in separating inflammatory spinal arthritis from mechanical low back pain in patients with IBD?

On the basis of history and physical examination, 95% of patients with inflammatory spinal arthritis can be differentiated from patients with mechanical low back pain.

Clinical Differentiation of Inflammatory Spinal Arthritis and Mechanical Low Back Pain

	INFLAMMATORY SPINAL ARTHRITIS	MECHANICAL LOW BACK PAIN
Onset of pain	Insidious	Acute
Duration of morning stiffness	> 60 min	< 30 min
Night-time pain	Yes	Infrequent
Effect of exercise on pain	Improvement	Worsening
Sacroiliac joint tenderness	Usually	No
Range of back motion	Global loss of motion	Abnormal flexion
Reduced chest expansion	Sometimes	No
Neurologic deficits	No	Possible
Duration of symptoms	> 3 mo	< 4 wk

10. Does the activity of inflammatory spinal arthritis correlate with the activity of the IBD?

No. The onset of sacroiliitis or spondylitis can precede by years, occur concurrently, or follow by years the onset of IBD. Furthermore, the course of the spinal arthritis is completely independent of the course of IBD.

11. Which human leukocyte antigen (HLA) occurs more commonly than expected with inflammatory arthritis secondary to IBD?

Frequency of HLA B27 in Inflammatory Bowel Disease

	CROHN'S DISEASE	ULCERATIVE COLITIS
Sacroiliitis/spondylitis	55%	70%
Peripheral arthritis	Same as normal healthy control populations	Same as normal healthy control populations

Eight percent of the normal healthy white population has the HLA B27 gene. Thus, a patient with IBD who possesses the HLA B27 gene has a 7–10 times increased risk of developing inflammatory sacroiliitis or spondylitis compared with IBD patients who are HLA B27-negative.

12. Describe the typical radiographic features of inflammatory sacroiliitis in IBD.

The radiographic abnormalities in IBD patients with inflammatory spinal arthritis are similar to those seen in ankylosing spondylitis. Patients with early inflammatory sacroiliitis frequently have normal plain radiographs, but magnetic resonance (MR) imaging of the sacroiliac joints demonstrates inflammation and edema. Over several months to years, patients develop sclerosis and erosions in the lower two-thirds of the sacroiliac joint. In some patients the joints may fuse completely.

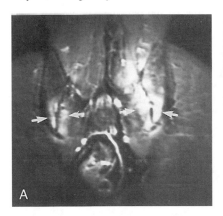 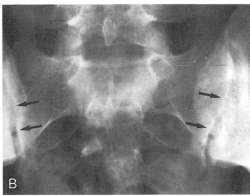

A, MR image of the sacroiliac joints showing inflammation *(arrows)* (T2-weighted image, TE50, TR2500). *B,* Radiograph showing early bilateral sacroiliitis *(arrows).*

13. Describe the typical radiographic features of spondylitis in IBD.

Patients with early spondylitis also may have normal radiographs. Later radiographs may show "shiny corners" at the insertion of the annulus fibrosus, anterior squaring of the vertebrae, and syndesmophyte formation. Syndesmophytes (calcification of annulous fibrosus) are thin, marginal, and bilateral. Some patients also show fusing of facet joints and calcification of the supraspinous ligament.

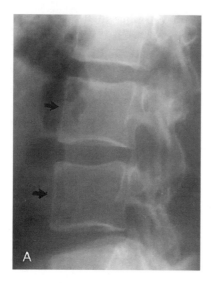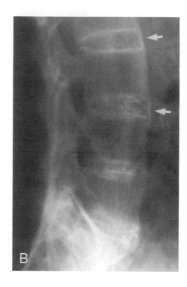

A, Radiograph showing anterior squaring of the vertebrae in a patient with early inflammatory spondylitis. B, Radiograph showing thin, marginal syndesmophytes *(arrows)* causing bamboo spine in a patient with Crohn's diseae with advanced inflammatory spondylitis.

14. Define bamboo spine.

Bamboo spine describes the radiographic appearance of a spine that demonstrates bilateral syndesmophytes traversing the entire spine (lumbar, thoracic, and cervical) (see Fig. B above). This phenomenon occurs in only 10% of patients with sacroiliitis or spondylitis. Patients who develop inflammatory hip disease may be at increased risk for developing bamboo spine.

15. What other rheumatic problems occur with increased frequency in patients with IBD?
- Achilles tendinitis/plantar fasciitis
- Clubbing of fingernails (5%)
- Hypertrophic osteoarthropathy
- Psoas abscess or septic hip from fistula formation (Crohn's disease)
- Osteoporosis secondary to medications (i.e., prednisone)
- Vasculitis
- Amyloidosis

16. Can treatment alleviate the symptoms of inflammatory peripheral arthritis and/or spinal arthritis in IBD?

	PERIPHERAL ARTHRITIS	SACROILIITIS/SPONDYLITIS
Nonsteroidal anti-inflammatory drugs*	Yes	Yes
Intraarticular corticosteroids	Yes	Yes (sacroiliitis)
Sulfasalazine	Yes	Maybe
Immunosuppressives	Yes	No
Antitumor necrosis factor alpha	Yes	Yes
Bowel resection		
Ulcerative colitis	Yes	No
Crohn's disease	No	No

• NSAIDs may exacerbate IBD.

17. What rheumatic disorders are associated with pouchitis, microscopic (lymphocytic) colitis, and/or collagenous colitis?

	POUCHITIS	MICROSCOPIC COLITIS	COLLAGENOUS COLITIS
IBD-like peripheral inflammatory arthritis	Yes	Yes	Yes (10%)
Rheumatoid arthritis	No	Yes	Yes
Ankylosing spondylitis*	No	Yes*	No
Thyroiditis/other autoimmune disease	No	Yes	Yes

* Up to 50% of patients with ankylosing spondylitis have asymptomatic MC/Crohn's-like lesions on right-sided colon biopsies.

CONTROVERSY

18. Why are patients with IBD more prone to develop an inflammatory arthritis?
Environmental antigens capable of inciting rheumatic disorders enter the body's circulation by traversing the respiratory mucosa, skin, or GI mucosa. The human GI tract has an estimated surface area of 1000 m^2 and functions not only to absorb nutrients but also to exclude potentially harmful antigens. Gut-associated lymphoid tissue (GALT), which includes Peyer's patches, the lamina propria, and intraepithelial T cells, constitutes 25% of the GI mucosa and helps to exclude entry of bacteria and other foreign antigens. Although the upper GI tract is normally not exposed to microbes, the lower GI tract is constantly in contact with millions of bacteria (up to 10^{12}/gm of feces).

Inflammation, whether from idiopathic IBD or infection with pathogenic microorganisms, can disrupt the normal integrity and function of the bowel, leading to increased gut permeability. This increased permeability may allow nonviable bacterial antigens in the gut lumen to enter the circulation more easily. These microbial antigens can either deposit directly in the joint synovia, leading to a local inflammatory reaction, or cause a systemic immune response, resulting in immune complexes that then deposit in joints and other tissues.

REACTIVE ARTHRITIS

19. What is reactive arthritis?
Reactive arthritis is a sterile inflammatory arthritis that occurs within 1–3 weeks after an extra-articular infection (usually of the GI or genitourinary tract).

20. What GI pathogens are implicated most commonly as causes of reactive arthritis?
- *Yersinia enterocolitica* or *Y. pseudotuberculosis*
- *Salmonella enteritidis* or *S. typhimurium*
- *Shigella dysenteriae* or *S. flexneri*
- *Campylobacter jejuni*

21. How common is reactive arthritis after an epidemic outbreak of infectious gastroenteritis?
Approximately 1–3% of patients who get infectious gastroenteritis during an epidemic subsequently develop reactive arthritis. The rate may be as high as 20% in *Yersinia*-infected people.

22. Which joints are most commonly involved in reactive arthritis after a bowel infection (i.e., postenteritic reactive arthritis)?
See figure at top of following page.

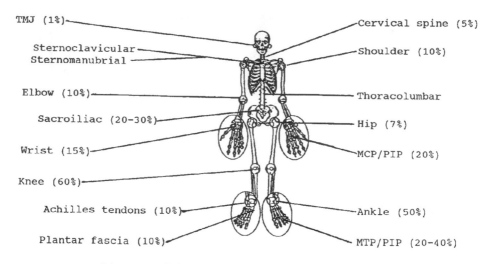

TMJ (1%)

Cervical spine (5%)

Sternoclavicular
Sternomanubrial

Shoulder (10%)

Elbow (10%)

Thoracolumbar

Sacroiliac (20-30%)

Hip (7%)

Wrist (15%)

MCP/PIP (20%)

Knee (60%)

Achilles tendons (10%)

Ankle (50%)

Plantar fascia (10%)

MTP/PIP (20-40%)

Joints commonly involved in reactive arthritis after bowel infection.

23. Describe the clinical characteristics of postenteritic reactive arthritis.

Demographics: males more often than females; average age = 30 yr
Onset of arthritis: abrupt, acute
Distribution of joints: asymmetric, pauciarticular; lower extremity involved in 80–90% of cases, sacroiliitis in 30%.
Synovial fluid analysis: inflammatory fluid (usually 10,000–50,000 white blood cells/mm^3), no crystals, negative cultures
Course and prognosis: 80% of cases resolve in 1–6 mo; 20% of patients have chronic arthritis with radiographic changes of peripheral and/or sacroiliac joints

24. What extraarticular manifestations may be seen in postenteritic reactive arthritis?

- Sterile urethritis (15–70%)
- Conjunctivitis
- Acute anterior uveitis
- Oral ulcers (painless or painful)
- Erythema nodosum (5% of *Yersinia* infections)
- Circinate balanitis (25% of *Shigella* infections)
- Keratoderma blennorrhagicum

25. How commonly do patients with postenteritic reactive arthritis have the clinical features of Reiter's syndrome?

The inflammatory arthritis, urethritis, conjunctivitis/uveitis, and mucocutaneous lesions that characterize Reiter's syndrome may develop 2–4 weeks after acute urethritis or diarrheal illness. The frequency varies with the causative enteric organism:

Shigella	85%	*Yersinia*	10%
Salmonella	10–15%	*Campylobacter*	10%

26. How do the radiographic features of inflammatory sacroiliitis and spondylitis due to postenteritic reactive arthritis differ from those of IBD?

	REACTIVE ARTHRITIS	INFLAMMATORY BOWEL DISEASE
Sacroiliitis	Unilateral, asymmetric	Bilateral, sacroiliac involvement
Spondylitis	Asymmetric, nonmarginal, jug-handle syndesmophytes	Bilateral, thin, marginal syndesmophytes

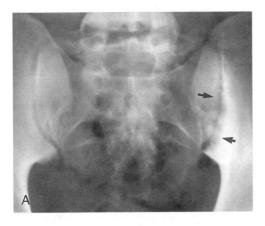

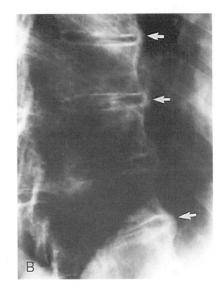

A, Radiograph showing unilateral sacroiliitis *(arrows)* in a patient with reactive arthritis. *B*, Radiograph showing large, nonmarginal syndesmophytes *(arrows)* of the spine in a patient with reactive arthritis.

27. Discuss the relationship of HLA-B27 positivity in patients with postenteritic reactive arthritis compared with a normal healthy population.

- Of patients with reactive arthritis, 70–80% are HLA-B27–positive; of normal healthy controls, 4–8% are HLA-B27–positive.
- Whites and patients with radiographic sacroiliitis are more likely to be HLA-B27–positive.
- People who are HLA-B27–positive have a 30–50-fold increased risk of developing reactive arthritis after infectious gastroenteritis compared with people without the HLA-B27 gene.
- Only 20–25% of all HLA-B27–positive people who get infectious gastroenteritis due to *Shigella, Salmonella,* or *Yersinia* develop postenteritic reactive arthritis.

28. Explain the current theory for the pathogenesis of a postenteritic reactive arthritis.

Bacterial lipopolysaccharide antigens from the pathogens (*Yersinia, Shigella, Salmonella*) causing the infectious gastroenteritis are deposited in the joints of patients who develop postenteritic reactive arthritis. These bacterial cell-wall components are believed to incite inflammation in the joint. The role of HLA-B27 in the pathogenesis is debated. One possibility is that the HLA-B27 molecule presents bacterial antigens to the immune system in a unique way, leading to inflammation. Another postulate is that molecular mimicry between the HLA-B27 molecule and bacterial antigens causes an aberrant immune response. Intact viable organisms cannot be cultured from the joint of a patient with reactive arthritis. However, chronic persistence of bacterial antigen is an important part of the pathogenesis of reactive arthritis.

29. How is postenteritic reactive arthritis treated?

| TREATMENT | PERIPHERAL ARTHRITIS | | SACROILIITIS |
	ACUTE	CHRONIC	
NSAIDs	Yes	Yes	Yes
Corticosteroids			
Intraarticular	Yes	Yes	Yes
Oral	Only if used in high doses		No
Antibiotics			
2-week course	No	No	No
3-month course	NA	No	No

Table continued on following page

| TREATMENT | PERIPHERAL ARTHRITIS | | SACROILIITIS |
	ACUTE	CHRONIC	
Sulfasalazine	NA	Yes	Maybe
Methotrexate	NA	Yes	No
Antitumor necrosis factor alpha	NA	Yes	Yes

NA = not applicable.

WHIPPLE'S DISEASE

30. Who was Whipple?

In 1907 George Hoyt Whipple reported the case of a 36-year-old medical missionary with diarrhea, malabsorption with weight loss, mesenteric lymphadenopathy, and migratory polyarthritis. He named the disease intestinal lipodystrophy, but it is now known as Whipple's disease. Whipple also became a Nobel Laureate in Physiology in 1934 and was founder of the University of Rochester Medical School.

31. What are the multisystem manifestations of Whipple's disease?

W = Wasting/weight loss   D = Diarrhea
H = Hyperpigmentation (skin)   I = Interstitial nephritis
I = Intestinal pain   S = Skin rashes
P = Pleurisy   E = Eye inflammation
P = Pneumonitis   A = Arthritis
L = Lymphadenopathy   S = Subcutaneous nodules
E = Encephalopathy   E = Endocarditis
S = Steatorrhea

32. Describe the clinical characteristics of arthritis associated with Whipple's disease.

Whipple's disease occurs most commonly in middle-aged white men. Seronegative oligoarthritis or polyarthritis is the presenting symptom in 60% of patients and may precede the intestinal symptoms by years. Over 90% of patients develop arthritis at some time during the disease course. Arthritis is inflammatory and often migratory and does not correlate with intestinal symptoms. Sacroiliitis or spondylitis occurs in 5–10% of patients, especially those who are HLA-B27–positive (33% of patients). Synovial fluid analysis shows an inflammatory fluid with 5000–100,000 cells/mm^3. Radiographs usually remain unremarkable.

33. What causes Whipple's disease?

Multiple tissues show deposits that stain with periodic acid-Shiff (PAS). These deposits contain rod-shaped free bacilli seen by electron microscopy. Recently, these bacilli have been shown to be a new organism, a gram-positive actinomycete called *Tropheryma whippelii*.

34. How is Whipple's disease best treated?

Tetracycline, penicillin, erythromycin, or trimethoprim/sulfamethoxazole (TMP/SMX) is given for > 1 year. Relapses occur in about 30% of cases. Chloramphenicol or TMP/SMX is recommended if the central nervous system is involved.

OTHER RHEUMATIC DISEASES

35. What rheumatic manifestations have been described in patients with celiac disease (gluten-sensitive enteropathy)?

Arthritis: symmetric polyarthritis involving predominantly large joints (knees and ankles > hips and shoulders); may precede enteropathic symptoms in 50% of cases.

Osteomalacia: due to steatorrhea from severe enteropathy.
Dermatitis herpetiformis

36. Which HLA type is more common in patients with celiac disease than in normal healthy controls?
HLA-DR3, frequently in association with HLA-B8, is seen in 95% of patients with celiac disease compared with 12% of the normal population.

37. What is the treatment for the arthritis secondary to celiac disease?
The arthritis responds dramatically to a gluten-free diet.

38. Describe the intestinal bypass arthritis-dermatitis syndrome.
This syndrome occurs in 20–80% of patients who have undergone intestinal bypass (jejunoileal or jejunocolic) surgery for morbid obesity. The arthritis is inflammatory, polyarticular, symmetric, and frequently migratory; it affects both upper and lower extremity joints. Radiographic findings usually remain normal, although 25% of patients have chronic recurring episodes of arthritis. Up to 80% develop dermatologic abnormalities, the most characteristic of which is a maculopapular or vesiculopustular rash.

39. Describe the pathogenesis of the intestinal bypass arthritis-dermatitis syndrome.
The pathogenesis involves bacterial overgrowth in the blind loop, resulting in antigenic stimulation that purportedly causes immune complex formation (frequently cryoprecipitates containing bacterial antigens), which deposits in the joints and skin. Treatment includes NSAIDs and oral antibiotics, which usually improve symptoms. Only surgical reanastomosis of the blind loop can result in complete elimination of symptoms.

40. What types of arthritis can be associated with carcinomas of the esophagus and colon?
Carcinomatous polyarthritis can be the presenting feature of an occult malignancy of the GI tract. The arthritis is typically acute in onset and asymmetric and predominantly involves lower extremity joints while sparing the small joints of the hands and wrists. Patients have an elevated erythrocyte sedimentation rate and a negative rheumatoid factor. Another type of arthritis associated with colorectal malignancy is septic arthritis due to *Streptococcus bovis*.

RHEUMATIC SYNDROMES AND PANCREATIC DISEASE

41. What pancreatic diseases have been associated with rheumatic syndromes?
Pancreatitis, pancreatic carcinoma, and pancreatic insufficiency.

42. What are the clinical features of pancreatic panniculitis syndrome?
Pancreatic panniculitis is a systemic syndrome occurring in some patients with pancreatitis or pancreatic acinar cell carcinoma. Its clinical manifestations include:
 • Tender, red nodules, usually on the extremities, which are frequently misdiagnosed as erythema nodosum but in fact are areas of panniculitis with fat necrosis.
 • Arthritis (60%) and arthralgias, usually of the ankles and knees. Synovial fluid is typically noninflammatory and creamy in color and contains lipid droplets that stain with Sudan black or oil red O.
 • Eosinophilia
 • Osteolytic bone lesions from bone marrow necrosis (10%), pleuropericarditis, fever

43. How can I remember the manifestations of pancreatic panniculitis syndrome?
A good mnenomic is **PANCREAS**:
 P = **P**ancreatitis
 A = **A**rthritis

N = Nodules secondary to fat necrosis
C = Cancer of the pancreas
R = Radiographic abnormalities (osteolytic lesions of bone)
E = Eosinophilia
A = Amylase, lipase, and trypsin elevations
S = Serositis, including pleuropericarditis

44. What causes pancreatic panniculitis syndrome?

Skin and synovial biopsies show fat necrosis, which is caused by release of trypsin, amylase, and lipase from the diseased pancreas.

45. What musculoskeletal problem can occur with pancreatic insufficiency?

Osteomalacia due to fat-soluble vitamin D malabsorption.

BIBLIOGRAPHY

1. Abibotol V, Roux C, Chaussade S, et al: Metabolic bone assessment in patients with inflammatory bowel disease. Gastroenterology 108:417–422, 1995.
2. Clegg CO, Reda DJ, Weisman MH, et al: Comparison of sulfasalazine and placebo in the treatment of reactive arthritis. Arthritis Rheum 39:2021–2027, 1996.
3. Dahl PR, Su WPD, Cullimore KC, Dicken CH: Pancreatic panniculitis. J Am Acad Dermatol 33:413–417, 1995.
4. Fomberstein B, Yerra N, Pitchumoni CS: Rheumatological complications of GI disorders. Amer J Gastroenterol 91:1090–1103, 1996.
5. Keyser FD, Elewaut D, DeVos M, et al: Bowel inflammation and the spondyloarthropathies. Rheumatic Dis Clin North Am 24:785–814, 1998.
6. Lubrano E, Cicacci C, Amers PR, et al: The arthritis of coeliac disease: Prevalence and pattern in 200 adult patients. Br J Rheumatol 35:1314–1318, 1996.
7. Naschitz JE, Rosner I, Rozenbaum M, et al: Cancer associated rheumatoid disorders: Clues to occult neoplasia. Semin Arthritis Rheum 24:231–241, 1995.
8. Nikkari S, Rantakokko K, Ekman P, et al: Salmonella-triggered reactive arthritis: Use of polymerase chain reaction, immunocytochemical staining, and gas chromatography-mass spectrometry in the detection of bacterial components from synovial fluid. Arthritis Rheum 42:84–89, 1999.
9. Relman DA, Schmidt TM, MacDermott RP, et al: Identification of the uncultured bacillus of Whipple's disease. N Engl J Med 327:293–301, 1992.
10. Roubenoff R, Ratain J, Giardiello I, et al: Collagenous colitis, enteropathic arthritis, and autoimmune diseases: Results of a patient survey. J Rheumatol 16:1229–1232, 1989.
11. Scofield RH, Warren WL, Koelsch G, et al: A hypothesis for the HLA B27 immune dysregulation in spondyloarthropathy: Contributions from enteric organisms, B27 structure, peptides bound by B27, and convergent evolution. Proc Natl Acad Sci USA 90:9330–9334, 1993.
12. Sieper J, Fendler C. Latiko S, et al: No benefit of long-term ciprofloxacin treatment in patients with reactive arthritis and undifferentiated oligoarthritis. Arthritis Rheum 42:1386–1396, 1999.
13. Schnabel A, Csernok E, Schultz H, et al: Bactericidal permeability increasing protein (BPI)-ANCA marked chronic inflammatory bowel diseases and hepatobiliary diseases. Med Klin 92:389–393, 1997.
14. Thomson GTD, DeRubeis DA, Hodge MA, et al: Post-Salmonella reactive arthritis: Late clinical sequelae in a point source cohort. Am J Med 98:13–21, 1995.
15. Utsinger PD, Weiner SR, Utsinger JH: Human models: Whipple's disease, coeliac disease, and jejunoileal bypass. Ballieres Clin Rheumatol 10:77–103, 1996.
16. Veloso FT, Carvalho J, Magro F: Immune-related systemic manifestations of inflammatory bowel disease: A prospective study of 792 patients. J Clin Gastroenterol 23:29–34, 1996.
17. Yu DT: Pathogenesis of reactive arthritis. Intern Med 38:97–101, 1999.

70. HEMATOLOGIC MANIFESTATIONS OF GASTROINTESTINAL DISEASE

Arlene J. Zaloznik, M.D.

1. Describe the etiology of postgastrectomy iron-deficiency anemia.

Iron-deficiency anemia is a frequent postoperative complication of gastric surgery, including both total and partial gastrectomy. In the early postoperative period, anemia results from the depletion of iron stores secondary to preoperative blood loss. Chronic iron deficiency develops later as a result of reduced gastric acidity and impaired iron absorption. Both ferrous and ferric iron are soluble in an acid pH. As the pH increases, ferric iron is converted to insoluble ferric hydroxide. Because iron is actively absorbed in the duodenum, the rapid intestinal transit that follows the loss of the reservoir function of the stomach may lead to decreased absorption. Iron deficiency is more common when the duodenum is surgically bypassed. Recurrent bleeding at the anastomotic site also may contribute to the development of the postgastrectomy iron-deficiency anemia.

2. What is the mechanism of vitamin B12 deficiency after a total or subtotal gastrectomy?

After **total gastrectomy**, vitamin B12 deficiency is inevitable over time. The loss of the intrinsic factor-secreting cells and the hydrochloric acid- and pepsin-secreting cells leads to an inability to absorb cobalamin (vitamin B12). The average time to develop the anemia is 5 years (range = 2–10 yr).

During the first several years after **partial gastrectom**y, vitamin B12 deficiency is uncommon. With time, atrophic gastritis develops in the gastric remnant and is the cause of late vitamin B12 deficiency.

Vitamin B12 deficiency is commonly seen in patients after **Billroth II surgery** who develop bacterial overgrowth syndrome. The bacteria take up cobalamin and reduce the amount available for absorption in the ileum. Small bowel bacterial overgrowth has the opposite effect on folate levels; abundant bacteria produce folate. High serum or red cell folate levels in the absence of folate supplements suggest small bowel bacterial overgrowth.

3. How should patients with postgastrectomy anemia be evaluated?

The evaluation of anemia in patients after surgery for peptic ulcer disease requires the measurement of serum ferritin and vitamin B12 levels. The stool should be examined for occult blood. The administration of intramuscular vitamin B12 and oral or intravenous iron may be required if deficiencies are documented. Antibiotic therapy may be necessary to eliminate excessive bacteria and reverse vitamin B12 deficiency in patients with small bowel overgrowth after Billroth II surgery.

4. What are the causes of anemia in the small intestinal malabsorption syndromes?

Celiac disease, tropical sprue, Whipple's disease, regional enteritis, and any other disorder that alters the integrity of the small bowel can lead to a malabsorption of iron, folate, and vitamin B12. Folate deficiency is the most common cause of anemia in the small intestinal malabsorption syndromes involving the proximal small bowel. Vitamin B12 deficiency is uncommon except with extensive involvement of the distal ileum. Iron-deficiency anemia secondary to chronic gastrointestinal blood loss is commonly seen in inflammatory bowel diseases. The hematologic consequences of small bowel resection depend on the area resected. If 100 cm of ileum is removed, vitamin B12 deficiency results. Although the duodenum is the primary site of iron absorption, the distal small bowel also can absorb iron to a limited degree. Iron deficiency usually does not occur except with extensive small bowel resection. Folate deficiency rarely occurs unless a large portion of the small intestine is removed.

DISEASE STATE	SMALL BOWEL INVOLVED	VITAMIN DEFICIENCY
Celiac disease	Duodenum and jejunum	Iron (most common) and folate (if jejunum is involved)
Tropical sprue	Jejunum (ileum in severe cases)	Folate and B-12 if ileum is involved
Whipple's disease	Duodenum and proximal jejunum	Iron and/or folate
Crohn's regional enteritis	Ileum	B12
Surgical resection	Ileum > 100 cm	B12

5. What is a potentially life-threatening sequela of acute viral hepatitis?

Pancytopenia with an aplastic or hypoplastic marrow is a rare, potentially fatal complication of viral hepatitis, occurring in 0.1–0.2% of patients. The risk of aplastic anemia appears to be greatest after non-A, non-B, non-C hepatitis. The average age of onset is 18 years, and males are affected more often than females. The aplastic anemia occurs within 6 months of the onset of hepatitis, often developing as the hepatitis is improved or resolved. There is no relation between the severity of the hepatitis and the occurrence of the aplasia. Although the pathogenesis of the aplasia is unknown, the most plausible explanation is an irreversible viral-induced hematopoietic stem cell injury. Fatality rates in posthepatitis aplastic anemia are > 80%, with a mean survival after the onset of pancytopenia of 10 weeks. Bone marrow transplantation is the treatment of choice for severe aplasia.

6. What is spur cell anemia?

The syndrome of spur cell anemia represents an abnormality of red cell changes in membrane lipids. Spur cells contain increased amounts of cholesterol and lecithin, resulting in an increased cholesterol:phospholipid ratio that persists 2–4 weeks after complete abstinence from alcohol. The red cells are bizarrely spiculated and undergo premature destruction in the spleen. Spur cell anemia, usually associated with hemolysis, is estimated to occur in 3% of patients with cirrhosis. Splenomegaly is a constant feature of this disorder and often associated with ascites and hepatic encephalopathy. In many patients, spur cell anemia occurs within weeks or months of death. Transfusion therapy is of limited value because transfused cells acquire the spur cell abnormality. Splenectomy may lead to the slowing of the hemolytic process but carries a high surgical risk in patients with end-stage liver disease, portal hypertension, and coagulopathy.

7. What etiologic factors (other than hemolysis) are involved in the development of anemia in patients with chronic liver disease?

Anemia is a frequent manifestation of chronic liver disease. Hypervolemia secondary to an increased plasma volume is frequently seen in patients with cirrhosis and results in a dilutional anemia. Hematocrit values may be as low as 20% in the presence of a normal red cell mass. The anemia of chronic liver disease is usually normochromic and normocytic. Gastrointesintal bleeding is a frequent cause of iron deficiency anemia in cirrhotic patients. Chronic alcoholics can develop megaloblastic anemia as a result of impaired folate metabolism or folic acid deficiency.

8. What is the cause of macrocytosis in alcoholic patients?

The presence of macrocytic red cells on blood smears and an elevated erythrocyte mean cell volume (MCV) are common findings in alcoholic patients. The macrocytosis may be the result of:
- Folate-deficiency megaloblastic anemia
- Reticulocytosis
- Macrocytosis of liver disease
- Macrocytosis of alcoholism

9. What are the findings in patients with folate-deficiency megaloblastic anemia?

Folate-deficiency megaloblastic anemia is the most common cause of macrocytosis in chronic alcoholics, occurring in almost 40%. Classic findings include an elevated erythrocyte

MCV, hypersegmented neutrophils (one 6-lobed neutrophil or > 5% of neutrophils with 5 lobes) and macro-ovalocytes on the peripheral smear, increased serum unconjugated bilirubin, markedly elevated serum lactic dehydrogenase (LDH), and megaloblastic erythroid and myeloid precursors in the bone marrow associated with low serum and erythrocyte folate concentrations. Folate deficiency develops commonly in drinkers of wine and whiskey, which contain little or none of the vitamin. It is seen less frequently in those who prefer beer, which is rich in the vitamin.

10. What are the findings in patients with macrocytosis of alcoholism?

Ethanol ingestion directly affects the bone marrow, causing megaloblastic changes. The degree of macrocytosis is typically modest, with MCVs no higher than 110 fl. Anemia is frequently absent or very slight. On the blood smear, the macrocytes are characteristically round and neutrophil hypersegmentation is absent. With abstention, the macrocytosis clears in 1–4 months.

11. Describe the diagnostic approach to anemia in alcoholic patients.

The most common causes of anemia in patients with cirrhosis are folate deficiency, iron deficiency, blood loss, and spur cell hemolytic anemia. The initial diagnostic approach should include the MCV, reticulocyte count, serum ferritin, and peripheral blood smear. Folate and vitamin B12 deficiency should be ruled out if the MCV is > 110 fl, if neutrophil hypersegmentation is present, and if > 3% macro-ovalocytes are present. If reticulocytosis is present with no evidence of intestinal bleeding or recovery from megaloblastic anemia, the patient should be evaluated for hemolysis. Serum ferritin levels are frequently increased in patients with alcoholic liver disease. When iron-deficiency anemia is present, serum ferritin levels are at the lower end of normal range rather than decreased. Serum ferritin is the best noninvasive screening test for iron-deficiency anemia in alcoholics.

12. What is the function of the liver in normal coagulation?

The liver is the principal site of synthesis and regulation of all coagulation proteins (fibrinogen and the vitamin K-dependent factors II, VII, IX, and X; factors V and VIII; contact factors XI and XII; and fibrin-stabilizing factor XIII), with the exception of von Willebrand factor and the fibrolytic proteins (tissue plasminogen activator and urokinase-type plasminogen activator). The liver also synthesizes protease inhibitors, such as antithrombin III, protein C, and heparin cofactor II, which modulate the coagulation cascade. In addition, the liver clears activated clotting factors, activation complexes, and end-products of the fibrinogen-to-fibrin conversion from the blood.

13. What coagulation abnormalities are associated with chronic liver disease?

Cholestatic liver disease leads to an inadequate excretion of bile salts into the gut, with malabsorption of vitamin K and consequent deficient hepatic synthesis of factors II, VII, IX, and X. In fulminant hepatic failure or decompensated cirrhosis, blood levels of all factors fall in proportion to their biologic half-life. Factor VII, with a half-life of 2–6 hours, drops first. As the liver disease progresses, the other factor levels also decrease. Only von Willebrand factor and factor VIII:C levels are unaffected. Fibrinogen concentrations are usually lower than normal. These changes result in prolongation of the activated partial thromboplastin time, prothrombin time, and thrombin clotting time. An increase in fibrinolytic activity may be manifest as disseminated intravascular clotting. Both qualitative and quantitative platelet abnormalities occur. Defective platelet aggregation correlates with the severity of the liver disease and results in prolonged bleeding times. Thrombocytopenia is often the result of increased platelet pooling in an enlarged spleen associated with portal hypertension.

14. How should the hemostatic defects of chronic liver disease be managed?

The management of patients with cirrhosis and a hemostatic defect depends on the nature of the defect and the degree and site of bleeding. Patients with a prolonged prothrombin time should receive parenteral vitamin K. Fresh frozen plasma (FFP) contains all components of the clotting and fibrinolytic system except platelets. Although FFP is the best treatment modality, volume overload may become a problem. Six to eight units of FFP are sufficient in most cases to correct severe clotting factor defects. Cryoprecipitate should be considered for patients with low fibrinogen concentrations. Platelet concentrates are indicated in patients with quantitative or qualitative platelet defects.

15. What are the causes of thrombocytopenia in alcoholic liver disease?

Thrombocytopenia occurs in both acutely ill, hospitalized alcoholic patients and chronic alcoholics. Megakaryocytes are typically normal to increased in numbers in the bone marrow. A rapid return to normal typically occurs within 1 week of alcohol withdrawal. Failure of the platelet count to increase within 5–7 days indicates the presence of an underlying disorder. Rebound thrombocytosis usually occurs during the second week of abstinence. The pathogenesis of the thrombocytopenia is most likely due to ineffective thrombopoiesis and a decrease in platelet survival. In addition, folate deficiency, hypersplenism, sepsis, and disseminated intravascular coagulation associated with shock, sepsis, or cirrhosis also may cause thrombocytopenia. Bone marrow aspiration for estimation of megakaryocyte numbers is not helpful, because all of the listed conditions are associated with normal to increased numbers of megakaryocytes. Most cases of alcohol-induced thrombocytopenia can be managed by expectant observation of the platelet count. Patients with serious hemorrhage and platelet counts < 20,000/ml should be given platelet transfusions.

16. Do hepatobiliary complications occur in sickle cell disease?

Yes. Hepatic crisis, gallstones, viral hepatitis, and hepatic failure may occur in patients with sickle cell disease. Patients also may have abnormal liver function tests in the absence of hepatic crisis, viral hepatitis, biliary disease, or other known causes of liver disease. Hepatomegaly develops in early childhood, with progression to cirrhosis in adults. Patients with sickle cell trait are not at an increased risk for hepatobiliary disease.

17. What is the clinical picture of hepatic crisis in patients with sickle cell disease?

The most common hepatic complication of sickle cell disease is the hepatic crisis, which occurs in 10% of patients. This syndrome, which resembles acute cholecystitis, presents with right upper quadrant (RUQ) pain, fever, leukocytosis, and variable elevations in serum transaminases and bilirubin levels. Often the patient has a preceding upper respiratory infection or vaso-occlusive crisis without hepatic involvement. The liver is enlarged and tender in most instances. The course is variable, but the disorder usually resolves in 1–2 weeks. Patients are managed with intravenous fluids, pain medications, and red cell transfusions on an individual basis. Each hepatic crisis leaves patches of ischemic necrosis, fibrosis, and nodular regeneration. An uncommon but virulent form of hepatic crisis is diffuse intrahepatic cholestasis. Massive intrasinusoidal sickling precipitates severe RUQ pain, hepatomegaly, and liver failure with hepatic encephalopathy. Treatment includes exchange transfusions, but patients usually die of hepatic failure.

18. How should gallstones be managed in patients with sickle cell disease?

Gallstones are found in 50–70% of adults with homozygous sickle cell disease and are asymptomatic in two-thirds of adults. The incidence increases with age. The diagnosis of acute cholecystitis is often difficult because the clinical picture resembles hepatic crisis. The management of asymptomatic gallstones remains controversial. The risk of surgery must be considered in determining the benefit. Complications of elective surgery, including pneumonia, pulmonary infiltrates, and atelectasis, are significant but not prohibitive. Emergency surgery for patients in crisis carries high morbidity and mortality rates. The course of asymptomatic gallstones in sickle cell disease is unknown, and cholecystectomy does not prevent future hepatic crisis. Cholecystectomy should be reserved for patients with demonstrated gallstones in whom it is difficult to differentiate recurrent abdominal crisis from cholecystitis and patients whose abdominal symptoms are clearly related to biliary disease.

19. What hematologic paraneoplastic syndromes are associated with gastrointestinal malignancies?

Mucin-producing adenocarcinomas, such as gastric cancer, have been associated with microangiopathic hemolytic anemia (MAHA). The anemia is characterized by red blood cell fragments in the peripheral blood, thrombocytopenia, and disseminated intravascular coagulation. The prognosis of patients who have MAHA and cancer is poor, with an average survival time of 3 weeks. There is no effective therapy. Tumor-associated erythrocytosis is uncommon but has been reported with hepatocellular carcinomas. Migratory superficial thrombophlebitis (Trousseau's syndrome) is characterized by recurrent thrombophlebitis in the absence of apparent predisposing factors. Mucin-producing adenocarcinomas of the gastrointestinal tract, particularly pancreatic cancer, are most frequently associated with this thrombosis. Trousseau's syndrome mainly involves multiple superficial and unusual vessels. The migratory thrombophlebitis may occur before or after the diagnosis of malignancy. Although acute episodes require heparin therapy, treatment of the underlying malignancy is the mainstay of therapy.

20. What are indications for red blood cell transfusion?

The goals of blood transfusion are to increase the red cell mass and, as a result, to increase oxygen transport while restoring and maintaining blood volume. The decision to transfuse a patient with red blood cells should be made after careful consideration of the cause and severity of anemia, physiologic adjustments to anemia, hemodynamic status, available alternatives to blood transfusion, and possible risks of transfusion therapy. Patients with acute blood loss can develop hypotension, tachycardia, and shock. Patients with chronic stable anemia or gradually developing anemia often tolerate very low levels of hemoglobin.

Patients with a hemoglobin > 10 gm/dl and no symptoms rarely need a transfusion. If the hemoglobin is 6–10 gm/dl, transfusion is indicated when symptoms are present; the asymptomatic patient may not need a transfusion. Once the hemoglobin is < 6 gm/dl, symptoms are almost always present, and red blood cells are usually needed. An exception is patients with chronic stable anemia, such as the anemia of chronic disease or pernicious anemia.

21. What are the nonhematologic adverse effects of blood transfusion?

Transfusion of red blood cells or plasma products may result in circulatory overload. In elderly patients with limited cardiac reserve or severely anemic patients in congestive heart failure, transfusion may lead to fatal pulmonary edema. Prevention of volume overload is preferable to treatment. In such patients, packed red blood cells are preferable to whole blood transfusion. Transfusions should be given at a rate of 1–2 ml of blood/kg of body weight/hr.

22. Define massive blood transfusion.

Several definitions for massive blood transfusion have been proposed: the replacement of a patient's entire blood volume in a 24-hour period; the transfusion of more than 10 units of whole blood or 20 units of paced red blood cells; or the replacement of more than 50% of the circulating blood volume in 3 hours or less.

23. How should hemorrhagic shock be managed in a patient with massive gastrointestinal bleeding?

The goal of resuscitation for hemorrhagic shock is prompt restoration of adequate perfusion and oxygen transportation. Lactated Ringer's solution is recommended as the initial therapy, until packed red blood cells are available. If cross-matched blood is not immediately available, a patient may be safely transfused with type O packed red blood cells until type-specific red cells are obtained. Massive transfusions of citrated blood products can lead to transient decreased levels of calcium. Most normothermic adults can withstand the transfusion of 20 units of packed red blood cells per hour without requiring calcium supplements. Close monitoring of calcium levels is advised instead of the indiscriminant infusion of calcium. Likewise, the concern of dilutional effects on plasma coagulation factors and platelets may be more theoretical than real. Patients without an underlying coagulopathy or thrombocytopenia may not need routine supplementation with fresh frozen plasma or platelets. However, in the setting of liver disease, in which the patient may have underlying coagulation factor deficiencies and thrombocytopenia, fresh frozen plasma and platelets need to be replaced. Like calcium supplementation, close monitoring of platelet levels and coagulation studies is recommended. Replacement products should be given as necessary.

BIBLIOGRAPHY

1. Cooper R: Hemolytic syndromes and red cell membrane abnormalities in liver disease. Semin Hematol 17:103–112, 1980.
2. Doll DC, Weiss RB: Neoplasia and the erythron. J Clin Oncol 3:429–446, 1985.
3. Jain R: Use of blood transfusion in management of anemia. Med Clin North Am 76:727–744, 1992.
4. Lindenbaum J: Hematologic complications of alcohol abuse. Semin Liver Dis 7:169–181, 1987.
5. Luzzatto G, Schafer AI: The prethrombotic state in cancer. Semin Oncol 17:147–159, 1990.
6. Mammen EF: Coagulation defects in liver disease. Med Clin North Am 78:545–554, 1994.
7. Phillips DL, Keefe EB: Hematologic manifestations of gastrointestinal disease. Hematol/Oncol Clin North Am 1:207–228, 1987.
8. Schubert TT: Hepatobiliary system in sickle cell disease. Gastroenterology 90:2013–2021, 1986.
9. Young, NS: Acquired aplastic anemia. JAMA 282:271–278, 1999.
10. Fakhry SM, Messick WJ, Shelton GF: Metabolic effects of massive transfusion. In Fakhry SM, Messick WJ, Shelton GF (eds): Principles of Transfusion Medicine, 2nd ed. Baltimore, Williams & Wilkins, 1996, pp 615–625.

71. DERMATOLOGIC MANIFESTATIONS OF GASTROINTESTINAL DISEASE

James E. Fitzpatrick, M.D.

1. List the most common skin manifestations of hepatic and biliary disease?
- Dilated abdominal wall veins
- Hyperpigmentation
- Jaundice
- Palmar erythema (liver palms)
- Peripheral edema
- Pruritus
- Purpura
- Spider hemangiomas

2. At what serum level of bilirubin do adults and infants develop clinically noticeable jaundice?

Adults develop clinically detectable jaundice when serum levels of bilirubin reach 2.5–3.0 mg/dl, whereas infants may not demonstrate visually detectable jaundice until serum levels reach 6.0–8.0 mg/dl. Hyperbilirubinemia typically precedes jaundice by several days because the bilirubin has not yet bound to tissue. Patients may remain visually jaundiced after serum levels of bilirubin normalize, because it takes several days for tissue-bound bilirubin to be released. Bilirubin has a strong affinity for elastin, which accounts for its early appearance in the sclera of the eye.

3. What is the differential diagnosis of yellowish discoloration of the skin?

Jaundice, carotenoderma due to excessive ingestion of carotene (e.g., yellow and orange vegetables such as carrots and squash), lycopenoderma due to excessive ingestion of lycopenes (e.g., red vegetables such as tomatoes and rose hips), and systemic administration of quinacrine. The skin also may demonstrate a sallow, subtle yellowish hue in patients with profound hypothyroidism.

4. What are spider angiomas? Why are they associated with liver disease?

Spider angiomas (nevus araneus) are vascular lesions characterized by a central arteriole and horizontal radiating thin-walled vessels that produce the "legs" of the vascular spider. The pulsation of the central vertically oriented arteriole in larger lesions can be visualized with diascopy (observation through a glass slide firmly pressed on the lesion). The mechanism is not proven, but the high incidence of spider angiomas in pregnancy and alcohol-associated hepatitis suggest that elevated levels of estrogens due to higher production or decreased metabolism are responsible. In the case of alcohol-associated liver disease, a direct effect on blood vessels of the skin or alteration of central vasomotor control mechanisms also has been postulated.

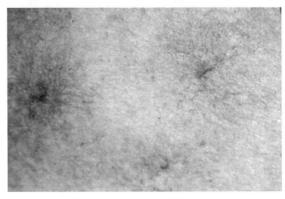

Three spider angiomas demonstrate central arteriole and radiating dilated blood vessels.

503

5. Does the number of spider angiomas correlate with the severity of alcohol-induced liver disease?

Yes, although there is some degree of individual susceptibility to spider angiomas. However, the correlation is high enough that barmaids in New York used to guess the severity of liver cirrhosis based on the number of visible spider angiomas! The number of spider angiomas also correlates with the presence of esophageal varices. One study demonstrated that more than 20 spider angiomas correlated with a 50% chance of esophageal bleeding.

6. Why do many patients with hepatobiliary disease itch?

Approximately 40% of patients with hepatic cirrhosis demonstrate moderate-to-severe pruritus. The mechanism of pruritus associated with hepatobiliary disease has not been firmly established, but it is believed to be due to elevated levels of bile acids secondary to cholestasis. Serum bile acids are frequently but not always elevated in patients with hepatobiliary disease and pruritus. Other mechanisms or chemical mediators may be involved because not all patients demonstrate this finding. Support for elevated bile acids comes from the observation that bile acid-binding resins relieve the pruritus. Studies of purified bile salts placed on blister bases demonstrated that all bile salts produce pruritus, but unconjugated chenodeoxycholate is the most potent.

7. A 25-year-old woman presents with painful, tender, red-to-violaceous subcutaneous nodules of the pretibial skin associated with diarrhea. What is the skin lesion?

The patient most likely has erythema nodosum, although the differential diagnosis includes other types of panniculitis (e.g., erythema induratum, pancreatitis-associated panniculitis), infection, and deep vasculitis (e.g., periarteritis nodosum). Erythema nodosum is a form of hypersensitivity panniculitis that preferentially affects the fibrous septae between the fat lobules. Clinically erythema nodosum most commonly presents on the anterior surface of the legs, less commonly on the forearms, as painful red-to-violaceous nodules without overlying scale. Lesions are typically bilateral, but unilateral and even annular variants exist. Typical lesions resolve over 3–6 weeks, but atypical lesions may persist for months. The diagnosis usually is made clinically, but occasional cases require biopsy. The histologic findings are characteristic if enough representative tissue is submitted. The mechanism is not understood.

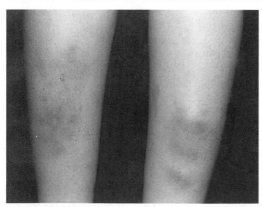

Typical lesions of erythema nodosum demonstrate bilateral, red, tender subcutaneous nodules on the anterior lower legs.

7. List the three most common GI disorders associated with erythema nodosum.

Ulcerative colitis, Crohn's disease, and infectious colitis (e.g., *Salmonella* spp. and *Yersinia enterocolitis*). In patients with inflammatory bowel disease, erythema nodosum is most commonly associated with ulcerative colitis (up to 7% of patients) and less commonly with Crohn's disease. The disease activity of erythema nodosum often parallels the activity of the bowel disease.

8. A 22-year-old woman presents with low-grade fever and an oozing ulcer of the hand that is rapidly expanding despite aggressive surgical debridement and intravenous antibiotics? What does she have?

The patient most likely has pyoderma gangrenosum, which usually affects the lower legs but may affect any cutaneous surface as well as mucosal surfaces of the eye and oral cavity. The lesions begin as a tender red papule or pustule that rapidly increases in size to form an ulcer with an undermined border. Lesions may remain fixed or expand rapidly at a rate of >1 cm/day. Pyoderma gangrenosum often demonstrates **pathergy**, which is the development of skin lesions at the site of trauma. Pyoderma gangrenosum mistaken for bacterial pyodermas may be treated with surgical debridement, which often makes the lesion worse. The pathogenesis of pyoderma gangrenosum is controversial. Histologically, the predominant effector cells are neutrophils. Some authorities have even considered it a form of vasculitis. Recent evidence suggests that it is probably lymphocyte-mediated, which accounts for the marked response to cyclosporine.

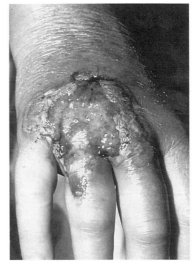

Typical lesion of pyoderma gangrenosum demonstrates tender, rapidly expanding ulcer with undermined edge.

9. List the GI diseases most commonly associated with pyoderma gangrenosum.

Ulcerative colitis (most common), Crohn's disease, and chronic infectious hepatitis. One study reported that 50% all cases of pyoderma gangrenosum are associated with ulcerative colitis, but < 10% of all patients with ulcerative colitis develop pyoderma gangrenosum. A separate study reported that one-third of patients with pyoderma gangrenosum had inflammatory bowel disease; ulcerative colitis and Crohn's disease were equally represented.

10. Describe the cutaneous manifestations of pancreatitis.

Cutaneous manifestations of pancreatitis include Cullen's sign, Grey Turner's sign, and pancreatic fat necrosis. Cullen's sign is a hemorrhagic discoloration of the umbilical area due to intraperitoneal hemorrhage from any cause; one of the more frequent causes is acute hemorrhagic panniculitis. Grey Turner's sign is a discoloration of the left flank associated with acute hemorrhagic pancreatitis. Acute and chronic pancreatitis and pancreatic carcinoma also may produce pancreatic fat necrosis, which presents as very tender, erythematous nodules of the subcutaneous fat that may spontaneously drain necrotic material. Patients also often have associated acute arthritis that may be crippling. Histologically pancreatic fat necrosis demonstrate necrosis and saponification of the fat associated with acute inflammation. The histologic findings are diagnostic. The fat necrosis is thought to be due to release of lipase and amylase, which have been demonstrated to be elevated within lesions.

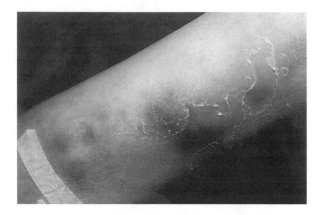

Pancreatic fat necrosis in a patient with alcohol-associated pancreatitis. Unlike erythema nodosum, epidermal changes (note scale) and ulceration are common.

11. A 32-year-old woman presents with recurrent blisters, primarily over the dorsum aspects of the hands. She reports two episodes of severe abdominal pain. One episode was associated with stupor. What disease does she have?

She most likely has variegate porphyria, which is inherited in an autosomal dominant fashion. A mutation in the protogen oxidase gene results in a reduction in the enzyme, protogen oxidase. Patients clinically resemble a cross between porphyria cutanea tarda (PCT) and acute intermittent porphyria (AIP). The skin lesions consist mainly of tense blisters, erosions, or scars, localized primarily to the dorsum of the hands. As in the case of PCT, patients also may demonstrate increased skin fragility, milia (small, white epidermoid cysts), hyperpigmentation, and hypertrichosis. As in the case of AIP, patients demonstrate intermittent abdominal pain that often is precipitated by drugs such as barbiturates or sulfonamides. The skin findings do not necessarily correlate with the abdominal attacks.

12. A 32-year-old man presents with a 2-year history of recurrent blisters that are intensely pruritic and recalcitrant to antihistamines and topical corticosteroids. They are located primarily on the elbows, knees, and buttocks. What does he most likely have?

Dermatitis herpetiformis, which is an autoimmune vesiculobullous disease characterized by intensely pruritic blisters that are often grouped (herpetiform) or may be plaques studded most commonly with vesicles and less commonly bullae. Dermatitis herpetiformis has a classic symmetric distribution; the characteristic sites are the elbows, knees, buttocks, and scalp. Because of the intense pruritus, patients often present to dermatologists with excoriations only. The diagnosis usually is established by demonstrating the presence of IgA autoantibodies along the dermoepidermal junction by direct immunofluorescence.

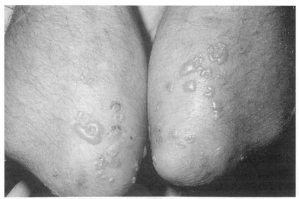

Grouped vesicles and bullae on the elbows of a patient with dermatitis herpetiformis.

13. What GI disease is most commonly associated with dermatitis hepertiformis?

Celiac disease (gluten-sensitive enteropathy). Although almost all patients demonstrate histologic findings of celiac disease, only one-third demonstrate clinical symptoms of celiac disease. Both celiac disease and dermatitis herpetiformis respond to a gluten-free diet.

14. A 30-year-old man presents with acute GI bleeding. He has yellowish, pebbly papules that coalesce into plaques on the neck, antecubital fossae, and axillae. Similar lesions are also present on his lower lip. What does the have?

The patient has pseudoxanthoma elasticum (PXE), a disorder characterized by progressive calcification of elastic fibers. It is inherited most commonly in an autosomal dominant fashion, but autosomal recessive variants have been described. The mucocutaneous manifestations often are described as looking like "plucked chicken skin." The histologic findings are diagnostic and demonstrate fragmentation of abnormal elastic fibers in the dermis associated with calcification. Identical yellowish papules are seen in the GI mucosa, including the mouth, esophagus, and stomach. Involvement of the elastic fibers in gastric arteries may result in acute and sometimes massive hemorrhage. Additional findings associated with PXE include angioid streaks of the retina, claudication, premature angina, and hypertension.

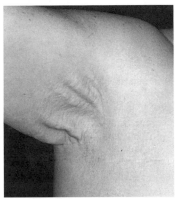

Confluent yellowish papules with appearance of "plucked chicken skin" in a patient with pseudoxanthoma elasticum.

15. A 24-year-old man presents with a history of unexplained melena, nose bleeds, and red macular lesions of the lips and fingers. What does he have?

The patient most likely has hereditary hemorrhagic telangiectasia (HHT), also known as Osler-Weber-Rendu disease. This uncommon genetic disorder is inherited in an autosomal dominant fashion. The cutaneous lesions typically present at puberty or later and manifest as linear, punctate, or macular lesions that most commonly affect the skin surfaces of the face, finger, and toes. Similar lesions also are found in many types of mucosal surfaces, including the nasal mucosa, lips, entire GI tract, and urinary tract. Arteriovenous malformations also may develop in the central nervous system, eye, lungs, and liver. Patients continue to develop new lesions during their lifetime and may experience chronic iron-deficiency anemia due to chronic low-grade blood loss from the GI tract.

16. During evaluation for GI bleeding, a 25-year-old man is noted to have 2–4-mm pigmented macules of the lips and buccal mucosa. What does he most likely have?

The patient most likely has Peutz-Jeghers syndrome, an autosomal dominant disorder characterized by round-to-oval pigmented macules that vary from brown to blue-brown in color and small intestine hamartomatous polyps. The pigmented macules are usually present at birth or develop during infancy. The most commonly affected areas are the lips, buccal mucosa, hard palate, gingival, anus, palms, and soles (see figure on page 389). Because pigmented macular lesions may be seen in these areas in normal individuals and in association with other syndromes, clinical and historical correlation is necessary to make a diagnosis of Peutz-Jeghers syndrome.

17. What is the risk of developing malignancy in the polyps associated with Peutz-Jeghers syndrome?

The lifetime risk of developing adenocarcinoma is calculated at 2–13%. Patients with Peutz-Jeghers syndrome also demonstrate an increased incidence of other types of neoplasia. The most common types are breast carcinoma, cervical adenocarcinoma, and both benign and malignant tumors of the ovary and testes.

18. During evaluation for numerous polyps of the colon, a 19-year-old man is noted to have multiple cysts of the skin and an osteoma. What does he most likely have?

Gardner's syndrome, which is inherited in an autosomal dominant fashion. This rare disorder occurs in 1 of every 14,000 births. The polyps resemble the polyps of familial adenomatous polyposis. All patients have colonic polyps, and 10% have small intestine polyps. The cutaneous manifestations consist of epidermoid cysts (epidermal inclusion cysts), lipomas, fibromas, desmoid tumors, and rarely, pilomatricomas (uncommon hair follicle tumors). Patient often have bone tumors, most of which are osteomas; supernumerary teeth; and congenital hypertrophy of the retinal pigmented epithelium.

19. What is the risk of developing malignancy in the polyps found in Gardner's syndrome?

The lifetime risk of colon cancer in Gardner's syndrome approaches 100%. Protocolectomy is recommended for all patients, followed by periodic monitoring of the rectal mucosal remnant and the upper GI tract. Patients with Gardner's syndrome also have a higher incidence of extracolonic malignancies, including papillary thyroid carcinoma, adrenal carcinoma, hepatoblastoma, periampullary carcinoma, and duodenal carcinoma.

20. A 44-year-old man presents with multiple hamartomatous polyps of the small and large bowel. Cutaneous examination reveals "cobblestoning" of the oral mucosa and multiple small papules and verrucous papules of the face. What does he most likely have?

Cowden's disease, also known as multiple hamartoma syndrome. This rare syndrome is inherited in an autosomal fashion. The mucocutaneous manifestations include small papules of the oral mucosa that are usually most prominent on the gingiva, are often numerous, and have been described as resembling cobblestones; papules and verrucous papules, usually located on the face, that histologically are trichilemmomas (benign follicular tumors); hyperkeratotic papules of the extremities; and firm nodules called sclerotic fibromas. Sclerotic fibromas are uncommon benign fibrous tumors that are typically solitary. Multiple sclerotic fibromas are considered to be a specific marker for Cowden's disease; the incidence approaches 100% if two or more are present. Polyps are present in the GI tract in approximately 30% of patients and may be present at any site.

21. What is the risk of developing malignancy in the polyps associated with Cowden's syndrome?

The polyps associated with Cowden's syndrome do not demonstrate an increased risk of malignancy. However, patients with Cowden's syndrome demonstrate an increased incidence of thyroid disease; up to two-thirds demonstrate goiter and 10% develop thyroid carcinoma. Seventy-five percent of female patients demonstrate breast neoplasia manifesting as fibrocystic breast disease, fibroadenomas, and breast carcinoma.

22. What is Trousseau's sign?

Trousseau's sign consists of superficial migratory thrombophlebitis associated with an underlying malignancy. Clinically it presents as erythematous linear cords that affect the superficial veins of the extremities and trunk. Patients typically continue to develop new lesions at multiple sites that may appear to "migrate." Trousseau's sign may be seen in association with many types of GI malignancies (e.g., gastric carcinoma, pancreatic adenocarcinoma) in addition to lung carcinoma, multiple myeloma, and Hodgkin's disease. The pathogenesis is not understood, and the thrombophlebitis is notoriously resistant to anticoagulant therapy. It is a cruel coincidence that

Trousseau, the physician who described the sign, developed it as a result of underlying gastric carcinoma, which ultimately was fatal.

23. A 50-year-old woman presents with alopecia, unexplained 20-lb weight loss, and superficial, flaccid vesicles and erosions on an erythematous base that preferentially involve the perioral and perianal areas. What does she most likely have?

The cutaneous lesions are consistent with necrolytic migratory erythema, a paraneoplastic cutaneous finding associated with $alpha_2$-glucagon-producing islet cell tumors of the pancreas. The cutaneous lesions characteristically start as broad areas of erythema that preferentially affect the face, intertriginous areas, ankles, and feet. The skin often appears to peel or demonstrate superficial vesicles. Patients also may demonstrate stomatitis, glossitis, alopecia, nail dystrophy, weight loss, diabetes mellitus, and anemia. Resection of the glucagon-producing tumor produces prompt resolution of the skin lesions.

24. What is Sister Mary Joseph's nodule?

Sister Mary Joseph's nodule is an umbilical metastasis of an internal malignancy. In the largest reported series, the most common primary malignancies were stomach (20%), large bowel (14%), ovary (14%), and pancreas (11%). In 20% of cases, the primary tumor could not be established. In 14% of cases, Sister Mary Joseph's nodule was the initial presentation of the internal malignancy. Umbilical metastasis usually indicates advanced disease. The average survival time is 10 months.

25. Who was Sister Mary Joseph?

Sister Mary Joseph was the first surgical assistant to W. J. Mayo. Although it was Mayo who described the clinical features of nodular umbilical metastases, she is credited with being the first to appreciate that patients with this finding have a poor prognosis. Sister Mary Joseph eventually became the superintendent of St. Mary's Hospital in Rochester, Minnesota.

BIBIOGRAPHY

1. Dahl PR, Su WPD, Cullimore KC, et al: Pancreatic panniculitis. J Am Acad Dermatol 33:413–417, 1995.
2. Foutch PG, Sullivan JA, Gaines JA: Cutaneous vascular spiders in cirrhotic patients: Correlation with hemorrhage from esophageal varices. Am J Gastroenterol 83:723–726, 1988.
3. Gregory B, Ho VC: Cutaneous manifestations of gastrointestinal disorders: Parts I and II. J Am Acad Dermatol 26:153–166, 371–383, 1992.
4. Powell FC, Cooper AJ, Massa MC, et al: Sister Mary Joseph's nodule: A clinical and histologic study. J Am Acad Dermatol 10:610–615, 1984.
5. Reilly PJ, Nostrant TT: Clinical manifestations of hereditary hemorrhagic telangiectasia. Am J Gastroenterol 79:363–367, 1984.
6. Smith KE, Fenske NA: Cutaneous manifestations of alcohol abuse. J Am Acad Dermatol 43:1–16, 2000.
7. Ward SK, Roenigk HH, Gordon KB: Dermatologic manifestations of gastrointestinal disorders. Gastroenterol Clin North Am 27:615–636, 1998.

72. ENDOCRINE DISORDERS AND THE GASTROINTESTINAL TRACT

John A. Merenich, M.D., and William J. Georgitis, M.D.

1. What are the common gastrointestinal (GI) complaints of patients with diabetes mellitus?

Common GI Symptoms in Diabetes Mellitus

Constipation	60%
Nausea and vomiting	30%
Abdominal pain	30%
Diarrhea	20%
Fecal incontinence	20%
Dysphagia	5%

GI complaints are reported by as many as 75% of patients with diabetes mellitus. Women report symptoms more often than men do. Although hyperglycemia, altered hormone production, increased susceptibility to secondary infections, and microangiopathy contribute to the development of alterations in GI tract function, visceral autonomic neuropathy appears to play a critical role in most disorders. Indeed, GI symptoms occur most often in patients with neuropathy and usually are not correlated with duration of diabetes, body mass index, glycosylated hemoglobin, or insulin dose.

2. Are esophageal motility abnormalities a common source of complaints in patients with diabetes mellitus?

Although specialized tests to assess esophageal function are rarely required in the clinical setting, manometry and scintigraphy reveal abnormalities of the esophagus in most patients with diabetes mellitus. Clinical symptoms, however, appear no more frequent than in patients of similar weight and age without diabetes. Symptomatic gastroesophageal reflux, when it occurs, is observed most often in patients with peripheral/sensory neuropathy or symptomatic diabetic gastroparesis. Dysphagia and odynophagia are also distinctly unusual; their occurrence in patients with diabetes should prompt further evaluation for another source. There is one notable exception to this generalization: because of their impaired immune status, patients with diabetes are more prone to candidal esophagitis, which occasionally causes difficulty or pain with swallowing. Fiberoptic esophagoscopy is often required to make the diagnosis because the presence or absence of oral *Candida* sp. does not predict or rule out esophageal infection.

3. What are the causes of gastroparesis in diabetic patients? How should it be treated?

Reduced amplitude of fundic contractions, decreased amplitude and frequency of antral contractions, and pylorospasm contribute to a delay in gastric emptying (solids > liquids) in patients with diabetes. In addition to worsening nausea and vomiting and early satiety, delayed gastric emptying may contribute to erratic glucose control in some individuals.

Treatment of Gastroparesis in Diabetes Mellitus

MANEUVER	COMMENTS
Avoid agents that impair gastric emptying	Especially anticholinergics and antidepressants: if needed, use agents with minimal anticholinergic properties, such as desipramine and fluoxetine

Table continued on following page

Treatment of Gastroparesis in Diabetes Mellitus (Continued)

MANEUVER	COMMENTS
Adjust diet	Decrease fat intake and avoid uncooked vegetables and fruits with hard-to-digest skins (e.g., apples, grapes, peas); give frequent small meals; increase liquid supplements
Use prokinetic agents (30 min before meals and at bedtime)	Metoclopramide, 5–20 mg Erythromycin, 250–500 mg Domperidone, 20 mg
Consider feeding jejunostomy	For refractory patients with severe malnutrition and volume depletion

4. Describe the mechanisms of chronic diarrhea in diabetes mellitus and their treatments.

Chronic diarrhea in patients with diabetes mellitus usually is related to either chronic autonomic dysfunction or associated diseases that are more prevalent in the diabetic population. The most common cause of nondiabetic diarrhea in diabetics is drug therapy with metformin.

Causes and Treatment of Chronic Diarrhea in Diabetes Mellitus

CAUSES OF DIABETIC DIARRHEA	TREATMENT
Intestinal bacterial overgrowth	Tetracycline, metronidazole, cephalosporins, quinolones, amoxicillin-clavulanic acid (10–14 days each month on rotating basis)
Celiac disease	Gluten-free diet
Use of dietetic foods	Avoid sorbitol products
Pancreatic exocrine deficiency	Pancreatic enzyme
Bile acid malabsorption	Cholestyramine (4–16 gm/day) or aluminum hydroxide
Abnormal colonic motility	Loperamide, diphenoxylate, clonidine (0.1–0.6 mg/day)
Altered intestinal secretion	Octreotide (50–75 µg subcutaneously before meals)
Anorectal dysfunction	Biofeedback

5. Explain the clinical implications of impaired GI motility in patients with hypothyroidism.

Delayed gastric emptying, prolonged intestinal transit time, and decreased amplitude and frequency of sigmoid colon and rectal muscular contractions have been documented in patients with hypothyroidism. Intestinal ischemia, myopathy, and neuropathy may contribute to dysmotility. Decreased frequency of bowel movements (< 1 every 48 hours) is reported in about 12% of patients with hypothyroidism. Elderly patients especially may complain of severe constipation refractory to laxatives; in severe cases, ileus progressing to pseudo-obstruction has been observed. Because of its insidious onset, intestinal dysmotility of hypothyroidism is sometimes misdiagnosed as functional bowel disease.

6. What autoimmune GI abnormalities are more prevalent in patients with autoimmune thyroiditis?

Immune gastritis and pernicious anemia coexist with hypothyroidism in about 10% of patients with autoimmune thyroiditis (Hashimoto's disease). Moreover, antiparietal cell antibodies are detected in up to one-third of patients with primary hypothyroidism. Autoimmune liver disease is also more prevalent in patients with thyroid disease. Hypothyroidism occurs in 16%, and thyroid antibody titers are elevated in 26% of patients with primary biliary cirrhosis. Indeed, primary biliary cirrhosis and chronic active hepatitis should be considered if the serum transaminase elevation commonly observed in hypothyroid patients is severe (> 2–3 times normal) or persists after thyroid hormone replacement. Celiac disease occurs frequently in patients with autoimmune thyroiditis, Addison's disease, and type 1 diabetes mellitus than in the general population. About 6% of patients with type 1 diabetes have celiac disease.

7. What are the GI manifestations of thyrotoxic storm?

Thyrotoxic storm refers to a rare, life-threatening syndrome resulting from extreme accentuation of the usual manifestations of thyrotoxicosis. The diagnosis is entirely clinical, but the disorder almost always includes some evidence of severe GI dysfunction. Nausea, vomiting, and abdominal pain are common. Hyperdefecation commonly observed in many patients with thyrotoxicosis may progress to severe diarrhea that can significantly compromise volume status. Hepatic dysfunction characterized by hepatomegaly, abdominal tenderness, and elevated serum transaminase concentrations is also a frequent component of thyroid storm; hyperbilirubinemia and jaundice indicate advanced disease and are associated with a high rate of mortality. The exact nature of hepatic inflammation, steatosis, necrosis, and cirrhosis described at autopsy in patients dying from thyrotoxicosis is unclear. The combination of increased metabolic demand without compensatory increase in hepatic blood flow results in relative ischemia that may account for some of the clinical and histologic findings.

8. Name the two metabolic causes of acute pancreatitis.

Hypertriglyceridemia and hypercalcemia are the two metabolic disturbances that can cause acute pancreatitis. Triglyceride concentration in excess of 1000 mg/dl has been reported in one-fourth to one-third of patients presenting with acute pancreatitis. Although excessive ethanol use may account for both pancreatitis and secondary triglyceride elevation, a direct causative or exacerbating role of hypertriglyceridemia in the development of pancreatic inflammation in many patients has been postulated. Acute pancreatitis has been reported in association with hypercalcemia of any cause, but it is observed most often in patients with hyperparathyroidism. Less than 1% of patients with acute pancreatitis, however, have documented hyperparathyroidism.

9. Discuss the three key steps in the management of pancreatitis associated with hypertriglyceridemia.

1. **Recognition.** Hypertriglyceridema should be considered in all patients with pancreatitis, especially those with "idiopathic" pancreatitis or recurrent episodes of inflammation. Serum triglyceride concentrations should be measured early in the course of pancreatitis, because clearance of chylomicrons (triglyceride-rich lipoprotein particles believed responsible for the syndrome) may be cleared within a few days of an acute attack, especially in fasting patients.

2. **Management of the acute attack.** Decreasing the triglyceride concentration to < 500 mg/dl is a primary concern and usually is associated with prompt cessation of abdominal pain. Initial fasting, followed by low-fat diet, is absolutely necessary to achieve this goal. Lipid-lowering agents, such as fibrates and nicotinic acid, are usually ineffective until serum triglyceride levels are reduced to 1000–1500 mg/dl. Administration of large doses of pancreatic enzymes also may help to suppress nausea and abdominal pain. Because excessive glucose serves as substrate for endogenous triglyceride production, appropriate insulin therapy to achieve euglycemia should be instituted as soon as possible in patients with diabetes mellitus.

3. **Prevention of recurrent hyperchylomicronemia.** Restricted fat intake, avoidance of alcohol, weight loss, and exercise help to prevent redevelopment of excessive chylomicrons. Patients should avoid agents known to increase serum triglycerides, including estrogens, vitamin A, retinoic acid, beta blockers, and thiazide diuretics. Patients with diabetes should be evaluated regularly to ensure adequate glycemic control. Triglyceride-lowering agents, such as niacin (3–6 gm/day), gemfibrozil (600 mg twice daily), fenofibrate (200 mg/day), and fish oils (3–15 gm/day), are prescribed if fasting triglyceride concentrations remain elevated. Although rarely required and poorly tolerated by patients, dietary medium-chain triacylglycerol also may be beneficial in patients whose serum triglycerides remain persistently elevated despite conventional maneuvers.

10. Define hypoglycemia and pathologic hypoglycemia.

Textbook definitions for hypoglycemia commonly cite a plasma glucose of less than 50 mg/dl (2.7 mmol/L). Experimental evidence in humans shows that lowering glucose levels provokes measurable physiologic responses at threshold glucose values well above 50 mg/dl. Glycemic thresholds for arterialized venous blood appear in the figure below. A practical dictum derived from these thresholds is that glucose levels below 75 mg/dl should be avoided during management of type 1 and type 2 diabetes mellitus to avoid creating hypoglycemic awareness from overly zealous glycemic control. Defining the cutoff value for pathologic hypoglycemia is complicated by the finding that a substantial minority of normal young women and young men have glucose levels below 50 mg/dl without neuroglycopenic symptoms when they are fasted.

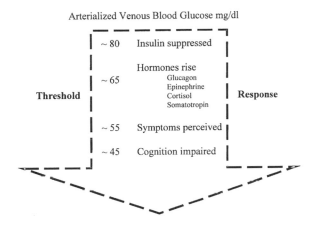

Glycemic thresholds for arterialized venous blood.

11. What are the two general classes of symptoms of hypoglycemia?

1. Neurogenic symptoms from autonomic nervous system discharge provoked by hypoglycemia include adrenergic symptoms of tremulousness, anxiety, and palpitations and cholinergic symptoms of sweating, hunger, and paresthesias.

2. Neuroglycopenic symptoms due to cerebral glucose deprivation range from confusion, difficulty in thinking, a sense of increased warmth, weakness, or fatigue to bizarre behavior, seizures, coma, and death.

12. What is Whipple's triad? Why is it important?

Whipple's triad should be present before insulin levels are measured in pursuit of the rare insulinoma:

1. Presence of symptoms consistent with hypoglycemia.
2. Documentation of a low plasma glucose.
3. Relief of symptoms after the plasma glucose is restored to normal.

13. How can GI and hepatic disturbances cause hypoglycemia?

Hypoglycemia (< 50 mg/dl) may occur in both the absorptive and postabsorptive state. Postabsorptive (fasting) hypoglycemia includes processes characterized by underproduction or overutilization of glucose; overutilizaion may be either insulin-dependent or insulin-independent. GI and hepatic disturbances, therefore, may result in or contribute to the development of hypoglycemia at many levels.

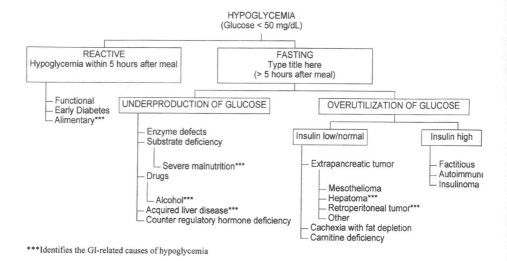

Contributions of GI and hepatic disturbances to the development of hypoglycemia.

14. How does ethanol cause hypoglycemia?

Ethanol impairs gluconeogenesis but not glycogenolysis. The sites of inhibition are shown in the figure below. Glycogen stores must be depleted for alcohol-induced hypoglycemia to occur. As ethanol is metabolized by alcohol dehydrogenase to acetaldehyde and then to acetic acid, hydrogen ions raise the cofactor ratio of nicotinamide adenine dinculeotide (NAD) to its reduced form (NADH). The falling cofactor ratio downregulates multiple hepatic gluconeogenic enzymes. Studies in humans and dogs also show that net uptake of hepatic lactate decreases in response to ethanol administration. Alcohol also dampens the release of glucose counterregulatory hormones. Levels attainable with social drinking diminish growth hormone, cortiocotropin, cortisol, and glucagon responses to induced hypoglycemia. This effect may be important in blunting recovery from low blood sugar.

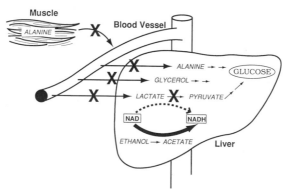

Ethanol inhibition of gluconeogenesis.

15. Is the frequency of GI neoplasms increased in acromegaly?

An increased incidence of tumors of various types has been reported in patients with acromegaly, including tumors of the thyroid, breast, and GI tract. Recent articles express skepticism due to the limited number of cases reported relative to comparison cohorts. Multiple articles report increased prevalence of colon polyps, prompting recommendations for colonoscopy at diagnosis or during follow-up of patients with acromegaly.

16. What GI symptoms may be seen with high serum calcium levels?

Hyperrcalcemic patients often present with gastrointestinal symptoms. Anorexia, nausea, and vomiting are early symptoms in hypercalcemic crisis. Poor oral intake and accelerated water loss from nephrogenic diabetes insipidus due to hypercalcemia lead to total body fluid depletion and decreased renal blood flow. The resulting fall in glomerular filtration rate leads to increased proximal tubular sodium reabsorption. Enhanced calcium reabsorption exacerbates the hypercalcemia. This vicious cycle can result in stupor, coma, and even death. Additional GI manifestations of hypercalcemia include constipation, pancreatitis, and peptic ulceration stemming from enhanced gastric acid secretion mediated in part by calcium-stimulated hypergastrinemia.

17. Weight loss, malaise, nausea, anorexia, vomiting and hyperpigmentation of the skin should prompt evaluation for what endocrine disorder? What United States president had this disease?

These signs and symptoms are present in primary adrenal insufficiency (Addison's disease), a malady diagnosed at an early age in President John F. Kennedy.

18. When is GI surgery warranted for the treatment of obesity?

A National Institutes of Health consensus conference concluded that surgical treatment for morbid obesity is acceptable in patients with a body mass index (BMI) exceeding 40 kg/m^2 and in patients with a BMI exceeding 35 kg/m^2 who have serious medical problems that can be expected to improve with weight loss achievable by surgery but not by medical therapy alone. BMI is calculated by dividing the patient's weight in kilograms by the patient's height in meters squared. Weight losses average from 30–40% of preoperative weight at 6–12 months after surgery. Losses are attributable primarily to decreased caloric consumption, not malabsorption. Surgical treatment of obesity is expensive and associated with some operative morbidity and mortality

19. What complications are specific to operations for obesity?

Numerous operations have been devised for weight loss. Jejunoileal bypass eventually achieved about a 1% operative mortality by the end of the 1970s but was fraught with complications, including diarrhea, bile acid malabsorption, fat-soluble vitamin deficiencies, calcium oxalate nephrolithiasis, inflammatory arthritis, and liver disease ranging from steatosis to fibrosis and even frank cirrhosis with hepatic failure. Gastric bypass or plication operations have mortality risks of approximately 1%. Deficiencies in iron, thiamine, and B12 are common.

20. What is MEN-1?

Multiple endocrine neoplasia syndrome type 1 (MEN-1), described by Wermer in 1954, is one of the pluriglandular disorders characterized by hyperplastic or neoplastic transformation of endocrine glands. Evolution of the syndrome involves the loss of a tumor suppressor gene encoded on the long arm of chromosome 11. A germ cell line mutant allele is inherited. Later, a somatic mutation leads to loss of the gene product menin, which results first in hyperplasia and later in neoplasia. Prevalence is estimated to range from 2 to 20/100,000.

21. List the MEN-1 pancreatic tumors in order of frequency.

In Wermer syndrome, the "three P" glands are involved in the following order of decreasing frequency: parathyroid, pancreas, and pituitary. Hyperparathyroidism is both the earliest to appear and the most prevalent manifestation (80–95% of cases). Parathyroid hyperplasia is treated by 3 and ½ parathyroidectomy. Pancreatic islet cell tumors occur in 80% and pituitary tumors in 50–71% of cases. Both may be multicentric in the affected glands. Islet cell tumors include gastrinomas and insulinomas, but they also may be associated with secretion of vasoactive intestinal peptide (VIP), somatostatin, and other peptide hormones or releasing factors. Prolactinomas are the most prevalent pituitary adenomas, but excessive secretion of growth hormone, corticotropin, and other anterior pituitary tumors can occur. In some cases, a hypersecretory tumor of one type presents initially and years later another hypersecretory tumor of pancreatic islet cell origin manifests itself. The distribution of islet cell hypersecretory tumors is as follows:

Gastrinoma	60%	Somatostatinoma	1%
Insulinoma	30%	Glucagonoma	5%
VIPoma	3%	Other	1%

22. Match the major clinical manifestations of the pancreatic endocrine tumors with their respective neoplasms:

Tumor	Clinical Manifestations
A. Pancreatic polypeptidoma	1. Hyperglycemia, anorexia, glossitis, anemia, migratory necrolytic erythema
B. Insulinoma	2. Recurrent peptic ulcer, refractory
C. Glucagonoma	3. Hypoglycemia, weight gain, neuroglycopenia, esophagitis, diarrhea
D. VIPoma	4. Diabetes mellitus, diarrhea, steatorrhea, cholelithiasis
E. Somatostatinoma	5. Water diarrhea, hypokalemia, hypercalcemia, hypochloremic metabolic alkalosis
F. Gastrinoma	6. None

Answers: A-6, B-3, C-1, D-5, E-4, and F-2.

23. Define carcinoid syndrome.

Carcinoid tumors can present with features of a syndrome, including flushing, diarrhea, abdominal cramping, eventual development of right-sided valvular heart disease, bronchospasm, and fibrosis of the pleura, peritoneum, or retroperitoneum. Tumors can be subdivided by origin into foregut, midgut, hindgut, and other sites (e.g., gonads or thymus). Secretory products include hormones and biogenic amine (e.g., serotonin, histamine, kallikrein, neurotensin, substance P, corticotropin, prostaglandins). Only 5–10% of patients harboring carcinoid tumors manifest the syndrome. Small tumors and those with venous drainage into the portal system may be clinically silent because of effective breakdown of tumor products. Large tumors, extensive hepatic metastases, or small tumors secreting directly into the systemic venous circulation (e.g., bronchial carcinoid tumors) most often manifest features of the carcinoid syndrome.

24. Describe the characteristic features of carcinoid tumors by site of origin.

Gastric carcinoids account for less than 1% of stomach neoplasms. Three quarters of gastric carcinoids are associated with chronic atrophic gastritis type A; the remainder appear in Zollinger-Ellison syndrome and in a sporadic form. One-half of gastric carcinoids are multifocal. Less than 10% metastasize, consistent with their usual indolent course.

Small intestinal carcinoids, which account for one-third of small bowel tumors, frequently are located in the distal ileum and present in patients in their 60s and 70s with small bowel obstruction or chronic abdominal pain, which often is present for years before diagnosis. Most patients have lymph node or hepatic metastases, and 5–7% manifest carcinoid syndrome. Tumor size correlates poorly with presence of metastases.

Appendiceal carcinoids are the most common tumor of the appendix. They present in the fourth or fifth decade of life. Less than 10% cause symptoms, metastases are rare, and prognosis is excellent and correlated with size.

Colonic carcinoids account for less than 1% of colon tumors. Most often they present in the seventh decade of life. Less than 5% present with carcinoid syndrome.

Rectal carcinoids account for only 1–2% of all rectal tumors. They usually contain glucagon- and glicentin-related peptides rather than serotonin. One-half are asymptomatic, and the rest present with rectal bleeding, pain, or constipation.

25. What general measures are used in the treatment of carcinoid syndrome?
    1. Niacin supplementation to compensate for accelerated conversion of tryptophan to serotonin
    2. High-protein diet
    3. Avoidance of precipitants for spells, such as sympathomimetics, alcohol, and stress

26. What agents are used to treat the flushing associated with carcinoid syndrome?
- Somatostatin analogs
- Interferon
- H1 and H2 blockers (e.g., gastric carcinoids)
- Phenoxybenzamine

27. List the agents used to treat diarrhea in patients with carcinoid syndrome.
- Loperamide and diphenoxylate
- Somatostatin analogs
- Antiserotonin agents (methysergide, cryproheptadine)
- Cholestyramine

28. How are asthma and bronchospasm treated in patients with carcinoid syndrome?
    Methylxanthines and glucocorticoids are the most commonly used agents. Beta agonists and epinephrine should be avoided because they may precipitate attacks.

29. What measures are used to reduce tumor burden in patients with carcinoid syndrome?
- Surgery
- Hepatic artery embolization or ligation
- Chemotherapy (streptoxocin and fluorouracil; methotrexate and cyclophosphamide; interferon; doxorubicin; cisplatinum; etoposide)
- Radiolabeled somatostatin analogs

30. What GI symptoms may be present in patients with pheochromocytoma?
    Weight loss, anorexia, and abdominal pain due to cholelithiasis are presenting features in some cases of pheochromocytoma.

31. What is the most prominent GI manifestation of medullary cancer of the thyroid?
    Diarrhea, sometimes severe, occurs in 30–50% of patients. Vasoactive intestinal polypeptide, kinins, and prostaglandins (not calcitonin) account for the diarrhea in most patients. Adrednocorticotropic hormone and serotonin also may be elaborated by the tumor, causing Cushing's syndrome and carcinoid syndrome, respectively.

32. What is the "rule of 10s" in regard to insulinoma?
- 10% of insulinomas are associated with MEN 1 syndrome
- 10% are malignant
- 10% are bilateral
- 10% are < 2 cm in size
- 10% occur in patients < 30 years of age

BIBLIOGRAPHY

1. Annese V, Bassotti G, Caruso N, et al: Gastrointestinal motor dysfunction, symptoms, and neuropathy in noninsulin-dependent (type 2) diabetes mellitus. J Clin Gastroenterol 29:171, 1999.
2. Arky RA: Hypoglycemia associated with liver disease and ethanol. Endocrinol Metab Clin North Am 18:75, 1989.
3. Asakura L, Lottenberg AM, Neves MQ, et al: Dietary medium-chain triacylglycerol prevents the postprandial rise of plasma triacylglycerols but induces hypercholesterolemia in primary hypertriglyceridemic subjects. Am J Clin Nutr 71:701, 2000.
4. Braverman LE, Utiger RD: The Thyroid, 6th ed. Philadelphia, J.B. Lippincott, 1991.
5. Bravo EL: Evolving concepts in the pathophysiology, diagnosis, and treatment of pheochromocytoma. Endocrine Rev 15:356, 1994.
6. Camilleri M: Gastrointestinal problems in diabetes. Endocrinol Metab Clin North Am 25:361, 1996.
7. Delcore R, Friesen SR: Gastrointestinal neuroendocrine tumors: J Am Coll Surg 178:187, 1994.
8. Greenway FL: Surgery for obesity. Endocrinol Metab Clin North Am 25:1005, 1999.

9. Kahn CR, Weir GC: Joslin's Diabetes Mellitus, 18th ed. Philadelphia, Lea & Febiger, 1994.
10. Kulke MH, Mayer RJ: Carcinoid tumors. N Engl J Med 18:858, 1999.
11. Lauffer JM, Zang T, Modlin IM: Current status of gastrointestinal carcinoids. Aliment Pharmacol Ther 13:271, 1999.
12. Lysy J, Israeli E, Goldin E: The prevalence of chronic diarrhea among diabetic patients. Am J Gastroenterol 94:2165, 1999.
13. Marks V, Teale J: Drug-induced hypoglycemia. Endocrinol Metab Clin North Am 28:555, 1999.
14. Modlin IM, Basson MD: Clinical applications of gastrointestinal hormones. Endocrinol Metab Clin North Am 22:823, 1993.
15. Molitch ME: Clinical manifestations of acromegaly. Endocrinol Metab Clin North Am 21:597, 1992.
16. Rensch MJ, Merenich JA, Lieberman M, et al: Gluten-sensitive enteropathy in patients with insulin-dependent diabetes mellitus. Ann Intern Med 124:564, 1996.
17. Scialpi C, Mosca S, Malguti A: Acromegaly and intestinal neoplasms. Panminerva Med 41:157, 1999.
18. Shulkes A, Wilson JS: Somatostatin in gastroenterology. BMJ 308:1381, 1994.
19. Spangeus A, El-Salhy M, Suhr O, Eriksson J, Lithner F: Prevalence of gastrointestinal symptoms in young and middle-aged diabetic patients. Scand J Gastroenterol 34:1196, 1999.
20. Steinberg W, Tenner S: Acute pancreatitis. N Engl J Med 330:1198, 1994.
21. Toskes PP: Hyperlipidemic pancreatitis. Gastroenterol Clin North Am 19:783, 1990.
22. Vassilopoulou-Sellin R, Ajani J: Neuroendocrine tumors of the pancreas. Endocrinol Metab Clin North Am 23:53, 1994.
23. Veldhuis JD, Norton JA, Wells SA: Surgical versus medical management of multiple endocrine neoplasia (MEN) Type 1. J Clin Endocrinol Metab 82:357, 1997.
24. Wilson JD, Foster DW: Williams Textbook of Endocrinology, 8th ed. Philadelphia, W.B. Saunders, 1992.
25. Yang R, Arem R, Chan L: Gastrointestinal tract complications of diabetes mellitus. Arch Intern Med 144:1251, 1984.

VII. Gastrointestinal Radiology

73. RADIOGRAPHY AND RADIOGRAPHIC-FLUOROSCOPIC CONTRAST STUDIES

Bernard E. Zeligman, M.D.

1. When you request an imaging examination, what information should you communicate to the radiologist?

By communicating the following information, a clinician helps ensure that imaging will be accomplished and images interpreted optimally for each patient:

1. Specify known major medical diagnoses.

2. Include all clinical information pertinent to the examination: (1) key findings from clincal history, physical examination, and laboratory tests that suggest the diagnosis and (2) any surgical alteration of anatomy that will be examined radiologically.

3. Specify the purpose of the examination: diagnoses, postprocedural complications, or radiologic findings to check for—or the known diagnosis or finding to follow for change.

4. Name the requested examination precisely. In particular, for fluoroscopic-radiographic gastrointestinal (GI) contrast examinations, terminology should clearly communicate the structures to evaluate. *Barium swallow* should not be added to *upper GI series* or *small bowel follow-through*— unless detailed evaluation of swallowing, an additional examination, is also indicated. Similarly, *upper GI series* should not be added to *small bowel follow-through* —unless detailed evaluation of the stomach and duodenum, an additional examination, is also indicated.

ABDOMINAL RADIOGRAPHY

2. Which radiographs should constitute an acute abdominal series?

The optimal series, sometimes called a *three-way abdomen*, includes:

1. Posteroanterior (PA) upright chest
2. Supine abdomen
3. Upright abdomen

If limited patient mobility precludes the upright position, the best series is:

1. Anteroposterior (AP) chest
2. Supine abdomen
3. Left lateral decubitus abdomen

To investigate the cause of an acute abdomen, the entire acute abdominal series should be requested. An upright abdominal radiograph is both less diagnostic than either an upright chest or left lateral decubitus abdomen for pneumoperitoneum, and also less diagnostic than a supine abdomen for bowel obstruction—and should never be the *only* image to evaluate for perforation or obstruction of the gut. A chest radiograph, the most sensitive image for pneumoperitoneum if the patient is upright, is important even if the patient is supine because thoracic abnormalities—especially if from pneumonia (Fig. 1) or pulmonary embolism, either of which may present as an acute abdomen—may be decisive.

3. What is the key abdominal radiographic finding of bowel obstruction?

The hallmark of obstruction is *dilatation*. If the bowel is dilated all of the way downstream to the anorectal junction, obstruction is functional (except for a newborn with anorectal malformation).

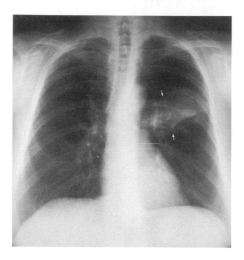

FIGURE 1.   Pneumonia presenting clinically as an acute abdomen. Abdominal radiographs were normal, but this posteroanterior upright chest radiograph shows an ill-defined opacity *(arrows)* in the left upper lobe.

Alternatively, if the bowel is dilated only down to a point of transition, downstream of which caliber appears normal or smaller than normal, obstruction is probably mechanical (Figs. 2 and 3) but may be functional (Fig. 4). The presence or absence of gas-fluid levels means little. Two old axioms—that gas in the lumen of the duodenal loop, jejunum, or ileum is abnormal and that gas-fluid levels in any of those locations or in the colon are abnormal—are excessively strict. Gas, with or without fluid levels, can be normal in any segment of intestine. Normal abdominal radiographs cannot exclude even high-grade small bowel obstruction.

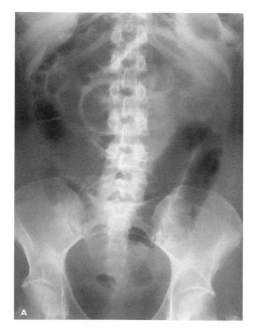

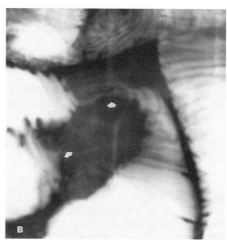

FIGURE 2.   Mechanical small bowel obstruction. *A,* Supine abdominal radiograph. Because small bowel dilatation does not reach the right lower quadrant, high-grade mechanical obstruction of the upper small bowel (above the lower ileum) is likely. *B,* The appropriate fluoroscopic examination, a small bowel follow-through, shows partial obstruction of two closely contiguous segments of jejunum *(arrows)* by adhesions.

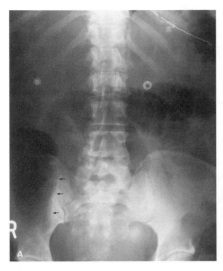 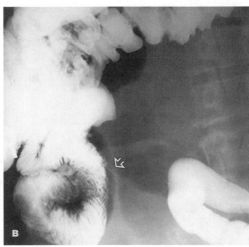

FIGURE 3.   Mechanical small bowel obstruction. *A,* Supine abdominal radiograph. Because small bowel is dilated even in the right lower quadrant *(arrows)* but the colon is not dilated, high-grade mechanical obstruction of lower ileum is likely. *B,* The appropriate fluoroscopic examination, a single-contrast barium enema, not only excluded obstruction of the colon but showed, in the right lower quadrant, complete obstruction to further retrograde flow of barium at a tapered narrowing *(arrow)* of ileum caused by an adhesion.

4. What are causes of pneumatosis intestinalis?

Reported causes of pneumatosis (Figs. 5 and 6B) are numerous, but a logical approach based on pathophysiology can bring common causes to mind:

1. Remember the two potential sites of origin of the gas: the lungs and the gut lumen (where gas and gas-producing bacteria exist).

2. Consider mechanisms by which gas may reach the wall of the gut from each site. (Increased intraluminal pressure, although it probably must cause mucosal tears for pneumatosis to develop, is a mechanism basically different from loss of mucosal integrity).

3. Think of possible causes for each mechanism. Because of its urgency, loss of mucosal integrity caused by bowel ischemia is the most important possible cause.

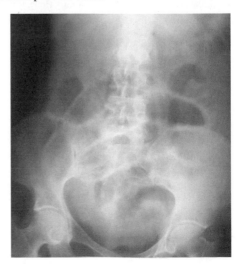

FIGURE 4.   Portable supine abdominal radiograph. Because dilatation of small bowel does not reach the right lower quadrant, mechanical obstruction of upper small bowel is likely. This obstruction, however, was functional as a result of acute pancreatitis.

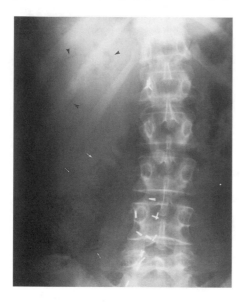

FIGURE 5. Supine abdominal radiograph. These two patterns of pneumatosis intestinalis—linear and bubbly *(arrows)*— suggest but are not diagnostic of bowel ischemia. A third possible pattern not shown here (cystic gas collections in the colonic wall) is characteristic of pneumatosis *Cystoides coli* and rarely, if ever, is due to ischemia. A second abnormal gas collection, branching and tapering in the liver *(arrowheads)*, is, as its predominantly peripheral location favors, not biliary but portal venous.

Major Causes of Pneumatosis Intestinalis

SOURCE OF GAS: LUNGS	SOURCE OF GAS: GUT LUMEN
Barotrauma	Mechanism: increased intraluminal pressure
Chronic obstructive pulmonary disease	Air insufflation (endoscopy)
	Bowel obstruction (mechanical or functional)
	Mechanism: loss of mucosal integrity
	Ischemia
	Inflammation (infectious or noninfectious)
	Drugs (e.g., glucocorticoids)

5. What distinguishes portal venous gas from pneumobilia?

Location usually distinguishes portal venous gas from the generally less serious pneumobilia. Because portal venous blood normally flows toward the periphery of the liver, portal venous gas tends to accumulate peripherally (Fig. 5). Because bile normally flows toward the liver hilum, biliary gas tends to accumulate near the hilum (Fig. 6A). These rules fail occasionally, however, because a radiograph shows the constantly moving gas only at one instant, when its location may be transiently atypical (Fig. 6B).

CONTRAST AGENTS

6. What is the role of barium to opacify the lumen of the GI tract?

Barium contrast agents consist of barium sulfate particles suspended in water. Because it produces better images, is less costly, and rarely does harm, barium is generally far superior to iodinated contrast. This superiority applies to examinations for possible bowel obstruction, except in one situation. At least in theory, barium may worsen a partial obstruction of one part of the gut, the *colon*; if a large volume of contrast medium may progress from upstream to a partial mechanical obstruction of the colon, barium possibly could do harm. Adequate assessment of oral and pharyngeal swallowing dysfunction requires barium. Barium aspirated in small volume during some of these examinations, although occasionally conspicuous on chest radiographs for months thereafter, does little or no harm.

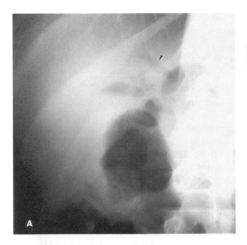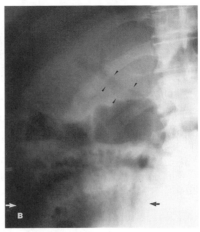

FIGURE 6. A branching and tapering gas collection in the liver, if predominantly near the hilum (*arrowheads*), usually is biliary *(A)* but occasionally is portal venous *(B)*. *B,* Below the liver, bubbly and linear patterns of pneumatosis raise the possibility of bowel ischemia.

7. What is the role of iodinated (water-soluble) contrast for luminal opacification?

The major indication for these media is examination for intra- or retroperitoneal perforation of gut. If extravasated into these spaces, iodinated media are apparently safer than barium. Because of its lower contrast resolution, however, an iodinated agent is less likely than barium to show a small or walled-off perforation. If no extravasation of iodinated water-soluble contrast is evident, examination with barium should follow; the importance of detecting a small or walled-off perforation that is inconspicuous with iodinated contrast far outweighs the risk of extravasation of a small volume of barium. To examine the esophagus for perforation, some radiologists begin with iodinated contrast. Others, because extravasation of barium into the mediastinum and pleural cavity has not been proved harmful, begin with barium.

8. Which type of iodinated contrast agent is best?

The two classes of iodinated contrast media are *high osmolality* and *low osmolality*. High osmolality contrast, if a substantial volume reaches the lungs, may precipitate potentially fatal pulmonary edema. If the route of administration and the patient's condition indicate a substantial possibility that contrast will reach the lungs by aspiration or a tracheoesophageal or bronchoesophageal fistula, either low osmolality iodinated contrast or barium should be used. Otherwise, for oral administration, iodinated contrast may be either a high osmolality medium designed for oral use (that is, flavored) or a low osmolality medium (which is designed for intravascular use but for which flavoring is unnecessary). For introduction through a tube into the stomach or intestine, the best iodinated contrast is the least costly: a high osmolality medium designed for intravascular use.

SWALLOWING STUDIES

9. What are barium swallows?

Barium swallow is the general term for a fluoroscopic-radiologic examination of oral, pharyngeal, and/or esophageal swallowing. Each examination should be tailored to the patient. An examination of the esophagus (often called an esophagogram) is for symptoms, such as restrosternal dysphagia and chest pain, that suggest disease only of the esophagus. Symptoms, such as coughing and choking with swallowing and a sensation that swallowed boluses stick in the

throat, suggest abnormalities of oral and pharyngeal swallowing. Possible causes include disease of the central nervous system, cranial nerves, neuromuscular junction (myasthenia gravis), and muscle (dermatomyositis, polymyositis, or muscular dystrophy). (See Chapter 1.) Adequate evaluation for these symptoms requires examination not only of oral and pharyngeal but also *esophageal* swallowing—a c*omplete barium swallow*—because:
- Dysphagia perceived in the throat is often of esophageal origin and referred upward.
- Symptomatic abnormalities of pharyngeal swallowing may be caused by abnormalities of the esophagus.
- Esophageal abnormalities coexisting with but unrelated to oral and pharyngeal swallowing dysfunction may contribute to dysphagia and often are more treatable.

Examinations limited to oral and pharyngeal swallowing are indicated only occasionally, usually to follow known abnormalities or for limited assessment of patients thought to have oral and pharyngeal swallowing dysfunction and who are too ill for a complete barium swallow.

10. What can a barium swallow contribute to evaluation for dysphagia?

The many possible causes of dysphagia can be difficult to distinguish by history, and multiple coexisting causes—functional and/or structural of oral, pharyngeal, and/or esophageal swallowing—are common. Because only a barium swallow can show functional and structural abnormalities of all three phases of swallowing (Fig. 7), the first diagnostic procedure for dysphagia should be a barium swallow.

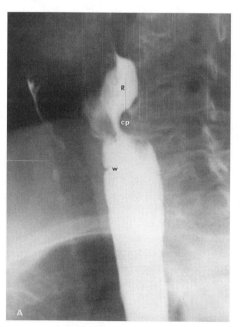
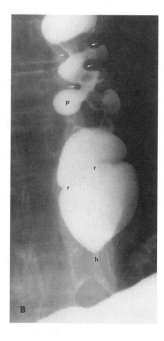

FIGURE 7.   Patient with dysphagia perceived in the throat. Abnormalities shown by barium swallow were numerous and widespread. *A,* Occasionally, before initiation of swallowing, portions of some boluses leaked from the mouth to the pharynx and were then aspirated. Weak pharyngeal muscle contraction and partial luminal obstruction from incomplete opening of the cricopharyngeus (cp) contributed to pharyngeal barium residue (R), which becomes apparent as this swallow progresses. A cervical esophageal web (w) is small. *B,* More inferiorly were marked spasm *(arrows)* and a pulsion diverticulum (p) of the lower esophagus; an incompletely reducing sliding hiatus hernia between a Schatzki ring (r) and the esophageal hiatus (h); and esophageal barium residue, resulting in part from weakness and breakup of peristalsis.

11. What may a barium swallow contribute to diagnosis and management of gastroesophageal reflux disease (GERD)?

Free gastroesophageal reflux of barium is diagnostic of, but uncommon in, GERD. A barium swallow can prove or exclude the common predisposing condition (sliding hiatus hernia), can show an uncommon predisposing condition (delayed gastric emptying), and sometimes shows esophagitis or suggests Barrett esophagus. However, a barium swallow cannot exclude GERD, esophagitis, or Barrett esophagus. For known or suspected GERD, these are the three major roles for a barium swallow:

1. **Investigation of dysphagia.** Possible causes related to GERD, often multiple in a single patient, are numerous: esophageal and pharyngeal, functional and morphologic.

2. **Evaluation for surgery.** Fluoroscopic evaluation for esophageal dysmotility, which is common in GERD, allows an estimate of the likelihood that a complete fundoplication will cause dysphagia and therefore should be avoided. In addition, whether or not a hiatus hernia remains substantial when maximally reduced helps some surgeons decide between an abdominal and thoracic surgical approach.

3. **Investigation of postoperative symptoms.** For dysphagia, a barium swallow can show, among other possible causes, whether or not a wrap excessively narrows the lower esophagus. For recurrent reflux symptoms, a barium swallow can show whether or not a fundoplication is intact and whether a hiatus hernia has developed.

12. What distinguishes achalasia from scleroderma?

When dysphagia is caused by one of these two conditions, esophagographic abnormalities—though often nonspecific if dysmotility is minimal—are ususally diagnostic if dysmotility is moderate or severe (Fig. 8).

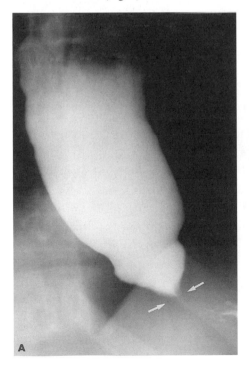
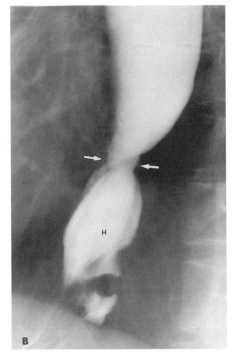

FIGURE 8. Lower esophagus. *A,* Achalasia. Dilatation is marked above a "birdbeak" *(arrows)* formed by the closed lower sphincter. *B,* Scleroderma. Dilatation is moderate above a cylindrical reflux esophagitis stricture *(arrows),* below which is a sliding hiatal hernia (H).

Achalasia vs. Scleroderma

	ESOPHAGEAL DILATATION	DIMINISHED PERISTALSIS	ESOPHAGOGASTRIC JUNCTION
Achalasia	May be marked	Entire esophagus	"Birdbeak": smooth concentric, tapered, flexible No hiatus hernia
Scleroderma	Minimal or moderate	Lower two-thirds	Stricture (from esophagitis): cylindrical, rigid, sometimes irregular or ulcerated Sliding hiatal hernia

UPPER GASTROINTESTINAL SERIES

13. Can benign and malignant ulcers be distinguished?

Images of a gastric ulcer shown by an upper GI series should be assessed for the likelihood of malignancy. Biphasic technique, which includes both double-contrast and single-contrast phases, usually shows benign and malignant signs better than either single-contrast or double-contrast technique alone. A malignant or possibly malignant appearance warrants gastroscopy and biopsy. For unequivocally benign radiographic features, however, radiologic follow-up is a less costly alternative. If follow-up shows complete healing and unequivocally benign features of any scar that may have developed, further evaluation for malignancy is unnecessary. If healing is partial but the appearance is still benign, a second follow-up radiologic examination is sufficient. If healing is then still incomplete, or if features of or equivocal for malignancy develop during follow-up, gastroscopy and biopsy are indicated.

Gastric Ulcers on Upper GI Series: Benign and Malignant Features

	BENIGN	MALIGNANT
Location in stomach	Other than greater curvature of fundus	Greater curvature of fundus
Profile view: relationship of ulcer to gastric lumen	Beyond expected lumen	Within expected lumen
Radiating folds	Regular To margin of ulcer or to ulcer mound (of edema)	Nodular, irregular, fused, clubbed, amputated, or nodular May not reach ulcer margin
Ulcer within a mass	Ulcer location: central Mass: smooth junction with wall: obtuse angle	Ulcer location: eccentric Mass: irregular junction with wall: acute angle
Pattern of surrounding mucosa	Intact	Distorted or obliterated
Ulcer shape	Round, oval, or linear	Angular
Other	Hampton's line	
Healing	Complete	Usually incomplete Occasionally complete but with scar: nodular radiating folds with malignant characteristics

EXAMINATION OF THE SMALL BOWEL

14. What are advantages and disadvantages of, and indications for, enteroclysis (small bowel enema)?

Advantages: For two reasons, enteroclysis usually provides more detail of small bowel anatomy than does a follow-through:

- Barium can be introduced into the lumen at whatever rate distends the bowel optimally.
- Double-contrast examination of the jejunum is possible—by instillation of methylcellulose through the tube immediately after barium. (Double-contrast examination of the ileum—sometimes called a *peroral pneumocolon* because air is introduced per rectum—is as likely to succeed during a follow-through as during enteroclysis.)

Disadvantages :

- Greater cost
- More patient discomfort
- More radiation exposure
- Nonphysiologic circumstances of examination

Indications: Opinions about the role of enteroclysis vary greatly, but the following guidelines are commonly used. A follow-through is the routine small bowel examination. Enteroclysis should be reserved for several situations in which superior anatomic information is especially advantageous because anatomic abnormalities may be subtle, the probability of a jejunal or ileal lesion is especially high, or both:

- Possible mechanical obstruction—if *low*-grade
- Gastrointestinal bleeding—if unexplained after evaluation of the upper GI tract and colon
- Malabsorption—if the suspected cause is not gluten enteropathy

15. When information from imaging beyond that provided by radiographs is important to manage suspected small bowel obstruction, which fluoroscopic-radiographic contrast examination is best?

Choice of Fluoroscopic Examination for Small Bowel Obstruction

CLINICAL SETTING	SUSPECTED OBSTRUCTION	BEST EXAMINATION
Illness too mild for hospitalization *and* small bowel dilatation is inconspicuous on radiographs	Low-grade	Enteroclysis
Radiographs show dilated small bowel, but not in right lower quadrant	High-grade Above lower ileum	Small bowel follow-through
Radiographs show dilated small bowel, including right lower quadrant	High-grade Near terminal ileum	Barium enema, single contrast, no preparation
Clinical picture characteristic of obstruction and severity suggests high-grade, but radiographs show no small bowel dilatation	High-grade Anywhere	Small bowel follow-through

For low-grade obstruction, enteroclysis is more likely than a follow-through to distend the bowel adequately to show minimal luminal narrowing. Alternatively, if obstruction is high-grade (Fig. 2), a follow-through is more likely than enteroclysis to be diagnostic (unless decompression of the small bowel by a long small bowel tube precedes enteroclysis).

For suspected obstruction far downstream in the small bowel, a single-contrast barium enema provides two advantages over other fluoroscopic studies:

1. If obstruction that on abdominal radiographs appears low in the ileum is actually colonic (a fairly common situation), the diagnosis will be obvious.

2. If the obstruction is in the lower ileum, the likelihood is substantial that barium will flow retrograde to the obstruction (Fig. 3) and establish the diagnosis much more quickly than is possible with oral barium.

16. When is computed tomography (CT) preferable to a fluoroscopic-radiographic contrast study for small bowel obstruction?

For suspected high-grade obstructions, some radiologists prefer CT to fluoroscopic contrast examination. In general, the clinical questions should determine the modality. For detection of a hernia (which may be the cause of or unrelated to an obstruction), strangulation, closed-loop obstruction, and abdominal abnormalities outside the gut, CT is better. Fluoroscopic examinations show more conclusively the presence or absence of, and degree of, luminal obstruction.

17. When is retrograde small bowel examination indicated?

A single-contrast barium enema for suspected high-grade obstruction of the lower ileum may be considered a limited retrograde small bowel study. Examination of the entire small bowel, however, is possible by introducing barium retrograde through an ileostomy. This examination is not only much faster than either enteroclysis or a follow-through but also demonstrates anatomy as well as single-contrast enteroclysis—with lower cost, less radiation exposure, and less discomfort. Examination of small bowel of most patients with an ileostomy should be retrograde. The most common indication is new symptoms suggesting Crohn's disease of small bowel months or years after total colectomy and ileostomy for known or suspected Crohn's colitis.

EXAMINATION OF THE COLON

18. What are the indications for single-contrast and double-contrast techniques of barium enema examination?

Double contrast: to evaluate for polyps, cancer, and colitis

Single contrast: to evaluate for fistula, sinus tract (including diverticulitis), or colon obstruction

Whatever the purpose of the examination, single-contrast technique must be used if patient mobility is inadequate for double-contrast technique. Detection of incidental adenomas and occasional carcinomas during barium enemas probably prevents some deaths from colon cancer. Because adenomas are significantly prevalent among people 40 years and older, double contrast is preferable in that age group without a special indication for single contrast.

19. What are advantages and disadvantages of using a barium enema instead of colonoscopy to screen for colon cancer?

Advantages

Lower cost

Greater safety

Greater likelihood that the entire colon will be examined

Disadvantages

Lower sensitivity for detection of polyps (especially diminutive ones)

Some false-positive examinations for polyps

Positive results (true and false) necessitate endoscopy for polypectomy or biopsy

20. Is a barium enema useful and safe for suspected diverticulitis?

If the purpose of imaging is to evaluate possible abdominal and pelvic abscesses, CT, not a barium enema, is indicated. For *intrinsic* disease of the colon, a barium enema tends to provide a more specific diagnosis than does CT. Preparation of the colon for the enema and the enema itself, however, may worsen moderate or severe diverticulitis. If the purpose of imaging is to determine if the diagnosis of diverticulitis and if the patient is only mildly ill, a single-contrast barium enema is unlikely to do harm and may be diagnostic.

21. What is the role of defecography (evacuation proctography)?

For symptoms that suggest anorectal dysfunction, such as difficult or painful rectal evacuation or incontinence, defecography may help to clarify the cause (Fig. 9). Barium contrast of paste consistency is introduced into the rectum. Subsequent imaging, predominantly videofluoroscopic in lateral projection, shows the speed and completeness of rectal evacuation and may show one or more of the following: rectocele, intussusception (rectorectal or intraanal), rectal prolapse, enterocele, sigmoidocele, excessive pelvic floor descent, and anismus. For optimal diagnosis and management, defecographic findings must be correlated with history, physical examination, and nonimaging tests of anorectal function.

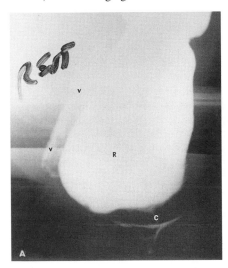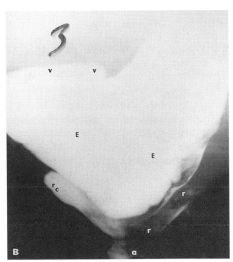

FIGURE 9.   Lateral views from a defecogram of a woman who complained of difficult and incomplete rectal evacuation. *A,* The appearance before evacuation was normal. Barium paste opacifies the rectum (R) and anal canal (C). A contrast-impregnated tampon is in the vagina (v). *B,* Evacuation was slow and incomplete. Intussuscepting rectal tissue (radiolucency demarcated anteriorly and posteriorly by linear barium) has descended into and now obstructs the lower rectum (r) and anal canal (a). A rectocele (rc) retains rectal contents. An enterocele (E) is very large: Numerous loops of ileum, opacified by barium swallowed earlier, have descended into the pelvis between the rectum and vagina (v), which they separate widely.

CHOLANGIOPANCREATOGRAPHY

22. List common causes of obstruction at various locations (Fig. 10) of the biliary tract.

Common Causes of Biliary Obstruction by Location

Hepatic ductal confluence
    Cholangiocarcinoma (Klatskin tumor)
    Gallbladder cancer
    Metastasis to porta hepatis lymph nodes
    Stricture from laparoscopic cholecystectomy
    Other
        Hepatocellular carcinoma (usually intraluminal masses)
        Oriental cholangiohepatitis (usually several strictures, often numerous stones)

Intrapancreatic common bile duct
    Cancer of head of pancreas
    Pancreatitis

Table continued on following page

Common Causes of Biliary Obstruction by Location (Continued)

Intraduodenal common bile duct
Neoplastic
Carcinoma of ampulla of Vater
Duodenal adenoma or carcinoma
Nonneoplastic
Stricture
Dyskinesiac
Inflammation
Acquired immunodeficiency (AIDS)
Acute pancreatitis
Iatrogenic

Multiple—intrahepatic and extrahepatic
Primary sclerosing cholangitis
AIDS cholangiopathy
Other
Secondary sclerosing cholangitis (including oriental cholangiohepatitis)
Cholangiocarcinoma (extensively infiltrating)

Possible at most locations

Stone	Other
Cholangiocarcinoma	Metastasis
	Lymphoma
	Iatrogenic

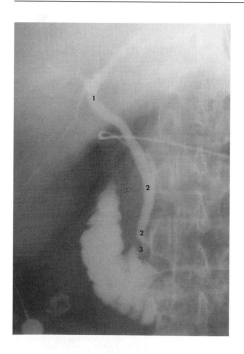

FIGURE 10.   Common sites of extrahepatic biliary obstruction are indicated on this operative cholangiogram. (1) Hepatic ductal confluence. (2) Intrapancreatic portion of common bile duct. (3) Intraduodenal portion of common bile duct (and/or the common channel for patients whose common bile and pancreatic ducts fuse before reaching the duodenal lumen).

23. What cholangiopancreatographic features distinguish pancreatitis from ductal adenocarcinoma of the pancreatic head?

The characteristics of abnormalities of both ductal systems (Figs. 11 and 12) are clues to this distinction.

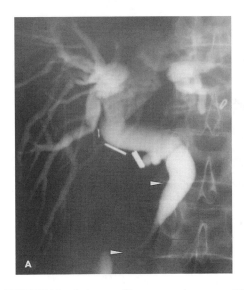
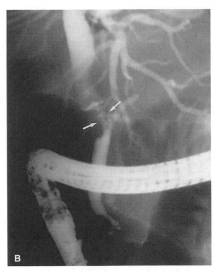

FIGURE 11. Strictures of intrapancreatic common bile duct. *A,* Percutaneous transhepatic cholangiogram. This stricture *(arrowheads),* showing benign characteristics, is due to pancreatitis. *B,* ERC. This stricture *(arrows),* showing all the characteristics of malignancy, is due to ductal adenocarcinoma of the pancreatic head.

Pancreatitis vs. Cancer of the Pancreatic Head: Cholangiopancreatographic Features

	PANCREATITIS	CARCINOMA
Pancreatogram	Acute pancreatitis: no abnormalities Chronic pancreatitis: widespread abnormalities (dilatations, narrowings, calcifications)	Focal abnormality of main duct in pancreatic head (obstruction, stricture, or disruption)
Cholangiogram (stricture of intrapancreatic common bile duct)	Long, smooth, tapered, concentric	Short, irregular, abrupt margins, eccentric

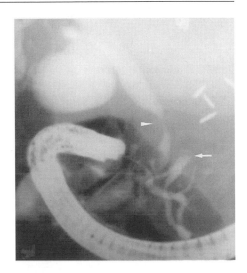

FIGURE 12. Double-duct sign. A stricture *(arrowhead)* of the intrapancreatic common bile duct, although smooth and predominantly tapered, may be malignant because it is short and eccentric. Nearby a complete obstruction *(arrow)* of the pancreatic duct is the only abnormality of this truncated segment of duct. Diagnosis: ductal adenocarcinoma of the pancreatic head.

24. What is the "double duct sign"?

One stricture or complete obstruction of the intrapancreatic common bile duct and another stricture or complete obstruction of the main pancreatic duct nearby (Fig. 12). The common benign cause is chronic pancreatitis. The most common malignant cause is ductal adenocarcinoma of the pancreatic head, but cholangiocarcinoma, lymphoma, and metastasis are occasional causes.

25. How do the pancreatographic appearances of pancreas divisum and complete obstruction of the main pancreatic duct differ?

Although the main duct opacified via the major papilla is shorter than normal in both conditions, they are usually distinguishable on the following basis:

With **obstruction** (Fig. 12), the main duct appears *truncated.* Caliber of the main duct and its branches is normal, and upstream termination of the main duct is abrupt. (Two other conditions—traumatic disruption of the main duct and excision of the pancreatic tail and body—can mimic obstruction.)

With **pancreas divisum** (Fig. 13), the ductal system appears *minified.* Caliber of the main duct and its branches is smaller than normal, and the main duct terminates upstream by branching and tapering.

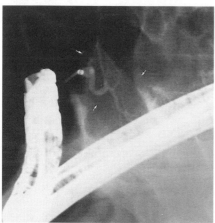

FIGURE 13.   Pancreas divisum. This short pancreatic ductal system *(arrows),* opacifed via the major papilla, is *minified.*

26. What are pancreatographic findings of traumatic perforation of the pancreatic duct?

The duct may have either of two appearances: (1) extravasation of contrast material from the site of disruption or (2) failure of contrast to flow upstream of the site of disruption.

27. What are advantages of fistulography?

For a suspected fistula between the skin and the lumen of the gut, a fistulagram is usually the most informative imaging examination. A fistulagram usually allows adequate assessment for intestinal obstruction downstream of a fistula. In addition, relative to barium studies of the gut:

- A fistulagram is more likely to show a fistula.
- A fistulagram usually demonstrates anatomy of a track in more detail and the site of gut in continuity with the track more precisely.
- A fistulagram is less likely to delay possible percutaneous therapy: drainage of an fistula or of an abscess communicating with the fistula or injection of collagen into the track.

BIBLIOGRAPHY

1. Levine MS, Rubesin SE, Laufer I: Double Contrast Gastrointestinal Radiography, 3rd ed. Philadelphia, W.B. Saunders, 2000.
2. Silvis SE, Rohrmann CA Jr, Ansel HJ: Text and Atlas of Endoscopic Retrograde Cholangiopancreatography. New York, Igaku-Shoin, 1995.
3. Somers S: Evacuation proctography. In Gore RM, Levine MS (eds): Textbook of Gastrointestinal Radiology, vol. 1, 2nd ed. Philadelphia, W.B. Saunders, 2000, pp 905–913.

74. INTERVENTIONAL RADIOLOGY

Paul D. Russ, M.D., Stephen W. Subber, M.D., Dale McCarter, M.D., and Keith Shonnard, M.D.

IMAGE-GUIDED INTERVENTIONS

1. What percutaneous procedures are performed using cross-sectional imaging guidance?

The two basic procedures performed in abdominal imaging are biopsies of masses and drainage of fluid collections. Masses and fluid collections of the solid viscera, peritoneum, retroperitoneum, vertebrae, psoas and paraspinous muscles are usually accessible.

Biopsies can be categorized as fine-needle aspiration (FNA), which yields clusters of cells and occasionally small tissue fragments for cytopathology, or core biopsy, which yields cylinders of tissue, 1–2 cm long, with preserved architecture for histopathologic analysis.

Fluid collections can be needled for Gram stain and culture and aspirated (sometimes repeatedly) for therapeutic decompression. They can be drained with percutaneous catheters for cure or for temporization and medical stabilization before surgery. Some cystic lesions and collections are catheterized for purposes of drainage and subsequent treatment (e.g., sclerotherapy).

2. What materials and equipment are used for FNAs, core biopsies, and percutaneous catheter drainages?

Most **FNAs** are performed using 20–22-gauge "skinny" needles. **Core biopsies** usually are obtained with 18-gauge disposable, spring-loaded, automated guns. In most situations, 18-gauge specimens are as diagnostic as those obtained with 14–16-gauge devices. Usually, better samples are obtained with 18-gauge than 20-gauge guns.

The vast majority of **fluid collections** can be drained and treated with 8-French self-retaining, pigtail catheters. Except for some percutaneous gallbladder and ascitic fluid drainages, catheters smaller than 8 French offer no advantages, are often more difficult to place, and are dislodged more frequently. The routine use of 10–28-French catheters is not necessary. However, multiple large catheters usually are required for percutaneous drainage of infected acute pancreatic necrosis.

3. What steps are taken in preparation for an image-guided procedure?

In all cases, the indications and risks of the procedure are discussed with the referring physician. The necessity for performing the procedure needs to be firmly established and documented. Plans for appropriate medical and surgical back-up must be in place, and postprocedure care must be determined.

Diagnostic images should be reviewed before the procedure is scheduled. This review allows the interventionalist to establish a presumptive diagnosis, assess the risks and benefits of the procedure, decide on the most appropriate procedure, choose the best imaging modality to guide the procedure, and plan a safe approach to the lesion.

4. What three conditions must be satisfied before a percutaneous procedure can be performed?

1. The patient or patient representative must provide written informed consent for both the procedure and anticipated intravenous conscious sedation.

2. The referring physician must order antibiotic coverage if there is any possibility that the lesion or fluid collection is infected.

3. The patient's coagulation profile must be determined.

5. What coagulation parameters are assessed before a percutaneous procedure?

Some literature suggests that the hemostatic evaluation can be stratified according to the patient's history and the predicted risk of the procedure. However, in a referral setting, the preprocedure assessment should be thorough. The patient history should be reviewed for bleeding risks, such as anticoagulant use or hepatocellular disease. At a minimum, prothrombin time (PT), international normalized ratio (INR), partial thromboplastin time (PTT), and platelet count should be assessed in all patients, regardless of the procedure. INR > 2.0, PTT > 1.5 times normal, or platelet count < 50,000–60,000/µl is a contraindication for most procedures. However, after the discontinuation or reversal of anticoagulants, administration of fresh frozen plasma, and/or platelet transfusion, many coagulopathies can be corrected temporarily to allow the intervention.

A history of antiplatelet drug use, uremia, or myeloproliferative disease may require measurement of the bleeding time. If the result is abnormal, consultation with a hematologist is recommended. The administration of platelets or 1-deamino-8-D-arginine vasopressin (DDAVP) may be necessary before proceeding.

6. Which imaging modalities are used to guide interventional procedures?

Fluoroscopy, ultrasound (US), computed tomography (CT) and magnetic resonance (MR) imaging can be used to guide interventions. On abdominal imaging services, US and CT are used most often (Fig. 1).

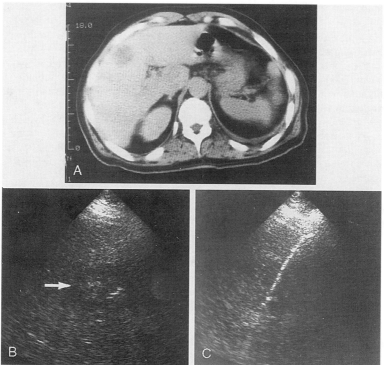

FIGURE 1.   Metastatic colon cancer to the liver. *A,* Contrast-enhanced CT of the liver demonstrates a 3-cm hypodense mass. *B,* Ultrasound of the liver reveals the mass to be primarily hypoechoic *(arrow). C,* The needle tract is conspicuously demonstrated during ultrasound-guided biopsy.

7. Summarize the advantages and disadvantages of US.

US is widely available and portable; it allows relatively easy scanning in nonorthogonal planes. The disadvantages of US are the inability to depict small deep lesions, to define bowel anatomy, to maintain a sterile field, and to use both hands with ease to perform the actual procedure as a single operator. In general, US often is selected for superficial and big lesions.

8. Summarize the advantages and disadvantages of CT.

CT provides excellent anatomic detail, allows safe needle passes into difficult locations, is more amenable to sterile technique, and permits a single operator to use both hands for performing the procedure (Fig. 2). The disadvantages of CT are that it is not portable and sick patients must be monitored by support personnel in the CT suite; needle localization can be slower than with US; and oblique sticks can be more difficult. CT is selected more often for deep and small abnormalities.

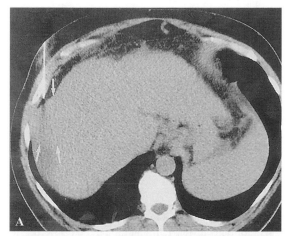

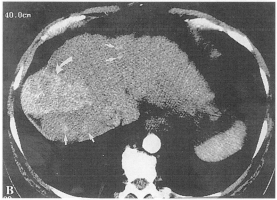

FIGURE 2. Biopsy of an hepatic mass in a 54-year-old man with end-stage alcoholic cirrhosis. *A,* Noncontrast CT performed during percutaneous biospy of a large solid liver lesion shows an isodense lobulation *(arrows)* of the right lobe corresponding to a tumor better demonstrated by previous dynamic CT. Two 21-gauge FNAs and two 18-gauge core biopsies of the lesion confirmed hepatocellular carcinoma. CT guidance allowed a tract to be selected that avoided aerated lung; thus a pneumothorax was avoided. *B,* After chemoembolization, the stained carcinoma is more conspicuously shown with CT *(curved arrow)*. Small satellite foci are also depicted *(small straight arrows)*.

9. Discuss the standard uses of fluoroscopy.

Fluoroscopy is rarely used on abdominal imaging services. Sometimes it is used in conjunction with US to biopsy or drain large, superficial masses and fluid collections. It is used not infrequently for simple tube exchanges and can be helpful with complex tube manipulations. Fluoroscopy is used for sinograms and abscessograms, although these procedures are now performed less often. Fluoroscopy is recommended by many authors during hepatic and renal cyst sclerotherapy to check for communication with the biliary tree and urinary collecting system, respectively.

10. Summarize the advantages and disadvantages of MR.

Standard and particularly open-sided MR systems are being used more frequently for interventional procedures. MR may be necessary if it is the only modality that depicts the lesion. MR can scan oblique planes. Interventions on high-field equipment are analogous to those done with

CT. Open-sided MRs allow easier access to the patient, facilitate patient monitoring, and decrease procedure time. Heat-sensitive pulse sequences available for both standard and open-sided MRs provide unique information during thermal ablations. Working in static and fluctuating electro-magnetic fields remains the major drawback to MR-guided interventional procedures.

11. What techniques have been developed for lesion localization?

For US, CT, and MR, various trigonometric, mechanical, electronic, and computer-assisted techniques and devices have been developed for lesion localization and guidance. They are used to facilitate procedures that require oblique punctures. Although not necessary in most cases, they have the potential to facilitate the approach to small lesions and lesions in difficult locations, such as the dome of the liver.

12. Why is it prudent to begin every biopsy of a suspected neoplasm with FNA?

FNA allows an initial approach with a "skinny" needle and provides the operator with a test pass before a large needle is used. If the interventionalist has inadvertently chosen an unsafe route, it is better to discover this error using a small rather than a large needle. If a lesion turns out to be exceptionally hypervascular (e.g., an unexpected hemangioma), this problem usually becomes obvious when the aspirating syringe fills quickly with blood. The procedure can be ter-minated before severe consequences are encountered with a cutting needle. Finally, if a cy-topathologist is present during the procedure (as is strongly recommended), 1–3 initial FNAs can be diagnostic, obviating subsequent core biopsy.

13. Why is FNA advantageous for initial aspiration of a suspected fluid collection?

In addition to establishing the safety of the percutaneous approach before a much larger catheter is placed, FNA can confirm that the lesion is in fact a fluid collection and not a solid mass. If necessary, a small aliquot can be sent for immediate Gram stain. If the fluid is sterile, the interventionalist, in consultation with the referring physician, has the opportunity to abort the procedure to avoid the small chance of superinfecting the collection with subsequent catheter placement. If the fluid is infected on Gram stain or by visual inspection of the aspirated material, the operator can proceed with catheter drainage. FNAs of the lesion should be sent for cytology to avoid the pitfall of draining a cystic, necrotic, or superinfected tumor without recognizing the nature of the underlying lesion.

14. What two techniques can be used to drain fluid collections?

1. With the **Seldinger technique**, a drainage catheter is placed after needle placement, guidewire insertion, and tract dilatation.

2. With the **trocar technique**, the fluid collection is punctured directly with the catheter mounted on a removable sharp-tipped trocar.

15. Which technique is used most often?

The Seldinger technique is used most often, because it starts with a smaller needle and be-cause catheter insertion over a guidewire is more controlled. The trocar technique is a faster, one-step procedure, but some control may be lost during catheter insertion compared with the Seldinger method. The trocar technique usually is reserved for large, superficial fluid collections or draining a large volume of ascites.

16. What are the major complications of percutaneous procedures?

The major complications of percutaneous procedures are hemorrhage, infection, sepsis, solid organ injury, bowel perforation, and pneumothorax. The complication rate of "skinny" needle in-terventions is about 0.06–0.6%. The complication rate of catheter drainage is 3–4%. The in-creased risk of large needle procedures compared with "skinny" needle procedures is the subject of some debate. However, it seems intuitive that the smallest adequate needle or catheter should be used for every procedure.

17. How common is seeding of the needle tract during routine tumor biopsy?

Seeding the needle tract is rare with 20–22-gauge aspiration needles and 18-gauge core biopsy guns. However, even with these devices, suspected cystadenomas or cystadenocarcinomas of the ovary or pancreas should not be sampled percutaneously because they are associated with an increased risk of postprocedure needle-tract seeding and subsequent pseudomyxoma peritonei or peritoneal carcinomatosis. Of interest, percutaneous thermal ablation (radiofrequency, microwave, laser) of hepatocellular carcinoma and hepatic colorectal cancer metastases, which uses probes as large as 14 gauge, are associated with tumor seeding of the tracts in about 2–3% of patients.

HEPATIC INTERVENTIONS

18. What image-guided procedures are performed in the liver?

Cross-sectional imaging is used to perform: (1) FNAs and core biopsies of primary and metastatic tumors, (2) catheter drainage of abscesses and other fluid collections, and (3) sclerotherapy of hepatic cysts.

19. How is hepatic metastic disease diagnosed?

FNAs are a simple and quick way to diagnose hepatic metastatic disease. Because of the marked difference between metastatic neoplastic cells and background hepatocytes, cytology alone is frequently diagnostic and core biopsies unnecessary. In difficult cases, comparison with previously obtained specimens of the primary tumor can help to establish the diagnosis.

20. How is primary hepatic neoplasm diagnosed?

Primary hepatic neoplasm may be diagnosed with FNA alone, depending on tumor type and skill of the cytopathologist. However, because many primary hepatic tumors require histologic evaluation, core biopsies are requisite (see Fig. 2). With current biopsy gun technology, 18 gauge cores are recommended. Core biopsy of background liver is helpful to the pathologist in cases of well-differentiated neoplasm and assists the hepatologist to choose among treatment options by detecting the presence and severity of underlying hepatocellular disease.

21. How are pyogenic hepatic or parahepatic abscesses treated?

Ninety percent of pyogenic hepatic or parahepatic abscesses can be successfully drained percutaneously (Fig. 3). Almost all pyogenic abscesses can be drained with an 8-French, self-retaining, pigtail catheter. After needle puncture, caution should be exercised during wire placement, dilatation, and catheter insertion; frequent imaging is necessary to ensure that the drainage devices have not migrated beyond the soft margin of the abscess, which can result in significant complications.

22. Describe the treatment of epithelialized hepatic cysts.

Epithelialized hepatic cysts can be drained successfully and obliterated with alcohol sclerotherapy. An 8-French, self-retaining, pigtail catheter can be used. After placement with US or CT guidance, most authors advocate contrast injection through the catheter under fluoroscopic guidance to ensure that there is no communication with the biliary tree. After complete cyst aspiration, samples are sent for culture and cytology. About 33–50% of the original cyst volume is replaced with sterile, absolute alcohol (not to exceed 100 ml). Dwell time is at least 20–30 minutes with the patient rotated several times to coat the entirety of the cyst wall. Patients receive prophylactic antibiotic coverage and are hospitalized for overnight drainage. The sclerosis is repeated 24 hours later, and then the catheter is removed.

Solitary congenital or acquired hepatic cysts are more often successfully sclerosed than cysts in patients with polycystic liver disease. In polycystic liver disease, cysts tend not to collapse, presumably because the surrounding liver is less pliable, making wall apposition and subsequent scarring of the cavity less likely (Fig. 4). In cases of polycystic liver disease, laparoscopic unroofing of multiple cysts is replacing alcohol sclerotherapy.

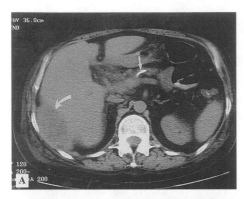

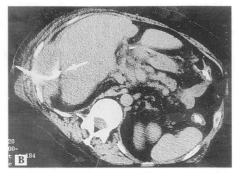

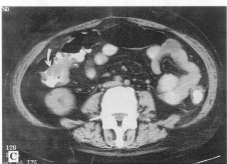

FIGURE 3. Parahepatic abscess in a 60-year-old woman at first diagnosed with acute pancreatitis. *A,* After she failed to respond to initial management, including pancreatic duct stenting *(straight arrow),* CT revealed a fluid collection *(curved arrow)* adjacent to the liver. *B,* An 8-French pigtail catheter successfully drained the *Streptococcus milleri* abscess *(straight arrow). C,* An hepatic flexure mass *(curved arrow)* was suspected to be the site of origin of the parahepatic abscess.

23. Is FNA or biopsy safe in all hepatic lesions?

FNA or biopsy of some hepatic lesions should be approached with extreme caution, if at all. Carcinoid crisis characterized by profound hypotension can be precipitated by FNA of hepatic carcinoid metastases. Intentional needling of hemangiomas is controversial at best. Because of the ability to characterize most hemangiomas noninvasively with cross-sectional imaging, obtaining specimens for cytology or histology is unnecessary in the management of most patients with typical hemangiomas (Fig. 5). Amebic abscesses do not require catheter drainage and usually respond well to medical treatment with metronidazole. Aspiration and drainage of echinococcal cysts is quite controversial; all options should be considered carefully before proceeding with percutaneous aspiration and drainage of a known echinococcal lesion.

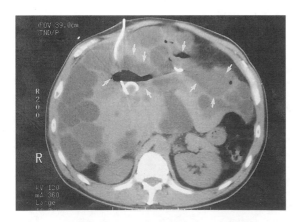

FIGURE 4. Alcohol sclerosis of hepatic cysts in a middle-aged man with polycystic liver disease who complained of abdominal distention and early satiety. Two large, dominant cysts *(small straight arrows)* have both been drained with 8-French pigtail catheters. Despite aggressive aspiration of cyst contents and sclerotherapy with sterile absolute alcohol, neither cyst completely collapsed; air was entrained into each cyst and wall coaptation did not occur. The patient subsequently required laparoscopic unroofing of multiple cysts for symptomatic relief.

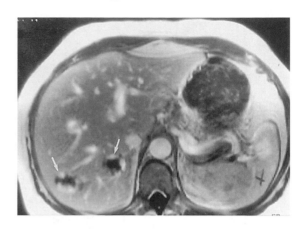

FIGURE 5. Dynamic, gadolinium-enhanced, T1-weighted MR scan of the liver shows two lesions *(arrows)* with perfusion patterns characteristic of hemangiomas. Their distinctive MR features allow conservative management with surveillance imaging, obviating biopsy. Incidental note is made of a nonspecific hyperintensity in the spleen.

SPLENIC INTERVENTIONS

24. What interventions are possible in the spleen?

Performance of percutaneous procedures in the spleen remains controversial. Scattered reports suggest that FNAs and catheter drainages of the spleen are possible. Although these procedures can be performed successfully, their overall risk is relatively high. Serious complications are estimated to occur in about 7% of cases (roughly 2–10 times more often than in other abdominal interventions). Uncontrolled hemorrhage necessitating emergency splenectomy is not uncommon. Therefore, the procedure should be clearly indicated; its risks and benefits need to be thoroughly discussed with the patient and the referring physician. The possibility of emergency splenectomy must be emphasized. Surgical back-up must be immediately available. If a percutaneous procedure is attempted, the size of the needle or catheter should be conservative, and the lesion should be approached through the least amount of normal splenic parenchyma (Fig. 6).

PANCREATIC PROCEDURES

25. What procedures are appropriate for solid pancreatic masses?

Solid masses, usually suspected tumors, can be aspirated percutaneously (Fig. 7). Only FNAs should be performed; core biopsies should be avoided, because the use of cutting needles can result in severe pancreatitis. If a "skinny" needle is used and the lesion is solid, any organ, including the stomach, small bowel, and colon, can be traversed. Antibiotic coverage is recommended for procedures through the bowel. Major blood vessels should be avoided. The diagnosis of pancreatic adenocarcinoma often can be established by cytopathology alone; a negative result must be interpreted cautiously and assumed to be a sampling error until proved otherwise. As noted above, percutaneous biopsy of suspected cystadenomas or cystadenocarcinomas should be avoided.

26. What procecedures are used for pancreatic fluid collections?

Various acute and chronic pancreatic fluid collections can be aspirated and drained. Fluid collections should be defined according to the classification system adopted by the International Symposium on Acute Pancreatitis. Pancreatic-related collections can be aspirated with "skinny" needles to determine whether they are sterile or infected (Fig. 8). In this setting, bowel should not be crossed with the aspiration needle to avoid contaminating and superinfecting otherwise sterile fluid.

27. What precautions apply to percutaneous drainage of pancreatic fluid collections?

If endoscopic internal drainage is not possible, percutaneous drainage of most sterile and infected pancreatic collections can be undertaken, if clinically indicated. The drainage of infected

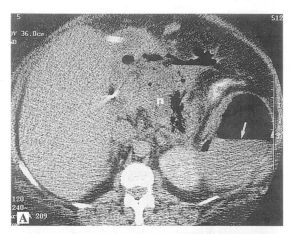

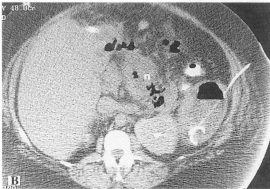

FIGURE 6. Percutaneous catheter drainage of a splenic abscess that developed after gastric bypass surgery. *A,* Diagnostic CT scan shows a large air-fluid level in the spleen *(arrow).* Although contained by the splenic capsule, virtually the entire spleen is suppurated. Note associated infected acute pancreatic necrosis (n). *B,* An 8-French catheter placed into the splenic abscess drained a large volume of purulent material. No hemorrhagic complication occurred, probably because only the splenic capsule was traversed. The infected pancreatic necrosis (n) was drained separately.

collections requires coverage with antibiotics. Routine techniques with 8-French catheters are often adequate. Unlike other fluid collections and abscesses, which can be successfully drained in 7–10 days, pancreatic collections may require straight catheter drainage for 30–120 days. Concomitant endoscopic stenting of obstructing pancreatic duct pathology can facilitate drainage and obviate pancreaticocutaneous fistula as a complication. Attempts at draining infected pancreatic necrosis may require aggressive treatment with multiple, large-bore, sump catheters. To prevent superinfection, percutaneous drains should be avoided in cases of sterile pancreatic necrosis.

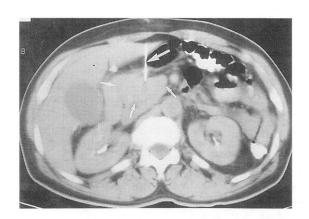

FIGURE 7. Fine-needle aspiration of pancreatic head carcinoma. CT shows mild fullness of the pancreatic uncinate process *(small straight arrows).* A "skinny" needle *(large straight arrow)* passed through the liver and bowel wall without complication was used to obtain cellular material diagnostic of pancreatic adenocarcinoma.

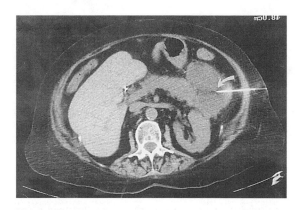

FIGURE 8. Aspiration of an acute pancreatic fluid collection associated with pancreatitis that occurred after lung transplantation. CT shows placement of a 20-gauge needle *(curved arrow)* into the collection. Withdrawn fluid was sterile; all cultures were negative for the growth of microorganisms.

ADRENAL BIOPSY

28. What is the role of adrenal gland biopsy?

Because incidental adrenal gland adenomas can be better characterized with thin-section, dynamic CT and in-phase vs. out-of-phase MR pulse sequences, fewer adrenal lesions need to be biopsied. Because of the risk of hypertensive crisis, possible pheochromocytomas should not be needled. FNA of other adrenal masses is usually sufficient for cytopathologic diagnosis. Approaching either adrenal gland can be difficult. Transhepatic access, decubitus positioning with the lesion-side down to elevate the adjacent hemidiaphragm, and angled routes may be necessary.

RENAL AND PERINEPHRIC INTERVENTIONS

29. Can renal masses be biopsied?

Given the high frequency and typical imaging features of renal cell carcinoma, most urologists are unwilling to risk the small chance of needle-tract seeding for preoperative diagnostic confirmation. In cases that are inoperable for cure or when renal lymphoma or metastatic disease is highly suspected, FNAs are performed. Cytopathology usually can distinquish among renal cell carcinoma, lymphoma, and metastasis. In difficult cases, 18-gauge core biopsies can be performed. Aggressive correction of any coagulopathy is recommended because of the hypervascularity of most renal cell carcinomas.

30. Can renal and perirenal abscesses and other fluid collections be drained percutaneously?

Renal and perirenal abscesses and other fluid collections can be drained using routine 8-French catheter techniques. Gram-negative antibiotic coverage is absolutely essential to prevent urosepsis during or after the procedure. To effect cure, a separate procedure to relieve an associated urinary tract obstruction, if present, is virtually always necessary.

31. What other intraabdominal or retroperitoneal fluid collections can be treated percutaneously?

Most other intraabdominal and retroperitioneal abscesses and fluid collections can be cured or palliated with routine 8-French catheter drainage. Pericholecystic, periappendiceal, diverticular, Crohn's-related, and postoperative abscesses can be managed percutaneously (Fig. 9). Percutaneous catheter drainage can allow subsequent one-stage interval surgery in cases of cholecystitis, appendicitis, and diverticulitis. Most postoperative abscesses and fluid collections can be cured percutaneously, obviating the need for reoperation. Even enteric fistulas can be closed with aggressive, although sometimes prolonged, catheter drainage.

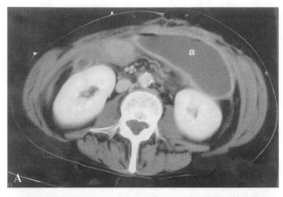

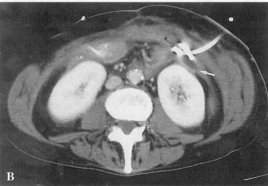

FIGURE 9. Postoperative fluid collection in a 55-year-old man who had undergone left colonic pull-up after esophagectomy for strictures. *A,* CT scan through the patient's midabdomen shows an abscess (a) in the left paracolic gutter. *B,* A 10-French catheter was placed into the collection using ultrasound guidance (not shown). Follow-up CT demonstrates almost complete decompression of the abscess cavity *(straight arrow)* after short-term catheter drainage.

HEPATIC CHEMOEMBOLIZATION

32. Define hepatic chemoembolization.
Hepatic chemoembolization (HCE) is a regional treatment for unresectable primary and secondary hepatic malignancies (Fig. 10). This procedure combines the intraarterial infusion of chemotherapeutic agents with embolization of the blood vessel supplying the tumor, a combination that leads to high local drug concentrations and tumor ischemia while decreasing systemic toxicity.

33. How safe is HCE?
HCE is a relatively safe therapy because liver tumors derive most of their blood supply from the hepatic artery. The unique dual blood supply to the liver (hepatic artery and portal vein) allows safe embolization of this vessel with little risk of hepatic ischemia.

34. Why would HCE be used to treat patients with hepatic malignancy?
Surgical resection is the optimal treatment for patients with hepatic malignancy. Unfortunately, many patients are not surgical candidates because of tumor extent, invasion of blood vessels, associated liver dysfunction, or distant metastases. Response to conventional treatments, such as systemic chemotherapy or radiation therapy, is also poor.

35. How effective is HCE?
Response rates are encouraging for hepatocellular carcinoma as well as metastatic carcinoid and islet cell tumors, but less promising for colorectal metastases. HCE has been effective in the palliation of symptoms, but increased survival rates have not been clearly shown.

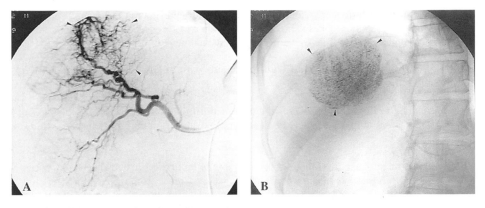

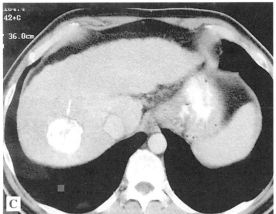

FIGURE 10. Chemoembolization of an hepatocellular carcinoma. *A,* Hepatic arteriogram demonstrates a hypervascular mass *(black arrowheads)* in the posterior segment of the right lobe. *B,* Angiographic image of the stained tumor *(black arrowheads)* after embolization with ethiodol/chemotherapeutic drug emulsion and particles. *C,* Postembolization CT scan shows persistent dense uptake and retention of ethiodol in the lesion *(arrow).* Complete tumor staining results in tumor necrosis and possibly longer patient survival.

BILIARY PROCEDURES

36. Is percutaneous transhepatic biliary drainage the primary method to treat biliary obstruction?

The role of percutaneous transhepatic biliary drainage (PTBD) in the management of benign and malignant biliary disease has diminished significantly with the advancement of interventional endoscopy. Currently, endoscopic drainage is the primary method for biliary decompression because of its relative lack of complications and better patient tolerance compared with the transhepatic approach. However, not all endoscopic drainages are successful, and PTBD continues to play an important role in the management of biliary disease. Biliary disease is best managed by a team that includes an endoscopist, interventional radiologist, and surgeon.

37. What are the indications for PTBD?

- Unsuccessful endoscopic drainage
- Biliary obstruction at or above the level of the porta hepatis
- Biliary obstruction following biliary-enteric anastomosis
- Bile duct injuries after laparoscopic cholecystectomy

The most common of these indications is failed endoscopic drainage for any reason.

38. What particular problems are involved in treatment of hilar obstruction?

Hilar obstruction is a difficult area to treat for both endoscopists and interventionalists. Usually it is secondary to cholangiocarcinoma or metastatic disease that involves the left and right biliary ducts, with frequent occlusion of intrahepatic segmental ducts. The multisegmental nature of these obstructions makes them difficult to drain by the endoscopist; in general, drainage is better accomplished by PTBD. Bilateral drains may be required.

39. Why is endoscopic drainage difficult in patients with biliary obstruction after biliary-enteric anastomosis?

The success rate for endoscopic drainage in patients with biliary obstruction after biliary-enteric anastomosis is < 50% because of the technical difficulty of negotiating the endoscope through the afferent loop. PTBD may be necessary to evaluate for recurrent disease or anastomotic stricture.

40. Describe the approach to bile duct injuries due to laparoscopic cholecystectomy.

Bile duct injuries due to laparoscopic cholecystectomy result from inadvertent laceration or ligation of the biliary system. PTBD is directed at relieving the obstruction or, in patients with a bile leak, diverting the bile and stenting the injury. This procedure allows healing and may be curative. Otherwise, elective surgery is performed once the patient's condition stabilizes. Endoscopic drainage can be difficult because the bile duct may be severed.

41. Explain the advantages and disadvantages of using metallic stents for the treatment of biliary obstruction.

Metallic stents have supplanted plastic endoprostheses in the percutaneous treatment of malignant biliary obstructions for palliation (Fig. 11). Their primary advantage is the smaller-sized catheter used to deliver the stent compared with the much larger plastic endoprosthesis, thus decreasing patient discomfort and liver complications. In addition, metallic stents expand to larger internal diameters (up to 12 mm or larger), affording better drainage and longer patency rates. A major disadvantage is the high cost; morever, if they occlude because of tumor overgrowth, epithelial hyperplasia, or inspissated bile, reintervention is necessary.

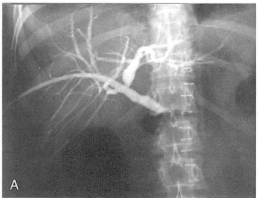
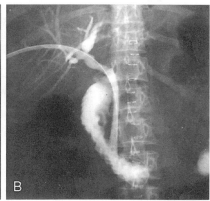
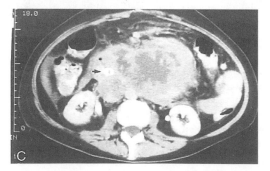

FIGURE 11.   A 58-year-old woman presented with jaundice and an abdominal mass. *A,* A cholangiogram performed after percutaneous transhepatic biliary drainage shows complete obstruction of the common bile duct. *B,* After placement of a metallic stent, the common bile duct is widely patent. *C,* CT scan of the abdomen shows the large, poorly differentiated lymphoma encasing the biliary stent *(arrow).*

42. What are the indications for percutaneous cholecystostomy?

Percutaneous placement of a drainage catheter into the gallbladder is a well-established technique. Its two primary indications are (1) persistent and unexplained sepsis in critically ill patients with acalculous cholecystitis and (2) acute cholecystitis in patients too ill to undergo surgery. In unstable patients, it can be performed at the bedside, if necessary. Less frequent indications include temporary treatment for gallbladder perforation, drainage for distant malignant biliary obstruction, and transcholecystic biliary intervention.

GASTROINTESTINAL BLEEDING

43. When do diagnostic angiography and percutaneous transcatheter therapy play a role in the management of gastrointestinal (GI) bleeding?

Acute GI bleeding that is refractory to conservative management or invasive endoscopic techniques requires angiographic evaluation. For the interventional radiologist to identify the bleeding site, the following conditions must be met:

1. The patient must be actively bleeding at the time of the study.
2. The bleeding must be brisk enough to be detectable during the angiogram, usually 1.5–2.0 ml/min. GI bleeding at lower rates is difficult to detect angiographically.

Once the bleeding site is identified, transcatheter embolization is a treatment option.

44. How important is localization of the bleeding site before angiography?

Preangiographic localization of the GI bleeding site is extremely helpful. A visceral angiogram involves evaluation of the celiac, superior mesenteric, and inferior mesenteric arteries; selective catheterization of these vessels and the multiple angiographic projections needed when looking for a bleeding site can make this a tedious and time-consuming procedure, requiring large contrast volumes. If the preangiographic endoscopy has localized and failed to treat the bleeding, the vessel supplying this region should be studied first to shorten the procedure. If the exact site of bleeding is not known, distinguishing an upper from a lower GI source is helpful and can guide the interventionalist in choosing which vessel should be studied first. A technetium 99m-labeled red blood cell study may provide localizing information; the procedure may be repeated after 12 hours if no bleeding is demonstrated initially.

45. What two types of transcatheter therapy are used for GI bleeding?

Pharmacologic agents and embolic materials.

46. Which pharmacologic agent is preferred? How is it used?

The pharmacologic agent of choice is vasopressin (Pitressin). This pituitary hormone acts directly on the smooth muscle of arterioles and capillaries to cause vasoconstriction. The superior mesenteric, gastroduodenal, left gastric, and gastroepiploic arteries are particularly sensitive to intraarterial administration. After selective catheterization of the bleeding vessel, vasopressin is infused at 0.2 units/min (Fig. 12). A repeat arteriogram is performed after 30 minutes to assess the effectiveness of treatment, and the dose may be increased to 0.4 units/min, if necessary. With excessive vasoconstriction, the dose is reduced to 0.1 units/min. The infusion is continued for 12–24 hours, during which time the patient is monitored closely for side effects (myocardial, bowel, and extremity ischemia, water retention, hyponatremia, and cardiac arrhythmias), which may prematurely terminate the therapy. The patient is reevaluated clinically and angiographically. If the bleeding has stopped, the vasopressin is slowly tapered to normal saline with subsequent catheter removal.

47. How is emoblization of the bleeding vessel achieved?

The catheter is selectively placed near the bleeding site for delivery of the embolic material. The embolic agents most commonly used are polyvinyl alcohol (PVA), gelfoam, and coils. The availability of coaxial systems and microcatheters permits superselective catheterization with accurate deposition of embolic material at the bleeding site. These advances have decreased the risk of bowel infarction, making this a relatively safe procedure even in the small bowel and colon.

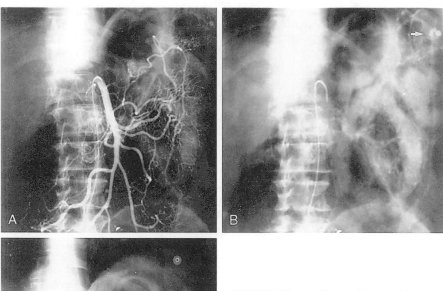

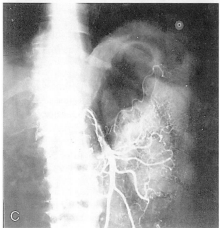

FIGURE 12. A 60-year-old man with lower GI bleeding. *A*, Diagnostic angiogram with selective injection into the superior mesenteric artery. Early arterial films show no bleeding. *B*, Later images reveal puddling of contrast in the proximal left colon consistent with a bleeding diverticulum *(arrow)*. *C*, After a 30-minute infusion of vasopressin (0.2 units/min), the bleeding has stopped. Note the vasoconstriction of the superior mesenteric artery and its branches.

TRANSJUGULAR INTRAHEPATIC PORTOSYSTEMIC SHUNT

48. What is TIPS? How is it performed?

Transjugular intrahepatic portosystemic shunt (TIPS) is a percutaneous technique that creates a shunt within the liver between the portal and hepatic veins to treat variceal bleeding or ascites, complications of portal hypertension (Fig. 13). The procedure is performed by accessing the hepatic venous system, usually the right hepatic vein, via the right internal jugular vein. A 16-gauge Colapinto transjugular needle is used to puncture through the liver from the hepatic vein into the portal vein. The transhepatic tract is dilated with a balloon catheter, followed by placement of a flexible metallic stent, usually 10–12 mm in diameter.

49. What are the benefits of successful TIPS?

Successful TIPS results in a reduction of the portosystemic pressure gradient (PSG) to 8–12 mmHg (bleeding from varices is rare in patients with a PSG < 12 mmHg), and the stent is dilated until this goal is reached. If the PSG cannot be reduced sufficiently, parallel shunts may be necessary. Esophageal and gastric varices usually decompress once the TIPS has been created. If the varices continue to fill at portal venography, the interventionalist may elect to embolize them.

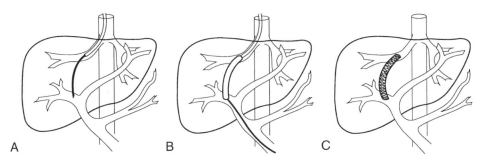

FIGURE 13. Transjugular intrahepatic portosystemic shunt procedure. *A,* After placement of a sheath in the right hepatic vein, a Colapinto needle is used to puncture through the liver to the portal vein. *B,* The liver parenchyma is dilated with a balloon catheter. *C,* A metallic stent is placed across the transhepatic tract, bridging the hepatic and portal veins.

50. What are the indications for TIPS?

The most important and frequent indication for TIPS is refractory variceal hemorrhage (Fig. 14), either acute (bleeding not controlled with sclerotherapy or pharmacotherapy) or chronic (recurrent major hemorrhage despite a course of sclerotherapy). TIPS is particularly helpful with bleeding from inaccessible intestinal or gastric varices and bleeding due to portal hypertensive gastropathy. Additional promising indications for TIPS include refractory ascites, refractory hepatic hydrothorax, and Budd-Chiari syndrome or other veno-occlusive diseases. TIPS is not indicated for the initial therapy of acute variceal bleeding, as a bridge to transplantation to reduce intraoperative morbidity, or for treatment of hepatopulmonary syndrome.

51. What are the contraindications to performing the TIPS procedure?

There are few absolute contraindications to TIPS. Because it is a portosystemic shunt, TIPS increases right-sided heart pressures and should not be performed in patients with right heart failure. It should not be performed in patients with polycystic liver disease, in whom the risk of hemorrhage is significantly increased because the shunt tract may traverse the cysts rather than be contained by hepatic parenchyma. If diversion of hepatic blood flow exacerbates hepatic dysfunction and severe hepatic failure, TIPS is also precluded. Exceptions include cases of variceal bleeding or fulminant Budd-Chiari syndrome. Relative contraindications include systemic infection, portal vein thrombosis, biliary obstruction, and severe hepatic encephalopathy.

52. What is the technical success rate for TIPS? What are the most common causes of a failed procedure?

TIPS is one of the more technically challenging procedures performed by the interventional radiologist. Nonetheless, the technical success rate is > 90%. Most failures are due to portal vein occlusion, when the occluded segment of portal vein cannot be catheterized from the transjugular approach.

53. How effective is the TIPS procedure for controlling variceal hemorrhage?

TIPS is extremely effective in controlling acute variceal hemorrhage. It appears to be as effective as a surgical portacaval shunt without the added risk of hepatic injury from general anesthesia. Mid-term studies have found the rate of recurrent variceal bleeding after TIPS to be < 10%. Nearly all patients with recurrent bleeding were found to have shunt abnormalities, either stenosis or occlusion. Angiographic reevaluation with shunt revision (balloon dilatation or additional stent placement) or placement of a second TIPS nearly always controls bleeding.

54. What are the morbidity and mortality rates for TIPS?

TIPS is generally accepted to have lower morbidity and mortality rates than surgically created portacaval shunts. Published series show a 30-day mortality rate of 3–15%. Most deaths are

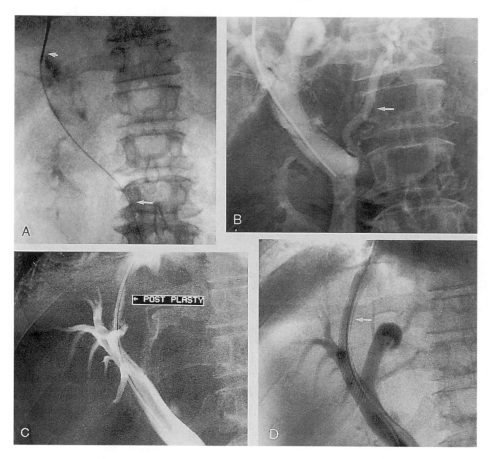

FIGURE 14. Transjugular intrahepatic portosystemic shunt in a 52-year-old woman with cryptogenic cirrhosis and refractory variceal bleeding. *A,* The portal vein has been punctured with a Colapinto needle *(arrowhead)* and a guidewire placed into the superior mesenteric vein *(arrow).* The portosystemic gradient (PSG) was 28 mmHg. *B,* Portal venogram shows a large cardiac vein and esophageal varices *(arrow). C,* After balloon dilation of the transhepatic tract, a suboptimal portosystemic shunt is shown. *D,* A metallic stent *(arrow)* has been deployed across the transhepatic tract, allowing greater luminal diameter. Postprocedural PSG was 10 mmHg.

in Child-Pugh class C patients. The direct procedure-related mortality rate is 2–5%. Procedure-related deaths are due predominantly to intraprocedural cardiac events or intraperitoneal hemorrhage after puncture through the liver capsule. Serious procedural complications, which occur in < 10% of patients, include self-limited peritoneal hemorrhage, myocardial infarction, transient renal failure, hepatic arterial injury, hepatic infarction, and pulmonary edema.

55. Describe the major short-term complications of TIPS.

The two main short-term complications of TIPS are shunt malfunction and hepatic encephalopathy. Acute thrombosis of the stent is infrequent but may occur immediately or shortly after the procedure. The interventionalist can treat this complication by removing or displacing the thrombus from the stent (i.e., shunt thrombectomy). Delayed shunt stenosis or occlusion usually results from pseudointimal proliferation within the stent or incomplete coverage of the parenchymal tract with the stent; treatment is shunt revision. Primary shunt patency is 70% at 1 year and 40% at 2 years. Secondary patency rates (patency after shunt revision) are > 90% at 2 years.

56. Describe the major long-term complication of TIPS. How is it treated?

The most significant long-term complication of TIPS is hepatic encephalopathy. New or worsened encephalopathy is seen in about 25% of patients after TIPS. Usually it can be treated with diet and lactulose administration. Clinical variables associated with increased risk for developing post-TIPS encephalopathy include an etiology of liver disease other than alcohol, female gender, increasing age, and prior history of encephalopathy. Severe encephalopathy may require complete or partial occlusion of the shunt.

57. How is shunt patency followed?

Shunt patency can be followed noninvasively by color Doppler ultrasound or venography. Protocols differ among institutions. A baseline study is obtained 24 hours after the procedure. In asymptomatic patients, routine follow-up is performed at 3 and 6 months after TIPS, then at 6-month intervals. If the patient becomes symptomatic (e.g., variceal bleeding or ascites) or if significant interval change is demonstrated by ultrasound, venography with therapeutic intervention should be performed to restore normal shunt function.

BIBLIOGRAPHY

1. Bissonnette RT, Gibney RG, Berry BR, Buckley AR: Fatal carcinoid crisis after percutaneous fine-needle biopsy of hepatic metastasis: Case report and literature review. Radiology 174:751–752, 1990.
2. Bradley EL III: A clinically based classification system for acute pancreatitis: Summary of the International Symposium on Acute Pancreatitis, Atlanta, September 11–13, 1992. Arch Surg 128:586–590, 1993.
3. Casola G, Nicolet V, van Sonnenberg E, et al: Unsuspected pheochromocytoma: Risk of blood-pressure alterations during percutaneous adrenal biopsy. Radiology 159:733–735, 1986.
4. Castaneda-Zuniga WR (ed): Interventional Radiology. Baltimore, Williams & Wilkins, 1997.
5. del Pilar Fernandez M, Murphy FB: Hepatic biopsies and fluid drainages. Radiol Clin North Am 29:1311–1328, 1991.
6. Dodd GD III, Soulen MC, Kane RA, et al: Minimally invasive treatment of malignant hepatic tumors: At the threshold of a major breakthrough. Radiographics 20:9–27, 2000.
7. Freeny PC, Hauptmann E, Althaus SJ, et al: Percutaneous CT-guided catheter drainage of infected acute necrotizing pancreatitis: Techniques and results. AJR 170:969–977, 1998.
8. Gerzof SG: Triangulation: Indirect CT guidance for abscess drainage. AJR 137:1080–1081, 1981.
9. Gerzof SG, Gale ME: Computed tomography and ultrasonography for diagnosis and treatment of renal and retroperitoneal abscesses. Urol Clin North Am 9:185–193, 1982.
10. Hariri M, Slivka A, Carr-Locke DL, Banks PA: Pseudocyst drainage predisposes to infection when pancreatic necrosis is unrecognized. Am J Gastroenterol 89:1781–1784, 1994.
11. Hopper KD, Baird DE, Reddy VV, et al: Efficacy of automated biopsy guns versus conventional biopsy needles in the pygmy pig. Radiology 176:671–676, 1990.
12. Kerlan RK, LaBerge JM, Gordon RL, Ring EJ: Transjugular intrahepatic portosystemic shunts: Current status. AJR 164:1059–1066, 1995.
13. Laberge J, Ring E, Gordon R, et al: Creation of transjugular intrahepatic portosystemic shunts with the Wallstent endoprosthesis: Results in 100 patients. Radiology 187:413–420, 1993.
14. Mannucci PM, Remuzzi G, Pusineri F, et al: Deamino-8-D-arginine vasopressin shortens the bleeding time in uremia. N Engl J Med 308:8–12, 1983.
15. Ong JP, Sands M, Younossi ZM: Transjugular intrahepatic portosystemic shunts (TIPS): A decade later. J Clin Gastroenterol 30:14–28, 2000.
16. Peck DJ, McLoughlin RF, Hughson MN, Rankin RN: Percutaneous embolization of lower gastrointestinal hemorrhage. J Vasc Interv Radiol 9:747–751, 1998.
17. Price RB, Bernardino ME, Berkman WA, et al: Biopsy of the right adrenal gland by the transhepatic approach. Radiology 148:566, 1983.
18. Quinn SF, van Sonnenberg E, Casola G, et al: Interventional radiology in the spleen. Radiology 161: 289–291, 1986.
19. Rosen RJ, Sanchez G: Angiographic diagnosis and management of gastrointestinal hemorrhage: Current concepts. Radiol Clin North Am 32:951–967, 1994.
20. Sheafor DH, Paulson EK, Kliewer MA, DeLong DM, Nelson RC: Comparison of sonographic and CT guidance techniques: Does CT fluoroscopy decrease procedure time? AJR 174:939–942, 2000.
21. Silverman SG, Mueller PR, Pfister RC: Hemostatic evaluation before abdominal interventions: An overview and proposal. AJR 154:233–238, 1990
22. Soulen MC: Chemoembolization of hepatic malignancies. Semin Interv Radiol 14:305–311, 1997.
23. Valji K: Vascular and Interventional Radiology. Philadelphia, W.B. Saunders, 1999.
24. van Sonnenberg E, D'Agostino HB, Casola G, et al: Percutaneous abscess drainage: Current concepts. Radiology 181:617–626, 1991.
25. van Sonnenberg E, Wittich GR, Casola G, et al: Percutaneous drainage of infected and noninfected pancreatic pseudocysts: experience in 101 cases. Radiology 170:757–776, 1981.
26. van Sonnenberg E, Wroblicka JT, D'Agostino HB, et al: Symptomatic hepatic cysts: Percutaneous drainage and sclerosis. Radiology 190:387–392, 1994.

75. NONIVASIVE GI IMAGING: ULTRASOUND, COMPUTED TOMOGRAPHY, MAGNETIC RESONANCE SCANNING

Michael G. Fox, M.D., David W. Bean, Jr., M.D., Steven H. Peck, M.D., and Kevin M. Rak, M.D.

LIVER IMAGING

1. How is segmental liver anatomy defined?

Early descriptions of liver anatomy divided the organ into four lobes based on the surface configuration. Recently, the segmental anatomy has been based on the vasculature, primarily involving the hepatic veins (Fig. 1). The different hepatic segments are divided by intersegmental fissures, which are traversed or are in the same plane as the hepatic veins.

The main lobar fissure divides the right and left lobes of the liver and is represented by a line extending from the gallbladder recess through the inferior vena cava (IVC). In the liver, it is represented by the middle hepatic vein. The right intersegmental fissure divides the anterior and posterior segments of the right lobe of the liver and is approximated by the right hepatic vein.

The left intersegmental fissure divides the medial and lateral segments of the left lobe of the liver. It is marked on the external liver margin by the falciform ligament, and internally the ligamentum teres runs within it. In the liver, it is represented by the left hepatic vein. The caudate lobe is the portion of liver located between the IVC and the fissure of the ligamentum venosum.

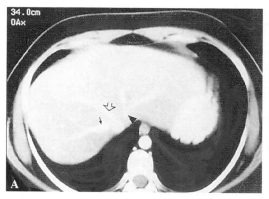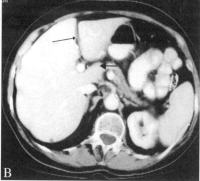

FIGURE 1.   CT scans showing vascular anatomy of the liver. *A*, The right hepatic vein *(black arrow)* divides the anterior and posterior segments of the right lobe of the liver. The middle hepatic vein *(open arrow)* divides the right lobe from the left lobe. The left hepatic vein *(arrowhead)* divides the medial and lateral segments of the left lobe of the liver. *B*, The falciform ligament *(small black arrow)* divides the medial and lateral segments of the left lobe of the liver. The caudate lobe is marked by the *large black arrow.*

2. What are the typical imaging features of liver metastases?

On CT, most liver metastases are of low attenuation compared with the surrounding parenchyma (Fig. 2); however, high attenuation metastases can be seen with pancreatic islet cell carcinoma, renal cell carcinoma, carcinoid tumor, or thyroid carcinoma.

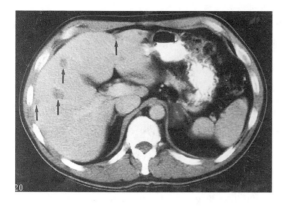

FIGURE 2. Liver metastases *(arrows)* in a patient with colon carcinoma present as hypodense lesions in the surrounding normal liver parenchyma.

3. How does vasculature determine the detection of liver metastases on CT?

Branches of the hepatic artery supply liver metastases, and their detection is based on the timing of the contrast bolus and the vascularity of the lesions. The liver parenchyma receives 75% of its blood flow from the portal vein and 25% from the hepatic artery. Immediately after peripheral injection of intravenous contrast, organs with only an arterial supply (e.g., spleen, kidney) enhance brightly, but the liver enhances little, because the contrast from the hepatic artery is diluted by blood from the portal vein. Only after contrast circulates through the spleen and mesentery to reach the portal vein does the dominant contrast effect occur. This takes about 60 seconds; the spleen and kidney enhance 30 seconds earlier. CT imaging usually is best performed during the portal venous contrast phase, when the contrast between the enhancing liver and low-density metastases is greatest.

The exception to this rule is imaging of hypervascular metastases. Imaging during the arterial phase, 30–40 seconds after injection, should be added to portal phase imaging. Triple-phase imaging—before contrast and 30 and 70 seconds after contrast—is helpful for evaluating metastases from renal cell, breast, thyroid, melanoma, and neuroendocrine tumors. This technique also should be used for evaluating other vascular lesions, such as hepatocellular carcinoma, focal nodular hyperplasia, and hepatic adenomas.

4. What is CT arterial portography?

To increase liver enhancement, many medical centers place a catheter in the superior mesenteric artery for contrast injection during CT scanning. This technique, called CT arterial portography (CTAP), can increase the sensitivity of lesion detection to 91%. A standard contrast-enhanced CT scan has a sensitivity of 63–71% ; triple-phase imaging has a sensitivity of 80%. The improved vascular contrast also improves localization of metastases to a specific subsegment. Improved localization and sensitivity are particularly helpful when partial hepatic resection is contemplated for metastases secondary to colorectal carcinoma. By detecting more lesions, needless surgery can be avoided. Other CT techniques such as delayed contrast-enhanced CT, noncontrast enhanced CT (NCCT), and CT scanning during contrast injection through a hepatic artery catheter, have failed to match the success of CTAP in clinical trials. About 5% of metastases contain calcification, usually from mucinous adenocarcinomas of the ovary or GI tract. Cystic metastatic lesions can arise from tumors of the pancreas and ovary or from necrotic squamous cell carcinoma metastases.

5. Describe the appearance of liver metastases on ultrasound (US).

It varies greatly. GI and more vascular tumors (e.g., islet cell, carcinoid, renal cell carcinomas) tend to produce hyperechoic metastases, but hypoechoic lesions are also common, particularly with lymphoma and cystic or necrotic metastases. Hypoechoic halos of edema surrounding hyperechoic metastases produce the common "bull's-eye" appearance. The sensitivity of US for detecting metastases is about 61%; however, intraoperative US can increase the sensitivity to 96% and may be the most sensitive modality available.

6. What is the role of magnetic resonance (MR) scanning in detection of liver metastases?

Researchers continue to evaluate the use of various MR pulse sequences for detection of liver metastases. The sensitivity of MR is less than that of contrast-enhanced CT. In general, metastases are hypointense on T1-weighted images and hyperintense on T2-weighted images. Exceptions occur with hemorrhagic and malignant melanoma metastases, which are hyperintense to varying degrees on T1-weighted images. Imaging with MRI contrast agents has shown promise in matching the sensitivity of CTAP.

7. What MRI contrast agents are available for use in hepatobiliary imaging?

The two main categories of MRI contrast agents used in hepatobiliary imaging are hepatobiliary and ferrous oxide agents. **Manganese dipyridoxyl diphosphate (Mn-DPDP)** is a hepatobiliary agent that is taken up by hepatocytes and excreted in the bile. It is convenient because it has a long (up to 10 hours) imaging window. On T1 images, Mn-DPDP causes increased signal in the normal liver. Therefore, lesions not of hepatocellular origin do not enhance. Examples include metastases, cholangiocarcinoma, and lymphoma. However, lesions that are of hepatocellular origin (hepatocellular carcinoma [HCC], focal nodular hyperplasia [FNH], and regenerating nodules) do enhance.

Superparamagnetic ferrous oxide agents (SPIOs) were approved by the FDA for commercial use in 1997. They are used primarily to evaluate for metastases, particularly in patients with colon carcinoma. They are taken up by the reticuloendothelial system, primarily by Kupffer cells, and result in a decreased T2 signal. Lesions that do not have reticuloendothelial elements, such as metastases and cysts, do not take up the agent and remain hyperintense on T2. Early studies with SPIOs, such as ferumoxide, detected 27% more lesions than unenhanced MR and 40% more lesions than noncontrast CT. They can improve the detection of HCC but are limited in severe cases of cirrhosis. A limited study reported a similar detection rate of metastases with both SPIO agents and CTAP, but additional study is needed. Limitations of SPIOs include lack of effectiveness at characterizing lesions smaller than 1–2 cm and dose-related toxicity.

8. What are the three growth patterns of HCC?

(1) Large solitary mass, (2) multifocal HCC with a dominant mass and satellite lesions, and (3) diffuse infiltration. In North America, underlying cirrhosis is seen in 60% and hemochromatosis in 20% of patients with HCC. HCC arising in normal livers tends to occur at a younger age (fibrolamellar HCC) and typically presents as a solitary, well-circumscribed mass.

9. Describe the sonographic characteristics of HCC.

They are variable and may simulate metastatic disease. HCCs < 3 cm are often hypoechoic, whereas larger lesions have mixed echogenicity. Fatty metamorphosis within the tumor may cause internal hyperechoic foci. Vascular invasion is common and suggestive of HCC, which invades portal veins more frequently than hepatic veins. Such tumor thrombus can be demonstrated with Doppler ultrasound and typically has an arterial waveform. Detecting malignant tumor thrombus is important, because it is the worst prognostic factor for tumor recurrence after surgery.

10. How does HCC appear on CT?

Underlying cirrhotic or hemochromatotic changes are commonly seen, and 7–10% of HCCs demonstrate calcification. Tumors are typically hypodense on noncontrast CT but may appear hyperdense in fatty livers. They typically are hypodense during portal venous phase imaging but may appear isodense. Because small HCCs may enhance much like liver parenchyma during portal phase imaging, making contour deformity or mass effect the only means of detection, arterial phase imaging should be used. Hepatic arterial phase imaging usually demonstrates a hyperdense lesion and increases detection by 10%. Central necrotic areas of low attenuation are common (Fig. 3). Hemoperitoneum, due to rare spontaneous rupture, and vascular invasion can be documented with CT. A hyperdense, enhancing capsule is common. CTAP increases sensitivity, especially in detecting small lesions.

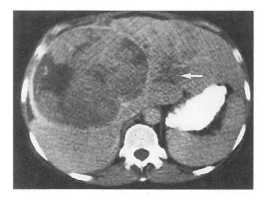

FIGURE 3. CT shows large necrotic hepato-cellular carcinoma. The area of lower attenuation in the left lobe *(arrow)* is a separate focus of multifocal HCC.

11. How does HCC appear on MR?

HCC is usually hypointense on T1 images but may be iso- or hyperintense, depending on the degree of fatty change and internal fibrosis. It is usually hyperintense on T2 images. Encapsulated HCC typically has a hypointense rim on T1 and T2 images. Fibrolamellar HCC appears somewhat similar to FNH. Both have a central scar with multiple fibrous septa. However, fibrolamellar HCC has a high prevalence of calcification, and the central scar is typically hypointense on T2 images, whereas it is hyperintense in FNH. The addition of dynamic enhanced gadolinium (Gd-DTPA) T1 imaging increases the detection of HCC.

12. What is the most common benign neoplasm of the liver?

Cavernous hemangiomas. Most are < 5 cm in size and solitary, although they can be multiple. They typically are located in a peripheral subcapsular location, commonly in the right lobe of the liver. Blood flow within cavernous hemangiomas is usually very slow, which accounts for some of its imaging characteristics.

13. Describe the imaging characteristics of hepatic hemangiomas.

US: Cavernous hemangiomas appear as well-defined hyperechoic masses. Doppler and color flow imaging show no detectable flow within the mass, but they may demonstrate a feeding vessel. Occasionally hemangiomas have a mixed or hypoechoic appearance.

CT: On unenhanced CT, hemangiomas are usually hypodense, well-defined lesions; 20% have calcifications. They may appear iso- or hyperdense if they arise in an area of focal fatty infiltration. Triple-phase imaging may reveal a characteristic enhancement pattern, initially showing peripheral enhancement isodense to the aorta followed by slow filling of the center of the lesion. This pattern has been described as nodular or fingerlike and can take from 5 to 60 minutes to fill completely. Up to one-fourth of lesions do not show this characteristic pattern; they may show initial central or uniform enhancement, which also may be seen in malignant lesions.

MRI: A typical hemangioma is well defined and has decreased signal intensity relative to normal liver on T1-weighted images. On T2-weighted images, hemangiomas have increased signal compared with the liver because of their high water content. The signal is equal to or greater than the signal of bile within the gallbladder and should continue to increase with greater T2 weighting. Using fast-scanning techniques and Gd-DTPA, a similar enhancement pattern can be seen on MRI and CT, with an accuracy approaching 95%.

14. Outline the work-up for a suspected cavernous hemangioma.

If a lesion has the typical US findings of a cavernous hemangioma and is < 3 cm, and if the patient has normal liver function tests (LFTs) and no history of a malignancy that may metastasize to the liver, follow-up US in 3–6 months is appropriate. If the lesion is atypical on US or if the patient has a known primary neoplasm or abnormal LFTs, further work-up is warranted. If the lesion is > 2 cm, a 99mTc-tagged red blood cell (RBC) scan is the next step. This procedure is highly sensitive and specific for lesions > 2 cm. If the lesion is < 2 cm, the RBC scan can be attempted, but sensitivity and specificity decrease as the size of the lesion decreases. If the RBC scan is equivocal, the next study is MRI, preferably with heavily T2-weighted and gadolinium enhanced T1 imaging. In this scenario, CT should be a third-line choice or used if MRI is not available.

If the initial lesion is found by CT and follows the strict criteria of a hemangioma (a well-defined, low-density lesion on unenhanced images, with peripheral enhancement followed by complete filling of the lesion), further work-up is probably not necessary. If the diagnosis needs confirmation, a tagged RBC study or ultrasound is a good choice. If the initial CT scan does not meet the strict criteria or the patient has abnormal LFTs, a confirmatory nuclear medicine or MRI scan is appropriate. If the CT criteria are not met, it is typically due to incomplete filling of the lesion.

If these different studies do not confirm that the lesion is a cavernous hemangioma, biopsy may be necessary for the final diagnosis.

15. How can FNH and hepatocellular adenoma (HCA) be differentiated?

Hepatic adenomas and FNH are more common in women, and both, particularly HCA, are associated with oral contraceptive use. FNH is benign, whereas HCA can cause morbidity and mortality because of its propensity for hemorrhage and rare malignant degeneration to HCC. Particularly in smaller lesions without hemorrhage, biopsy may be required for differentiation.

16. Describe the appearance of FNH on imaging modalitites.

FNH contains all of the normal liver elements in an abnormal arrangement. The characteristic feature is the central scar, containing radiating fibrous tissue with vascular and biliary elements. However, the central scar is nonspecific and may be seen with fibrolamellar HCC, hemangioma, and other lesions. On **US**, FNH is a well-demarcated hypo- to isoechoic mass, possibly demonstrating a central scar. On **triple-phase CT**, a central low-density scar may be seen in 20–40% of cases. The scar should be somewhat linear or branching to help distinguish it from central necrosis in a mass. On **noncontrast CT**, FNH is hypo- to isodense without calcification. FNH is hyperdense on arterial phase images, because it is supplied by the hepatic artery. On **portal phase images**, it commonly enhances much like normal liver, except for the persisting central scar, which may become hyperdense on delayed images. Thus, if no central scar is seen, FNH may be missed on CT or seen only as a deformity of the liver contour. On **MR**, FNH is hypo- to isointense on T1 and iso- to hyperintense on T2. The central scar is hypointense on T1 and hyperintense on T2 images and enhances with Gd-DTPA. Because of the presence of Kupffer cells, **sulfur-colloid scintigraphy** demonstrates normal uptake in 50%, decreased uptake in 40%, and increased uptake or "hot-spots" in 10%. However, HCA also may show normal sulfur colloid uptake in 20%.

17. How does HCA appear on imaging modalities?

Sonography typically shows a heterogeneous mass due to areas of internal hemorrhage; however, the mass may be hyperechoic because of the high lipid content. On **noncontrast CT**, a hypodense mass is typically seen; however, internal areas of higher attenuation may be present due to recent hemorrhage. Hemorrhage is a key distinguishing feature from FNH. **Contrast CT** may show centripetal enhancement similar to that in hemangiomas, though this enhancement does not persist in adenomas. On **MR**, HCA may be hyperintense on T1 because of internal fat/glycogen, although similar findings may be seen in HCC. The lesions are commonly heterogeneous as a result of necrosis and internal hemorrhage.

18. Describe the appearance of a hepatic abscess on imaging.

US: On ultrasound, a hepatic abscess appears as a complex fluid collection, typically with septations, an irregular wall, and debris or air within the fluid. Air is seen as a focal area of echogenicity with posterior shadowing. Abscesses also can appear as simple fluid collections similar to a cyst.

CT: CT is the most sensitive imaging modality (95–98%). CT findings vary with the size and age of the abscess. Generally, the abscess appears as a low-density, well-defined mass and may be uni- or multilocular and contain internal septations. It usually has a well-defined wall, with either smooth or irregular margins, that may enhance. Density values of the fluid range from

2–40 Hounsfield units (HU) depending on the protein content. The most specific sign is air bubbles within the abscess cavity, although this sign is seen in only 20% of cases.

MRI: An abscess appears as a well-defined lesion of low signal intensity on T1 images and bright signal intensity on T2 images. The cavity may have homogeneous or heterogeneous signal, and septations may be seen. The capsule appears as a low-signal rim and may enhance with gadolinium.

Other causes of complex cysts, such as a focal hematoma, and necrotic or hemorrhagic neoplasm, may have similar appearances.

19. What causes fatty filtration of the liver?

Fatty infiltration of the liver is due to deposition of triglycerides within the hepatocytes and is associated with many disorders, including ethanol abuse, obesity, excessive steroids, hyperalimentation, diabetes, radiation or chemotherapy, and glycogen storage disease. It can cause slightly abnormal LFTs and hepatomegaly. Fatty infiltration may be diffuse or focal.

20. Describe the imaging findings of fatty infiltration of the liver.

US: Fatty infiltration is seen as a focal or diffuse area of increased echogenicity. There is decreased visualization or nonvisualization of intrahepatic vessels, the deeper posterior portions of the liver, and the diaphragm posterior to the liver. US does not show any mass effect on adjacent biliary structures or blood vessels. The finding of diffusely increased echogenicity of the liver is nonspecific and can be seen in hepatitis or cirrhosis.

CT: Fatty infiltration is seen as an area of decreased attenuation, which is easier to appreciate in the focal form with adjacent normal liver (Fig. 4). On noncontrast CT scan, the normal liver is usually 8 HU greater in density than the spleen, but in fatty infiltration it is less dense than the spleen by 10 HU or more. However, other lesions may appear as an area of decreased density on noncontrast CT, such as hepatomas and metastatic disease. In fatty infiltration, the hepatic vessels stand out and may appear as if they contain contrast on an unenhanced scan. In focal fatty infiltration, the normal hepatic vessels traverse the area of decreased attenuation, a finding not seen in a malignant mass. Focal fatty infiltration tends to have linear margins and to be in a lobar distribution.

MRI: Fat tissue typically has increased signal on T1 images and decreased signal on T2 images. Signal differences in focal fatty infiltration of the liver usually are not as dramatic as those seen in subcutaneous fat; in fact, the signal changes may be quite subtle. As with CT, it is important to see normal vessels in the area of signal abnormality and no mass effect on adjacent structures. Fat-suppression MRI scans are more sensitive than routine T1 and T2 scans and show fatty infiltration as areas of decreased signal intensity compared with normal liver. With chemical shift techniques, such as opposed-phase imaging, fatty areas demonstrate decreased signal.

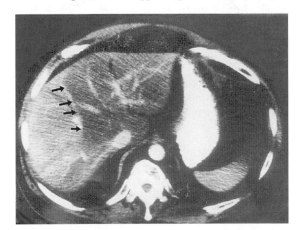

FIGURE 4. Focal fatty infiltration of the liver shown as a low-attenuation area next to normal liver *(arrows)*.

21. Which imaging techniques are used to detect cirrhosis?

US: Cirrhosis is characterized by abnormal echotexture. The hepatic parenchyma is typically hyperechoic with "coarsened" echoes, making the liver somewhat heterogeneous, and the intrahepatic vasculature is poorly defined. Unfortunately, these findings are nonspecific. Increased parenchymal echogenicity also is seen in fatty infiltration, and heterogeneity may be due to infiltrating neoplasm. Furthermore, no direct correlation exists between degree of hepatic dysfunction and sonographic appearance. More specific sonographic features of cirrhosis include nodularity of the liver surface and selective enlargement of the caudate lobe (Fig. 5A). A caudate-to-right lobe volume ratio > 96% allows 96% confidence in diagnosing cirrhosis. In portal hypertension, the normal portal venous velocity is highly variable, but the Doppler detection of hepatofugal flow is diagnostic. Doppler also provides improved identification of portal collateral vessels, particularly the recanalized umbilical vein.

CT: Although early parenchymal changes may not be visible on CT, fatty infiltration, the initial manifestation of alcoholic liver disease, is well seen. The liver enlarges, and its attenuation becomes abnormally lower than that of the spleen. In later stages of cirrhosis, liver volume typically decreases. A nodular contour (due to regenerating nodules, scarring, and atrophy) may be seen, with somewhat heterogeneous enhancement. Regenerating nodules are isodense with liver and can be inferred only from contour deformity. The caudate lobe and lateral-segment left lobe are typically enlarged, and atrophy of the right lobe and medial-segment left lobe is seen. Mesenteric fat develops a higher attenuation than retroperitoneal or subcutaneous fat. CT demonstrates varices, ascites, and splenomegaly associated with portal hypertension (Fig. 5B). Unlike sonography, CT cannot determine the direction of vascular flow, but it is superior in delineating the full extent of varices and collateral vessels.

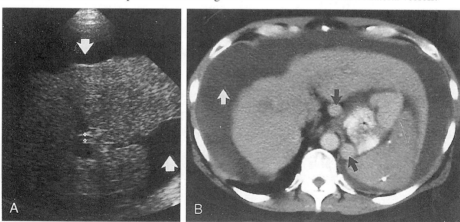

FIGURE 5. Cirrhosis. *A,* Ultrasound shows small, echogenic liver with nodular contour, compatible with cirrhosis. Low echogenicity ascites surrounds the liver *(arrows)*. *B,* CT demonstrates small liver with nodular contour and enhancing varices *(black arrows)* and extensive ascites *(white arrow)*.

MR: MR has little role in the diagnosis of cirrhosis but can help to distinguish cirrhotic nodules from HCC. Regenerating nodules are hypointense on T2 because of hemosiderin deposits, whereas HCC is hyperintense. Hyperplastic adenomatous nodules without atypia are hyperintense on T1 and hypointense on T2, again allowing differentiation from carcinoma.

22. Define primary and secondary hemochromatosis.

Primary hemochromatosis is an autosomal recessive disease in which patients absorb excessive amounts of dietary iron that accumulate in the parenchymal cells of the liver, heart, and pancreas. Patients with primary hemochromatosis are at increased risk of developing HCC. HCC appears hyperintense to the background of a low intensity liver. **Secondary hemochromatosis,** caused by multiple blood transfusions, results in iron deposition in the reticuloendothelial cells of primarily the liver and spleen. In cirrhosis or intravascular hemolysis, iron level in the hepato-cytes is mildly increased. Neither MR nor CT can distinguish which cells of a particular organ are overloaded with iron. However, the organ distribution of imaging abnormalities can some-times provide valuable information.

23. Which is the most sensitive exam in detecting hemochromatosis?

MR and CT imaging rely on the increased iron content of the liver and other organs to diag-nose hemochromatosis. US of the liver is normal despite iron deposition unless underlying cir-rhosis exists. Increased attenuation of the liver on CT is due to the high atomic number of iron, but it is not a specific finding; amiodarone, chemotherapy agents, gold therapy, and glycogen de-posits can produce similar findings. The attenuation of the liver on noncontrast CT scans is typi-cally > 85 HU in hemochromatosis, compared with a normal attenuation of ~ 60 HU. With MR, the iron deposition causes decreased intensity compared with the paraspinal muscles because of paramagnetic effects. The findings are most striking on T2 images but can be seen to a lesser extent on T1 images. MR appears to be more sensitive and specific than CT, and MR quantifica-tion in the future may eliminate the need for some liver biopsies.

24. What is a normal Doppler waveform?

The changing frequency of reflected sound waves from flowing blood allows US to calculate the velocity and direction of blood flow. A "normal" Doppler waveform is different for each artery or vein of the body. Veins have continuous low-velocity flow that frequently varies with respira-tion. In the portal vein, flow is hepatopedal and generally ranges from 15–25 cm/sec (Fig. 6A). Flow velocity normally decreases during inspiration and increases during expiration. Arterial flow does not vary with respiration but varies dramatically with the cardiac cycle, showing high-veloc-ity flow during systole and relatively high flow (i.e., low resistance) during diastole (Fig. 6B) In fasting patients, the superior mesenteric artery has equally high systolic velocity but minimal flow and even flow reversal during diastole (i.e., high resistance). Ingestion of a meal creates a lower re-sistance system by increasing the diastolic flow to the bowel with end arterial dilatation.

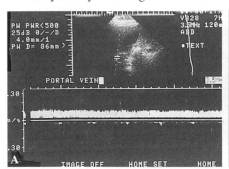 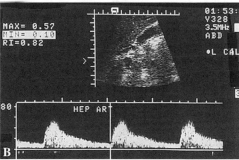

FIGURE 6. Doppler ultrasound. *A,* Normal blood flow in the portal vein. Flow registers above the baseline because it is traveling toward the ultrasound probe. *B,* Normal hepatic artery blood flow. Again, flow is toward the ultrasound probe. High-velocity flow represents systole, and lower-velocity flow represents diastole.

In both arteries and veins, color Doppler can be used to verify the presence and direction of flow. The operator determines whether blood flowing toward the transducer is blue or red, and blood flowing away from the transducer takes on the other color. Therefore, flow in arteries and veins normally is assigned a different color. Arteries also demonstrate color pulsation due to rapidly changing speed of flow.

25. How are Doppler waveforms altered in portal vein thrombosis?

In acute portal vein thrombosis, flow in the portal vein is markedly diminished or absent. In most instances, echogenic material is seen in the portal vein (Fig. 7A), although in a few cases the portal vein may appear normal. Doppler analysis yields no waveform, and with color imaging, no color is seen in the vessel. In the more chronic condition of cavernous transformation of the portal vein, the portal vein cannot be seen, but an echogenic structure in the porta hepatis represents a fibrotic remnant. The presence of multiple tubular channels in the porta hepatis with demonstrable flow by color imaging or Doppler evaluation is virtually diagnostic of cavernous transformation.

26. Describe the effect of portal hypertension on Doppler waveforms.

Portal hypertension can be suggested on US by a portal vein > 13 mm with decreased flow velocity, although portal vein size is so variable that specific measurements are unreliable. Retrograde (hepatofugal) flow in the portal vein indicates advanced disease and is a useful but late finding (Figs. 7B and C). Detection of portosystemic collaterals aids greatly in detecting portal hypertension. The easiest collateral to detect by US is the recanalized paraumbilical vein (Fig. 7D), which drains the left portal vein as it travels through the ligamentum teres to the abdominal wall. The coronary (left gastric) vein, another collateral vessel, originates at the portosplenic confluence and ascends to the gastroesophageal junction to feed esophageal varices. Detection of hepatofugal flow in the coronary vein is one of the best indicators of portal hypertension. Splenic varices are easily

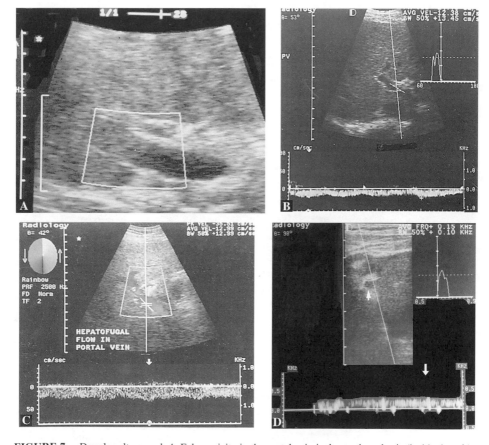

FIGURE 7. Doppler ultrasound. *A,* Echogenicity in the portal vein is due to thrombosis (inside the *white square*) in a patient with HCC invading the portal vein. *B,* Hepatofugal blood flow registers below the baseline in the portal vein of a patient with known portal hypertension. *C,* Color Doppler images registers blue (retrograde) flow in the portal vein in a patient with hypertension and hepatofugal flow. If direction of flow were normal, it would be red. (Courtesy of Patrick Meyers, RT). *D,* Doppler-identified blood flow in the falciform ligament (in *white arrow*) is due to recanalized paraumbilical veins in a patient with portal hypertension. Note subhepatic ascites.

detected as tubular structures with flow in the splenic hilum. Other portosystemic collaterals include splenorenal shunts and retroperitoneal veins.

27. How does Budd-Chiari syndrome affect Doppler waveforms?

Budd-Chiari syndrome refers to obstruction of hepatic venous outflow. It can occur at a number of levels, from the small hepatic venules to the inferior vena cava (IVC). Typically, the liver parenchyma is diffusely heterogeneous, but to make the diagnosis, one must observe echogenic thrombus or absent flow in one or more of the hepatic veins or the suprahepatic IVC. Twenty percent of patients have associated portal vein thrombosis, and many others have ascites.

28. Discuss the role of US in the evaluation of transjugular intrahepatic portosystemic shunts (TIPS).

Ultrasound is used for preprocedure evaluation and to assess shunt patency after the procedure. The preprocedure examination is obtained 24–48 hours before the TIPS. It assesses the size and parenchyma of the liver and spleen, flow characteristics of the hepatic and portal vessels, patency of the internal jugular veins, and presence or absence of varices and ascites.

A new baseline examination, documenting flow within the shunt and determining velocity measurements in the middle and at both ends of the shunt, is obtained 24–48 hours after the procedure. The flow is usually of high velocity and turbulent; however, there is a wide range of peak velocities in patent, well-functioning shunts (Fig. 8). A decrease in peak velocity, along with other signs of shunt failure, should prompt a portagram for further evaluation. Signs of a failing shunt include decreased velocity in the shunt, reaccumulation of ascites, reappearance or increased size of varices, and flow of blood away from the shunt. A peak shunt velocity of 50–60 cm/sec should prompt an angiographic study of the shunt to evaluate for stenosis. Routine follow-up imaging is recommended every 3 months.

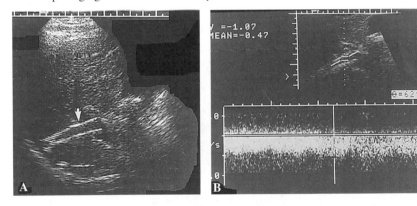

FIGURE 8.   *A,* Ultrasound appearance of a TIPS. *B,* Doppler ultrasound showing flow within a patent TIPS.

BILIARY TRACT IMAGING

29. What is the significance of gallbladder wall thickening on US?

A wall thickness > 3 mm in a distended gallbladder is abnormal and must be explained. Abnormal wall thickness, combined with a sonographic Murphy's sign and gallstones, has a positive predictive value of > 90% for acute cholecystitis, the most common cause of pathologic wall thickening. Many other conditions can cause gallbladder wall thickening. Congestive heart failure and constrictive pericarditis cause congestive hepatomegaly, which often is accompanied by a thickened, edematous gallbladder wall. Hypoalbuminemia, secondary to chronic liver dysfunction or nephrotic syndrome, results in a decrease in plasma oncotic pressure that produces generalized tissue edema, including edema of the gallbladder wall. Portal venous congestion from portal hypertension of any cause and hepatic veno-occlusive disease can produce gallbladder wall thickening. Inflammation of the gallbladder from nearby hepatitis or AIDS-related cholangitis may produce wall thickening. Chronic cholecystitis, adenomyomatosis, primary sclerosing cholangitis, and leukemic infiltration are additional causes of wall thickening. Gallbladder carcinoma also causes wall thickening but is easily differentiated by its mass-like appearance and association with adenopathy and liver metastases.

30. Describe the radiologic work-up of suspected biliary tree obstruction.

US is the screening examination of choice when biliary ductal disease is suspected. Normal nondilated intrahepatic ducts are 1–2 mm in diameter and usually are not visualized. The size of the common hepatic duct (CHD) is a sensitive indicator of the presence of biliary obstruction; it is more sensitive than intrahepatic ducts in assessing early or partial biliary obstruction. The normal CHD is 4–5 mm in diameter; a diameter > 6 mm indicates ductal dilatation (Fig. 9A). However, extrahepatic ductal diameter increases with age and may be increased after cholecystectomy or resolved obstruction. Thus, dilated ducts are not the equivalent of obstruction. Repeat scanning after an oral fatty meal or intravenous cholecystokinin may help to distinguish dilatation due to obstruction. A dilated CHD that fails to decrease in size or increases after this provocative test indicates obstruction. In complicated cases, Doppler examination can readily differentiate the biliary ducts from vasculature in the portal triad. With intrahepatic ductal dilatation, tubular low-echogenicity structures are seen to parallel the portal veins, producing the "too many tubes" sign.

Although US is the best screening exam for biliary disease, once disease is detected, CT is more efficacious in depicting the degree, site, and cause of obstruction. CT provides more complete delineation of the full length of the CBD, because bowel gas commonly obscures sonographic visualization of the distal CBD. The normal CBD is up to 6 mm, whereas a 9-mm CBD is considered dilated (Fig. 9B).

Newer techniques allow the diagnosis of biliary ductal dilatation by MR. ERCP or percutaneous transhepatic cholangiography provides a more detailed evaluation than US or CT but is invasive.

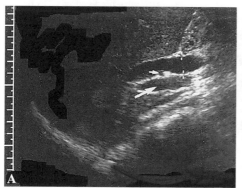 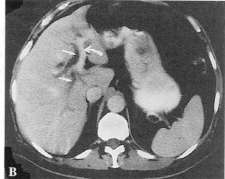

FIGURE 9. *A,* Ultrasound demonstrates a dilated common biliary duct, marked by calipers, measuring 15.7 mm in a patient with a CBD stricture. A hypoechoic portal vein *(long arrow)* and hepatic artery *(short arrow)* are seen posterior to the CBD. *B,* CT demonstrates a dilated intrahepatic biliary tree *(straight arrow)* adjacent to an enhancing portal vein *(curved arrow)* in a patient with pancreatic carcinoma.

31. What is MR cholangiopancreatography (MRCP)? What advantages does it have compared with ERCP?

MRCP is a noninvasive way to evaluate the hepatobiliary tract. MRCP can demonstrate the common bile duct in 98% of patients and can evaluate the pancreatic duct in the head, body, and tail in 97%, 97%, and 83% of patients, respectively. It can differentiate dilated from normal ducts in 95% of patients and is comparable to ERCP and exceeds the accuracy of CT and US in detecting choledocholithiasis. It is comparable to ERCP in detecting extrahepatic strictures, and it is 98% accurate in detecting aberrant hepatic ducts and 95% accurate in demonstrating the cystic duct.

MRCP is comparable to ERCP in diagnosing extrahepatic bile and pancreatic duct abnormalities, and it is the modality of choice for imaging patients with biliary-enteric anastomoses. It is more sensitive than ERCP in detecting pseudocysts and is potentially more accurate in evaluating biliary cystadenomas and cystadenocarcinomas.

The advantages of MRCP over ERCP are that it is noninvasive and less expensive, does not require radiation or sedation, can detect extraductal pathology, and better visualizes ducts proximal to an obstruction. The drawbacks of MRCP are that it has decreased spatial resolution and difficulty with imaging nondilated, peripheral intrahepatic or side ducts. However, the main drawback of MRCP is that it may delay therapeutic intervention in patients with a high clinical suspicion of bile duct obstruction.

32. Describe the differential imaging features seen in the common causes of biliary obstruction.

1. Biliary obstruction may be related to biliary (choledocholithiasis, cholangitis, cholangiocarcinoma) or extrabiliary disease (pancreatitis, periampullary carcinoma). Intrahepatic ductal dilatation with a normal CBD suggests an intrahepatic mass or abnormality. Dilatation of the pancreatic duct typically localizes the obstruction to the pancreatic or ampullary level.

2. An abrupt transition from a dilated CBD to a narrowed or obliterated duct is more characteristic of a neoplasm or stone, whereas a gradual tapering of the CBD at the pancreatic head is typical of fibrosis associated with chronic pancreatitis.

3. US is 60–70% accurate in detecting common duct stones; unlike gallbladder calculi, CBD stones do not necessarily cause acoustic shadowing. CT detection requires thin-section (3-mm) acquisition. Depending on their composition, stones may be seen as soft tissue or calcific intraluminal densities.

4. Cholangiocarcinoma should be suspected in patients with abrupt biliary obstruction but no visualized mass or stone. The primary mass is commonly difficult to identify by US or CT. Because cholangiocarcinoma often arises near or at the liver hilum (Klatskin tumor), it commonly presents with dilated intrahepatic ducts and normal-sized extrahepatic ducts. MR imaging with a hepatobiliary agent may be beneficial if the diagnosis remains in doubt.

5. An abrupt vs. tapered appearance of the CBD helps to differentiate pancreatic carcinoma from chronic pancreatitis. However, chronic pancreatitis also can present as a focal mass, and, biopsy may be required for differentiation.

PANCREATIC IMAGING

33. How can acute pancreatitis be distinguished from chronic pancreatitis on imaging?

Acute: The classic sonographic appearance of acute pancreatitis is a hypoechoic, diffusely enlarged pancreas, although focal involvement may be seen in 18% of cases. US is inferior to CT in evaluating acute pancreatitis for several reasons: (1) overlying bowel gas frequently limits complete visualization of the gland; (2) definition of extent of peripancreatic fluid collections is inferior to that of CT; and (3) US cannot diagnose pancreatic necrosis. Therefore, CT is the preferred study in patients with clinically severe pancreatitis. However, US is effective in follow-up of pseudocysts, which may be echo-free or have internal echogenicity due to hemorrhage or debris.

CT is typically performed with intravenous contrast, but if hemorrhagic pancreatitis is suspected, noncontrast images should be performed first to detect high-attenuation hemorrhage. CT may be normal in **mild** cases of pancreatitis, whereas with **moderate** disease the gland becomes enlarged and slightly heterogeneous, with inflammation causing peripancreatic fat to have higher attenuation ("dirty fat"). With **severe** disease, intraglandular intravasation of pancreatic fluid causes intrapancreatic fluid collections, and extravasation causes peripancreatic fluid collections, peripancreatic inflammation, and thickened fascial planes (Fig. 10A). Fluid collections are most common in the anterior pararenal space and lesser sac but may have wide extension.

Chronic: Sonography is 60–80% accurate in diagnosing chronic pancreatitis, and dilatation of the pancreatic duct is the most specific sonographic abnormality. Calcifications are seen as echogenic, shadowing foci within the gland. The gland may be enlarged early in the disease but atrophic or focally enlarged later. Parenchymal echogenicity is variable.

Similar findings are noted with CT. Alteration of gland size is variable, and focal enlargement due to a chronic inflammatory mass may necessitate biopsy to exclude carcinoma. The pancreatic duct can be dilated (> 3 mm) to the level of the papilla and may appear beaded, irregular, or smooth. Calcifications are the most reliable CT indicator of chronic pancreatitis and are seen in 50% of cases (Fig. 10B). Pseudocysts may be seen within or adjacent to the gland.

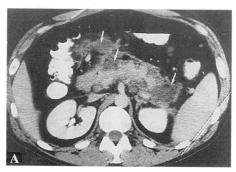 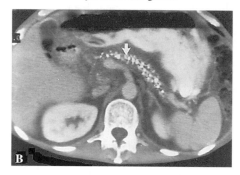

FIGURE 10.   Pancreatitis. *A,* CT in acute pancreatitis demonstrates extensive peripancreatic fluid collections *(arrows). B,* CT shows multiple pancreatic calcifications *(arrows)* in a patient with chronic pancreatitis.

34. Describe the role of CT and US in assessing the complications of pancreatitis.

1. **Pseudocysts** evolve from fluid collections in about 30–50% of patients with acute pancreatitis. The development of a pseudocyst requires at least 4 weeks. More than half of those measuring < 5 cm regress spontaneously. Pseudocysts failing to resolve or causing symptoms (pain, infection, hemorrhage, GI obstruction or fistula) require drainage. On CT, a pseudocyst appears as an oval fluid collection with a nonepithelialized, enhancing wall. US demonstrates an anechoic fluid collection with or without internal debris surrounded by a thin wall. Gas bubbles inside a pseudocyst relate to infection or fistula formation within the bowel.

2. **Pancreatic ascites** presents as free intraperitoneal fluid with high amylase levels in about 7% of patients with acute pancreatitis. Patients tend to have severe disease with obvious additional CT abnormalities, but in rare patients, the pancreas appears normal; in such cases, percutaneous drainage of fluid and evaluation of amylase level is needed to establish the diagnosis.

3. In acute pancreatitis, CT can detect **necrosis** with a sensitivity of about 75–80%. Necrosis is defined as a lack of contrast enhancement in the expected location of pancreatic tissue, and it can develop early or late in the course of the illness. The degree of necrosis is an important prognostic factor. Patients with no CT evidence of necrosis have no mortality and a morbidity rate of only 6%. Patients with mild necrosis (< 30% of the total gland) exhibit no mortality but have a rate of complications of 40%, and patients with more severe necrosis (> 50%) have a morbidity rate of 75–100% and a mortality rate of 11–25%. Necrotic tissue can become secondarily infected, which is recognized on CT as gas bubbles within areas of pancreatic gland necrosis (i.e., emphysematous pancreatitis). More commonly, infected areas do not contain gas, and a culture of a percutaneous aspirate is needed to verify the diagnosis and identify the organism.

4. **Pancreatic abscesses** result from liquefactive necrosis with subsequent infection. CT shows a focal low-attenuation fluid collection with thick enhancing walls. Gas bubbles may be present. US shows a hypoechoic or even anechoic mass with a surrounding hyperechoic wall. Rates of abscess formation vary with the amount of pancreatic necrosis. Abscesses usually occur 4 weeks after the onset of acute pancreatitis. The distinction between abscess and infected necrosis can be difficult, but it is an important one because the treatment alternatives are quite different.

5. **Pseudoaneurysms**, resulting from enzymatic breakdown of the arterial wall, most commonly involve the splenic artery, followed by the gastroduodenal and pancreaticoduodenal arteries. Pseudoaneurysm rupture can cause massive hemorrhage and may occur into the retroperitoneum, peritoneal cavity, pancreatic duct, pseudocyst, or bowel, causing a GI tract bleed. CT is probably best for identifying pseudoaneurysms. High-density areas in or around a pseudoaneurysm represent either acute thrombus or hemorrhage. US with color Doppler can be just as sensitive in detecting pseudoaneurysms and their complications, provided that there is no overlying bowel gas.

6. **Splenic vein thrombosis** is detected by lack of normal enhancement in the expected region of the splenic vein on CT. Color Doppler can be used to make the same diagnosis. Thrombosis of the portal and superior mesenteric veins, although less common, is also well imaged by both modalities.

35. What are the imaging findings of pancreatic ductal adenocarcinoma?

1. **Pancreatic enlargement.** Although enlargement may be focal or diffuse, focal enlargement is more common. Diffuse enlargement is often secondary to pancreatitis caused by the neoplasm. Focal enlargement is better appreciated in the body and tail of the pancreas.

2. **Distortion of the pancreatic contour or shape.** Pancreatic cancer also may cause a focal bulge or irregularity of the organ surface. Involvement of the uncinate process of the pancreas may cause it to have a focal bulge or rounded appearance. Enlargement and contour distortion are the most frequent findings of pancreatic cancer.

3. **Difference in density or echogenicity.** On US pancreatic cancer tends to be hypoechoic compared with normal pancreas; however, it also may appear isoechoic compared with normal pancreas. On CT, it is usually hypodense in comparison with normal pancreas; this distinction is better demonstrated with the use of intravenous contrast.

4. **Pancreatic duct dilatation** can be an important clue of a small neoplasm that may not be appreciated otherwise. It is more common when the neoplasm is located in the pancreatic head.

5. **Biliary tract dilatation.** Bile duct dilatation is more commonly seen with a neoplasm in the head of the pancreas. Isolated intrahepatic biliary ductal dilatation may be seen with pancreatic cancer that has spread to the porta hepatis.

6. **Local invasion** into the peripancreatic fat is most commonly seen, but invasion into the porta hepatis, stomach, spleen, and adjacent bowel loops also may occur.

7. **Regional lymph node enlargement.** Pancreatic cancer may spread to the nodes in the porta hepatis, para-aortic region, and region around the celiac and superior mesenteric artery axis.

8. **Liver metastasis.** The liver is a common site of metastasis for pancreatic cancer. Metastases appear as low-density lesions and may be single or multiple.

36. Which imaging modality is best for detecting and evaluating pancreatic cancer?

The two primary modalities to evaluate suspected pancreatic cancer are US and CT. Triple-phase CT is probably the best first-line imaging modality. CT is better at evaluating adjacent spread or nodal involvement than US, and it does not have the problem of incomplete evaluation of the body and tail of the pancreas, which occurs in up to 25% of US examinations. Overlying bowel gas can obscure these areas on US. In patients who present with biliary obstruction, both US and CT are good first-line examinations. MR imaging with gadolinium can be performed in patients with iodine contrast allergy.

37. What are the common cystic pancreatic neoplasms?

Serous (microcystic) and mucinous (macrocystic) cystic neoplasms are the most common. Serous tumors are more common in women, and 82% occur in people aged 60 years or older. They are almost always benign and predominate in the pancreatic head. Serous tumors calcify more commonly (50%) than any other pancreatic tumors and are typified by a central stellate scar, that frequently calcifies. They typically comprise numerous < 2-cm cysts. On US, the mass is often hyperechoic because the multiple small cysts may not be individually resolved. The hyperechoic central stellate scar and calcifications suggest the diagnosis and may be seen on US or CT. The CT appearance is also varied; innumerable minute cysts may appear as a solid tumor, whereas multiple small but visible cysts have a honeycomb or "Swiss-cheese" appearance. Soft-tissue components enhance with contrast, and the pancreatic contour may be lobulated.

Mucinous cystic neoplasms also have a strong female predominance but tend to occur in younger patients. They have a strong predilection for the pancreatic tail (85%), calcify in 30% of cases, and must be considered malignant. They are larger lesions, averaging 12 cm, and are composed of unilocular or multilocular cysts > 2 cm. US demonstrates internal septations that may be few or many, thick or thin. These septations are thicker than those in microcystic tumors, and the septations may calcify, which is better seen with CT. The tumor wall and organ of origin are better demonstrated with CT, whereas internal septations and solid excrescences are better seen by US. Differential diagnostic considerations include papillary cystic tumor, cystic islet cell tumor, cystic metastasis, pseudocysts, and abscess.

ABDOMINAL AND PELVIC IMAGING

38. How is simple ascites distinguished from complicated ascites?

Simple ascites is a watery transudate that is usually secondary to major organ system failure (i.e., hepatic, renal, or cardiac failure). Because it is a transudate, simple ascites has a CT density similar to water (0–20 HU). In general, as the protein content of the fluid increases, so do the Hounsfield units. By US, simple ascites is anechoic, without internal echoes or septations, and demonstrates increased through transmission. Simple ascites is "free-flowing" and located in the dependent portions of the abdomen and pelvis. It is often found in Morison's pouch, paracolic gutters, and the pelvis. With large amounts of ascites, the bowel seems to float within the fluid, usually in the center of the abdomen. Simple ascites also has a sharp, smooth interface with other intra-abdominal contents (Fig. 11A and B).

Loculated ascites is not a "simple" fluid collection, because it indicates the presence of adhesions. The adhesions may be due to benign causes (e.g., prior surgery) or an infectious or malignant process. Loculated ascites is typically located in nondependent portions of the abdomen, does not move when the patient is scanned in a different position, and often displaces adjacent bowel loops.

Complex ascites is usually secondary to an infectious, hemorrhagic, or neoplastic process. The findings of complex ascites include density greater than water, internal debris or septations, air bubbles within the collection, or a thick or nodular border or capsule (Fig. 11C and D). Usually, the density measurements must be > 20 HU to be considered complex, reflecting the increased protein content. Some complex fluid collections do not have these findings and may appear simple. Often aspiration is the only way to confirm whether a collection is simple.

39. How do you differentiate abdominal fluid from pleural fluid?

Both US and CT are good modalities to ascertain whether a collection is intra-abdominal or pleural. If the collection can be seen by US, it usually outlines the diaphragm, making the determination less confusing. Certain signs have been described to make this differentiation on CT:

1. Ascites is located anterior or lateral to the diaphragmatic crus, whereas pleural fluid is located posterior or medial to the crus.
2. Pleural effusion can extend medial to the crus and appear to touch the spine or aorta.
3. Abdominal fluid is often contiguous with other abdominal fluid collections.
4. Ascites has a sharp interface with intra-abdominal organs such as the liver and spleen. Pleural fluid has a less sharp interface because the diaphragm lies between the fluid and abdominal organs.
5. Ascitic fluid spares the bare area of the liver, which lies between the left and right coronary ligaments along the posterior border of the right lobe of the liver. These bare areas are peritoneal reflections that suspend the liver from the diaphragm; peritoneal fluid cannot pass through these ligaments to accumulate in the bare area. However, because bare area is in contact with the diaphragm, pleural fluid can accumulate behind the bare area.

40. When is CT used to evaluate the small bowel?

Conventional barium examinations remain superior to CT for evaluating intraluminal and mucosal disease, but CT is far better for evaluating the intramural component of small bowel as

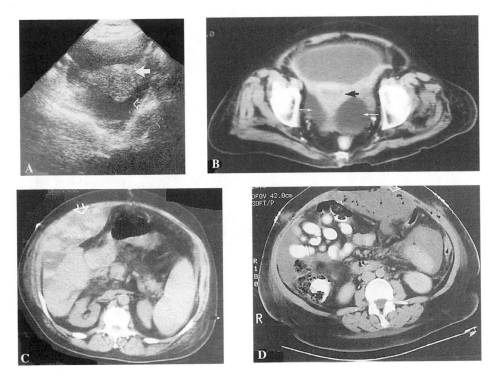

FIGURE 11.   Ascites. *A* and *B*, Ultrasound and CT scan showing simple ascites *(arrows)* in the pelvis adjacent to the uterus *(arrowhead)*. *C*, Intra-abdominal hemorrhage presenting as a complex fluid collection, *D*, Intra-abdominal abscess presenting as a complex fluid collection with multiple air bubbles.

well as the adjacent mesentery, omentum, retroperitoneum, peritoneal cavity, and viscera. Optimal evaluation requires opacification and distention with oral and intravenous contrast. With adequate distention, the thickness of the bowel wall is about 2 mm.

Smooth and concentric thickening of the bowel wall (7–11 mm) is a typical appearance for nonmalignant disease (e.g., Crohn's, ulcerative colitis, Shönlein-Henoch purpura, intramural hemorrhage, bowel edema from portal hypertension, and ischemic, infectious, or radiation enteritis). Extraintestinal findings are an important part of the exam. For example, with Crohn's disease, one should look for associated abscesses, fibrofatty proliferation, fistulas, and inflammation of the mesentery. Thickening of the skin and increased density of the mesenteric and subcutaneous fat can accompany radiation enteritis, which typically involves bowel in the pelvis. Severe cases of ischemic enteritis can demonstrate portal venous gas, intramural hemorrhage, or blood elsewhere in the peritoneal cavity (Fig. 12).

Eccentric and irregular bowel wall thickening > 2 cm is suspicious for carcinoma, especially if confined to a short segment. Lymphoma should be considered if this finding is associated with massive mesenteric or retroperitoneal adenopathy; adenocarcinoma should be considered in the presence of associated liver lesions. Most benign small bowel tumors, such as neurofibromas and leiomyomas, are difficult to distinguish from malignant tumors. Lipomas are the exception. They are easily recognized by their low attenuation (–90 to –120 HU). Small bowel carcinoids are typically located in the right lower quadrant, characteristically contain calcification, and have a surrounding desmoplastic reaction.

Enteroenteric intussusception is easily defined by the invaginated low-density mesenteric fat situated between the higher density of the inner intussusceptum and the outer intussuscipiens. The underlying neoplasm may not be seen.

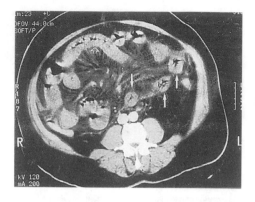

FIGURE 12. Thickening of multiple loops of small bowel due to ischemia in a patient with mesenteric infarction. Thickened loops are best seen in both longitudinal *(open arrow)* and cross-sectional *(arrows)* planes.

CT is also a useful tool in the evaluation of **small bowel obstruction**, especially when the diagnosis is in doubt or the patient has certain medical conditions (e.g., inflammatory bowel disease, known abdominal tumor). It can determine the cause and level of obstruction in up to 95% of cases, particularly those cases with a high-grade obstruction. CT findings can play a role in patient management by helping to separate patients requiring immediate surgery from patients who can be observed. It is also able to diagnose closed-loop obstruction and bowel strangulation.

41. How is CT used to evaluate the large bowel?

Optimal evaluation of the colon requires bowel preparation and luminal distention with rectal contrast or air to evaluate the true wall thickness. Normal wall thickness of a distended colon is < 3 mm. Inflammatory bowel disease, diverticulitis, appendicitis, and staging of colorectal or pelvic cancer are indications for optimal colonic distention. The addition of intravenous contrast facilitates the evaluation of the bowel wall and improves the evaluation of solid organs and vascular structures.

Diverticulitis is well suited for evaluation with CT because it is a pericolic process rather than a disease of the lumen. Acute findings include increased density in the pericolic fat, thickening of the bowel wall, and diverticula. CT is excellent for imaging complications of diverticulitis (e.g., abscess, fistula formation). It can be difficult to differentiate between perforated sigmoid carcinoma and diverticulitis with CT alone. Wall thickening that is excessive (> 3 cm) or eccentric favors sigmoid carcinoma.

Circumferential wall thickening (Fig. 13A) is a nonspecific finding in numerous conditions, including Crohn's disease, ischemic colitis, pseudomembranous colitis, radiation colitis, neutropenic colitis, and inflammatory colitis due to cytomegalovirus or *Campylobacter* infection. Benign intestinal wall thickening of an involved segment can present either as homogeneous enhancing soft-tissue density or, less commonly, as concentric rings of high and low attenuation-termed the "double halo" or target sign (Fig. 13B). Concentric rings result from hyperemic enhancement of the mucosa and serosa (high attenuation) and submucosal edema (low attenuation).

The cause of wall thickening sometimes can be determined by location or associated findings. For example, bowel wall thickening in the region of the splenic flexure suggests ischemic disease from occlusion of the superior mesenteric artery. Thickening of the rectosigmoid colon and pelvic small bowel loops suggest radiation enteritis. Inflammation from a ruptured appendix can produce wall thickening mimicking a primary cecal process, and a severe episode of pancreatitis can cause thickening of the transverse colon if inflammatory changes spread through the transverse mesocolon (Fig. 13C).

Irregular, eccentric, or lobulated wall thickening is suggestive of **adenocarcinoma**. In some cases, an intraluminal polypoid mass can be seen. CT is only 50% accurate in staging the tumor by the Dukes system. However, findings of regional adenopathy, retroperitoneal adenopathy, or liver metastases help to confirm the diagnosis of carcinoma. The large tumor mass usually enhances

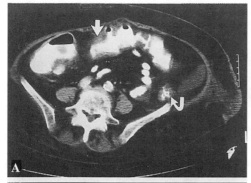

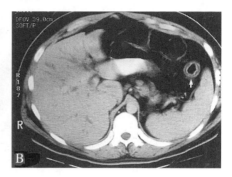

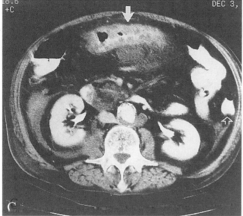

FIGURE 13. Large bowel. *A,* Large bowel wall thickening involves both the transverse *(straight arrow)* and descending colon *(curved arrow)* on an axial image of the lower abdomen in a patient with pseudomembranous colitis. *B,* Thickening of the left colon wall *(arrow)* displays the "double halo" sign in a patient with Crohn's disease. The dilated intrahepatic ducts are due to primary sclerosing cholangitis. *C,* Wall thickening of the transverse colon *(arrows)* in both longitudinal and cross-sectional planes in a patient with severe pancreatitis.

heterogeneously secondary to regions of necrosis, and local tumor extension is usually masslike. In the absence of perforation, the surrounding pericolic fat maintains its homogeneous low attenuation in contrast to inflammatory conditions. CT is useful in evaluating anastamotic recurrence from colorectal carcinoma, which can occur in the serosa beyond the reach of the endoscope.

Lymphoma of the colon presents differently from adenocarcinoma. It thickens the wall to a much greater degree, often up to 4 cm. Lymphoma is rarely isolated to the colon, and additional sites of involvement should be sought.

42. Describe the optimal radiographic work-up of diverticulitis.

CT is generally considered the most efficacious method for the radiologic diagnosis of diverticulitis. Abdominal plain films are typically noncontributory. The barium enema depicts diverticula and may demonstrate fistulous tracts or extrinsic luminal defects related to the adjacent inflammatory process. CT is superior because it directly depicts the severity of the pericolic inflammation and the full degree of intraperitoneal or retroperitoneal extension. It is more sensitive than a barium study in detecting abscesses and fistulas.

The hallmark of acute diverticulitis on CT is increased attenuation in the pericolic fat (so-called **dirty fat**; Fig. 14). With greater degrees of inflammation, a soft tissue phlegmon or a fluid- and occasionally air-containing abscess may be seen. With free perforation, air bubbles may be seen in the peritoneal cavity or retroperitoneum. Diverticula and a thickened bowel wall (> 4 mm) are usually present, but these findings are nonspecific and also may be seen with diverticulosis. The bowel wall thickening occasionally may be difficult to distinguish from that seen in colon cancer; however, an abrupt transition zone is more suggestive of tumor, and pericolic fatty inflammation suggests diverticulitis.

The assessment of the colon by CT is greatly improved with adequate colonic opacification or distention, which can be achieved with oral contrast or, if the patient has no peritoneal signs, with rectal air insufflation or water-soluble contrast per rectum.

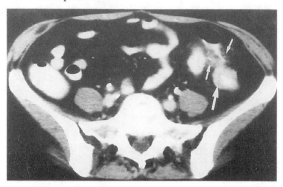

FIGURE 14. Typical CT appearance of diverticulitis, with stranding and increased density of the pericolic fat *(short arrows)* and thickening of the descending colon *(long arrow)*.

43. What are the CT and US findings of acute appendicitis?

US: Findings of acute appendicitis include a distended and noncompressible appendix, appendicolith, adjacent fluid collection, peritoneal fluid, and a focal mixed echogenic mass representing a phlegmon or abscess. The normal anterior-posterior dimension of the appendix is 5–6 mm; larger dimensions are considered abnormal (Fig. 15).

CT: The hallmark finding is a distended (> 6 mm) and thick-walled appendix. An appendicolith may be seen in one-fourth of cases. Local signs of inflammation include increased density or stranding in the adjacent fat tissue, focal thickening of adjacent fascia, focal fluid collections, and adjacent phlegmon or abscess.

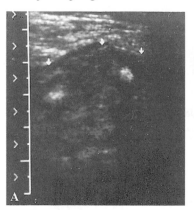
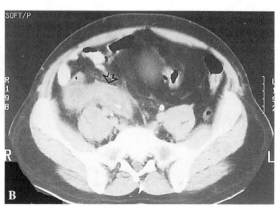

FIGURE 15. Acute appendicitis. *A,* Ultrasound shows a thickened appendix wall *(arrows)* and echogenic appendicolitis. *B,* CT shows a distal fluid-filled appendix and a calcified appendicolith.

44. Which examination is better for diagnosing acute appendicitis?

The 96% sensitivity of CT is superior to that of ultrasound (85–90%). The specificity is comparable at 90%. CT is better at showing a normal appendix and at showing the extent of adjacent inflammatory changes. The disadvantages of CT are its higher cost, use of ionizing radiation, and use of contrast material. US is highly operator-dependent but is usually a good first choice in children, pregnant women, and thin people. CT should be used for all other types of patients and is highly effective in heavier patients.

45. Discuss the role of imaging in the assessment of intra-abdominal abscess.

US: In suspected intra-abdominal abscess, US has the advantage of being performed at the patient's bedside. It is best suited for evaluation of abscesses in the pelvis and right and left upper quadrants, where the bladder, liver, and spleen, respectively, provide acoustic windows for sound transmission. However, assessment of the midabdomen is commonly impossible because of overlying bowel gas. Abscesses have a varied appearance but commonly are irregularly marginated and primarily hypoechoic, with internal areas of increased echogenicity.

CT: The entire abdomen and pelvis should be scanned after the administration of sufficient oral contrast to opacify the bowel, because fluid-filled bowel loops can easily simulate an abscess. Rectal contrast also may be helpful. The CT appearance of an abscess depends on its maturity. Initially, an abscess may appear as a soft-tissue density mass. As it matures and undergoes liquefactive necrosis, the central region develops a near-water attenuation, possibly with internal air bubbles or an air-fluid level (Fig. 16). Granulation tissue forming the wall of the abscess typically enhances with intravenous contrast, providing a higher attenuation rim. Mass effect with displacement of surrounding structures may be seen, and increased density in the adjacent fat is common.

Scintigraphy: Radionuclide imaging may be performed with gallium-67 citrate or indium-111-labeled white blood cells (WBCs). The advantage of scintigraphy is that it provides whole-body images and may detect infection in unsuspected sites. Gallium images, however, may require 48–72 hours for optimal interpretation, and normal colonic excretion of gallium may cause confusion in interpretation. Indium-labeled WBC imaging is more rapid than Ga-67, but uptake is somewhat nonspecific, and the liver and spleen are difficult to evaluate because of normal uptake in these organs.

Recommendations: CT is the first choice for detecting abscess in acutely ill patients. US can be used as the initial exam if the abscess is suspected in the right or left upper quadrant or pelvis and in patients with suspected appendiceal abscess. Radionuclide scintigraphy can be considered the initial screening technique in patients without localizing signs and acute illness.

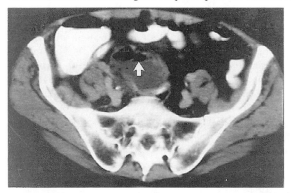

FIGURE 16. Abdominal abscess with air-fluid level *(arrow)* and internal debris.

AIDS-RELATED DISORDERS

46. What characteristic features of AIDS are seen in the biliary system?

Gallbladder and bile duct abnormalities, including gallbladder wall thickening, sludge, cholelithiasis, bile duct dilatation, bile duct wall thickening, pericholecystic fluid, and a sonographic Murphy's sign, can be seen in as many as 20% of AIDS patients during US. The most common abnormality, **gallbladder wall thickening**, is often asymptomatic and not related to intrinsic gallbladder disease but rather to edema from hepatitis or hypoproteinemia. Gallbladder wall thickening associated with a positive Murphy's sign is suggestive of acalculous cholecystitis, either secondary to cytomegalovirus or *Cryptosporidium* infection.

AIDS-related cholangitis is usually secondary to cytomegalovirus or *Cryptosporidium* infection. US is the best noninvasive test for evaluating the extrahepatic ducts, but CT is better for evaluating the intrahepatic ducts. ERCP displays the morphologic appearance of the entire ductal system better than either modality, and the findings of dilated ducts, papillary narrowing, diffuse intrahepatic strictures, extrahepatic strictures, or any combination of these findings seen in AIDS-related cholangitis mimic those of sclerosing cholangitis, papillary stenosis, or both. Patients with papillary stenosis or isolated extrahepatic ductal involvement benefit most from sphinctero-tomy or common bile duct stents.

Biliary ductal dilatation can also be caused by obstruction from enlarged lymph nodes in the porta hepatis from **Kaposi's sarcoma** or **lymphoma**. Non–AIDS-related conditions, such as bil-iary calculi, cholangiocarcinoma, or pancreatic carcinoma, also may be a consideration. A search for these entities should be made in the appropriate clinical setting.

47. Describe the imaging features of AIDS in the liver.

Hepatomegaly is seen in nearly 20% of patients with AIDS. It is usually a nonspecific re-sponse to infection, hepatitis, fatty infiltration, or neoplastic infiltration from lymphoma or Kaposi's sarcoma. Approximately 10% of AIDS patients have diffusely increased liver echogenic-ity on US due to either **fatty infiltration** caused by malnutrition (a fatty liver has decreased atten-uation on CT) or **hepatic granulomatosis** caused by *Mycobacterium avium-intracellulare, M. tuberculosis, Cryptococcus* spp., histoplasmosis, cytomegalovirus, toxoplasmosis, or a drug reac-tion from sulfonamides. Infection in the liver also can take the form of single or multiple liver ab-scesses. On US, such lesions may have increased, decreased, or mixed echogenicity, but with CT they are generally low in attenuation. Microscopic involvement of the liver may show few changes on CT and US, and a core biopsy may be the only method of diagnosis. When infection involves the liver, it is almost always secondary to disseminated disease, and one should search for associ-ated abnormalities such as cholangitis, adenopathy, splenomegaly, and ascites.

Kaposi's sarcoma (KS) is the most common neoplasm in AIDS; however, the diagnosis of liver involvement is rarely made antemortem. The findings are variable because the tumor is mul-tifocal. US shows hepatomegaly and hyperechoic lesions in the parenchyma (often adjacent to the portal veins), whereas on contrast-enhanced CT, lesions are initially low in attenuation but enhance after time (4–7 min) to become either homogeneous with or more attenuated than the surrounding liver parenchyma. KS is more likely to present as adenopathy in the retroperi-toneum, mesentery, or mediastinum than as lesions in the liver.

Lymphoma is more commonly extranodal in patients with AIDS than in the general popula-tion, and the liver and spleen are two of the more common extranodal sites. Both CT and US show one or more visceral lesions. With US, lesions are usually hypoechoic, whereas on CT they are generally low in attenuation. Organ involvement may be the sole manifestation, yet normally lym-phoma is associated with bulky adenopathy of the retroperitoneum, mesentery, or mediastinum.

48. What extrahepatic manifestations of AIDS in the GI tract can be noted by imaging?

HIV-positive patients often demonstrate hepatosplenomegaly, and CT may show multiple, small (< 5-mm) mesenteric or retroperitoneal nodes. Proctitis may be seen as a thickened rectal wall with increased attenuation of perirectal fat. Patients with clinical AIDS often demonstrate an opportunistic infection or tumor on CT or US. Enlargement of lymph nodes suggests AIDS rather than HIV disease, and focal defects in solid organs suggest either abscess or tumor infiltration.

GI tract involvement with KS is common (as is skin involvement), and submucosal nodules may be seen with barium studies anywhere in the GI tract. When the nodules become larger, they can be seen on CT, and nodular mural thickening of the gut suggests KS. Lymphadenopathy is usually absent or mild in KS, unlike lymphoma.

Lymphoma in AIDS is usually of B-cell type and aggressive, with a propensity for extran-odal distribution. Lymphadenopathy is usually bulky, but an isolated node may be involved. Hepatic and splenic lesions have low attenuation on CT and are hypoechoic by US. Bowel wall thickening may be a manifestation of GI tract involvement.

Opportunistic infections are manifold: Candida sp., herpes simplex, or cytomegalovirus (CMV) may cause esophagitis, possibly delineated with barium studies. CMV may involve any area of the gut, but most commonly the cecal region. CT may demonstrate thick-walled bowel with enhancing serosa and mucosa. *M. tuberculosis* may involve the ileocecal region, and wall thickening and low-density lymph nodes in the RLQ are typical on CT.

M. avium-intracellulare usually involves the small bowel. Multiple nodes have central low attenuation due to liquefaction. *Cryptosporidium* infection is characterized by profuse watery small bowel contents on CT. *Pneumocystis carinii* abscesses are seen as small multifocal areas of low attenuation in the liver, spleen, pancreas, kidneys, or lymph nodes. Calcifications are common early as well as late in abscess formation.

BIBLIOGRAPHY

1. Balthazar EJ: CT of the gastrointestinal tract: Principles and interpretation. AJR 156:23–32, 1991.
2. Balthazar EJ, Freeny PC, vanSonnenberg E: Imaging and intervention in acute pancreatitis. Radiology 193:297–306, 1994.
3. Dolmatch BL, Lang FC, Federle MP, et al: AIDS-related cholangitis: Radiographic findings in nine patients. Radiology 14:143–147, 1987.
4. Federle MP (ed): Radiology of the immunocompromised host. Radiol Clin North Am 27:507–662, 1989.
5. Ferrucci JT: Advances in abdominal MR imaging. Radiographics 18:1569–1586, 1998.
6. Freeny PC: Radiologic diagnosis and staging of pancreatic ductal adenocarcinoma. Radiol Clin North Am 27:121–128, 1989.
7. Foshager MC, Ferral H, Finlay DE, et al: Color Doppler sonography of transjugular intrahepatic portosystemic shunts (TIPS). AJR 163:105–111, 1994.
8. Gore RM, Levine MS, Laufer I (eds): Textbook of Gastrointestinal Radiology. Philadelphia, W.B. Saunders, 1994.
9. Lee JKT, Sagel SS, Stanley RJ, et al (eds): Computed Body Tomography with MRI, 3rd ed. Philadelphia, Lippincott-Raven, 1998.
10. Lee MJ, et al: Differential diagnosis of hyperintense liver lesions on T1-weighted MR images. AJR 159:1017–1020, 1992.
11. Maglinte DDT, Balthazar EJ, Kelvin FM, et al: The role of radiology in the diagnosis of small-Bowel obstruction. AJR 168: 1171–1180, 1997.
12. Moss AA, Gamsu G, Genant HK: Computed Tomography of the Body with Magnetic Resonance Imaging, 2nd ed. Philadelphia, W.B. Saunders, 1992.
13. Putnam CE, Ravin CE: Textbook of Diagnostic Imaging, 2nd ed. Philadelphia, W.B. Saunders, 1994.
14. Redvanly RD, Silverstein JE: Intra-abdominal manifestations of AIDS. Radiol Clin North Am 35:1083 1125, 1997.
15. Ros PR (ed): Hepatic Imaging. Radiol Clin North Am 36: 237–375, 1998.
16. Ros PR, Bidgood WD: Abdominal Magnetic Resonance Imaging. St. Louis, Mosby, 1993.
17. Schneiderman DJ: Hepatobiliary abnormalities of AIDS. Gastroenterol Clin North Am 17:615–630, 1988.
18. Smith FJ, et al: Abdominal abnormalities in AIDS: Detection at US in a large population. Radiology 192:691– 695, 1994.
19. Teixidor HS, Godwin TA, Ramirez EA: Cryptosporidiosis of the biliary tract in AIDS. Radiology 180:51–56, 1991.

76. NUCLEAR MEDICINE STUDIES

Colonel Mike McBiles, II, M.D.

1. Outline the general advantages of nuclear medicine procedures compared with other imaging modalities.

1. They provide functional information that either is not available by other modalities or is obtained at greater expense or patient risk.

2. High contrast (target-to-background ratio) can be achieved in many instances by nuclear medicine techniques, allowing diagnostic studies despite poor spatial resolution.

3. Relatively noninvasive studies are the rule in nuclear medicine. They require only injection of a radioactive dose or swallowing of a substance, followed by imaging.

2. What are the disadvantages of nuclear medicine procedures compared with other radiographic studies?

1. Spatial resolution, usually on the order of 1–2 cm, is inferior to that of other imaging modalities.

2. Imaging times can be long, sometimes up to 1 hour or more.

3. Radiation risk is obviously greater than with magnetic resonance (MR) or ultrasound (US). However, the radiation risk from most nuclear medicine studies is equal to or less than that of an average computed tomographic (CT) study. Gallium-67 and indium-111 white blood cell studies are the exceptions; they involve an average of 2–4 times more radiation exposure than other nuclear medicine studies. In some studies, such as gastric emptying and esophageal transit studies, radiation risk is insignificant compared with traditional imaging methods, such as fluoroscopy.

4. Availability may be limited. Specialized procedures require radiopharmaceuticals or interpretive expertise not available in all centers.

3. What nuclear medicine tests are most helpful in GI medicine?

Nuclear medicine procedures have been used in the evaluation of practically every GI problem. However, improvements in and widespread use of endoscopy, manometry, pH monitoring, and traditional imaging techniques (CT, MRI, US) have limited their application to specific clinical problems.

Uses of Nuclear Medicine Procedures in GI Diseases

TEST/STUDY	USEFUL IN DIAGNOSIS/EVALUATION
Cholescintigraphy (hepatobiliary imaging)	Acute cholecystitis
	Gallbladder dyskinesis
	Common duct obstruction
	Biliary atresia
	Sphincter of Oddi dysfunction
	Mass lesions
	Biliary leak
	Choleangiointestinal anastomosis patency
	Gastroenterostomy, afferent loop patency
Gastric emptying	Quantification of gastric motility
Esophageal motility/transit	Quantificaiton of esophageal transit
	Evaluation/detection of reflux
	Aspiration detection
Liver/spleen scan	Hepatic mass lesions
	Accessory spleen/splenosis

Table continued on following page

Uses of Nuclear Medicine Procedures in GI Diseases

TEST/STUDY	USEFUL IN DIAGNOSIS/EVALUATION
Heat-damaged RBC scan	Accessory spleen/splenosis
Gallium scanning	Staging of many abdominal malignancies
	Abdominal abscess
^{131}I-MIBG, ^{111}In-pentetreotide (Octreo-scan), ^{99m}Tc-depreotide (Neotect)	Neural crest tumor staging/recurrence
[111]In-satumomab pentetide (Oncoscint)	Colorectal/ovarian cancer staging/recurrence
[99m]Tc-arcitumomab (CEA-scan)	Colorectal cancer staging/recurrence
In WBC scanning	Evaluation of abdominal infection/abscess
^{99m}Tc-HMPAO WBC scanning	Evaluation of sites of active inflammatory bowel disease
^{99m}Tc-RBC scanning	GI bleeding localization
	Hepatic hemangiomas
Pertechnetate scanning	Meckel diverticulum
	Retained gastric antrum
Sulfur-colloid injections	GI bleeding localization
Peritoneovenous shunt study	Peritoneovenous shunt patency
Hepatic arterial perfusion	Territory perfused by hepatic intraarterial catheters
Shilling test	Vitamin B12 malabsorption

RBC = red blood cell, MIBG = m-iodobenzylguanidine, Tc = technetium, In = indium, HM-PAO = hexamethyl-propyleneamineoxime, WBC = white blood cell.

4. How is cholescintigraphy (hepatobiliary imaging) performed? What is a normal study?

The conduct of the basic cholescintigraphic study is the same for nearly all of its clinical indications (see question 3). The patient is injected with a technetium-99m–labeled imidodiacetic acid (IDA) derivative. Currently, commonly used compounds are DISIDA, mebrofenin, and HIDA (hepato-IDA; the term used among clinicians for all of these tests). Despite their excretion by the same mechanism as bilirubin, current compounds can provide diagnostic studies at high bilirubin levels (> 20 mg/dl).

After injection, sequential images, usually 1 minute in duration, are obtained for 60 minutes or longer. Normally, the liver rapidly clears the IDA compound. On images displayed at normal intensity, blood pool activity in the heart is faint or not discernible by 5 minutes after injection. Persistent blood pool activity and poor liver uptake are indications of hepatocellular dysfunction. Right and left hepatic ducts often are seen by 10 minutes and the common bile duct and small bowel by 20 minutes. The gallbladder usually is seen at the same time but normally can be visualized for up to 1 hour, provided the patient has not eaten within 4 hours. By 1 hour, almost all activity is in the bile ducts, gallbladder, and bowel; the liver is seen faintly or not at all.

In all of the studies listed in question 3, failure to see an expected structure at 1 hour (e.g., gallbladder in acute cholecystitis, small bowel in biliary atresia) requires delayed imaging for up to 4 hours. In some cases, various manipulations, such as sincalide or morphine infusions, are performed after the initial 60-minute images and imaging is continued for another 30–60 minutes.

5. How should patients with acute cholecystitis be prepared? What manipulations are used to shorten the study or increase its reliability?

Traditionally, acute cholecystitis is diagnosed on functional cholescintigraphy by noting a lack of filling of the gallbladder (usually due to a cystic duct stone) on the initial 60-minute study and on 4-hour images. Manipulations and preparations are designed to ensure that lack of gallbladder visualization is a true-positive finding or to shorten this long, sometimes tedious study. Because food is a potent and long-lasting stimulus for endogenous cholecystokinin (CCK) release and subsequent gallbladder contraction, the patient should not eat for 4 hours before the study; otherwise a false-positive study may result. Prolonged fasting causes viscous bile formation in the normal gallbladder, which may impair its filling by the radiopharmaceutical and cause a false-positive study. Most clinics give the short-acting CCK analog sincalide, 0.01–0.04 μg/kg intravenously over 3 minutes, one-half hour before cholescintigraphy, if the patient has fasted > 24 hours, receives hyperalimentation, or is severely ill.

Despite these manipulations, the gallbladder may not fill during the 60-minute cholescintigraphic study. Rather than reimage at 4 hours, morphine, 0.01 mg/kg intravenously, may be given if the gallbladder is not seen but the small bowel is seen at 60 minutes. After morphine administration, imaging is continued for 30 additional minutes. Because morphine causes sphincter of Oddi contraction, which results in increased biliary tree pressure, this manipulation overcomes functional obstruction of the cystic duct. If the gallbladder still is not seen, delayed imaging is not necessary and acute cholecystitis is diagnosed (Fig. 1).

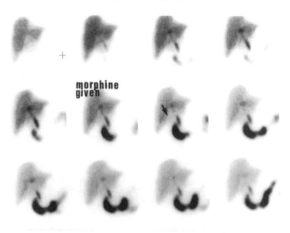

FIGURE 1.   Acute cholecystitis. Hepatobiliary study with 99mTc-mebrofenin, acquired every 5 minutes after injection, shows rapid clearance and uptake by the liver, with rapid excretion into the common bile duct and small bowel. Morphine, 1 mg IV given at the 30-minute image, failed to fill the gallbladder in an additional 30 minutes of imaging. Alternatively, a 4-hour delayed image may be obtained instead of injecting morphine, but this step prolongs the study unnecessarily.

6. If acute cholecystitis is a possibility, when should hepatobiliary scintigraphy be used?

Hepatobiliary scintigraphy is the most accurate imaging method to diagnose acute cholecystitis, with a sensitivity and specificity of 95%. However, it should not be used in every instance when acute cholecystitis is suspected. If, for example, the pretest clinical probability of acute cholecystitis is low (< 10%), a positive study in a screening population is likely to be false. Likewise, if the pretest probability is high (> 90%), a negative study is likely to be false. The same admonitions apply to CT and US, which are even less sensitive and specific.

In the absence of obvious clinical acute cholecystitis, both US and CT are frequently the initial studies of choice, because not only the gallbladder but also adjacent structures causing the symptoms can be easily evaluated. CT is notoriously insensitive for acute cholecystitis, although the presence of inflammatory changes around the gallbladder should strongly raise this possibility. Although US is frequently the initial study of choice, only in the presence of all of the classic signs of cholecystitis (gallbladder wall thickening, gallstones, common duct dilation, and sonographic Murphy sign) does the sensitivity of US approach cholescintigraphy. Similarly, if only a few of these US signs are present, specificity suffers.

7. How is cholescintigraphy used to diagnose and manage biliary leak?

Cholescintigraphy is highly sensitive and specific for detecting biliary leak (Fig. 2). Because non-bile fluid collections are common after surgery, anatomic studies have a poor specificity.

Because cholescintigraphy has poor spatial resolution, the exact site of the leak may not be documented; endoscopic retrograde cholangiopancreatography (ERCP) or percutaneous transhepatic cholangiography (PTC) may be necessary for anatomic definition. Cholescintigraphy also can be used noninvasively to document resolution of a bile leak.

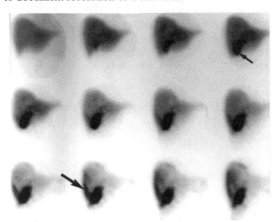

FIGURE 2. Bile leak. After percutaneous liver biopsy, the patient developed severe right upper quadrant pain. US was not helpful. Sequential 5-minute images after ^{99m}Tc-mebrofenin injection show leakage of a thin rim of bile along the inferior and lateral liver edge *(large arrow)*. Note gallbladder filling early in the study *(small arrow)* and the lack of small bowel activity, implying preferential flow of bile to the gallbladder and site of leakage.

8. How is cholescintigraphy used in diagnosing common bile duct obstruction?

Ductal dilatation seen on US may be a nonspecific finding in patients with previous biliary surgery, and acute obstruction (< 24–48 hours old) may not show ductal dilatation. Cholescintigraphy shows a lack of gallbladder and small bowel visualization and often a lack of biliary tree visualization on the 4-hour delayed images in common duct obstruction. Sensitivity and specificity are high (Fig. 3). Cholescintigraphy is reliable even at high bilirubin levels. It can be used to distinguish obstructive from nonobstructive jaundice.

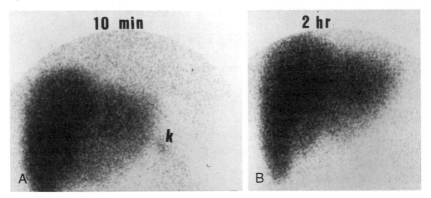

FIGURE 3. Common bile duct obstruction. After injection of the hepatobiliary agent, there is no visible activity in the intrahepatic ducts or small bowel on 10-minute *(A)* or 2-hour *(B)* images. US did not show dilated ducts, and a common duct stone was not seen, a common finding in acute common duct obstruction. Activity to left of liver *(k)* is the radiopharmaceutical agent excreted in the urine in an alternate pathway to biliary excretion.

9. What is cholescintigraphy's role in diagnosing biliary atresia?

By the same rationale outlined in question 8, cholescintigraphy is sensitive and highly specific for the diagnosis of biliary atresia if the patient is properly prepared. The major differential diagnostic possibility in neonates is severe neonatal hepatitis. US findings are insensitive. US may show ductal dilatation or gallbladder absence in biliary atresia, but dilatation is usually absent, and the gallbladder is usually present. The main scintigraphic problem is a false-positive study caused by a lack of biliary secretion in severe hepatitis. Premedication of the neonate with oral phenobarbital, 5 mg/kg/day for 5 days, stimulates bile flow and eliminates this problem. The importance of therapeutic serum levels of phenobarbital cannot be overemphasized. If radioactivity in the small bowel is seen on delayed images, biliary atresia is ruled out (Fig. 4).

10. How is sphincter of Oddi dysfunction assessed by cholescintigraphy?

A significant number of patients continue to have pain after cholescintigraphy, and sphincter of Oddi dysfunction may be the cause. Although manometry during ERCP is diagnostic, this study is invasive and not without complications. An empiric scintigraphic scoring system looking at quantitative parameters of bile movement and liver function has been developed. High correlation with biliary tree manometric findings has been demonstrated.

11. When can cholescintigraphy help to evaluate obstruction in gastroenterostomies?

Afferent loops are difficult to evaluate with barium studies because the afferent loop must be filled retrograde with barium. By cholescintigraphy, afferent loop obstruction can be reliably excluded if activity is seen in the afferent and efferent loops 1 hour after radiopharmaceutical injection. Persistent accumulation in the afferent loop with little or no efferent loop activity at 2 hours establishes the diagnosis of afferent loop obstruction.

12. What is gallbladder dyskinesia? How does cholescintigraphy evaluate the emptying of the gallbladder?

A significant number of patients with normal imaging and clinical work-ups have pain referable to the gallbladder, as evidenced by relief of symptoms after cholecystectomy. The poorly understood and heterogeneous entity of gallbladder dyskinesia has been proposed as the cause of this pain. It is thought that poorly coordinated contractions between the gallbladder and cystic duct can cause pain. Gallbladder dyskinesia may be manifested by an abnormally low ejection of bile under the stimulus of cholecystokinin (sincalide).

After the gallbladder is filled during traditional cholescintigraphy, gallbladder contraction is stimulated by an infusion of sincalide, 0.01 mg/kg. The amount of gallbladder emptying over 30 minutes reflects the gallbladder ejection fraction (GBEF; normal > 35–40%). This protocol has demonstrated correlation of both normal and abnormal GBEF with surgical and medical follow-up.

13. What is a nuclear medicine gastric emptying study?

Both liquid and solid gastric emptying studies can be performed with nuclear medicine. Liquid studies usually are performed on infants. After the infant receives a mixture of ^{99m}Tc-sulfur colloid with milk or formula at normal feeding time, imaging is done every 15 minutes for 60 minutes, and an emptying half-time is calculated. In adults, a solid-phase emptying study usually is performed after an overnight fast by mixing ^{99m}Tc-sulfur colloid-labeled scrambled eggs with a standard meal, performing anterior and posterior imaging every 15 minutes for 90 minutes, and calculating the percentage of emptying. The meal has not been standardized, and normal values depend on the meal composition. Using a 300-calorie meal of scrambled eggs, bread, and butter, solid gastric emptying is 63% at 1 hour (standard deviation of 11%).

14. In what clinical situations is a nuclear medicine gastric emptying study useful?

Symptoms related to problems of abnormal gastric motility may be nonspecific, and barium studies are neither quantifiable nor physiologic. Although gastric emptying studies are semiqualitative, show less than optimal reproducibility, and are not standardized, a rough estimate of emptying

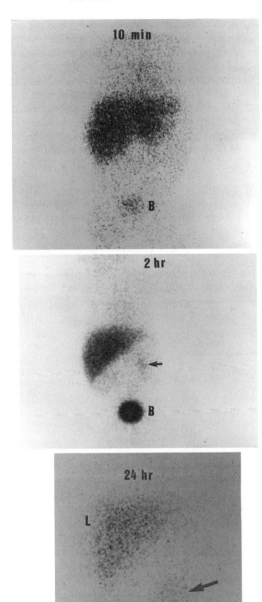

FIGURE 4. Neonatal hepatitis with suspected biliary atresia. This difficult diagnosis can be made with a hepatobiliary agent. In this case, ^{99m}Tc-mebrofenin was injected after a 5-day preparation with phenobarbital. Note the continued blood pool activity in the heart on the 2-hour image and excretion into the baldder *(B)*, suggesting hepatocellular dysfunction with abnormal excretion of the hepatobiliary agent into the alternate urinary pathway. At 4 hours there is a subtle focus *(arrow)* in the abdomen that may be in the bowel or radiopharmaceutical agent excreted by the alternate urinary pathway. In the 24-hour image with the bladder catheterized, ill-defined activity in the left lower quadrant *(arrow)*, inferolateral to the liver *(L)*, confirms excretion of the radiopharmaceutical agent into the bowel and rules out biliary atresia.

in clinically important groups (such as diabetics and patients with partial gastrectomy) can help
to explain nonspecific symptoms or suggest another etiology if the results are clearly normal or
abnormal (Fig. 5).

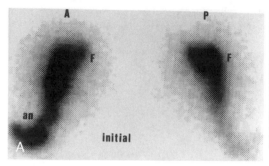

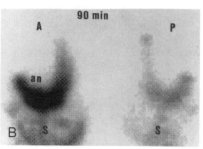

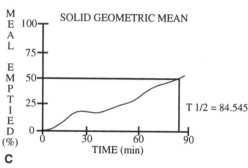

FIGURE 5. Normal gastric emptying study. *A,* Initial anterior (A) and posterior (P) images after ingestion of ^{99m}Tc-sulfur colloid-labeled scrambled eggs in beef stew show activity in the fundus (F) on posterior imagges and extending to the antrum *(an). B,* At 90 minutes, little radiopharmaceutical agent is left in the fundus, but a significant amount is seen in the antrum (an), and noticeable activity is distributed throughout the smallbowel (S). *C,* At 84.5 minutes, 50% of the meal had emptied (normal = 35–60% with this type of meal).

15. What nuclear medicine esophageal studies are available? How are they used?

Esophageal motility study. This study is performed by rapid sequential imaging of the
esophagus during swallowing of ^{99m}Tc-colloid in water. Although it provides a precise and reproducible quantitation of esophageal function, barium studies usually provide adequate definition
of the anatomic or functional problem. Esophageal motility studies are useful as an easily performed study in the noninvasive follow-up of therapy for dysmotility and achalasia.

Esophageal reflux study. This study is performed by serial imaging of the esophagus after
the patient drinks acidified orange juice containing ^{99m}Tc-colloid and during serial inflation of an
abdominal binder. Although less sensitive than 24-hour pH monitoring, the test is more sensitive
than barium studies and can be used for screening study or evaluation of response to therapy.

Pulmonary aspiration studies. These studies are performed by imaging the chest after oral
administration of ^{99m}Tc-colloid in water. Activity in the lungs is diagnostic of aspiration.
Although sensitivity is low, it is probably higher than that of radiographic contrast studies. The
test has the advantage of easy serial imaging to detect intermittent aspiration.

16. What is the role for nuclear medicine studies in evaluating hepatic mass lesions?

The traditional liver/spleen scan using an intravenous injection of the Kupffer cell-seeking
^{99m}Tc-sulfur has largely been replaced by US and dynamic multiphase CT and MRI. Because of
superior resolution with CT and MRI, lesion blood flow characteristics are evident, and adjacent
structures can be evaluated.

Virtually all neoplasms, including metastasis, focal inflammatory and infectious diseases of
the liver, and vascular malformations, manifest as decreased radionuclide activity ("cold") on
both liver-spleen and hepatobiliary imaging. However, **focal nodular hyperplasia** (FNH) often
has a nonspecific appearance on CT, MRI, and US but appears warm (isointense with the rest of

the liver) or hot on liver/spleen imaging because of the predominance of Kupffer cells. Liver-spleen scanning, therefore, has a limited role in evaluating this rare lesion. **Hepatic adenomas** usually are composed mostly of hepatocytes and appear warm or hot on hepatobiliary imaging and cold on liver/spleen imaging. This unique combination is not always seen, but its presence is diagnostic. Because focal fatty replacement does not affect Kupffer cell distribution or the kinetics of hepatobiliary scintigraphy, a normal liver-spleen strongly suggests this diagnosis (Fig 6).

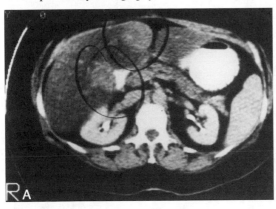 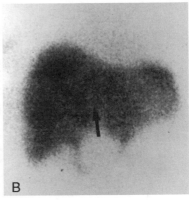

FIGURE 6. Evaluation of mass lesions. *A*, Contrast-enhanced CT scan of the liver shows diffuse fatty infiltration with two areas of relatively normal-appearing liver *(circles)* in this patient with colon cancer treated with 5-fluorouracil. Regenerating liver nodules and metastatic disease are the diagnostic possibilities. *B*, Given the large size of these lesions and their anterior location, metastatic lesions would be readily seen as a photopenic defect on hepatobiliary imaging *(arrows)*. Because no defects are seen, the diagnosis is regenerating nodules.

Most **hepatomas** avidly accumulate gallium-67; in the absence of a known gallium-67–avid primary tumor elsewhere, a gallium-avid liver lesion is highly suspicious for hepatoma. Occasionally, certain kinds of metastatic lesions (see question 25) may be occult, or CT, MRI, or US may not distinguish benign or malignant nature. Radionuclide receptor or antibody imaging may be helpful.

With dynamic multiphase imaging, CT and MRI are diagnostic for **hepatic hemangioma**. Delayed imaging with single-photon emission computed tomography (SPECT), which produces three-dimensional scintigraphic images similar to CT, with ^{99m}Tc-labeled red blood cells provides comparable sensitivity and specificity in the diagnosis of hemangiomas > 2 cm (Fig. 7), frequently at lower cost and without contrast injection. The positive predictive value of SPECT for hemangiomata < 1 cm is also high because of the high target-to-background ratio in such lesions, a result of their uniquely high proportion of blood to other tissue, at 2-hour delayed SPECT imaging. In lesions near large vessels, however, it may be difficult to differentiate the vessel from the hemangioma, and other imaging modalities should be used. The unusual clot-filled or fibrotic lesions are not detected with high sensitivity

17. Describe the vitamin B12 absorption (Schilling) test and its use.

The Schilling test measures the ability of the body to absorb and excrete vitamin B12. Because there are many causes of vitamin B12 malabsorption, the work-up usually is performed in stages. Each stage is designed to evaluate in sequence the most clinically prevalent causes of vitamin B12 deficiency. Although some clinicians treat all B12-deficient patients without searching for a cause, the etiology can be important because of associated or unsuspected problems that should be recognized.

It is not necessary, or in fact desirable, for the patient with severe vitamin B12 deficiency to abstain from vitamin B12 therapy before the Schilling test. In stage 1 and all subsequent stages, nonradiolabeled vitamin B12, 1 mg intramuscularly, is given to bind B12 receptors 2 hours after the patient takes a pill containing radioactive-cobalt-labeled vitamin B12. It is extremely important that

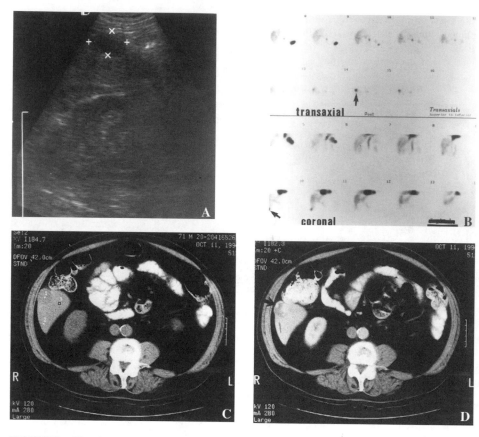

FIGURE 7.   Liver hemangioma. *A,* Ultrasound shows a 3-cm hypoechoic lesion with internal echoes, consistent with hemangioma but a nonpsecific finding. *B,* A ^{99m}Tc-RBC study obtained at 2 hours with SPECT shows an intense focus in the inferior right lobe of the liver on transaxial and coronal images *(arrows). C,* CT scan without contrast shows a lesion in this same area *(box 1). D,* CT with contrast shows centripetal, nodular filling of this lesion *(arrow),* confirming the diagnosis of hemangioma made on the ^{99m}Tc-RBC study.

the patient not eat for 3 hours before and after taking the pill (to prevent the radiolabeled B12 from being bound by food) and that a 24- to 48-hour urine sample be accurately collected. Urinary creatinine and volume should be determined. Less-than-normal 24-hour urinary creatinine levels suggest inadequate collection, which artifactually decreases the amount of vitamin B12 excreted in the urine. The collected urine is analyzed for radioactive cobalt. Normally, > 10% of the radioactive oral dose is excreted by 24 hours. If the excretion of vitamin B12 at 24 hours is normal, normal GI absorption is implied.

If the results of stage 1 are abnormal, the patient undergoes stage 2, which is a repeat of stage 1 except that oral intrinsic factor is given together with the radioactive B12 pill. Stage 3 has several variations that depend on the clinical suspicion of the etiology of B12 malabsorption (Fig. 8). A normal stage-2 excretion of vitamin B12 after an abnormal stage-1 excretion implies the diagnosis of pernicious anemia.

18. How can nuclear medicine procedures assist in detecting ectopic gastric tissue?

As a source of pediatric GI bleeding, Meckel diverticulum almost always contains gastric tissue. Because ^{99m}Tc-pertechnetate is concentrated and extracted by gastric tissue, it is an ideal agent to localize sources of GI bleeding, which can be difficult to detect with traditional contrast studies.

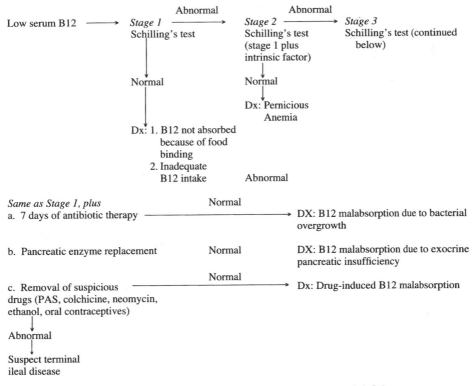

FIGURE 8. Algorithm for determining the cause of vitamin B12 deficiency.

The study is performed by injecting pertechnetate intravenously and imaging the abdomen for 45 minutes. Typically, ectopic gastric mucosa appears at the same time as stomach tissue and does not move during imaging. The test's sensitivity is 85% for detection of bleeding Meckel diverticula. Manipulations to increase the sensitivity of the study include pretreatment with cimetidine (to block pertechnetate excretion into the bowel lumen) and/or glucagon (to inhibit bowel motility so that ^{99m}Tc-pertechnetate is not washed away). A similar procedure can be performed to identify a retained gastric antrum after surgery for peptic ulcer disease and has a sensitivity of 73% and specificity of 100%.

19. Can accessory splenic tissue or splenosis be detected via nuclear medicine procedures?

After splenectomy as treatment of idiopathic thrombocytopenia, treatment failure is associated with unremoved accessory spleen. Unrecognized splenosis also may be a cause of unexplained abdominal pain. The most sensitive imaging procedure for localization of small foci of splenic tissue is the heat-damaged ^{99m}Tc-RBC scan, because damaged red blood cells localize in splenic tissue intensely and specifically. This is the procedure of choice, especially if SPECT is used. However, the RBC-damaging process requires exquisite laboratory technique and may not be readily available in many centers. It is therefore reasonable to perform a liver/spleen scan as an initial study and, if it is positive for splenic tissue, to institute appropriate therapy (Fig. 9). If it is negative, a heat-damaged RBC study should be performed.

20. What nuclear medicine studies help in the management of inflammatory bowel disease and abdominal abscesses?

Gallium-67 is normally excreted into the bowel, and a small amount of ^{99m}Tc-HMPAO dissociates from the WBCs and is excreted into the bowel; therefore, these agents are less useful for

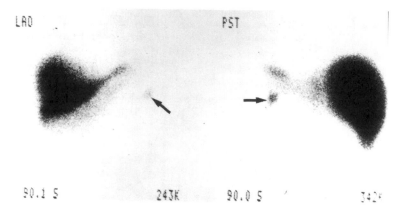

FIGURE 9.   Accessory spleen in a patient after splenectomy for idiopathic thrombocytopenic purpura. The high contrast achieved with ^{99m}Tc-suflur colloid can detect a small remnant *(arrow)* and direct surgical exploration. Left anterior oblique (LAO) and posterior (PST) images of the abdomen are shown. If ^{99m}Tc-sulfur colloid studies are negative, even higher contrast, specificity, and target-to-background ratios can be obtained by using scanning with heat-damaged RBCs, which preferentially accumulate in splenic tissue and demonstrate an almost identical scintigraphic pattern, as does ^{99m}Tc-sulfur colloid.

imaging abdominal inflammation. With **gallium-67**, it may be necessary to image for up to 1 week to allow bowel activity to move so that suspicious abdominal foci can be adequately characterized. This disadvantage is offset slightly by the low cost of gallium-67, despite its higher dosimetry (equal to the radiation of 2–4 abdominal CT scans). ^{99m}Tc-HMPAO and ^{111}In-labeled WBC studies are expensive and require special labeling expertise.

   ^{111}**In-labeled WBCs**, which normally accumulate only in the liver, spleen, and bone marrow, are the agent of choice in localizing abdominal infection in cases in which CT, MRI, and US are nondiagnostic. The normal WBC uptake in the liver and spleen is a minor drawback and can be overcome by dual-isotope imaging with ^{99m}Tc-colloid (liver/spleen scanning), because intra- and perisplenic or liver abscess is cold on liver/spleen scanning and hot on the ^{111}In-WBC study. The necessity for delayed 24-hour imaging to maximize sensitivity is also a drawback.

   One-hour post-injection ^{99m}**Tc-HMPAO WBC imaging** also correlates well with the degree of inflammation and localization of inflammatory bowel disease seen on other imaging modalities; thus it can be used for noninvasive follow-up. This agent is preferable to ^{111}In-WBC studies because of higher sensitivity and lower radiation dosimetry.

21. Which nuclear medicine procedures are useful in localizing lower GI bleeding?

   The difficulty of localizing acute lower GI bleeding is well recognized. The precise nature of the bleeding lesion is frequently immaterial to patient management, because the final common therapeutic pathway often involves partial bowel resection. Even acute and rapid bleeding is intermittent and frequently not detected on angiography, or the culprit lesion is obscured by luminal blood during endoscopy. Small bowel bleeding distal to areas reachable by upper endoscopy is notoriously difficult to localize.

   Two nuclear procedures have been used to localize GI bleeding sources: short-term imaging after ^{99m}Tc-colloid injection, and extended imaging after ^{99m}Tc-tagged RBC injection. Despite the theoretical advantage of ^{99m}Tc-colloids in being able to detect smaller bleeds, this technique shares the limitation of angiography: short intravascular residence time (few minutes) of the contrast material. ^{99m}Tc-RBC imaging has assumed dominance because the long intravascular residence time (limited by radioactive decay) allows detection of intraluminal radioactive blood accumulation if extended imaging is used.

The study is begun by performing an in vitro tag of RBCs with ^{99m}Tc-pertechnetate. The radiolabeled RBCs are injected, and multiple sequential computer images are obtained for 90 minutes or longer. Computer acquisition is important because sensitivity for localization is higher when the study is displayed in a cine-loop.

22. Are nuclear medicine procedures clinically useful in localizing GI bleeding, or are simpler techniques adequate?

^{99m}Tc-RBC studies are more sensitive, in general, than angiography in detecting intermittent bleeding (Fig. 10). Early claims that the nuclear medicine GI bleeding study should be used as a screening study prior to angiography may not be defensible. However, with rigorous technique and attention to rigid diagnostic criteria for bleeding localization, the bleeding study is helpful in many difficult cases. Knowledge of the advantages and disadvantages of each technique allows the clinician to select the most appropriate study for the specific situation.

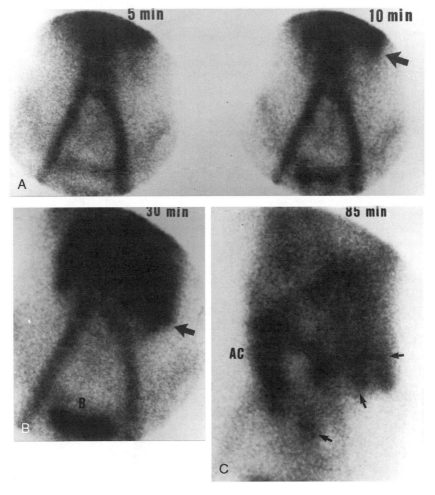

FIGURE 10. GI bleeding from the small bowel. After negative upper endoscopy and continued bleeding, a ^{99m}Tc-labeled RBC scan shows a focus of bleeding near the spleen *(large arrows)*. Continued imaging at 85 minutes demonstrates serpiginous transit time through the small bowel *(small arrows)* toward the right lower quadrant, confirming a proximal small bowel origin. At surgery, a bleeding distal duodenal ulcer was found (B, bladder; AC, ascending colon).

23. Is nuclear medicine helpful in placement of arterial perfusion catheters?

Occasional unrecognized systemic shunting, catheter dislodgment, and unintended perfusion of an area not suitable for highly toxic chemotherapeutic drugs hamper placement of hepatic arterial perfusion catheters. Arterial catheter injection of ^{99m}Tc-macroaggregated albumin (MAA) results in microembolization at the arteriolar level and provides an imaging map of the true area of perfusion of the catheter, especially if SPECT is used. This imaging cannot be done reliably with radiographic contrast because of its rapid dilution at the arteriolar level.

24. How can nuclear medicine assess peritoneovenous shunt patency?

Increasing abdominal girth in the presence of a peritoneovenous shunt can be a diagnostic challenge because it may be due to shunt obstruction, increased ascites production, or loculation. Radiographic studies are not possible if the shunt is radioopaque; in any event, such studies require shunt cannulation. Because a one-way valve is located at the abdominal origin of the shunt, it is difficult to evaluate the shunt in a retrograde manner. Patency can be readily evaluated by injecting ^{99m}Tc-MAA intraperitoneally and imaging the chest for 30 minutes. The shunt tube may not be visualized, but trapping of the ^{99m}Tc-MAA in lung arterioles is de facto evidence of shunt patency.

25. Can abdominal malignancies be evaluated with nuclear medicine studies?

Traditionally, **gallium-67**, a nonspecific tumor and infection marker, has been used to evaluate suspicious malignancy. It is not useful in staging of tumors but rather in evaluating recurrence of hepatomas and Hodgkin's and non-Hodgkin's lymphomas. Anatomic studies have difficulty separating necrosis and scar from recurrent tumor. Its utility is hampered by variable tumor avidity and by interference from GI activity caused by its excretion into the large bowel. The problem of separating GI activity from target lesion activity can be partially overcome by SPECT and serial imaging for up to 1 week to allow elimination of gallium-67 excreted into the bowel.

Recent FDA approval of ^{111}In-pentetreotide, ^{99m}Tc-depreotide and ^{131}I-MIBG for imaging of neural crest tumors has opened new possibilities in evaluating these difficult-to-image tumors. ^{131}**I-MIBG**, a dopamine analog, is a particularly useful complement to CT and MRI in staging and detecting carcinoid tumors, neuroblastoma, paragangliomas, and pheochromocytomas. ^{111}**In-octreotide** and possibly ^{99m}**Tc-depreotide**, both of which are somatostatin analogs and therefore accumulate in tissues with somatostatin receptors, are also highly sensitive and specific for a variety of neural chest tumors that express somatostatin receptors (Fig. 11). They frequently detect

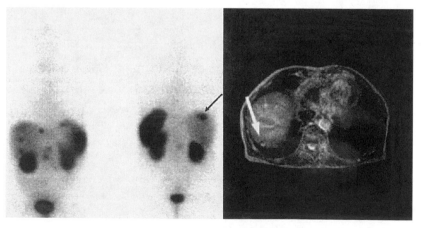

FIGURE 11.   Left image shows an ^{111}In-pentetreotide scan in a patient with multiple metastases of gastrinoma to the liver. Two foci consistent with gastrinoma are seen in the pancreas. The black arrow points to one of the metastases in the dome of the liver. Note the normal homogenous distribution of the radiopharmaceutical agent in the spleen, kidneys, and bladder. The right image is a T2-weighted transaxial MR scan at the level of the subtle metastasis in the dome of the liver *(white arrow)* seen in the nuclear medicine study.

occult lesions not seen by other modalities and can lend specificity to questionable GI lesions found on MRI and CT, including gastrinoma, glucagonoma, paraganglioma, pheochromocytoma, carcinoid, and Hodgkin's and non-Hodgkin's lymphoma.

The radiolabeled antibody [111]**In-satumomab** also has been approved recently by the FDA and is extremely useful in evaluating colon and ovarian cancer in patients with an elevated CEA level and an otherwise negative diagnostic evaluation; patients with known recurrent disease presumed to be isolated and amenable to surgical resection; and patients in whom the standard diagnostic work-up provides equivocal information. ^{111}In-satumomab frequently detects occult disease and significantly affects therapy in almost one-fourth of these patients.

26. What are the advantages and drawbacks of radioactive receptor and antibody imaging?

Many tumors express either unique antigens or high concentrations of peptide receptors. The table in question 3 lists only the radiopharmaceuticals approved by the FDA at the time of this printing; promising new agents are under development. Tumors with peptide receptors are ideally suited for radionuclide imaging with radiolabeled peptides or antibodies because of high theoretic target-to-background ratios despite extremely low receptor or antigen concentrations. In clinical trials, these radiopharmaceuticals often have outperformed CT and MRI in both sensitivity and specificity. Nevertheless, sensitivity and specificity frequently are less than optimal (70–80%), although in certain tumor/radiopharmaceutical combinations they may be even higher. These radiopharmaceuticals may be helpful when other imaging and/or biopsy results are inconclusive, when detection of multiple lesions would affect treatment, and when a residual mass after treatment cannot be adequately characterized by CT, MRI, or US.

Several drawbacks have become evident. Radiopharmaceuticals can be expensive, and their preparation requires some expertise. The best results require state-of-the-art equipment, careful attention to imaging protocol details, and interpretive expertise not available at all imaging centers. Nonspecific accumulation of the radiopharmaceutical or its breakdown products in the liver, kidney, and bowel is a common finding and sometimes necessitates complex dual isotope subtraction techniques, multi-day imaging, or bladder catheterization or bowel cleansing. Imaging times may be long, which increases the chance of motion artifacts. Some drugs may interfere with radiopharmaceutical localization. Some monoclonal antibodies derived from mouse hybrid cells may cause unwanted immune response. Careful consultation with the nuclear medicine physician is necessary for selection of the proper test, patient preparation, and statement of the clinical questions needing an answer.

BIBLIOGRAPHY

1. Arndt J, Van der Sluys, Veer A, Blok D, et al: Prospective comparative study of technetuim-99m-WBCs and indium-111-granulocytes for the examination of patients with inflammatory bowel disease. J Nucl Med 34:1052–1057, 1993.
1a. Corman M, Galandiak S, Block G, et al: Immunoscintigraphy with ^{111}In-satumomab pentetide in patients with colorectal adenocarcinoma: Performance and impact on clinical management. Dis Colon Rectum 37:129–137, 1994.
2. Davis L, McCarroll K: Correlative imaging of the liver and hepatobiliary system. Semin Nucl Med 26:208–216, 1994.
3. Drane W: Scintigraphic techniques for hepatic imaging: Update for 2000. Radiol Clin of North Am 36:309–318, 1999.
4. Fischman A, Babich J: Radiolabeled peptides: A new class of imaging agents. In Freeman L (ed): Nuclear Medicine Annual. Philadelphia, Lippincott-Raven, 1997, pp 103–131.
5. Mettler F, Guiberteau M: Essentials of Nuclear Medicine Imaging, 4th ed. Philadelphia, W.B. Saunders, 2000.
6. Pawels S, Leners N, Fiasse R, Jamar F: Localization of gastroenteropancreatic neuroendocrine tumors with 111indium-pentetreotide scintigraphy. Semin Oncol 12(Suppl 13):15–20, 1994.
7. Shapiro M: The role of the radiologist in the management of gastrointestinal bleeding. Gastroenterol Clin North Am 1994;23:123–181, 1994.
8. Sodee D, Velchik M, Noto R, et al: Gastrointestinal system. In Early P, Sodee D (eds): Principles and Practice of Nuclear Medicine. St. Louis, Mosby, 1995, pp 476–579.
9. Sostre S, Kalloo A, Spiegler E, et al: A noninvasive test of sphincter of Oddi dysfunction in postcholecystectomy patients: The scintigraphic score. J Nucl Med 33:1216–1222, 1992.
10. Weissmann H, Gliedman M, Wilk P, et al: Evaluation of the postoperative patient with ^{99m}Tc-IDA cholescintigraphy. Semin Nucl Med 12:27–52, 1982.
11. Yap L, Wycherley, Morphett A, Toouli J: Acalculous biliary pain: Cholecystectomy alleviates symptoms in patients with abnormal cholescintigraphy. Gastroenterology 101:786–793, 1991.

77. ENDOSCOPIC ULTRASOUND

Peter R. McNally, D.O.

1. When was intraluminal gastrointestinal (GI) ultrasound first performed?

Wild and Reid performed the first ultrasound (rectal) in 1956. For the past decade, interest in the use of GI ultrasound has been revitalized. Intraluminal ultrasound permits precise definition of the gut wall layers and examination of adjacent structures of the chest and abdomen. The proximity of the ultrasound transducer and the high scanning frequencies provide incomparable morphologic detail of the gut wall and extraintestinal anatomy.

2. How do ultrasound waves visualize the GI tract?

Ultrasound pulses represent longitudinal waves that are propagated through soft tissues or fluid by motion of molecules within the conducting media. The ultrasound wavelength is the distance between two waves of compression and rarefaction. Ultrasound is defined as frequency > 20,000 cycles/sec (20 Hz); most diagnostic ultrasound uses frequencies ranging from 2–20 million cycles/sec (2–20 MHz). The velocity of sound transmission through soft tissues is a constant 1540 m/sec and is independent of frequency. Transmission of ultrasound within a medium depends on the compressibility and density of the medium, two properties that tend to be inversely proportional. Because ultrasound power is diminished as it traverses tissue, the intensity of the returning echo, when related to the original echo, is expressed in negative terms.

3. How does the frequency of the ultrasound beam influence the depth of beam penetration and image resolution?

For maximal resolution of ultrasound, the transmitted waves should be parallel. If the target of interest is too close or too far from the transducer, divergence of the wavelength causes distortion of the image. Hence, proper positioning of the ultrasound (US) transducer and use of the appropriate frequency are essential to provide maximal resolution.

US FREQUENCIES	PENETRATION	AXIAL RESOLUTION
5 MHz	8 cm	0.8 mm
10 MHz	4 cm	0.4 mm
20 MHz	2 cm	0.2 mm

4. What are the ultrasonographic properties of the common structures of the body?

Water/blood	Echo poor (black)
Collagen	Echo rich (white)
Air	Reflection (reverberation echoes)
Bone	Reflection (reverberation echoes)
Muscle	Echo poor (black)

NORMAL ANATOMY

5. What determines the thickness of the echosonographic layer visualized? What is the normal endosonographic anatomy of the intestinal wall?

The thickness of the intraluminal ultrasound image of the intestinal wall does not equal the total thickness of a histologic section. Kimmey et al. hypothesized that the overall appearance of the ultrasound image is determined by a combination of echoes from two sources: those created at interfaces between tissue layers with different acoustic impedances and those created within the internal structures of the tissue layer. Using 5–12-MHz scanning frequencies, the intestinal wall has five sonographic layers (Fig. 1).

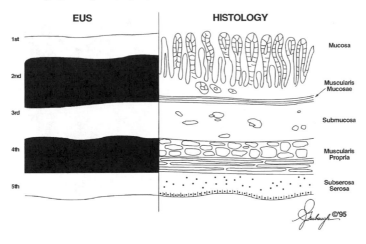

FIGURE 1. Correlation of endoscopic ultrasound image to the histologic composition of the bowel wall.

6. What are the imaging characteristics of normal and malignant lymph nodes on endoscopic ultrasound (EUS)?

The high resolution of EUS imaging allows even normal lymph nodes to be visualized. Normal lymph nodes are characterized by the presence of internal echoes, a bean-like shape, and size < 1 cm. Malignant lymph nodes tend to be hypoechoic, rounded, and > 1 cm; they exhibit distinct margins.

7. How are blood vessels distinguished from lymph nodes on EUS?

Blood vessels generally appear as anechoic, curvilinear structures that often branch. Branching and posterior wall enhancement (hyperechoic) are helpful in distinguishing paraluminal vessels from hypoechoic lymph nodes.

8. Describe the normal EUS anatomy of the retroperitoneum. What are its major landmarks?

The pancreas and retroperitoneum are the most challenging and difficult areas to examine with intraluminal US. Familiarity with the gross and US anatomy is essential. The examination begins with the echoendoscope at the level of the duodenal ampulla. Antimotility agents, such as glucagon, are frequently necessary. The US examination usually is conducted with a 7.5-MHz scanning frequency. The normal paraduodenal anatomy is shown in Figure 2. The normal pancreas has a homogeneous echo pattern, usually slightly more hyperechoic than the liver. There is considerable interobserver variation in measurement of the head of the pancreas, probably due to variations in the angle of view. The remainder of the pancreas is examined from a paragastric position. In the stomach, the water-filled lumen method is used.

9. What are the indications for EUS examination?
Staging of GI tumors

Esophageal carcinoma	Ampullary tumors
Gastric carcinoma	Biliary tract carcinoma
Gastric lymphoma (non-	Colorectal carcinoma
Hodgkin's lymphoma)	Colorectal adenoma
Pancreatic lymphoma	Submucosal tumors
Pancreatic endocrine tumors	

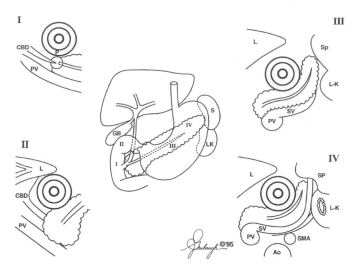

FIGURE 2. Four commonly used positions to examine the pancreas by EUS. *I,* Transverse section at the level of the ampulla. *II,* Sagittal section near the duodenal bulb. *III,* Transverse section of the pancreatic body through the posterior wall of the stomach. *IV,* Transverse section of the body and tail of the pancreas from the proximal stomach. A = ampulla, CBD = common bile duct, L-K = left kidney, PV = portal vein, SV = splenic vein, L = liver, Sp = spleen, SA = superior mesenteric artery, Ao = aorta.

Evaluation of nonneoplastic disease

Reflux esophagitis	Portal hypertension
Achalasia	Chronic pancreatitis
Gastric ulcer	Common bile duct stones
Giant gastric folds	Inflammatory bowel disease

10. How is EUS used in the clinical evaluation of esophageal cancer?

Currently, EUS has no role in the diagnosis of esophageal cancer. Findings from EUS provide morphologic staging but do not supplant the need for histologic diagnosis of malignancy. EUS has not been shown to be helpful in differentiating malignant from inflammatory strictures. It is not sufficiently sensitive to use as a screening test for cancer (i.e., in Barrett's esophagus with dysplasia). Combined EUS with or without fine-needle aspiration (FNA) and computed tomographic (CT) scanning provide the most accurate method of TNM staging for esophageal cancer. CT should be performed first to exclude distant metastasis (M stage), followed by EUS for precise T and N staging.

TNM Staging for Esophageal Carcinoma

Primary tumor (T)		Regional lymph nodes (N)	
Tx	Primary tumor cannot be assessed	Nx	Regional lymph nodes cannot be assessed
T0	No evidence of primary tumor	N0	No regional lymph node metastasis
Tis	Carcinoma in situ	N1	Regional lymph node metastasis
T1	Tumor invades lamina propria or submucosa	**Distant metastasis (M)**	
T2	Tumor invades muscularis propria	Mx	Presence of distant metastasis
T3	Tumor invades the adventitia	M0	No distant metastasis
T4	Tumor invades adjacent structures	M1	Distant metastasis

11. How can EUS findings affect clinical management of esophageal carcinoma?

- Direct stage-dependent treatment decisions
- Preoperative assessment of tumor resectability
- More accurate pretreatment prognosis

12. Compare the staging accuracies of EUS and CT for esophageal malignancy.

STAGE	NO.	ACCURACY (%) EUS	CT
T1	12	92	—
T2	15	73	11
T3	42	93	69
T4	46	91	59
N0	42	64	67
N1	80	84	36

13. What are the problematic areas for EUS in the staging of esophageal cancer?

• At presentation, 25–50% of esophageal cancers are so advanced that passage of the echoendoscope beyond the cancer is prohibited. Wallace and others recently showed that obstructing malignant esophageal strictures can be safely dilated to permit EUS with fine-needle aspiration (FNA) in ~90% of such patients.
• Accurate T1 staging is difficult, and overstaging is common.
• EUS features cannot accurately distinguish between malignant and inflammatory lymph nodes. Only about 25% of patients with nodal metastasis exhibit the four characteristic EUS features: round shape, size > 1 cm, hypoechoic and distinct margins. EUS-FNA of suspicious lymph nodes can be done safely and significantly improves staging accuracy.
• EUS does not accurately stage esophageal cancer after chemoradiation.

14. Does EUS have a role in the evaluation of gastric cancer?

EUS has no role in the initial diagnosis of gastric cancer and should not be used as a screening tool in patients at risk for this disease. However, in patients where the suspicion of linitis plastica is not confirmed by biopsy, identification of the typical EUS pattern of this cancer contributes significantly to the correct diagnosis (Fig. 3). Radial sector scanning in the region of the pylorus and proximal fundus can be technically difficult. If stage-dependent treatment protocols are employed, then EUS is indicated when CT shows no metastasis (M0). EUS appears to be reliable in predicting stages T1-3 which are surgically resectable (R0).

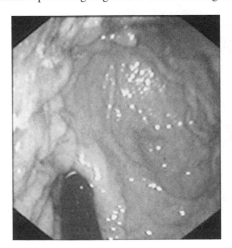 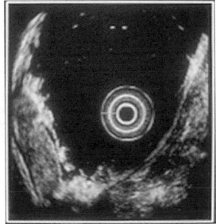

FIGURE 3. Endoscopic view of a gastric adenocarcinoma *(left)* compared with EUS findings *(right)* of a thickened tumor involving the first three echo layers, from 7–9 o-clock. The echoendoscope is located in the center of the water-filled stomach.

15. What are the problematic areas for EUS staging of gastric malignancy?

1. Overstaging of 20–30%, mainly in T2 lesions, is partly due to the peculiar histopathologic definition of stage T2 (infiltration into the submucosa) vs. T3 (invasion of the serosa), a differentiation that cannot be made by EUS. Also, portions of the stomach are not covered by serosa.

2. Differentiation of gastric cancer confined to the mucosa (and therefore amenable to endoscopic treatment) from cancer involving the submucosa (with an attendant increase in the incidence of lymph node metastasis) is relatively inaccurate (60–70%°). Small lesions that are flat, slightly depressed, or elevated at endoscopy and cancerous on biopsy can be assumed to be confined to the mucosa if EUS shows no abnormality of the gastric wall in relation to the tumor. Overstaging occurs predominantly with ulcerating, early carcinomas, because EUS cannot differentiate malignancy from ulcer-related fibrosis and inflammation.

3. Distinguishing inflammatory from malignant lymph nodes is problematic and requires EUS-FNA sampling.

16. Summarize the TNM staging classification for gastric malignancy.

Primary tumor (T)

Tx	Primary tumor cannot be assessed
T0	No evidence of primary tumor
T1	Tumor confined to mucosa or submucosa
T2	Tumor invades muscularis propria or subserosa
T3	Tumor invades serosa without invasion into adjacent structures
T4	Tumor invades adjacent structures

Regional lymph nodes (N)

Nx	Regional lymph nodes cannot be assessed
N0	No regional lymph node metastasis
N1	Positive perigastric lymph nodes, 3 cm from the tumor edge
N2	Positive perigastric lymph nodes, 3 cm from the tumor edge or positive lymph nodes along the gastric, common hepatic, splenic, or celiac arteries

Distant metastasis (M)

Mx	Presence of distant metastasis
M0	No distant metastasis
M1	Distant metastasis

17. How does staging affect treatment?

Resectable tumors (R0) = stages T1–T3. Chemotherapy is used for stage T4.

18. Is EUS helpful in the evaluation of gastric lymphoma?

Yes. Unlike gastric adenocarcinoma, gastric lymphoma has a highly characteristic pattern of horizontal extension. EUS is quite accurate in determining the T and N stage for gastric lymphoma and helps to select the most appropriate medical or surgical treatment (Fig. 4). Low-grade mucosa-associated lymphoid tissue (MALT) lymphoma often is associated with *Helicobacter pylori* and may regress with antibiotic eradication of the infection. When antibiotic treatment fails to reverse the malignant process or if *H. pylori* is absent, EUS is helpful in staging and guiding treatment.

19. How is EUS helpful in evaluating pancreatic neoplasms?

The introduction of EUS-FNA has greatly advanced the role of EUS in the management of suspected pancreatic neoplasms. Organ-preserving pancreatic resections can be performed when tumors of low malignant potential, such as cystadenomas and neuroendocrine tumors, are diagnosed. Erickson and Carza showed that EUS-FNA is superior to CT-FNA for the diagnosis of pancreatic cancer. In their hands EUS-FNA decreased the need for operative staging by 75%.

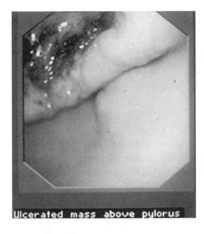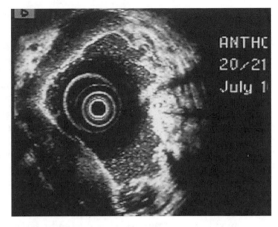

FIGURE 4. Endoscopic view of a gastric lymphoma *(left)* compared with EUS findings of a thickened hypoechoic tumor with foot-like extensions (pseudopodia) into the fourth echogenic layer at the 9 o'clock position. The echoendoscope is located in the center of the water-filled stomach *(right)*.

20. What are the problematic areas of EUS evaluation and staging of pancreatic cancer?
- EUS depth of penetration may be insufficient to visualize the entire margin of large tumors.
- EUS diagnosis of vascular invasion may be < 80%.
- Tumors that infiltrate the uncinate process are difficult to define by EUS.
- A recent report from a tertiary center suggests that overall accuracy of EUS for T and N staging is 69% and 49% and does not predict resectability in stage T3 or T4 pancreatic malignancy.

21. Neuroendocrine tumors of the pancreas and peripancreas are often difficult to localize by conventional CT, ultrasound, and angiography. Does EUS examination offer any value in localizing these tumors?
Yes. EUS is the most accurate imaging method available for the localization of pancreatic endocrine tumors. When CT and sonographic findings are negative, EUS remains > 90% accurate. However, EUS fails to detect up to 50% of extrapancreatic neuroendocrine tumors; either transabdominal ultrasound or CT remains the preferred first test. One needs considerable experience with EUS of the pancreas to achieve this accuracy rate.

22. Can EUS assist in the evaluation of ampullary tumors?
EUS is highly accurate in staging ampullary tumors, especially in determining intrapancreatic spread. Until the role of local tumor resection for ampullary adenomas and T1 carcinoma of the ampulla is defined and accepted as a treatment option vs. Whipple's procedure for more advanced cancers (T2–T4), the clinical utility of EUS is uncertain.

23. Is EUS helpful in evaluating biliary malignancies?
Gallbladder cancer is a highly malignant tumor with poor 5-year survival rate. Risk factors include race (Native Americans and Chileans), cholelithiasis (especially large stones), gallbladder polyps (> 1 cm, single, sessile, and echopenic are associated with higher risk), anomalous junction of pancreatobiliary ducts (AJPBD), and porcelain gallbladder. Cholecystectomy is recommended for patients with AJPBD or porcelain gallbladder. The utility of EUS in gallbladder polyps and large gallstones is under evaluation. The use of EUS miniprobes to stage bile duct tumors is promising.

24. Describe the use of EUS in the evaluation of colon malignancy.
Advances in laparoscopic and endoscopic surgical techniques provide alternatives to conventional exploratory laparotomy and segmental colonic resection for patients diagnosed with

early-stage colon cancer. Studies are under way to evaluate the utility of colonoscopic EUS for accurate staging and selection of patients suitable for minimal access surgery and endoscopic muscosal resection.

25. Describe the use of EUS in the evaluation of rectal malignancy.

EUS is highly accurate in determining the T and N stage and superior to CT scanning. The combination of EUS and CT provides the most practical and accurate approach to staging rectal cancers, and the results of both tests should be considered in treatment planning. The surgical options are largely determined by the tumor stage: T1 is appropriate for local resection, whereas T2–T4 require radical extirpation with or without adjuvant radiation/chemotherapy. A recent comparison of endorectal surface coil magnetic resonance imaging (ERSCMRI) with EUS showed that MR and EUS tumor staging are equal, but MR is more accurate in node staging. Further studies comparing the staging accuracy of ERSCMRI and EUS with FNA are needed.

26. Can submucosal tumors be evaluated by EUS?

Endoscopic ultrasound is 95% accurate in distinguishing true submucosal tumors from extraluminal compression by normal or pathologic structures. Once the submucosal nature of the tumor is established, signs and symptoms guide treatment. Submucosal lesions that cause obstruction and/or bleeding require treatment regardless of the EUS findings. Palazzo et al. suggest the following EUS characteristics to discriminate between benign and malignant leiomyomas or stomal cell tumors (SCTs).

	Benign	**Malignant**
Margins	Regular	Irregular
Size	< 30 mm	> 30 mm
Echo pattern	Homogeneous	Cystic spaces

When all three benign features are present, 100% of SCTs are benign. The combination of 2–3 malignant features has a positive predictive value of 100%.

27. Summarize the EUS characteristics of submucosal tumors.

Aberrant pancreas	Submucosal; similar in echogenicity to the pancreas; hypoechoic ductular structure may be present
Bronchogenic carcinoma	Hypoechoic; disrupts submucosa and muscularis propria; usually irregular outer margin
Breast cancer	Metastatic; same as bronchogenic cancer
Carcinoid	Mucosal; hypoechoic (Fig. 5)
Fibrovascular polyp	Submucosal; mixed echogenicity (Fig. 6)
Gastric cyst	Anechoic; smooth border; submucosal

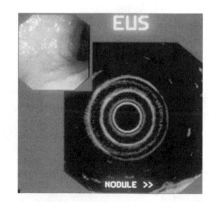

FIGURE 5.   EUS finding of a mucosal hypoechoic carcinoid tumor and endoscopic findings.

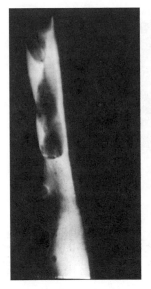
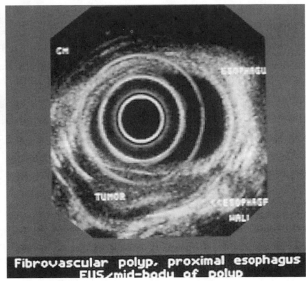

FIGURE 6. Esophageal fibrovascular polyp seen on barium swallow radiograph *(left)* and EUS findings *(right).*

Granular cell tumors	Hypoechoic; submucosal; smooth margin
Lipoma	Hyperechoic; submucosal (Fig. 7)
Leiomyoma	Hypoechoic; contiguous with muscularis propria; smooth outer margin (Fig. 8)
Leiomyosarcoma	Hypoechoic; contiguous with muscularis propria; large lesions may have irregular outer margin; adenopathy; small lesions identical to leiomyoma
Lymphoma	Hypoechoic; may disrupt submucosa; muscularis propria and adenopathy
Pancreatic pseudocyst	Anechoic; smooth margin; compress N1 wall
Varices	Anechoic; submucosal serpentine
Vessels	Anechoic; curvilinear branching; often with through-penetration enhancement of the posterior wall

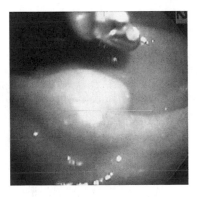
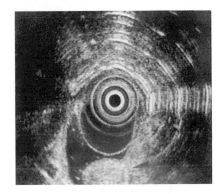

FIGURE 7. Endoscopic finding of a soft submucosal tumor *(left)* and EUS findings of a hyperechoic lipoma *(right).*

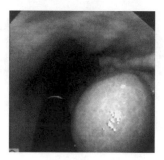 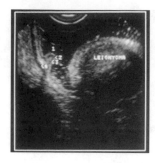

FIGURE 8.   Endoscopic view of a submucosal tumor *(left)*, confirmed to be a leiomyoma, arising from the fourth hyperechoic layer *(right)*.

28. Is EUS useful in the evaluation of nonneoplastic disease?

Preliminary studies of EUS in the evaluation of reflux esophagitis, achalasia, and gastric ulcer have not shown EUS to be clinically important. EUS evaluation of enlarged gastric folds can determine the safety of large-particle biopsy devices and exclude the presence of intramural vascular structures. EUS findings contribute to the characterization of the cause of the process. Thickening of the first two layers is characteristic of inflammation, Ménétrier's disease, and lymphoma; large-particle biopsies should be safe and diagnostic. Thickening of all layers suggests lymphoma or linitis plastica. If biopsy findings are still equivocal, laparoscopy/ laparotomy may be indicated.

29. How is EUS used in the evaluation of patients with portal hypertension?

EUS can demonstrate fundal varices when endoscopic results are equivocal and define the vascular patency of the splenic vein. Some authorities suggest that intramural vessel enlargement can be detected in patients with portal hypertensive gastropathy. Faigel et al. determined that EUS identification of large paraesoaphegal varices > 5 mm was predictive of variceal hemorrhage. Others have shown that EUS can guide treatment of esophageal varices and facilitate treatment of bleeding gastric varices with injection of cyanoacrylate glue.

30. Does EUS have a role in the evaluation of recurrent idiopathic pancreatitis?

Yes. When ERCP fails to detect the anatomic cause of recurrent idiopathic pancreatitis (e.g., choledocolithiasis, microlithiasis, sphincter of Oddi dysfunction, pancreatic divism), EUS should be performed. Lui et al. showed that EUS detects stones in the gallbladder and/or common bile duct in 77% of patients with recurrent idiopathic pancreatitis and negative results with previous CT, US, or ERCP.

31. What is the stack sign? Does it have clinical significance?

The stack sign refers to a characteristic view of the bile and pancreatic ducts. The view is obtained by positioning the echoendoscope in the long scope position with the transducer in the duodenal bulb. The balloon is inflated and advanced snugly into the apex of the bulb. From this position, the bile duct (closest to the transducer) and pancreatic duct can be seen to run parallel through the pancreatic head. The absence of the stack sign may suggest pancreatic divism.

32. Describe the role of EUS in the evaluation of chronic pancreatitis.

EUS is more sensitive than CT in detection of early chronic pancreatitis. Its role in monitoring for neoplastic change in patients with hereditary or chronic alcoholic pancreatitis is under evaluation. EUS-guided celiac block appears to be superior to CT-guided block in terms of pain control and cost. EUS features of chronic pancreatitis include parenchymal and ductal abnormalities:

Parenchymal abnormalities
- Hyperechoic foci (distinct 1–2-mm hyperechoic points)
- Hyperechoic strands (hyperechoic irregular lines)

- Lobularity (2–5-mm lobules)
- Cysts (thin-walled, round, anechoic structures > 2 mm in diameter within the pancreatic parenchyma)
- Shadowing calcifications

Ductal abnormalities
- Dilation (head > 3 mm, body > 2 mm, and tail > 1 mm)
- Irregular duct
- Hyperechoic duct margins (duct wall visible as a distinct, hyperechoic structure)
- Visible side branches (anechoic structures budding from the main pancreatic duct)

33. Summarize the EUS criteria for chronic pancreatitis.

Mild chronic pancreatitis: 1–2 abnormal features
Moderate chronic pancreatitis: 3–5 abnormal features
Severe chronic pancreatitis: > 5 abnormal features

34. Discuss the role of EUS in evaluating patients with common bile duct stones.

A recent study of patients with choledocholithiasis found EUS to be superior to magnetic resonance cholangiopancreatography (MRCP), but both are highly accurate (96.9% and 82.2%, respectively). However, in most hospitals extracorporeal ultrasound will continue to be the most cost-effective first test to evaluate for choledocholithiasis. When the patient is too obese to permit diagnostic extracorporeal ultrasound, MRCP is the most accurate noninvasive test. The ~5% risk of pancreatitis with ERCP increases the appeal of EUS for evaluation of choledocholithiasis in high-risk patients.

BIBLIOGRAPHY

1. Anderson MA, Carpenter S, Thompson NW, et al: Endoscopic ultrasound is highly accurate and directs management in patients with neuroendocrine tumors of the pancreas. Am J Gastroenterol 95:2271–2277, 2000.
2. Ahmad NA, Lewis JD, Ginsberg GG, et al: EUS in preoperative staging of pancreatic cancer. Gastrointest Endosc 52:463–468, 2000.
3. Antillon MR, Chang KJ. Endoscopic and endosonographic guided fine-needle aspiration. Gastrointest Endosc Clin North Am 10:619–636, 2000.
4. Armengol Miro JR, Benjamin S, Binmoeller K, et al: Clinical applications of endoscopic ultrasound in gastroenterology—State of the art 1993 (consensus conference). Endoscopy 25:358–366, 1993.
5. Beseth BD, Bedford R, Isacoff WH, et al: Endoscopic ultrasound does not accurately assess pathologic stage of esophageal cancer after neoadjuvant chemoradiation. Am Surg 66:827–831, 2000.
6. Botet JF, Lightdale CJ, Zauber AG, et al: Preoperative staging of esophageal cancer: Comparison of endoscopic US and dynamic CT. Radiology 181:419–425, 1991.
7. Boyce GA, Sivak MV, Lavery IC, et al: Endoscopic ultrasound in pre-operative staging of rectal carcinoma. Gastrointest Endosc 38:468–471, 1992.
8. Boyce GA, Sivak MV, Rosch T, et al: Evaluation of submucosal upper gastrointestinal tract lesions by endoscopic ultrasound. Gastrointest Endosc 37:449–454, 1991.
9. Bhutani MS, Hoffman BJ, Hawes RH: Diagnosis of pancreas divism by endoscopic ultrasonography. Endoscopy 31:167–169, 1999.
10. Caletti GC, Fusaroli P, Togliani T, Roda E: Endosonography in gastric lymphoma and large gastric folds. Eur J Ultrasound 11:31–40, 2000.
11. Caletti GC, Zani L, Bolondi L, et al: Endoscopic ultrasonography in the diagnosis of gastric submucosal tumor. Gastrointest Endosc 35:413–418, 1989.
12. Catalano MF, Lahoti S, Geenen JE, Hogan WJ: Prospective evaluation of endoscopic ultrasonography, endoscopic retrograde pancreatography, and secretin test in the diagnosis of chronic pancreatitis. Gastrointest Endosc 48:11–17, 1998.
13. de Ledinghen V, Lecesne R, Raymond JM, et al: Diagnosis of choledocholithiasis: EUS or magnetic resonance cholangiography? A prospective controlled study. Gastrointest Endosc 49:26–31, 1999.
14. Dittler HJ, Siewert JR: Role of endoscopic ultrasonography in esophageal carcinoma. Endoscopy 25:156–161, 1993.
15. Dittler HJ, Siewert JR: Role of endoscopic ultrasonography in gastric carcinoma. Endoscopy 25:162–166, 1993.
16. Erickson RA, Garza AA. Impact of endoscopic ultrasound on the management and outcome of pancreatic carcinoma. Am J Gastroenterol 95:2248–2254, 2000.
17. Frucht H, Norton JA, London JF, et al: Detection of duodenal gastrinomas by operative endoscopic transillumination. Gastroenterology 99:162–1627, 1990.
18. Gress F, Schmitt C, Sherman S, et al: A prospective randomized comparison of endoscopic ultrasound- and computed tomography-guided celiac plexus block for managing chronic pancreatitis pain. Am J Gastroenterol 94:900–905, 1999.

19. Lahoti S, Catalano MF, Alcocer E, et al: Obliteration of esophageal varices using EUS-guided sclerotherapy with color Doppler. Gastrointest Endosc 51:331–333, 2000.
20. Lambert R, Caletti G, Cho E, et al: International workshop on the clinical impact of endoscopic ultrasound in gastroenterology. Endoscopy 32:549–584, 2000.
21. Lee YT, Chan FK, Ng EK, et al: EUS-guided injection of cyanoacrylate for bleeding gastric varices. Gastrointest Endosc 52:168–174, 2000.
22. Lightdale C: Endoscopic ultrasonograpy. Gastrointest Endosc Clin North Am 2:557–749, 1992.
23. Lui C, Lo C, Chan JKF, et al: EUS for detection of occult cholelithiasis in patients with idiopathic pancreatitis. Gastrointest Endosc 51:28–32, 2000.
24. Martin SP, Ulrich CD II: Pancreatic cancer surveillance in a high-risk cohort. Is it worth the cost? Med Clin North Am 84:739–747, 2000.
25. Maldjian C, Smith R, Kilger A, et al: Endorectal surface coil MR imaging as a staging technique for rectal carcinoma: A comparison study to rectal endosonography. Abdom Imag 25:75–80, 2000.
26. Norton SA, Thomas MG: Staging of rectosigmoid neoplasia with colonoscopic endoluminal ultrasonography. Br J Surg 86:942–946, 1999.
27. Powis ME, Chang KJ: Endoscopic ultrasound in the clinical staging and management of pancreatic cancer: Its impact on cost of treatment. Cancer Control 7:413–420, 2000.
28. Rosch T, Dittler HK, Strobel K, et al: Endoscopic ultrasound criteria for vascular invasion in the staging of cancer of the head of the pancreas: A blind reevaluation of videotapes. Gastrointest Endosc 52:469–477, 2000.
29. Sandy H, Cooperman A, Siegel JH: Endoscopic ultrasonography compared with computed tomography with ERCP in patients with obstructive jaundice or small peripancreatic mass. Gastrointest Endosc 38:27–34, 1992.
30. Schechter NR, Yahalom J: Low-grade MALT lymphoma of the stomach: A review of treatment options. Int J Radiat Oncol Biol Phys 46:1093-1103, 2000.
31. Sheth S, Bedford A, Chopra S: Primary gallbladder cancer: Recognition of risk factors and role of prophylactic cholecystectomy. Am J Gastroenterol 95:1402–1410, 2000.
32. Wallace MB, Hawes EH, Sahai AV, et al: Dilation of malignant esophageal stenosis to allow EUS guided fine-needle aspiration: Safety and effect on patient management. Gastrointest Endosc 51:309–313, 2000.
33. Yasuda K, Cho E, Nakajima M, Kawai K: Diagnosis of submucosal lesions of the upper gastrointestinal tract by endoscopic ultrasonography. Gastrointest Endosc 36:S17–S20, 1990.

78. ENDOSCOPIC RETROGRADE CHOLANGIOPANCREATOGRAPHY

John A. Dumot, D.O., and Gregory Zuccaro, Jr., M.D.

1. What is the distinction between diagnostic and therapeutic ERCP?

The goal of diagnostic endoscopic retrograde cholangiopancreatography (ERCP) is to inject contrast material into the biliary tree and pancreatic duct. ERCP allows radiographic visualization of the biliary tree and pancreatic duct, which can aid in the diagnosis of several pancreatic and biliary diseases. Adjunctive maneuvers of diagnostic ERCP include endoscopic biopsy of an abnormal papilla and brush cytology or biopsy of ductal strictures. Skills necessary to perform diagnostic ERCP include those of all diagnostic endoscopy: knowledge of sedation and analgesia and ability to maneuver the endoscope. Therapeutic ERCP involves all of the requisite elements of the diagnostic procedure as well as additional maneuvers necessary to provide definitive therapy and/or palliation, including papillotomy, stone extraction, stricture dilation, and placement of plastic or metal stents.

2. What training is required to perform ERCP?

ERCP is an advanced procedure, not part of the core endoscopic procedures expected of every gastroenterologist. Recent guidelines from the American Society for Gastrointestinal Endoscopy (ASGE) recommend an additional year of training beyond the standard 3-year fellowship. The advanced training should be offered to interested trainees with an aptitude for endoscopic procedures. Training must be provided in a center with adequate patient volume and faculty expertise. Previously, the ASGE assigned threshold numbers of procedures for assessing competence in standard and advanced endoscopic procedures (75 for diagnostic ERCP and an additional 25 for therapeutic ERCP), implying that training in diagnostic ERCP alone is an acceptable goal. Some programs graduate trainees with only diagnostic ERCP skills, assuming that they will gain experience and training in therapeutic skills through proctoring or other relationships developed in their professional practice. The most recent ASGE guidelines state that the completion of advanced training in private practice after brief exposure to therapeutic ERCP (30–40 procedures) during standard gastroenterology training is no longer appropriate. The role of endoscopy simulators remains to be determined.

3. Should all endoscopists performing ERCP possess therapeutic skills?

A strong case can be made that only persons competent in therapeutic interventions should perform ERCP. With continued improvements in noninvasive imaging techniques such as CT and MRI scanning (Fig. 1), the necessity of ERCP to diagnose pancreatic and biliary disorders has decreased (see Chapter 75). Indications for therapeutic retrograde cholangiography have increased, particularly as a complement to laparoscopic cholecystectomy. Diagnosis of choledocholithiasis by an endoscopist untrained in papillotomy and stone extraction necessitates another ERCP for therapy, exposing the patient to additional risk(s) of endoscopy, pancreatitis, and cost. Injection of contrast material above a biliary stricture by an endoscopist unable to provide prompt drainage increases the risk of cholangitis.

4. Discuss the special considerations for sedation and analgesia during ERCP.

For most standard endoscopy, a single GI assistant is sufficient to monitor the patient and assist with minor ancillary tasks. For ERCP, the first assistant (at the head of the bed) is often completely occupied with the preparation and movement of catheters, guidewires, and other accessories necessary for procedure completion. Therefore, a second assistant is needed to monitor the patient.

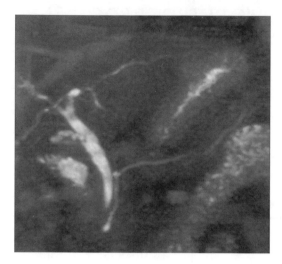

FIGURE 1. Magnetic resonance cholangiopancreatography (MRCP) of a patient with abdominal pain and suspected choledocholithiasis several years after cholecystectomy revealed mild bile duct dilation, which was attributed to surgical removal of the gallbladder.

Whereas a diagnostic upper endoscopy is typically brief, ERCP takes considerably longer. The length and complexity of the procedure often require administration of higher cumulative doses of sedative/analgesics, which may become problematic in elderly patients or those taking daily narcotics for pain relief. For special cases, including extremes in age and patients with conditions such as severe cardiopulmonary disease, chronic narcotic use, morbid obesity, or inability to cooperate, consultation with an anesthesiologist is advisable. In most cases, ERCP can be accomplished safely with standard sedative/analgesic agents prudently administered by the endoscopist. Careful monitoring, including the use of pulse oximetry in all cases and cardiac monitoring for patients with a recent history of significant cardiac disease, is essential. Supplemental oxygen is not a must at the beginning of each case but should be used if hypoxemia occurs. Reversal agents for narcotics and benzodiazepines should be present, as should all equipment necessary to maintain a patent airway and provide cardiopulmonary resuscitation. Emergency medical services and extended recovery with monitoring should be immediately available.

5. What are the common indications for retrograde cholangiography?

Common indications include the investigation of obstructive jaundice or abdominal pain in which a mechanical cause, such as stone, tumor, or biliary stricture, is suspected. In virtually all cases, identification of such abnormalities leads to therapeutic intervention (e.g., stone extraction, stent placement). Other indications include investigation of patients with recurrent acute pancreatitis, identification of sclerosing cholangitis in patients with predisposing factors (e.g., inflammatory bowel disease, AIDS), obtaining bile for crystal or other analyses, and performance of ancillary tasks such as biliary manometry. For assessment of patients with right upper quadrant abdominal pain suspected to be due to sphincter of Oddi dysfunction, see Chapter 37.

6. How has laparoscopic cholecystectomy affected the use of retrograde cholangiography?

It has led to increased use. During cholecystectomy, a cholangiogram usually can be obtained via the cystic duct. However, techniques for laparoscopic-guided extraction of common bile duct stones or common duct exploration are difficult to perform and not widely available. Therefore, the surgeon often requests retrograde cholangiography for stone extraction prior to laparoscopic cholecystectomy when choledocholithiasis is strongly suspected or after surgery when the operative cholangiogram reveals unexpected retained stones. Complications of laparoscopic cholecystectomy appear higher than with open cholecystectomy, particularly early in the surgeon's experience. Endoscopic papillotomy with or without stent placement hastens closure of the postoperative biliary leaks into the bed of the gallbladder from either the cystic duct remnant or the transhepatic ducts of Luschka. Retrograde cholangiography can identify the rare bile duct transection. Postoperative strictures can be identified and dilated and/or stented.

7. How successful is retrograde cholangiography?
In experienced hands, the success rate is 85–95%.

8. What techniques may increase the success rate?
Successful opacification and/or cannulation of the desired duct can be achieved using a variety of catheters, papillotomes, and guidewires. Standard catheters accept specially coated guidewires that may "slip" up the bile duct and facilitate cannulation. One useful technique is to use a guidewire with a single-lumen catheter to achieve free cannulation, then advance the catheter freely up the biliary tree. The guidewire is removed, and the assistant aspirates air from the catheter until free flow of bile is noted in the syringe before contrast injection. This strategy reduces the likelihood of introducing air bubbles into the duct. If the tip is occluded, the endoscopist may need to reposition the catheter away from the bile duct wall while trying to clear the air from the catheter's lumen. Many endoscopists prefer a papillotome to achieve selective bile duct cannulation and thereby avoid the pancreatic duct, where a pancreatogram is undesirable. Variable tension on the cutting wire to bow the catheter toward the 10–11 o'clock positions on the ampulla aligns the catheter with the orientation of the intraduodenal segment of the common bile duct. Simultaneous manipulation of endoscope, papillotome cutting-wire, and guidewire allows selective cannulation of the biliary tree in most cases.

9. Discuss the role of tapered-tip catheters with reduced diameter.
Some commercially available tapered-tip catheters have a reduced diameter compared with standard catheters to allow cannulation of small orifices, such as the minor papilla. Many of these catheters do not accept the standard 0.035-in guidewires, which is a potential drawback because catheter exchanges over the smaller 0.018-in guidewires can be technically difficult. Guidewires of intermediate size (0.021 and 0.025 inches) are stiff enough for catheter exchanges or stent placements and compatible with tapered-tip catheters. An even smaller end on the needle tip catheters provides pinpoint accuracy for contrast injections, but such catheters are too small to allow passage of a guidewire.

10. What is a precut papillotomy?
A precut papillotomy involves creation of an incision with special catheters in the papillary area when free, selective cannulation of the bile duct cannot be achieved. It may be performed using a bare wire "needle knife" papillotome or a more conventional papillotome with a cutting wire that extends to the catheter tip.

11. What two approaches have been used for precut papillotomy?
1. Place either of the catheters into the meatus, and cut upward in the direction of the bile duct with the hope of locating the bile duct.
2. Use the needle-knife to create a fistula between the duodenum and the common bile duct by cutting directly into the intraduodenal segment of the most distal bile duct, approximately 5–10 mm above the ampullary orifice. This approach has a theoretical advantage of avoiding the pancreatic orifice, thereby reducing the incidence of ERCP-induced pancreatitis. Cannulation after the small incision is made should be performed with a papillotome and guidewire combination. Injection of contrast after a precut papillotomy commonly results in submucosal infiltration and edema, which lead to a more difficult cannulation.

12. Should precut papillotomy be used in diagnostic cholangiography?
Although this technique does appear to increase the rate of successful retrograde cholangiography in experienced hands, the complication rate is 2–3 times that of conventional papillotomy. Therefore, experienced endoscopists should perform a precut only when there is a strong indication for cholangiography and/or endoscopic papillotomy.

Stent placement into the pancreatic duct before the precut is performed appears to decrease the rate of postpapillotomy pancreatitis. One relatively strong indication for a precut is a large biliary calculus impacted at the level of the papilla, where free cannulation of the biliary tree is precluded (Fig. 2). Even in these circumstances, however, a concerted attempt to achieve a free biliary

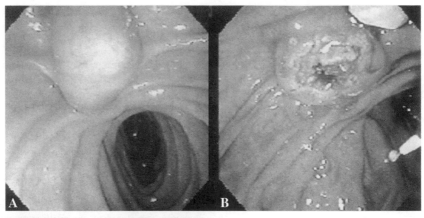

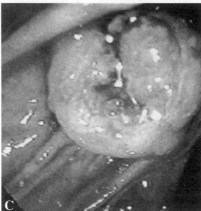

FIGURE 2. A patient with gallstone pancreatitis was found to have a biliary calculus impacted at the level of the main duodenal papilla *(A)*. Free cannulation failed, and stone removal required a precut or "needle-knife" sphincterotomy, which dislodged the stone *(B)*. The sphincterotomy was completed with a standard wire-guided sphincterotome *(C)*.

cannulation using guidewires and other techniques should precede precut papillotomy because of the inherent risks of perforation, edema, and hemorrhage, which can prevent a successful procedure.

When cholangiography is clearly indicated and the above measures fail, the interventional radiologist often can obtain a transhepatic cholangiogram. If indicated, the radiologist may pass a wire into the duodenum, which can be used by the endoscopist to guide papillotomy and therapeutic procedures such as stone extraction. Most procedures such as stone extraction and stent placement can be performed via the percutaneous route, but usually the tract must mature before extensive manipulation is attempted.

13. Discuss the common indications for diagnostic endoscopic retrograde pancreatography.

A common indication is to clarify findings on noninvasive imaging of the pancreas. When a mass lesion suspicious for cancer is identified on transabdominal ultrasound or CT scan, a tissue diagnosis is desirable. A mass lesion in the pancreatic head may lead to stricture or obstruction of both the pancreatic duct and distal common bile duct, the so-called double-duct sign (Fig. 3). ERCP may afford a cytologic diagnosis and palliation of the biliary obstruction during the same procedure. Improvements in CT and ultrasound-guided aspiration and biopsy, as well as endoscopic ultrasound (EUS)-guided fine needle aspiration (FNA), have reduced the use of retrograde pancreatography simply to characterize or obtain brushings from pancreatic masses, especially in the body and tail.

Another common indication is to provide anatomic detail before surgery for chronic pancreatitis. The presence or absence of ductal dilation, obstruction due to strictures, and/or a calculus and the communication of pseudocysts with the main pancreatic duct are relevant to the likelihood

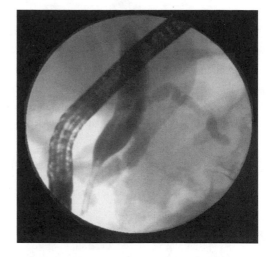

FIGURE 3. A mass lesion in the pancreatic head may lead to stricture or obstruction of both the pancreatic duct and the distal common duct, the so-called double-duct sign. A stent was placed into the bile duct.

of successful surgical intervention. Patients with acute, recurrent pancreatitis often undergo retrograde pancreatography to exclude anatomic abnormalities, such as pancreas divisum, neoplastic obstruction, and chronic pancreatitis, as well as cholangiography to exclude choledocholithiasis.

14. List five guidelines that help the beginner endoscopist to obtain a successful, uncomplicated biliary papillotomy.

1. Accept only optimal cutting-wire orientation. The bile duct papillotomy is carried out along the maximal impression of the intraduodenal segment of the common bile duct (the 10 o'clock to 1 o'clock position). If the cutting wire does not orient in this fashion, the endoscopist should remove the catheter and try to reorient the cutting wire by gently bending the tip. If the attempt at reorientation does not succeed, request another papillotome. If this happens with two papillotomes, particularly if the cutting wires are relatively short, request a papillotome with a long cutting wire, which orients more favorably in a variety of circumstances.

2. Do not overreach. The new endoscopist wants to demonstrate a high skill level and earn a reputation. However, this desire should not lead to continuing unsuccessful procedures for inordinate amounts of time (increasing the risk of complications of sedation/analgesia), repeated filling of the pancreatic duct in attempts at bile duct cannulation, or an imprudent attempt at precut papillotomy. Alternative interventions such as a more experienced colleague, percutaneous approach by a radiologist, or surgical intervention are far preferable.

3. Perform bile duct papillotomy only after free, selective cannulation. Experienced endoscopists often begin therapeutic cases with a papillotome rather than a standard diagnostic catheter. A soft-tipped guidewire and the gentle hand of your assistant can facilitate bile duct cannulation when repeated injections of contrast provide only pancreatic duct opacification.

4. Use one model of papillotome, and know its every mark. Most experienced endoscopists prefer the cutting wire to be one-half to one-third the way out of the papilla to ensure controlled cutting. They can achieve this placement by sight and feel. An alternative is to memorize each mark on the papillotome, particularly those coincident with the proximal and distal ends of the cutting wire, and the point halfway between. This knowledge allows the endoscopist to maneuver the catheter by following the marks and increases confidence that the cutting wire is properly situated.

5. Use a guidewire that can be left in place during papillotomy. Some guidewires must be removed before the papillotomy is performed. However, special "protected" wires that can be left safely in place are readily available from various manufacturers. They provide an extra measure of confidence in withdrawal of the papillotome to its proper position, because the endoscopist need not fear loss of selective cannulation.

15. What are the common complications of ERCP?

The most frequent complication of diagnostic and therapeutic ERCP is pancreatitis (1–9%). Postpapillotomy bleeding (2%), cholangitis (1%), cholecystitis (0.5%), perforation (< 1%), infection, and oversedation occur less frequently.

16. What causes ERCP-induced pancreatitis?

The cause is likely multifactorial. The amount of contrast infused into the main pancreatic duct may be one precipitating factor. Experience of the endoscopist, difficulty with cannulation, sphincter of Oddi manometry, and sphincterotomy are clearly related to the incidence of ERCP-induced pancreatitis.

17. What are the risk factors for ERCP-induced pancreatitis?

Risk factors include an inexperienced endoscopist, young patients, patients with a nondilated bile duct, multiple pancreatic duct contrast injections, difficult cannulation with multiple attempts, and performing precut sphincterotomy, pancreatic duct sphincterotomy, and manometry.

18. List strategies for reducing the risk of ERCP-induced pancreatitis.

1. Have the procedure indication in mind before beginning. If there is no reason to obtain a pancreatogram, attempt a selective free cannulation of the bile duct. If the main pancreatic duct is inadvertently filled with contrast, cease the injection immediately and use a soft-tip guidewire for subsequent cannulation attempts.

2. Use the minimum contrast volume necessary to establish the diagnosis during pancreatography. Overinjection increases hydrostatic pressure and disrupts the pancreatic acinar units. This complication is called acinarization and appears as a blush of contrast on fluoroscopy.

3. Do not ignore the head of the pancreas when focusing fluoroscopic attention on the pancreatic tail or proximal biliary tree. Overfilling of side branches or acinarization in the pancreatic head can occur unbeknownst to the endoscopist and assistants.

4. Listen to your assistant. If the injection can be made only with force, take the time to readjust catheter position for a smoother, controlled injection.

19. When does bleeding occur? How is the risk reduced?

Bleeding may be recognized at the time of papillotomy or occur several days after an apparently unremarkable procedure. Using a generator with a "blended" current (part cutting current and part coagulation) and a slow, controlled cut with scrupulous attention to orientation of the cutting wire may decrease the likelihood of bleeding.

20. What causes ERCP-induced cholangitis and cholecystitis?

Cholangitis occurs after instillation of contrast into an obstructed biliary tree without adequate drainage. Patients are more likely to develop cholangitis with proximal malignant strictures than distal obstructions. Giving broad-spectrum antibiotics before cholangiography is performed for obstructive jaundice is prudent but not a substitute for definitive drainage. In addition, pancreatic pseudocysts communicating with the ductal system may be infected after contrast injection of the pancreatic duct.

21. Where does perforation occur? How is it managed?

Perforation often is recognized during the procedure. It may occur at the cervical esophagus (usually in the piriform sinus), gastroesophageal junction, and duodenal bulb as a result of either passage of the duodenoscope or papillotomy. Management must be individualized, but not all perforations require immediate surgical exploration. Placement of a biliary stent or nasobiliary drain should be strongly considered in suspected or confirmed perforations during papillotomy. Presumably, the papillotomy was done to remedy a structural abnormality. Placement of the biliary stent or nasobiliary tube allows drainage of biliary contents and may limit retroperitoneal infection. Conservative management of perforations should be attempted only in consultation with surgeons experienced in diseases of the biliary tract.

22. How is infection prevented?

Infection from the duodenoscope is extremely rare and does not warrant prophylactic antibiotic use in routine diagnostic ERCP. Proper disinfecting and handling of endoscopes and accessories are essential. Biliary sepsis related to *Pseudomonas* spp. has been traced to contaminated water bottles.

23. What are the potential consequences of oversedation?

Oversedation is a potential complication of all GI endoscopic procedures in which sedation or analgesia is administered. Aspiration of gastric contents resulting in pneumonia can occur because the patient is prone for long periods. If significant gastric contents are noted, the risks of continuing the procedure must be weighed against the potential benefits. In extreme cases, lavage of the stomach contents and increased vigilance of the assistant may be beneficial.

24. Are balloon catheters or basket catheters preferable for extraction of bile duct stones after papillotomy?

Both are effective and may complement one another. Stone extraction balloons of varied diameters are available and can be selected as appropriate for the size of the papillotomy and degree of ductal dilation. After creation of an adequate papillotomy, a balloon catheter can be passed above the most proximal stone and inflated with air. The inflated balloon catheter is then pulled gradually into the duodenum. Gentle insertion and clockwise rotation of the endoscope, along with movement of the tip away from the medial wall (using the large wheel), may facilitate delivery of the balloon through the papilla. Basket catheters are used to grasp and extract individual stones (Fig. 4).

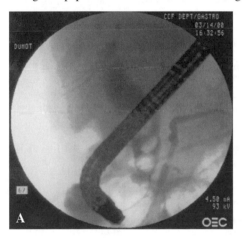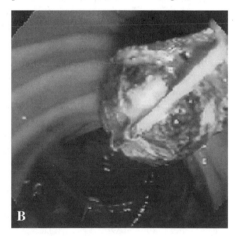

FIGURE 4.   *A,* Cholangiogram revealing three large common bile duct stones. *B,* Basket catheters are used to grasp and extract or crush individual stones.

25. List the advantages and disadvantages of balloon catheters.

Advantages include obtaining an occlusion cholangiogram during stone extraction, guidewire compatibility, and low frequency of a "trapped" catheter among large hard stones.

Disadvantages include the inability to remove extremely large stones, which have a tendency to impact into the distal common bile duct. At times it is difficult to visualize the passage of stones because the balloons tend to be delivered from the bile duct across the papillotomy quickly. Balloons may fail in patients with a capacious biliary tree. Even the largest of balloons can be drawn past small stones and fragments without delivering them into the duodenum.

26. List the advantages and disadvantages of basket cathers.

Advantages include direct tactile and visual confirmation of stone extraction. The basket is opened and closed by the assistant, who manipulates the catheter's handle. A few commercial stone extraction baskets are wire-guided, but manipulation of these dual-lumen devices is cumbersome.

Disadvantages include the inability to perform occlusion cholangiography during or after stone extraction. Some endoscopists are concerned about impacting the basket around a stone that cannot be delivered through the papilla, but ancillary techniques, such as mechanical lithotripsy, often remedy this infrequent occurrence.

27. Should patients with cholelithiasis or choledocholithiasis and acute pancreatitis undergo emergent ERCP?

Most patients with gallstone pancreatitis show signs of improvement early in their hospital stay, and emergent ERCP is not warranted. Patients with more severe gallstone pancreatitis or patients in whom clear progressive improvement is not obvious are more likely candidates for urgent ERCP. In many patients with severe or ongoing pancreatitis, choledocholithiasis is identified. A gallstone impacted at the level of the papilla may be the culprit. *Early ERCP is clearly warranted in patients with gallstone pancreatitis complicated by cholangitis because it lowers the overall mortality rate.* In this circumstance, an experienced endoscopist is essential. Many such patients are quite ill. The endoscopic intervention should be carried out with all deliberate speed. Selective free cannulation of the biliary tree is important; opacification of the main pancreatic duct theoretically may worsen the pancreatitis. Precut papillotomy may be necessary for extraction of a stone impacted at the level of the papilla, and placement of a biliary drain or stent to augment biliary drainage is usually recommended. Occasionally, patients may require intensive care monitoring; if such a patient is transported to the endoscopy suite, all necessary monitoring should accompany them. Consultation and an anesthesiologist to administer sedation/analgesia may be appropriate for the most acutely ill.

28. Describe the management of retained stones.

Retained choledocholithiasis should be addressed in a timely fashion to prevent further episodes of pancreatitis. Intraoperative cholangiography during cholecystectomy or noninvasive imaging such as magnetic resonance cholangiography is preferable to routine diagnostic ERCP for patients without a high probability of retained stones.

29. Compare the use of plastic vs. metals stents in the endoscopic management of malignant biliary obstruction.

Polyethylene or plastic stents are subject to clogging due to biofilm, and most endoscopists recommend regular stent changes approximately every 3 months to prevent cholangitis. They provide adequate drainage and are easily placed in most cases. Plastic stents are easily removed, but metal ones are not; therefore, palliation for a patient in whom surgical resection is still possible is better managed with a plastic stent. If subsequently surgery is ruled out, a metal stent can still be placed at the time of the first scheduled stent change.

Several types of **self-expanding metal stents** are commercially available and may be placed by the endoscopist or radiologist in a similar fashion. Clogging and obstruction are less frequent with metal stents than with polyethylene stents but can occur when patients outlive the patency of the devices. Tumor ingrowth and overgrowth are the principal causes of stent malfunction in malignant obstructions. In addition, epithelial or mucosal hyperplasia (foreign body reaction), and sludge can cause metal stents to fail. Metal stents are permanent and cannot be removed in the vast majority of cases. For these reasons, metal stents should *not* be placed in patients with benign strictures. Placing polyethylene stents within the larger metal stents treats metal stent failure due to tumor ingrowth or overgrowth. Routine stent changes every 2–3 months should be performed thereafter.

30. Are metal stents cost-effective?

The initial cost of metal stent placement exceeds that of the polyethylene stent, but the long-term costs may be lower. Both the need for subsequent endoscopy for polyethylene stent change and total hospital days for cholangitis due to stent obstruction are reduced with metal stents. Metal stents are not cost-effective for patients with an extremely short life expectancy (< 4 months).

31. Describe the role of therapeutic endoscopic retrograde pancreatography.

Endoscopic therapy may be used for acute, recurrent pancreatitis attributed to pancreas divisum. There appears to be an association between divisum (failed fusion of the dorsal and ventral pancreatic ducts) and pancreatitis. It is theorized that the volume of pancreatic drainage via the dorsal duct through the smaller accessory papilla exceeds their capacity, leading to episodic pancreatitis. Surgical sphincteroplasty of the accessory papilla appears to decrease or eliminate further attacks. In endoscopic therapy, the accessory papilla may be cannulated using special tapered or fine-tipped catheters. Both dorsal duct stent placement and stent placement with papillotomy of the accessory papilla have provided benefit to patients with acute recurrent pancreatitis in controlled clinical trials with short-term follow-up. Pancreatic stents can induce strictures, which has tempered the enthusiasm for long-term management of pancreatic strictures. Experience with endoscopic pancreatic duct sphincterotomy, stent placement, stone extraction, and pseudocyst drainage as therapy for sequelae of chronic pancreatitis is growing. Long-term studies are needed to determine the circumstances under which these interventions are most beneficial and to assess their efficacy compared with standard surgical and radiologic interventions.

32. Does cholangioscopy have a role in the diagnosis and management of biliary tract disorders?

Direct visualization of the bile duct or main pancreatic duct can be accomplished with special small-caliber endoscopes passed through a duodenoscope with a large operating channel or special small optical fibers. The information gained during routine ERCP is sufficient to establish diagnosis and management for most patients. In rare circumstances, cholangioscopy or pancreatoscopy may add relevant information. Occasionally, it may be difficult to distinguish a mass lesion in the biliary tree from an adherent calculus. Direct visualization of a bile duct stricture may add to the information gained from cytology or noninvasive imaging; directed cytology or biopsy may be possible with some cholangioscopes.

33. How is cholangioscopy used with laser therapy?

Cholangioscopy can direct laser therapy for large stones that fail routine mechanical lithotripsy. One of the most successful applications of intracorporeal lithotripsy is the holmium laser because of its ability to vaporize stone material. This laser operates in the infrared wavelength spectrum within an aqueous environment. The working channel of the cholangioscope is less than 2 mm but easily handles a perfusion of saline and the 365-μm fiber for contact lithotripsy.

34. What is the role of tumor ablation during ERCP?

The use of high-energy lasers within the bile duct is limited by the ease of perforation through normal tissue. One prospective trial of laser ablation of nonresectable cholangiocarcinoma with photodynamic therapy (PDT) suggested an improvement in overall survival and quality of life. This case series suggests that PDT may have a role in patients with persistent jaundice after endoscopic stent placement. PDT involves administering a photosensitizing agent, which is activated by an intense light source that causes tissue destruction in the area radiated by the light. Problems associated with this off-label use of PDT within the biliary tree include prolonged photosensitivity and technical problems associated with delivering the laser light to the tumor stricture with currently available laser fibers. Controlled trials are necessary before widespread use can be recommended.

35. Discuss the role of the radiologist in ERCP.

The radiologist's role varies with the institution. In many practices, ERCP is performed in the radiology suite rather than in the endoscopy unit. Often a member of the radiology staff (attending physician, resident physician, or technician) is in attendance. When the attending radiologist is present, interpretation of hard copy films is straightforward, because the radiologist knows the relevant history, results of correlative imaging, and sequence of procedural events. When the radiologist is not present, the endoscopist must take responsibility to identify the relevant findings and document them on hard copy film for later reference.

BIBLIOGRAPHY

1. American Society for Gastrointestinal Endoscopy: Principles of training in gastrointestinal endoscopy. Gastrointest Endosc 49:845–853, 1999.
2. American Society for Gastrointestinal Endoscopy: The role of ERCP in diseases of the biliary tract and pancreas: Guidelines for clinical application. Gastrointest Endosc 50:915–920, 1999.
3. Bromley MJK, Nicholson DA, Bartal G, et al: Holmiun-YAG laser for gallstone fragmentation: An endoscopic tool. Gut 36:442–445, 1995.
4. Classen DC, Jacobson JA, Burke JP, et al: Serious pseudomonal infections associated with endoscopic retrograde cholangiopancreatography. Am J Med 84:590–596, 1988.
5. Cotton PB: Precut papillotomy: A risky technique for experts only. Gastrointest Endosc 35:578–579, 1989.
6. Cotton PB, Lehman G, Vennes J, et al: Endoscopic sphincterotomy complications and their management: An attempt at consensus. Gastrointest Endosc 37:383–393, 1991.
7. Deviere J, Motte S, Dumonceau JM, et al: Septicemia after endoscopic retrograde cholangiopancreatography. Endoscopy 22:72–75, 1990.
8. Fan ST, Lai EC, Mok FP, et al: Early treatment of acute biliary pancreatitis by endoscopic papillotomy. N Engl J Med 328:228–232, 1993.
9. Freeman ML, Nelson DB, Sherman S, et al: Complications of endoscopic biliary sphincterotomy. N Engl J Med 335;909–918, 1996.
10. Geenen JE, Vennes JA, Silvis SE: Resume of a seminar on endoscopic retrograde sphincterotomy (ERS). Gastrointest Endosc 7:31–38, 1981.
11. Huibregtse K, Smits ME: Endoscopic management of diseases of the pancreas. Am J Gastroenterol 88(Suppl):S66–S77, 1994.
12. Knyrim K, Wagner HJ, Pausch J, et al: A prospective, randomized, controlled trial of metal stents for malignant obstruction of the common bile duct. Endoscopy 25:207–212, 1993.
13. Lans JI, Geenen JE, Johanson JF, Hogan WJ: Endoscopic therapy in patients with pancreas divisum and acute pancreatitis: A prospective, randomized, controlled clinical trial. Gastrointest Endosc 38:430–434, 1992.
14. Loperfido S, Angelini G, Benedetti G, et al: Major early complications from diagnostic and therapeutic ERCP: A prospective multicenter study. Gastrointest Endosc 48:1–10, 1998.
15. Lehman GA, Sherman S, Hisi R, Hawes RH: Pancreas divisum: Results of minor papilla sphincterotomy. Gastrointest Endosc 39:1–8, 1993.
16. Motte S, Deviere J, Dumonceau JM, et al: Risk factors for septicemia following endoscopic biliary stenting. Gastroenterology 101:1374–1381, 1991.
17. Ortner MJ, Liebetruth J, Schreiber S, et al: Photodynamic therapy of nonresectable cholangiocarcinoma. Gastroenterology 114:536–542, 1998.
18. Richter JM, Schapiro RH, Mulley AG, Warshaw AL: Association of pancreas divisum and pancreatitis, and its treatment by sphincteroplasty of the accessory ampulla. Gastroenterology 81:1104–1110, 1981.
19. Roszler MH, Campbell WL: Post-ERCP pancreatitis: Association with urographic visualization during ERCP. Radiology 157:595–598, 1985.
20. Sherman S, Lehman GA: ERCP-and endoscopic sphincterotomy-induced pancreatitis. Pancreas 6:350–367, 1991.
21. Sherman S, Ruffolo TA, Hawes R, Lehman G: Complications of endoscopic sphincterotomy: A prospective series with emphasis on the increased risk associated with sphincter of Oddi dysfunction and nondilated bile ducts. Gastroenterology 101:1068–1075, 1991.
22. Tweedle DEF, Martin DF: Needle knife papillotomy for endoscopic sphincterotomy and cholangiography. Gastrointest Endosc 37:518–521, 1991.
23. Yeoh KG, Zimmerman MJ, Cunningham JT, Cotton PB: Comparative costs of metal versus plastic biliary stent strategies for malignant obstructive jaundice by decision analysis. Gastrointest Endosc 49:466–471, 1999.

VIII. Surgery and the GI Tract

79. SURGERY OF THE ESOPHAGUS

Amjad Ali, M.D., and Carlos A. Pellegrini, M.D.

GASTROESOPHAGEAL REFLUX DISEASE

1. Define gastroesophageal reflux disease (GERD).

GERD is best defined as symptoms and/or esophageal mucosal injury due to the abnormal reflux of gastric contents into the esophagus. One-third of the U.S. population suffers from symptoms of GERD at least once monthly, and 4–7% experience daily symptoms. Although there is a high prevalance of heartburn, not everyone with heartburn has GERD.

2. What is the natural history of reflux esophagitis?

Reflux esophagitis is the damage (visible on endoscopy) that occurs to the mucosa of the esophagus as a consequence of abnormal (high) amounts of gastroesophageal reflux. Although all patients with reflux esophagitis have GERD, not all patients with GERD have reflux esophagitis. The few studies of the natural history of reflux esophagitis involve patients who received some form of therapy. In one of the most detailed studies, Monnier et al. did an intensive endoscopic follow-up of a defined population of 959 patients over a 30-year period. They included only patients who had esophagitis on endoscopy and excluded patients who had symptoms without mucosal injury. In about 45% of patients esophagitis developed as an isolated episode and did not recur as long as the patient was taking acid suppression therapy. In the remaining patients, esophagitis intermittently recurred during acid suppression therapy. Esophagitis progressed during therapy to more severe mucosal injury in 42% of patients. The study also showed that 18% of the initial population, while on therapy and within as short a period as 6 weeks, acquired Barrett's esophagus with intestinal metaplasia.

3. Describe the typical and atypical symptoms of GERD.

The **most common complaints** in patients with GERD are heartburn, regurgitation, and occasionally, dysphagia (more precisely, the sensation of blockage to the passage of food in the lower substernal area).

Atypical or extraesophageal symptoms include cough, asthma, hoarseness, and noncardiac chest pain, which may manifest with or without associated heartburn and regurgitation. Atypical symptoms are the primary complaint in 20–25% of patients with GERD and are secondarily associated with heartburn and regurgitation in many more. Studies have shown that nearly 50% of patients with chest pain and negative coronary angiograms, 75% of patients with chronic hoarseness, and up to 80% of patients with asthma have a positive 24-hour esophageal pH test, indicating abnormal acid reflux into the esophagus. However, it is considerably more difficult to prove a cause-and-effect relationship between atypical symptoms and gastroesophageal reflux than it is for the typical symptoms. Many patients with atypical symptoms benefit from antireflux surgery, but surgery results are not as good as for patients with typical symptoms. A trial of proton-pump inhibitors (PPIs) helps to determine which patients will benefit from antireflux surgery. Those whose symptoms are controlled by PPIs are more likely to benefit from antireflux surgery.

4. What is Barrett's esophagus? What are the risk factors for Barrett's esophagus?

Barrett's esophagus is metaplasia of the normally squamous endothelium of the esophagus into columnar endothelium with intestinal metaplasia (goblet cells). It is a premalignant condition.

Prospective studies have determined that the risk of developing esophageal adenocarcinoma in the presence of long-segment Barrett's esophagus is approximately 1 per 100 patient years or 1% per year. This translates into a 5-10% lifetime risk. Factors leading to Barrett's esophagus include (1) early-onset GERD, (2) abnormal lower esophageal sphincter (LES) and low amplitude of esophageal peristalsis, and (3) mixed reflux of gastric and duodenal contents into the esophagus. Direct measurement of esophageal bilirubin exposure as a marker for duodenal juice indicates positive results in 58% of patients with GERD. This finding is related most closely to Barrett's esophagus.

5. What factors play a primary role in altering the gastroesophageal (GE) barrier?

Although several factors have been identified, the two most important are hypotension of the LES and loss of the angle of His due to hiatal hernia. Either may contribute to loss of competency and thus abnormal reflux. Hypotension of the LES may take the form of transient loss of the high-pressure zone due to relaxation of the LES. Gastroesophageal reflux results from the loss of the high-pressure zone normally created by the tonic contraction of the smooth muscle fibers of the LES. Physiologic reflux or reflux in early diseases result from this transient relaxation. In severe GERD, the high-pressure zone is permanently reduced or nonexistent.

A large hiatal hernia alters the geometry of the GE junction, and the angle of His is lost. There is a close relationship between the degree of gastric distention necessary to overcome the high-pressure zone and the morphology of the gastric cardia. In patients with an intact angle of His, more gastric dilatation and higher intragastric pressure are necessary to "open" the sphincter than in patients with a hiatal hernia. This explains the association of hiatal hernia with gastroesophageal reflux. A hiatal hernia also may result in hypotension of the LES. Therefore, hiatal hernia may alter the geometry of the GE junction and also the competence of the LES. However, every patient with a hiatal hernia does not have gastroesophageal reflux, and the presence of a small sliding hiatal hernia without gastroesophageal reflux is not an indication for medical or surgical intervention.

6. Describe the role of 24-hour pH monitoring in the management of patients with GERD.

It provides the most direct method of assessing the presence and severity of GERD and, because it has the highest sensitivity and specificity of all available tests, has become the gold standard for the diagnosis of GERD. It is especially useful in the evaluation of patients with atypical symptoms and patients with typical symptoms but no evidence of esophagitis on endoscopy. The test also measures the correlation between symptoms and episodes of reflux. This information can be used to predict the success of treatment.

7. What is the role of esophageal manometry in the management of patients with GERD?

Esophageal manometry evaluates the peristaltic function of the esophagus and the pressure of the LES. It is not a diagnostic test but provides information about the severity of the underlying physiologic defects of the LES and esophageal body. It also determines the location of the LES for proper placement of 24-hour pH probes (i.e., 5 cm above the LES.)

8. Describe the role of radiology in the management of GERD.

Barium swallow can be used to diagnose the complications of advanced GERD, including peptic strictures, but its most important role is in preoperative evaluation. The study is used to assess the size and reducibility of a hiatal hernia and the presence of esophageal shortening. It also evaluates the propulsive action of the esophagus for both liquids and solids. A large, fixed hiatal hernia and a short esophagus are evidence of advanced disease and may predict a long, difficult operation.

9. What is the role of upper endoscopy in the management of GERD?

Endoscopic visualization of the esophagus helps to identify the presence of esophagitis and Barrett's esophagus. It also can be used to evaluate response to treatment and to detect complications of GERD, including a peptic stricture and shortened esophagus. These findings influence therapeutic decisions. Finally, endoscopy provides valuable information about the absence of other lesions in the upper GI tract that can produce symptoms identical to those of GERD.

10. What is the significance of a defective LES?

The finding of a permanently defective LES (LES pressure < 6 mmHg) has several implications. First, it is almost always associated with esophageal mucosal injury and predicts that symptoms will be difficult to control with medical therapy. It is a signal that surgical therapy is probably needed for consistent, long-term control. When the LES is permanently defective, the condition is irreversible even when the associated esophagitis has healed. The worse the esophageal injury, the more likely it is that the LES is defective. Approximately 40% of patients with pH-positive GERD and no mucosal injury have a mechanically defective LES, whereas nearly 100% of patients with long-segment Barrett's esophagus have a defective LES.

11. What is the significance of abnormal esophageal motility in patients with GERD?

Longstanding, severe GERD can lead to deterioration of esophageal body function. Abnormalities of esophageal body function can present as a lack of peristalsis, severely disordered peristalsis (> 50% simultaneous contractions), or ineffective peristalsis (the amplitude of the contractions in one or more of the lower esophageal segments is < 20 mmHg). Dysphagia is a prominent symptom in patients with defective peristalsis. A partial fundoplication may be preferable in patients with poor esophageal motility. A poor result after fundoplication may be due to defective emptying of the esophagus secondary to persistence of poor esophageal propulsive function.

12. Summarize the principles of medical treatment of GERD.

Initial therapy for GERD includes lifestyle changes. Patients should be advised to elevate the head of the bed; avoid tight clothing; eat small, frequent meals; avoid eating the nighttime meal shortly before retiring; lose weight; and avoid alcohol, coffee, chocolate, and peppermints, all of which may aggravate symptoms. Alginic acid, in combination with simple antacids, may give symptomatic relief by creating a physical barrier to reflux as well as by acid reduction.

Patients with moderate-to-severe disease need more intensive pharmacotherapy. The mainstay of medical therapy is acid suppression. Esophageal acid exposure is reduced by up to 80% with H_2-receptor antagonists and up to 95% with PPIs. In patients with persistent symptoms, PPIs such as omeprazole, in doses as high as 40 mg/day, may be needed to cause an 80–90% reduction in gastric acidity. This is usually sufficient to heal mild esophagitis. The rate of healing is influenced by the degree of esophagitis and the dose of the drug. In general, the dose needed to heal esophagitis and relieve symptoms is the dose required to maintain remission. Healing may occur in only three-fourths of patients with severe esophagitis. Even with PPI therapy, periods of acid breakthrough can occur, most commonly during the night time. For this reason, it often is best to split the dose. Acid breakthrough may occur in the absence of symptoms and may be responsible for persistent esophagitis in some patients.

13. What are the indications for an antireflux operation?

• Complications of GERD, including erosive esophagitis, stricture, and Barrett's esophagus
• Dependent on proton pump inhibitors for symptom relief, even without mucosal injury
• Atypical or respiratory symptoms that respond well to intensive medical treatment
• Need for long-term medical therapy, particularly if escalating doses of PPIs are needed to control symptoms
• Young age with onset of disease in infancy

The operation also is indicated for younger patients (< 50 years of age) who are noncompliant with a drug regimen or for whom medications are a financial burden and for patients who prefer a single intervention to long-term drug treatment. Surgery may be the treatment of choice in patients who are at high risk of progression despite medical therapy. Although this population is not well defined, risk factors that predict progressive disease and poor response to medical therapy include:

• Nocturnal reflux on 24-hour esophageal pH study
• Structurally deficient LES (LES pressure < 6 mmHg)
• Mixed reflux of gastric and duodenal juice
• Mucosal injury at presentation

14. What are the important technical steps of an antireflux operation?

Most antireflux operations are now performed through a laparoscopic technique. Five trocars are inserted in the upper abdomen to provide access to the laparoscope and instruments. The short gastric vessels are divided in the proximal part of the stomach, and the fundus of the stomach is mobilized so that it can be placed around the distal esophagus without tension. Dissection is performed to identify the right and left crura of the diaphragm. The distal esophagus is mobilized so that at least 3 cm of the distal esophagus lies without tension in the abdomen. The crura are approximated with nonabsorbable sutures, and the fundoplication is constructed around the distal esophagus. A 52-French bougie is placed in the esophagus to prevent a tight fundoplication. Some surgeons anchor the wrap to the crura of the diaphragm and to the esophagus to prevent it from slipping into the chest.

15. List the predictors of successful antireflux surgery.

1. Abnormal score on 24-hour esophageal pH monitoring
2. Typical symptoms of GERD (heartburn and regurgitation)
3. Symptomatic improvement in response to acid suppression therapy before surgery

Each of these factors helps to establish that GERD is the cause of the symptoms. They have little to do with severity of the disease.

16. What are the predictors of poor outcome after antireflux surgery?

Most patients with GERD have relatively mild disease and normal esophageal body function and length without stricture or scarring. They do well. The presence of GI symptoms other than typical GERD symptoms predicts less than optimal results. A large hiatal hernia, stricture with persistent dysphagia, and Barrett's are characteristics of advanced GERD and predict less than ideal results.

17. Explain the benefits of surgical treatment of GERD.

Antireflux procedures provide several benefits that cannot be accomplished with antacid medications. A successful operation augments the LES and repairs the hiatal hernia. It prevents the reflux of both gastric and duodenal juice, thus preventing aspiration. Antireflux operations also improve esophageal body motility and speed gastric emptying, which often is subclinically delayed in patients with GERD. Most patients (> 90%) are relieved of symptoms, eat unrestricted diets, and are satisfied with the outcome of surgery. These results have been shown to hold true on long-term follow-up.

18. Discuss the complications of laparoscopic fundoplication.

Improvements in technology have led to the successful application of the laparoscopic surgical approach for the treatment of GERD over the past 10 years. A laparoscopic antireflux operation is associated with significantly reduced postoperative pain, shorter hospitalization, quicker recovery, and improved cosmesis. The overall incidence of complications after laparoscopic Nissen fundoplication is 8% (range: 2–13%). Most complications are minor and include urinary retention, postoperative gastric distention, and superficial wound infections. Mild early dysphagia is common (15–20% of patients), but the incidence of residual dysphagia after 3 months is < 5%. Fewer than 1% of these patients need intervention to treat dysphagia. The incidence of serious complications is < 1%, and mortality is extremely rare (< 1%).

19. Is antireflux surgery cost-effective?

Yes. Three cost-utility analyses from the U.S. and Europe have shown that the cost of open or laparoscopic surgery is less than the cost of lifelong daily therapy with PPIs. Even for men as old as 65–69 years, the cost of lifelong omeprazole (20 or 40 mg/day) exceeds the costs of either open or laparoscopic surgery. The point at which the cost of medical therapy equals the cost of surgical treatment is 4 years for open surgery and 17 months for laparoscopic fundoplication. Laparoscopic fundoplication is the most cost-effective treatment for patients likely to need lifelong therapy.

ACHALASIA

20. Define achalasia. What are the classic findings of esophageal achalasia?

Achalasia means "failure to relax" in Greek. The disease is characterized by the triad of (1) incomplete or absent relaxation in the LES, (2) progressive loss of peristalsis in the body of the esophagus, and (3) resultant esophageal dilatation.

21. What are the most common symptoms of achalasia?

All patients with achalasia have a history of **dysphagia**. Many patients describe exacerbation of dysphagia when they drink cold liquids or are under emotional stress. Patients accumulate food in the esophagus until the hydrostatic pressure at the bottom of the column overcomes the resistance of the LES and pushes some food into the stomach. The sensation of dysphagia disappears over time in some patients as the esophagus becomes distended and food collects in the distended esophagus instead of passing into the stomach. At that stage patients may develop **heartburn** due to bacterial fermentation of retained food in the esophagus. Two-thirds of patients with achalasia experience **regurgitation** and may present with aspiration pneumonia. Distinguishing regurgitation from vomiting may be difficult at times. Regurgitation generally occurs during or at the end of a meal, and the regurgitated material tastes bland rather than sour or bitter. Such patients are usually slow eaters and frequently have to leave the table to regurgitate. Regurgitation during sleep may cause coughing and in some instances staining of the pillows. It often leads to aspiration. One-third to one-half of patients suffer from **chest pain**. Symptoms usually are present for several years before the diagnosis is made. Some patients develop a distal esophageal diverticulum as a result of chronic distal obstruction and are at a higher risk of esophageal perforation with pneumatic dilatation.

22. Describe the radiologic findings in achalasia.

Radiologic findings depend on the stage of the disease. Nonspecific findings on chest x-ray include mediastinal widening, presence of an air-fluid level in the mid-esophagus, absence of a gastric air bubble, and abnormal pulmonary markings due to chronic aspiration. The barium upper GI study is normal in the early stages, but as the disease progresses it shows a dilated, tortuous or sigmoid esophagus with air-fluid level. When the cardia is well visualized, it typically has a narrow, tapering bird's beak appearance. This appearance also may be seen in patients with pseudoachalasia. The inability to push swallowed air into the stomach leads to the absence of a gastric air bubble.

23. What is the role of endoscopy in the diagnosis of achalasia?

Endoscopy reveals a dilated tortuous esophagus with residual liquid or food in the lumen. Esophagitis discovered during endoscopy is usually a result of fermentation of esophageal contents in untreated cases or of gastroesophageal reflux in patients previously treated for achalasia. The LES appears puckered and does not open with air insufflation; however, unlike a stricture, it permits the passage of the endoscope with a characteristic popping sensation. Endoscopy also picks up yeast esophagitis, which can obliterate the submucosal plane due to inflammation and scarring and can contaminate the mediastinum in case of an accidental perforation of the esophagus. Therefore, yeast esophagitis should be treated aggressively with oral antifungal agents before achalasia is treated. Endoscopy also identifies patients at a higher risk of esophageal perforation with balloon dilatation due to the presence of a hiatal hernia or an epiphrenic diverticulum.

24. Discuss the role of esophageal manometry in the diagnosis of achalasia.

Manometry is the gold standard for diagnosing achalasia. There are four classic features of achalasia on manometry, but all four are *not* always present:

1. **Incomplete relaxation of the LES** is the most characteristic finding (80% of patients). Normally the LES relaxes 100% (i.e., to the level of the gastric baseline) during swallowing. In patients with achalasia relaxation is incomplete. However, interpretation of LES relaxation may be misleading if the tip of the manometry catheter is placed in the lower part of the LES. Upward movement of the LES during swallowing brings the tip of the catheter briefly into the stomach and gives a false impression of relaxation. It is important to place the transducer in the proximal part of the LES.

2. **Lack of peristalsis** in the distal (smooth-muscle) segment of the esophagus. Typical peristaltic waves are of very low amplitude, and peristalsis is absent in patients with a massively distended esophagus. It may be impossible to pass the manometry catheter through the LES even under fluoroscopy. In such patients an esophageal body study demonstrating lack of peristalsis is sufficient documentation to proceed with treatment.

3. **Elevated LES pressure.** Most patients have elevated (> 25 mmHg) LES pressure. Although LES pressure may be normal, it is usually not subnormal in untreated achalasia.

4. **Positive intraesophageal body pressure.** Normal intraesophageal pressure is subatmospheric. But in patients with achalasia it is positive as a result of outflow obstruction and retention of food and secretions.

25. What is pseudoachalasia? How is it diagnosed?

Characteristic manometric and radiologic findings of achalasia occasionally may be seen in patients with distal esophageal obstruction from an infiltrating tumor. Such patients have a local tumor that may directly compress the esophagus or a remote tumor (causing paraneoplastic syndrome). Endoscopy helps to rule out the possibility of pseudoachalasia, but careful examination of the GE junction with the scope retroflexed is required to avoid missing a small cancer. However, endoscopy cannot rule out pseudoachalasia caused by a mural or extramural tumor. When this is suspected based on the history (rapid weight loss, weight loss > 20 lb, or symptoms with duration < 6 months), endoscopic ultrasonography is recommended.

26. Explain vigorous achalasia.

Chest pain is a common complaint in patients with a variant of the disease called vigorous achalasia. Such patients have high-amplitude, simultaneous esophageal contractions. They usually are younger and have chest pain as a prominent symptom. Most investigators believe that vigorous achalasia is an early form of the disease. The cut-off pressure for esophageal contractions used by most experts is 40 mmHg. Patients with nonreduced pressure waves > 40 mmHg are classified as having vigorous achalasia, whereas those with esophageal body pressure waves < 40 mm Hg are said to have classic achalasia.

27. What studies other than esophageal manometry can be used to diagnose achalasia?

In many patients, the esophageal manometry catheter cannot negotiate the tight LES, and some patients cannot tolerate esophageal intubations. In such patients, a radio-labeled semisolid meal has been used to assess esophageal emptying and peristalsis. This study is less specific than manometry but is noninvasive and also can be used to assess treatment response. A timed barium swallow has been suggested by de Oliveira et al. as a simple and reproducible alternative. The patient ingests 100–200 ml of low-density barium over 30–45 seconds. Three-on-one spot x-ray films are obtained at 1, 2, and 5 minutes after ingestion. The degree of emptying is estimated qualitatively by comparing the 1- and 5-minute films. The degree of emptying also may be estimated quantitatively by measuring the height and width of the barium column for both films, calculating the area for both, and determining the percentage of change in the area. Both qualitative and quantitative assessments are accurate methods of estimating esophageal emptying.

28. Describe the role of smooth muscle relaxants in the treatment of achalasia.

Smooth muscle relaxants, including long-acting nitrates and calcium channel blockers, are the mainstay of medical treatment. They act by reducing the LES tone. A number of non–placebo-controlled trials based on small patient populations have shown satisfactory response to long-acting nitrates and calcium channel blockers. However, because these results have not been reproduced by other investigators, their use is limited to mild cases or patients unsuitable for mechanical or surgical therapies. Recently sildenafil (Viagra) has been shown to reduce LES pressure in patients with achalasia. Sildenafil augments the smooth muscle relaxation caused by nitric oxide. The role of this new modality in the treatment of achalasia remains to be defined.

29. What is the role of mechanical esophageal dilatation in achalasia?

Dilatation of the LES is widely used for treatment of achalasia. The type of dilators and the technique of dilatation have improved considerably over the past 4 decades. A comparison of pneumatic dilatation with the mercury bougie in patients with Chagas' disease who were followed for 1 year after dilatation showed a 65% decrease in LES pressure after pneumatic dilatation vs. a 15% decrease after dilatation with the mercury bougie. Other studies have shown similar results and have established pneumatic dilatation as the standard for treating achalasia.

Dilatation to a diameter of at least 3 cm (> 90 French) is recommended to achieve long-term results. Low-compliance balloon (LCB) dilators such as the Rigiflex and Witzel systems are preferred over high-compliance balloons (HCB) to minimize the risk of esophageal rupture. LCB dilators have a maximal designated diameter, and further inflation results in an increase in the pressure within the balloon lumen only. Because HCB dilators adapt to the surrounding esophagus, esophageal wall tension increases in the more dilated esophagus proximal to the obstruction, thus increasing the risk of perforation. However, a recent trial comparing LCB and HCB dilators found no significant difference in complication rate or clinical outcome. The Rigiflex pneumatic dilatation is performed under fluoroscopic guidance; the Witzel balloon dilator allows endoscopic positioning of the balloon without fluoroscopy.

30. Discuss the complications of mechanical esophageal dilatation.

Immediate complications include intramural hematoma, GI bleeding, and esophageal perforation. Because most complications occur within 6 hours after the procedure, patients should be closely observed during that period. The most feared complication is esophageal perforation (reported incidence: 1–13%). Factors that increase the risk of esophageal perforation include massively dilated esophagus, large hiatal hernia, and an epiphrenic diverticulum. Other factors include the aggressiveness with which dilatation is performed and the size of the balloon. Patients with suspected esophageal perforation should undergo a gastrografin swallow, followed by a barium swallow if no leak is identified. Some patients with localized perforation may be managed conservatively with bowel rest and broad-spectrum antibiotics, but most patients need an emergency thoracotomy.

31. What are the long-term results of mechanical esophageal dilatation?

The reported success rate in terms of resolution of dysphagia is 60–80%. Relief is immediate for most patients. However, long-term results show that only 60% of patients are in remission at 1 year and more than one-half develop recurrent symptoms by 5 years. A second session of esophageal dilatation is equally effective in patients who respond to the first dilatation, but the chance of success in patients who did not respond to the first dilatation is < 20%. The success rate of esophageal myotomy is no different in patients with prior pneumatic dilatation, but dissection and myotomy may occasionally be technically more challenging. Patients younger than 40 years have a lower success rate with esophageal dilatation. Postprocedure gastroesophageal reflux has been reported in 2–30% of patients but responds well to medical therapy.

32. What is the role of botulinum toxim (Botox) in the treatment of achalasia?

Botox injection of the LES sphincter is a newer adaptation of successful treatment of skeletal muscle disorders. Botox is a potent inhibitor of acetylcholine release from presynaptic nerve terminals. The proposed mechanism of action is reduction in cholinergic excitation. Early clinical trial results were encouraging. Pasricha et al. reported an immediate clinical response in 28 of 31 (90%) patients. However, the results were not nearly as good on follow-up. Treatment failure (lack of initial response or rapid relapse) was observed in 14 patients. Sustained remission at 6-month follow-up was seen in only 20 of 31 (65%). Among patients who responded to the treatment, the probability of remaining in remission at 1 year was 68%, and the average duration of sustained response was 1.3 years. Patients who were older and had symptoms characteristic of vigorous achalasia were found to respond significantly better than younger patients and patients with classic achalasia. Other studies have reported similar results. At this point Botox therapy is an option for debilitated patients who are unable to tolerate balloon dilatation or surgical myotomy.

33. How is botulinum toxin useful in patients with an unclear presentation?

Botulinum toxin recently has been used in the diagnosis and management of three groups of patients with an unclear presentation: (1) patients with symptoms consistent with achalasia but insufficient manometric criteria to make the diagnosis; (2) patients in whom factors in addition to achalasia contribute to symptoms, and (3) patients with advanced achalasia in whom it is not clear whether sphincter-directed therapy would be of benefit before consideration of esophagectomy. The short duration of the action of Botox can be used to the advantage of such patients because little harm is done if the injection does not help to relieve symptoms. Other advantages include minimal morbidity and ease of administration.

34. What are the disadvantages of botulinum toxin for treatment of achalasia?

Preoperative use of Botox increases the technical difficulties of esophagomyotomy and thus its potential risks. Because successful dilatation disrupts the muscularis in only one area, healing and scarring are limited to that area of the esophageal wall. Botox, on the other hand, is injected at multiple sites, and injections are frequently repeated. This repeated injury causes the muscularis and the mucosa to seal the area and eliminate the plane that the surgeon needs to developed for a satisfactory esophageal myotomy.

35. Describe the role of esophageal myotomy in the treatment of achalasia.

Surgical treatment of achalasia consists of a longitudinal myotomy of the distal esophagus and GE junction. Most myotomies were performed through the chest in the U.S. before the advent of minimally invasive surgery. A transabdominal laparoscopic approach is gaining wider acceptance. Both laparoscopic and thoracoscopic approaches are well established and offer the benefits of minimally invasive surgery. However, the thoracoscopic approach requires double-lumen endotracheal intubation with collapse of the left lung. The rigid nature of the chest wall obviates the need for gas insufflation, but thoracoscopy does not offer an axial alignment of the operating instruments with the esophagus (as in the laparoscopic approach) and makes dissection and suturing more difficult. This problem is increased at the most distal part of the dissection, which is seen less clearly during a thoracoscopic myotomy. Finally, conversion to an open procedure is associated with much more morbidity in the chest than in the abdomen.

36. What are the basic components of laparoscopic Heller myotomy for achalasia?

Five trocars are placed in the upper abdomen in an arrangement similar to that of a laparoscopic antireflux operation. A myotomy roughly 6–8 cm in length is performed, with 2–3 cm below the GE junction. The myotomy is carried down to the level of the mucosa. A partial antireflux wrap is performed after the completion of the myotomy around a 52-French bougie.

There is a general consensus that a complete 360° wrap may cause significant obstruction at the distal end of esophagus and lead to worsening of esophageal function in patients who already have impaired peristalsis. Therefore, most experts favor a partial fundoplication after laparoscopic Heller myotomy. The two types of partial wraps—partial posterior wrap (Toupet fundoplication) and partial anterior wrap (Dor fundoplication)—are equally popular among surgeons performing a laparoscopic transabdominal myotomy. The incidence of gastroesophageal reflux after surgery for achalasia is 25–48% but with the addition of an antireflux wrap the rate decreases to 5–10%. Most of these patients have mild-to-moderate reflux and can be managed medically.

37. How do the long-term results of Heller myotomy compare with mechanical esophageal dilatation?

Many retrospective studies have compared the outcome of surgery (open or minimally invasive) with balloon dilatation. Most have shown superior long-term results with surgery. Repeat pneumatic dilatations increase the effectiveness of dilatation from 66% to 80%, but they also increase the risk of esophageal perforation by 2–3-fold. Younger patients (< 30 years) should be treated primarily with myotomy because pneumatic dilatation is < 50% effective.

38. Describe the complications of Heller myotomy.

Laparoscopic Heller myotomy is a very low-risk operation. The most common complication is perforation of the mucosa, which can be solved by immediate closure. The most feared early complication is an unrecognized esophageal perforation, but the incidence is < 1%. Perforation should be suspected in a patient with persistent fever and left-sided pleural effusion.

Early postoperative dysphagia usually results from an incomplete myotomy. Late dysphagia results from an incomplete myotomy, healing of the myotomy, or, more rarely, a reflux-induced peptic stricture. Incomplete myotomy usually responds to extension of the myotomy. Patients with late dysphagia are difficult to treat, especially in the presence of LES pressure < 10 mmHg. The cause of dysphagia is extremely poor esophageal body function or a peptic stricture. Further division of the LES may be of benefit; pneumatic dilatation or even Botox injection also may be effective. Takedown of the wrap may be useful as well. A second myotomy is less likely to be successful; such patients often need esophageal resection.

29. Describe the association between achalasia and cancer of the esophagus.

Achalasia is a premalignant condition. One study found that 5% of patients develop squamous cell cancer of the esophagus within 20 years after the diagnosis of achalasia. Tumors develop at an age 10 years younger than in the general population and carry a worse prognosis because of late diagnosis. Surveillance endoscopy is recommended every 2 years by some authors. A change in the esophageal mucosa to a "tree bark" appearance should increase the suspicion of cancer. The effect of treatments on the incidence of cancer is not known.

30. Summarize the approach to patients with symptoms of achalasia.

Most patients with achalasia are seen by gastroenterologists and referred for surgery after failure of pneumatic dilatation or Botox injections. Every patient with suspicion of achalasia should undergo (1) esophageal manometry, (2) barium upper GI study, and (3) upper endoscopy. Patients with shorter duration of symptoms and a history of substantial weight loss (> 20 lbs in 6 months) also should undergo endoscopic ultrasonography to rule out the possibility of pseudo achalasia. Laparoscopic Heller myotomy should be offered as early as possible to young patients (< 40 years old) with achalasia. They have a higher incidence of failure with dilatation and Botox injections, and early surgery is recommended to avoid long-term complications.

The laparoscopic approach to esophageal myotomy provides a magnified view of the operative field and allows precise division of the muscle fibers with excellent results. Laparoscopic Heller myotomy results in reduced postoperative pain, shorter hospitalization, and better cosmetic results. Pneumatic dilatation may be offered once or twice to patients with mild-to-moderate disease. However, superior long-term results after surgical myotomy argue strongly for surgery in any patient who is fit enough to undergo general anesthesia. Botox therapy should be reserved for patients who are unable to tolerate surgery because of significant comorbidities or whose clinical presentation is complicated and the diagnosis of achalasia is in doubt.

BIBLIOGRAPHY

Gastroesophageal Reflux Disease
1. Allen CJ, Anvari M: Gastro-oesophageal reflux related cough and its response to laparoscopic fundoplication. Thorax 53:963–968, 1998.
2. Andersen LI, et al: Validity of clinical symptoms in benign esophageal disease, assessed by questionnaire. Acta Med Scand 221:171–177, 1987.
3. Becker DJ, et al: A comparison of high and low fat meals on postprandial esophageal acid exposure. Am J Gastroenterol 84:782–786, 1989.
4. Reference deleted.
5. Campos GM, et al: The pattern of esophageal acid exposure in gastroesophageal reflux disease influences the severity of the disease. Arch Surg 134:882–887; discussion, 887–888, 1999.
6. Campos GM, et al: Multivariate analysis of factors predicting outcome after laparoscopic Nissen fundoplication. J Gastrointest Surg 3:292–300, 1999.
7. Castel DO: Management of gastroesophageal reflux disease. Maintenance medical therapy of gastroesophageal reflux–which drugs, how long? Dis Esophagus 7:230–233, 1994.

8. Collet D, Cadiere GB: Conversions and complications of laparoscopic treatment of gastroesophageal reflux disease. Formation for the Development of Laparoscopic Surgery for Gastroesophageal Reflux Disease Group. Am J Surg 169:622–626, 1995.
9. Costantini M, et al: The role of a defective lower esophageal sphincter in the clinical outcome of treatment for gastroesophageal reflux disease. Arch Surg 131:655–659, 1996.
10. DeMeester TR, Ireland AP: Gastric pathology as an initiator and potentiator of gastroesophageal reflux disease. Dis Esophagus 10:1–8, 1997.
11. DeVault KR, Castell DO: Guidelines for the diagnosis and treatment of gastroesophageal reflux disease. Practice Parameters Committee of the American College of Gastroenterology. Arch Intern Med 155:2165–2173, 1995.
12. Fein M, et al: Role of the lower esophageal sphincter and hiatal hernia in the pathogenesis of gastroesophageal reflux disease. J Gastrointest Surg 3:405–410, 1999.
13. Heudebert GR, et al: Choice of long-term strategy for the management of patients with severe esophagitis: A cost-utility analysis. Gastroenterology 112:1078–1086, 1997.
14. Hinder RA, et al: Laparoscopic Nissen fundoplication is an effective treatment for gastroesophageal reflux disease. Ann Surg 220:472–481; discussion, 481–483., 1994.
15. Hunter JG, et al:A physiologic approach to laparoscopic fundoplication for gastroesophageal reflux disease. Ann Surg 223:673–685; discussion, 685–687, 1996.
16. Ismail T, Bancewicz J, Barlow J: Yield pressure, anatomy of the cardia and gastro-oesophageal reflux. Br J Surg 82:943–947, 1995.
17. Johnson WE, et al: Outcome of respiratory symptoms after antireflux surgery on patients with gastroesophageal reflux disease. Arch Surg 131:489–492, 1996.
18. Johnson LF, DeMeester TR: Evaluation of elevation of the head of the bed, bethanechol, and antacid form tablets on gastroesophageal reflux. Dig Dis Sci 26:673–680, 1981.
19. Katzka DA, et al: Prolonged ambulatory pH monitoring in patients with persistent gastroesophageal reflux disease symptoms: Testing while on therapy identifies the need for more aggressive anti-reflux therapy. Am J Gastroenterol 91:2110–2113, 1996.
20. Klauser AG, Schindlbeck NE, Muller-Lissner SA: Symptoms in gastro-oesophageal reflux disease. Lancet 335:205–208, 1990.
21. Klinkenberg-Knol EC, et al: Long-term treatment with omeprazole for refractory reflux esophagitis: Efficacy and safety. Ann Intern Med 121(3):161–167, 1994.
22. Kuster E, et al: Predictive factors of the long term outcome in gastro-oesophageal reflux disease: Six year follow up of 107 patients. Gut 35:8–14, 1994.
23. Mittal RK, McCallum RW: Characteristics and frequency of transient relaxations of the lower esophageal sphincter in patients with reflux esophagitis. Gastroenterology 95:593–599, 1988.
24. Monnier OH, Fontolliet C, et al: Epidemiology and natural history of reflux esophagitis. Semin Laparosc Surg 2:2–9, 1995.
25. Nehra D, et al: Toxic bile acids in gastro-oesophageal reflux disease: Influence of gastric acidity. Gut 44:598–602, 1999.
26. Oberg S, et al: Endoscopic grading of the gastroesophageal valve in patients with symptoms of gastroesophageal reflux disease (GERD). Surg Endosc 13:1184–1188, 1999.
27. Peghini PL, et al: Nocturnal recovery of gastric acid secretion with twice-daily dosing of proton pump inhibitors. Am J Gastroenterol 93:763–767, 1998.
28. Perdikis G, et al: Laparoscopic Nissen fundoplication: Where do we stand? Surg Laparosc Endosc 7:17–21, 1997.
29. Peters JH: The surgical management of Barrett's esophagus. Gastroenterol Clin North Am 26:647–668, 1997.
30. Richter JE: Extraesophageal presentations of gastroesophageal reflux disease: The case for aggressive diagnosis and treatment. Cleve Clin J Med 64:37–45, 1997.
31. Singh P, et al: Oesophageal motor function before and after healing of oesophagitis. Gut 33:1590–1596, 1992.
32. So JB, Zeitels SM, Rattner DW: Outcomes of atypical symptoms attributed to gastroesophageal reflux treated by laparoscopic fundoplication. Surgery 124:28–32, 1998.
33. Stein HJ, et al: Complications of gastroesophageal reflux disease. Role of the lower esophageal sphincter, esophageal acid and acid/alkaline exposure, and duodenogastric reflux. Ann Surg 216:35–43, 1992.
34. Stein, HJ, et al: Circadian esophageal motor function in patients with gastroesophageal reflux disease. Surgery 108(4):769–777; discussion, 777–778, 1990.
35. Van Den Boom G, et al: Cost effectiveness of medical versus surgical treatment in patients with severe or refractory gastroesophageal reflux disease in the Netherlands. Scand J Gastroenterol 31:1–9, 1996.
36. Vigneri S, et al: A comparison of five maintenance therapies for reflux esophagitis. N Engl J Med 333: 1106–1110, 1995.
37. Viljakka M, Nevalainen J, Isolauri J: Lifetime costs of surgical versus medical treatment of severe gastro-oesophageal reflux disease in Finland. Scand J Gastroenterol 32:766–772, 1997.

Achalasia
38. Bortolotti MM, Lopilato C, Porrazzo C, et al: Effects of sildenafil on esophageal motility of patients with idiopathic achalasia. Gastroenterology118:253–257, 2000.
39. Csendes A, et al: Late results of a prospective randomised study comparing forceful dilatation and oesophagomyotomy in patients with achalasia [see comments]. Gut 30:299–304, 1989.
40. de Oliveira JM, et al: Timed barium swallow: A simple technique for evaluating esophageal emptying in patients with achalasia. AJR 169:473–479, 1997.
41. Eckardt VF, Bernhard G: Predictors of outcome in patients with achalasia treated by pneumatic dilation. Gastroenterology 103:1732, 1992.
42. Horgan S, Pellegrini CA: Botulinum toxin injections for achalasia symptoms [editorial; comment]. Am J Gastroenterol 94:300–301, 1999.
43. Hunter JG, Richardson WS: Surgical management of achalasia. Surg Clin North Am 77:993–1015, 1997.

44. Katzka DA, Castell DO: Use of botulinum toxin as a diagnostic/therapeutic trial to help clarify an indication for defini-
    tive therapy in patients with achalasia. Am J Gastroenterol 94:637–642, 1999.
45. Meijssen MAC, Van Blakenstein M, et al: Achalasia complicated by esophageal squamous cell carcinoma. A prospective
    study in 195 patients. Gut 33(155), 1992.
46. Moonka R, et al: Clinical presentation and evaluation of malignant pseudoachalasia. J Gastrointest Surg 3:456–461, 1999.
47. Moonka R, Pellegrini CA: Malignant pseudoachalasia. Surg Endosc 13:273–275, 1999.
48. Muehldorfer SM, Hahn EG, Ell C: High- and low-compliance balloon dilators in patients with achalasia: A randomized
    prospective comparative trial. Gastrointest Endosc 44:398–403, 1996.
49. Paricio PP, Ortiz A, Aguayo JL: Achalasia of the cardia: Long-term results of esophagomyotomy and posterior partial
    fundoplication. Br J Surg 77:1371–1374, 1990.
50. Parkman HP, Ouyang A, et al: Pneumatic dilatation or esophagomyotomy treatment for idiopathic achalasia: Clinical
    outcomes and cost analysis. Dig Dis Sci 38:75, 1993.
51. Pasricha PJ, et al: Treatment of achalasia with intrasphincteric injection of botulinum toxin. A pilot trial. Ann Intern Med
    121:590–591, 1994.
52. Pasricha PJ, Hendrix TR, et al: Intrasphincteric botulinum toxin for the treatment of achalasia. N Engl J Med 322:774, 1995.
53. Pasricha PJ, Kalloo AN: Effects of intrasphincteric botulinum toxin on the lower esophageal sphincter in piglets.
    Gastroenterology 105:1045, 1993.
54. Pasricha PJ, Ravich WJ, et al: Botulinum toxin for achalasia: Long term outcome and predictors of response.
    Gastroenterology 110:1410, 1996.
55. Pellegrini C, et al: Thoracoscopic esophagomyotomy. Initial experience with a new approach for the treatment of achala-
    sia. Ann Surg 216:291–296; discussion, 296–299, 1992.
56. Raizman RE, Neva FA: A clinical trial with pre and post treatment manometry comparing pneumatic dilation with
    bougienage for treatment of achalasia. Am J Gastroenterol 74:405, 1980.
57. Spiess AE, Kahrilas PJ: Treating achalasia: from whalebone to laparoscope. JAMA 280:638–642, 1998.
58. Vaezi MF, et al: Botulinum toxin versus pneumatic dilatation in the treatment of achalasia: A randomised trial. Gut
    44:231–239, 1999.
59. Vaezi MF, Baker ME, Richter JE: Assessment of esophageal emptying post-pneumatic dilation: Use of the timed barium
    esophagram. Am J Gastroenterol 94:1802–1807, 1999.

80. SURGERY FOR PEPTIC ULCER DISEASE

Jaimie D. Nathan, M.D., and Theodore N. Pappas, M.D.

1. Describe the classic indications and goals for peptic ulcer surgery.

Since the introduction of H_2 receptor antagonists and proton pump inhibitors and the identification of *Helicobacter pylori* as an ulcerogenic cofactor, the frequency of elective operations for peptic ulcer disease (PUD) has decreased. Operative surgery for duodenal and gastric ulcers is generally reserved for the management of complications of PUD. The classic indications for peptic ulcer surgery are intractability, perforation, bleeding, and obstruction. The three goals of surgery are (1) to eliminate the factors that contribute to ulcer occurrence, (2) to treat any complications of peptic ulcer disease, and (3) to minimize the incidence of surgical side effects.

2. Define intractability in terms of the medical treatment of PUD.

Intractability is defined as mucosal healing refractory to maximal medical therapy. The following three criteria define a refractory ulcer and are indications for operative intervention: (1) ulcer persistence after 3 months of medical therapy, (2) ulcer recurrence within 1 year despite maintenance medical therapy, and (3) ulcer disease in which cycles of prolonged activity are interrupted by brief or absent remissions.

3. What are the three most widely used operations for PUD?
1. Truncal vagotomy and drainage
2. Truncal vagotomy and antrectomy
3. Highly selective vagotomy (parietal cell vagotomy, or proximal gastric vagotomy)

4. What are the surgical options for reconstruction after antrectomy?

1. The Billroth I reconstruction consists of a gastroduodenostomy in which the anastomosis is created between the gastric remnant and the duodenum.

2. The Billroth II reconstruction consists of a gastrojejunostomy in which a side-to-side anastomosis is created between the gastric remnant and a loop of jejunum with closure of the duodenal stump.

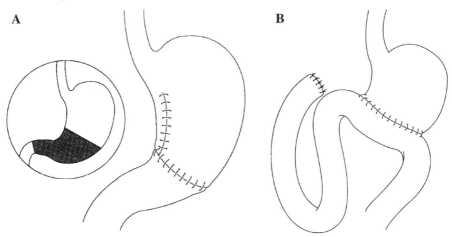

Billroth I gastroduodenostomy *(A)* and Billroth II gastrojejunostomy *(B)* reconstructions following antral resection (shaded area in inset). (From Greenfield LJ: Surgery: Scientific Principles and Practice. Philadelphia, Lippincott-Raven, 1997, p 768, with permission.)

3. The Roux-en-Y reconstruction involves the creation of a jejunojejunostomy (forming a Y-shaped figure of small bowel) downstream from the anastomosis of the free jejunal end to the gastric remnant (gastrojejunostomy).

5. How do you decide which option to use for a given patient?

The decision of which type of reconstruction to perform is determined, in part, by the extent of duodenal scarring due to PUD. Severely scarred duodenum cannot be used for an anastomosis. The Billroth I reconstruction is the most physiologic anastomosis because it restores normal continuity of the GI tract. The Billroth II reconstruction may be complicated by the afferent loop syndrome in which obstruction of the afferent limb results in accumulation of bile and pancreatic secretions, causing right upper quadrant abdominal pain that is alleviated by bilious vomiting. The Roux-en-Y reconstruction allows diversion of bile and pancreatic secretions away from the gastric outlet, thereby reducing the risk of bile reflux gastritis.

6. Why is an outlet or "drainage" procedure added to truncal vagotomy? What are the surgical options?

Truncal vagotomy involves division of both anterior and posterior vagal trunks at the esophageal hiatus. This procedure results in denervation of the acid-producing mucosa of the gastric fundus as well as the pylorus and antrum, causing alteration of normal pyloric coordination and impaired gastric emptying. Thus, a procedure to eliminate function of the pyloric sphincter must be performed to allow gastric drainage. There are four primary options for an outlet procedure:

1. **Heineke-Mikulicz pyloroplasty**, in which a longitudinal incision of the pyloric sphincter extending into the duodenum and antrum is closed transversely.

2. **Finney pyloroplasty**, which is used in cases of extensive duodenal scarring to create a wider gastroduodenal opening. A U-shaped incision crossing the pylorus is made and a gastroduodenostomy is created.

3. **Jaboulay gastroduodenostomy**, which is used when severe pyloric scarring precludes safe division of the pyloric channel. A side-to-side gastroduodenostomy is created in which the incision does not cross the pyloric sphincter.

4. **Gastrojejunostomy**

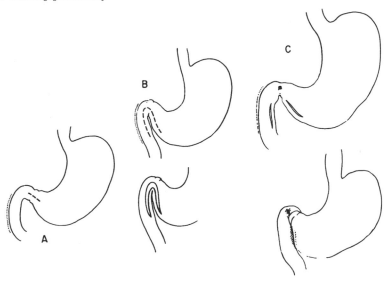

Heineke-Mikulicz pyloroplasty *(A)*, Finney pyloroplasty *(B)*, and Jaboulay gastroduodenostomy *(C)* are the primary options for an outlet or "drainage" procedure after truncal vagotomy. (From Zollinger RM: Atlas of Surgical Operations. New York, McGraw-Hill, 1993, p 41, with permission.)

7. **Describe the truncal vagotomy, selective vagotomy, and highly selective vagotomy (parietal cell vagotomy, or proximal gastric vagotomy).**

Truncal vagotomy involves division of both anterior and posterior vagal trunks at the esophageal hiatus above the origins of the hepatic and celiac branches. Periesophageal dissection must include the distal 6–8 cm of the esophagus to ensure division of gastric vagal branches that arise from the trunks above the level of the hiatus, including the "criminal nerve of Grassi," the first and highest posterior branch supplying the fundus. Thus, truncal vagotomy results in denervation of all vagally supplied viscera. A drainage procedure, usually a pyloroplasty, must be performed with truncal vagotomy, because denervation of the pylorus results in impaired gastric emptying.

Selective vagotomy involves division of the vagal trunks distal to the hepatic and celiac branches, thereby preserving vagal innervation to the gallbladder and celiac plexus and reducing the incidence of gallbladder dysmotility, gallstones, and diarrhea. Selective vagotomy also results in complete gastric vagotomy, necessitating a drainage procedure. Selective vagotomy is not the operation of choice. Most surgeons find it needlessly complex and not superior to truncal vagotomy.

Highly selective vagotomy (parietal cell vagotomy or proximal gastric vagotomy) involves selective division of the vagal fibers to the acid-producing parietal cell mass of the gastric fundus, while maintaining vagal fibers to the antrum and distal gut. The anterior and posterior neurovascular attachments are divided along the lesser curvature of the stomach, beginning approximately 7 cm from the pylorus and progressing to the gastroesophageal junction, with additional skeletalization of the distal 6–8 cm of the esophagus to ensure division of the "criminal nerve of Grassi." Innervation of the antrum and pylorus is maintained because the two terminal branches of the anterior and posterior nerves of Latarjet are left intact.

8. **What are the relative indications and contraindications to highly selective vagotomy?**

Highly selective vagotomy is indicated for the treatment of intractable duodenal ulcers because, unlike truncal vagotomy, it does not require a drainage procedure. It is also the procedure of choice in the emergent treatment of bleeding or perforated duodenal ulcers in stable patients. Highly selective vagotomy is contraindicated in patients with prepyloric ulcers or with gastric outlet obstruction, because they demonstrate high rates of recurrent ulceration. Cigarette smokers are also at high risk for recurrence and should not undergo highly selective vagotomy.

9. **Describe the five types of gastric ulcer in terms of location, gastric acid secretory status, incidence, and complications.**

Type I: located on the gastric body, typically along the lesser curvature; associated with low-to-normal acid output; about 55% of gastric ulcers. Bleeding is relatively uncommon.

Type II: located on the gastric body in combination with a duodenal ulcer; typically associated with acid hypersecretion; about 20% of gastric ulcers. Bleeding, perforation, and obstruction are frequent complications.

Type III: prepyloric ulcer; associated with acid hypersecretion; about 20% of gastric ulcers. Bleeding and perforation are frequent complications.

Type IV: located high on the lesser curvature in proximity to the gastroesophageal junction; associated with low acid secretion; < 10% of gastric ulcers. Bleeding is a frequent complication.

Type V: may be located anywhere in the stomach; secondary to chronic use of aspirin or nonsteroidal anti-inflammatory drugs; highly prone to bleeding and perforation.

10. **Describe the most appropriate operative procedure for each type of gastric ulcer.**

The choice of operation for gastric ulcers depends on several factors: ulcer location, acid secretory status, and presence of a coexistent duodenal ulcer. The operation of choice for **type I gastric ulcer** is antrectomy with inclusion of the ulcer in the resected specimen and reconstruction with a gastroduodenostomy (Billroth I). Alternatively, a gastrojejunostomy (Billroth II) may be created. Although type I gastric ulcers are associated with low-to-normal acid output, most surgeons now include a truncal vagotomy, unless achlorhydria is demonstrated. Highly selective vagotomy with ulcer excision is an alternative operation, although the rate of recurrence is significantly higher.

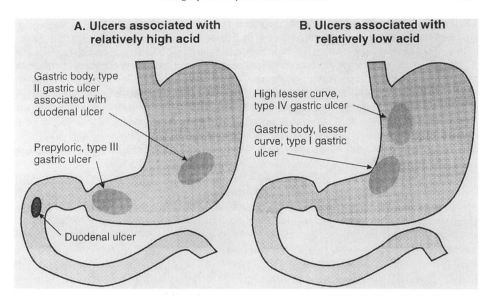

The four major types of gastric ulcers and their association with either high acid *(A)* or low acid *(B)*. (From Sabiston DC Jr: Textbook of Surgery: The Biological Basis of Modern Surgical Practice. Philadelphia, W.B. Saunders, 1997, p 854, with permission.)

Type II gastric ulcers are associated with high rates of acid secretion. Thus, the goal of operation is removal of the gastric mucosa at risk for ulceration (with inclusion of the gastric ulcer itself) and reduction of acid secretion. The procedure of choice is antrectomy with Billroth I reconstruction (with inclusion of the gastric ulcer in the resection) and truncal vagotomy. Truncal vagotomy with drainage procedure and excision of the ulcer is an acceptable alternative.

Patients with **type III gastric ulcers** are also acid hypersecretors. Truncal vagotomy and antrectomy (with inclusion of the ulcer) is the operation of choice and carries a recurrence rate of < 2%.

Type IV gastric ulcers present a challenge, because they are located high on the lesser curvature near the gastroesophageal junction. Other factors to be considered in surgical management are size and degree of adjacent inflammation. A distal gastrectomy may be performed with extension of the resection vertically to include the lesser curvature (with the ulcer), followed by a gastroduodenal anastomosis.

Type V gastric ulcers generally heal rapidly with cessation of aspirin or NSAID and institution of an H_2 receptor antagonist or proton pump inhibitor. An intractable type V gastric ulcer should raise suspicion for underlying malignancy. Surgical intervention for benign type V gastric ulcers is reserved for the treatment of complications, such as perforation or bleeding.

11. Describe the presentation of a patient with a perforated peptic ulcer.

Patients usually describe a prodrome of gnawing abdominal pain in the epigastric region prior to perforation. With acute perforation the epigastric pain becomes diffuse and often is associated with fever, tachycardia, tachypnea, and hypotension. Some patients present with GI bleeding. On examination, the patient with peptic ulcer perforation lies immobile. Bowel sounds are typically absent, and the abdomen is diffusely tender and rigid. The white blood cell count is elevated, and in 70% of cases free intraperitoneal air is found on upright abdominal x-rays. Although CT scan is the most sensitive radiologic test for free intraperitoneal air, it is rarely indicated because patients with perforated peptic ulcer usually present with classic signs and symptoms.

12. Why do almost all perforated gastric ulcers require operation?

1. Perforated gastric ulcers usually fail to heal spontaneously.

2. They are associated with a risk of adenocarcinoma.

3. Gastric ulcer disease produces a hypoacidic environment with resultant bacterial overgrowth and abscess formation after perforation.

Occasionally patients with perforated duodenal ulcer may be managed medically, particularly if the ulcer has been perforated for longer than 24 hours and a contrast study indicates that the perforation is contained.

13. What are three additional contraindications to medical management of perforated peptic ulcer disease?

1. Concurrent use of steroids, which makes healing unlikely.

2. Continued leak, as demonstrated by a contrast radiograph.

3. Perforation in a patient taking an H_2 receptor antagonist or a proton pump inhibitor. A definitive ulcer operation is required to allow ulcer healing and to reduce the risk of recurrence.

14. What are the three risk factors for mortality in the surgical treatment of perforated PUD?

(1) Severe co-morbidities, (2) perforation present for longer than 24 hours, and (3) hemodynamic instability on presentation. Patients with one of these risk factors have a mortality rate of approximately 10%; with two risk factors, the mortality rate increases to 46%. Patients with all three risk factors have a mortality rate of nearly 100%. Thus, nonsurgical management of perforated PUD should be considered strongly in elderly patients with any of these risk factors.

15. What are the three major goals of operation for perforated PUD?

(1) Closure of the perforation, which is usually performed by suturing omental fat into the defect as a patch (Graham patch); (2) copious irrigation of the abdominal cavity; and (3) definitive ulcer operation, as necessary. A patient who has had a perforation for < 24 hours and is hemodynamically stable without significant comorbidities should undergo a definitive ulcer operation if he or she has known PUD, has been receiving medical therapy for PUD, or is taking medications that increase the risk of PUD.

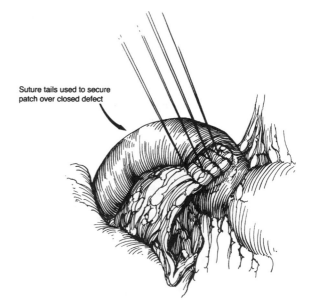

Suture tails used to secure patch over closed defect

Omental patching of a perforated peptic ulcer. (From Sabiston DC Jr: Atlas of General Surgery. Philadelphia, W.B. Saunders, 1994, p 327, with permission.)

16. What is the preferred operation for treatment of a perforated duodenal ulcer?

In patients who have undergone medical therapy to eradicate *H. pylori*, the classic operation for a perforated duodenal ulcer is truncal vagotomy and pyloroplasty with incorporation of the perforation into the pyloroplasty closure. This relatively simple procedure requires a short operative time. In the ideal surgical candidate, highly selective vagotomy with patch closure of the perforation is recommended, although this procedure requires a high degree of surgical expertise. Patients who have not been treated for *H. pylori* should undergo patch closure of a perforated duodenal ulcer with postoperative *H. pylori* eradication therapy.

17. What is the preferred operation for treatment of perforated gastric ulcer?

The major distinction between surgical management of perforated duodenal and perforated gastric ulcers is that in all cases of perforated gastric ulcers, carcinoma must be excluded. Thus, all perforated gastric ulcers must be biopsied or resected. One option is to perform a wedge resection and diagnostic biopsy. Controversy exists as to whether a definitive ulcer operation should be added to this procedure, but most surgeons perform an ulcer operation if the ulcer is a type II or type III variant. An alternative for perforated antral ulcers is antrectomy (with inclusion of the ulcer in the resection), to which truncal vagotomy may be added if the patient is an acid hypersecretor.

18. Explain the role for laparoscopy in the management of perforated PUD.

The surgical goals in the laparoscopic management of a perforated peptic ulcer are similar to those of open surgical management: (1) closure of the perforation, which is most easily performed in the setting of an anterior duodenal perforation; (2) copious irrigation and removal of enteric soilage; and (3) addition of a definitive ulcer operation, which depends on the skill of the surgeon and may involve either laparoscopic truncal vagotomy and pyloroplasty or a highly selective laparoscopic vagotomy.

19. In patients presenting with GI bleeding due to PUD, what are the predictors for rebleeding in the hospital?

- Hemodynamic instability
- Multiple comorbidities
- Hematemesis
- Hematocrit < 30
- Documented coagulopathy
- Inability to clear the stomach with aggressive lavage

Findings at endoscopy help to predict which patients are at highest risk for continued bleeding or rebleeding. Active bleeding on endoscopy is a good predictor of rebleeding. A spurting artery is associated with a rebleeding rate of 70–90%; a visible nonbleeding vessel in the ulcer bed with a rebleeding rate of 40–50%; and an adherent clot with a rebleeding rate of 10–20%.

20. What is the classic indication for operation for rebleeding after endoscopic therapy?

After endoscopic therapy for a bleeding peptic ulcer, patients who require further resuscitation with 6 units of blood should be strongly considered for surgical intervention. In general, the indications for surgical treatment of a bleeding peptic ulcer are (1) hemodynamic instability as a result of massive hemorrhage, although cardiovascular stabilization must precede surgery; (2) need for multiple transfusions due to continued bleeding; and (3) failure of nonsurgical therapy to prevent rebleeding.

21. What is the most appropriate surgical procedure for a bleeding duodenal ulcer?

Control of the ulcer bed is attained by performing a duodenotomy with direct ligation of the bleeding vessel or complete plication of the ulcer bed. If the ulcer has eroded into the gastroduodenal artery, bleeding may be profuse. A definitive ulcer operation is then performed, which may consist of either a truncal vagotomy and pyloroplasty or a truncal vagotomy and antrectomy. An alternative approach is to attain control of the bleeding duodenal ulcer via a pyloroplasty incision, in which case a truncal vagotomy completes the definitive ulcer operation. Evidence indicates no difference in mortality rates between local procedures (ulcer underrunning or vessel oversewing) and radical operations (partial gastrectomy). Reports suggest that the rate of rebleeding may be higher in patients treated with local procedures, but most of these studies have not been properly controlled.

22. What are the operative options for control of a bleeding gastric ulcer?

Bleeding gastric ulcers require excision and biopsy to rule out malignancy. Small gastric ulcers (< 2 cm) usually can be excised easily and safely, with the addition of an ulcer operation for patients who are acid hypersecretors. Large gastric ulcers, lesser curvature ulcers, bleeding ulcers associated with gastritis, and gastric ulcers that penetrate into the pancreas often require a more radical and technically demanding operation (subtotal or near-total gastrectomy) to control hemorrhage.

23. How is gastric outlet obstruction due to PUD surgically managed?

Gastric outlet obstruction can result from an acute exacerbation of PUD in the setting of chronic pyloric and duodenal scarring. Classically, such patients present with nausea, emesis, early satiety, and weight loss. Although radiologic contrast studies are useful in evaluation, upper endoscopy is critical to rule out a malignant cause of the obstruction. Operative intervention is necessary in 75% of patients presenting with gastric outlet obstruction. The two main goals of surgery are to relieve the obstruction and to perform a definitive ulcer operation. Truncal vagotomy and antrectomy with Billroth II reconstruction is performed if the duodenal stump can be safely closed. If the stump cannot be closed, a tube duodenostomy is left in place for control of secretions until the stump closes by secondary intention. An alternative is to perform a truncal vagotomy and pyloroplasty, which often requires the Finney pyloroplasty or Jaboulay gastroduodenostomy because of severe scarring. Truncal vagotomy and gastrojejunostomy may be performed if the severe scarring precludes an adequate drainage procedure via the duodenum.

24. What are the long-term outcomes and risks for complications after truncal vagotomy and drainage, truncal vagotomy and antrectomy, and highly selective vagotomy?

	TRUNCAL VAGOTOMY AND DRAINAGE (%)	TRUNCAL VAGOTOMY AND ANTRECTOMY (%)	HIGHLY SELECTIVE VAGOTOMY (%)
Mortality rate	0.5–0.8	1.5	0.05
Recurrence rate	12	1–2	10–15
Dumping	10	10–15	1–5
Diarrhea	25	20	1–5

25. How should postoperative gastroparesis be managed?

Postoperative gastroparesis typically occurs in patients who undergo surgery for gastric outlet obstruction. Such patients should receive prolonged nonoperative management. Prokinetic agents (e.g., erythromycin, metaclopramide) may be useful. The indications for reoperation are (1) early marginal ulcers refractory to medical management, (2) anatomic abnormalities of the gastric outlet, and (3) recurrent bezoar associated with weight loss.

26. Describe the management of duodenal stump disruption ("blow-out") after truncal vagotomy, antrectomy, and Billroth II reconstruction.

Patients presenting with low-grade right upper quadrant sepsis may be managed by percutaneous drainage of the abscess under radiologic guidance. An acute abdomen suggests free perforation with leakage of duodenal contents into the peritoneal cavity. Management requires reoperation for reclosure of the duodenal stump over a tube duodenostomy as well as an external drain around the tube. Mortality from stump blow-out approaches 10%.

27. What are the Visick criteria?

The Visick criteria are used to grade outcome after surgery for PUD:

Grade I   No symptoms
Grade II   Mild symptoms that do not affect daily life
Grade III Moderate symptoms that affect daily life, require treatment but are not disabling
Grade IV   Recurrent ulceration or disabling symptoms

Grades I and II are considered adequate results. Most poor outcomes fall into grade III.

28. What is the dumping syndrome? Describe its pathophysiology and treatment.

The dumping syndrome consists of tachycardia, diaphoresis, hypotension, and abdominal pain after meals in patients who have undergone ulcer operations, such as vagotomy. Its pathophysiology is loss of receptive relaxation of the fundus in response to a gastric load. Thus, gastric pressure increases during a meal, and rapid decompression through the gastric outlet procedure causes the classic signs and symptoms. Symptoms typically improve with time and can be alleviated in some patients by separation of solids and liquids during meals. Conversion of a Billroth II reconstruction to a Billroth I or a Billroth operation to a Roux-en-Y reconstruction can improve symptoms. Octreotide, a somatostatin analog, also has been used to alleviate symptoms.

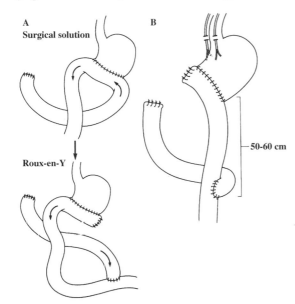

Technique for conversion of a Billroth II reconstruction to a Roux-en-Y gastrojejunostomy. After division of the afferent limb *(A)*, a jejunojejunal anastomosis is created approximately 50–60 cm distal to the original Billroth II gastrojejunostomy *(B)*. (From Greenfield LJ: Surgery: Scientific Principles and Practice. Philadelphia, Lippincott-Raven, 1997, p 772, with permission.)

29. Describe the pathophysiology of bile reflux gastritis. How is it managed?

Bile reflux gastritis occurs when ablation of the pylorus in a gastric ulcer operation results in stasis of bile in the stomach. The diagnosis is made with the following triad of findings: (1) postprandial epigastric pain accompanied by nausea and bilious emesis; (2) evidence of bile reflux into the stomach or gastric remnant; and (3) biopsy-proven gastritis. Bile reflux gastritis can occur after truncal vagotomy and pyloroplasty or truncal vagotomy and antrectomy with Billroth reconstruction. Although up to 20% of patients who undergo these operations may have transient bile reflux gastritis postoperatively, symptoms resolve in all but 1–2%.

Treatment of bile reflux gastritis requires revision of the pyloroplasty or the Billroth reconstruction to a Roux-en-Y gastrojejunostomy with a 50–60 cm limb (see figure above). Bilious emesis resolves in nearly 100% of patients who undergo revision. The symptoms of bile reflux gastritis may be indistinguishable from those of gastroparesis. Because the Roux-en-Y gastrojejunostomy worsens the symptoms of gastroparesis, care must be taken to exclude the diagnosis of gastroparesis preoperatively.

30. How do patients with Zollinger-Ellison syndrome present?

Most patients with Zollinger-Ellison syndrome present with PUD and/or diarrhea. Ulcers are typically duodenal. The diarrhea resembles steatorrhea and results from a combination of high volumes of acid and neutralization of pancreatic enzymes. In patients with Zollinger-Ellison syndrome associated with multiple endocrine neoplasia (MEN) syndrome I, signs and symptoms at presentation may be related to parathyroid or pituitary disease.

31. How is Zollinger-Ellison syndrome diagnosed?

A high level of suspicion is required for the diagnosis of gastrinoma. Serum gastrin should be measured in all patients undergoing peptic ulcer surgery. If the gastrin level is in the range of 1000–2000 pg/ml, gastric pH analysis demonstrating acid production confirms the diagnosis. If the gastrin level is minimally elevated, the patient should undergo gastric pH analysis and a secretin test. The secretin test is performed by comparison of basal serum gastrin level with gastrin level after the administration of secretin. Gastrinoma is suspected in patients with further elevation of serum gastrin. Normal patients have no change or a reduction in serum gastrin after secretin administration.

32. For which patients with Zollinger-Ellison syndrome is operative intervention indicated?

Patients with nonmetastatic sporadic gastrinoma and patients who are unable to tolerate or are refractory to medical management should be considered for operative intervention. The gastrinoma seen as part of the multiple endocrine neoplasia (MEN) syndrome differs from sporadic gastrinomas. Sporadic gastrinomas are often solitary and located in the pancreas or duodenum, but not both, and are amenable to surgical resection and cure. Although gastrinomas seen with MEN syndrome are usually multiple, virtually always in the duodenum, and often multicentric, they are also found in the pancreas and are more difficult to cure surgically. Gastrinoma associated with hypercalcemia should suggest MEN syndrome complicated by hyperparathyroidism, and parathyroidectomy is essential for management of gastric acid hypersecretion. Elevated serum gastrin levels postoperatively indicate residual gastrinoma(s) that should be treated medically. Medical management also is indicated for patients with metastatic gastrinoma. Medical management consists of high-dose proton pump inhibitors (60–80 mg/day), with the goal of reducing gastric acid output to < 10 mEq/hr for the hour that immediately precedes the next scheduled dose of antisecretory medication.

33. Describe the preoperative evaluation for gastrinoma.

CT scan with intravenous and oral contrast is routine in the preoperative evaluation for gastrinoma resection to rule out metastatic disease. In some cases, MRI is used because it is more sensitive than CT scan for liver metastasis. Rarely, partial venous sampling for gastrin has been successful in localizing gastrinoma. A newer technique that has shown promise for improving preoperative localization of gastrinomas is somatostatin receptor scintigraphy (octreotide scan). This study relies on the high density of somatostatin receptors on gastrinomas and uses the radio-labeled synthetic somatostatin analog, 125-iodine [^{125}I]-octreotide, to identify primary as well as metastatic gastrinomas. Recent studies have demonstrated that somatostatin receptor scintigraphy has high sensitivity and specificity for detection of primary and metastatic gastrinomas and may be more cost-effective as the initial imaging modality. Intraoperative localization of the tumor remains the standard of care. A modification of octreotide scanning is currently under evaluation as an adjunct to intraoperative localization. A hand-held gamma-detecting probe is used intraoperatively to localize gastrinomas after the injection of [^{125}I]-octreotide.

34. Where is the gastrinoma triangle? What percentage of tumors occur in this area?

The apex of the gastrinoma triangle is at the cystic duct-common bile duct junction and the base is located along the third portion of the duodenum (see figure at top of following page). Approximately 60–75% of gastrinomas are found in this triangle.

35. Describe the operative scheme for exploration, localization, and removal of gastrinoma.

If no tumor is obvious on preoperative CT scan and other preoperative localization studies have failed, exploration begins with exposure of the anterior surface of the pancreas by mobilization of the transverse colon. A Kocher maneuver is then performed to mobilize the duodenum, allowing complete palpation of the pancreas. Intraoperative ultrasound is concentrated in the gastrinoma triangle. Biopsy of lymph nodes should be performed, because occasionally the gastrinoma is localized to a solitary node. If ultrasound of the pancreas does not reveal the tumor, duodenal gastrinoma should be suspected. A pyloroplasty incision is made, and the duodenal wall is palpated with the index finger. Gastrinomas in the duodenal wall or pancreas may be enucleated, but solitary lesions in the pancreatic tail are often treated by pancreatic tail resection.

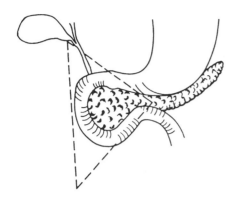

The gastrinoma triangle. (From Tzu-Ming C, Stabile BE, Passaro E: Gastrinoma: Current medical and surgical therapy. Contemp Surg 29:34, 1986, with permission.)

If no lesion is found or if the disease is found to be multicentric or metastatic, an ulcer operation may be performed as palliation. This procedure often consists of addition of a truncal vagotomy to the pyloroplasty. Alternatively, the patient may be maintained on a proton pump inhibitor. In patients who are refractory to medical therapy or unable to tolerate the side effects, a total gastrectomy may be performed for control of acid production.

36. What is a giant gastric ulcer? How is it managed?

A giant gastric ulcer is an ulcer with diameter ≥ 3 cm. Typically it is located along the lesser curvature and carries a high risk of bleeding, perforation, and obstruction. Although some studies have documented that giant peptic ulcers can be successfully treated medically, giant gastric ulcers carry an incidence of malignancy of up to 30%. Risk increases with size. Because of the high risk of complications and malignancy, the treatment of choice is early surgical intervention if the ulcer does not completely resolve with an initial course of medical therapy. Giant ulcers are treated by resection, with the addition of a truncal vagotomy for type II or type III variants.

37. Describe the risk of gastric stump cancer after partial gastrectomy for duodenal and gastric ulcer.

Gastric stump carcinoma is defined as adenocarcinoma of the stomach that occurs at least 5 years after partial gastric resection for benign disease. In patients who have undergone partial distal gastrectomy for duodenal ulcer, the relative risk of developing stump carcinoma is low in the first 20 years postoperatively but rises to 2.0 after 20 years. In patients who have had a partial distal gastrectomy for gastric ulcer, the relative risk is no different than in the general population in the first 20 years but rises to 3.0 after 20 years. Multivariate analysis has indicated that the most important risk factor in the development of gastric stump cancer is the time interval since surgery. Annual screening gastroscopy and biopsy should be performed in patients who underwent gastric resection at least 15 years ago and have moderate-to-severe dysplasia on biopsy.

38. What is the proposed mechanism for the development of stump carcinoma?

Post-partial gastrectomy hypochlorhydria results in bacterial overgrowth in the gastric remnant. The bacteria convert nitrates to nitrites, allowing the production of carcinogenic N-nitroso compounds. It is also believed that bile reflux into the gastric remnant increases the permeability of the gastric mucosal barrier to carcinogens. A final factor believed to promote the development of stump carcinoma is the presence of gastric mucosal atrophy, which results because the trophic effects of the antrum-produced peptide gastrin are absent after antrectomy.

BIBLIOGRAPHY

1. Arai R, Barkin JS: Managing recurrent peptic ulcer bleeding: The scalpel or the scope? Am J Gastroenterol 94:3365–3367, 1999.
2. Benevento A, Dominioni L, Carcano G, Dionigi R: Intraoperative localization of gut endocrine tumors with radiolabeled somatostatin analogs and a gamma-detecting probe. Semin Surg Oncol 15:239–244, 1998.

3. Bulut O, Rasmussen C, Fischer A: Acute surgical treatment of complicated peptic ulcers with special reference to the elderly. World J Surg 20:574–577, 1996.
4. Casas AT, Gadacz TR: Laparoscopic management of peptic ulcer disease. Surg Clin North Am 76:515–522, 1996.
5. Chung SCS, Li AKC: *Helicobacter pylori* and peptic ulcer surgery. Br J Surg 84:1489–1490, 1997.
6. Donahue PE: Ulcer surgery and highly selective vagotomy-Y2K. Arch Surg 134:1373–1377, 1999.
7. Donahue PE: Parietal cell vagotomy versus vagotomy-antrectomy: Ulcer surgery in the modern era. World J Surg 24:264–269, 2000.
8. Dubois F: New surgical strategy for gastroduodenal ulcer: Laparoscopic approach. World J Surg 24:270–276, 2000.
9. Greene FL: Discovery of early gastric remnant carcinoma: Results of a 14-year endoscopic screening program. Surg Endosc 9:1199–1203, 1995.
10. Hansson L-E: Risk of stomach cancer in patients with peptic ulcer disease. World J Surg 24:315–320, 2000.
11. Jamieson GG: Recent developments in upper gastrointestinal surgery. Aust N Z J Surg 66:46-49, 1996.
12. Jamieson GG: Current status of indications for surgery for peptic ulcer disease. World J Surg 24:256–258, 2000.
13. Jensen RT, Gibril F: Somatostatin receptor scintigraphy in gastrinomas. Ital J Gastroenterol Hepatol 31(Suppl):S179–185, 1999.
14. Johnson AG: Proximal gastric vagotomy: Does it have a place in the future management of peptic ulcer? World J Surg 24:259–263, 2000.
15. Kauffman GL, Conter RL: Stress ulcer and gastric ulcer. In Greenfield LJ (ed): Surgery: Scientific Principles and Practice, 2nd ed. Philadelphia, Lippincott-Raven, 1997, pp 773–788.
16. Livingstone AS, Sosa JL: Surgical laparoscopy: Impact on the management of abdominal disorders. Dig Dis 13:56–67, 1995.
17. Millat B, Fingerhut A, Borie F: Surgical treatment of complicated duodenal ulcers: Controlled trials. World J Surg 24:299–306, 2000.
18. Mulholland MW: Duodenal ulcer. In Greenfield LJ (ed): Surgery: Scientific Principles and Practice, 2nd ed. Philadelphia, Lippincott-Raven, 1997, pp 759–773.
19. Ohmann C, Imhof M, Roher H-D: Trends in peptic ulcer bleeding and surgical treatment. World J Surg 24:284–293, 2000.
20. Pappas TN: The stomach and duodenum. In Sabiston DC Jr (ed): Textbook of Surgery: The Biological Basis of Modern Surgical Practice, 15th ed. Philadelphia, W.B. Saunders, 1997, pp 847–868.
21. Sabiston DC Jr: Atlas of General Surgery. Philadelphia, W.B. Saunders, 1994.
22. Simeone DM, Hassan A, Scheiman JM: Giant peptic ulcer: A surgical or medical disease? Surgery 126:474–478, 1999.
23. Soper NJ, Brunt LM, Kerbl K: Laparoscopic general surgery. N Engl J Med 330:409–419., 1994
24. Stael von Holstein C: Long-term prognosis after partial gastrectomy for gastroduodenal ulcer. World J Surg 24:307–314, 2000.
25. Svanes C: Trends in perforated peptic ulcer: Incidence, etiology, treatment, and prognosis. World J Surg 24:277–283, 2000.
26. Termanini B, Gibril F, Reynolds JC, et al: Value of somatostatin receptor scintigraphy: A prospective study in gastrinoma of its effects on clinical management. Gastroenterology 112:335–347, 1997.
27. Tersmette AC, Giardiello FM, Tytgat GNJ, Offerhaus GJA: Carcinogenesis after remote peptic ulcer surgery: The long-term prognosis of partial gastrectomy. Scand J Gastroenterol 30(Suppl):96–99, 1995.
28. Tzu-Ming C, Stabile BE, Passaro E: Gastrinoma: Current medical and surgical therapy. Contemp Surg 29:34, 1986.
29. Yeo CJ: Neoplasms of the endocrine pancreas. In Greenfield LJ (ed): Surgery: Scientific Principles and Practice, 2nd ed. Philadelphia, Lippincott-Raven, 1997, pp 918–929.
30. Zollinger RM: Atlas of Surgical Operations. New York, McGraw-Hill, 1993.

81. SURGICAL APPROACH TO THE ACUTE ABDOMEN

Frank H. Chae, M.D.

1. What are the two main goals of a surgeon consulted for an acute abdomen?
(1) To determine whether the patient requires surgery and (2) if so, whether the patient has time for adequate resuscitation and diagnostic work-up before the general anesthesia.

2. What are the critical factors in the history of present illness?
Age, location, duration of pain, and associated problems.

3. Which disorders are associated with specific age groups?
Neonates: intussusception, appendicitis, Meckel's diverticulitis, mesenteric adenitis, midgut volvulus, malrotation, hypertrophic pyloric stenosis, small bowel atresia, annular pancreas
Adults: cholecystitis, gynecologic disorders, peptic ulcer disease, incarcerated hernia, ruptured spleen, renal or biliary stone, pancreatitis, small bowel obstruction
Elderly patients: diverticulitis, colon cancer, appendicitis, ruptured aneurysm, volvulus, bowel ischemia, pseudo-obstruction

4. Summarize the significance of location.
Right upper quadrant: biliary tract disease, peptic ulcer disease
Right flank: hepatitis, pyelonephritis
Right lower quadrant: appendicitis (see Chapter 53), ectopic pregnancy, incarcerated hernia
  rectus hematoma, torsion of ovary, Meckel's diverticulitis
Epigastrium: pancreatitis, peptic ulcer disease
Left upper quadrant: ruptured spleen, subdiaphragmatic abscess, leaking aneurysm
Central abdomen: bowel obstruction, mesenteric infarction, midgut volvulus
Left lower quadrant: diverticulitis, incarcerated hernia, torsion of ovary, perforated colon
  cancer.

5. How does duration of pain help in making a diagnosis?
Pain is sudden with a perforated ulcer or diverticulum, renal stones, and ruptured ectopic pregnancy and intermittent in bowel obstruction; it is gradual in appendicitis or pyelonephritis.

6. What associated problems help to pinpoint the diagnosis?
Past surgical and medical history. In premenopausal women, pelvic inflammatory disease and pregnancy-related problems must be screened as part of the initial assessment.

7. What are peritoneal signs?
Inflammation of the parietal peritoneum causes localized tenderness, involuntary guarding, rebound tenderness, and referred pain.

8. Is acute abdomen ruled out by absence of fever or leukocytosis?
No. Fever and leukocytosis are late occurrences. Elderly and immunocompromised patients often are unable to mount these responses despite significant abdominal disease.

9. What is the significance of bowel sounds?
Bowel sounds are not highly reliable in surgical evaluation of the abdomen. Their absence may indicate ileus, whereas high-pitched rushes may indicate small bowel obstruction.

10. What is the most important part of the abdominal examination?

Palpation, which permits assessment of localized tenderness, guarding, or diffuse peritonitis. Rectal exam is also essential. A pelvic exam must be performed in all female patients with abdominal pain.

11. What are psoas and obturator signs?

Inflammation of the psoas muscle causes pain on hip flexion-extension, whereas inflammation of the internal obturator muscle causes pain on internal rotation and flexion of the hip. Retrocecal appendicitis or, on occasion, diverticulitis may be responsible for these signs.

12. What is Rovsing's sign?

Palpation of the *left* lower quadrant causes pain in the *right* lower quadrant, indicating appendicitis.

13. What is Kehr's sign?

Pain in the left upper quadrant radiates to the left shoulder because of diaphragmatic irritation. Kehr's sign usually indicates hematoma from splenic injury.

14. Define mittelschmerz.

Pain in the middle of the menstrual cycle from ovulation.

15. How does urinalysis help in the assessment?

White blood cells in the urine may indicate urinary tract infection. Hematuria may suggest ureteral stones or tumor. Glucose or ketones may reveal diabetic ketoacidosis. An inflamed appendix abutting an adjacent ureter may lead to the fiinding of white and/or red blood cells in the urine.

16. What should be the first x-ray studies obtained?

Upright chest radiograph may reveal free air under the diaphragm or suggest a pulmonary process. Free air also may be seen over the liver in a left lateral decubitus abdominal film. Air-fluid levels on the upright abdominal film may suggest bowel obstruction. Only 10% of gallstones are radiopaque, but 90% of ureteral calculi are visualized. An appendiceal fecalith may suggest appendicitis. Absence of rectal air may indicate complete bowel obstruction. Air in the biliary system indicates biliary-enteric fistula.

17. How is ultrasound (US) used?

US helps to evaluate the gallbladder, biliary tree, free peritoneal fluid collection, and female adnexa (to assess for ectopic pregnancy or ovarian cyst/mass). Unfortunately, US abdominal exam is limited in the setting of obesity, bowel distention from obstruction, and poorly prepped bowel. The usefulness of ultrasound is limited when the appendix appears "normal" or is not visualized.

18. What additional x-ray studies may help in the diagnosis?

CT of the abdomen and pelvis with oral and intravenous contrast is useful for intra-abdominal abscess, pancreatitis, aortic, hepatic, splenic, retroperitoneal, and renal disorders. Upper and lower GI series may pinpoint the level of bowel obstruction if CT scan is inconclusive.

19. If the diagnosis is in doubt, what other tests should be done?

Surgical exploration (laparotomy) of the abdomen is the next step if CT scan cannot confirm a diagnosis and mandatory when the patient's condition worsens despite aggressive resuscitation.

20. Is exploratory laparotomy justified even it produces no significant findings?

Yes. Despite pain from postoperative incisions, risk of wound infection, and a small life-time risk of bowel obstruction (< 5%) from adhesions, it is still safer to undergo an exploratory laparotomy than to miss the diagnosis of developing appendicitis or bowel infarction.

21. Discuss the role of exploratory laparoscopy.

Laparoscopy is useful only when it provides a positive pathologic finding. If the exam is negative, the next appropriate step is conversion to laparotomy. In the setting of distended abdomen from bowel obstruction, laparoscopy is not advised; thus, its role is very limited. When the presumptive diagnosis is acute appendicitis but the appendix appears normal, it should be removed anyway to eliminate future confusion for the cause of right lower quadrant pain. Meckel's diverticulum, inflammatory bowel disease, mesenteric adenitis, and pelvic disorders may be adequately assessed via laparoscopy.

22. In blunt trauma, CT scan of the abdomen and pelvis reveals free peritoneal fluid collections. When is observation appropriate instead of immediate surgical exploration?

First and foremost, the patient must be hemodynamically stable and the identified injury must be confined to the liver and spleen. Small lacerations to the liver and spleen may be managed by aggressive resuscitation. Immediate access to the operating room must be available at all times in case the patient's condition deteriorates. Evidence on CT scan that suggests biliary or bowel injury requires surgical exploration.

23. Do all penetrating injuries to the abdomen require laparotomy?

No. If the patient is hemodynamically stable and the stab wound(s) or a low-velocity tangential bullet wound does not penetrate the fascia, observation and resuscitation suffice after a negative CT scan. Immediate surgery is recommended with a high index of suspicion for abdominal injury. In case of multiple trauma victims, surgical exploration may be safer than observation of a penetrating wound because adequate and frequent exams during the observation period may be impossible due to shortage of health care personnel. High-velocity bullet wounds almost always require surgery. The transmission of explosive energy on impact usually delivers severe injury to adjacent organs.

24. Does laparoscopy have any role in trauma?

Laparoscopy is appropriate when diaphragmatic injury is suspected or when penetration of abdominal fascia cannot be ascertained. Otherwise, its use in major trauma is not advised.

25. When is surgery indicated for peptic ulcer disease (PUD)?

Perforation. Closure with an omental patch (Graham patch) is acceptable for patients without previous history of PUD and hemodynamically unstable patients. Definitive antiulcer surgery is indicated for patients with a history of chronic PUD and hemodynamic stability. Resection of the ulcer crater with adequate margins should be performed for gastric ulcers. Definitive gastrectomy is performed after recovery if carcinoma is found on the specimen.

Obstruction. If duodenal obstruction from ulcer is not relieved by medical therapy in 7 days, surgery should be performed. Balloon dilatation is an option in patients who are not surgical candidates.

Bleeding. If more than 6 units of packed red blood cells within 24 hours are required for resuscitation, surgery should be performed.

Intractability. Despite benign biopsies, if gastric ulcers do not heal after medical therapy, surgery is recommended for suspected gastric carcinoma.

26. When is cholecystectomy optimal for acute pancreatitis presumably due to gallbladder disease?

Cholecystectomy should be performed before discharge from hospital after resolution of acute pancreatitis. Recurrence rates for pancreatitis may be as high as 60% within 6 months if the source of the gallstone is not treated.

27. How should acute pancreatitis due to biliary tract stone be managed?

The stone should be extracted as soon as possible. Endoscopic retrograde cholangiopancreatography (ERCP) should be tried first; if it is unsuccessful, surgery is necessary.

28. When is surgery indicated for severe acute pancreatitis?

Patients with progressively hemorrhagic or necrotizing pancreatitis and infected debris should undergo surgery when resuscitative measures fail. CT-guided catheter drainage may be an option for well-localized pancreatic abscess. Despite aggressive surgery, mortality rates are still as high as 40%. The impact of surgery on long-term survival is still debatable.

29. Describe treatment for a pancreatic pseudocyst.

An asymptomatic cyst < 2 cm in diameter on CT scan should be followed. Larger cysts with symptoms or infected cysts should be drained by endoscopy, CT-guided catheterization, or surgery. Patients with an isolated pancreatic cyst and no previous history of pancreatitis should undergo partial pancreatic resection for suspicion of cystadenocarcinoma.

30. How can you diagnose small bowel ischemia due to vascular obstruction?

Despite advances in technology, a high index of suspicion based on history and physical exam remains the best indicator. Pain out of proportion with abdominal exam, atrial fibrillation, recent cardiac surgery, and hypercoagulable state should arouse suspicion of bowel infarction. Base deficit from arterial blood gas may reflect a late and fulminant course of bowel infarction, but a normal blood gas should not delay surgery. Immediate surgical exploration based on high index of suspicion is not only justified but also mandatory.

31. Describe the surgical strategy for the treatment of Crohn's disease.

The goal is to preserve as much small bowel as possible. Only segments with complete obstruction should be excised. Partial obstruction may be repaired by stricturoplasty. Diseased appearance by itself at the time of surgery is not an indication for resection.

32. When should surgery be offered for uncomplicated acute diverticulitis?

After more than two recurrent episodes, although the risk of recurrence after the first episode may be as high as 30–40%. Age less than 50 years is a relative, not an absolute, indication. Complications such as perforation, bowel obstruction, fistula formation, or severe bleeding require immediate surgery.

33. Should elderly patients with sigmoid or cecal volvulus undergo surgery?

Yes. After immediate reduction with barium enema or endoscopy, the recurrence rate may be as high as 50–90%. If the patient is not in a moribund state, surgery should be offered.

34. How do you manage toxic megacolon in the setting of ulcerative colitis?

Aggressive resuscitation in the intensive care unit with frequent abdominal exam and serial abdominal radiographs to monitor colonic distension. If there is no improvement after 48 hours, total abdominal colectomy with ileostomy may be the only course available.

35. How should Ogilvie's syndrome be managed?

The vast majority of cases may be treated by colonoscopic decompression, with or without addition of prokinetic agents. Surgical resection should be offered when signs of ischemia or peritonitis are noted or when cecal diameter reaches 12 cm of distention. Ileostomy with mucous fistula is established after bowel resection. Decompression by tube cecostomy should be reserved for moribund patients.

36. After ERCP, a patient develops upper abdominal and back pain. What steps should be considered?

CT scan and/or repeat ERCP usually reveals the injury. The main focus should be the location of leak: is it the biliary-pancreatic system or the duodenum? Bile duct injury may be treated by endoscopic stent placement with percutaneous drainage of intra-abdominal collection or surgery, if the injury is complex. Pancreatitis should be treated expectantly. A contained, small leak in the posterior wall of the duodenum may be treated with bowel rest and gastric decompression;

however, ongoing leakage should be repaired immediately, before onset of inflammatory tissue response. Late manifestation of duodenal leak requires extensive drainage and possible duodenal exclusion. Perforation involving the ampulla of Vater usually requires surgical repair.

37. How should esophageal perforation after endoscopy be managed? What if the patient has achalasia? Esophageal carcinoma?

Small, contained leaks may be treated with avoidance of oral ingestion and antibiotics, although decompression with chest tubes usually is required. More extensive leaks require surgical repair. In the setting of achalasia, concomitant Heller myotomy with fundoplication should be performed. In the presence of esophageal carcinoma, the tumor, including the area of injury, should be resected, followed by an esophagogastrostomy at the same time.

38. How should colonic perforation be managed after colonoscopy?

With well-prepped bowel, patients may be treated with bowel rest, antibiotics, and observation for a small perforation. Immediate laparoscopic repair is a viable, minimally invasive alternative. With extensive laceration or with signs of diffuse peritonitis, surgery is required.

39. How should colonic perforation be managed after barium enema?

Unlike colonoscopic injuries, colonic perforation after a barium contrast study requires immediate surgery. As much barium contaminant as possible must be removed from the peritoneal cavity to minimize the risk of chemical peritonitis. Fluid resuscitation is delivered to offset third-space fluid shift. Diverting proximal colostomy and resection of perforated segment usually are required.

BIBLIOGRAPHY

1. Boyd WP, Nord HJ: Diagnostic laparoscopy. Endoscopy 32:153–158, 2000.
2. Simic O, Strathausen S, Hess W, Ostermeyer J: Incidence and prognosis of abdominal complications after cardiopulmonary bypass. Cardiovasc Surg 7:419–424, 1999.
3. Mindelzun RE, Jeffrey RB: The acute abdomen: Current CT imaging techniques. Semin Ultrasound CT MR 20(2):63–67, 1999.
4. Marco CA, Schoenfeld CN, Keyl PM, et al: Abdominal pain in geriatric emergency patients: variables associated adverse outcomes. Acad Emerg Med 5:1163–1168, 1998.
5. Chae FH, Stiegmann GV: Current laparoscopic gastrointestinal surgery. Gastroint Endosc 47:500–511, 1998.
6. McKellar DP, Reiling RB, Eiseman B: Prognosis and Outcomes in Surgical Disease. St. Louis, Quality Medical Publishing, 1999.
7. Norton LW, Stiegmann GV, Eiseman B: Surgical Decision Making. Philadelphia, W.B. Saunders, 2000.
8. Heaton KW: Diagnosis of acute non-specific abdominal pain. Lancet 355:1644, 2000.

82. COLORECTAL SURGERY

Bradley G. Bute, M.D., FACS, FASCRS

POLYPOSIS SYNDROMES AND INFLAMMATORY BOWEL DISEASE

1. What are the different types of intestinal polyps?
Neoplastic, hamartomatous, inflammatory/lymphoid, and hyperplastic.

2. What is a hamartoma?
A hamartoma is an exuberant growth of normal tissue in an abnormal amount or location. An isolated hamartomatous polyp has no malignant potential.

3. Which intestinal polyposis syndromes are associated with hamartomatous polyps?
- Peutz-Jeghers syndrome
- Juvenile polyposis (familial or generalized)
- Cronkhite-Canada syndrome (hamartomatous polyps with alopecia, cutaneous pigmentation, and toenail and fingernail atrophy)
- Intestinal ganglioneuromatosis (isolated or with von Recklinghausen's disease or multiple endocrine neoplasia type 2)
- Ruvalcaba-Myrhe-Smith syndrome (polyps of colon and tongue, macrocephaly, retardation, unique facies, pigmented penile macules)
- Cowden's disease (GI polyps with oral and cutaneous verrucous papules [tricholemmomas], associated with breast cancer, thyroid neoplasia, and ovarian cysts)

4. How is Peutz-Jeghers syndrome manifest?
This autosomal dominant trait is often heralded by the presence of melanin spots on the lips and buccal mucosa (see Chapter 71). Hamartomas are almost always present on the small intestine and occasionally on the stomach and colon.

5. Do the hamartomatous polyposis diseases have malignant potential?
In the past, the malignant potential for hamartomatous polyps was considered nil. Recent reviews suggest an increased incidence of GI cancers in patients with multiple hamartomatous polyposis syndromes. A hamartoma-adenoma-carcinoma sequence has been postulated for Peutz-Jeghers syndrome, and patients also seem to be at increased risk for extraintestinal cancers, including sex cord tumors and pancreatic and breast cancer. Generalized juvenile polyposis is now considered to be a premalignant state, with associated malignant degeneration of the polyps.

6. Describe familial adenomatous polyposis (FAP).
FAP is a mendelian-dominant, non–sex-linked disease in which > 100 adenomatous polyps affect the colon and rectum. One-third of patients present as the propositus case (presumed mutation) with no prior family history. The disease invariably leads to invasive colon cancer if not treated. The average age at diagnosis of colon cancer is 39 years compared with 65 years for routine colon cancer.

7. What extracolonic abnormalities are associated with FAP?

BENIGN	MALIGNANT
Congenital hypertrophy of retinal pigment epithelium (CHRPE)	Gastric cancer
	Periampullary carcinoma
Gastric fundic gland polyps	Duodenal adenocarcinoma
Antral adenomas	Pancreatic adenocarcinoma

Table continued on following page

BENIGN	MALIGNANT
Duodenal adenomas	Cholangiocarcinoma
Jejunoileal adenomas	Small intestinal carcinoma
Desmoid tumors	Ileal carcinoids
Adrenal adenomas	Adrenal adenocarcinoma
Pituitary adenomas	Medulloblastoma
	Turcot's syndrome or glioblastoma
	Thyroid carcinoma
	Osteogenic sarcoma
	Hepatoblastoma

8. What is Gardner's syndrome?

FAP plus fibromas of the skin, osteomas (typically of the mandible, maxilla, and skull), epidermoid cysts, desmoid tumors, and extra dentition.

9. How does one screen for FAP?

When family history is positive, children should undergo annual sigmoidoscopic surveillance beginning at age 10–12 years. When polyps are identified, a full colonoscopy is recommended. Once multiple adenomas are documented, colectomy is recommended. State-of-the-art presymptomatic detection uses molecular genetic screening. FAP is caused by mutation in the adenomatous polyposis coli (APC) gene on the long arm of chromosome 5 at the 5q21–q22 locus. Restrictive fragment length polymorphism linkage analysis can determine whether a person is affected with 95–99% certainty if genetic material is available from affected and unaffected members of the kindred. Direct determination of somatic mutations in the APC gene may be detectable in spontaneous cases of FAP. Ophthalmoscopic exam for CHRPE can detect involved patients as early as 3 months of age with a 97% positive predictive value for developing FAP. CHRPE is present in 55–100% of FAP patients and is documented with wide-angle fundus photography.

10. What is Crohn's disease?

A nonspecific inflammatory disease that may involve any portion of the GI tract; regional enteritis commonly causes abdominal pain and diarrhea. The distribution of disease in the GI tract may be discontinuous. Presenting patterns are ileocolic in about 40%, colonic Crohn's alone in 30%, small bowel involvement alone in 25%, and anorectal disease alone in 5%.

11. What is ulcerative colitis?

A nonspecific inflammatory bowel disease that involves the colon and rectum. Bloody diarrhea is the classic presenting symptom. Disease may be limited to the rectum (proctitis), left colon (proctosigmoiditis), or entire colon (pancolitis). The rectum is always involved; the disease process is one of continuous inflammation (no skip areas).

12. How is Crohn's disease differentiated from ulcerative colitis?

	ULCERATIVE COLITIS	CROHN'S COLITIS
Clinical manifestations		
Bleeding per rectum	3+	1+
Diarrhea	3+	3+
Abdominal pain	1+	3+ (especially with ileal involvement)
Fever	R	2+
Palpable abdominal mass	R	2+
Internal fistula	R	4+
Intestinal obstruction (stricture or infection)	0	4+

Table continued on following page

	ULCERATIVE COLITIS	CROHN'S COLITIS
Clinical manifestations *(cont.)*		
Rectal involvement	4+	1+
Small bowel involvement	0	4+
Anal and perianal involvement	R	4+
Thumbprinting sign on barium enema	R	1+
Risk of cancer	2+	1+
Clinical course	Relapses/ remissions	Slowly progressive
Gross appearance		
Thickened bowel wall	0	4+
Shortening of bowel	2+	R
Fat creeping onto serosa	0	4+
Segmental involvement	0	4+
Aphthous ulcer	0	4+
Linear ulcer	0	4+
Microscopic picture		
Depth of involvement	Mucosa and submucosa	Full thickness
Lymphoid aggregation	0	4+
Sarcoid-type granuloma	0	4+
Fissuring	0	2+
Surgical treatment		
Total proctocolectomy	Gold standard	Indicated in total large bowel involvement
Segmental resection	Infrequent	Frequent
Ileal pouch procedure	Excellent option in selected patients	Contraindicated
Recurrence after surgery	0	3+

R = rare, 0 = not found, 1+ = may be present, 2+ = common, 3+ = usual finding, 4+ = characteristic (not necessarily common).
From Nivatvongs S: The colon, rectum and anal canal. In James EC, Corry RJ, Perry JF Jr (eds): Basic Surgical Practice. Philadelphia, Hanley & Belfus, 1987, p 325.

13. What are the surgical indications for ulcerative colitis?
- Intractability or failure of medical management
- Fulminant colitis
- Toxic megacolon
- Massive bleeding
- Prophylaxis of carcinoma (presence of high-grade dysplasia)
- Treatment of carcinoma
- Palliation of cutaneous and systemic (extracolonic) manifestations

14. Identify the extracolonic manifestations of ulcerative colitis.

Skin: Pyoderma gangrenosum, erythema nodosum
Liver: Fatty infiltration of the liver, pericholangitis, cirrhosis
Biliary: Primary sclerosing cholangitis, bile duct carcinoma
Eye: Uveitis, episcleritis, conjunctivitis, retrobulbar neuritis
Joints: Monoarticular arthritis, ankylosing spondylitis, sacroiliitis
Mouth: Aphthous ulcers, stomatitis
Renal: Pyelonephritis, nephrolithiasis
Systemic: Amyloidosis, thromboembolic disease, hypercoaguability, vasculitis, pericarditis

15 What are the elective surgical options for FAP and chronic ulcerative colitis?
- Total proctocolectomy with end (Brooke) ileostomy
- Total proctocolectomy with continent ileostomy reservoir (Kock pouch)

- Abdominal colectomy with ileorectal anastomosis
- Near-total proctocolectomy ± rectal mucosectomy and ileal pouch-anal anastomosis (IPAA) with J, S, W, or H pouch

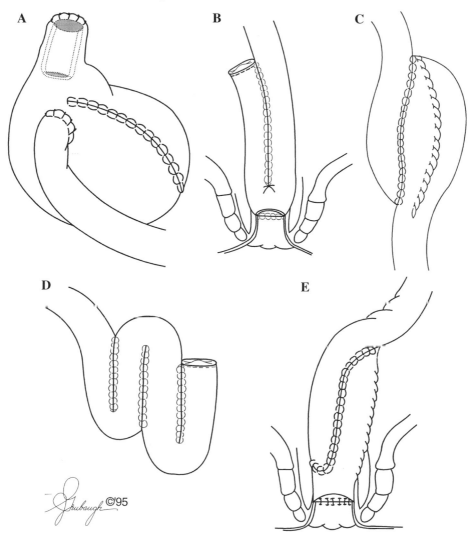

A, Kock pouch. *B,* J pouch. *C,* S pouch. *D,* W pouch. *E,* H pouch.

16. Why should one not perform ileal pouch-anal anastomosis for colonic Crohn's disease?

The high rate of recurrence of disease in the pouch, with resultant inflammation and fistulas, requires eventual excision of the pouch in 24–30% of cases. Fifty percent or more of patients suffer postoperative complications.

17. Can one always tell the difference between Crohn's disease and ulcerative colitis?

No. Colitis that cannot be categorized as definitely Crohn's or ulcerative colitis is called indeterminate colitis and may account for 5–10% of cases referred for surgical consideration. The postoperative result when IPAA is performed for indeterminate colitis has generally been held to be the same as that obtained with definite ulcerative colitis. However, a recent Mayo Clinic review notes that pouch failure is twice as common in indeterminate colitis as in ulcerative colitis, (18% and 9%, respectively).

18. What is pouchitis? How is it treated?

Pouchitis, one of the most frequent long-term complications of IPAA, is a nonspecific acute and/or chronic inflammation of the reservoir. Pouchitis is found in 7–44% of patients with IPAA; it presents with watery, bloody stools, urgency, frequency, abdominal pain, fever, malaise, and possible exacerbation of extraintestinal manifestations of inflammatory bowel disease. The cause is uncertain, but the risk is greater in chronic ulcerative colitis than in familial polyposis. Pouch stasis, bacterial overgrowth, colonification of ileal mucosa, ischemia, pelvic sepsis, oxygen-derived free radicals, altered immune status, and lack of mucosal trophic factors have been proposed as etiologies.

Successful treatment regimensinclude metronidazole and other antianaerobic antibiotics as well as steroid or 5- aminosalicylate enemas. Topical volatile fatty acids and glutamine have been used with variable success. Although half of patients with pouchitis at some time suffer a recurrence, very few develop intractable involvement requiring pouch excision.

19. Does a defunctionalized colon develop colitis?

Yes. Perhaps 30% of patients with a portion or all of the colon out of the fecal stream develop an inflammation difficult to distinguish from ulcerative colitis on biopsy. The diagnosis of diversion colitis is suggested when bloody mucopus is passed from the separate colorectal segment. The colon may be isolated by diverting ileostomy, end or loop colostomy, mucous fistula, or Hartmann's procedure. It is believed that short-chain fatty acids normally produced by anaerobic bacteria serve as a trophic factor for the colonocytes. The diversion colitis quickly resolves on restoration of intestinal continuity; when restoration is not possible, the administration of short-chain fatty acid enemas is beneficial.

Controversies

20. Should the anorectum be everted to allow a more complete or longer rectal mucosal stripping in IPAA?

Eversion of the anorectum to ensure complete removal of the mucosa was common in the past. However, the pudendal nerves may be damaged by stretching during eversion, leading to continence problems. Shorter rectal muscle cuffs are now used to avoid abscesses between the pouch and cuff; adequate stripped cuff length can be obtained without eversion. Several rectal retractors that facilitate transanal mucosectomy are now available.

21. Should the rectal mucosectomy be done transanally or abdominally?

The dissection can be done from either direction. The shorter rectal cuffs now in vogue are easily performed from the perineal (transanal) approach.

22. Should a mucosectomy be done at all?

Mucosectomy removes part or all of the anal transition zone, a highly sensitive area that may be important for critical discrimination of pouch content and continence. Studies can be found favoring either leaving or removing this mucosa. Mucosa left in place is at risk for persistent inflammation, dysplasia, or development of carcinoma in ulcerative colitis or FAP. No mucosectomy may be preferable in the elderly (with less time at risk to develop a carcinoma and a relatively greater need for all maneuvers to preserve continence).

23. Should the IPAA be stapled or hand-sewn?

If a mucosectomy is performed, a hand-sewn anastomosis of the pouch to the dentate line is created. If the anal transition zone mucosa is preserved, a stapled anastomosis may be performed at the top of the anorectal ring.

24. Should IPAA be a one- or two-stage operation?

The procedure has classically been two-staged, with construction of a temporary ileostomy followed at an interval by ileostomy takedown. Recent experience has shown that the morbidity of a one-stage IPAA may be less if the patient is taking no or low-dose steroids and the operation is performed without complication. Because there is really only "one shot" at getting it right, intraoperative judgment is at a premium.

25. What type of pouch should be used?

Higher-volume pouches are advocated. W (quadruplicated) pouches have a greater capacity than S (triplicated) and J (two-limbed) pouches. The functional results may not be all that different. Shorter efferent limbs (for S pouches) are also used to avoid outlet obstruction. The author prefers a noneverted, triple stapled anastomosis of a 15-cm long J pouch in a one-stage approach, when feasible, preserving the anal transition zone.

ANORECTAL DISEASE

26. What are anal fissures?

A generally painful rip or tear in the sensitive anoderm of the anal canal. Most anal fissures are located in the posterior (90%) or anterior (10%) midline of the anal canal.

27. What disorders should be considered in patients with laterally situated anal fissures?

Crohn's disease, ulcerative colitis, syphilis, tuberculosis, leukemia, carcinoma, and AIDS.

28. What does anorectal manometry demonstrate in patients with an anal fissure?

After transient relaxation, the internal sphincter shows a prolonged elevation in pressure above the normal baseline—the "overshoot" phenomenon associated with the pain/spasm cycle of fissure disease.

29. How are acute fissures managed?

Conservative treatment consists of stool softeners and bulk agents to avoid hard bowel movements, sitz baths to help decrease sphincter spasm, topical anesthetics, and topical steroids. Suppositories generally should be avoided because they may induce anal spasm. Topical nitroglycerine or nifedipine ointment reduces anal spasm. Injection of botulinum toxin also has been used.

30. How does nitroglycerine ointment work?

Nitroglycerine ointment breaks down into the active moiety nitric oxide, an inhibitory neurotransmitter for the internal sphincter. Thus it allows relaxation of the muscle, relief of spasm, and, ultimately, increased blood flow and increased oxygen delivery through the microcapillaries to the area of anoderm breakdown. To avoid the common side effect of headache seen with the use of 2% nitroglycerine ointment used for angina, 0.2% strength should be used for anal fissure.

31. What are the signs of a chronic anal fissure? What do they imply?

A chronic anal fissure can be identified by the presence of a sentinel pile (skin tag or hemorrhoid), anal ulcer (with fibropurulent material or visible internal sphincter muscle in the base), and a hypertrophied anal papilla arising from the dentate line. A chronic anal fissure usually does not respond to conservative treatment, and surgical intervention is in order.

32. Which surgical procedures are available for treatment of a chronic anal fissure?

Open or closed lateral internal sphincterotomy, excision (ulcerectomy), excision and Y-V or other anoplasty, or anal dilation.

33. Why has posterior anal sphincterotomy fallen out of favor?

It can result in a posterior anal canal "keyhole" defect with anal seepage.

34. What are hemorrhoids?

Hemorrhoids are difficult to define precisely. Everyone has vascular cushions in the anal canal that contain veins (and arteries), elastic and connective tissue, and smooth muscle. Hemorrhoids are not "varicose veins of the anus;" they may play a role in fine control of anal continence. It has been suggested that the term "hemorrhoid" be reserved for symptomatic involvement of these structures.

35. How are hemorrhoids classified?

External hemorrhoids originate distal to the dentate line of the anus and are covered by squamous epithelium. External hemorrhoids may thrombose or become filled with clotted blood.

Internal hemorrhoids arise above (proximal to) the dentate line and are covered with transitional and columnar epithelium. First-degree hemorrhoids swell and bleed. Second-degree hemorrhoids prolapse and spontaneously reduce. Third-degree hemorrhoids prolapse and can be manually reduced, whereas fourth-degree hemorrhoids are irreducible.

36. What are acute hemorrhoids?

Internal hemorrhoids that protrude suddenly and painfully, becoming incarcerated in the prolapsed position. A single quadrant or the entire circumference of the anal orifice may be involved.

37. How are acute hemorrhoids treated?

Topical medicines: anesthetics, hydrocortisone preparations, astringents (witch hazel, glycerine, magnesium sulfate).

Emergency hemorrhoidectomy (*ouch!*) requires 2 weeks of recovery time.

Office treatment: local anesthesia with or without hyaluronidase, manual reduction of hemorrhoids, rubber band ligation to maintain reduction and prevent recurrent edema, compressive bandaging.

38. Where in the anal canal are hemorrhoids classically found?

Left lateral, right anterior, and right posterior locations are typical. The use of clockface times as descriptions of hemorrhoids (e.g., "large bundle at 9 o'clock") is confusing and should be avoided, because patients may be examined in lithotomy, jackknife, or decubitus positions by different examiners with resulting confusion.

39. List several minimally invasive outpatient treatments of internal hemorrhoids.

Rubber band ligation, bipolar cautery, direct current electrical therapy, infrared coagulation, sclerotherapy, and cryotherapy.

40. What is the dreaded complication of rubber band ligation of internal hemorrhoids?

Postligation pelvic sepsis. Although exceedingly rare (perhaps approaching the order of one in a million), this problem has often proved fatal. Seen in otherwise healthy middle-aged men, it presents with severe pain, marked perianal edema, fever, and difficulty with urination. Pelvic edema may progress rapidly to fulminant sepsis unresponsive to any treatment.

41. Who is the patron saint of hemorrhoid sufferers?

Fiachra (Irish), Fiacre (French), or Fiacrius (Latin). An Irish holy man famed for cures of such less desirable maladies, he died in France on August 30, 670 A.D.

42. How is an acute thrombosed external hemorrhoid best treated?

Excision of the clot and involved hemorrhoidal complex (as opposed to incision alone) better prevents future recurrence at the same site.

43. Explain the cause of anorectal abscesses and fistulas.

A cryptoglandular origin seems to provide the best explantion. Four to ten anal glands enter the anal canal at the level of the crypts in the dentate line. The glands extend back into the internal sphincter two-thirds of the time and into the intersphincteric space half the time. Blockage of the gland leads to an overgrowth of bacteria with resultant pressure necrosis and abscess formation.

An abscess or infection that causes an abnormal communication between two surfaces (such as the anal canal and perianal skin) creates a fistula. Infections can extend in fairly standard fashion along anatomic planes to produce clinical abscesses and potentially related fistulas.

44. List the various types of anorectal abscesses.
Submucosal, intersphincteric, perianal (anal verge), ischiorectal (perirectal), and supralevator.

45. What is a horseshoe abscess?
A perirectal abscess that connects the ischiorectal fossae bilaterally through the deep postanal space posteriorly or anteriorly.

46. What is the best treatment for an anorectal abscess?
Prompt incision and drainage! There is little or no role for antibiotics (exceptions are immunocompromised patients and patients with prosthetic heart valves or severe cellulitis) and no reason to wait for the abscess to "point" or become fluctuant before surgical treatment.

47. What is Goodsall's rule?
This rule helps predict the location of the internal opening of an anal fistula based on the site of its external opening. Accurately determining the "criminal crypt" of fistula origin on the dentate line is important at the time of surgical treatment, generally fistulotomy. If the anus is divided into imaginary anterior and posterior halves in the coronal plane, posterior fistulas tend to curve into the posterior midline. Anterior fistulas shorter than 3 cm tend to proceed radially to the dentate line, whereas anterior fistulas longer than 3 cm may track back to the posterior midline.

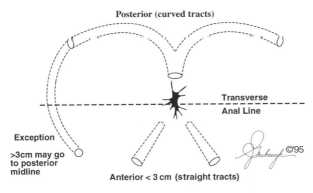

Goodsall's rule.

48. What is a seton?
A drainage device used to control and treat an anal fistulous abscess. It is inserted through and through a fistula tract and secured to itself, thus making a circle about some portion of the anal sphincter muscle. Typical setons are Penrose drains, silastic "vessel loops," or silk sutures.

49. Why is a seton used?
- To provide permanent drainage, as in perianal Crohn's disease with multiple fistulae
- To serve as a cutting device to exteriorize the fistula slowly
- To act as a temporizing agent while awaiting a staged fistulotomy
- To treat primarily by sequential down-sizing of the seton material until eventually all drains are removed

50. What are the common indications for inserting a seton?
- High fistulous abscesses involving greater than one-half the length of the anal canal muscle
- Anterior fistulas in a woman

• Inflammatory bowel disease
• Elderly patients or patients with multiple previous anorectal surgeries

51. List new developments for treatment of anorectal fistulae.

• Fibrin sealant glues
• Monoclonal anti-tumor necrosis factor antibodies for Crohn's fistulae
• Revival of Park's fistulotomy procedure, with excision/debridement of the fistula tract, muscle repair, advancement flap coverage of the internal opening, and drainage of the external portion of the fistula tract

52. When is anorectal suppurative disease especially dangerous?

In the presence of neutropenia, as associated with chemotherapy, the mortality at 1 month may approach 50%. Unfortunately, surgery and even anorectal digital examination may be contraindicated. Often bacterial infection is widespread without formation of purulence or a classic abscess.

53. What treatment may be used to augment antibiotics in treating an infected neutropenic patient?

Low-dose radiation may help to "sterilize" an otherwise uncontrolled septic perineum.

54. How does one differentiate true rectal prolapse from a circumferential hemorrhoidal mucosal enlargement?

The folds of tissue are concentric rings in rectal prolapse, whereas they are radially oriented in hemorrhoidal disease.

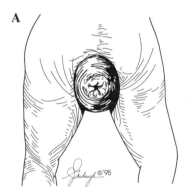 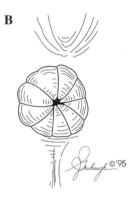

A, Rectal prolapse shows concentric rings of tissue. *B*, tissue folds in hemorrhoids are radially oriented.

55. Which patient characteristics are associated with rectal prolapse?

According to Corman:

Chronic constipation	Deep pouch of Douglas
Neurologic disease	Patulous anus
Female sex	Diastasis of the levator ani muscles
Nulliparity	Lack of fixation of the rectum to the sacrum
Redundant rectosigmoid colon	Previous anorectal surgery

56. How can a patient demonstrate rectal prolapse during physical exam?

It is possible for some patients to prolapse the rectum voluntarily with Valsalva maneuvers and straining as if to defecate. However, this maneuver may be impossible in the commonly used jackknife or decubitus examination position. A useful technique is to examine after the patient has strained while sitting on a toilet or, better yet, observe through a transparent elevated toilet.

57. What radiologic procedure may document a prolapse that cannot be reproduced in the office?

(Cine)defecography may reveal an internal intussusception beginning on the anterior rectal wall several centimeters above the anal verge, which may progress to complete prolapse.

58. What is the relationship between rectal prolapse and anal continence?

Some degree of incontinence almost always accompanies rectal prolapse. Surgical repair may not correct incontinence problems. Abdominal approaches tend to have higher success rates for continence than perineal operations, but the results vary widely.

59. What surgical options are available for rectal prolapse?

In general, procedures can narrow the anal orifice (Thiersch operation), obliterate the pouch of Douglas (Moschcowitz procedure), restore the condition of the pelvic floor (levator plication), excise (abdominally or perineally) the excess rectosigmoid colon, and/or fixate or suspend the rectum. Combinations of these options are often used.

60. How is rectal prolapse handled in pediatric patients?

Most prolapse in children is a mucosal prolapse alone. It is usually handled with a bowel management program to reduce constipation and straining. Surgical or invasive methods, such as sclerosis, encirclement, or excision, are rarely necessary.

BENIGN COLON AND SMALL BOWEL DISEASE

61. Which type of colonic volvulus is most common?

Sigmoid volvulus accounts for 75% of cases seen in the United States. It is far more common than cecal volvulus.

62. Is volvulus a "constant" disease worldwide?

No. In the United States, volvulus causes only 10% of colonic obstruction cases. In the past, more than 50% of colonic obstructions in Iran, Ethiopia, and Russia have been attributed to volvulus. The disease process tends to present at an older age in the U.S. than in more rural countries.

63. List the characteristics of a typical American patient with colonic volvulus.

Male, black, elderly, and possibly from a nursing home or mental institution.

64. What are the findings of sigmoid volvulus on plain abdominal film and contrast enema?

The plain film demonstrates a "bent inner tube" or "coffee-bean" sign of massively dilated, air-filled sigmoid colon arising out of the pelvis. The contrast enema shows a "bird's beak" appearance as the colon narrows at the twist at the rectosigmoid junction.

65. How is a nonstrangulated sigmoid volvulus treated?

Rigid or flexible sigmoidoscopic or colonoscopic decompression, followed by elective sigmoid resection.

66. Why should elective surgery be performed after a successful endoscopic detorsion and decompression of a sigmoid volvulus?

Recurrence is the rule with sigmoid volvulus. Elective sigmoid resection of prepped and decompressed bowel generally can be accomplished with a mortality rate < 5%. Emergency operation for a sigmoid volvulus involves a mortality rate of 35–80%.

67. Name the two types of large bowel obstruction.

Dynamic (mechanical) and adynamic.

68. What is the most common cause of mechanical large bowel obstruction in western society?

Carcinoma far outnumbers diverticular causes and volvulus.

69. What does plain x-ray study of the abdomen reveal in large bowel obstruction?

Differential air-fluid levels (stair steps) of the small intestine or a massively dilated colon. The colon is identified by the presence of haustral folds, as compared to the valvulae conniventes of the small intestine. The rectum is usually gasless, although gas distal to a colonic obstruction may not have completely cleared the distal colon. A picture resembling small bowel obstruction alone may appear in a very proximal colon obstruction. Colonic pseudo-obstruction also may give a roentgenographic picture similar to true obstruction.

70. How can one safely differentiate true from false colonic obstruction?

A water-soluble enema contrast study reveals the presence or absence of an organic obstructing lesion. It is best to avoid barium, because a perforation during the study or a leak of colonic contents and barium at the time of surgery may lead to a severe barium peritonitis.

71. List the classes of prokinetic agents and give an example of each.

Cholinergic agonists (bethanechol)
Benzamides (metoclopramide, cisapride [needs special FDA approval])
Dopamine antagonists: domperidone
Macrolide antibiotics (erythromycin)
Opiate antagonists (naloxone)
Somatostatin analogs (octreotide)

72. Which lower intestinal motility disorders may respond to prokinetic agents?

Irritable bowel syndrome, acute colonic psuedo-obstruction, chronic intestinal pseudo-obstruction, idiopathic constipation, chronic constipation associated with neurologic causes, and idiopathic megacolon/megarectum.

73. What is a bezoar?

A concretion formed in the alimentary tract that may produce an obstruction. It can be caused by vegetable matter (phytobezoar), hair (trichobezoar), or a combination of hair and food (trichophytobezoar).

74. Which food is most commonly associated with the development of phytobezoars?

Persimmons.

75. What antecedent surgical history accompanies most cases of small intestinal bezoars?

A recent review found that 76% of patients had previous peptic ulcer disease surgery. A vagotomy and pyloroplasty or antrectomy is believed to allow a large bolus of relatively undigested food to pass into the small intestine, where obstruction is possible.

76. What does endometriosis have to do with the alimentary system?

Endometriosis is the presence of functioning endometrial tissue outside the uterus. When this hormonally active tissue implants on intestinal surfaces, it can cause pain, cyclical bleeding, and obstructive symptoms.

77. What common symptoms are seen in women requiring surgery for endometriosis?

Pelvic pain (85%), dyspareunia (64%), and rectal pain (52%).

78. Which area of the GI tract is most often involved with endometriosis?

The rectum/cul de sac is involved in over 90% of cases requiring surgery.

79. How is postoperative ileus differentiated from postoperative small bowel obstruction?

This distinction can be extremely difficult. Postoperative ileus generally occurs up to 1 week after operation, whereas postoperative small bowel obstruction (SBO) may last 7–30 days or longer. SBO is associated with nausea, vomiting, distention, and abdominal pain, whereas an ileus may be associated with painless failure to pass bowel movements. The radiographic picture may or may not include differential air-fluid levels in each disorder.

80. Is treatment of postoperative SBO different from treatment of SBO remote from surgery?

Yes. Generally, one waits out a postoperative obstruction for an indefinite period, as long as there is no evidence of strangulation or impending perforation. Approximately 80% resolve without surgery. Nasogastric suction is the mainstay of treatment for postoperative SBO, whereas "the sun never sets" on a suspected mechanical SBO remote from surgery; one generally operates as soon as the diagnosis of complete obstruction is made.

81. What is the leading cause of SBO?

Adhesions.

82. Can adhesions be prevented?

Absorbable hyaluronate and carboxymethylcellulose membranes lead to a statistically significant reduction in the number and severity of intra-abdominal adhesions.

83. What are the pathologic findings of late radiation enteritis?

Obliterative arteritis. Severe fibrosis commonly is accompanied by telangiectasia formation. The pelvis may be "frozen" because of incredibly dense adhesions and fibrosis.

84. What are general principles of managing radiation enteritis?

Medical management options are generally exhausted before surgery is contemplated or attempted. Cholestyramine, elemental diets, and total parenteral nutrition are commonly used. Although surgery is not withheld for urgent indications (complete obstruction, perforation, abscess not amenable to percutaneous drainage, bleeding, or unresponsive fistulas), it carries significant morbidity (up to 65%) and mortality (up to 45%) rates. Enterolysis, or separating of adhesions, in radiated bowel is associated with a high rate of fistula formation. Anastomosis can be performed safely if at least one end of bowel to be connected has not been radiated. Intestinal bypass procedures without resection may be necessary.

85. What treatments are available for bleeding radiation proctitis?

Topical anti-inflammatories (steroids, mesalamine enemas or suppositories), laser ablation of telangectasias, and application of 4% formaldehyde solutions (under controlled situations in the operating room).

BIBLIOGRAPHY

1. Altomare DF, Rinaldi M, Milito G, et al: Glyceryl trinitrate for chronic anal fissure—healing or headache? Dis Colon Rectum 43:174, 2000.
2. Bailey HR, Ott MT, Hartendorp P: Aggressive surgical management for advanced colorectal endometriosis. Dis Colon Rectum 37:747, 1994.
3. Bapat BP, Parker JA, Berk T, et al: Combined use of molecular and biomarkers for presymptomatic carrier risk assessment in familial adenomatous polyposis: Implications for screening guidelines. Dis Colon Rectum 37:165, 1994.
4. Becker JM, Dayton MT, Fazio VW, et al: Prevention of postoperative abdominal adhesions by a sodium hyaluronate-based bioresorbable membrane. J Am Coll Surg 183:297, 1996.
5. Bute BG, Hoexter B: Pelvic sepsis after rubber band ligation [unpublished data from ASCRS membership questionnaire]. 2001.
6. Corman ML: Colon and Rectal Surgery. Philadelphia, J.B. Lippincott, 1998.
7. Escamilla C, Robles-Campos R, Parrilla-Paricio P, et al: Intestinal obstruction and bezoars. J Am Coll Surg 179:285, 1994.
8. Gordon PH, Nivatvongs S: Principles and Practice of Surgery for the Colon, Rectum and Anus. St. Louis, Quality Medical Publishing, 1999.
9. Hizawa K, Iida M, Matsumoto T, et al: Neoplastic transformation arising in Peutz-Jeghers polyposis. Dis Colon Rectum 36:953, 1993.
10. Jagelman DG: Familial polyposis coli. In Fazio VW (ed): Current Therapy in Colon and Rectal Surgery. Philadelphia, B.C. Decker, 1990.
11. Keighley MR, Williams NS: Surgery of the Anus, Rectum and Colon. London, W.B. Saunders, 1993.
12. Longo WE, Vernava AM III: Prokinetic agents for lower gastrointestinal motility disorders. Dis Colon Rectum 36:696, 1993.
13. McIntyre PB, Pemberton JH, Wolff BG, et al: Indeterminate colitis: Long term outcome in patients after ileal pouch-anal anastomosis. Dis Colon Rectum 38:51, 1995.
14. Mignon M, Stettler C, Phillips SF: Pouchitis-a poorly understood entity. Dis Colon Rectum 38:100, 1995.
15. Saclarides TJ, King DG, Franklin H, et al: Formalin instillation for refractory radiation-induced hemorrhagic proctitis. Dis Colon Rectum 39:196, 1996.
16. Sudduth RH, Bute BG, Schoelkopf L, et al: Small bowel obstruction in a patient with Peutz-Jeghers syndrome: The role of intra-operative endoscopy. Gastrointest Endosc 38:69, 1992.

83. PANCREATIC SURGERY

Jeffrey R. Clark, M.D., F.A.C.S.

A certain mystique surrounds the pancreas because of several unique circumstances:
1. The pancreas is responsible for one of humankind's most common afflictions–diabetes mellitus.
2. The etiology of many pancreatic diseases defies logical explanation (pancreatitis).
3. Appropriate therapy for all pancreatic diseases is surrounded by considerable controversy. (Controversy is a polite way of saying we do not know what we are doing.)
4. Surgical intervention frequently is associated with high mortality and morbidity rates because the pancreas has a retroperitoneal location and close proximity to vital structures (aorta, vena cava, superior mesenteric vein and artery, hilum of kidneys); shares a common blood supply with the duodenum, necessitating removal of both when resecting either; contains potent indiscriminate digestive enzymes that will just as readily digest the host if uncontained; and has a fragile parenchyma that is difficult to suture, resulting in anastomotic leaks, fistulas, and bleeding.
5. Questions about the pancreas are the resident's worst nightmare. Numerous exotic endocrine tumors give rise to a disproportionate number of questions far in excess of the prevalence of the diseases that such tumors produce.
6. The pancreas is unjust and unpredictable. Operations performed in close proximity with considerable care occasionally elicit its wrath (splenectomy), and even remote operations (open heart) may elicit pancreatitis.

ACUTE PANCREATITIS

1. What is acute pancreatitis?
Inflammation of the pancreas with variable involvement of regional tissues and remote organ systems. Mild acute pancreatitis is accompanied by minimal organ dysfunction and has an uncomplicated recovery. Severe acute pancreatitis is associated with distant organ failure and defined as follows:

Pulmonary	Partial pressure of oxygen (PO_2) < 60 mmHg
Renal	Creatinine > 2 mg/dl
Cardiac	Blood pressure < 90 mm Hg
Hematopoietic	Disseminated intravascular coagulation
Metabolic	Hypocalcemia and hyperglycemia
Gastrointestinal	Bleeding > 500 ml/24 hr
Complications	Pancreatic necrosis, abscess, pseudocyst, others

2. How common is acute pancreatitis?
Acute pancreatitis is responsible for > 100,000 hospital admissions and > 2000 deaths each year in the United States.

3. What are the causes of acute pancreatitis?

Alcohol	40%
Gallstones	40%
Miscellaneous (e.g., drugs, toxins, trauma, hyperlipidemia, hypercalcemia)	10%
Idiopathic	10%

4. Describe the pathogenesis of acute pancreatitis.
The pathogenesis of acute pancreatitis remains unclear, but current hypotheses suggest that pancreatic enzymes (trypsin) are activated intracellularly by lysosomal enzymes secondary to the

646

direct action of toxins (alcohol) and/or pancreatic ductal obstruction (gallstones). The result is ductal hypertension, which overwhelms the natural trypsin inhibitors. The process is enhanced by the presence of bile, bile salts, and duodenal contents refluxing into the pancreatic duct. Trypsin activates the other potent digestive enzymes (phospholipase A, elastase, lipase), and the gland is autodigested. The damage is immediate. Necrosis occurs quickly, and inflammatory mediators (cytokines and acute-phase reactants) are activated and released systemically.

5. How is the diagnosis of acute pancreatitis established?

History: sudden onset of constant and unrelenting epigastric pain ranging from mild to catastrophic and radiating straight through to the back; pain is relieved by sitting and leaning forward.

Physical findings: Upper abdominal pain and tenderness, including rigidity and rebound. (The presence of acute surgical abdomen with acute pancreatitis does not indicate emergency surgical exploration.)

Laboratory findings: Elevations of serum amylase (half-life, hours) and lipase (half-life, days) remain the gold standards. Diagnostic accuracy increases with rising levels so that amylase levels > 1000 IU/l are virtually diagnostic of acute pancreatitis.

Surgical findings: Diagnosis of acute pancreatitis may be made unexpectedly during surgery, when the abdomen is explored for another reason (e.g., appendicitis, cholecystitis).

6. List the differential diagnosis of acute pancreatitis.

- Small bowel obstruction, especially closed loop (rule out with Gastrograffin upper GI series)
- Perforated viscus, especially duodenal ulcer (rule out with upright chest radiograph for free air)
- Bowel infarction (rule out with arteriogram)

7. What tests help to determine severity and predict outcome?

Ranson's criteria. Ranson's original description of prognostic indicators was published in 1974, but significant improvements in intensive care, operative management techniques, and antibiotics have lowered the high mortality rate originally reported. Nevertheless, the criteria continue to reflect accurately the severity of acute pancreatitis.

APACHE II (Acute Physiology and Chronic Health Evaluation). Patients are assigned points for advancing age, abnormal physiology, and presence of severe organ dysfunction. Scores > 10 are associated with increased morbidity and mortality rates.

Pancreatic necrosis. Presence of 30% necrosis on dynamic computed tomographic (CT) scan (performed on patients with > 3 Ranson's criteria or APACHE II scores > 10).

8. List Ranson's prognostic indicators for severity of acute pancreatitis.

Initial findings	Findings that develop during first 48 hr
• Age > 55 yr	• Hematocrit fall > 10%
• White blood count > 16,000/mm^3	• Blood urea nitrogen > 8 mg/dl
• Glucose > 200 mg/dl	• Calcium < 8 mg/dl
• Lactate dehydrogenase > 350 IU/dl	• PO$_2$ < 60 mmHg
• Aspartate aminotransferase > 250 IU/dl	• Base deficit > 6 mEq/L
	• Fluid sequestration > 6 L

9. What mortality rates are associated with Ranson's criteria?

< 3 = 10%	5–6 = 40%
3–4 = 15%	> 7 = 100%

10. Describe the APACHE II scoring system for severity of acute pancreatitis.

1. **Age > 45 years:** assigned ascending points to age 75 (6-point maximum)
2. **Acute physiology score:** points are assigned for abnormal values (50-point maximum)
   - Vital signs
   - Arterial blood gases
   - Electrolytes
   - Glasgow Coma Scale (actual score)

3. **Chronic health score:** 2 points for each of the following conditions:
    - Cirrhosis of the liver
    - Severe chronic obstructive pulmonary disease
    - Renal dialysis
    - Congestive heart failure or angina at rest
    - Immunocompromise (chemotherapy, radiation therapy, AIDS)

11. **What physical and radiologic signs are associated with pancreatitis?**
    - Grey Turner sign: hemoglobin dissecting through tissue causes a bruise to the flank 3–5 days after acute necrotizing pancreatitis with hemorrhage
    - Cullen's sign: same as Gray Turner sign except bruise appears around the umbilicus
    - Colon cut-off sign: distended transverse colon with overlying inflammatory process in pancreas seen on upright abdominal radiograph
    - Sentinel loop: same as colon cut-off sign except radiographs show paralytic loop of air-filled jejunum.

12. **What steps are appropriate in managing acute pancreatitis?**
    - Admission to the hospital for all initial attacks. Recurrent mild attacks of pancreatitis may be managed on an outpatient basis.
    - Admission to intensive care unit (ICU) for all patients with severe acute pancreatitis.
    - Gallbladder ultrasound to rule out gallstones as the cause.
    - Dynamic computed tomography (CT) scan is indicated in patients with > 3 Ranson's criteria or APACHE II scores >10. CT scan should be performed to determine the extent of necrosis.
    - Laboratory studies include complete blood count, blood urea nitrogen, creatinine, calcium, lactate dehydrogenase, aspartate aminotransferase, bilirubin, glucose, and arterial blood gases. All used to determine Ranson's prognostic criteria.
    - Narcotics are given as necessary. Use meperidine; morphine causes contraction of the sphincter of Oddi.

13. **Which steps are *not* necessary initially?**
    - A nasogastric tube is needed only for severe cases, not for routine cases.
    - The prophylactic use of antibiotics has inconclusive benefits. Therapeutic use is indicated only when superinfection is definitely established.
    - Somatostatin analog has no proven benefit.

14. **When should a surgeon be consulted about a case of acute pancreatitis?**
    When gallstones are discovered, when significant pancreatic necrosis is present, when infection is suspected, or when the patient requires admission to ICU.

15. **List the complications of pancreatitis.**
    - Superinfection
    - Pseudocyst
    - Pancreatic ascites and pancreatic pleural effusion
    - Endocrine malfunction (diabetes)
    - Exocrine malfunction (steatorrhea and malabsorption)

16. **Is there any way to predict which patients will have superinfected pancreatitis?**
    Infection is unusual unless necrosis is present. The more extensive the necrosis, the higher the chances of infection (up to 80%).

17. **How is superinfection diagnosed?**
    CT-guided fine-needle aspiration with Gram stain, culture, and sensitivity tests.

18. What are the three types of infection? How is each treated?

    1. **Infected pancreatic pseudocyst.** Treatment is external drainage via exploratory laparotomy (open) or percutaneous drainage (closed).

    2. **Pancreatic abscess** (well-defined loculated cavity). Treatment is external drainage, open or closed.

    3. **Infected pancreatic necrosis.** Treatment is open operation only, with removal of the necrotic pancreas. The abdomen is either left open and reexplored to remove additional necrotic pancreas via multiple "second-look" procedures or large-bore sump catheters are left in place through which large-volume peritoneal lavage is performed. Total pancreatectomy is no longer indicated; the morbidity and mortality rates are too high.

19. What are the indications for surgery in acute severe pancreatitis with necrosis?
- When superinfection has been diagnosed.
- When the patient is nonresponsive to intensive care management techniques and is dying despite all efforts

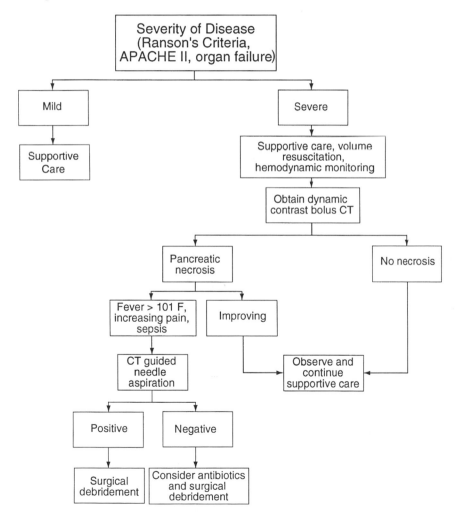

Treatment algorithm for acute pancreatitis.

20. What is the prognosis when aggressive surgical techniques are used for pancreatic necrosis and superinfection?
The mortality rate is decreased from > 80% to < 25%.

21. Describe acute fluid collections in patients with acute severe pancreatitis.
Acute fluid collections are located in or near the pancreas, occur early in the disease course, lack a defined wall, and usually resolve spontaneously. Pancreatic pseudocysts are collections of pancreatic juice confined by a discrete wall of fibrous tissue; they occur later in the course of the disease (average time = 4–6 weeks). Pancreatic abscess is a well-defined pus-filled cavity in proximity to the pancreas, usually without pancreatic juice and without necrosis. Pancreatic necrosis is nonviable pancreatic tissue caused by enzymatic autodigestion.

22. How often do pseudocysts form?
Fluid collections associated with acute pancreatitis are common and usually resolve spontaneously. Only 1–2% of all patients with pancreatitis develop pseudocysts that persist beyond 6 weeks.

23. What symptoms are associated with pseudocysts?
Chronic pain and persistently elevated amylase level.

24. How is the diagnosis made?
CT scan or ultrasound.

25. What are the indications for pseudocyst therapy?
Symptomatic pseudocyst > 5 cm that persists beyond 6 weeks.

26. What procedures are available for treatment of chronic pseudocysts?
- Percutaneous external catheter drainage. Length of treatment is prolonged; secondary infection rate is high.
- Excision: for a pseudocyst located in the tail of the pancreas.
- Internal drainage: into stomach, duodenum or roux-en-Y limb of jejunum—usual choice.
- Endoscopic cystogastrostomy

27. What complications do neglected pseudocysts cause? Describe the therapy for each.
- Superinfection: external drainage, open or closed, with or without somatostatin analog.
- Erosion into adjacent blood vessels: arteriographic embolization.
- Free rupture into abdominal cavity: emergency laparotomy with external drainage and/or pancreatic resection.
- Obstruction via compression of bile ducts, stomach, or intestinal tract: internal drainage into duodenum or stomach or roux-en-Y limb of jejunum.

28. What factors are considered in determining the correct timing of surgery for gallstone pancreatitis?
1. The gallstone usually obstructs the pancreatic duct only transiently and then passes into the duodenum. Amylase levels quickly return to normal, and 90% of patients recover rapidly.
2. Pancreatic necrosis is unusual in gallstone pancreatitis.
3. Early operations (within 48 hours) do not improve survival or enhance recovery.
4. Operations delayed beyond 6 weeks result in 50% recurrence of gallstone pancreatitis.
5. Most surgeons prefer to remove the gallbladder laparoscopically during the initial hospitalization (3–8 days) after the amylase level has returned to normal. If necrotizing pancreatitis is present, most surgeons delay cholecystectomy until the pancreatitis is totally resolved.

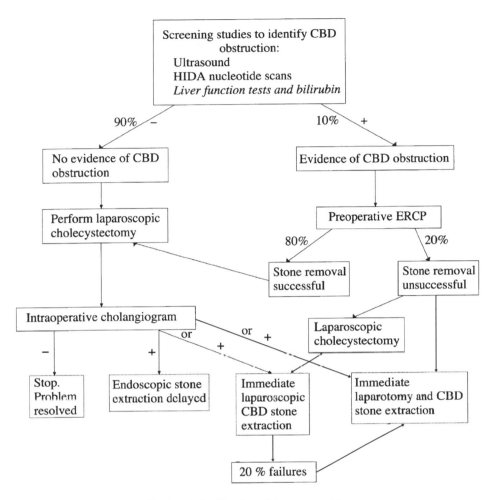

Treatment algorithm for gallstone pancreatitis.

29. What is pancreas divisum? How is it implicated in pancreatitis?

The dorsal pancreatic duct of Santorini fails to fuse with the ventral pancreatic duct of Wirsung in approximately 5% of the population. Obstruction of the minor pancreatic ampulla (Santorini duct) may result in recurrent episodes of pancreatitis. Sphincterotomy of the minor ampulla may be curative.

CHRONIC PANCREATITIS

30. What are the characteristic features of chronic pancreatitis?
- Recurrent attacks
- Mild elevation of amylase
- Destruction and fibrous replacement of parenchyma
- Loss of exocrine and endocrine function
- Disabling pain.

652   Pancreatic Surgery

31. How does chronic pancreatitis differ from acute pancreatitis?

	ACUTE	CHRONIC
Recurrent "attacks"	Rare	Classic
Reversible parenchymal changes	Yes	No
Fibrosis	No	Yes
Ductal dilations and obstructions	Rare	Common
Pancreatic calcifications	Never	Common
Peripancreatic digestion	Yes	No
Diabetes	Rare	Common
Exocrine dysfunction	Rare	Common
Etiology	Gallstones	Alcohol
Pseudocysts	1+	4+
Secondary infection	Common	Almost never
Amylase elevation	Higher	Lower
Surgical procedure	Debride and drain	Resect/drain duct

32. How is diagnosis of chronic pancreatitis established?
History of recurrent episodes of disabling pain with mild elevations of amylase, abdominal films showing calcifications, and endoscopic retrograde cholangiopancreatography (ERCP) revealing duct dilations and obstructions (chain of lakes). Not all cases of chronic pancreatitis have calcifications and ductal abnormalities, but their presence is diagnostic of the disease.

33. What is the medical therapy for chronic pancreatitis?
Symptomatic treatment only is the rule, with pain control, alcohol abstinence, and insulin and pancreatic enzyme replacement as necessary. Antibiotics, nasogastric tubes, and somatostatin analogs are of no value. Chronic pancreatitis is not as life-threatening as acute pancreatitis. Management is frustrating, palliative, and noncurative.

34. Who is a candidate for surgical therapy?
Patients with recurrent attacks who require repeated hospitalizations and have disabling pain that disrupts employment or narcotic addiction are legitimate surgical candidates.

35. What is role of ERCP in chronic pancreatitis?
1. It is used to establish the diagnosis by visualizing the dilated duct with obstructions (chain of lakes).
2. It is used preoperatively to define pancreatic duct anatomy and help plan surgery. ERCP is done within 12–24 hours of the planned surgery with antibiotic coverage.

36. What are the surgical options in chronic pancreatitis?
- Anastomoses of the pancreatic duct side-to-side with roux-en-Y limb of jejunum (Puestow procedure) are used when the pancreatic duct is a "chain of lakes" (see figure on following page).
- Distal resection and drainage to roux-en-Y limb of jejunum are used when the pancreatic duct is dilated with proximal obstruction.
- Total pancreatectomy should be performed only rarely (i.e., in patients who have previously failed other procedures and are already exocrine- and endocrine-deficient).
- Nerve ablation procedures, such as celiac ganglionectomy, are infrequently combined with the other approaches to alleviate pain.

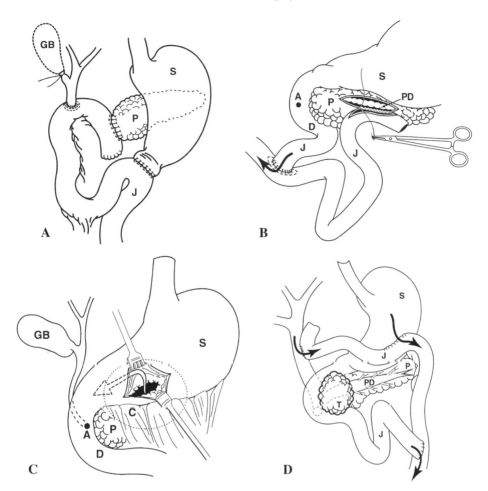

Surgical procedures on the pancreas. A, Pylorus-preserving pancreaticoduodenectomy (Whipple procedure). B, Roux-en-Y side-to-side pancreaticojejunostomy. C, Pancreatic pseudocystogastrostomy. D, Roux-en-Y choledochogastrojejunostomy (palliative gastric bypass) for a tumor of the head of the pancreas. S= stomach, D = duodenum, J = jejunum, P = pancreas, C = pseudocyst of the pancreas, T = tumor of the head of the pancreas, GB = gallbladder, A = ampulla, PD = pancreatic duct.

37. What is pancreatic ascites?

When pancreatic ductal disruption occurs in chronic pancreatitis secondary to alcoholism and trauma (rare), the pancreatic juice leaks into the free peritoneal cavity. Pancreatic ascites differs from ascites secondary to cirrhosis in two ways:

1. The amylase content is very high (in the thousands).
2. The protein concentration is > 2.5 gm/dl.

Even more rarely, a pleural effusion with the same characteristics may result when the pancreatic ductal disruption communicates with the pleural space. Because the digestive enzymes in pancreatic ascites are not activated, digestion of surrounding tissues does not occur.

38. How is the diagnosis of pancreatic ascites or pancreatic pleural effusion made?

Tap fluid and measure amylase and protein.

39. How is pancreatic ascites treated?

Conservative therapy resolves 50% of cases within 4–6 weeks. The patient must avoid oral ingestion and take somatostatin to decrease pancreatic secretions; total parenteral nutrition corrects the malnutrition; and peritoneal or pleural taps are used to relieve the pressure (as necessary).

If conservative therapy fails, preoperative endoscopic pancreatography is performed to localize the leak, and pancreatic resection and/or anastomosis of the leaking duct to a roux-en-Y limb of jejunum is performed. The mortality rate for these conditions remains high (20%) because underlying cirrhosis, alcoholism, and cachexia are common.

CANCER OF PANCREAS AND PERIAMPULLARY REGION

40. What are the cancers of the periampullary region? Why are they lumped together?

Cancers of the pancreas (70%), ampulla of Vater (10%), duodenum (10%), and distal common bile duct (10%) present with similar features:
- Obstructive jaundice
- Weight loss
- Abdominal pain
- Palpable gallbladder (30%)

41. How are cancers of the periampullary region diagnosed and treated?
Diagnosis
- Laboratory data: elevated obstructive enzymes (alkaline phosphatase and gamma-glutamyl transpeptidase) and direct bilirubin
- Imaging procedures: ultrasound, CT scan, ERCP (in that order)

Treatment: Whipple procedure (pancreaticoduodenectomy)

42. What are the 5-year survival rates when periampullary cancers are resected with Whipple procedure for cure?

Pancreas	< 10% if nodes positive; as high as 50% if nodes are negative
Ampulla	30–40%
Duodenum	15–30%
Distal common bile duct	30–40%

43. Describe the typical patient with pancreatic cancer.

The typical patient is a middle-aged black man who smokes and has diabetes as well as a history of alcoholism and pancreatitis. He presents with a dull aching pain, weight loss, and palpable gallbladder. Obstructive enzymes are elevated, and hepatocellular enzymes are normal; direct bilirubin is elevated.

44. What is the best serum marker for cancer of the pancreas?

CA 19-9. Both sensitivity and specificity are about 90%.

45. What is the "double duct" sign?

On ERCP, when both the distal common bile duct and proximal pancreatic duct are obstructed and dilated, the probability of pancreatic cancer is very high.

46. What is Courvoisier's sign?

Palpable gallbladder in a jaundiced patient secondary to malignant obstruction of the common bile duct. It is present in 25–40% of patients with periampullary cancers.

47. What percentage of patients with pancreatic cancer present with localized disease that can be cured by surgery?

Of 30,000 cases diagnosed annually in the United States, only about 1500 Whipple procedures are performed (5%). Eighty percent of cases have positive nodes, 50% have distant disease, and 40% have locally advanced disease. Almost all patients eventually die of the disease, 95% within a few months. In over 90% of patients who have surgical exploration, tumors are unresectable for cure.

48. Should all patients with pancreatic cancer be referred for surgical exploration to determine resectability or to bypass the GI tract and biliary tree when the tumor is unresectable?

No. CT scan, endoscopic ultrasound, or arteriography may reveal unresectability (liver metastases, malignant ascites, invasion of the portal vein or inferior vena cava, or bulky lymphadenopathy). In such cases, fine-needle aspiration to confirm the diagnosis precedes endoscopic or transhepatic percutaneous stent decompression of the common duct obstruction.

49. Does laparoscopy have a role in the management of periampullary cancer?

Yes. Not for resection but for determination of resectability without open surgical exploration.

50. When cancer arises in the body and tail of the pancreas, what is the prognosis?

Incurable. Virtually all tumors are unresectable.

51. What is the standard operative approach to periampullary cancer?

Exploratory laparotomy is used initially. In patients with no evidence of distant positive lymph nodes or metastases and no invasion into the inferior vena cava, portal vein, or adjacent organs, a Whipple procedure is performed to remove the distal stomach, duodenum, head of the pancreas, and distal common bile duct.

52. What is a pylorus-preserving Whipple procedure? When should it be performed?

When the cancer does not involve the stomach and the first 2.0 cm of the duodenum, these structures can be preserved. Thus, the complications of partial gastrectomy are avoided and long-term survival is preserved.

53. When should preoperative biliary decompression be performed?

Rarely. When ascending cholangitis is present or delay for nutritional support is deemed important, decompression is indicated. Most often surgery can be performed in the presence of obstructive jaundice without increasing mortality and morbidity rates.

54. At the time of surgery, should the pancreas be biopsied to verify cancer?

This question probably will never be settled. Surgeons who favor biopsy argue that because the operative mortality of a Whipple procedure is 10–20% (community practice) and the 5-year survival rate is low (<5%), pathologic confirmation of cancer is mandatory. Furthermore, biopsy is harmless, with a low complication rate (especially with fine-needle aspiration), and roux-en-Y choledochojejunostomy and gastrojejunostomy provide respectable long-term palliation.

Surgeons who proceed with a "blind" Whipple procedure argue that the clinical accuracy of the detection of pancreatic cancer by the experienced surgeon is > 95%. Thus delay for pathologic confirmation is avoided. Mortality rates at large centers performing many Whipple procedures is < 5%, and palliation is best when the cancer is resected.

A word of caution is appropriate. Although the mortality rate of pancreaticoduodenectomy at several centers of excellence has been lowered to 1%, the same mortality rate is not necessarily duplicated in community hospitals. Interpret these data within the context and results of your own hospital and staff. Certainly, attempts to duplicate these results are most appropriate when feasible, but the safe surgeon acknowledges the limits of his or her ability and hospital and refers complex cases to a center of excellence.

55. Because pancreatic cancer is multicentric and many complications are related to pancreatic anastomosis, why not remove the entire pancreas?

Survival rates are not improved, and the resultant diabetes is difficult to control. The combination of loss of insulin and glucagon and the presence of malabsorption requiring pancreatic enzymes entails erratic glucose metabolism.

56. What can be done to prevent pancreatic anastomotic complications?

Somatostatin analog, 100 mg subcutaneously every 8 hours, decreases the incidence.

57. Is advanced age a contraindication to Whipple resection?

No. This view is controversial, but recent experience in larger centers indicates that age is no contraindication. Common sense suggests that the elderly patient should be in excellent health without comorbid conditions and that the surgeon's results should be superlative to escape criticism.

58. Should the Whipple procedure be performed if regional lymph nodes are positive?

Probably not. Prognosis is dismal in this setting, and palliation is the most logical approach.

59. Describe the role of arteriography in periampullary cancer.

Arteriography is routinely performed by some surgeons to identify anomalous anatomy and determine whether the blood vessels are encased by cancer (evidence of unresectability).

60. When resection for cure is not possible, should biliary and stomach bypass procedures be performed?

Always bypass the biliary tree, and, if intestinal obstruction appears imminent, bypass the stomach also because up to 30% of tumors eventually obstruct the GI tract.

61. Is adjuvant therapy helpful in pancreatic cancer?

Yes. Use of chemotherapy and radiation therapy after all gross cancer is removed (adjuvant therapy) doubles the 2-year survival rate in patients with pancreatic cancer (43% vs. 18%).

ENDOCRINE TUMORS OF THE PANCREAS

62. What is the incidence of endocrine tumors of pancreas?

Functioning pancreatic endocrine tumors occur in 5 per million population per year. Nonfunctioning pancreatic endocrine tumors are more common. Autopsy reports indicate a prevalence as high as 1%. Insulinomas are the most common type of functional endocrine tumors (~1 per million population per year).

63. What are amine precursor uptake and decarboxylate (APUD) cells?

Some 40 endocrine cell types can take up amino acids and decarboxylate the molecules to synthesize functional endocrine, paracrine, or neurotransmitters. Many but not all adrenal cells (examples include islet cells and C cells of thyroid) migrate embryologically from the neural crest ectoderm. Kulchitsky cells (carcinoid) and enterochromaffin cells (adrenal) are other examples. High concentrations of these neuroendrocrine cells are found in the central nervous system, endocrine glands and gastrointestinal tract. Neoplastic proliferation of these cell lines results in the neuroendocrine syndromes (e.g., Zollinger-Ellison syndrome).

64. How do nonfunctioning tumors present?

As large bulky malignant masses. Small, benign, nonfunctioning tumors usually remain undiagnosed. Because of their protean manifestations, a delay in diagnosis is common for many islet cell tumors. The most common functioning islet cell tumor is an insulinoma.

Islet Cell Tumors

TUMOR	CELL TYPE	HORMONE	SYMPTOMS	% MALIGNANT	% MEN
Insulinoma	B	Insulin	Hypoglycemia	10	10
Gastrinoma	G	Gastrin	Peptic ulcers, diarrhea	60–80	25
Glucagonoma	A	Glucagon	Hyperglycemia Anemia, cachexia Necrolytic migratory erythema	70	1
Somatostatinoma	D	Somatostatin	Gallstones, diabetes	75	0

Table continued on following page

Islet Cell Tumors (Continued)

TUMOR	CELL TYPE	HORMONE	SYMPTOMS	%MALIGNANT	% MEN
VIPoma (pancreatic cholera, Verner-Morrison syndrome, WDHA syndrome)	H	Vasoactive intestinal peptide (VIP)	Watery diarrhea Hypokalemia Achlorhydria	50	5

MEN = multiple endocrine neoplasia type I, WDHA = watery diarrhea, hypokalemia, achlorhydria.

65. What is an insulinoma?

A rare tumor of pancreatic islet B cells that produces excessive insulin, causing either symptoms related to CNS hypoglycemia (confusion, erratic behavior, seizures, coma) or to excessive compensatory catecholamine release (sweating, tachycardia, palpitations).

66. Define Whipple's triad.

Whipple's triad refers to the three cardinal features of an insulinoma:
1. Symptoms precipitated by fasting.
2. Blood sugar < 50 mg/dl.
3. Symptoms relieved by glucose.

67. How is the diagnosis of insulinoma established?

An in-hospital, observed 72-hour fast with simultaneous blood glucose and insulin measurements diagnoses all patients with insulinoma, usually within the first 24 hours. An insulin/glucose ratio > 0.3 is diagnostic (μg/ml insulin to mg/dl glucose).

68. What is the rule of 10s?

Roughly 10% of insulinomas are malignant, 10% are multiple, 10% are associated with multiple endocrine neoplasia type I (MEN I), and most are about 10 mm in size.

69. What is MEN I syndrome?

An autosomal dominant, genetic defect of the long arm of chromosome 11. Remember the 3 Ps: tumor of the pituitary, pancreas, and parathyroid characterize MEN I. Whenever one type of tumor is found, screening should be done for the other types, even though they may not be found simultaneously. Islet cell tumors associated with MEN are treated differently from sporadic islet cell tumors.

70. Can the pathologist diagnose endocrine malignancy by cellular appearance alone?

Usually not, because all endocrine tumors can manifest bizarre nuclear atypia and may still behave in a benign fashion. The only proof of endocrine malignancy is metastasis.

71. Define factitious hypoglycemia.

Hypoglycemia induced by taking insulin or sulfonylureas, usually in health care workers. Diagnosis is based on detection of insulin antibodies or sulfonylureas in the blood.

72. What medications are used to control hypoglycemia in patients with an insulinoma?

Diazoxide and somatostatin analog (octreotide) with or without glucose drip.

73. How are insulinomas localized in the pancreas?

Because insulinomas are seldom malignant and usually small and solitary, they are highly curable. Thus, preoperative localization is important. CT, MRI, or US alone or in combination reveals approximately 50% of tumors, especially those > 1 cm. Because localization is so important, various creative preoperative tests have been devised. Angiography with injection of calcium promotes tumor release of insulin, which is simultaneously sampled in the hepatic venous return and may identify the general area of pancreatic involvement in 60–80% of cases. Indium[111]-labeled octreotide nuclear scan with or without use of an intraoperative hand-held isotope detector has limited use because only one-half of insulinomas have somatostatin receptors. By far the most sensitive localization technique is intraoperative US by the surgeon (> 90% effective, even when other techniques fail). Most surgeons use preoperative arteriograms and intraoperative US.

74. Who should be explored?

Any patient with a confirmed insulinoma who does not have bulky, advanced metastatic disease. A simple enucleation of the tumor suffices in most cases. Occasionally large metastatic lesions are debulked to reduce insulin load and enhance efficacy of medications. A subtotal pancreatectomy or Whipple procedure is occasionally necessary for large bulky tumors. Suspicious lymph nodes are also removed. In patients with MEN I, the insulinomas are multiple, microscopic, and macroscopic; a subtotal pancreatectomy is advisable.

75. What is the second most common islet tumor?

Gastrinoma or Zollinger-Ellison (ZE) syndrome, in which the tumor causes hypersecretion of stomach acid via the hormone gastrin. The only way to treat the syndrome until cimetidine was introduced in the 1980s was to remove the stomach (total gastrectomy).

76. What is the ZE or gastrinoma triangle?

The anatomic area in which 90% of all gastrinomas are located. The gastrinoma triangle is defined by the junction of the cystic and common bile ducts superiorly, the second and third portions of the duodenum inferiorly, and the junction of the neck and body of the pancreas medially. Technically gastrinomas are considered islet cell tumors, but more than 50% are found outside the pancreas, usually in the duodenal wall. Gastrinomas are the islet cell tumor most often associated with MEN.

77. How do patients with ZE syndrome present?

With refractory peptic ulcer disease, usually with ulcers in the duodenum but also with ulcers in the third and fourth portions of the duodenum or jejunum. Patients may have severe esophagitis and frequently screen negative for *Helicobacter pylori*. Some patients present with perforation of ulcers in the duodenum or even perforated esophagitis, before or after ulcer surgery (i.e., vagotomy, antrectomy). Most patients have diarrhea secondary to high acid irritation of small bowel mucosa and acid interference with lipase and bile salt metabolism, resulting in high bile salt and fat concentrations in the colon. Some patients, however, present with neither ulcers nor diarrhea.

78. How is the diagnosis of ZE syndrome established?

The diagnosis is delayed by an average of 6 years. Ninety-nine percent of patients have fasting gastrin > 100 pg/ml; a fasting gastrin level > 1000 pg/ml is diagnostic. Basal acid output (BAO) is > 15 mEq/hr, or BAO/maximal acid output is > 75%. Parietal stomach acid cells work at full capacity virtually all of the time because of increased basal level of gastrin. Calcium, protein meal, and glucagon have been used as provocative tests, but the secretin stimulation test is the gold standard to rule out other causes of elevated gastrin and to confirm indeterminate cases (gastrin = 100–1000 pg/ml). After administration of secretin, 2 U/kg IV, gastrin is measured every 5 minutes × 4. An increase of gastrin > 200 pg/ml is diagnostic of gastrinoma.

79. What may cause increased serum gastrin besides ZE syndrome?

- Achlorhydria (most common cause)
- Retained antrum after vagotomy and Billroth II procedure (the antrum must be attached to the duodenum and continuously bathed with alkaline duodenal secretions)
- Gastrectomy or massive small bowel resection
- Gastric outlet obstruction
- So-called G cell hyperplasia syndrome (ask your gastroenterologist to explain this one)

Patients with these disorders have indeterminate levels of gastrin (100–1000 pg/ml) and negative secretin stimulation tests.

80. Can gastric acid hypersecretion be medically controlled?

Yes, in virtually 100% of patients with ZE syndrome. A combination of H_2 blockers and proton pump inhibitors can be titrated to achieve endoscopically verified mucosal healing. Doses ranging from 3–5 times the usual dose are given to maintain BAO at 1–5 mEq/hr without producing achlorhydria.

81. What localization studies should be done before surgery?

CT should be ordered to look for liver metastasis and large pancreatic tumors. Endoscopic US is particularly helpful to localize small duodenal wall tumors. Angiograms with or without secretin injections into the gastroduodenal, splenic, and superior mesenteric arteries with simultaneous hepatic vein sampling for gastrin are more sophisticated tests. Gastrinomas have a bright vascular blush on angiography. As in insulinoma, indium-labeled somatostatin analog is occasionally useful in detecting gastinomas. These tests should be discussed with the endocrine surgeon, many of whom believe that they are expensive, inaccurate, and unnecessary and that intraoperative techniques are best. Most surgeons do preoperative angiograms and intraoperative US.

82. If complications of ZE syndrome can be prevented by medications, why refer anyone for surgery?

Long-term survival depends on curative resection of both malignant and benign lesions. Total gastrectomy is no longer indicated, but careful systematic resection of all disease may offer 5-year cure rates as high as 75%. Unfortunately, most gastrinomas recur (usually 6 years after surgery); thus the 10-year cure rate is < 50%.

83. Who should undergo surgical exploration?

Everyone except possibly patients with MEN I and patients with extensive unresectable metastatic disease.

84. Why is surgery not done for gastrinomas associated with MEN syndrome?

These gastrinomas are usually multiple (sometimes dozens) and microscopic. Surgical procedures do not cure MEN gastrinomas. If the gastrinoma is associated with hyperparathyroidism, however, a parathyroidectomy should be done because calcium is a secretogogue for gastrinomas and many of the symptoms can be ameliorated with subtotal parathyroidectomy.

85. Describe the surgical strategy.

Intraoperative ultrasound and open duodenotomy with careful bimanual palpation of the duodenal wall remain the mainstay of surgical exploration. Successful identification occurs in 80–90% of cases, even without preoperative localization. Pancreatic and duodenal tumors are enucleated and excised; large bulky tumors may require pancreatic resections. All palpable lymph nodes are excised in the area of the gastroduodenal triangle. Other types of islet cell tumors are so rare as to represent a medical curiosity.

BIBLIOGRAPHY

1. Bradley EL: Classification for acute pancreatitis. Arch Surg 128:586–590, 1993.
2. Bradley EL: Experience with open drainage for infected pancreatic necroses. Surg Gynecol Obstet 177:215–222, 1993.
3. Buchler M: Role of octreotide in the prevention of postoperative complications following pancreatic resections. Am J Surg 163:125, 1992.
4. Cameron JL: Factors influencing survival after pancreaticoduodenectomy for pancreatic cancer. Am J Surg 161:120–125, 1991.
5. Cameron JL, et al: One hundred and forty–five consecutive pancreaticoduodenectomies without mortality. Am Surg 217:430–435, 1993.
6. Grace PA: Pylorus preserving pancreaticoduodenectomy: An overview. Br J Surg 77:968–974, 1990.
7. Gumaste VV: Diagnostic tests for acute pancreatitis. Gastroenterologist 2:119–130, 1994.
8. Imric CW, et al: Predictions of outcome in acute pancreatitis. Br J Surg 77:1260–1264, 1990.
9. Marshall JB: Acute pancreatitis: A review. Arch Intern Med 153:1185–1198, 1993.
8. Pellegrini CA: Surgery for gallstone pancreatitis. Am J Surg 165:515–518, 1993.
11. Posner MR, et al: The use of serologic markers in gastrointestinal malignancies. Hematol/Oncol Clin North Am 8:533–553, 1994.
12. Ranson JHC: Prognostic signs and the role of surgery in acute pancreatitis. Surg Gynecol Obstet 139:69–81, 1974.
13. Ranson JHC: The role of surgery in acute pancreatitis. Am Surg 211:382–393, 1990.
14. Warshaw AL, et al:Early debridement of pancreatic necroses is beneficial. Am J Surg 163:105–110, 1992.
15. Whittington R, et al: Adjuvant therapy for cancer of pancreas. Int J Radiat Oncol Biol Phys 21(5):1137–1143, 1991.

84. HEPATOBILIARY SURGERY

Anthony J. Canfield, M.D, FACS, John D. Moffat, M.D., FACS, Michael C. Hotard, M.D., FACS, and F. Calvin Bigler, M.D., FACS

BILIARY DISEASE

1. What are the clinical manifestations of acute cholecystitis?

Acute cholecystitis usually occurs in patients 40–80 years old. The female-to-male ratio is 3:1. Most patients complain of severe right upper quadrant (RUQ) pain that radiates to the right scapula or midback, which often is accompanied by nausea and occasionally by vomiting. Physical findings include fever, RUQ tenderness, and Murphy's sign (inspiratory arrest with steady palpation of the right upper quadrant). Presence of a mass in the RUQ implies omental inflammation or gallbladder dilation.

2. How is acute cholecystitis diagnosed?

Laboratory tests demonstrate elevated WBC count and occasionally a mild increase in bilirubin. Plain abdominal films may show radiopaque gallstones (15–20% of cases). Ultrasound (US) findings include thickened gallbladder wall with pericholecystic fluid. A hepatobiliary (HIDA) scan shows nonvisualization of the gallbladder. HIDA scan is highly accurate for the diagnosis of acute cholecystitis (sensitivity, 95–100%; specificity, 95%).

3. Describe the treatment of acute cholecystitis.

Surgical intervention includes hydration, antibiotic therapy and prompt cholecystectomy. The laparoscopic approach is preferred, but conversion to a conventional open cholecystectomy is required when the inflammation is severe. Percutaneous cholecystostomy is useful when the patient is too ill to tolerate surgery.

4. Explain "hydrops" of the gallbladder.

Hydrops refers to the accumulation of clear mucus within a chronically obstructed and inflamed gallbladder. The gallbladder often is dilated and palpable on physical exam. Outlet obstruction of the cystic duct usually is caused by an impacted stone but may be due to chronic inflammation of the gallbladder neck or congenital stenosis of the cystic duct. The mucus is produced by the secretory epithelium of the gallbladder.

5. What bacteria are commonly found within the gallbladder with acute cholecystitis?

Escherichia coli, Pseudomonas aeruginosa, anaerobic streptococci, *Streptococcus fecalis,* and species of *Klebsiella, Clostridium, Proteus,* and *Enterobacter.* Antibiotic coverage includes either ampicillin/sulbactam (Unasyn), piperacillin (Pipracil), or ticarcillin (Timentin).

6. A 36-year-old woman presents with a 4-month history of postprandial right upper quadrant pain with radiation to the right scapula, accompanied by nausea and occasional emesis. US shows no gallstones, and the white blood cell count is normal. What further work-up should be obtained?

Patients with "typical" symptoms of biliary colic but without demonstrable gallstones frequently have chronic inflammation of the gallbladder, known as chronic acalculous cholecystitis or biliary dyskinesia. The diagnosis can be confirmed by CCK-HIDA scan, which determines cystic duct patency (accumulation of radionuleotide in the gallbladder) and the gallbladder's capacity to contract (referred to as the ejection fraction). An ejection fraction < 35% correlates strongly with chronic acalculous cholecystitis and predicts a 95% probability of symptomatic cure after cholecystectomy.

7. A 53-year-old American Indian woman with RUQ pain undergoes laparoscopic cholecys-tectomy for a 3.1-cm. gallstone. During the surgery you find nodular indentation at the gall-bladder fundus that appears to be extending into the liver bed. What should you do next?

This finding may represent gallbladder carcinoma. Biopsy with frozen section should be per-formed. When gallbladder carcinoma is identified, the surgery should be converted to an open la-parotomy and intraoperative staging performed.

8. Summarize the tumor-node-metastasis (TNM) classification of gallbladder cancer.

SIZE OF PRIMARY TUMOR (T)	REGIONAL LYMPH NODE METASTASIS
Tis: carcinoma in situ	N0: no lymph node metastasis
T1: tumor invades mucosa	N1: metastasis to cystic duct, pericholedochal,
T2: tumor invades perimuscular connective tissue	and/or hilar lymph nodes
T3: tumor perforates serosa or invades into one	N2: metastasis to peripancreatic, periduodenal,
adjacent organ (< 2m of liver)	periportal celiac, and/or superior mesenteric
T4: tumor extends more than 2 cm into liver or into	lymph nodes
two or more adjacent organs	

9. How is gallbladder cancer staged?

Stage I	T1, N0, M0	Stage IVA	T4, N0, or N1, M0
Stage II	T2, N0, M0	Stage IVB	Any T, N2, M0 or any T, any N, M1
Stage III	T1, T2, or T3, N0, or N1, M0		

10. How does stage affect treatment?

Treatment for stage I and carcinoma in situ requires only cholecystectomy. Stages II, III, and IVA require radical cholecystectomy with lymph node dissection and end-block segmental exci-sion of lobes IV and V of the liver. For stage IVB, the mortality and morbidity rates of surgery are excessively high, and surgery offers no clinical benefit. Response rates to chemotherapy and radiation therapy are generally poor. The 5-year survival rate is approximately 5%.

11. List the major risk factors for gallbladder carcinoma.

Race: The highest incidence of gallbladder carcinoma is seen among Native American Indians, Mexican Americans, and Native Alaskans.

Gallstones: Most gallbladder cancer (90%) is associated with cholelithiasis, and the pres-ence of large gallstones (> 2.5 cm) increases the risk for cancer significantly.

"Porcelain" gallbladder: 12–61% risk for gallbladder cancer.

12. A 67-year-old woman with a history of intermittent RUQ pain for several years com-plains of nausea and bilious emesis for 2 days, with crampy mid-abdominal pain and bloat-ing. She denies passing flatus. The abdomen is distended and nontender, and abdominal x-rays show distended loops of small bowel with air-fluid levels. What is the likely cause?

Gallstone ileus is the cause of nonstrangulated small bowel mechanical obstruction in 25% of patients older than 65 years. The usual mechanism involves acute cholecystitis with adherence of the duodenum or jejunum to the gallbladder, followed by subsequent erosion of the gallstone into the duodenum or jejunum. The gallstones are usually > 2.5 cm. Of importance, only 20% of stones are radiopaque and visible on plain abdominal radiographs.

13. Describe the surgical management of gallstone ileus.

Stage 1: removal of gallstone to relieve bowel obstruction and antibiotic therapy.

Stage 2: elective surgery to repair the cholecystoenteric fistula.

14. Why is the two-stage approach preferred?

The mortality rate for simultaneous surgery of the small bowel obstruction and cholecys-toenteric fistula is approximately 20%, whereas the mortality rate for the two-stage surgery is about 11%. Most cholecystoenteric fistulas close spontaneously with conservative management.

CYSTIC DISEASE OF THE LIVER (see ch. 35)

15. In a patient with atypical RUQ abdominal pain, CT reveals a hepatic cyst. Discuss the symptoms and characteristics of the cyst that warrant surgical treatment.

The simple cyst is the most common cystic lesion of the liver. It often is discovered by radiologic tests performed to evaluate unrelated symptoms or during surgery for unrelated reasons. Small, asymptomatic simple cysts do not require treatment. However, simple hepatic cysts > 5 cm tend to enlarge slowly and become symptomatic. Symptoms may range from mild discomfort to debilitating pain. Hepatic cysts also may become infected, obstruct the biliary tree, rupture, and even hemorrhage. Although hepatic cysts generally consist of biliary epithelium, they do not communicate with the biliary system. Internal cyst hemorrhage, decompression into the biliary tree, and cholangitis are rare complications that may warrant emergent surgical intervention.

16. Discuss the nonsurgical treatment options for benign hepatic cysts.

Treatment options vary widely and may be tailored to the patient's presentation and medical condition. Simple percutaneous aspiration is generally ineffective and associated with a high recurrence rate. Most centers limit this technique to a diagnostic role (i.e., to determine whether symptoms are related to the cyst). Percutaneous cyst aspiration combined with cyst sclerosis is gaining popularity because it is technically simple and minimally invasive and can be performed on an outpatient basis. Contraindications to cyst sclerosis include communication of the cyst with the biliary tree and systemic coagulopathy. Complications of the technique include hemorrhage, sepsis, bile duct injury, and biliary leak. Repeated attempts at sclerotherapy do not preclude subsequent surgical treatment.

17. What are the goals of surgical treatment?

Successful surgery for simple hepatic cysts requires complete excision and wide exposure of the superficial cyst wall. This technique permits free flow of cyst secretions into the peritoneal cavity and cyst decompression. Surgically applied coagulation or sclerosants can treat hepatic cysts that are inaccessible to complete excision of the cyst epithelium. Partial excision with fenestration, involving wide unroofing of the superficial cyst surface, is also effective when cysts are multilocular but communicate with each other. Advantages of surgical treatment include lowest recurrence rate and ability to repair cystobiliary communications and control hemorrhage.

18. Discuss differences in presentation of adult polycystic liver disease and simple liver cysts.

Adult polycystic liver disease is an inherited disorder that tends to progress slowly after late onset of symptoms. It is characterized by cystic transformation of both lobes of the liver. The most common symptoms include abdominal swelling, abdominal pain, pain with bending, and shortness of breath. Physical findings include increasing abdominal girth and enlarged nodular liver; tenderness is rare.

19. How is adult polycystic liver disease treated?

Treatment options are more limited. Aspiration and sclerosis are generally used to provide symptomatic relief of larger lesions. Surgical resection of larger cysts, with or without combined fenestration of multiple adjacent cysts, has been the mainstay of treatment to relieve symptoms. Postoperative treatment with H_2 receptor blockade and octreotide has been effective in reducing hepatic drainage. Hepatic resection of polycystic liver disease can be dangerous, but recent studies have shown that combined anatomic resection of the diffusely cystic portion of the liver, with fenestration of a less involved portion of the liver, produces good long-term results.

PARASITIC AND OTHER INFECTIOUS DISEASES OF THE LIVER (see ch. 32)

20. What are the important considerations in both presentation and management of hydatid diseases of the liver?

The tapeworm, *Echinococcus granulosus*, causes hepatic hydatid disease. A long latent period is typical, and painless hepatomegaly may be the only sign of disease. Free peritoneal rupture of the cyst can cause fatal anaphylaxis. Preoperative administration of steroids and diphenhydramine and cyst injection with hypertonic saline and scolicidal agents may decrease the risk of fatal anaphylaxis associated with operative leak of cyst contents. Recent studies have shown that complete pericystectomy is more effective at reducing recurrence and improves resolution of the hepatic defect.

21. Describe the changes in etiology, diagnosis, and treatment of pyogenic liver abscess over the past 40 years.

Earlier in the twentieth century, pyogenic liver abscess was caused primarily by pylephlebitis due to complicated appendicitis or diverticulitis. For the past 40 years, biliary tract obstruction and cholangitis from either benign or malignant causes has become the most common cause of pyogenic liver abscess. Abdominal imaging with US, CT, and percutaneous FNA and cholangiography have greatly improved the ability to diagnosis pyogenic abscess. Treatment options include antibiotics alone, antibiotics in combination with drainage procedures (e.g., percutaneous aspiration or indwelling catheter drainage), and surgical drainage. Recent studies have shown that percutaneous indwelling catheter drainage and antibiotic therapy are superior to surgical cyst drainage. Simple aspiration has a high recurrence rate and often requires repeated aspiration. Antibiotic treatment alone has a high mortality rate (up to 25%).

22. A patient has been treated appropriately with broad-spectrum antibiotics and drainage for pyogenic hepatic abscess but fails to improve. What is a possible explanation? What treatment options should be entertained?

The patient with a presumptive pyogenic liver abscess that fails indwelling catheter drainage and antibiotics should be carefully evaluated for a mixed fungal/pyogenic abscess. Fungal hepatic abscesses are recognized with increasing frequency, especially in immunocompromised patients.

23. How does amebic abscess of the liver differ from pyogenic abscess of the liver in diagnosis and treatment?

An amebic abscess is less likely to perforate than a pyogenic abscess. Circulating amebic antibody is detected by indirect hemagglutination test in > 95% of cases and is sufficient to initiate treatment when a liver abscess is identified. Primary treatment for amebic abscess is metronidazole, 750 mg 3 times/day for 10 days, plus an intraluminal agent (e.g., iodoquinol) for cyst passers. Most amebic liver abscesses respond to metronidazole treatment alone. Mixed amebic/pyogenic abscesses occur in 15% of cases and should be considered when metronidazole treatment fails. Surgical treatment is rarely necessary.

BENIGN HEPATIC TUMORS (see ch. 24)

24. What are the most common benign hepatic tumors? Discuss briefly their distinguishing characteristics, and recommended treatment.

The increased use of US and CT to evaluate abdominal complaints has led to increased detection of coincidental, asymptomatic benign hepatic tumors, including cavernous hemangiomas, hepatic adenomas, and focal nodular hyperplasia (FNH).

25. Describe cavernous hemangiomas.

Cavernous hemangiomas are the most common benign liver tumor and occur more often in women than in men. They are usually small (< 3 cm) and asymptomatic and can be safely followed radiographically. When mass effect produces symptoms or spontaneous rupture occurs, surgical excision is indicated. Preoperative biopsy is often complicated by hemorrhage and is not necessary.

26. What causes hepatic adenomas? How are they treated?

Hepatic adenomas generally occur in women of menstrual age and are associated with oral contraceptive use. Discontinuation of oral contraceptives may lead to regression of small, asymptomatic lesions within several months. Larger lesions are less likely to regress, and resection should be considered, especially when pregnancy is contemplated. Needle biopsy may be effective in distinguishing hepatic adenoma from other benign lesions and hepatocellular carcinoma. Symptoms from hepatic adenoma are mostly due to mass effect and include abdominal pain, early satiety, nausea, and vomiting. Hepatic adenomas are more likely to hemorrhage and may undergo malignant degeneration. Hepatic adenomas should be resected when they produce symptoms or when the diagnosis is uncertain.

27. How is FNH diagnosed and treated?

FNH primarily affects women of menstrual age but has not been associated with oral contraceptive use. Most (90%) of patients with FNH are asymptomatic; work-up is usually initiated when it is difficult to distinguish the presence of malignancy or other benign tumors. Focal nodular hyperplasia has a highly characteristic intraoperative appearance: usually tan-to-dark brown, smaller than 5 cm, and usually located in the periphery of the liver. Specific radiologic imaging tests, and needle biopsy are helpful in establishing the diagnosis. Once the diagnosis is established, FNH can be managed expectantly; it has no malignant potential. Wedge resection is the treatment of choice when the diagnosis is in doubt or significant enlargement occurs.

MALIGNANT HEPATIC TUMORS

28. What is the only treatment of hepatocellular carcinoma (HCC) that can significantly prolong survival?

Surgical resection. Unfortunately the presence of cirrhosis and decreased hepatic reserve precludes significant liver resection in most patients. A limited disease-free margin of 1 cm has been shown to improve survival. Intraoperative US at the time of operative exploration is useful in detecting more extensive disease and avoids unnecessary and unhelpful resection. Some transplant centers offer liver transplantation for small (< 5 cm), solitary HCC after preoperative chemotherapy.

29. What is the differential diagnosis of obstructive jaundice?

Benign: choledocholithiasis or biliary stricture (usually of surgical etiology)

Malignant: extrinsic: primary or metastatic pancreatic head tumor or gallbladder cancer; intrinsic: cholangiocarcinoma

30. What is a Klatskin's tumor?

A primary biliary or metastatic malignancy at the bifurcation of the left and right hepatic duct. A Klatskin tumor should be suspected when US or CT shows dilation of the right and left intrahepatic bile ducts but a small to normal-sized common bile duct and gallbladder.

31. What clues may help to define the nature of the biliary obstruction?

The history and physical exam often provide important clues to the diagnosis. Biliary tract pain develops as a consequence of sudden biliary distention, as seen clinically with migration of a gallstone. Insidious and slow obstruction frequently is painless; hence, painless jaundice is often of malignant etiology. Weight loss may suggest underlying malignancy, whereas fever, chills, and rigors may suggest a diagnosis of biliary infection, which is more commonly seen with gallstones. Recent biliary surgery suggests surgical misadventure or complication.

Physical exam frequently demonstrates jaundice and scleral icterus. A nontender, palpable gallbladder (Courvoisier's gallbladder) suggests distal biliary obstruction. A painful distended gallbladder is more often due to an impacted stone in the neck of the gallbladder that produces acute hydrops. Compression of the common bile duct by an inflamed Hartman's pouch or large cystic duct stone may produce a picture of obstructive jaundice known as Mirizzi's syndrome. Spiking fevers suggest a diagnosis of ascending cholangitis, which is more often seen with choledocholithiasis.

32. What investigations should be undertaken in a jaundiced patient?

Laboratory tests: complete blood count, liver panel, and coagulation studies.

Radiology: US is the best first test; dilation of the bile ducts implies obstruction. Important findings include gallstones and the size of the common bile duct and intrahepatic ducts. On occasion, common bile duct stones are identified on US. Intravenous cholangiography is of historical interest only. Endoscopic retrograde cholangiography is the gold standard for investigating patients with obstructive jaundice. Magnetic resonance cholangiography is a new, accurate, and noninvasive method, but its availability is limited.

33. Can obstructive jaundice constitute a surgical emergency?

Yes. Jaundice, fever and RUQ pain (Charcot's triad) suggest a diagnosis of ascending cholangitis. Untreated, the disease can progress rapidly to septic shock with the added features of hypotension and confusion (Reynold's pentad). Complete cardiovascular collapse and death may ensue without prompt intervention.

34. Describe the treatment of ascending cholangitis.

Immediate institution of broad-spectrum antibiotics may abort the progression of ascending cholangitis, but biliary decompression is still necessary. It can be accomplished by ERCP with sphincterotomy and internal drainage or via either laparoscopic or open cholecystectomy.

35. Is ERCP the gold standard for the investigation and treatment of obstructive jaundice?

Yes. In expert hands ERCP can determine the cause of biliary obstruction and provide internal biliary decompression in 90–95% of cases.

36. What is postcholecystectomy syndrome?

Patients who continue to complain of upper abdominal discomfort suggestive of biliary tract pain after removal of the gallbladder have been labeled as suffering from the post cholecystectomy syndrome. Unrelated factors (e.g., hiatal hernia, gastroesophageal reflux disease, duodenal ulcer, colon cancer) may be the underlying cause of symptoms.

Biliary manometry has demonstrated that some patients have high resting sphincter of Oddi (SO) pressures that may be caused by fibrosis or SO spasm. When biliary manometry identifies SO pressures > 40 mmHg, sphincterotomy may relieve pain.

37. List some uncommon causes of jaundice.

Primary sclerosing cholangitis (PSC) is an inflammatory and fibrotic process that can involve part or all of the biliary tree. PSC has an insidious and progresses to liver failure or cholangiocarcinoma. The cause is uncertain but may be related to viral infection and altered immune function. Coincident inflammatory bowel disease is seen in 80% of cases. PSC is diagnosed by ERCP.

Choledochal cysts are relatively rare and have a five-part subclassification. They may not present until adulthood, when the patient develops recurrent bouts of cholangitis. Choledochal cysts are associated with an increased risk of bile duct cancer and should be treated with resection and reconstitution.

BIBLIOGRAPHY

1. Cameron JL, et al: Current Surgical Therapy, 6th ed. St. Louis, Mosby, 1998.
2. Caporale A, Guiliani A, Teneriello FL, et al: Surgical management of nonparasitic cysts of the liver: Report of 17 cases. Dig Surg 10:249–253, 1994.
3. Fong Y, Kemenly N, Paty P, et al: Treatment of colorectal cancer: Hepatic metastasis. Cohen Semin Surg Oncol 12:219–252, 1996.
4. Huang C-J, Pitt HA, Lipsett PA, et al: Pyogenic hepatic abscess: Changing trends over 42 years. Ann Surg 223:600–609, 1996.
5. Huguier M, Hobeika J, Houry S: Hydatid cysts of the liver: Surgical treatment. Dig Surg 12:314–317, 1995.
6. Lipsett PA, Huang C-J, Lillemoe KD, et al: Fungal hepatic abscesses: Characterization and management. J Gastrointest Surg 1:78–84, 1997.
7. Madariaga JR, Shunzaburo I, Starzl TE, et al: Hepatic resection for cystic lesions of the liver. Ann Surg 218:610–614, 1993.
8. Marcos-Alvarez A, Jenkins R, Washburn WK, et al: Multimodality treatment of hepatocellular carcinoma in a hepatobiliary specialty center. Arch Surg 131:292–298, 1996.
9. Meng X-J, Wu, J-X: Perforated amebic liver abscess: Clinical analysis of 110 cases. South Med J 87:988–990, 1994.
10. Moskal TL, Charnsangavej C, Ellis LM: Workup, diagnosis, and treatment of benign hepatic tumors. Cancer Bull 47:385-391, 1995.
11. Sabiston DC Jr, et al: Textbook of Surgery, 14th ed. Philadelphia, W.B. Saunders, 1991.
12. Seeto RK, Rockey DC: Pyogenic liver abscess: Changes in etiology, management, and outcome. Medicine 75(2):99-113, 1996.
13. Soravia C, Mentha G, Giostra E, et al: Surgery for adult polycystic liver disease. Surgery 117:272–275, 1995.
14. Vauthey J-N, Maddern GJ, Blumgart LH: Adult polycystic disease of the liver. Br J Surg 78:524–527, 1991.
15. Yamanaka N, Okamoto E, Tsuyosi O, et al: A prediction scoring system to select the surgical treatment of liver cancer: Further refinement based on 10 years of use. Ann Surg 219:342–346, 1994.

85. LAPAROSCOPIC SURGERY

Anthony J. LaPorta, M.D., and Bernard Kopchinski, M.D.

1. You are evaluating a patient who may require surgery. During your work-up, the patient tells you that he is taking ginseng. What recommendations should you make?

Ginseng is a common herbal preparation taken by many people to increase energy levels and improve memory. Ginseng has been reported to cause tachycardia and hypertension. An interaction with ginseng and estrogens or warfarin also has been reported. Recently, the American Society of Anesthesiologists recommended that all herbal preparations be stopped 2–3 weeks before surgery.

2. What is the difference between the hepatocystic triangle and the triangle of Calot?

To avoid major biliary tract injury, knowledge of the hepatocystic triangle and Calot's triangle is essential. Lateral inferior retraction of the gallbladder at the infundibulum (Hartman's pouch) with cephaled retraction at the dome facilitates the identification of both. Dissection for laparoscopic cholecystitis should start at the gallbladder neck (Hartman's pouch) and proceed to the cystic duct, followed by dissection of the cystic artery. Excessive dissection toward the common bile duct is fraught with danger and may result in inadvertent injury to the common hepatic duct or an aberrant right hepatic artery (seen in 10% of cases). Identification of the hepatocystic triangle (cystic duct, common hepatic duct, and border of the liver) avoids injury to the common hepatic duct.

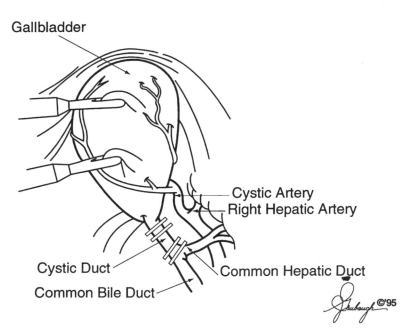

Calot's triangle, formed by the cystic duct, cystic artery, and common hepatic duct, is essential for dissection in laparoscopic cholecystectomy. The hepatocystic triangle is defined as the area between the cystic duct, common hepatic duct, and border of the liver.

3. Summarize the key strategies for safe laparoscopic cholecystectomy.

1. Dissection from the infundibulum down toward the cystic duct
2. Dissection from lateral to medial
3. Adequate inferolateral traction to open the triangle of Calot
4. Dissection to develop continuity both laterally and medially from the neck of the gallbladder onto the cystic duct
5. Divide no structure unless you are certain about its identity

4. Is there any clearly defined benefit to laparoscopic appendectomy?

No. Most studies have shown no benefit for laparoscopic appendectomy over open appendectomy in hospital length of stay, total hospital charges, operative time, recovery time or return to work, or postoperative pain. However, the false diagnosis rate for appendicitis is four times higher among females. For young women, the laparoscopic approach has a clear advantage because gynecologic disorders (ectopic pregnancy, pelvic inflammatory disease, ovarian cysts, and endometriosis) may mimic appendicitis.

5. What is the harmonic scalpel? How does it work?

The ultrasonic scalpel utilizes ultrasonic energy that causes the blade to vibrate up to 55,000 times per second. By adjusting the power level and selecting the appropriate blade, both cutting and coagulation functions are possible.

	STRAIGHT TIP	HOOK TIP
Setting 1 (55,000/sec)	Cutting	Cutting and coagulation
Setting 2	Cutting > coagulation	Coagulation
Setting 3	Coagulation	Coagulation

Vibration of the tip causes intracellular water to vaporize, allowing for the cutting function. The coagulation function allows the operator to achieve homeostasis in vessels as large as 3 mm. When the instrument contacts human tissue, high-frequency vibrations generate heat secondary to the friction created between the cells. This effectively seals the ends of the vessels by denaturing the protein and producing a sticky coagulum.

6. What are the major outcome factors in evaluating patients for the laparoscopic approach to a colonic malignancy?

It has been feared that laparoscopic surgery for colon cancer would be associated with metastatic seeding of trocar insertion sites. Technically, the laparoscopic approach can provide an adequate operation, with adequate cancer-free margins, nodal dissection, and primary anastomosis. Conversion to an open procedure is more prevalent in obese patients or when the malignancy is adherent to local structures. It has been speculated that carbon dioxide pneumoperitoneum may enhance liver metastasis. A prospective National Cancer Institute study of laparoscopic colectomy for colon cancer (Clinical Outcome of Surgical Therapy [COST]) is under way to answer these questions.

7. Does laparoscopic surgery preserve immune function?

Yes. Both human and animal studies have shown that laparoscopy preserves immune function. In contrast, open surgery causes a reduction in lymphocyte and neutrophil chemotaxis, killer cell activity, and lymphocyte and macrophage interactions as well as delayed hypersensitivity responses. After open surgery immunosuppression persists for 6–9 days.

8. Elder surgical statesmen are fond of saying that the incision heals from side to side and that the length of the incision does not matter. Is this true? What is the evidence for or against?

A large portion of the recent research on immune function and surgery has been performed by Bessler and Whelan. Their series of experiments show that the immune depression is directly related to incision length. No more is the longer incision acceptable because it heals from side to side. Although adequate exposure is crucial, we must learn to perform laparoscopic surgery through smaller incisions that preserve the immune response.

9. A 9-year-old girl presents with a 2-month history of right upper quadrant abdominal pain that most commonly occurs after eating fatty foods and usually resolves in 30 minutes. The pain radiates to the right shoulder. It is not associated with nausea or vomiting. She has no prior medical or surgical history. She is afebrile, and the physical exam is unremarkable. Laboratory values, including complete blood count and biliary panel, are normal. An abdominal ultrasound of the right upper quadrant demonstrates no evidence of cholelithiasis, gallbladder wall thickening, or pericholecystic fluid. What should be the next step in your evaluation?

The history is consistent with biliary colic. An initial diagnosis of cholelithiasis was not demonstrated by ultrasound. An upper gastrointestinal (GI) series or esophagogastroduodenoscopy (EGD) would demonstrate possible gastric pathology but would not evaluate the biliary system. A computed tomography (CT) scan is less sensitive than ultrasound for detection of gallstones and would not be helpful. Because the history points toward a biliary etiology, a hepatoiminodiacetic acid (HIDA) scan should be the next step in the evaluation.

10. The HIDA scan demonstrated rapid filling of the gallbladder and unobstructed flow into the duodenum. Cholecystikinin (CCK) is administered, and the gallbladder ejection fraction (EF) is calculated at 30%. What is the most likely diagnosis?

The most likely diagnosis is biliary dyskinesia, which is defined as the presence of symptoms of typical biliary colic without evidence of cholelithiasis and a gallbladder ejection fraction < 35–50 %. Typical symptoms of biliary colic include right upper quadrant or epigastric pain, which may radiate to the right scapula. The pain is often aggravated by eating, especially fatty foods. The cause of biliary dyskinesia is unknown.

11. How should the patient be treated?

Cholecystectomy is successful in 85% of patients with typical symptoms of colic and gallbladder EF < 35–50%. A recent study by Gollin et al. demonstrated that children with biliary dyskinesia characterized by typical biliary colic and a gallbladder EF < 40% respond equally well to cholecystectomy (about 79% success rate).

12. What percentage of patients have free intraabdominal air on upright radiograph 24 hours after laparoscopic procedure?

In the nonpostoperative state, the presence of subdiaphragmatic free air on upright chest radiograph is diagnostic of intraabdominal perforation. After an open abdominal or laparoscopic procedure the significance of free intraabdominal air is less clear. Nonpathologic subdiaphragmatic air may be seen in 24–39% of patients after laparoscopic surgery and in 60% of patients after open surgical procedures. The difference relates to the solubility of carbon dioxide used in laparoscopy vs. the solubility of trapped room air within the abdominal cavity. Carbon dioxide is more soluble in serum than room air and is absorbed 32 times more quickly.

13. Describe the cause and incidence of electrocautery injuries to the small bowel during laparoscopic surgery.

Electrocautery injuries during laparoscopic surgery most commonly occur during the lysis of adhesions and dissection of Calot's triangle. The causes can be separated into two types: contact or conductive. **Contact injuries** occur when the electrocautery instrument directly touches the tissue. Such injuries are more likely to be recognized intraoperatively. The most common location of contact injury is the common bile duct.

Conductive injuries are secondary to the conversion of electrical energy into thermal energy by passing through high-resistance tissue. Conductive injuries to the bowel are rare

(0.07–0.7% of laparoscopic cholecystectomies) and usually present 2–21 days postoperatively as delayed perforations. The duodenum is the most common site of bowel injury (58%), and most are *not* recognized at the time of surgery.

14. How do electrocautery injuries to the small bowel present?
Patients with bowel or bile duct cautery injuries commonly present with fever, abdominal pain, nausea, and vomiting. Common clinical findings include temperature > 38° Celsius, tachycardia, ileus, leukocytosis, and possibly free subdiaphragmatic air on upright chest radiograph. A recent study by Bishoff et al. demonstrated that the symptom of pain at the trocar site closest to the perforation was the most reliable clinical finding. Clinical evidence of peritonitis and sepsis after surgery require immediate evaluation. When findings indicate visceral injury, exploration by laparoscopy or celiotomy is necessary.

15. List the advantages and disadvantages of using carbon dioxide (CO_2) as an insufflation gas instead of other gases.

ADVANTAGES	DISADVANTAGES
CO_2 suppresses combustion and therefore is believed to be ideal for operative laparoscopy.	CO_2 is rapidly absorbed and thus can raise the arterial partial pressure of CO_2 and lower pH, with adverse potential metabolic and hemodynamic consequences in susceptible patients.
CO_2 has a high diffusion coefficient, reducing the risk of a serious gas embolism. Up to 100 ml/min of CO_2 can be injected directly into the bloodstream of animals without adverse outcome.	Insufflation of cold CO_2 (0.3°C), especially in high-flow systems or long procedures, can result in a drop in core temperature with resultant hypothermia.
CO_2 is safely absorbed and can be effectively eliminated by the lungs with moderate hyperventilation.	Tension CO_2 pneumothorax, either from occult defects in the diaphragm or in the absence of diaphragmatic injury (typically in subhiatal laparoscopic surgery), has been reported.
CO_2 is inexpensive and readily available.	CO_2 gas embolism can occur, even without direct insufflation into mesenteric veins.

16. Which alternative gases can be used for laparoscopy?
Room air, oxygen, nitrous oxide, helium, and carbon dioxide have been used to create the pneumoperitoneum needed for laparoscopy, but CO_2 is the most commonly used. Research is ongoing to identify alternative gases for pneumoperitoneum. Helium shows promise in an experimental animal model of chronic obstructive pulmonary disease, in which helium compared with CO_2 pneumoperitoneum showed far less arterial CO_2 retention.

17. What are the respiratory effects of pneumoperitoneum (planned intraabdominal hypertension)?
Pnuemoperitoneum alters respiratory mechanics. Intraabdominal hypertension results in elevation of the diaphragm, decreases in functional residual capacity and total lung volume, ventilation-perfusion inequalities and atelectasis. Some patients may require increased peak inspiratory pressure to compensate for decreased respiratory compliance. No significant change occurs in arterial oxygenation in healthy patients under pneumoperitoneum, but in patients with cardiopulmonary compromise, arterial oxygen desaturation has been reported, presumably secondary to mechanical pulmonary dysfunction.

18. What are the hemodynamic effects?
Mean arterial blood pressure (MAP) and systemic peripheral resistance are increased (up to 35% and 160%, respectively) at operative levels of pneumoperitoneum (12–15 mmHg), presumably as a result of sympathetic vasoconstriction from hypercarbia. Cardiac index may increase

20%. As intraabdominal pressure increases more than 20 mmHg, cardiac output falls and abdominal venous compliance decreases, reaching a point at which effective Trendelenberg position and higher pneumoperitoneum can combine in patients with preexisting cardiopulmonary disease to produce potential hemodynamic compromise. Portal venous blood flow is reduced by 70% when intraabdominal pressure reaches 25 mmHg. Many workers believe that renal blood flow and therefore glomerular filtration rate also decrease with pneumoperitoneum > 12–15 mmHg, although this phenomenon has not been well documented.

In summary, intraabdominal hypertension > 15 mmHg can result in significant changes in central hemodynamics and even more pronounced changes in splanchnic circulation.

19. What is recommended as the maximal safe pressure setting for a CO_2 insufflator?

Based on the potential adverse cardiopulmonary effects of intraabdominal hypertension, the maximal recommended insufflation pressure setting is 15 mmHg.

20. What are the current contraindications to laparoscopic surgery?

There are no absolute contraindications to laparoscopic surgery. However, the Society of American Gastrointestinal Endoscopic Surgeons (SAGES) suggests that possible contraindications include known ruptured diaphragm, hemodynamic instability, uncooperative patient, mechanical or paralytic ileus, large hiatal hernia, abdominal wall infection, multiple previous abdominal procedures, and pregnancy.

Fundamental to safe laparoscopic surgery is patient selection and the surgeon's skill. More difficult surgeries require advanced skills and carry higher anticipated rates of conversion to an open procedure. The decision to convert a closed procedure to open surgery should not be viewed as surgeon failure but as good judgment to ensure patient safety.

21. A thin, 68-year-old woman with chronic obstructive pulmonary disease from 52 years of smoking undergoes laparoscopic cholecystectomy for acute cholecystitis. Because she has had a previous lower midline abdominal incision, you choose the "open" Hasson technique for initial trocar placement and have no difficulties with access to the peritoneal cavity. You immediately insufflate with a flow rate of 10 L/min to a pneumoperitoneum of 15 mmHg and then proceed with laparoscopic cholecystectomy. Fifteen minutes into the procedure, the anesthesiologist observes that the patient's end-tidal CO_2 is elevated and plans to draw an arterial blood gas. Before he can do so, the patient experiences several episodes of ventricular tachycardia and arrests. What is the pathophysiology behind these events?

Insufflated CO_2 is directly absorbed through the peritoneum into the capillary bed and bloodstream. Typically, the partial pressure of CO_2 (PCO_2) and end-tidal CO_2 increase only slightly, but in certain circumstances the PCO_2 can rise dramatically, causing a significant drop in pH. The resulting acidemia aggravates any preexisting cardiac condition. Most patients adapt to the absorbed CO_2 by maximizing plasma and intracellular buffering systems and accelerating CO_2 transport and elimination with mild hyperventilation, but some patients have impaired CO_2 clearance mechanisms. Patients who cannot handle an acute change in PCO_2 are those with high metabolic and cellular respiratory rates (e.g., septic patients), those with large ventilatory deadspace (e.g., patients with chronic obstructive pulmonary disease [COPD]), and those with poor cardiac output (e.g., patients with cardiac failure).

During laparoscopy, special care and monitoring should be provided to prevent significant hypercarbia and acidemia. Rapid shifts in intraabdominal pressure (with attendant PCO_2 absorption gradients) should be avoided, such as those that follow initial insufflation at a high rate with a resultant sudden large gradient between intraabdominal CO_2 pressure and PCO_2. Equilibrium between CO_2 pressure in blood and tissues occurs at about 20 minutes. After initial insufflation, arterial PCO_2 steadily rises for about 20 minutes, then plateaus.

This septic patient with preexisting COPD was subjected to rapid CO_2 insufflation, which resulted in hypercarbia, peaking 15–20 minutes after rapid insufflation, and consequent acidemia, triggering ventricular irritability and arrest.

22. Who introduced electrocautery? Why is the alternating cycle (AC) frequency used?

The "Bovie" nickname for electrosurgical units in most operating rooms acknowledges the introduction in 1929 of electrocautery by William Bovie and Harvey Cushing. In most American homes, the alternating current (AC) that powers appliances and lights alternates at 60 cycles/sec. In the operating room or endoscopy suite, however, the electrosurgical unit alternates between 400,000 and 2,000,000 cycles/sec. This high-frequency electrical current is essential to avoid neuromuscular stimulation. Lower-frequency currents, such as the standard 60-cycle AC current, can cause tetany and electrocution.

23. How do electrocautery units work?

Electrosurgery units work by producing heat at the cellular level. When the electrosurgical unit is set on **cut**, the current is "on" nearly 100% of the time, but at a lower voltage (e.g., 100 V) than during **coagulation** (e.g., 600 V), when the current typically is "on" in bursts 5–10% of the time and "off" 90% of the time. The various blends of cut and coagulation modes combine lower voltages than those used with coagulation (but higher than those used with cut) with varying percentages of time that the current is "on" for optimal effect.

24. Describe the mechanisms by which the cut and coagulation modes work.

Although the precise mechanisms are not known, the **cut** mode of electrosurgery generates an uninterrupted current with movement of ions within the cell, vaporizing the cell. The release of vaporized (boiled) cell content from the disrupted cell dissipates the heat, accounting for the lack of damage to surrounding tissue.

In the **coagulation** mode, the higher-voltage but short-duration energy "bursts" lead to cellular insult but not vaporization. The drying effect on the cells during the "off" part of the cycle (i.e., cellular desiccation) leaves an area of increased resistance to electron flow and thus allows more heat dissipation and progressive insult to deeper tissue layers. This can be explained partially by the formula $p = I^2R$, where p (power, or relative heat per unit of time) is equal to a given current (I) through a certain resistance (R). The issue is more complex than this simple formula suggests, because various body tissues have different levels of conductivity and resistance. Thus some structures may be affected by electrosurgical energy while others are spared injury.

25. Morbid obesity, defined as > 100 lb above ideal body weight, is no longer a contraindication to laparoscopic cholecystectomy. Describe the technical changes necessary for successful laparoscopic cholecystectomy in morbidly obese patients.

1. Safe access and adequate visualization of the porta hepatis structures are the major concerns for safe laparoscopic cholecystectomy in morbidly obese patients. In patients with normal body habitus, the umbilicus typically is the optimal site for the telescope trocar. In obese patients, particularly those who are taller, shifting the trocar site 1–5 inches cephalad from the umbilicus allows optimal visualization of the portal structures with a 0° telescope. Visualization from an umbilical port is often obscured by the bowel horizon in the upper abdomen or by the heavy pannus, which the insufflation cannot sufficiently elevate.

2. Some physicians prefer to gain access to the peritoneum in obese patients by using the "closed" Verress needle approach through the umbilicus. After insufflation they pass an extra-long trocar from the skin level at a previously determined supraumbilical position. Preperitoneal insufflation is a common problem in obese patients because, even with mechanical elevation of the interior abdominal wall, the posterior fascia often does not become elevated. We favor an "open" Hasson approach at a supraumbilical location.

3. Another technique to improve visualization of the porta hepatis in morbidly obese patients involves use of a 30°-angled telescope, which may obviate the need for a supraumbilical trocar site selection. Care must be taken with placement of lateral trochars to avoid skiving the trocar to a preperitoneal position and not entering the abdominal cavity.

4. Placement of a fifth 5-mm subcostal trocar either medially or laterally may be necessary to facilitate adequate retraction and exposure. Some surgeons employ a 5-mm, fan-type retractor

to press down the duodenum or transverse colon. Such retractors should be used with care, particularly if they are positioned off camera.

26. How does morbid obesity affect operative times?
Operative times for laparoscopic cholecystectomy are longer in morbidly obese patients than in patients of normal weight. No increases in conversion rates or complication rates have been reported. Laparoscopic cholecystectomy has become the treatment of choice for morbidly obese patients with symptomatic cholelithiasis, but special skills and techniques are required.

27. Compare the rate of conversion from laparoscopic cholecystectomy to open cholecystectomy in patients with acute vs. chronic cholecystitis.
The rate of conversion from laparoscopic cholecystectomy to open cholecystectomy is 2–4 times higher for acute cholecystitis than for chronic cholecystitis (typically reported at 3–5%) among experienced laparoscopic surgeons.

28. What pathophysiologic features of acute cholecystitis increase the likelihood of technical difficulties?
  1. Distended, inflamed, thick-walled gallbladder
  2. Increased likelihood of bile spill
  3. Inflammation of cystic duct and cystic artery

29. What techniques are used to decompress the distended gallbladder?
Decompression of the distended gallbladder with a special trocar, or even percutaneously (under direct visualization) with a central venous pressure catheter, makes it easier to grasp the gallbladder with laparoscopic forceps. It may be necessary to use traumatic/toothed forceps, but because they tend to puncture the gallbladder wall, they should be left in place to minimize bile spillage. When there is an area of bile leakage, from either the percutaneous drainage site or a tear from a traumatic grasper in the gallbladder wall, a suture or loop ligature can be used to close a small rent in the gallbladder wall. Some acutely inflamed gallbladders cannot be grasped with conventional graspers. In such cases, one solution is to use commercial screw-like devices, such as the Reddick screw, which facilitate retraction of the gallbladder.

30. How are bile spills managed?
Despite the best efforts by experienced surgeons, bile spill is seen in 30–50% of laparoscopic cholecystectomies. Sterile laparoscopic specimen bags are indicated to retrieve lost gallstones, to remove a friable, disrupted gallbladder, or to remove detached, necrotic tissue. Use of closed suction drains should follow the same guidelines used at open surgery.

31. How is inflammation of the cystic duct and cystic artery managed?
The degree of inflammation may make utilization of laparoscopic clip devices inadequate. In such cases, pre-tied loop ligatures can be used to control the cystic duct or cystic artery.

32. Should we routinely use prophylactic antibiotics for laparoscopic cholecystectomy?
Yes, for the following reasons:
  1. Bile spills during laparoscopic cholecystectomy occur in 30–50% of cases
  2. Normal bile is often colonized with bacteria (30–40% of patients).
  3. Acute cholecystitis is associated with a 60% rate of bacterbilia after the first 24 hours of inflammation.

33. Which antibiotic should be used?
For routine laparoscopic cholecystectomies, a first-generation cephalosporin should provide adequate prophylaxis for most common organisms, although many surgeons use a second-generation cephalosporin.

34. At 24 hours after open upper abdominal surgery using subcostal incisions, patients show a decrease in pulmonary function tests of nearly 50%. What decreases should be expected at 24 hours after laparoscopic cholecystectomy?

Postoperative Pulmonary Function Tests: Open versus Laparoscopic Surgery

	PERCENTAGE OF PREOPERATIVE VALUE	
MEASUREMENT AT 24 HR AFTER SURGERY	OPEN SURGERY	LAPAROSCOPIC SURGERY
Forced vital capacity (FVC)	54%	73%
Forced expiratory volume at 1 sec (FEV_1)	52%	72%
Forced expiratory flow at 25–75% (FEF_{25-75})	53%	81%

In one study, the decrease in pulmonary function measured at 24 hours after laparoscopic cholecystectomy was approximately one-half of that seen with open surgery. In a related study, age-, gender-, and size-matched patients were randomized prospectively to open vs. laparoscopic cholecystectomy, and pulmonary function tests were measured pre- and postoperatively. FVC and FEV_1 were similarly decreased, but less so with laparoscopic than with open surgery. Functional residual capacity was significantly higher at 72 hours after laparoscopic than after open surgery. Respiratory function is less impaired and recovery is improved after laparoscopic surgery compared with open surgery.

35. An 18-year-old woman with a hemoglobinopathy is admitted for elective laparoscopic cholecystectomy. The procedure was performed uneventfully, but after surgery her umbilical dressing is persistently wet. Chemical analysis of the fluid demonstrates a creatinine value of 20 mg/dl. A Foley urinary catheter was placed during the procedure, making the surgeon confident that no urinary bladder injury had occurred. What is the diagnosis? What key historical fact may have prevented this complication?

The patient has a persistent congenital anomaly, a vesicoumbilical fistula or persistent urachal sinus/diverticulum, that was injured during trocar placement. The easily obtainable history of chronic or episodic drainage from the umbilicus would have prompted an investigation into the possibility of a urachal remnant and allowed repair in conjunction with the laparoscopic cholecystectomy. In general, it is not uncommon for patients to have some trocar-site leakage of irrigation fluid for up to 8–12 hours postoperatively, but persistence of fluid drainage beyond 24 hours warrants further evaluation to rule out an occult intraabdominal injury.

36. What are the indications and contraindications for laparoscopic adrenalectomy?

Adrenal masses can be divided into functioning, nonfunctioning, and malignant tumors. Functioning or hormonally active tumors (e.g., pheochromocytoma, aldosteronoma, androgen-producing adenoma, glucocorticoid-producing adenoma, bilateral adrenal hyperplasia) should be resected. Studies have shown that tumors as large as 10 cm can be resected laparoscopically. Nonfunctioning or hormonally inactive adrenal tumors > 4 cm or tumors > 3 cm that have grown on serial studies should be resected. The risk of malignancy increases with size; most adrenal cancers measure > 6 cm. Laparoscopic resection of andrenocortical cancer is controversial. If the tumor is confined to the adrenal gland, laparoscopic resection may be possible. The need for clear surgical margins may necessitate conversion to an open procedure if direct extension of tumor involves surrounding structures.

The contraindications to laparoscopic resection of adrenal tumors are based on the surgeon's clinical judgment and laparoscopic abilities. Radiographic imaging aids the surgeon in determining laparoscopic resectability.

37. What are the advantages of laparoscopic adrenalectomy?

Studies have demonstrated that laparoscopic adrenalectomy is a safe and beneficial alternative to an open procedure. Patients who undergo laparoscopic adrenalectomy have less operative blood loss, lower transfusion requirements, fewer admissions to intensive care, decreased use of pain medication, quicker return of bowel function, and decreased hospital stay. In some studies, however, operative times were significantly longer for laparoscopic surgery.

BIBLIOGRAPHY

1. Allendorf JDF, Bessler M, et al: Postoperative immune function varies inversely with the degree of surgical trauma in a murine model. Surg Endosc 11:427–430, 1997.
2. Berry SM, Ose RH, et al: Thermal injury of the posterior duodenum during laparoscopic cholecystectomy. Surg Endosc 8:197–200, 1984.
3. Bishoff, JT, Allaf ME, et al: Laparoscopic bowel injury: Incidence and clinical presentation. J Urol 161:887–890, 1999.
4. Brunt LM, et al: Laparoscopic adrenalectomy compared to open adrenalectomy for benign adrenal neoplasms. J Am Coll Surg 183:1–10, 1996.
5. Cameron J: Current Surgical Therapy, 6th ed. St. Louis, Mosby, 1998.
6. Cho JM, LaPorta AJ, Clark JR, et al: Response of serum cytokines in patients undergoing laparoscopic cholecystectomy. Surg Endosc 8:1380–1384, 1994.
7. Crist DW, Gadacz TR: Complications in laparoscopic surgery. Surg Clin North Am 3:265–289, 1993.
8. Deziel DJ, Millikan KW, et al: Scientific papers: Complications of laparoscopic cholecystectomy. A national survey of 4,292 hospitals and an analysis of 77,604 cases. Am J Surg 165:9–14, 1993.
9. Farooqui MO, Bazzoli JM: Significance of radiologic evidence of free air following laparoscopy. J Reprod Med 16(3):119–125, 1976.
10. Fitzgerald SD, Andrus CH, Baudendistel DF, et al: Hypercarbia during carbon dioxide pneumoperitoneum. Am J Surg 163:186–190, 1992.
11. Fleshman JW, Nelson H, et al: Early results of laparoscopic surgery for colorectal cancer: Retrospective analysis of 372 patients treated by Clinical Outcomes of Surgery Therapy (COST) study group. Dis Colon Rectum 39(Suppl): S53–S58, 1996.
12. Frazee RC, Roberts JW, Okeson GC, et al: Open versus laparoscopic cholecystectomy: A comparison of operative pulmonary functions. Ann Surg 213:651–653, 1991.
13. Gollin G, Raschbaum GR, et al: Cholecystectomy for suspected biliary dyskinesia in children with chronic abdominal pain. J Pediatr Surg 34:854–857, 1999.
14. Greene FL: The impact of laparoscopy on cancer management. Surg Endosc 14(3):217–218, 2000.
15. Hammer JH, Neilsen HJ, Moesgaard F, et al: Duration of post-operative immunosuppression assessed by repeated delayed typed hypersensitivity skin test. Eur Surg Res 24:133, 1992.
16. Ishida H, Murata N, et al: Pneumoperitoneum with carbon dioxide enhances liver metastases of cancer cells implanted into the portal vein in rabbits. Surg Endosc 4:239–242, 1999.
17. Jones DM, Weintraub PS: Anesthesiologists warn if you're taking herbal products, tell your doctor before surgery. ASA Publ Educ, 1999.
18. Joris JL, Noirot DP, Legrand MJ, et al: Hemodynamic changes during laparoscopic cholecystectomy. Anesth Analg 76:106–107, 1992.
19. Lee SW, Southall JC, Gleason NR, et al: Lymphocyte proliferation in mice after full laparotomy is the same whether performed in a sealed carbon dioxide chamber or room air. Surg Endosc 14:235–238, 2000.
20. McCahill, LE, Pellegrini, CA, et al: A clinical outcome and cost analysis of laparoscopic versus open appendectomy. Am J Surg 171:533–537, 1996.
21. McLucas B, March C: Urachal sinus perforation during laparoscopy: A case report. J Reprod Med 35:573–574, 1990.
22. McVay CB, Anson BJ (eds): Surgical Anatomy1 6:622–628, 1984 [entire issue].
23. Miller LG: Herbal medicinals selected clinical considerations focusing on known or potential drug-herb interactions. Arch Intern Med 1998;158(20): 2200-2211.
24. Minne L, Varner D, et al: Laparoscopic vs. open appendectomy. Arch Surg 132:708–712, 1997.
25. Prinz RA: A comparison of laparoscopic and open adrenalectomies. Arch Surg 30:489–494, 1995.
26. Rattner DW, Ferguson C, et al: Factors associated with successful laparoscopic cholecystectomy for acute cholecystitis. Ann Surg 217:233–236, 1993.
27. Reddick EJ, Olsen DO, Daniell JF, et al: Laparoscopic laser cholecystectomy. Laser Med Surg News Adv 7:38–40, 1989 [first U.S. report].
28. Reich H: Laparoscopic bowel injury. Surg Laparosc Endosc 2:74–78, 1992.
29. SAGES Committee on Standards of Practice: Guidelines for Diagnostic Laparoscopy. Santa Monica, CA, SAGES Guidelines, 1998.
30. Schauer PR, Page CP, et al: Incidence and significance of subdiaphragmatic air following laparoscopic cholecystectomy. Am Surg 63:132–136, 1997.
31. Schirmer BD, Dix J, Edge SB, et al: Laparoscopic cholecystectomy in the obese patient. Ann Surg 216:146–152, 1992.
32. Schren P, Woisetschlager R, et al: Mechanism, management, and prevention of laparoscopic bowel injuries. Gastrol Endosc 43:572–574, 1996.
33. Stocchi L, Nelson H: Laparoscopic colectomy for colon cancer: Trial update. Surg Oncol 68:255–267, 1998.
34. Talamini MA, Gadacz TR: Equipment and instrumentation. In Zuker KA, Bailey RW, Reddick EJ (eds): Surgical Laparoscopy Update. St. Louis, Quality Medical Publishing, 1993, pp 4–5.
35. Voyles CR, Tucker RD: Education and engineering solutions for potential problems with monopolar electrosurgery at laparoscopy. Am J Surg 164:57–62, 1992.
36. Yost, F, Margenthaler, J, et al: Cholecystectomy is an effective treatment for biliary dyskinesia. Am J Surg 178(6):462–465, 1999.

INDEX

Page numbers in **boldface type** indicate complete chapters.